£1·50

Anaesthesia

Commissioning Editor: Michael Parkinson
Development Editor: Barbara Simmons
Project Manager: Alan Nicholson
Design Direction: Sarah Russell

TEXTBOOK OF
Anaesthesia

FIFTH EDITION

Edited by

Alan R **Aitkenhead**
BSc MD FRCA

Professor of Anaesthesia
University Department of Anaesthesia and Intensive Care
Queen's Medical Centre
Nottingham
UK

Graham **Smith**
BSc(Hons) MD FRCA

Emeritus Professor of Anaesthesia
University Division of Anaesthesia, Critical Care and Pain Management
Leicester Royal Infirmary
Leicester
UK

David J **Rowbotham**
MD FRCP MRCP FRCA

Professor of Anaesthesia and Pain Management
University Division of Anaesthesia, Critical Care and Pain Management
Leicester Royal Infirmary
Leicester
UK

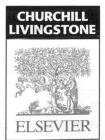

EDINBURGH   LONDON   NEW YORK   OXFORD   PHILADELPHIA   ST LOUIS   SYDNEY   TORONTO   2007

CHURCHILL LIVINGSTONE
ELSEVIER

An imprint of Elsevier Limited

First published 1985
Second edition 1990
Third edition 1996
Fourth edition 2001
Fifth edition 2007

Main edition
ISBN 10: 0-443-10078-0
ISBN 13: 978-0-443-10078-9

International edition
ISBN 10: 0-443-10085-3
ISBN 13: 978-0-443-10085-7

British Library Cataloguing in Publication Data
A catalogue record for this book is available from the British Library

Library of Congress Cataloging in Publication Data
A catalog record for this book is available from the Library of Congress

Note
Knowledge and best practice in this field are constantly changing. As new research and experience broaden our knowledge, changes in practice, treatment and drug therapy may become necessary or appropriate. Readers are advised to check the most current information provided (i) on procedures featured or (ii) by the manufacturer of each product to be administered, to verify the recommended dose or formula, the method and duration of administration, and contraindications. It is the responsibility of the practitioner, relying on their own experience and knowledge of the patient, to make diagnoses, to determine dosages and the best treatment for each individual patient, and to take all appropriate safety precautions. To the fullest extent of the law, neither the Publisher nor the Editors assumes any liability for any injury and/or damage to persons or property arising out of or related to any use of the material contained in this book.

The Publisher

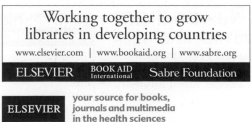

The Publisher's policy is to use **paper manufactured from sustainable forests**

Printed in the Netherlands

Preface

The objective of the 5th edition of *Textbook of Anaesthesia* remains the same as that of previous editions; namely, to provide a concise, easy-to-read text for beginners in anaesthesia and an essential resource for those preparing for the Primary Examination of the Royal College of Anaesthetists. Candidates for this examination require an extensive knowledge of the basic sciences underpinning anaesthesia, critical care and pain management, and the clinical knowledge and skills expected in those who have completed at least 12–18 months in a full-time training post.

In order to respond to changes in the syllabus of this examination, the 4th edition of *Textbook of Anaesthesia* incorporated a large number of chapters devoted entirely to basic science. The intention was to produce a single book suitable as an introduction to clinical anaesthesia and a learning resource for the basic science component of the Primary FRCA Examination. Although the book was received well by its readers and reviewers, it was impossible within a single book of acceptable size to achieve the second objective effectively. Furthermore, between the planning and publication of the 4th edition, several excellent books emerged which are devoted specifically to the physiology and pharmacology of anaesthesia. Consequent to this development and our feeling that the 4th edition had become too large to be conveniently portable, we have reverted in this 5th edition to the principles on which earlier editions were based, in a more concise format.

In preparing the present edition, we have made many significant modifications. After extensive and careful review, we felt that it was essential to continue to cover in some detail all basic science that has direct and close clinical relevance. Indeed, without this information, it is not possible to understand the clinical material described in the book. The contents have been reorganised completely resulting in a book of more reasonable size. Seamless integration of basic science and clinical practice remains a feature of this new edition and we anticipate that, in common with earlier smaller editions, it may be a constant companion of the novice anaesthetist during clinical work.

We asked a number of senior, experienced authors with expertise in their subject area to modify or completely re-write their contributions. We have also recruited many new authors ensuring the invigoration of the text by fresh younger minds. We are grateful to all the authors for their contributions and we also thank our reviewers and readers who have made helpful suggestions, many of which have influenced planning of the new edition. We are grateful to the publishers who have cooperated in our desire to make fundamental changes. We are indebted to all our proof readers and our secretaries Christine Gethins (Leicester) and Sunita Gupta (Nottingham) for their considerable assistance.

We hope that the 5th edition will be as popular as previous editions and remain the book of choice for trainees embarking upon a career in anaesthesia. Although this book is aimed primarily at the beginner, we are aware that many anaesthetists studying for the Final FRCA examination use *Textbook of Anaesthesia* when revising the basics; we hope that this will continue. We also believe that this is more than a book suitable for examination preparation; it continues to be a practical guide for all anaesthetists and other health care professionals involved in the care of patients in the perioperative period.

AR Aitkenhead, Nottingham
G Smith, Leicester
DJ Rowbotham, Leicester

Contributors

Alan R Aitkenhead BSc MD FRCA
Professor of Anaesthesia, University Department of
Anaesthesia and Intensive Care, Queen's Medical
Centre, Nottingham, UK

Robert Atcheson MD FRCA
Consultant Anaesthetist, Royal Hallamshire Hospital,
Sheffield, UK

Bryn R Baxendale MBChB FRCA
Consultant Anaesthetist, Department of Anaesthesia,
Queen's Medical Centre, Nottingham, UK

Nigel M Bedforth BMedSci BMBS FRCA
Consultant Anaesthetist, Department of Anaesthesia,
Queen's Medical Centre, Nottingham, UK

Mark C Bellamy MA MBBS FRCA
Consultant Anaesthetist, St James's University
Hospital, Leeds, UK

Timothy Bourne MBBS FRCA
Consultant Anaesthetist, Department of Anaesthesia
Leicester Royal Infirmary, Leicester, UK

Donal J Buggy MD MSc DipMedELD FRCIP FCAI FRCA
Honorary Senior Lecturer in Anaesthesia, National
University of Ireland, Dublin; Consultant
Anaesthetist, Mater Misericordiae Hospital, Dublin,
Ireland

Aiden J Byrne MD MRCP FRCA
Consultant Anaesthetist, Senior Clinical Tutor,
Swansea Clinical School, Morriston Hospital,
Swansea, UK

Beverly J Collett MBBS FRCA
Consultant in Pain Management and Anaesthesia,
Pain Management Service, Leicester Royal Infirmary,
University Hospitals of Leicester, Leicester, UK

Lesley A Colvin MBChB FRCA PhD
Consultant and Senior Lecturer in Anaesthesia and
Pain Management, Department of Anaesthesia,
Critical Care and Pain Management, Western General
Hospital, Edinburgh, UK

David M Coventry MBChB FRCA
Consultant Anaesthetist and Honorary Senior
Lecturer, Department of Anaesthesia, Ninewells
Hospital and Medical School, Dundee, UK

Eric de Melo FRCA
Consultant Anaesthetist, Department of Anaesthesia,
University Hospitals of Leicester, Leicester Royal
Infirmary, Leicester, UK

David R Derbyshire MBChB FRCA
Consultant in Anaesthesia, Warwick Hospital,
Warwick, UK (Retired)

David J R Duthie MD FRCA
Consultant Cardiothoracic Anaesthetist,
Department of Anaesthesia, Leeds General Infirmary,
Leeds, UK

Christopher D Elton FRCA
Consultant Anaesthetist, Department of Anaesthesia,
University Hospitals of Leicester, Leicester Royal
Infirmary, Leicester, UK

Agota Ermenyi MD
Research Fellow, Department of Anaesthesia,
St James's University Hospital, Leeds, UK

David Fell FRCA
Consultant Anaesthetist, Department of Anaesthesia,
University Hospitals of Leicester, Leicester Royal
Infirmary, Leicester, UK

Thomas C E Gale BMedSci BMBS FRCA FANZCA
Consultant, Department of Anaesthesia, Derriford
Hospital, Plymouth, UK

Neville W Goodman MA DPhil BM BCh FRCA
Consultant Anaesthetist, Southmead Hospital, North
Bristol NHS Trust, Bristol, UK

Ian S Grant MBChB FRCP(Edin) FFARCSI
Consultant in Intensive Care Management and
Anaesthesia, Western General Hospital, Edinburgh,
UK

Jonathan G Hardman BMedSci BM BS FANZCA DM FRCA
Clinical Senior Lecturer and Honorary Consultant,
Department of Anaesthesia, University Hospital,
Nottingham, UK

Jennifer M Hunter MBChB PhD FRCA
Professor of Anaesthesia, University of Liverpool,
Liverpool, UK

Gareth W Jones BSc MRCP FRCA
Consultant Anaesthetist, University Hospitals of
Leicester, Leicester Royal Infirmary,
Leicester, UK

Judith Kendell MBBS FRCA
SpR Anaesthesia and Intensive Care, Ninewells
Hospital and Medical School, Dundee, UK

David Kirkbride FRCA
Consultant Anaesthetist, Department of Anaesthesia,
University Hospitals of Leicester, Leicester Royal
Infirmary, Leicester, UK

Nisha Kumar MSc BM FRCA
Consultant Anaesthetist, Department of Anaesthesia,
University Hospitals of Leicester, Leicester Royal
Infirmary, Leicester, UK

J M Lamb MBBS FRCA
Consultant Anaesthetist, University Hospital,
Queen's Medical Centre, Nottingham, UK

Jeremy A Langton MBBS MD FRCA ILTM
Clinical Director, Consultant Anaesthetist and
Honorary Reader, Department of Anaesthesia,
Critical Care and Pain Management, Plymouth
Hospitals, Devon, UK

Ravi P Mahajan MD FRCA
Professor of Anaesthesia and Intensive Care,
University Department of Anaesthesia and Intensive
Care, Queen's Medical Centre and City Hospital,
Nottingham, UK

Peter F Mahoney MSc FRCA FIMC RCSEdin DMCC FAMC
Lieutenant Colonel, Royal Army Medical Corps;
Senior Lecturer (Military), Leonard Cheshire Centre
of Conflict Recovery, University College London;
Honorary Consultant in Anaesthesia, Lincoln County
Hospital, UK

Anne May MBBS FRCA
Consultant Anaesthetist, Leicester Royal Infirmary,
Honorary Senior Lecturer, Department of
Anaesthesia, University of Leicester, Leicester, UK

Mary C Mushambi MBChB
Consultant Anaesthetist, Leicester Royal Infirmary,
Leicester, UK

Michael H Nathanson MBBS MRCP FRCA
Consultant Anaesthetist, University Hospital,
Queen's Medical Centre, Nottingham, UK

Martin Nicoll FFA (South Africa)
Consultant Anaesthetist, Queen's Medical Centre,
University Hospital, Nottingham, UK

Graham R Nimmo MD FRCP(Edin) FFARCSI
Consultant Physician, Medicine and Intensive Care,
Western General Hospital, Edinburgh, UK

Susan Nimmo MBChB MRCP FRCA
Consultant Anaesthetist, Western General Hospital,
Edinburgh, UK

Ian Power
BSC(Hons) MD FRCA FFPMANZCA FANZCA FRCSEd FRCPEdin
Professor, Clinical and Surgical Sciences (Anaesthesia,
Critical Care and Pain Medicine), School of Clinical
Sciences and Community Health, University of
Edinburgh, Royal Infirmary, Edinburgh, UK

Charles S Reilly MD FRCA
Professor of Anaesthesia, University of Sheffield,
Sheffield, UK

Bernard Riley MBE BSc MBBS FRCA
Consultant in Adult Critical Care Medicine and
Anaesthesia, University Hospital, Nottingham, UK

David J Rowbotham MD FRCP MRCP FRCA
Professor of Anaesthesia and Pain Management,
University Division of Anaesthesia, Critical Care and
Pain Management, Leicester Royal Infirmary,
Leicester, UK

Colin J Runcie FRCA FRCP(Glas)
Consultant Anaesthetist, Western Infirmary, Glasgow,
UK

A R A Rushton BM BCh FRCA
Consultant Anaesthetist, Derriford Hospital,
Plymouth, UK

Peter J Simpson MD FRCA
Consultant Anaesthetist, Frenchay Hospital, Bristol,
UK

Graham Smith BSc(Hons) MD FRCA
Emeritus Professor of Anaesthesia, University
Division of Anaesthesia, Critical Care and Pain
Management, Leicester Royal Infirmary, Leicester, UK

Justiaan L C Swanevelder MBChB MMed(Anes) FRCA
Consultant Anaesthetist, Department of Anaesthesia,
University Hospitals of Leicester, Glenfield General
Hospital, Leicester, UK

Jonathan P Thompson BSc(Hons) MBChB MD FRCA
Senior Lecturer in Anaesthesia and Critical Care,
University of Leicester; Honorary Consultant,
University Hospitals of Leicester, Leicester Royal
Infirmary, Leicester, UK

Douglas A B Turner MBBS FRCA
Consultant in Anaesthesia and Intensive Care,
University Hospitals of Leicester, Leicester, UK

Jennifer Warner MBBS FRCA
Consultant Anaesthetist, Nottingham City Hospital,
Nottingham, UK

J A W Wildsmith MD FRCA FRCPEd
Foundation Professor of Anaesthesia, Ninewells
Hospital and Medical School, Dundee, UK

Contents

Appendices

General principles of pharmacology

HOW DO DRUGS ACT?

Drugs produce their effects on biological systems by several mechanisms; these include physicochemical action, activity at receptors and inhibition of reactions mediated by enzymes.

PHYSICOCHEMICAL PROPERTIES

Sodium citrate is an alkali and neutralizes acid; it is often administered orally to reduce the likelihood of pneumonitis after regurgitation of gastric contents. Chelating agents (*chel* is the Greek word for a crab's claw) combine chemically with metal ions, reducing their toxicity and enhancing elimination, usually in the urine. Such drugs include desferrioxamine (chelates iron and aluminium), dicobalt edetate (cyanide toxicity), sodium calcium edetate (lead) and penicillamine (copper and lead). Stored blood contains a citrate-based anticoagulant that prevents clotting; this chelates calcium ions and may cause hypocalcaemia after massive blood transfusion. Phenol and alcohol denature proteins; they are used occasionally to produce prolonged or permanent nerve blockade.

ACTION ON RECEPTORS

A receptor is a complex structure on the cell membrane which can bind selectively with endogenous compounds or drugs, resulting in changes within the cell which modify its function. These include changes in selective ion channel permeability (e.g. acetylcholine, glutamate, GABA receptors), cyclic adenosine monophosphate (e.g. opioid, β, α_2 and dopamine receptors), cyclic guanosine monophosphate (e.g. atrial natriuretic peptide receptor), inositol phosphate and diacylglycerol (e.g. α_1, angiotensin AT_1, endothelin, histamine H_1 and vasopressin V_1 receptors) and nitric oxide (e.g. muscarinic M_3 receptor).

A compound which binds to a receptor and changes intracellular function is termed an agonist. The classic dose–response relationship of an agonist is shown in Figure 1.1. As the concentration of the agonist increases, a maximum effect is reached as the receptors in the system become saturated (Fig. 1.1A). Conventionally, log dose is plotted against effect, resulting in a sigmoid curve which is approximately linear between 20 and 80% of maximum effect (Fig. 1.1B). Three agonists are shown in Figure 1.2. Agonist A produces 100% effect at a lower concentration than agonist B. Therefore, compared with A, agonist B is less potent but has similar efficacy. Drug C is termed a partial agonist as the maximum effect is less than that of A or B. Buprenorphine is a partial agonist (at the μ-opioid receptor), as are some of the β-blockers with intrinsic activity, e.g. oxprenolol, pindolol, acebutalol, celiprolol.

Antagonists combine selectively with the receptor but produce no effect. They may interact with the receptor in a competitive (reversible) or non-competitive (irreversible) fashion. In the presence of a competitive antagonist, the dose–response curve of an agonist is shifted to the right but the maximum effect remains unaltered (Fig. 1.3A). Examples of this effect include the displacement of morphine by naloxone and endogenous catecholamines by β-blockers.

A non-competitive (irreversible) antagonist shifts the dose–response curve to the right also but, with increasing concentrations, reduces the maximum effect (Fig. 1.3B). For example, the α_1-antagonist phenoxybenzamine, used in the preoperative preparation of patients with phaeochromocytoma, has a long duration of action because of the formation of stable chemical bonds between drug and receptor.

The relationship between drug dose and response is often described by a Hill plot (Fig. 1.4). A typical agonist such as that shown in Figure 1.1 produces a straight line with a slope (i.e. Hill coefficient) of +1.

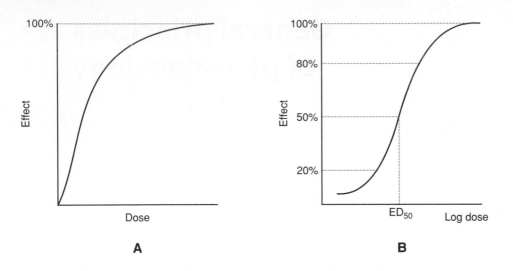

A

B

Fig. 1.1
(**A**) The effect of an agonist peaks when all the receptors are occupied. (**B**) A semilog plot produces a sigmoid curve which is linear between 20 and 80% effect. ED_{50} is the dose which produces 50% of maximum effect.

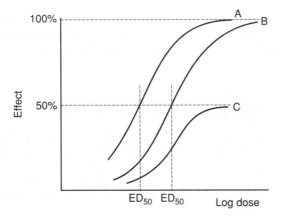

Fig. 1.2
Agonist B has a similar dose–response curve to A but is displaced to the right. A is more potent than B (smaller ED_{50}) but has the same efficacy. C is a partial agonist which is less potent than A and B and less efficacious (maximum effect 50% of A and B).

ACTION ON ENZYMES

Drugs may act by inhibiting the action of an enzyme or competing for its endogenous substrate. Reversible inhibition is the mechanism of action of edrophonium (acetylcholinesterase), aminophylline (phosphodiesterase) and captopril (angiotensin-converting enzyme). Irreversible enzyme inhibition occurs when a stable chemical bond is formed between drug and enzyme, resulting in prolonged or permanent inactivity, e.g. omeprazole (gastric hydrogen-potassium ATPase), aspirin (cyclo-oxygenase) and organophosphorus compounds (acetylcholinesterase).

However, the interaction between drug and enzyme may be more complex than this simple classification implies. For example, neostigmine inhibits acetylcholinesterase in a reversible manner, but the mechanism of action is more akin to that of an irreversible drug as neostigmine forms covalent chemical bonds with the enzyme.

THE BLOOD–BRAIN BARRIER AND PLACENTA

Many drugs used in anaesthetic practice must cross the blood–brain barrier in order to reach their site of action. The brain is protected from most potentially toxic agents by tightly overlapping endothelial cells which surround the capillaries and interfere with passive diffusion. Enzyme systems are present in the endothelium which may also break down many potential toxins. Consequently, only relatively small, highly lipid-soluble molecules (e.g. intravenous and volatile anaesthetic agents, opioids, local anaesthetics) have access to the central nervous system (CNS). Compared with most opioids, morphine takes some time to reach its site of action because it has a relatively low lipid solubility. Highly ionized drugs (e.g. muscle relaxants, glycopyrronium) do not cross the blood–brain barrier.

The chemoreceptor trigger zone is situated in the area postrema near the base of the fourth ventricle (see

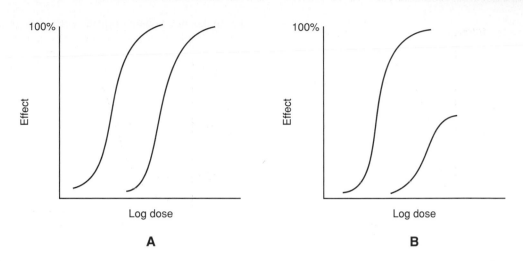

Fig. 1.3
(**A**) The dose–response curve of an agonist is displaced to the right in the presence of a reversible antagonist. There is no change in maximum effect but the ED$_{50}$ is increased. (**B**) The dose–response curve is displaced to the right also in the presence of an irreversible antagonist but the maximum effect is reduced.

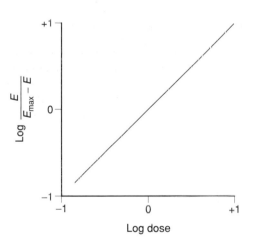

Fig. 1.4
A Hill plot. The Hill coefficient is the slope of the line (+1 for this drug). E_{max} = maximum effect, E = effect at different doses.

Ch. 26). It is not protected by the blood–brain barrier as the capillary endothelial cells are not bound tightly in this area and allow relatively free passage of large molecules. This is an important afferent limb of the vomiting reflex and stimulation of this area by toxins or drugs in the blood or cerebrospinal fluid often leads to vomiting. Many antiemetics act at this site.

The transfer of drugs across the placenta is of considerable importance in obstetric anaesthesia (see Ch. 35). In general, all drugs which affect the CNS cross the placenta and affect the fetus. Highly ionized drugs (e.g. muscle relaxants) pass across less readily.

PLASMA PROTEIN BINDING

Many drugs are bound to proteins in the plasma. This is important as only the unbound portion of the drug is available for diffusion to its site of action. Changes in protein binding may have significant effects on the active unbound concentration of a drug and therefore its actions.

Albumin is the most important protein in this regard and is responsible mainly for the binding of acidic and neutral drugs. Globulins, especially α_1-glycoprotein, bind mainly basic drugs. If a drug is highly protein bound (>80%), any change in plasma protein concentration or displacement of the drug by another with similar binding properties may have clinically significant effects. For example, most NSAIDs displace warfarin, phenytoin and lithium from plasma binding sites, leading to potential toxicity.

Plasma albumin concentration often decreased in the elderly, in neonates and in the presence of malnutrition, liver, renal or cardiac failure and malignancy. α_1-Glycoprotein concentration is decreased during pregnancy and in the neonate but may be increased in the postoperative period and other conditions such as infection, trauma, burns and malignancy.

METABOLISM

Most drugs are lipid-soluble and many are metabolized in the liver into more ionized compounds which are inactive pharmacologically and excreted by the kidneys. However, metabolites may be active (Table 1.1). The liver is not the only site of metabolism. For example, succinylcholine and mivacurium are metabolized by plasma cholinesterase, esmolol by erythrocyte esterases, remifentanil by tissue esterases and, in part, dopamine by the kidney and prilocaine by the lungs.

A substance is termed a *prodrug* if it is inactive in the form in which it is administered, pharmacological effects being dependent on the formation of active metabolites. Examples of this are codeine (morphine), diamorphine (6-monoacetylmorphine, morphine), chloral hydrate (trichlorethanol) and parecoxib (valdecoxib). Midazolam is ionized and dissolved in an acidic solution in the ampoule; after intravenous injection and exposure in the blood to pH 7.4, the molecule becomes lipid-soluble.

Drugs undergo two types of reactions during metabolism: phase I and phase II. Phase I reactions include reduction, oxidation and hydrolysis. Drug oxidation occurs in the smooth endoplasmic reticulum, primarily by the cytochrome P450 enzyme system. This system and other enzymes also perform reduction reactions. Hydrolysis is a common phase I reaction in the metabolism of drugs with ester groups (e.g. remifentanil, succinylcholine, atracurium, mivacurium). Amide drugs often undergo hydrolysis and oxidative N-dealkylation (e.g. lidocaine, bupivacaine).

Phase II reactions involve conjugation of a metabolite or the drug itself with an endogenous substrate. Conjugation with glucuronic acid is a major metabolic pathway, but others include acetylation, methylation and conjugation with sulphate or glycine.

ENZYME INDUCTION AND INHIBITION

Some drugs may enhance the activity of enzymes responsible for drug metabolism, particularly the cytochrome P450 enzymes and glucuronyl transferase. Such drugs include phenytoin, carbamazepine, phenylbutazone, barbiturates, ethanol, steroids and some inhalation anaesthetic agents (halothane, enflurane). Cigarette smoking also induces cytochrome P450 enzymes.

Drugs with mechanisms of action other than on enzymes may also interfere significantly with enzyme systems. For example, etomidate inhibits the synthesis of cortisol and aldosterone – an effect which may explain the increased mortality in critically ill patients which occurred when it was used as a sedative in intensive care. Cimetidine is a potent enzyme inhibitor and may prolong the elimination of drugs such as diazepam, propranolol, oral anticoagulants, phenytoin and lidocaine. Troublesome interactions with enzyme systems are less of a problem with new drugs; if significant enzyme interaction is discovered in the early stages of development, the drug is usually abandoned.

DRUG EXCRETION

Ionized compounds, with a low molecular weight (MW), are excreted mainly by the kidneys. Most drugs and metabolites diffuse passively into the proximal renal tubules by the process of glomerular filtration, but some are secreted actively (e.g. penicillins, aspirin, many diuretics, morphine, lidocaine and glucuronides). Ionization is a significant barrier to reabsorption at the distal tubule. Consequently, basic drugs or metabolites are excreted more efficiently in acid urine and acidic compounds in alkaline urine.

Some drugs and metabolites, particularly those with larger molecules (MW > 400 D), are excreted in the bile (e.g. glycopyrronium, vecuronium, pancuronium and the metabolites of morphine and buprenorphine). Ventilation is responsible for excretion of volatile agents.

Table 1.1 Examples of active metabolites

Drug	Metabolite	Action
Morphine	Morphine-6-glucuronide	Potent opioid agonist
Diamorphine	6-Monoacetylmorphine Morphine	Opioid agonist
Meperidine (pethidine)	Normeperidine (norpethidine)	Epileptogenic
Codeine	Morphine	Opioid agonist
Diazepam	Desmethyldiazepam Temazepam Oxazepam	Sedative
Tramadol	O-desmethyltramadol	Opioid agonist
Parecoxib	Valdecoxib	COX 2 specific inhibitor

PHARMACOKINETIC PRINCIPLES

Pharmacokinetics is the study of what happens to drugs after they have been administered. By contrast, pharmacodynamics is concerned with their effects on biological systems. An understanding of the basic principles of pharmacokinetics is an important aid to the safe use of drugs in anaesthesia, pain management and intensive care medicine. Pharmacokinetics is an attempt to fit observed changes in plasma concentration of drugs into mathematical equations which may then be used to predict concentrations under various circumstances.

Derived values describing volume of distribution (V), clearance (Cl) and half-life ($t_{1/2}$) give an indication of the likely properties of a drug. However, even in healthy individuals of the same sex, weight and age, there is significant variability which makes precise prediction very difficult. It is important to remember that the accepted pharmacokinetic values of drugs are usually the mean of a wide range of observations.

VOLUME OF DISTRIBUTION

Volume of distribution is a good example of the abstract nature of pharmacokinetics; it is not a real volume but merely a concept which helps us to understand what we observe. Nevertheless, it is a very useful notion which enables us to predict certain properties of a drug and also calculate other pharmacokinetic values.

Imagine that a patient receiving an intravenous dose of an anaesthetic induction agent is a bucket of water and that the drug is distributed evenly throughout the water immediately after injection. The volume of water represents the initial volume of distribution (V). It may be calculated easily:

$$C_0 = \frac{\text{dose}}{V} \qquad (1)$$

where C_0 is the initial concentration. Therefore:

$$V = \frac{\text{dose}}{C_0} \qquad (2)$$

A more accurate measurement of V is possible during constant rate infusion when the distribution of the drug in the tissues has time to equilibrate; this is termed volume of distribution at steady state (V_{ss}).

Drugs which remain in the plasma and do not pass easily to other tissues have a small V and therefore a large C_0. Relatively ionized drugs (e.g. muscle relaxants) or drugs highly bound to plasma proteins (e.g. NSAIDs) often have a small V. Drugs with a large V are often lipid-soluble and therefore penetrate and accumulate in tissues outside the plasma (e.g. intravenous induction agents). Some drugs accumulate outside the plasma, making values for V greater than total body volume (a reminder of the abstract nature of pharmacokinetics). Large V values are often observed for drugs highly bound to proteins outside plasma (e.g. local anaesthetics, digoxin).

Several factors may affect V and therefore C_0 on bolus injection of a drug. Patients who are dehydrated, or have lost blood, have a significantly greater plasma C_0 after a normal dose of intravenous induction agent, increasing the likelihood of severe side-effects, especially hypotension. Neonates have a proportionally greater volume of extracellular fluid compared with adults, and water-soluble drugs (e.g. muscle relaxants) tend to have a proportionally greater V. Factors affecting plasma protein binding (see above) may also affect V.

Finally, V can give some indication as to the half-life. A large V is often associated with a relatively slow decline in plasma concentration; this relationship is expressed below in a useful pharmacokinetic equation (eqn 4).

CLEARANCE

Clearance is defined as the volume of blood or plasma from which the drug is removed completely in unit time. Drugs may be eliminated from the blood by the liver, kidney or occasionally other routes (see above). The relative proportion of hepatic and renal clearance of a drug is important. Most drugs used in anaesthetic practice are cleared predominantly by the liver, but some rely on renal or non-organ-dependent clearance. Excessive accumulation of a drug occurs in patients in renal failure if its renal clearance is significant. For example, morphine is metabolized primarily in the liver and this is not affected significantly in renal impairment. However, the active metabolite morphine-6-glucuronide is excreted predominantly by the kidney. This accumulates in renal insufficiency and is responsible for increased morphine sensitivity in these patients.

As with volume of distribution, clearance may suggest likely properties of a drug. For example, if clearance is greater than hepatic blood flow, factors other than hepatic metabolism must account for its total clearance. Values greater than cardiac output may indicate metabolism in the plasma (e.g. succinylcholine) or other tissues (e.g. remifentanil). Clearance is an important (but not the only) factor affecting $t_{1/2}$ and steady-state plasma concentrations achieved during constant rate infusions (see below).

ELIMINATION HALF-LIFE

Methods of administration of a drug are influenced considerably by its plasma $t_{1/2}$, as this often reflects duration of action. It is important to remember that $t_{1/2}$ is influenced not only by clearance (Cl) but also by V:

$$t_{1/2} \propto \frac{V}{Cl} \qquad (3)$$

or

$$t_{1/2} = \text{constant} \times \frac{V}{Cl}$$

The constant in this equation (elimination rate constant) is the natural logarithm of 2 (ln 2) i.e. 0.693. Therefore:

$$t_{1/2} = 0.693 \times \frac{V}{Cl} \qquad (4)$$

Half-life often reflects duration of action but not if the drug acts irreversibly (e.g. some NSAIDs, omeprazole, phenoxybenzamine) or if active metabolites are formed (Table 1.1).

So far, we have considered metabolic or elimination $t_{1/2}$ only. The initial decrease in plasma concentrations after administration of many drugs, especially if given intravenously, occurs primarily because of redistribution into tissues. Therefore, the simple relationship between elimination $t_{1/2}$ and duration of action does not apply in many situations (see below, 'two-compartment models').

CALCULATING $t_{1/2}$, V AND CLEARANCE

It is a simple exercise to calculate these values for a drug after intravenous bolus administration. A known dose is given and regular blood samples for plasma concentration measurements are taken. In this example, we assume that the drug remains in the plasma and is removed only by metabolism; this is a called a one-compartment model. After achieving C_0, plasma concentration (C_p) declines in a simple exponential manner as shown in Figure 1.5A. If the natural logs of the concentrations are plotted against time (semilog plot), a straight line is produced (Fig. 1.5B). The gradient of this line is the elimination rate constant k, which is related to $t_{1/2}$ in the following equation:

$$k = \frac{\ln 2}{t_{1/2}} \qquad (5)$$

We may calculate V using equation (2) and then clearance from equation (4). C_p may be predicted at any time from the following equation:

$$C_p = C_0 e^{-kt} \qquad (6)$$

where t is the time after administration.

Clearance may be derived also by calculation of the area under the concentration–time curve extrapolated to infinity (AUC_∞) and substitution in the following equation:

$$Cl = \frac{\text{dose}}{AUC_\infty} \qquad (7)$$

TWO-COMPARTMENT MODELS

The body is not, of course, a single homogeneous compartment; drug plasma concentrations are the result of elimination by metabolism and redistribution to and from tissues such as brain, heart, liver, muscles and fat. The mathematics describing this real situation are extremely complex. However, plasma concentrations of many drugs behave approximately as if they were distributed in two or three compartments. Applying these mathematical models is a reasonable compromise.

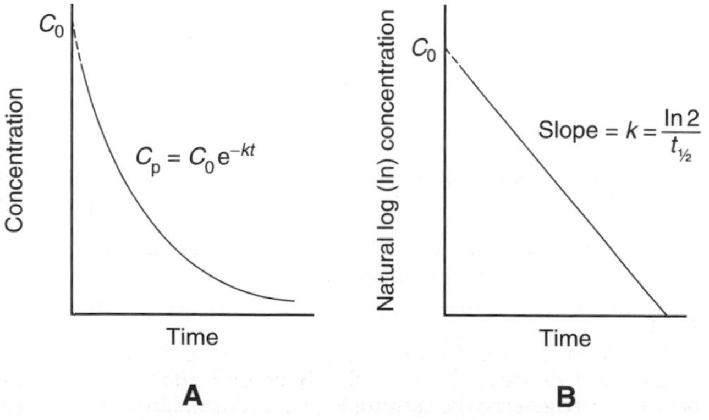

Fig. 1.5
(**A**) Exponential decline in plasma drug concentration (C_p) in a one-compartment model. The equation predicts C_p at any time (t). (**B**) Semilog plot enables easy calculation of $t_{1/2}$. Extrapolation of this line enables C_0 and AUC_∞ to be derived easily.

Let us consider a two-compartment model; one compartment may be thought of as representing the plasma and the other, the remainder of the body. When an intravenous bolus is injected into this system, C_p decreases because of an exponential decay resulting from elimination and another exponential decay resulting from redistribution into the tissues. Therefore, when C_p is plotted against time, the curve may be described by a biexponential equation. If plotted on a semilogarithmic plot (Fig. 1.6), two straight lines can be identified and derived. Their gradients are the elimination rate constants dependent on elimination (β) and redistribution (α).

Redistribution kinetics are not only of theoretical interest, because it is often the decline in C_p resulting from redistribution which is responsible for the cessation of an observed effect of a drug; intravenous induction agents and *initial* doses of intravenous fentanyl are good examples of this. Patients wake up after a bolus administration of propofol because of redistribution, not metabolism.

Calculating the separate pharmacokinetic values is easy; one curve is simply subtracted from the other. Consider Figure 1.6 where natural log concentration is plotted against time and two slopes are seen. The second and less steep slope represents decline in plasma concentration caused by elimination of the drug by metabolism. From this, the elimination half-life ($t^{\beta}_{1/2}$)

may be calculated. In order to calculate the half-life of the redistribution phase ($t^{\alpha}_{1/2}$), the elimination slope is extrapolated back to time 0. If data on this imaginary part of the elimination slope are subtracted from those on the real line above it, another imaginary line may be constructed which represents that part of the decline in plasma concentration which is the result of redistribution. From this line, the redistribution half-life ($t^{\alpha}_{1/2}$) may be calculated.

The equation for C_p at any time in a two-compartment model after bolus intravenous administration is therefore:

$$C_p = Ae^{-\alpha t} + Be^{-\beta t} \qquad (8)$$

where α and β are the redistribution and elimination rate constants, respectively, and A and B are values derived by back extrapolation of the redistribution and elimination slopes to the y-axis.

Some drugs, e.g. propofol, are best fitted to a triexponential, three-compartment model which reveals half-lives for two processes of redistribution (conventionally $t^{\alpha}_{1/2}$ and $t^{\beta}_{1/2}$) and one for elimination ($t^{\gamma}_{1/2}$). Equations developed from these basic concepts are contained in the software of target-controlled infusion pumps.

CONTEXT-SENSITIVE HALF-LIFE

This concept refers to plasma half-life (time for plasma concentration to decline by 50%) after an intravenous drug infusion is stopped; 'context' refers to the duration of infusion. The amount of drug accumulating in body tissues increases with duration of infusion for most drugs. Consequently, on stopping the infusion, time for the plasma concentration to decline by 50%

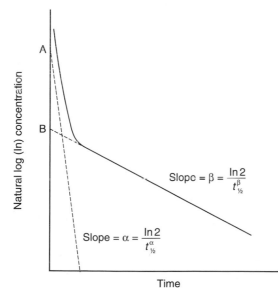

Fig. 1.6
Semilog plot of a two-compartment model: α = rate constant for exponential decay resulting from redistribution; β = rate constant for exponential decay resulting from elimination.

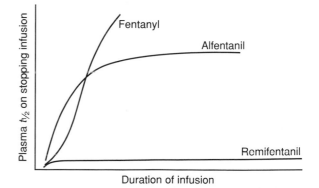

Fig. 1.7
Context-sensitive half-life. The time for plasma concentration to decline by 50% increases with duration of infusion for alfentanil and fentanyl. This is not the case for remifentanil.

depends on duration of infusion. The longer the infusion, the more drug accumulates and the longer the plasma half-life becomes, because there is more drug to enter the plasma on stopping the infusion.

Figure 1.7 shows the effect of infusion duration on half-life of alfentanil, fentanyl and remifentanil. Alfentanil, and especially fentanyl, accumulate during infusion, causing an increase in context-sensitive half-live as the duration of infusion increases. In other words, time to recovery from alfentanil- or fentanyl-based anaesthesia depends on duration of infusion. Remifentanil is metabolized by tissue esterases and does not accumulate. Therefore, time for plasma concentration of remifentanil to decline by 50% is independent of duration of infusion, i.e. recovery times after remifentanil-based anaesthesia are short and predictable, no matter how long the infusion has run.

METHODS OF DRUG ADMINISTRATION

ORAL

The oral route of drug administration is important in modern anaesthetic practice (e.g. premedication, post-operative analgesia). It is often necessary also to continue concurrent medication during the perioperative period (e.g. antihypertension therapy, anti-anginal medication). It is therefore important to appreciate the factors involved in the absorption of orally administered drugs.

The formulation of tablets or capsules is very precise, as their consistent dissolution is necessary before absorption can take place. The rate of absorption, and therefore effect of the drug, may be influenced significantly by this factor. Most preparations dissolve in the acidic gastric juices and the intact drug is absorbed in the upper intestine. However, some drugs are broken down by acids (e.g. omeprazole, benzylpenicillin) or are irritant to the stomach (e.g. aspirin, phenylbutazone) and may be given as enteric-coated preparations. Drugs given in solution are often absorbed more rapidly but this may induce nausea or vomiting immediately after anaesthesia. Some drugs used in anaesthetic practice are available in slow-release preparations (e.g. morphine, oxycontin, tramadol).

Gastric emptying

Most drugs are absorbed only when they have left the stomach; therefore, if gastric emptying is delayed, absorption is affected. Furthermore, if oral medication is given continuously during periods of impaired emptying, it may accumulate in the stomach, only to be delivered to the small intestine *en masse* when gastric function returns, resulting in overdose. Many factors influence the rate of gastric emptying and these are described in Chapter 26.

Any factor increasing upper intestinal motility (e.g. metoclopramide) reduces the time available for absorption and may reduce the total amount of drug absorbed.

First-pass effect

Before entering the systemic circulation, a drug must pass through the portal circulation and, if metabolized extensively by the liver or even the gut wall, absorption may be reduced significantly (i.e. first-pass effect). For example, compared with intramuscular administration, significantly larger doses of oral morphine are required for the same effect. In fact most opioids, except methadone, are susceptible to significant first-pass metabolism.

Bioavailability

Bioavailability is the percentage of the oral dose of a drug which is absorbed into the systemic circulation. It is calculated by giving the same individual, on two separate occasions, the same dose of a drug orally and intravenously. The resulting plasma drug concentrations are plotted against time and the area under the curve after oral administration is compared with that after intravenous administration.

LINGUAL AND BUCCAL

This is a useful method of administration if a drug is lipid-soluble and crosses the oral mucosa with relative ease. First-pass metabolism is avoided. Glyceryl trinitrate and buprenorphine are available as sublingual tablets and morphine as a buccal preparation.

INTRAMUSCULAR

Intramuscular administration is still used frequently in the perioperative period. It may avoid the problems associated with large initial plasma concentrations after rapid intravenous administration, is devoid of first-pass effects and may be administered relatively easily. However, absorption may be unpredictable, some preparations are particularly painful and irritant (e.g. diclofenac) and complications include damage to nervous and vascular tissue and inadvertent intravenous injection. It is disliked intensely by most adults and nearly all children.

Variations in absorption may be clinically relevant. For example, peak plasma concentrations of morphine may occur at any time from 5 to 60 min after intramuscular administration, an important factor in the failure of this method to produce good reliable analgesia (see Ch. 25).

SUBCUTANEOUS

Absorption is very susceptible to changes in skin perfusion, and tissue irritation may be a significant problem. However, this method is used in several centres for providing postoperative pain relief, particularly in children, and has the advantage that potentially difficult intravenous access is not required. A small cannula is placed subcutaneously during anaesthesia and can be replaced, if necessary, with relative ease. Even patient-controlled analgesia (PCA) has been used effectively by this route.

INTRAVENOUS

Bolus

The majority of drugs used in anaesthetic practice are given intravenously as boluses and the pharmacokinetics are described in some detail above. The major disadvantage of this method is that dangerously high drug concentrations may occur readily, particularly with drugs of narrow therapeutic index and large interpatient pharmacodynamic and pharmacokinetic variations (i.e. most drugs used in anaesthetic practice). Therefore, it is an important general rule that all drugs administered intravenously should be given slowly. Manufacturers' recommendations in this regard are often surprising; for example, a 10 mg dose of metoclopramide should be given over 1–2 min.

Only two factors have a major influence on the plasma concentrations achieved during a bolus intravenous injection: speed of injection and cardiac output. Therefore, an elderly, sick or hypovolaemic patient undergoing intravenous induction of anaesthesia is likely to suffer significant side-effects if the drug is given at the same rate as would be used in a normal, healthy young adult.

Infusion

Drugs may be given by constant-rate infusion, a method used frequently for propofol, neuromuscular blocking agents, opioids and many other drugs. Plasma concentrations achieved during infusions may

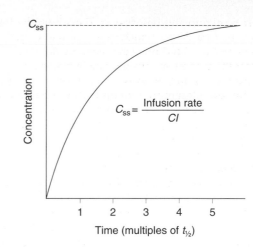

Fig. 1.8
Plasma concentrations during a constant-rate intravenous infusion against time expressed as multiples of $t_{1/2}$. C_{ss} = concentration at steady state, Cl = clearance.

be described by a simple wash-in exponential curve (Fig. 1.8). The only factor influencing time to reach steady-state concentration is $t_{1/2}$. Maximum concentration is achieved after approximately 4–5 half-lives. Therefore, this method of administration is best suited to drugs with short half-lives such as remifentanil, glyceryl trinitrate, epinephrine and dopamine. However, in practice, it is often used for drugs such as morphine. Assuming a morphine $t_{1/2}$ of 4 h, it will be about 20 h before steady-state concentration is reached. Therefore, vigilant observation is required with this method of delivery, especially if active metabolites are involved – in this example, morphine-6-glucuronide.

There is a simple equation describing the concentration achieved at steady state during a constant-rate infusion; this is based on the principle that, at steady state, the amount of drug cleared from the plasma is equal to that delivered:

$$\text{Rate of infusion} = Cl \times C_{ss} \qquad (9)$$

where C_{ss} is the concentration at steady state.

Many pathological conditions reduce drug clearance and may therefore result in unexpectedly large plasma concentrations during infusions. Half-life does not influence C_{ss}, only how quickly it is achieved.

Patient-controlled analgesia (PCA)

The use of PCA for the treatment of postoperative pain has become widespread and is described in detail in Chapter 25. The patient titrates opioid delivery to requirements by pressing a button on a PCA device which results in the delivery of a small bolus dose. A lockout time is set which does not allow another bolus to be delivered until the previous dose has had time to have an effect. There is an enormous interpatient variability in opioid requirement after surgery; effective and closely monitored PCA is able to cope with this.

RECTAL

This technique reduces the problems of first-pass metabolism and the need for injections. It is used in children and adults (paracetamol, diclofenac, ibuprofen) for postoperative analgesia.

TRANSDERMAL

Drugs with a high lipid solubility and potency may be given transdermally. The pharmacological properties of glyceryl trinitrate render it ideal for this technique (i.e. potent, highly lipid-soluble, short half-life). Transdermal hyoscine is used for travel and other causes of sickness. Fentanyl patches can be very effective, particularly in patients with cancer pain. Buprenorphine and lidocaine transdermal delivery systems are also available. The latter is used for post-herpetic neuralgia which has not responded to more conventional techniques.

It may take some time before a steady-state plasma concentration is achieved and many devices incorporate large amounts of drug in the adhesive layer in order to provide a loading dose which reduces this period. At steady-state, transdermal delivery has several similarities to intravenous infusion. However, on removing the adhesive patch, plasma concentrations may decline relatively slowly because of a depot of drug in the surrounding skin; this occurs with transdermal fentanyl systems.

INHALATION

The delivery of inhaled volatile anaesthetics is discussed below, but other drugs may be given by this route, especially bronchodilators and steroids. Atropine and epinephrine are absorbed if injected into the bronchial tree and this offers a route of administration in emergencies if no other method of delivery is possible. Opioids such as fentanyl and diamorphine have been given as nebulized solutions but this technique is not routine.

EPIDURAL

This is a common route of administration in anaesthetic practice. The epidural space is very vascular and significant amounts of drug may be absorbed systemically, even if any vessels are avoided by the needle or cannula. Opioids diffuse across the dura to act on spinal opioid receptors, but much of their action when given epidurally is the result of systemic absorption. Complications include haematoma and infection, inadvertent dural puncture with consequent headache or spinal administration of the drug.

SPINAL (SUBARACHNOID)

When given spinally, drugs have free access to the neural tissue of the spinal cord and small doses have profound rapid effects, an advantage and also disadvantage of the method. Protein binding is not a significant factor as CSF protein concentration is relatively low.

DRUG INTERACTIONS

There are three basic types of drug interaction; examples are listed in Table 1.2.

Pharmaceutical

In this type of interaction, drugs often mixed in the same syringe or infusion bag react chemically with adverse results. For example, mixing succinylcholine with thiopental (pH 10–11) hydrolyses the former, rendering it inactive. Before mixing drugs, data should be sought on their compatibility.

Pharmacokinetic

Absorption of a drug, particularly if given orally, may be affected by other drugs because of their action on gastric emptying (see above). Interference with protein binding (see above) is a common cause of drug interaction. We have discussed drug metabolism in some detail and there are many potential sites in this process where interactions can occur (e.g. competition for enzyme systems, enzyme inhibition or induction).

Pharmacodynamic

This is the most frequent type of interaction in anaesthetic practice. A typical anaesthetic is a series of pharmacodynamic interactions. These may be adverse (e.g. increased respiratory depression with opioids and volatile agents) or advantageous (e.g. reversal of muscle relaxation with neostigmine). An understanding of the many subtle pharmacodynamic interactions in modern anaesthesia accounts for much of the difference in the

Table 1.2   Examples of drug interactions in anaesthesia

Type	Drugs	Effect
Pharmaceutical	Thiopental: succinylcholine	Hydrolysis of succinylcholine
	Ampicillin: glucose, lactate	Reduced potency
	Blood: dextrans	Rouleaux formation
		Cross-matching difficulties
	Plastic: glyceryl trinitrate	Adsorption to plastic
	Sevoflurane: soda lime	Compound A
Pharmacokinetic	Opioids: most drugs	Delayed oral absorption
	Warfarin: NSAIDs	↑ Free warfarin
	Barbiturates: warfarin	↑ Warfarin metabolism
	Neostigmine: succinylcholine	↓ Succinylcholine metabolism
Pharmacodynamic	Volatiles: opioids	↓ MAC
	Volatiles: benzodiazepines	↓ MAC
	Volatiles: N_2O	↓ MAC
	Volatiles: muscle relaxants	↑ Relaxation
	Morphine: naloxone	Reversal (receptor antagonism)
	Muscle relaxants: neostigmine	↓ Relaxation

quality of anaesthesia and recovery associated with the experienced compared with the novice anaesthetist.

VOLATILE ANAESTHETIC AGENTS

MECHANISM OF ACTION

The exact mechanism of action of volatile anaesthetic agents is at present unknown. Potency is, in general, related to lipid solubility (Meyer–Overton relationship, Table 1.3) and this has given rise to the concept of volatile agents dissolving in the lipid cell membrane in a non-specific manner, disrupting membrane function and thereby influencing the function of proteins, e.g. ion channels. However, it is now appreciated that volatile agents may affect neuronal function as a consequence of binding to specific protein sites (e.g. $GABA_A$ receptor).

POTENCY

The potency of volatile agents is defined in terms of minimum alveolar concentration (MAC). MAC is the alveolar concentration of a volatile agent that produces no movement in 50% of spontaneously breathing patients after skin incision. MAC is inversely related to lipid solubility (Table 1.3).

Table 1.3   MAC in oxygen and lipid solubility (expressed as oil/gas solubility coefficient)

Agent	MAC (%) in O_2	Oil/gas solubility
N_2O	104	1.4
Desflurane	6.6	18.7
Sevoflurane	1.8	42
Isoflurane	1.17	97
Halothane	0.75	224

ONSET OF ACTION

When considering onset of action of volatile agents, there is a fundamental difference compared with intravenous agents. Effects of non-volatile drugs are related to plasma or tissue concentrations; this is not so with volatile agents. Partial pressure of the volatile agent is important, not concentration. If a volatile agent is highly soluble in blood, partial pressure increases slowly as large amounts dissolve in the blood. Consequently, onset of anaesthesia is slow with agents soluble in blood and rapid with agents which are relatively insoluble. The same applies to recovery from

Table 1.4   Solubility of inhaled anaesthetic agents in blood (expressed as blood/gas solubility coefficients)

Agent	Blood/gas solubility coefficient
Desflurane	0.42
N_2O	0.47
Sevoflurane	0.65
Isoflurane	1.4
Halothane	2.3

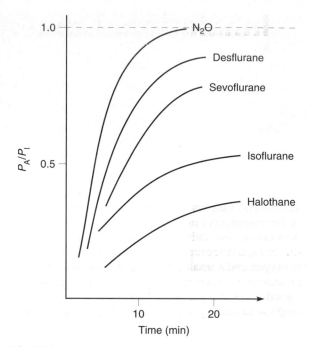

Fig. 1.9
The rate at which P_A reaches P_I is related to the speed of induction of anaesthesia. Agents insoluble in blood equilibrate more rapidly.

anaesthesia. Table 1.4 lists the most commonly used inhaled agents (in order of speed of onset) and their relative blood/gas solubilities.

Alveolar partial pressure (P_A) is assumed to be equivalent to cerebral artery partial pressure and therefore depth of anaesthesia. At a fixed inspired partial pressure (P_I), the rate at which P_A approaches P_I is related to speed of onset of effect (Fig. 1.9). This is rapid with agents of low blood solubility (e.g. sevoflurane) and relatively slow with more soluble agents (e.g. halothane).

Clearly, solubility of the agent in blood is a major determinant of the speed of onset of anaesthesia, but other factors can have significant effects. The rate of delivery of the agent to the alveoli is important; therefore increasing P_I by adjusting the vaporizer (a factor limited by irritant effects on the airway in spontaneously breathing patients), reducing apparatus dead space and increasing alveolar ventilation increase speed of induction of anaesthesia. If cardiac output is reduced, relatively less agent is removed from the alveolus and P_A increases towards P_I more rapidly. Consequently, induction of anaesthesia is more rapid in patients with reduced cardiac output. Both rate of delivery and cardiac output have particularly signifi-

cant effects with agents that are relatively soluble in blood but less so with insoluble agents.

Ventilation/perfusion mismatch may reduce the speed of induction, an effect more significant in agents of low solubility. For example, if one lung is collapsed (i.e. perfused but not ventilated) increasing ventilation or inspired concentration of agents such as halothane helps to compensate. However, this is not the case for agents such as sevoflurane.

FURTHER READING

Calvey T N, Williams N E 2001 Principles and practice of pharmacology for anaesthetists, 4th edn. Blackwell Scientific Publications, Oxford

Inhalational anaesthetic agents

2

Volatile and gaseous anaesthetic agents remain popular for maintenance of anaesthesia and, under some circumstances, for induction of anaesthesia. In many situations, it is appropriate to use a mixture of 66% N_2O in oxygen and a small concentration of a volatile agent to maintain anaesthesia, although for reasons discussed below there are occasions when an anaesthetist might wish actively to avoid the use of nitrous oxide.

PROPERTIES OF THE IDEAL INHALATIONAL ANAESTHETIC AGENT

- It should have a pleasant odour, be non-irritant to the respiratory tract and allow pleasant and rapid induction of anaesthesia.
- It should possess a low blood/gas solubility, which permits rapid induction of and rapid recovery from anaesthesia.
- It should be chemically stable in storage and should not interact with the material of anaesthetic circuits or with soda lime.
- It should be neither flammable nor explosive.
- It should be capable of producing unconsciousness with analgesia and preferably some degree of muscle relaxation.
- It should be sufficiently potent to allow the use of high inspired oxygen concentrations when necessary.
- It should not be metabolized in the body, be non-toxic and not provoke allergic reactions.
- It should produce minimal depression of the cardiovascular and respiratory systems and should not interact with other drugs used commonly during anaesthesia, e.g. pressor agents or catecholamines.
- It should be completely inert and eliminated completely and rapidly in an unchanged form via the lungs.

- It should be easy to administer using standard vaporizers.
- It should not be epileptogenic or raise intracranial pressure.

None of the inhalational anaesthetic agents approaches the standards required of the ideal agent.

MINIMUM ALVEOLAR CONCENTRATION (MAC)

MAC is the minimum alveolar concentration (in volumes per cent) of an anaesthetic at 1 atmosphere absolute (ata) that prevents movement of 50% of the population to a standard stimulus. Anaesthesia is related to the partial pressure of an inhalational agent in the brain rather than its percentage concentration in alveoli, but the term MAC has gained widespread acceptance as an index of anaesthetic potency because this can be measured. It may be applied to all inhalational anaesthetics and it permits comparison of different agents. However, it represents only one point on a dose–response curve; 1 MAC of one agent is equivalent in anaesthetic potency to 1 MAC of another, but it does not follow that the agents are equipotent at 2 MAC. Nevertheless, in general terms, 0.5 MAC of one agent in combination with 0.5 MAC of another approximates to 1 MAC in total.

The MAC values for the anaesthetic agents quoted in Table 2.1 (see p. 26) were determined experimentally in humans (volunteers) breathing a mixture of the agent in oxygen. MAC values vary under the following circumstances.

Factors which lead to a reduction in MAC

- sedative drugs such as premedication agents, analgesics
- nitrous oxide
- increasing age

- drugs which affect neurotransmitter release such as methyldopa, pancuronium and clonidine
- higher atmospheric pressure, as anaesthetic potency is related to partial pressure – e.g. MAC for enflurane is 1.68% (1.66 kPa) at a pressure of 1 ata, but 0.84% (still 1.66 kPa) at 2 ata
- hypotension
- hypothermia
- myxoedema
- pregnancy.

Factors which increase MAC

- decreasing age
- pyrexia
- induced sympathoadrenal stimulation, e.g. hypercapnia
- the presence of ephedrine, or amphetamine
- thyrotoxicosis
- chronic alcohol ingestion.

INDIVIDUAL ANAESTHETIC AGENTS

Physical properties of the inhalational anaesthetic agents are summarized in Appendix B, II. The structural formulae of the agents discussed in this chapter are shown in Figure 2.1.

AGENTS IN COMMON CLINICAL USE

In Western countries, it is customary to use one of the five modern volatile anaesthetic agents – desflurane, enflurane, halothane, isoflurane and sevoflurane – vaporized in a mixture of nitrous oxide in oxygen. In recent years, the use of halothane has declined because of medicolegal pressure relating to the very rare occurrence of hepatotoxicity and hence there has been a clear trend to avoidance of repeated halothane anaesthesia. The use of sevoflurane is increasing rapidly, particularly in paediatric anaesthesia because of its superior quality as an inhalational induction agent. Desflurane produces rapid recovery from anaesthesia, but it is very irritant to the airway and is therefore not used as an inhalational induction agent.

The following account of these agents, with a comparison of their pharmacological properties, may tend to exaggerate the differences between them. However, an equally satisfactory anaesthetic may be administered in the majority of patients with any of the five agents.

Ethers

Diethyl ether
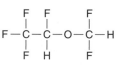

Desflurane
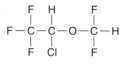

Enflurane

Isoflurane

Sevoflurane
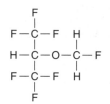

Halogenated hydrocarbons

Halothane
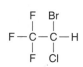

Fig. 2.1
Structural formulae of inhalational anaesthetic agents.

DESFLURANE

Between 1959 and 1966, Terrell and his associates at Ohio Medical Products synthesized more than 700 compounds to try to produce improved inhalational anaesthetic agents. Two of these products were the halogenated methyl ethyl ethers, isoflurane and enflurane, which have now been widely used. Some of the original 700 products were re-examined many years later. Many were discarded for a variety of reasons.

One of these (the 653rd) was difficult to synthesize because of a potentially explosive step using elemental fluorine and it had a vapour pressure close to 1 atm. However, because it was predicted to have a low solubility in blood and hence would allow rapid recovery, it was re-examined with heightened interest. This product became known as desflurane. Desflurane was first used in humans in 1988 and it became available for general clinical use in the UK in 1993. Its structure (CHF_2–O–CHF–CF_3) differs from that of isoflurane (CHF_2–O–CHCl–CF_3) only in the substitution of fluorine for chlorine.

Physical properties

It is a colourless agent, which is stored in amber-coloured bottles without preservative. It is not broken down by soda lime, light or metals. It is non-flammable.

Desflurane has a boiling point of 23.5°C and a vapour pressure of 88.5k Pa (664 mmHg) at 20°C and therefore it cannot be used in a standard vaporizer. A special vaporizer (the TEC-6) has been developed which requires a source of electric power to heat and pressurize it.

The MAC of desflurane is approximately 6% in oxygen (3% in 60% nitrous oxide). As with all volatile agents, its MAC is higher in children (9–10% in the neonate in oxygen, 7% in 60% nitrous oxide)

It has an ethereal but less pungent odour than isoflurane.

Uptake and distribution

Desflurane has a blood/gas partition coefficient of 0.42, almost the same as that of nitrous oxide. The rate of equilibration of alveolar with inspired concentrations of desflurane is virtually identical to that for nitrous oxide (Fig. 2.2). Induction of anaesthesia is therefore extremely rapid in theory but limited somewhat by its pungent nature. However, it is possible to alter the depth of anaesthesia very rapidly and the rate of recovery of anaesthesia is faster than that following any other volatile anaesthetic agent (Fig. 2.3).

Metabolism

There is very little defluorination of desflurane, and after prolonged anaesthesia there is only a very small increase in serum and urine trifluoroacetic acid concentrations. Approximately 0.02% of inhaled desflurane is metabolized in the body.

Respiratory system

Desflurane causes respiratory depression to a degree similar to that of isoflurane up to a MAC of 1.5. It increases P_aCO_2 (Fig. 2.4) and decreases the ventilatory response to imposed increases in P_aCO_2. It is irritant to the upper respiratory tract, particularly at concentrations greater than 6%. It is therefore not recommended for gaseous induction of anaesthesia because it causes coughing, breath-holding and laryngospasm.

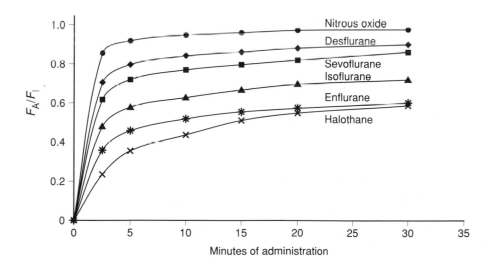

Fig. 2.2
Ratio of alveolar (F_A) to inspired (F_I) fractional concentration of nitrous oxide, desflurane, sevoflurane, isoflurane, enflurane and halothane in the first 30 min of anaesthesia. The plot of F_A/F_I expresses the rapidity with which alveolar concentration equilibrates with inspired concentration. It is most rapid for agents with a low blood/gas partition coefficient.

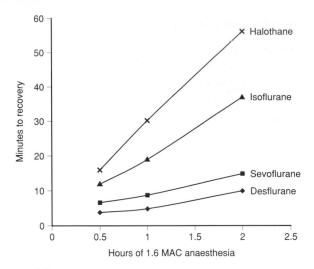

Fig. 2.3
Rapidity of recovery from anaesthesia is inversely proportional to the solubility of the anaesthetic: the most rapid recovery is with the least soluble anaesthetic (desflurane). The difference is amplified by duration of anaesthesia. Note that the difference in time of recovery between the least (desflurane) and most soluble anaesthetic (halothane) is greater after 2 h of anaesthesia than after 0.5 h of anaesthesia.

Cardiovascular effects

Desflurane appears to have two distinct actions on the cardiovascular system. Firstly, its main actions are those which are similar to isoflurane: dose-related decreases in systemic vascular resistance, myocardial contractility and mean arterial pressure (Figs 2.5–2.7). Heart rate is unchanged at lower steady-state concentrations, but increases with higher concentrations (Fig. 2.9). Addition of nitrous oxide maintains heart rate unchanged. Cardiac output tends to be maintained as with isoflurane. The second cardiovascular action occurs when its inspired concentration is increased rapidly to greater than 1 MAC. In the absence of premedication drugs, this increases sympathetic activity, leading to increased heart rate and mean arterial pressure. Preliminary experimental studies in animals have not detected a coronary steal phenomenon. Desflurane, in common with isoflurane and sevoflurane, does not sensitize the myocardium to catecholamines (Fig. 2.8).

Central nervous system

The effects of desflurane are similar to those of isoflurane. It depresses the EEG in a dose-related manner. It does not cause seizure activity at any level of anaesthesia, with or without hypocapnia. Desflurane decreases cerebrovascular resistance and increases intracranial pressure in a dose-related manner. In dogs, it increases cerebral blood flow at deep levels of anaesthesia if systemic arterial pressure is maintained.

Musculoskeletal system

Desflurane causes muscle relaxation in a dose-related manner. Concentrations exceeding 1 MAC produce fade in response to tetanic stimulation of the ulnar

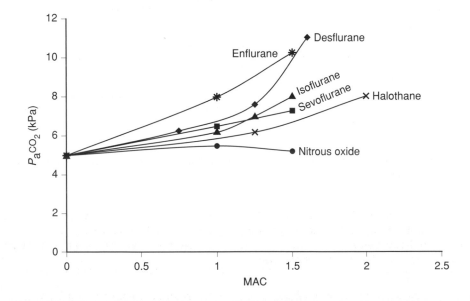

Fig. 2.4
Effects on $P_a\text{CO}_2$ of halothane, enflurane, isoflurane, sevoflurane, desflurane and nitrous oxide at equivalent MAC during spontaneous ventilation by healthy volunteers. (Nitrous oxide was administered in a hyperbaric chamber.)

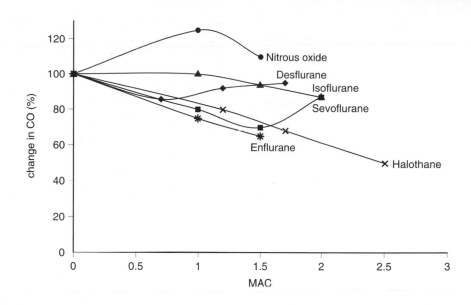

Fig. 2.5
Comparative effects of nitrous oxide, isoflurane, halothane, enflurane, desflurane and sevoflurane on cardiac output (CO) in healthy volunteers.

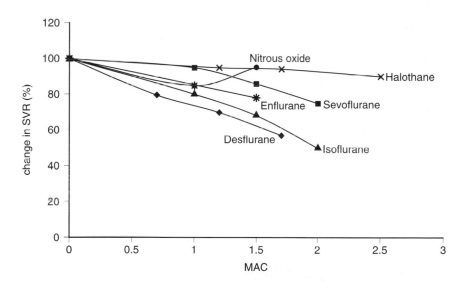

Fig. 2.6
Comparative effects of nitrous oxide, halothane, enflurane, isoflurane, sevoflurane and desflurane on systemic vascular resistance (SVR) in healthy volunteers.

nerve. It enhances the effect of muscle relaxants. Studies in susceptible swine indicate that desflurane may trigger malignant hyperthermia.

Therefore, in summary, desflurane offers some advantages over other agents:

- It has a low blood solubility; therefore it offers more precise control of maintenance of anaesthesia and rapid recovery.

- It is minimally biodegradable and therefore non-toxic to the liver and kidney.
- It does not cause convulsive activity on EEG.

However, it has some significant drawbacks:

- It cannot be used for inhalational induction because of its irritant effects on the airway.
- It causes tachycardia at higher concentrations.

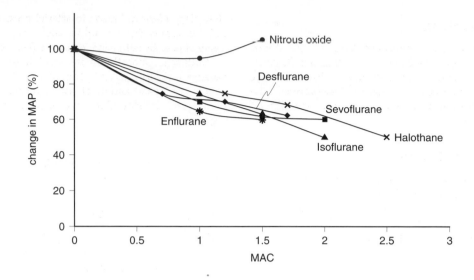

Fig. 2.7
Comparative effects of nitrous oxide, halothane, enflurane, isoflurane, sevoflurane and desflurane on mean arterial pressure (MAP) in healthy volunteers.

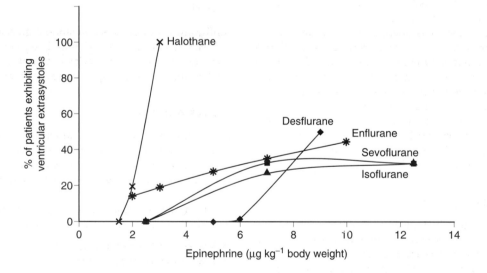

Fig. 2.8
Cumulative plots representing dose of subcutaneous epinephrine required to produce ventricular extrasystoles in normocapnic patients receiving 1.25 MAC of halothane, enflurane, isoflurane, sevoflurane or desflurane.

- It requires a special vaporizer. Although the TEC-6 vaporizer is reasonably easy to use, it is more complex than the more conventional vaporizers and the potential for failure may be higher.
- It is expensive.

ENFLURANE

Enflurane (2-chloro-1,1,2-trifluoroethyl difluoromethyl ether) was synthesized in 1963 and first evaluated clinically in 1966. It was introduced into clinical practice in the USA in 1971.

Physical properties

Enflurane is a clear, colourless, volatile anaesthetic agent with a pleasant ethereal smell. It is non-flammable in clinical concentrations, stable with soda lime and metals and does not require preservatives. The MAC of enflurane is 1.68% in oxygen and 0.57% in 70% nitrous oxide.

Uptake and distribution

Enflurane has a blood/gas solubility coefficient of 1.9, which is between that of halothane and isoflurane. Thus, induction of and recovery from anaesthesia are faster than halothane but slower than isoflurane, desflurane and sevoflurane (Fig. 2.2).

Metabolism

Approximately 2.5% of the absorbed dose is metabolized, predominantly to fluoride. In common with other ether anaesthetic agents, the presence of the ether bond imparts stability to the molecule.

Defluorination of enflurane is increased in patients treated with isoniazid, but not with a classic enzyme-inducing agent such as phenobarbital. Serum fluoride ion concentrations are greater after administration of enflurane to obese patients. To date, extensive studies have failed to demonstrate that the serum concentrations of fluoride ion reach toxic levels after enflurane anaesthesia. The plasma fluoride ion concentrations attained after enflurane anaesthesia are approximately 20 μmol L^{-1} (which is below the 50 μmol L^{-1} thought to be associated with renal damage after anaesthesia with methoxyflurane).

Respiratory system

Enflurane is non-irritant and does not increase salivary or bronchial secretions; thus inhalational induction is relatively pleasant and rapid.

In common with all other volatile anaesthetic agents, enflurane causes dose-dependent depression of alveolar ventilation with a reduction in tidal volume and an increase in ventilatory rate in the unpremedicated subject. This results in an increase in arterial partial pressure of CO_2 (Fig. 2.4).

Cardiovascular system

Enflurane causes dose-dependent depression of myocardial contractility, leading to a reduction in cardiac output (Fig. 2.5). In association with a small reduction in systemic vascular resistance, this leads to a dose-dependent reduction in arterial pressure (Figs 2.6, 2.7). Because enflurane (unlike halothane) has no central vagal effects, hypotension leads to reflex tachycardia.

Enflurane anaesthesia is associated with a much smaller incidence of arrhythmias than halothane and much less sensitization of the myocardium to catecholamines, either endogenous or exogenous (Fig. 2.8).

Uterus

Enflurane relaxes uterine muscle in a dose-related manner.

Central nervous system

Enflurane produces a dose-dependent depression of EEG activity, but at moderate to high concentrations (more than 3%) it produces epileptiform paroxysmal spike activity and burst suppression. These are accentuated by hypocapnia. Twitching of the face and arm muscles may occur occasionally. Enflurane should be avoided in the epileptic patient.

Muscle relaxation

Enflurane produces dose-dependent muscle relaxation with potentiation of non-depolarizing neuromuscular blocking drugs to a greater extent than that produced by halothane. It may trigger malignant hyperthermia.

Hepatotoxicity

There have been several case reports of jaundice attributable to the use of enflurane, and derangement of liver enzymes also occurs after enflurane anaesthesia, although to a lesser extent than after halothane.

In summary, enflurane is a useful alternative agent to halothane. Its main advantages are:

- low risk of hepatic dysfunction
- low incidence of arrhythmias.

Its disadvantages are:

- seizure activity on EEG
- its use in patients with pre-existing renal disease or in those taking enzyme-inducing drugs may be unwise.

HALOTHANE

Halothane (2-bromo-2-chloro-1,1,1-trifluoroethane) was synthesized in 1951 and introduced into clinical practice in the UK in 1956. It is a colourless liquid with a relatively pleasant smell. It is decomposed by light.

The addition of 0.01% thymol and storage in amber-coloured bottles renders it stable. Although it is decomposed by soda lime, it may be used safely with this mixture. It corrodes metals in vaporizers and breathing systems. In the presence of moisture, it corrodes aluminium, tin, lead, magnesium and alloys. It should be stored in a closed container away from light and heat.

Uptake and distribution

Halothane has a blood/gas solubility coefficient of 2.5, which is the highest of all the modern agents. It is not irritant to the airway and therefore inhalational induction with halothane is relatively fast compared with either desflurane or isoflurane. However, it may take at least 30 min for the alveolar inspired concentration to reach 50% of the inspired concentration (Fig. 2.2); this is slower than for the other agents. As with all the volatile agents, it is customary to use the technique of 'over-pressure' and induce halothane anaesthesia with concentrations two to three times higher than the MAC value; the inspired concentration is reduced when a stable level of anaesthesia has been achieved. The MAC of halothane in oxygen is approximately 1.1% in the neonate, 0.95% in the infant, 0.9% at 1–2 years, 0.75% at 40 years (0.29 in 70% nitrous oxide) and 0.65% at 80 years.

Recovery from halothane anaesthesia is slower than with the other agents because of its high blood/gas solubility, and recovery is prolonged with increasing duration of anaesthesia (Fig. 2.3).

Metabolism

Approximately 20% of halothane is metabolized in the liver, usually by oxidative pathways. The end products are excreted in the urine. The major metabolites are bromine, chlorine, trifluoroacetic acid and trifluoroacetylethanol amide.

A small proportion of halothane may undergo reductive metabolism, particularly in the presence of hypoxaemia and when the hepatic microsomal enzymes have been stimulated by enzyme-inducing agents such as phenobarbital. Reductive metabolism may result in the formation of reactive metabolites and fluoride, although normally serum fluoride ion concentrations are considerably lower than those likely to induce renal dysfunction.

Respiratory system

Halothane is non-irritant and pleasant to breathe during induction of anaesthesia. There is rapid loss of pharyngeal and laryngeal reflexes and inhibition of salivary and bronchial secretions. In the unpremed-

icated subject, halothane anaesthesia is associated with an increase in ventilatory rate and reduction in tidal volume. $P_a\mathrm{CO}_2$ increases as the depth of halothane anaesthesia increases (Fig. 2.4).

Halothane causes a dose-dependent decrease in mucociliary function, which may persist for several hours after anaesthesia. This may contribute to postoperative sputum retention.

Halothane antagonizes bronchospasm and reduces airway resistance in patients with bronchoconstriction, possibly by central inhibition of reflex bronchoconstriction and relaxation of bronchial smooth muscle. It has been suggested that halothane exerts a β-mimetic effect on bronchial muscle.

Cardiovascular system

Halothane is a potent depressant of myocardial contractility and myocardial metabolic activity as a result of inhibition of glucose uptake by myocardial cells. During controlled ventilation, halothane anaesthesia is associated with dose-related depression of cardiac output (by decrease in myocardial contractility) with little effect on peripheral resistance (Figs 2.5, 2.6). Thus, there is a reduction in arterial pressure (Fig. 2.7) and an increase in right atrial pressure. In spontaneously breathing patients, some of these effects may be offset by a small increase in $P_a\mathrm{CO}_2$ which leads to a reduction in systemic vascular resistance and a shift in cardiac output back towards baseline values as a result of indirect sympathoadrenal stimulation.

The hypotensive effect of halothane is augmented by a reduction in heart rate, which commonly accompanies halothane anaesthesia. Antagonism of the bradycardia by administration of atropine frequently leads to an increase in arterial pressure.

The reduction in myocardial contractility is associated with reductions in myocardial oxygen demand and coronary blood flow. Provided that undue elevations in left ventricular diastolic pressure and undue hypotension do not occur, halothane may be advantageous in patients with coronary artery disease because of the reduced oxygen demand caused by a low heart rate and decreased contractility.

The depressant effects of halothane on cardiac output are augmented in the presence of β-blockade.

Arrhythmias are very common during halothane anaesthesia and far more frequent than with any of the other agents. Arrhythmias are produced by:

- increased myocardial excitability augmented by the presence of hypercapnia, hypoxaemia or increased circulating catecholamines
- bradycardia caused by central vagal stimulation.

During local infiltration with local anaesthetic solutions containing epinephrine, multifocal ventricular extrasystoles and sinus tachycardia have been observed and cardiac arrest has been reported. Thus, caution should be exercised when these solutions are used. The following recommendations have been made:

- Avoid hypoxaemia and hypercapnia.
- Avoid concentrations of epinephrine greater than 1 in 100 000.
- Avoid a dosage in adults exceeding 10 ml of 1 in 100 000 epinephrine in 10 min (i.e. 100 μg) or 30 ml h^{-1} (300 μg).

Approximately 20% of patients breathing 1.25 MAC of halothane and who receive subcutaneous infiltration of 2 μg kg^{-1} epinephrine exhibit ventricular ectopics. This increases to 100% of patients receiving 2.5–3 μg kg^{-1} (Fig. 2.8).

Patients undergoing dental surgery with halothane anaesthesia are particularly prone to developing arrhythmias.

Central nervous system

Halothane produces anaesthesia without analgesia. Cerebral blood flow and intracranial pressure are raised. It does not cause seizure activity on EEG.

Gastrointestinal tract

Gastrointestinal motility is inhibited. Postoperative nausea and vomiting are seldom severe.

Uterus

Halothane relaxes uterine muscle and may cause postpartum haemorrhage. It is said that a concentration of less than 0.5% is not associated with increased blood loss during anaesthesia for Caesarean section, but this concentration causes increased blood loss during therapeutic abortion.

Skeletal muscle

Halothane causes skeletal muscle relaxation and potentiates non-depolarizing relaxants. Postoperatively, shivering is common; this increases oxygen requirements and results in hypoxaemia unless oxygen is administered. Halothane may trigger malignant hyperthermia in susceptible patients.

Halothane-associated hepatic dysfunction

There are two types of dysfunction which may occur after halothane anaesthesia. The first is mild and is associated with derangement in liver function tests. These changes are transient and generally resolve within a few days. Similar changes in liver function tests have also been reported after enflurane anaesthesia and, to a lesser extent, isoflurane anaesthesia.

This subclinical type of hepatic dysfunction, evidenced by an increase in glutathione-S-transferase (GST) concentrations, probably occurs as a result of metabolism of halothane in the liver, where it reacts with hepatic macromolecules, resulting in tissue necrosis, which is worsened by hypoxaemia.

The second type of hepatic dysfunction is extremely uncommon and takes the form of severe jaundice, progressing to fulminating hepatic necrosis. The mortality of this condition varies between 30 and 70%. The likelihood of this type of hepatic dysfunction is increased by repeated exposure to the drug. The mechanism of these changes is probably the formation of a hapten–protein complex. The hapten is probably one of the metabolites of halothane, notably trifluoroacetyl (TFA) halide, as antibodies to TFA proteins have been detected in patients who develop jaundice after halothane anaesthesia.

The incidence of type 2 liver dysfunction after halothane anaesthesia is extremely low — so low that it is extremely difficult to mount well-controlled studies of the condition, and consequently this whole subject has been an area of great controversy in the past. Nonetheless, as a result of this concern, the Committee on Safety of Medicines has made the following recommendations in respect of halothane anaesthesia:

- A careful anaesthetic history should be taken to determine previous exposure and any previous reaction to halothane.
- Repeated exposure to halothane within a period of 3 months should be avoided unless there are overriding clinical circumstances.
- A history of unexplained jaundice or pyrexia after previous exposure to halothane is an absolute contraindication to its future use in that patient.

The incidence of halothane hepatotoxicity in paediatric practice is extremely low, although there have been case reports in children. Nevertheless, halothane is still used in paediatric anaesthesia

In summary, halothane is a very useful inhalational anaesthetic agent. Its main advantages are:

- smooth induction
- minimal stimulation of salivary and bronchial secretions
- bronchodilatation.

The disadvantages are:

- arrhythmias
- possibility of liver toxicity, especially with repeated administrations
- slow recovery compared with other new agents (see Fig. 2.3).

ISOFLURANE

Isoflurane (1-chloro-2,2,2-trifluoroethyl difluoromethyl ether) is an isomer of enflurane and was synthesized in 1965. Clinical studies were undertaken in 1970, but because of early laboratory reports of carcinogenesis (which were not confirmed subsequently) it was not approved by the Food and Drug Administration in the United States until 1980.

Physical properties

Isoflurane is a colourless, volatile liquid with a slightly pungent odour. It is stable and does not react with metal or other substances. It does not require preservatives. Isoflurane is non-flammable in clinical concentrations. The MAC of isoflurane is 1.15% in oxygen and 0.56% in 70% nitrous oxide.

Uptake and distribution

Isoflurane has a low blood/gas solubility of 1.4 and thus alveolar concentrations equilibrate rapidly with inspired concentrations. The alveolar (or arterial) partial pressure of isoflurane increases to 50% of the inspired partial pressure within 4–8 min, and to 60% by 15 min (Fig. 2.2). However, the rate of induction is limited by the pungency of the vapour and clinically may be no faster than that which may be achieved with halothane. The incidence of coughing or breathholding on induction is significantly greater with isoflurane than with halothane. It is not an ideal agent to use for inhalational induction.

Metabolism

Approximately 0.17% of the absorbed dose is metabolized. Metabolism takes place predominantly in the form of oxidation to produce difluoromethanol and trifluoroacetic acid; the former breaks down to formic acid and fluoride. Because of the minimal metabolism, only very small concentrations of serum fluoride ions are found, even after prolonged administration. The minimal metabolism renders hepatic and renal toxicity most unlikely.

Respiratory system

In common with other modern volatile agents, it causes dose-dependent depression of ventilation (Fig. 2.4); there is a decrease in tidal volume but an increase in ventilatory rate in the absence of opioid drugs. Isoflurane causes some respiratory irritation. This makes inhalational induction with isoflurane difficult.

Cardiovascular system

In vitro, isoflurane is a myocardial depressant, but in clinical use there is less depression of cardiac output than with halothane or enflurane (Fig. 2.5). Systemic hypotension occurs predominantly as a result of reduction in systemic vascular resistance (Figs 2.6, 2.7). Arrhythmias are uncommon and there is little sensitization of the myocardium to catecholamines (Fig. 2.8).

In addition to dilating systemic arterioles, isoflurane causes coronary vasodilatation. In the past there has been some controversy regarding the safety of isoflurane in patients with coronary artery disease because of the possibility that the coronary steal syndrome may be induced; dilatation in normal coronary arteries offers a low resistance to flow and may reduce perfusion through stenosed vessels. It has been shown that isoflurane affects small arterioles (which makes coronary steal a theoretical possibility), but this does not appear to be of any clinical significance. Production of myocardial ischaemia in clinical practice may be a result of many factors in addition to coronary vasodilatation, including tachycardia, hypotension, increase in left ventricular end-diastolic pressure and reduced ventricular compliance. Attention should be directed to these factors before a diagnosis of isoflurane-induced coronary steal is considered.

Uterus

Isoflurane has an effect on the pregnant uterus similar to that of halothane and enflurane.

Central nervous system

Low concentrations of isoflurane do not cause any change in cerebral blood flow at normocapnia. In this respect, the drug is superior to enflurane and halothane, both of which cause cerebral vasodilatation. However, higher inspired concentrations of isoflurane cause vasodilatation and increase cerebral blood flow. It does not cause seizure activity on the EEG.

Muscle relaxation

Isoflurane causes dose-dependent depression of neuromuscular transmission with potentiation of non-depolarizing neuromuscular blocking drugs.

In summary, the advantages of isoflurane are:

- rapid recovery
- minimal biotransformation with little risk of hepatic or renal toxicity
- very low risk of arrhythmias
- muscle relaxation.

Its disadvantages are:

- a pungent odour which makes inhalational induction relatively unpleasant, particularly in children.

SEVOFLURANE

Sevoflurane (fluoromethyl-2,2,2-trifluoro-1-ethyl ether) was first synthesized in 1968 and its clinical use reported in 1971. The initial development was slow because of some apparent toxic effects, which were found later to be caused by flawed experimental design. After its first use in volunteers in 1981, further work was delayed again because of the problems of biotransformation and stability with soda lime. The drug has been available for general clinical use since 1990.

Physical properties

It is non-flammable and has a pleasant smell. The blood/gas partition coefficient of sevoflurane is 0.69, which is about half that of isoflurane (1.43) and closer to those of desflurane (0.42) and nitrous oxide (0.44). The MAC value of sevoflurane in adults is between 1.7 and 2% in oxygen and 0.66% in 60% nitrous oxide. The MAC, in common with other volatile agents, is higher in children (2.6% in oxygen and 2.0% in nitrous oxide) and neonates (3.3%) and it is reduced in the elderly (1.48%). It is stable and is stored in amber-coloured bottles. In the presence of water, it undergoes some hydrolysis and this reaction also occurs with soda lime.

Uptake and distribution

It has a low blood/gas partition coefficient and therefore the rate of equilibration between alveolar and inspired concentrations is faster than that for halothane, enflurane or isoflurane but slower than that for desflurane (Fig. 2.2). It is non-irritant to the upper respiratory tract and therefore the rate of induction of anaesthesia should be faster than that with any of the other agents.

Because of its higher partition coefficients in vessel-rich tissues, muscle and fat than corresponding values for desflurane, the rate of recovery is slower than that after desflurane anaesthesia (Fig. 2.3).

Metabolism

Approximately 5% of the absorbed dose is metabolized in the liver to two main metabolites. The major breakdown product is hexafluoroisopropanol, an organic fluoride molecule which is excreted in the urine as a glucuronide conjugate. Although this molecule is potentially hepatotoxic, conjugation of hexafluoroisopropanol occurs so rapidly that clinically significant liver damage seems theoretically impossible. The second breakdown product is inorganic fluoride ion. The mean peak fluoride ion concentration after 60 min of anaesthesia at 1 MAC is 22 μmol L^{-1}, which is similar to that produced after enflurane anaesthesia and significantly higher than that after an equivalent dose of isoflurane. The metabolism of sevoflurane is catalysed by the 2E1 isoform of cytochrome P450 which may be induced by phenobarbital, isoniazid and ethanol and inhibited by disulfiram.

Respiratory system

The drug is non-irritant to the upper respiratory tract. It produces dose-dependent ventilatory depression, reduces respiratory drive in response to hypoxia and increases carbon dioxide partial pressure comparable with levels achieved with other volatile agents (Fig. 2.4). The ventilatory depression associated with sevoflurane may result from a combination of central depression of medullary respiratory neurones and depression of diaphragmatic function and contractility. It relaxes bronchial smooth muscle but not as effectively as halothane.

Cardiovascular system

The properties of sevoflurane are similar to those of isoflurane with slightly smaller effects on heart rate (Fig. 2.9) and less coronary vasodilatation. It decreases arterial pressure (Fig. 2.7) mainly by reducing peripheral vascular resistance (Fig. 2.6), but cardiac output is well maintained over the normal anaesthetic maintenance doses (Fig. 2.5). There is mild myocardial depression resulting from its effect on calcium channels. Sevoflurane does not differ from isoflurane in its sensitization of the myocardium to exogenous catecholamines (Fig. 2.8). It is a less potent coronary arteriolar dilator and does not appear to cause 'coronary steal'. Sevoflurane is associated with a lower heart rate

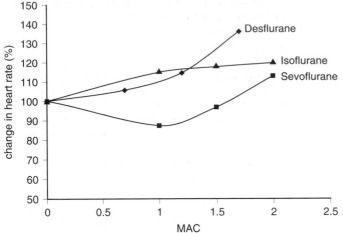

Fig. 2.9
Comparative effects of isoflurane, sevoflurane and desflurane on heart rate in healthy volunteers.

and therefore helps to reduce myocardial oxygen consumption.

Central nervous system

Its effects are similar to those of isoflurane and desflurane. Intracranial pressure increases at high inspired concentrations of sevoflurane but this effect is minimal over the 0.5–1.0 MAC range. It decreases cerebral vascular resistance and cerebral metabolic rate. It does not cause excitatory effects on the EEG.

Renal system

The peak concentration of inorganic fluoride after sevoflurane is similar to that after enflurane anaesthesia and there is a positive correlation between duration of exposure and the peak concentration of fluoride ions. Serum fluoride concentrations greater than 50 μmol L^{-1} have been reported. However, renal toxicity does not appear to be related to inorganic fluoride concentrations following anaesthesia with sevoflurane as opposed to that associated with methoxyflurane. The apparent lack of renal toxicity with sevoflurane may be related to its rapid elimination from the body. This reduces the total amount of drug available for in vivo metabolism.

Renal blood flow is well preserved with sevoflurane.

Musculoskeletal system

In common with isoflurane, the drug potentiates nondepolarizing muscle relaxants, and to a similar extent. Sevoflurane may trigger malignant hyperthermia in susceptible patients and there have been cases reported in the literature.

Obstetric use

There are limited data on the use of sevoflurane in the obstetric population.

Interaction with carbon dioxide absorbers

Sevoflurane is absorbed and degraded by both soda lime and Baralyme. When mixed with soda lime in artificial situations, five breakdown products are identified, which are termed compounds A, B, C, D and E. These products are thought to be toxic in rats, primarily causing renal, hepatic and cerebral damage. However, in clinical situations, it is mainly compound A and, to a lesser extent, compound B that are produced. The evidence suggests that the concentration of compound A produced is well below the level that is toxic to animals. The use of Baralyme is associated with production of higher concentrations of compound A and this may be related to the higher temperature which is attained when Baralyme is used. The presence of moisture reduces compound A formation. The concentration of compound A is highest during low-flow anaesthesia (<2 L min^{-1}) and is reduced by increasing fresh gas flow rate. The toxicity of sevoflurane in combination with carbon dioxide absorbers is possibly more a theoretical than a clinical problem but it may be wise to avoid its use with very low fresh gas flows and in patients with poor renal function.

In summary, sevoflurane is a newer inhalational anaesthetic agent which offers many advantages over other volatile agents. These are:

- smooth, fast induction
- rapid recovery
- ease of use, requiring conventional vaporizers (particularly when compared with desflurane).

Its disadvantages are:

- production of potentially toxic metabolites in the body (more a theoretical problem)
- instability with carbon dioxide absorbers
- relative expense.

COMPARISON OF HALOTHANE, ENFLURANE, ISOFLURANE, SEVOFLURANE AND DESFLURANE

Pharmacokinetics

The rate of equilibration of alveolar with inspired concentrations is related to blood/gas solubility. The rate of uptake of desflurane is faster than that of any of the other volatile agents and similar to that of nitrous oxide (Fig. 2.2). Despite its low blood/gas solubility, the rate of induction of anaesthesia with desflurane (and isoflurane) may be reduced because of the pungent odour compared with the more pleasant odours of sevoflurane, halothane and enflurane. Sevoflurane provides a smooth rapid induction and it has largely replaced halothane for induction in children. Potency, on the other hand, is related to the lower oil/water solubility. Sevoflurane and desflurane are less potent than the older agents as reflected by their higher MAC values.

On recovery from anaesthesia, the rate of elimination of desflurane is faster than that for the other agents (Fig. 2.3).

Respiratory system

All inhalational agents cause dose-related respiratory depression. This results in reduced tidal volume, increased respiratory rate and reduced minute ventilation. $P_a CO_2$ increases (Fig. 2.4). In unstimulated volunteers, enflurane and desflurane cause greater ventilatory depression than isoflurane, halothane or sevoflurane. Nitrous oxide does not cause hypercapnia. Thus the reduction in inspired volatile anaesthetic concentration permitted by addition of nitrous oxide is associated with less ventilatory depression. In addition, surgical stimulation is responsible for considerable antagonism of ventilatory depression during anaesthesia and $P_a CO_2$ does not normally reach the values shown in Figure 2.4 during surgery.

With all agents, depression of ventilation is associated with depression of whole body oxygen consumption and carbon dioxide production.

Halothane and, to a lesser extent, sevoflurane and enflurane cause bronchodilatation.

Cardiovascular system

All the agents reduce arterial pressure because of reduced systemic vascular resistance and myocardial depression to varying degrees. Desflurane and isoflurane tend to maintain cardiac output, decreasing arterial pressure mainly by decreasing systemic vascular resistance. Halothane reduces arterial pressure principally by decreasing cardiac output with little effect on systemic vascular resistance.

Isoflurane, enflurane and desflurane increase heart rate as a result of sympathetic stimulation, whereas halothane and sevoflurane reduce heart rate.

The data in Figures 2.5–2.7 and 2.9 were derived from studies in volunteers who were not subjected to surgical stimulation and in whom artificial ventilation was used to achieve normocapnia.

Some of the cardiovascular effects of these volatile agents are antagonized by the addition of nitrous oxide. In addition, during spontaneous ventilation, the modest hypercapnia which occurs with all agents also offsets some of the changes. With enflurane and isoflurane, for example, cardiac output may be increased compared with pre-anaesthesia levels, although there is little effect on systemic arterial pressure.

Desflurane, isoflurane and sevoflurane do not sensitize the myocardium to exogenous catecholamines, but halothane and, to a lesser extent, enflurane predispose to arrhythmias.

Isoflurane causes coronary vasodilatation and experimentally this was found to cause coronary steal syndrome but this has now been demonstrated to be of no clinical significance. Sevoflurane causes some coronary vasodilatation but does not appear to cause coronary steal syndrome. The other three agents do not cause any coronary vasodilatation.

Central nervous system

All agents cause dose-related depression of cerebral activity. Enflurane causes convulsive activity on the EEG. All the agents decrease cerebrovascular resistance and increase intracranial pressure in a dose-related manner.

Neuromuscular junction

All agents produce muscle relaxation sufficient to perform lower abdominal surgery in spontaneously breathing thin subjects. In addition, there is potentiation of non-depolarizing muscle relaxants. In this respect, isoflurane, sevoflurane and desflurane are similar and cause markedly greater potentiation than that produced by halothane or enflurane.

Uterus

Halothane, isoflurane and enflurane relax uterine muscle in a dose-related manner. There is limited experience with desflurane and sevoflurane in the obstetric population. Sevoflurane appears to have similar uterine effects to isoflurane. In practice, in the UK, isoflurane appears to be the standard volatile anaesthetic agent used for obstetric anaesthesia.

Metabolism

Halothane, enflurane and sevoflurane are metabolized to potentially toxic metabolites and desflurane is the most resistant to metabolism. Halothane is associated with liver toxicity, while sevoflurane and enflurane are associated with production of inorganic fluoride ion.

Carbon dioxide absorbers

Sevoflurane and halothane react with soda lime, while the other three do not.

A comparison of other characteristics of the five agents is shown in Tables 2.1 and 2.2.

AGENTS IN OCCASIONAL USE

DIETHYL ETHER

Because of its flammability, the use of ether has been abandoned in Western countries, but it remains an agent of widespread use in underdeveloped countries. It therefore warrants a brief description in this text.

It is a colourless, highly volatile liquid with a characteristic smell. It is flammable in air and explosive in oxygen. Ether is decomposed by air, light and heat, the most important products being acetaldehyde and ether peroxide. It should be stored in a cool environment in opaque containers.

Uptake and distribution

Ether has a high blood/gas solubility coefficient of 12 and thus the rate of equilibration of alveolar with inspired concentrations is slow. Therefore induction and recovery with ether are slow.

Central nervous system

In common with all general anaesthetic agents, there is depression of the cortex. Because induction of anaesthesia with ether is so slow, the classical stages of anaesthesia are seen; these are described in detail on page 301 and in Figure 16.2.

Ether anaesthesia is associated with stimulation of the sympathoadrenal system and increased levels of circulating catecholamines, which offset the direct myocardial depressant effect of the drug.

Respiratory system

Ether is irritant to the respiratory tract and provokes coughing, breath-holding and profuse secretions from all mucus-secreting glands. Premedication with an anticholinergic agent is therefore essential.

Ether stimulates ventilation and minute volume is maintained with increasing depth of anaesthesia until

Table 2.1 Comparison of modern volatile anaesthetic agents

	Halothane	Enflurane	Isoflurane	Desflurane	Sevoflurane
Molecular weight (Da)	197	184.5	184.5	168	200
Boiling point (°C)	50	56	49	23.5	58.5
Blood/gas partition coefficient	2.5	1.9	1.4	0.42	0.69
Oil/gas partition coefficient	220	98	91	18.7	55
MAC (in oxygen) %	0.75	1.68	1.15	6.3	1.7–2.0
Preservative	Thymol	None	None	None	None
Stability in CO_2 absorbers	?Unstable	Stable	Stable	Stable	Unstable

Table 2.2 Systemic effects of volatile agents

	Halothane	Enflurane	Isoflurane	Desflurane	Sevoflurane
Alveolar equilibration	Slow	Moderate	Moderate	Fast	Fast
Recovery	Slow	Moderate	Fast	Very fast	Fast
Cardiovascular system					
Heart rate	Reduced	Increased	Increased	Increased	Stable
Cardiac output	Reduced	Reduced	Slightly reduced	Stable to slightly reduced	Stable to slightly reduced
SVR	Stable	Slightly reduced	Reduced	Reduced	Reduced
MAP	Reduced	Reduced	Reduced	Reduced	Reduced
Sensitization of myocardium	Yes	Slight	No	No	No
Respiratory system					
Respiratory irritation	Nil	Minimal	Significant	Significant	Nil
Respiratory depression	Yes	Marked	Yes	Marked	Yes
Central nervous system					
Seizure activity on EEG	No	Yes	No	No	No
Renal system					
Renal toxic metabolites	No	Yes	No	No	Yes
Liver					
Hepatotoxicity	Yes	Yes	No	No	?Yes
Metabolism (%)	20	2.5	0.2	0.02	3–5
Musculoskeletal system					
Muscle weakness	Moderate	Moderate	Significant	Significant	Significant

SVR = systemic vascular resistance, MAP = mean arterial pressure.

surgical anaesthesia is achieved; thereafter, there is a gradual diminution in alveolar ventilation as plane 4 of stage 3 is approached (Fig. 16.2).

Because ether is irritant to the respiratory tract, laryngeal spasm is not uncommon during induction with ether, but during established anaesthesia there is dilatation of the bronchi and bronchioles; at one time, the drug was recommended for the treatment of bronchospasm.

Cardiovascular system

In vitro, ether is a direct myocardial depressant. However, during light planes of clinical anaesthesia, there is sympathetic stimulation and this often results in little change in cardiac output, arterial pressure or peripheral resistance. In deep planes of anaesthesia, cardiac output decreases as a result of myocardial depression.

Cardiac arrhythmias occur rarely with ether and there is no sensitization of the myocardium to circulating catecholamines.

Alimentary system

Salivary and gastric secretions are increased during light anaesthesia but decreased during deep anaesthesia. Ether causes a very high incidence of postoperative nausea and vomiting.

Skeletal muscle

Ether potentiates the effects of non-depolarizing muscle relaxants.

Uterus and placenta

The pregnant uterus is not affected during light anaesthesia, but relaxation occurs during deep anaesthesia.

Metabolism

At least 15% of ether is metabolized to carbon dioxide and water; approximately 4% is metabolized in the liver to acetaldehyde and ethanol.

Ether stimulates gluconeogenesis and therefore causes hyperglycaemia.

Clinical use of ether

Ether has a much higher therapeutic ratio than halothane, enflurane or isoflurane and is therefore safer for administration in the hands of unskilled individuals or from an uncalibrated vaporizer. Because of its high blood/gas solubility coefficient and irritant properties to the respiratory tract, induction of anaesthesia is very slow.

Administration of ether may be undertaken using an anaesthetic breathing system with a non-calibrated vaporizer (Boyle's bottle) or calibrated vaporizer (the EMO, which may be used as a draw-over or as a plenum vaporizer). It may be used safely in a closed circuit with soda lime absorption.

Vapour strengths of up to 20% are required for induction; light anaesthesia may be maintained with 3–5% and deep anaesthesia with 5–6% inspired concentrations.

ANAESTHETIC GASES

NITROUS OXIDE (N$_2$O)

Manufacture

Nitrous oxide is prepared commercially by heating ammonium nitrate to a temperature of 245–270°C. Various impurities are produced in this process, including ammonia, nitric acid, nitrogen, nitric oxide and nitrogen dioxide.

After cooling, ammonia and nitric acid are reconstituted to ammonium nitrate, which is returned to the beginning of the process. The remaining gases then pass through a series of scrubbers. The purified gases are compressed and dried in an aluminium dryer. The resultant gases are expanded in a liquefier, with the nitrogen escaping as gas. Nitrous oxide is then evaporated, compressed and passed through another aluminium dryer before being stored in cylinders.

The higher oxides of nitrogen dissolve in water to form nitrous and nitric acids. These substances are toxic and produce methaemoglobinaemia and pulmonary oedema if inhaled. In the past, there have been several reports of death occurring during anaesthesia as a result of the inhalation of nitrous oxide contaminated with higher oxides of nitrogen.

Storage

Nitrous oxide is stored in compressed form as a liquid in cylinders at a pressure of 44 bar (4400 kPa; 638 lb in^{-2}). In the UK, the cylinders are painted blue.

Because the cylinder contains liquid and vapour, the total quantity of nitrous oxide contained in a cylinder may be ascertained only by weighing. Thus, the cylinder weights, full and empty, are stamped on the shoulder. Nitrous oxide cylinders should be kept in a vertical position during use so that the liquid phase remains at the bottom of the cylinder. During continuous use, the cylinder may cool as a result of the latent heat of vaporization of liquid anaesthetic and ice may form on the lower part of the cylinder.

Physical properties

Nitrous oxide is a sweet-smelling, non-irritant colourless gas, with a molecular weight of 44, boiling point of –88°C, critical temperature of 36.5°C and critical pressure of 72.6 bar.

Nitrous oxide is not flammable but it supports combustion of fuels in the absence of oxygen.

Pharmacology

Nitrous oxide is frequently said to be a good analgesic but a weak anaesthetic. The latter refers to the fact that its MAC value is 105%. This value was calculated theoretically from its low oil/water solubility coefficient of 3.2 and has been confirmed experimentally in volunteers anaesthetized in a pressure chamber compressed to 2 ata, where the MAC value was found to be 52.5% N$_2$O.

As it is essential to administer a minimum F_1O_2 of 0.3 during anaesthesia, nitrous oxide alone is insufficient to produce an adequate depth of anaesthesia in all but the most seriously ill patients; therefore, nitrous oxide is used usually in combination with other agents. When using nitrous oxide in a relaxant technique, the inspired gas mixture should be supplemented with a low concentration of a volatile agent to eliminate the risk of awareness, which occurs in 1-2% of patients if nitrous oxide anaesthesia is supplemented only by the administration of opioids.

Nitrous oxide has a low blood/gas solubility coefficient (0.47 at 37°C) and therefore the rate of equilibration of alveolar with inspired concentrations is very fast (Fig. 2.2).

Because of the low solubility, a change in alveolar ventilation has less effect on the rate of uptake than occurs with the more soluble agents such as halothane and ether (Fig. 2.10). Similarly, changes in cardiac output have less effect with nitrous oxide (Fig. 2.11). Nitrous oxide does not undergo metabolism in the body and is excreted unchanged.

The concentration effect

The inspired concentration of nitrous oxide affects its rate of equilibration; the higher the inspired concentration, the faster is the rate of equilibration between alveolar and inspired concentrations. Nitrous oxide is more soluble in blood than is nitrogen. Thus, the volume of nitrous oxide entering pulmonary capillary blood from the alveolus is greater than the volume of nitrogen moving in the opposite direction. As a result, the total volume of gas in the alveolus diminishes and the fractional concentrations of the remaining gases increase. This has two consequences:

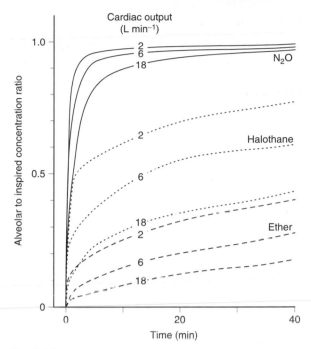

Fig. 2.11
Influence of cardiac output on the rate of equilibration between alveolar and inspired concentrations of nitrous oxide, halothane and ether. The effects of cardiac output are more marked on the agents with higher blood/gas solubility coefficients.

- The higher the inspired concentration of nitrous oxide, the greater is the concentrating effect on the nitrous oxide remaining in the alveolus.
- At high inspired concentrations of nitrous oxide, the reduction in alveolar gas volume causes an increase in $P_A\text{CO}_2$. Equilibration with pulmonary capillary blood results in an increase in $P_a\text{CO}_2$.

The result of the concentration effect on equilibration of nitrous oxide is illustrated in Figure 2.12.

The second gas effect

When nitrous oxide is administered in a high concentration with a second anaesthetic agent, e.g. halothane, the reduction in gas volume in the alveoli caused by absorption of nitrous oxide increases the alveolar concentration of halothane, thereby augmenting the rate of equilibration with inspired gas. This is illustrated in the lower part of Figure 2.12. The second gas effect results also in small increases in $P_A\text{O}_2$ and $P_a\text{O}_2$.

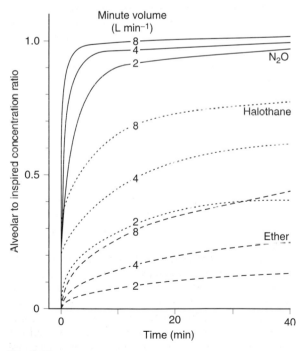

Fig. 2.10
Influence of minute volume on the rate of equilibration between alveolar and inspired concentrations of nitrous oxide, halothane and ether. The effects of ventilation are more marked on the agents with higher blood/gas solubility coefficients.

29

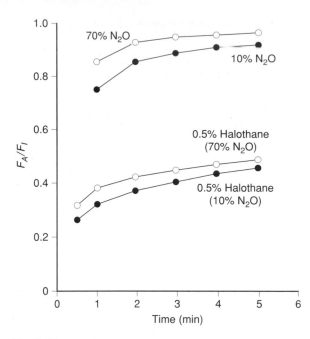

Fig. 2.12
The concentration and second gas effects. High concentrations of nitrous oxide increase the F_A/F_I ratio for nitrous oxide (the concentration effect) and for a volatile agent administered with nitrous oxide (the second gas effect). See text for details.

Side-effects of nitrous oxide

Diffusion hypoxia

At the end of an anaesthetic, when the inspired gas mixture is changed from nitrous oxide/oxygen to nitrogen/oxygen, hypoxaemia may occur as the volume of nitrous oxide diffusing from mixed venous blood into the alveolus is greater than the volume of nitrogen taken up from the alveolus into pulmonary capillary blood (the opposite of the concentration effect). Thus, the concentration of gases in the alveolus is diluted by nitrous oxide, leading to reductions in P_aO_2 and P_aCO_2. In the healthy individual, diffusion hypoxia is relatively transient, but may last for up to 10 min at the end of anaesthesia; the extent of reduction in P_aO_2 may be of the order of 0.5–1.5 kPa. Administration of oxygen during this period is essential in order to avoid desaturation.

Effect on closed gas spaces

When blood containing nitrous oxide equilibrates with closed air-containing spaces inside the body, the volume of nitrous oxide that diffuses into the cavity exceeds the volume of nitrogen diffusing out. Thus, in compliant spaces, such as the bowel lumen or the pleural or peritoneal cavities, there is an increase in volume of the space. If the space cannot expand (e.g. sinuses, middle ear) there is an increase in pressure. In the middle ear, this may cause problems with surgery on the tympanic membrane. When nitrous oxide is administered in a concentration of 75%, the volume of a cavity may increase to as much as three to four times the original volume within 30 min. If an air embolus occurs in a patient who is breathing nitrous oxide, equilibration with the gas bubble leads to expansion of the embolus within seconds; the volume of the embolus may double within a very short period of time. A similar problem arises during prolonged procedures where nitrous oxide diffuses into the cuff of the tracheal tube and may increase the pressure exerted on the tracheal mucosa. Either avoiding the use of nitrous oxide or inflating the cuff with saline or nitrous oxide may prevent this.

A complication of the effect of nitrous oxide on closed gas spaces which has been described recently is the loss of vision caused by expansion of intraocular perfluoropropane gas during nitrous oxide anaesthesia. Perfluoropropane is used in vitreoretinal surgery to provide long-acting gas tamponade. The visual loss is caused possibly by central retinal artery occlusion as a result of expansion of the gas by nitrous oxide, resulting in increased intraocular pressure. Therefore the use of nitrous oxide in these patients should be avoided. In order to aid identification of these patients by the anaesthetists preoperatively, it is recommended that the patients should be aware of this risk in order to warn the anaesthetist and also it may be prudent for them to wear an intraocular gas identity bracelet.

Cardiovascular depression

Nitrous oxide is a direct myocardial depressant, but in the normal individual this effect is antagonized by indirectly mediated sympathoadrenal stimulation (effects similar to those produced by carbon dioxide). Thus, healthy patients exhibit little change in the cardiovascular system during nitrous oxide anaesthesia. However, in patients with pre-existing high levels of sympathoadrenal activity and poor myocardial contractility, the administration of nitrous oxide may cause reductions in cardiac output and arterial pressure. For this reason (in addition to avoidance of the risk of doubling the size of air emboli), nitrous oxide is avoided in some centres during anaesthesia for cardiac surgery.

Toxicity

Nitrous oxide affects vitamin B_{12} synthesis by inhibiting the enzyme methionine synthetase. This effect is important if the duration of nitrous oxide anaesthesia exceeds 8 h. Nitrous oxide also interferes with folic acid metabolism and impairs synthesis of DNA; prolonged exposure may cause agranulocytosis and bone marrow aplasia. Exposure of patients to nitrous oxide for 6 h or longer may result in megaloblastic anaemia. Occupational exposure to nitrous oxide may result in myeloneuropathy. This condition is similar to subacute combined degeneration of the spinal cord and has been reported in some dentists and also in individuals addicted to inhalation of nitrous oxide.

Teratogenic changes

Teratogenic changes have been observed in pregnant rats exposed to nitrous oxide for prolonged periods. There is no evidence that similar effects occur in humans, but it has been suggested that nitrous oxide should be avoided in early pregnancy; however, this is not a generally held view at the present time.

OTHER GASES USED DURING ANAESTHESIA

OXYGEN

Manufacture

Oxygen is manufactured commercially by fractional distillation of liquid air. Before liquefaction of air, carbon dioxide is removed and liquid oxygen and nitrogen separated by means of their different boiling points (oxygen, –183°C; nitrogen, –195°C).

Oxygen is supplied in cylinders at a pressure of 137 bar (approximately 2000 lb in^{-2}) at 15°C. In the UK, the cylinders are painted black with a white shoulder.

Many institutions use piped oxygen and this is supplied either by a bank of oxygen cylinders, ensuring a continuous supply, or from liquid oxygen. Premises using in excess of 150 000 L of oxygen per week find the latter more economical. The pressure of oxygen in a hospital pipeline is approximately 4 bar (60 lb in^{-2}), which is the same as the pressure distal to the reducing valves of gas cylinders attached to anaesthetic machines.

Oxygen is tasteless, colourless and odourless, with a specific gravity of 1.105 and a molecular weight of 32. At atmospheric pressure, it liquefies at –183°C, but at 50 atm the liquefaction temperature increases to –119°C.

Oxygen supports combustion, although the gas itself is not flammable.

Oxygen concentrators

Oxygen concentrators produce oxygen from ambient air by absorption of nitrogen onto some types of alumina silicates. Oxygen concentrators are useful both in hospitals and in long-term domestic use in remote areas, in developing countries and in military surgery. The gas produced by oxygen concentrators contains small quantities of inert gases (e.g. argon) which are harmless.

Adverse effects of oxygen

Fire

Oxygen supports combustion of fuels. An increase in the concentration of oxygen from 21% up to 100% causes a progressive increase in the rate of combustion with the production of either conflagrations or explosions with appropriate fuels.

Cardiovascular depression

An increase in P_aO_2 leads to direct vasoconstriction, which occurs in peripheral vasculature and also in the cerebral, coronary, hepatic and renal circulations. This effect is not manifest at a P_aO_2 of less than 30 kPa and assumes clinical importance only at hyperbaric pressures of oxygen. Hyperbaric pressures of oxygen also cause direct myocardial depression. In patients with severe cardiovascular disease, elevation of P_aO_2 from the normal physiological range to 80 kPa may produce clinically evident cardiovascular depression.

Absorption atelectasis

Because oxygen is highly soluble in blood, the use of 100% oxygen as the inspired gas may lead to absorption atelectasis in lung units distal to the site of airway closure. Absorption collapse may occur in as short a time as 6 min with 100% oxygen, and 60 min with 85% oxygen. Thus, even small concentrations of nitrogen exert an important splinting effect and this accounts for current avoidance of 100% oxygen in estimation of pulmonary shunt ratio ($\dot{Q}_s/\dot{Q}_t$) in patients with lung pathology, in whom a greater degree of airway closure would result in greater areas of alveolar atelectasis. Absorption atelectasis has been demonstrated in volunteers breathing 100% oxygen at FRC; atelectasis is evident on chest radiography for a period of at least 24 h after exposure.

Pulmonary oxygen toxicity

Chronic inhalation of a high inspired concentration of oxygen may result in the condition termed pulmonary oxygen toxicity (Lorrain–Smith effect), which is manifest by hyaline membranes, thickening of the interlobular and alveolar septa by oedema and fibroplastic proliferation. The clinical and radiological appearance of these changes is almost identical to that of the acute respiratory distress syndrome. The biochemical mechanisms underlying pulmonary oxygen toxicity probably include:

- oxidation of SH groups on essential enzymes such as coenzyme A
- peroxidation of lipids; the resulting lipid peroxides inhibit the function of the cell
- inhibition of the pathway of reversed electron transport, possibly by inhibition of iron and SH-containing flavoproteins.

These changes lead to loss of synthesis of pulmonary surfactant, encouraging the development of absorption collapse and alveolar oedema. The onset of oxygen-induced lung pathology occurs after approximately 30 h exposure to a P_1O_2 of 100 kPa.

Central nervous system oxygen toxicity

Convulsions, similar to those of grand mal epilepsy, occur during exposure to hyperbaric pressures of oxygen.

Retrolental fibroplasia

Retrolental fibroplasia (RLF) is the result of oxygen-induced retinal vasoconstriction, with obliteration of the most immature retinal vessels and subsequent new vessel formation at the site of damage in the form of a proliferative retinopathy. Leakage of intravascular fluid leads to vitreoretinal adhesions and even retinal detachment. Retrolental fibroplasia occurs in infants exposed to hyperoxia in the paediatric intensive care unit and is related not to the F_1O_2 per se, but to an elevated retinal artery Po_2. It is not known what the threshold of P_aO_2 is for the development of retinal damage, but an umbilical arterial Po_2 of 8–12 kPa (60–90 mmHg) is associated with a very low incidence of RLF and no signs of systemic hypoxia. It should be stressed, however, that there are many factors involved in the development of RLF in addition to arterial hyperoxia.

Depressed haemopoiesis

Long-term exposure to elevated F_1O_2 leads to depression of haemopoiesis and anaemia.

CARBON DIOXIDE

Carbon dioxide is a colourless gas with a pungent odour. It has a molecular weight of 44, a critical temperature of –31°C and a critical pressure of 73.8 bar.

Carbon dioxide is obtained commercially from four sources:

- as a byproduct of fermentation in brewing of beer
- as a byproduct of the manufacture of hydrogen
- by heating magnesium and calcium carbonate in the presence of their oxides
- as a combustion gas from burning fuel.

In the UK, carbon dioxide is supplied in a liquid state in grey cylinders at a pressure of 50 bar. The liquid phase occupies approximately 90–95% of the cylinder capacity.

Physiological data

Variations in cardiovascular state induced by alterations in P_aCO_2 may be similar to those induced by pain or lightness of anaesthesia and the differential diagnosis is described in Table 24.2. The cardiovascular effects of CO_2 are summarized in Table 2.3.

Uses of carbon dioxide in anaesthesia

The use of carbon dioxide in anaesthetic practice has declined as appreciation of its disadvantages has increased. Because of reports of accidental administration of high concentrations of CO_2, it is not available on most modern anaesthetic machines. Carbon dioxide is used mainly by surgeons for insufflation during laparoscopic procedures.

Table 2.3 Cardiovascular effects of CO_2

Arterial pressure Cardiac output Heart rate	Biphasic response. Progressive increases in these variables with increase in P_aCO_2 up to approximately 10 kPa as a result of indirect sympathetic stimulation. At very high P_aCO_2, these variables decrease as a result of myocardial depression
Skin Coronary circulation Cerebral circulation Gastrointestinal circulation	Dilatation with hypercapnia Constriction with hypocapnia

MEDICAL AIR

Nitrous oxide is still commonly used in combination with a volatile agent to maintain anaesthesia. However, there is growing concern regarding its toxic effects and its cost. Consequently, medical air is being used more frequently in combination with oxygen during anaesthesia.

Medical air is obtained from the atmosphere near to the site of compression. Great care is taken to position the air intake in order to avoid contamination with pollutants such as carbon monoxide from car exhausts. Air is compressed to 137 bar and then passed through columns of activated alumina to remove water.

Air for medical purposes is supplied in cylinders (grey body and black and white shoulders in the UK) or as a piped system. A pressure of 4 bar is available for attachment to anaesthetic machines, and 7 bar for orthopaedic tools. Its composition varies slightly depending on location of compression and moisture content.

Uses of medical air

- driving gas for ventilators
- to operate power tools, e.g. orthopaedic drills
- together with oxygen and a volatile or intravenous agent to maintain anaesthesia.

Advantages of air

- readily available
- non-toxic.

XENON

Inert gases such as argon, krypton and xenon, which form crystalline hydrates, have been reported to exert anaesthetic actions. Cullen and Gross first reported the anaesthetic properties of xenon in humans in 1951. Xenon offers many advantages over nitrous oxide, for which it could theoretically be a suitable replacement. The reasons that it is not routinely available are that it is expensive, there are no commercially available anaesthetic machines in which to use xenon, its concentration in inspired gas cannot be measured with conventional anaesthetic gas analysers and there is still limited clinical experience with its use.

Physical properties

Xenon is a non-explosive, colourless and odourless gas. It is non-flammable and does not support combustion. Its blood/gas partition coefficient of 0.14–0.2 is lower than that of nitrous oxide (0.47). It therefore provides rapid induction of and recovery from anaesthesia. Xenon is more potent than nitrous oxide, with a MAC of 70%. It does not undergo biotransformation and it is harmless to the ozone layer.

Systemic effects

Studies so far have shown no cardiorespiratory side-effects or reduction in local organ perfusion. It is non-irritant to the respiratory tract. However, in common with nitrous oxide, xenon appears to be associated with postoperative nausea and vomiting.

FURTHER READING

Miller RD 2005 Miller's Anaesthesia, 6th edn. Elsevier, Edinburgh

Smith I, Nathanson M, White P F 1996 Sevoflurane – a long awaited volatile agent. Review article. British Journal of Anaesthesia 76: 435–445

3 Intravenous anaesthetic agents

General anaesthesia may be produced by many drugs which depress the CNS, including sedatives, tranquillizers and hypnotic agents. However, for some drugs the doses required to produce surgical anaesthesia are so large that cardiovascular and respiratory depression commonly occur, and recovery is delayed for hours or even days. Only a few drugs are suitable for use routinely to produce anaesthesia after intravenous (i.v.) injection.

Intravenous anaesthetic agents are used commonly to induce anaesthesia, as induction is usually smoother and more rapid than that associated with most of the inhalational agents. Intravenous anaesthetics may also be used for maintenance, either alone or in combination with nitrous oxide; they may be administered as repeated bolus doses or by continuous i.v. infusion. Other uses include sedation during regional anaesthesia, sedation in the intensive therapy unit (ITU) and treatment of status epilepticus.

PROPERTIES OF THE IDEAL INTRAVENOUS ANAESTHETIC AGENT

- Rapid onset – this is achieved by an agent which is mainly unionized at blood pH and which is highly soluble in lipid; these properties permit penetration of the blood–brain barrier
- Rapid recovery – early recovery of consciousness is usually produced by rapid redistribution of the drug from the brain into other well-perfused tissues, particularly muscle. The plasma concentration of the drug decreases, and the drug diffuses out of the brain along a concentration gradient. The quality of the later recovery period is related more to the rate of metabolism of the drug; drugs with slow metabolism are associated with a more prolonged 'hangover' effect and accumulate if used in repeated doses or by infusion for maintenance of anaesthesia
- Analgesia at subanaesthetic concentrations
- Minimal cardiovascular and respiratory depression

- No emetic effects
- No excitatory phenomena (e.g. coughing, hiccup, involuntary movement) on induction
- No emergence phenomena (e.g. nightmares)
- No interaction with neuromuscular blocking drugs
- No pain on injection
- No venous sequelae
- Safe if injected inadvertently into an artery
- No toxic effects on other organs
- No release of histamine
- No hypersensitivity reactions
- Water-soluble formulation
- Long shelf-life
- No stimulation of porphyria.

None of the agents available at present meets all these requirements. Features of the commonly used i.v. anaesthetic agents are compared in Table 3.1, and a classification of i.v. anaesthetic drugs is shown in Table 3.2.

PHARMACOKINETICS OF INTRAVENOUS ANAESTHETIC DRUGS

After i.v. administration of a drug, there is an immediate rapid increase in plasma concentration followed by a slower decline. Anaesthesia is produced by diffusion of drug from arterial blood across the blood–brain barrier into the brain. The rate of transfer into the brain, and therefore the anaesthetic effect, is regulated by the following factors:

Protein binding. Only unbound drug is free to cross the blood–brain barrier. Protein binding may be reduced by low plasma protein concentrations or displacement by other drugs, resulting in higher concentrations of free drug and an exaggerated anaesthetic effect. Protein binding is also affected by changes in blood pH. Hyperventilation decreases protein binding and increases the anaesthetic effect.

Blood flow to the brain. Reduced cerebral blood flow (CBF), e.g. carotid artery stenosis, results in reduced delivery of drug to the brain. However, if CBF is reduced

Table 3.1   Main properties of intravenous anaesthetics

	Thiopental	Methohexital	Propofol	Ketamine	Etomidate
Physical properties					
Water-soluble	+	+	−	+	+[a]
Stable in solution	−	−	+	+	+
Long shelf-life	−	−	+	+	+
Pain on i.v. injection	−	+	++[b]	−	++[b]
Non-irritant on s.c. injection	−	±	+	+	
Painful on arterial injection	+	+	−		
No sequelae from intra-arterial injection	−	±	+		
Low incidence of venous thrombosis	+	+	+	+	−
Effects on body					
Rapid onset	+	+	+	+	+
Recovery due to:					
Redistribution	+	+	+	+	
Detoxification	+	+			
Cumulation	++	+	−	−	−
Induction					
Excitatory effects	−	++	+	+	+++
Respiratory complications	−	+	+	−	−
Cardiovascular					
Hypotension	+	+	++	−	+
Analgesic	−	−	−	++	
Antanalgesic	+	+	−	−	?
Interaction with relaxants	−	−	−	−	−
Postoperative vomiting	−	−	−	++	+
Emergence delirium	−	−	−	++	−
Safe in porphyria	−	−	+	+	−

[a]Aqueous solution not commercially available.
[b]Pain may be reduced when emulsion with medium-chain triglycerides is used.

because of low cardiac output, initial blood concentrations are higher than normal after i.v. administration, and the anaesthetic effect may be delayed but enhanced.

Extracellular pH and pK_a of the drug. Only the non-ionized fraction of the drug penetrates the lipid blood–brain barrier; thus, the potency of the drug depends on the degree of ionization at the pH of extracellular fluid and the pK_a of the drug.

The relative solubilities of the drug in lipid and water. High lipid solubility enhances transfer into the brain.

Speed of injection. Rapid i.v. administration results in high initial concentrations of drug. This increases

Table 3.2 Classification of intravenous anaesthetics

Rapidly acting (primary induction) agents

Barbiturates:
  Methohexital
  Thiobarbiturates – thiopental, thiamylal

Imidazole compounds – etomidate

Sterically hindered alkyl phenols – propofol

Steroids – eltanolone, althesin, minaxolone (none currently available)

Eugenols – propanidid (not currently available)

Slower-acting (basal narcotic) agents

Ketamine

Benzodiazepines – diazepam, flunitrazepam, midazolam

Large-dose opioids – fentanyl, alfentanil, sufentanil, remifentanil

Neuroleptic combination – opioid + neuroleptic

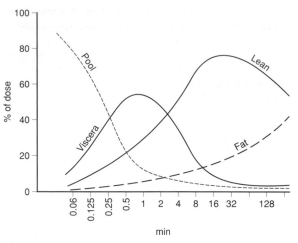

Fig. 3.1
Distribution of thiopental after intravenous bolus administration.

the speed of induction, but also the extent of cardiovascular and respiratory side-effects.

In general, any factor which increases the blood concentration of free drug, e.g. reduced protein binding or low cardiac output, also increases the intensity of side-effects.

Distribution to other tissues

The anaesthetic effect of all i.v. anaesthetic drugs in current use is terminated predominantly by distribution to other tissues. Figure 3.1 shows this distribution for thiopental. The percentage of the injected dose in each of four body compartments as time elapses is shown after i.v. injection. A large proportion of the drug is distributed initially into well-perfused organs (termed the vessel-rich group, or viscera – predominantly brain, liver and kidneys). Distribution into muscle (lean) is slower because of its low lipid content, but it is quantitatively important because of its relatively good blood supply and large mass. Despite their high lipid solubility, i.v. anaesthetic drugs distribute slowly to adipose tissue (fat) because of its poor blood supply. Fat contributes little to the initial redistribution or termination of action of i.v. anaesthetic agents, but fat depots contain a large proportion of the injected dose of thiopental at 90 min, and 65–75% of the total

remaining in the body at 24 h. There is also a small amount of redistribution to areas with a very poor blood supply, e.g. bone. Table 3.3 indicates some of the properties of the body compartments in respect of the distribution of i.v. anaesthetic agents.

After a single i.v. dose, the concentration of drug in blood decreases as distribution occurs into viscera, and particularly muscle. Drug diffuses from the brain into blood along the changing concentration gradient, and recovery of consciousness occurs. Metabolism of most i.v. anaesthetic drugs occurs predominantly in the liver. If metabolism is rapid (indicated by a short

Table 3.3 Factors influencing the distribution of thiopental in the body

	Viscera	Muscle	Fat	Others
Relative blood flow	Rich	Good	Poor	Very poor
Blood flow (L min^{-1})	4.5	1.1	0.32	0.08
Tissue volume (L; A)	6	33	15	13
Tissue/blood partition coefficient (B)	1.5	1.5	11.0	1.5
Potential capacity (L; $A \times B$)	9	50	160	20
Time constant (capacity/flow; min)	2	45	500	250

elimination half-life), it may contribute to some extent to the recovery of consciousness. However, because of the large distribution volume of i.v. anaesthetic drugs, total elimination takes many hours, or, in some instances, days. A small proportion of drug may be excreted unchanged in the urine; the amount depends on the degree of ionization and the pH of urine.

BARBITURATES

Amobarbital and pentobarbital were used i.v. to induce anaesthesia in the late 1920s, but their actions were unpredictable and recovery was prolonged. Manipulation of the barbituric acid ring (Fig. 3.2) enabled a short duration of action to be achieved by:

- substitution of a sulphur atom for oxygen at position 2
- substitution of a methyl group at position 1; this also confers potential convulsive activity and increases the incidence of excitatory phenomena.

An increased number of carbon atoms in the side chains at position 5 increases the potency of the agent. The presence of an aromatic nucleus in an alkyl group at position 5 produces compounds with convulsant properties; direct substitution with a phenyl group confers anticonvulsant activity.

The anaesthetically active barbiturates are classified chemically into four groups (Table 3.4). The methylated oxybarbiturate hexobarbital was moderately successful as an i.v. anaesthetic agent, but was superseded by the development in 1932 of thiopental. Although propofol has become very popular in a number of countries, thiopental remains one of the most commonly used i.v. anaesthetic agents through-

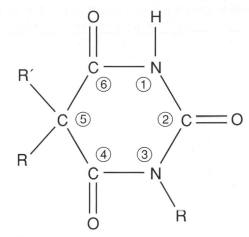

Fig. 3.2
Structure of barbiturate ring.

out the world. Its pharmacology is therefore described fully in this chapter. Many of its effects are shared by other i.v. anaesthetic agents and consequently the pharmacology of these drugs is described more briefly.

THIOPENTAL SODIUM

Chemical structure

Sodium 5-ethyl-5-(1-methylbutyl)-2-thiobarbiturate.

Physical properties and presentation

Thiopental sodium, the sulphur analogue of pentobarbital, is a yellowish powder with a bitter taste and a faint smell of garlic. It is stored in nitrogen to prevent chemical reaction with atmospheric carbon dioxide, and mixed with 6% anhydrous sodium carbonate to

Table 3.4   Relation of chemical grouping to clinical action of barbiturates

| Group | Substituents | | Group characteristics when given intravenously |
	Position 1	Position 2	
Oxybarbiturates	H	O	Delay in onset of action depending on 5 and 5' side chain. Useful as basal hypnotics. Prolonged action
Methyl barbiturates	CH$_3$	O	Usually rapid acting with fairly rapid recovery. High incidence of excitatory phenomena
Thiobarbiturates	H	S	Rapid-acting, usually smooth onset of sleep and fairly prompt recovery
Methyl thiobarbiturates	CH$_3$	S	Rapid onset of action and very rapid recovery but with so high an incidence of excitatory phenomena as to preclude use in clinical practice

increase its solubility in water. It is available in single-dose ampoules of 500 mg and is dissolved in distilled water to produce 2.5% (25 mg ml^{-1}) solution with a pH of 10.8; this solution is slightly hypotonic. Freshly prepared solution may be kept for 24 h. The oil/water partition coefficient of thiopental is 4.7, and the pK_a 7.6.

Central nervous system

Thiopental produces anaesthesia usually less than 30 s after i.v. injection, although there may be some delay in patients with a low cardiac output. There is progressive depression of the CNS, including spinal cord reflexes. The hypnotic action of thiopental is potent, but its analgesic effect is poor, and surgical anaesthesia is difficult to achieve unless large doses are used; these are associated with cardiorespiratory depression. The cerebral metabolic rate is reduced and there are secondary decreases in CBF, cerebral blood volume and intracranial pressure. Recovery of consciousness occurs at a higher blood concentration if a large dose is given, or if the drug is injected rapidly; this has been attributed to acute tolerance, but may represent only altered redistribution. Consciousness is usually regained in 5–10 min. At subanaesthetic blood concentrations (i.e. at low doses or during recovery), thiopental has an antanalgesic effect and reduces the pain threshold; this may result in restlessness in the postoperative period. Thiopental is a very potent anticonvulsant.

Sympathetic nervous system activity is depressed to a greater extent than parasympathetic; this may occasionally result in bradycardia. However, it is more usual for tachycardia to develop after induction of anaesthesia, partly because of baroreceptor inhibition caused by modest hypotension and partly because of loss of vagal tone which may predominate normally in young healthy adults.

Cardiovascular system

Myocardial contractility is depressed and peripheral vasodilatation occurs, particularly when large doses are administered or if injection is rapid. Arterial pressure decreases, and profound hypotension may occur in the patient with hypovolaemia or cardiac disease. Heart rate may decrease, but there is often a reflex tachycardia (see above).

Respiratory system

Ventilatory drive is decreased by thiopental as a result of reduced sensitivity of the respiratory centre to carbon dioxide. A short period of apnoea is common, frequently preceded by a few deep breaths. Respiratory depression is influenced by premedication and is more pronounced if opioids have been administered; assisted or controlled ventilation may be required. When spontaneous ventilation is resumed, ventilatory rate and tidal volume are usually lower than normal, but they increase in response to surgical stimulation. There is an increase in bronchial muscle tone, although frank bronchospasm is uncommon.

Laryngeal spasm may be precipitated by surgical stimulation or the presence of secretions, blood or foreign bodies (e.g. an oropharyngeal or laryngeal mask airway) in the region of the pharynx or larynx. Thiopental is less satisfactory in this respect than propofol, and appears to depress the parasympathetic laryngeal reflex arc to a lesser extent than other areas of the CNS.

Skeletal muscle

Skeletal muscle tone is reduced at high blood concentrations, partly as a result of suppression of spinal cord reflexes. There is no significant direct effect on the neuromuscular junction. When thiopental is used as the sole anaesthetic agent, there is poor muscle relaxation, and movement in response to surgical stimulation is common.

Uterus and placenta

There is little effect on resting uterine tone, but uterine contractions are suppressed at high doses. Thiopental crosses the placenta readily, although fetal blood concentrations do not reach the same levels as those observed in the mother.

Eye

Intraocular pressure is reduced by approximately 40%. The pupil dilates first, and then constricts; the light reflex remains present until surgical anaesthesia has been attained. The corneal, conjunctival, eyelash and eyelid reflexes are abolished.

Hepatorenal function

The functions of the liver and kidneys are impaired transiently after administration of thiopental. Hepatic microsomal enzymes are induced and this may increase the metabolism and elimination of other drugs.

Pharmacokinetics

Blood concentrations of thiopental increase rapidly after i.v. administration. Between 75 and 85% of the drug is bound to protein, mostly albumin; thus, more free drug is available if plasma protein concentrations are reduced by malnutrition or disease. Protein binding is affected by pH and is decreased by alkalaemia; thus the concentration of free drug is increased during hyperventilation. Some drugs, e.g. phenylbutazone, occupy the same binding sites, and protein binding of thiopental may be reduced in their presence.

Thiopental diffuses readily into the CNS because of its lipid solubility and predominantly unionized state (61%) at body pH. Consciousness returns when the brain concentration decreases to a threshold value, dependent on the individual patient, the dose of drug and its rate of administration, but at this time nearly all of the injected dose is still present in the body.

Metabolism of thiopental occurs predominantly in the liver, and the metabolites are excreted by the kidneys; a small proportion is excreted unchanged in the urine. The terminal elimination half-life is approximately 11.5 h. Metabolism is a zero-order process; 10–15% of the remaining drug is metabolized each hour. Thus, up to 30% of the original dose may remain in the body at 24 h. Consequently, a 'hangover' effect is common; in addition, further doses of thiopental administered within 1–2 days may result in cumulation. Elimination is impaired in the elderly. In obese patients, dosage should be based on an estimate of lean body mass, as distribution to fat is slow. However, elimination may be delayed in obese patients because of increased retention of the drug by adipose tissue.

Dosage and administration

Thiopental is administered i.v. as a 2.5% solution; the use of a 5% solution increases the likelihood of serious complications and is *not* recommended. A small volume, e.g. 1–2 mL in adults, should be administered initially; the patient should be asked if any pain is experienced in case of inadvertent intra-arterial injection (see below) before the remainder of the induction dose is given.

The dose required to produce anaesthesia varies, and the response of each patient must be assessed carefully; cardiovascular depression is exaggerated if excessive doses are given. In healthy adults, an initial dose of 4 mg kg^{-1} should be administered over 15–20 s; if loss of the eyelash reflex does not occur within 30 s, supplementary doses of 50–100 mg should be given slowly until consciousness is lost. In young children, a dose of 6 mg kg^{-1} is usually necessary. Elderly patients often require smaller doses (e.g. 2.5–3 mg kg^{-1}) than young adults.

Induction is usually smooth and may be preceded by a taste of garlic. Side-effects are related to peak blood concentrations, and in patients in whom cardiovascular depression may occur the drug should be administered more slowly; in very frail patients, as little as 50 mg may be sufficient to induce sleep.

No other drug should be mixed with thiopental. Muscle relaxants should *not* be given until it is certain that anaesthesia has been induced. The i.v. cannula should be flushed with saline before vecuronium or atracurium is administered, to obviate precipitation.

Supplementary doses of 25–100 mg may be given to augment nitrous oxide/oxygen anaesthesia during short surgical procedures. However, recovery may be prolonged considerably if large total doses are used (>10 mg kg^{-1}).

Adverse effects

Hypotension. The risk is increased if excessive doses are used, or if thiopental is administered to hypovolaemic, shocked or previously hypertensive patients. Hypotension is minimized by administering the drug slowly. Thiopental should not be administered to patients in the sitting position.

Respiratory depression. The risk is increased if excessive doses are used, or if opioid drugs have been administered. Facilities must be available to provide artificial ventilation.

Tissue necrosis. Local necrosis may follow perivenous injection. Median nerve damage may occur after extravasation in the antecubital fossa, and this site is *not* recommended. If perivenous injection occurs, the needle should be left in place and hyaluronidase injected.

Intra-arterial injection. This is usually the result of inadvertent injection into the brachial artery or an aberrant ulnar artery in the antecubital fossa but has occurred occasionally into aberrant arteries at the wrist. The patient usually complains of intense, burning pain, and this is an indication to stop injecting the drug immediately. The forearm and hand may become blanched and blisters may appear distally. Intra-arterial thiopental causes profound constriction of the artery accompanied by local release of norepinephrine. In addition, crystals of thiopental form in arterioles. In combination with thrombosis caused by endarteritis, adenosine triphosphate release from damaged red cells and aggregation of platelets, these result in emboli and may cause ischaemia or gangrene in parts of the forearm, hand or fingers.

The needle should be left in the artery and a vasodilator (e.g. papaverine 20 mg) administered. Stellate ganglion or brachial plexus block may reduce arterial spasm. Heparin should be given i.v. and oral anticoagulants should be prescribed after operation.

The risk of ischaemic damage after intra-arterial injection is much greater if a 5% solution of thiopental is used.

Laryngeal spasm. The causes have been discussed above.

Bronchospasm. This is unusual, but may be precipitated in asthmatic patients.

Allergic reactions. These range from cutaneous rashes to severe or fatal anaphylactic or anaphylactoid reactions with cardiovascular collapse. Severe reactions are rare (approximately 1 in 14 000–20 000). Hypersensitivity reactions to drugs administered during anaesthesia are discussed on page 50.

Thrombophlebitis. This is uncommon (Table 3.5) when the 2.5% solution is used.

Indications

- induction of anaesthesia
- maintenance of anaesthesia – thiopental is suitable only for short procedures because cumulation occurs with repeated doses
- treatment of status epilepticus
- reduction of intracranial pressure (see Ch. 38).

Absolute contraindications

- Airway obstruction – intravenous anaesthesia should not be used if there is anticipated difficulty in maintaining an adequate airway, e.g. epiglottitis, oral or pharyngeal tumours.
- Porphyria – barbiturates may precipitate lower motor neurone paralysis or severe cardiovascular collapse in patients with porphyria.
- Previous hypersensitivity reaction to a barbiturate.

Precautions

Special care is needed when thiopental is administered in the following circumstances:

Cardiovascular disease. Patients with hypovolaemia, myocardial disease, cardiac valvular stenosis or constrictive pericarditis are particularly sensitive to the hypotensive effects of thiopental. However, if the drug is administered with extreme caution, it is probably no more hazardous than other i.v. anaesthetic agents. Myocardial depression may be severe in patients with right-to-left intracardiac shunt because of high coronary artery concentrations of thiopental.

Severe hepatic disease. Reduced protein binding results in higher concentrations of free drug. Metabolism may be impaired, but this has little effect on early recovery. A normal dose may be administered, but very slowly.

Renal disease. In chronic renal failure, protein binding is reduced, but elimination is unaltered. A normal dose may be administered, but very slowly.

Muscle disease. Respiratory depression is exaggerated in patients with myasthenia gravis or dystrophia myotonica.

Reduced metabolic rate. Patients with myxoedema are exquisitely sensitive to the effects of thiopental.

Obstetrics. An adequate dose must be given to ensure that the mother is anaesthetized. However, excessive doses may result in respiratory or cardiovascular depression in the fetus, particularly if the interval between induction and delivery is short.

Outpatient anaesthesia. Early recovery is slow in comparison with other agents. This is seldom important unless rapid return of airway reflexes is essential, e.g. after oral or dental surgery. However, slow elimination of thiopental may result in persistent drowsiness for 24–36 h, and this impairs the ability to drive or use machinery. There is also potentiation of the effect of alcohol or sedative drugs ingested during that period. It is preferable to use a drug with more rapid elimination for patients who are ambulant within a few hours.

Adrenocortical insufficiency.
Extremes of age.
Asthma.

METHOHEXITAL SODIUM

Chemical structure

Sodium α-*dl*-5-allyl-1-methyl-5-(1-methyl-2-pentynyl) barbiturate.

Physical properties and presentation

Although no longer available in the United Kingdom, methohexital is still used in a number of other countries. The drug has two asymmetrical carbon atoms, and therefore four isomers. The α-*dl* isomers are clinically useful. The drug is presented as a white powder mixed with 6% anhydrous sodium carbonate and is readily soluble in distilled water. The resulting 1% ($10 \, mg \, mL^{-1}$) solution has a pH of 11.1 and pK_a of 7.9. Single-dose vials of 100 mg and multidose bottles containing 500 mg or 2.5 g are available in some countries. Although the solution is chemically stable for up to 6 weeks, the manufacturers recommend that it should not be stored for longer than 24 h because it does not contain antibacterial preservative.

Pharmacology

Central nervous system

Unconsciousness is usually induced in 15–30 s. Recovery is more rapid with methohexital than with thiopental, and occurs after 2–3 min; it is caused predominantly by redistribution. Drowsiness may persist for several hours until blood concentrations are decreased further by metabolism. Epileptiform activity has been demonstrated by EEG in epileptic patients. However, in sufficient doses, methohexital acts as an anticonvulsant.

Cardiovascular system

In general, there is less hypotension in otherwise healthy patients than occurs after thiopental; the decrease in arterial pressure is mediated predominantly by vasodilatation. Heart rate may increase slightly because of a decrease in baroreceptor activity. The cardiovascular effects are more pronounced in patients with cardiac disease or hypovolaemia.

Respiratory system

Moderate hypoventilation occurs. There may be a short period of apnoea after i.v. injection.

Pharmacokinetics

A greater proportion of methohexital than thiopental is in the unionized state at body pH (approximately 75%), although the drug is less lipid-soluble than the thiobarbiturate. Binding to plasma protein occurs to a similar degree. Clearance from plasma is higher than that of thiopental, and the elimination half-life is considerably shorter (approximately 4 h). Thus, cumulation is less likely to occur after repeated doses.

Dosage and administration

Methohexital is administered i.v. in a dose of 1–1.5 mg kg^{-1} to induce anaesthesia in healthy young adult patients; smaller doses are required in the elderly and infirm.

Adverse effects

Cardiovascular and respiratory depression. This is probably less than that associated with thiopental.

Excitatory phenomena during induction, including dyskinetic muscle movements, coughing and hiccups. Muscle movements are reduced by administration of an opioid; the incidence of cough and hiccups is reduced by premedication with an anticholinergic agent. The incidence of excitatory effects is dose-related.

Epileptiform activity on EEG in epileptic subjects.

Pain on injection (Table 3.5).

Tissue damage after perivenous injection is rare with 1% solution.

Intra-arterial injection may cause gangrene, but the risk with 1% solution is considerably less than with 2.5% thiopental.

Allergic reactions occur, but are uncommon.

Thrombophlebitis is a rare complication.

Indications

Induction of anaesthesia, particularly when a rapid recovery is desirable. Methohexital has been used commonly as the anaesthetic agent for electroconvulsive therapy (ECT) and for induction of anaesthesia for outpatient dental and other minor procedures.

Absolute contraindications

These are the same as for thiopental.

Precautions

These are similar to the precautions listed for thiopental. However, methohexital is a suitable agent for outpatients. It should not be used to induce anaesthesia in patients who are known to be epileptic.

THIAMYLAL SODIUM

This is a sulphur analogue of quinalbarbital. It is slightly more potent than thiopental, but otherwise almost identical in its properties. It is not available in the UK, but is used in some other countries.

NON-BARBITURATE INTRAVENOUS ANAESTHETIC AGENTS

PROPOFOL

This phenol derivative was identified as a potentially useful intravenous anaesthetic agent in 1980, and became available commercially in 1986. It has achieved great popularity because of its favourable recovery characteristics and its antiemetic effect.

Chemical structure

2,6–Di-isopropylphenol (Fig. 3.3).

Table 3.5 Percentage incidences of pain on injection and thrombophlebitis after intravenous administration of anaesthetic drugs into a large vein in the antecubital fossa or a small vein in the dorsum of the hand or wrist

	Pain		Thrombophlebitis	
Agent	Large	Small	Large	Small
Saline 0.9%	0	0	0	0
Thiopental 2.5%	0	12	1	0
Methohexital 1%	8	21	0	0
Propofol – LCT emulsion	10	40	0	0
Propofol – MCT emulsion	n/a	15	0	0
Etomidate – propylene glycol	8	80	15	20
Etomidate – MCT emulsion	n/a	4	0	0

MCT = medium-chain triglyceride, LCT = long-chain triglyceride.

Physical properties and presentation

Propofol is extremely lipid-soluble, but almost insoluble in water. The drug was formulated initially in Cremophor EL. However, several other drugs formulated in this solubilizing agent were associated with release of histamine and an unacceptably high incidence of anaphylactoid reactions, and similar reactions occurred with this formulation of propofol. Consequently, the drug was reformulated in a white, aqueous emulsion containing soyabean oil and purified egg phosphatide. Ampoules of the drug contain 200 mg of propofol in 20 mL (10 mg mL⁻¹), and 50 mL bottles containing 1% (10 mg mL⁻¹) or 2% (20 mg mL⁻¹) solution, and 100 mL bottles containing 1% solution, are available for infusion. In addition, 50 mL prefilled syringes of 1 and 2% solution are available and are designed for use in target-controlled infusion techniques (see below).

Pharmacology

Central nervous system

Anaesthesia is induced within 20–40 s after i.v. administration in otherwise healthy young adults. Transfer from blood to the sites of action in the brain is slower than with thiopental, and there is a delay in disappearance of the eyelash reflex, normally used as a sign of unconsciousness after administration of barbiturate anaesthetic agents. Overdosage of propofol, with exaggerated side-effects, may result if this clinical sign is used; loss of verbal contact is a better end-point. EEG frequency decreases, and amplitude increases. Propofol reduces the duration of seizures induced by ECT in humans. However, there have been reports of convulsions following the use of propofol and it is recommended that caution be exercised in the administration of propofol to epileptic patients. Normally cerebral metabolic rate, CBF and intracranial pressure are reduced.

Recovery of consciousness is rapid and there is a minimal 'hangover' effect even in the immediate postanaesthetic period.

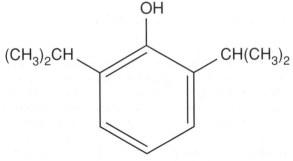

Fig. 3.3
Chemical structure of propofol (2,6-di-isopropylphenol).

Cardiovascular system

In healthy patients, arterial pressure decreases to a greater degree after induction of anaesthesia with propofol than with thiopental; the reduction results predominantly from vasodilatation although there is a slight negative inotropic effect. In some patients, large decreases (>40%) occur. The degree of hypotension is substantially reduced by decreasing the rate of administration of the drug and by appreciation of the kinetics of transfer from blood to brain (see above). The pressor response to tracheal intubation is attenuated to a greater degree by propofol than thiopental. Heart rate may increase slightly after induction of anaesthesia with propofol. However, there have been occasional reports of severe bradycardia and asystole during or shortly after administration of propofol, and it is recommended that a vagolytic agent (e.g. glycopyrronium or atropine) should be considered in patients with a pre-existing bradycardia or when propofol is used in conjunction with other drugs which are likely to cause bradycardia.

Respiratory system

After induction, apnoea occurs more commonly, and for a longer duration, than after thiopental. During infusion of propofol, tidal volume is lower and respiratory rate higher than in the conscious state. There is decreased ventilatory response to carbon dioxide. As with other agents, ventilatory depression is more marked if opioids are administered.

Propofol has no effect on bronchial muscle tone and laryngospasm is particularly uncommon. The suppression of laryngeal reflexes results in a low incidence of coughing or laryngospasm when a laryngeal mask airway (LMA) is introduced, and propofol is regarded by most anaesthetists as the drug of choice for induction of anaesthesia when the LMA is to be used.

Skeletal muscle

Tone is reduced, but movements may occur in response to surgical stimulation.

Gastrointestinal system

Propofol has no effect on gastrointestinal motility in animals. Its use is associated with a low incidence of postoperative nausea and vomiting.

Uterus and placenta

Propofol has been used extensively in patients undergoing gynaecological surgery, and it does not appear to have any clinically significant effect on uterine tone. Propofol crosses the placenta. Its safety to the neonate has not been established and its use in pregnancy (except for termination), in obstetric practice and in breast-feeding mothers is not recommended by the manufacturers.

Hepatorenal

There is a transient decrease in renal function, but the impairment is less than that associated with thiopental. Hepatic blood flow is decreased by the reductions in arterial pressure and cardiac output. Liver function tests are not deranged after infusion of propofol for 24 h.

Endocrine

Plasma concentrations of cortisol are decreased after administration of propofol, but a normal response occurs to the administration of Synacthen.

Pharmacokinetics

In common with other i.v. anaesthetic drugs, propofol is distributed rapidly, and blood concentrations decline exponentially. Clearance of the drug from plasma is greater than would be expected if the drug was metabolized only in the liver, and it is believed that extrahepatic sites of metabolism exist. The kidneys excrete the metabolites of propofol (mainly glucuronides); only 0.3% of the administered dose of propofol is excreted unchanged. The terminal elimination half-life of propofol is 3–4.8 h, although its effective half-life is much shorter (30–60 min). The distribution and clearance of propofol are altered by concomitant administration of fentanyl. Elimination of propofol remains relatively constant even after infusions lasting for several days.

Dosage and administration

In healthy, unpremedicated adults, a dose of 1.5–2.5 $mg\,kg^{-1}$ is required to induce anaesthesia. The dose should be reduced in the elderly; an initial dose of 1.25 $mg\,kg^{-1}$ is appropriate, with subsequent additional doses of 10 mg until consciousness is lost. In children, a dose of 3–3.5 $mg\,kg^{-1}$ is usually required; the drug is not recommended for use in children less than 1 month of age. Cardiovascular side-effects are reduced if the drug is injected slowly. Lower doses are required for induction in premedicated patients. Sedation during regional analgesia or endoscopy may be achieved with infusion rates of 1.5–4.5 $mg\,kg^{-1}\,h^{-1}$.

Infusion rates of up to $15\,mg\,kg^{-1}\,h^{-1}$ are required to supplement nitrous oxide/oxygen for surgical anaesthesia, although these may be reduced substantially if an opioid drug is administered. The average infusion rate is approximately $2\,mg\,kg^{-1}\,h^{-1}$ in conjunction with a slow infusion of morphine ($2\,mg\,h^{-1}$) for sedation of patients in ICU.

Adverse effects

Cardiovascular depression. Unless the drug is given very slowly, cardiovascular depression following a bolus dose of propofol is greater than that associated with a bolus dose of a barbiturate and is likely to cause profound hypotension in hypovolaemic or untreated hypertensive patients and in those with cardiac disease. Cardiovascular depression is modest if the drug is administered slowly or by infusion.

Respiratory depression. Apnoea is more common and of longer duration than after barbiturate administration.

Excitatory phenomena. These are more frequent on induction than with thiopental, but less than with methohexital. There have been occasional reports of convulsions and myoclonus during recovery from anaesthesia in which propofol has been used. Some of these reactions are delayed.

Pain on injection. This occurs in up to 40% of patients (Table 3.5). The incidence is greatly reduced if a large vein is used, if a small dose (10 mg) of lidocaine is injected shortly before propofol, or if lidocaine is mixed with propofol in the syringe (up to 1 mL of 0.5 or 1% lidocaine per 20 mL of propofol). A preparation of propofol in an emulsion of medium-chain triglycerides and soya (Propofol-Lipuro®) causes a lower incidence of pain, and less severe pain in those who still experience it, than other formulations (which use long-chain triglycerides) and may obviate the need for lidocaine. Accidental extravasation or intra-arterial injection of propofol does not appear to result in adverse effects.

Allergic reactions. Skin rashes occur occasionally. Anaphylactic reactions have also been reported, but appear to be less common than with thiopental.

Indications

Induction of anaesthesia. Propofol is indicated particularly when rapid early recovery of consciousness is required. Two hours after anaesthesia, there is no difference in psychomotor function between patients who have received propofol and those given thiopental or methohexital, but the former enjoy less drowsiness in the ensuing 12 h. The rapid recovery

characteristics are lost if induction is followed by maintenance with inhalational agents for longer than 10–15 min. The rapid redistribution and metabolism of propofol may increase the risks of awareness during tracheal intubation after the administration of non-depolarizing muscle relaxants, or at the start of surgery, unless the lungs are ventilated with an appropriate mixture of inhaled anaesthetics, or additional doses or an infusion of propofol administered.

Sedation during surgery. Propofol has been used successfully for sedation during regional analgesic techniques and during endoscopy. Control of the airway may be lost at any time, and patients must be supervised continuously by an anaesthetist.

Total i.v. anaesthesia (see below). Propofol is the most suitable of the agents currently available. Recovery time is increased after infusion of propofol compared with that after a single bolus dose, but cumulation is significantly less than with the barbiturates.

Sedation in ICU. Propofol has been used successfully by infusion to sedate adult patients for several days in ICU. The level of sedation is controlled easily, and recovery is rapid (usually < 30 min).

Absolute contraindications

Airway obstruction and known hypersensitivity to the drug are probably the only absolute contraindications. Propofol appears to be safe in porphyric patients. Propofol should not be used for long-term sedation of children (under 17 years of age) in the ICU because of a number of reports of adverse outcome.

Precautions

These are similar to those listed for thiopental. The side-effects of propofol make it less suitable than thiopental or methohexital for patients with existing cardiovascular compromise unless it is administered with great care. Propofol is more suitable than thiopental for outpatient anaesthesia, but its use does not obviate the need for an adequate period of recovery before discharge.

Solutions of propofol do not possess any antibacterial properties, and they support the growth of microorganisms. The drug must be drawn aseptically into a syringe and any unused solution should be discarded if not administered promptly. Propofol must not be administered via a microbiological filter.

ETOMIDATE

This carboxylated imidazole compound was introduced in 1972.

Chemical structure

D-Ethyl-1-(α-methylbenzyl)-imidazole-5-carboxylate.

Physical characteristics and presentation

Etomidate is soluble but unstable in water. It is presented as a clear aqueous solution containing 35% propylene glycol, or in an emulsion preparation with medium-chain tryglycerides and soya-bean oil. Ampoules contain 20 mg of etomidate in 10 mL ($2 \, mg \, mL^{-1}$). The pH of the propylene glycol solution is 8.1.

Pharmacology

Etomidate is a rapidly acting general anaesthetic agent with a short duration of action (2–3 min) resulting predominantly from redistribution, although it is also eliminated rapidly from the body. In healthy patients, it produces less cardiovascular depression than does thiopental; however, there is little evidence that this benefit is retained if the cardiovascular system is compromised. Large doses may produce tachycardia. Respiratory depression is less than with other agents.

Etomidate depresses the synthesis of cortisol by the adrenal gland and impairs the response to adrenocorticotrophic hormone. Long-term infusions of the drug in the ICU have been associated with increased infection and mortality, probably related to reduced immunological competence. Its effects on the adrenal gland occur also after a single bolus, and last for several hours.

Pharmacokinetics

Etomidate redistributes rapidly in the body. Approximately 76% is bound to protein. It is metabolized in the plasma and liver, mainly by esterase hydrolysis, and the metabolites are excreted in the urine; 2% is excreted unchanged. The terminal elimination half-life is 2.4–5 h. There is little cumulation when repeated doses are given. The distribution and clearance of etomidate may be altered by concomitant administration of fentanyl.

Dosage and administration

An average dose of $0.3 \, mg \, kg^{-1}$ i.v. induces anaesthesia. The propylene glycol preparation of the drug should be administered into a large vein to reduce the incidence of pain on injection.

Adverse effects

Suppression of synthesis of cortisol. See above.

Excitatory phenomena. Moderate or severe involuntary movements occur in up to 40% of patients during induction of anaesthesia. This incidence is reduced in patients premedicated with an opioid. Cough and hiccups occur in up to 10% of patients.

Pain on injection. This occurs in up to 80% of patients if the propylene glycol preparation is injected into a small vein, but in less than 10% when the drug is injected into a large vein in the antecubital fossa (Table 3.5). The incidence is reduced by prior injection of lidocaine 10 mg. The incidence of pain on injection has been reported to be as low as 4% when the emulsion formulation is injected.

Nausea and vomiting. The incidence of nausea and vomiting is approximately 30%. This is very much higher than after propofol.

Emergence phenomena. The incidence of severe restlessness and delirium during recovery is greater with etomidate than barbiturates or propofol.

Venous thrombosis is more common than with other agents.

Indications

Etomidate is used by many anaesthetists in patients with a compromised cardiovascular system. It is suitable for outpatient anaesthesia. The high incidence of pain on injection of the propylene glycol preparation of etomidate limited its use to patients in whom depression of the cardiovascular system was undesirable, but the preparation as an emulsion with medium-chain triglycerides has greatly reduced the incidence of pain on injection and is likely to result in increased use of the drug in all patient groups.

Absolute contraindications

- airway obstruction
- porphyria
- adrenal insufficiency
- long-term infusion in ITU.

Precautions

These are similar to the precautions listed for thiopental. Etomidate is suitable for outpatient anaesthesia. However, the incidence of excitatory phenomena is unacceptably high unless an opioid is administered; this delays recovery and is unsuitable for most outpatients.

KETAMINE HYDROCHLORIDE

This is a phencyclidine derivative and was introduced in 1965. It differs from other i.v. anaesthetic agents in many respects, and produces dissociative anaesthesia rather than generalized depression of the CNS.

Chemical structure

2-(o-Chlorophenyl)-2-(methylamino)-cyclohexanone hydrochloride.

Physical characteristics and presentation

Ketamine is soluble in water and is presented as solutions of 10 mg mL^{-1} containing sodium chloride to produce isotonicity, and 50 or 100 mg mL^{-1} in multidose vials which contain benzethonium chloride 0.1 mg mL^{-1} as preservative. The pH of the solutions is 3.5–5.5. The pK_a of ketamine is 7.5.

Pharmacology

Central nervous system

Ketamine is extremely lipid-soluble. After i.v. injection, it induces anaesthesia in 30–60 s. A single i.v. dose produces unconsciousness for 10–15 min. Ketamine is also effective within 3–4 min after i.m. injection and has a duration of action of 15–25 min. It is a potent somatic analgesic at subanaesthetic blood concentrations. Amnesia often persists for up to 1 h after recovery of consciousness. Induction of anaesthesia is smooth, but emergence delirium may occur, with restlessness, disorientation and agitation. Vivid and often unpleasant nightmares or hallucinations may occur during recovery and for up to 24 h. The incidences of emergence delirium and hallucinations are reduced by avoidance of verbal and tactile stimulation during the recovery period, or by concomitant administration of opioids, butyrophenones, benzodiazepines or physostigmine; however, unpleasant dreams may persist. Nightmares are reported less commonly by children and elderly patients.

The EEG changes associated with ketamine are unlike those seen with other i.v. anaesthetics, and consist of loss of alpha rhythm and predominant theta activity. Cerebral metabolic rate is increased in several regions of the brain, and CBF, cerebral blood volume and intracranial pressure increase.

Cardiovascular system

Arterial pressure increases by up to 25% and heart rate by approximately 20%. Cardiac output may increase, and myocardial oxygen consumption increases; the positive inotropic effect may be related to increased calcium influx mediated by cyclic adenosine monophosphate. There is increased myocardial sensitivity to epinephrine.

Sympathetic stimulation of the peripheral circulation is decreased, resulting in vasodilatation in tissues innervated predominantly by α-adrenergic receptors, and vasoconstriction in those with β-receptors.

Respiratory system

Transient apnoea may occur after i.v. injection, but ventilation is well maintained thereafter and may increase slightly unless high doses are given. Pharyngeal and laryngeal reflexes and a patent airway are maintained well in comparison with other i.v. agents; however, their presence cannot be guaranteed, and normal precautions must be taken to protect the airway and prevent aspiration. Bronchial muscle is dilated.

Skeletal muscle

Muscle tone is usually increased. Spontaneous movements may occur, but reflex movement in response to surgery is uncommon.

Gastrointestinal system

Salivation is increased.

Uterus and placenta

Ketamine crosses the placenta readily. Fetal concentrations are approximately equal to those in the mother.

The eye

Intraocular pressure increases, although this effect is often transient. Eye movements often persist during surgical anaesthesia.

Pharmacokinetics

Only approximately 12% of ketamine is bound to protein. The initial peak concentration after i.v. injection decreases as the drug is distributed, but this occurs more slowly than with other i.v. anaesthetic agents. Metabolism occurs predominantly in the liver by demethylation and hydroxylation of the cyclohexanone ring; among the metabolites is norketamine, which is pharmacologically active. Approximately 80% of the injected dose is excreted renally as glucuronides; only 2.5% is excreted unchanged. The elimination half-life is approximately 2.5 h. Distribution and elimination are slower if halothane, benzodiazepines or barbiturates are administered concurrently.

After i.m. injection, peak concentrations are achieved after approximately 20 min.

Dosage and administration

Induction of anaesthesia is achieved with an average dose of 2 mg kg^{-1} i.v.; larger doses may be required in some patients, and smaller doses in the elderly or shocked patient. In all cases, the drug should be administered slowly. Additional doses of 1–1.5 mg kg^{-1} are required every 5–10 min. Between 8 and 10 mg kg^{-1} is used i.m. A dose of 0.25–0.5 mg kg^{-1} or an infusion of 50 μg kg^{-1} min^{-1} may be used to produce analgesia without loss of consciousness.

Adverse effects

- emergence delirium, nightmares and hallucinations
- hypertension and tachycardia – this may be harmful in previously hypertensive patients and in those with ischaemic heart disease
- prolonged recovery
- salivation – anticholinergic premedication is essential
- increased intracranial pressure
- allergic reactions – skin rashes have been reported.

Indications

The high-risk patient. Ketamine is useful in the shocked patient. Arterial pressure may decrease if hypovolaemia is present, and the drug must be given cautiously. These patients are usually heavily sedated in the postoperative period, and the risk of nightmares is therefore minimized.

Paediatric anaesthesia. Children undergoing minor surgery, investigations (e.g. cardiac catheterization), ophthalmic examinations or radiotherapy may be managed successfully with ketamine administered either i.m. or i.v.

Difficult locations. Ketamine has been used successfully at the site of accidents, and for analgesia and anaesthesia in casualties of war.

Analgesia and sedation. The analgesic action of ketamine may be used when wound dressings are changed, or while positioning patients with pain before performing regional anaesthesia (e.g. fractured neck of femur). Ketamine has been used to sedate asthmatic patients in the ICU.

Developing countries. Ketamine is used extensively in countries where anaesthetic equipment and trained staff are in short supply.

Absolute contraindications

- Airway obstruction – although the airway is maintained better with ketamine than with other agents, its patency cannot be guaranteed. Inhalational agents should be used for induction of anaesthesia if airway obstruction is anticipated.
- Raised intracranial pressure.

Precautions

Cardiovascular disease. Ketamine is unsuitable for patients with pre-existing hypertension, ischaemic heart disease or severe cardiac decompensation.

Repeated administration. Because of the prolonged recovery period, ketamine is not the most suitable drug for frequent procedures, e.g. prolonged courses of radiotherapy, as it disrupts sleep and eating patterns.

Visceral stimulation. Ketamine suppresses poorly the response to visceral stimulation; supplementation, e.g. with an opioid, is indicated if visceral stimulation is anticipated.

Outpatient anaesthesia. The prolonged recovery period and emergence phenomena make ketamine unsuitable for adult outpatients.

OTHER DRUGS

Opioids and benzodiazepines may also be used to induce general anaesthesia. However, very large doses are required, and recovery is prolonged. Their use is confined to specialist areas, e.g. cardiac anaesthesia. The pharmacology of these drugs is described in Chapters 5 and 7, respectively.

INTRAVENOUS MAINTENANCE OF ANAESTHESIA

INDICATIONS FOR INTRAVENOUS MAINTENANCE OF ANAESTHESIA

There are several situations in which i.v. anaesthesia (IVA; the use of an i.v. anaesthetic to supplement nitrous oxide) or total i.v. anaesthesia (TIVA) may offer advantages over the traditional inhalational techniques. In the doses required to maintain clinical anaesthesia, i.v. agents cause minimal cardiovascular depression. In comparison with the most commonly used volatile anaesthetic agents, IVA with propofol (the only currently available i.v. anaesthetic with an appropriate pharmacokinetic profile) offers rapid recovery of consciousness and good recovery of psychomotor function, although the newer volatile anaesthetics desflurane and sevoflurane are also associated with rapid recovery and minimal hangover effects.

The use of TIVA allows a high inspired oxygen concentration in situations where hypoxaemia may otherwise occur, such as one-lung anaesthesia or in severely ill or traumatized patients, and has obvious advantages in procedures such as laryngoscopy or bronchoscopy, when delivery of inhaled anaesthetic agents to the lungs may be difficult. TIVA may also be used to provide anaesthesia in circumstances where there are clinical reasons to avoid nitrous oxide, such as middle-ear surgery, prolonged bowel surgery and in patients with raised intracranial pressure. There are few contraindications to the use of IVA, provided that the anaesthetist is aware of the wide variability in response (see below). For surgical anaesthesia, it is desirable either to use nitrous oxide supplemented by IVA or to infuse an opioid in addition to the i.v. anaesthetic.

PRINCIPLES OF IVA

The calibrated vaporizer allows the anaesthetist to establish stable conditions, usually with relatively few changes in delivered concentration of volatile anaesthetic agents during an operation. This is largely because the patient tends to come into equilibrium with the delivered concentration, irrespective of body size or physiological variations; the total dose of drug taken up by the body is variable, but is relatively unimportant, and is determined by the characteristics of the patient and the drug rather than by the anaesthetist. The task of achieving equilibrium with i.v. anaesthetic agents is more complex, as delivery must be matched to the size of the patient and also to the expected rates of distribution and metabolism of the drug. Conventional methods of delivering i.v. agents result in the total dose of drug being determined by the anaesthetist, and the concentration achieved in the brain depends on the volume and rate of distribution, the relative solubility of the agent in various tissues and the rate of elimination of the drug in the individual patient. Consequently, there is considerably more variability among patients in the infusion rate of an i.v. anaesthetic required to produce satisfactory anaesthesia than there is in the inspired concentration of an inhaled agent. There is concern among some anaesthetists that the difficulty in predicting the correct infusion rate for an individual patient may result in a higher risk of awareness in the paralysed patient, although the risks appear in practice to be similar, and related to inadvertent failure of delivery of the drug or the use of inappropriate infusion schemes rather than to an inherent flaw in the technique.

TECHNIQUES OF ADMINISTRATION

Intermittent injection

Although some anaesthetists are skilled in the delivery of i.v. anaesthetic agents by intermittent bolus injection, the plasma concentrations of drug and the anaesthetic effect fluctuate widely, and the technique is acceptable only for procedures of short duration in unparalysed patients.

Manual infusion techniques

The infusion rate required to achieve a predetermined concentration of an i.v. drug can be calculated if the clearance of the drug from plasma is known [infusion rate (μg min^{-1}) = steady-state plasma concentration (μg mL^{-1}) $\times$ clearance (mL min^{-1})]. One of the difficulties is that clearance is variable, and it is possible only to estimate the value by using population kinetics; depending on the patient's clearance in relation to the average, the actual plasma concentration achieved may be higher or lower than the intended concentration.

A fixed-rate infusion is inappropriate because the serum concentration of the drug increases only slowly, taking four to five times the elimination half-life of the drug to reach steady state (Fig. 3.4). A bolus injection followed by a continuous infusion results initially in achievement of an excessive concentration (with an increased incidence of side-effects), and this is followed by a prolonged dip below the intended plasma concentration (Fig. 3.5). In order to achieve a reasonably constant plasma concentration (other than in very long procedures), it is necessary to use a multistep infusion

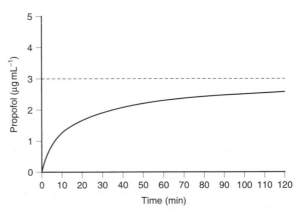

Fig. 3.4
Average blood concentration during the first 2 h of a continuous infusion of propofol at a rate of 6 mg kg^{-1} h^{-1}. Note that, even after 2 h, the equilibrium concentration of 3 μg mL^{-1} has not been achieved.

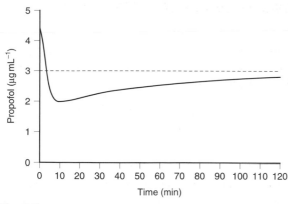

Fig. 3.5

Average blood propofol concentration following a bolus dose of propofol followed by a continuous infusion of 6 mg kg^{-1} h^{-1}. Note that the target concentration is initially exceeded, but that the blood concentration then decreases below the target concentration, which is not achieved within 2 h.

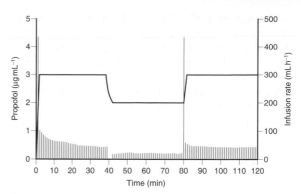

Fig. 3.6

Average blood concentrations of propofol achieved using a target-controlled infusion system. The narrow vertical lines represent the infusion rate calculated by the computer to achieve, and then to maintain, the target concentration in blood. A target concentration of 3 μg mL^{-1} was programmed initially. When the target concentration is reset to 2 μg mL^{-1}, the infusion is stopped and then restarted at a rate calculated to maintain that concentration. The target concentration is then increased to 3 μg mL^{-1}; the infusion pump delivers a rapid infusion rate to achieve the target concentration, and then gradually decreases the infusion rate to maintain a constant blood concentration.

regimen, a concept similar to that of overpressure for inhaled agents. A commonly used scheme for propofol is injection of a bolus dose of 1 mg kg^{-1} followed by infusion initially at a rate of 10 mg kg^{-1} h^{-1} for 10 min, then 8 mg kg^{-1} h^{-1} for the next 10 min, and a maintenance infusion rate of 6 mg kg^{-1} h^{-1} thereafter. This achieves, on average, a plasma concentration of propofol of 3 μg mL^{-1}, and this is effective in achieving satisfactory anaesthesia in unparalysed patients who *also* receive nitrous oxide and fentanyl; higher infusion rates are required if nitrous oxide and fentanyl are not administered. These infusion rates must be regarded only as a guide and must be adjusted as necessary according to clinical signs of anaesthesia.

Target-controlled infusion (TCI) techniques

By programming a computer with appropriate pharmacokinetic data and equations, it is possible at frequent intervals (several times a minute) to calculate the appropriate infusion rate required to produce a preset target plasma concentration of drug. The drug is infused by a syringe driver. To produce a step increase in plasma concentration, the syringe driver infuses drug very rapidly (a slow bolus) and then delivers drug at a progressively decreasing infusion rate (Fig. 3.6). To decrease the plasma concentration, the syringe driver stops infusing until the computer calculates that the target concentration has been achieved, and then infuses drug at an appropriate rate to maintain a constant level. The anaesthetist is required only to enter the desired target concentration and to change it when clinically indicated, in the same

way as a vaporizer might be manipulated according to clinical signs of anaesthesia.

The potential advantages of such a system are its simplicity, the rapidity with which plasma concentration can be changed (particularly upwards) and avoidance of the need for the anaesthetist to undertake any calculations (resulting in less potential for error). The actual concentration achieved may be >50% greater than or less than the predicted concentration, although this is not a major practical disadvantage provided that the anaesthetist adjusts the target concentration according to clinical signs relating to adequacy of anaesthesia, rather than assuming that a specific target concentration always results in the desired effect.

Using a TCI system in female patients, the target concentration of propofol required to prevent movement in response to surgical incision in 50% of subjects (the equivalent of minimum alveolar concentration; MAC) was 6 μg mL^{-1} when patients breathed oxygen, and 4.5 μg mL^{-1} when 67% nitrous oxide was administered simultaneously.

A TCI system for administration of propofol is available in many countries. The anaesthetist is required to input the weight and age of the patient, and then to select the desired target concentration. These devices can be used only with prefilled syringes, which contain an electronic tag that is recognized by the infusion pump. These TCI systems are currently suitable for use only in patients over the age of 16 years. Target concentrations selected for elderly patients should be lower than those for younger adults, in order to minimize the risk of side-effects.

The TCI infusion pumps assume that the patient is conscious when the infusion is started. Consequently, it is inappropriate to connect and start a TCI system in a patient who is already unconscious, as this results in an initial overdose.

In adult patients under 55 years of age, anaesthesia may be induced usually with a target propofol concentration of $4–8\,\mu g\,mL^{-1}$. An initial target concentration at the lower end of that range is suitable for premedicated patients. Induction time is usually between 1 and 2 min. The brain concentration of propofol increases more slowly than the blood concentration, and following induction it is usually appropriate to reduce the target concentration; target propofol concentrations in the range of $3–6\,\mu g\,mL^{-1}$ usually maintain satisfactory anaesthesia in patients who are also receiving an analgesic drug.

Later versions of the TCI infusion pumps show the predicted brain concentration, which may be used as a guide to the timing of alterations in the blood target concentration.

Closed-loop systems

Target-controlled infusion systems may be used as part of a closed-loop system to control depth of anaesthesia. Because there is no method of measuring blood concentrations of i.v. anaesthetics on-line, it is necessary to use some type of monitor of depth of anaesthesia (such as the auditory evoked response; see Ch. 18) on the input side of the system.

ADVERSE REACTIONS TO INTRAVENOUS ANAESTHETIC AGENTS

These may take the form of pain on injection, venous thrombosis, involuntary muscle movement, hiccup, hypotension and postoperative delirium. All of these reactions may be modified by the anaesthetic technique.

Hypersensitivity reactions, which resemble the effects of histamine release, are more rare and less predictable. Other vasoactive agents may also be released. Reactions to i.v. anaesthetic agents are caused usually by one of the following mechanisms:

Type I hypersensitivity response. The drug interacts with specific immunoglobulin E (IgE) antibodies, which are often bound to the surface of mast cells;

these become granulated and release histamine and other vasoactive amines.

Classic complement-mediated reaction. The classic complement pathway may be activated by type II (cell surface antigen) or type III (immune complex formation) hypersensitivity reactions. IgG or IgM antibodies are involved.

Alternate complement pathway activation. Preformed antibodies to an antigen are not necessary for activation of this pathway; these reactions may therefore occur without prior exposure to the drug.

Direct pharmacological effects of the drug. These anaphylactoid reactions result from a direct effect on mast cells and basophils. There may be local cutaneous signs only. In more severe reactions, there are signs of systemic release of histamine.

Clinical features

In a severe hypersensitivity reaction, a flush may develop over the upper part of the body. There is usually hypotension, which may be profound. Cutaneous and glottic oedema may develop and may result in hypovolaemia because of loss of fluid from the circulation. Very severe bronchospasm may also occur, although it is a feature in less than 50% of reactions. Diarrhoea often occurs some hours after the initial reaction.

Predisposing factors

Age. In general, adverse reactions are less common in children than in adults.

Pregnancy. There is an increased incidence of adverse reactions in pregnancy.

Gender. Anaphylactic reactions are more common in women.

Atopy. There may be an increased incidence of type IV (delayed hypersensitivity) reactions in non-atopic individuals, and a higher incidence of type I reactions in those with a history of extrinsic asthma, hay fever or penicillin allergy.

Previous exposure. Previous exposure to the drug, or to a drug with similar constituents, exerts a much greater influence on the incidence of reactions than does a history of atopy.

Solvents. Cremophor EL, which was used as a solvent for several i.v. anaesthetic agents, was associated with a high incidence of hypersensitivity reactions.

Incidence

The incidences of hypersensitivity reactions associated with i.v. anaesthetic agents are shown in Table 3.6.

Table 3.6 Incidences of adverse reactions to intravenous anaesthetic agents

Drug	Incidence
Thiopental	1:14 000–1:20 000
Methohexital	1:1600–1:7000
Etomidate	1:450 000
Propofol	1:50 000–100 000 (estimated)

Treatment

This is summarized in Table 3.7. Appropriate investigations should be undertaken after recovery to identify the drug responsible for the reaction.

FURTHER READING

Association of Anaesthetists of Great Britain and Ireland 2003 Suspected anaphylactic reactions associated with anaesthesia 3. AAGBI, London

McCaughey W, Clarke R S J, Fee J P H, Wallace W F M 1997 Anaesthetic physiology and pharmacology. Churchill Livingstone, Edinburgh

Sneyd J R 2004 Recent advances in intravenous anaesthesia. British Journal of Anaesthesia 93: 725–736

Table 3.7 Suggested management of suspected anaphylaxis during anaesthesia

Aims

- Correct arterial hypoxaemia

- Restore intravascular fluid volume

- Inhibit further release of chemical mediators

Immediate management

1. Stop administration of all agents likely to have caused the anaphylaxis

2. Call for help

3. Maintain airway, give 100% oxygen and lie patient supine with legs elevated

4. Give epinephrine (adrenaline). This may be given intramuscularly in a dose of 0.5–1 mg (0.5–1 mL of 1:1000) and may be repeated every 10 min according to the arterial pressure and pulse until improvement occurs
   Alternatively, 50–100 µg intravenously (0.5–1 mL of 1:10 000) over 1 min has been recommended for hypotension with titration of further doses as required
   Never give undiluted epinephrine 1:1000 intravenously
   In a patient with cardiovascular collapse, 0.5–1 mg (5–10 mL of 1:10 000) may be required intravenously in divided doses by titration. This should be given at a rate of 0.1 mg min^{-1} stopping when a response has been obtained
   Paediatric doses of epinephrine depend on the age of the child. Intramuscular epinephrine 1:1000 should be administered as follows:

>12 years	500 µg i.m. (0.5 mL)
6–12 years	250 µg i.m. (0.25 mL)
>6 months to 6 years	120 µg i.m. (0.12 mL)
<6 months	50 µg i.m. (0.05 mL)

5. Start rapid intravenous infusion of colloids or crystalloids. Adult patients may require 2–4 L of crystalloid

Secondary management

1. Give antihistamines (chlorpheniramine 10–20 mg by slow i.v. infusion)

2. Give corticosteroids (100–500 mg hydrocortisone slowly i.v.)

3. Bronchodilators may be required for persistent bronchospasm

4   Local anaesthetic agents

Local anaesthetic drugs act by producing a reversible block to the transmission of peripheral nerve impulses. A reversible block may also be produced by physical factors, including pressure and cold. Although nerve compression is of purely historical interest, cold (produced by the evaporation of ethyl chloride, the application of ice packs or the use of a cryoprobe) still has a limited use.

Many types of drug have local anaesthetic actions (e.g. β-blockers and antihistamines), but all those known and used as local anaesthetics have originated from cocaine, the alkaloid found in the leaves of the South American bush *Erythroxylum coca*. Its local anaesthetic action was demonstrated first by Koller, an ophthalmic surgeon working in Vienna. Although most of the major local anaesthetic techniques were described within a few years of that discovery, the drug was not used widely other than as a topical agent because of its systemic toxicity, central nervous stimulant and addictive properties and tendency to produce allergic reactions.

The demonstration of the physical structure of cocaine as an ester of benzoic acid permitted the production of safer agents, all with the same general structure of an aromatic group joined to an amine by an intermediate chain containing either an ester or an amide link (Fig. 4.1). Procaine, an ester synthesized in 1904, was the first significant advance and it allowed wider use of local anaesthetic techniques. Many other drugs were introduced, but none displaced procaine as the standard until the synthesis of the standard amide, lidocaine, in the 1940s. The intermediate chain in lidocaine contains an amide bond and this obviated many of the problems associated with the ester group present in the older drugs. The subsequent production of other amide agents with varying clinical profiles has greatly extended the scope of modern local anaesthesia.

Local anaesthetics act by blocking membrane depolarization in all excitable tissues. As local anaesthetics are injected at their site of action, only peripheral nerve is usually exposed to concentrations high enough to have a significant effect. However, when sufficient drug reaches other organs via the circulation, more widespread effects occur.

MODE OF ACTION

NEURAL TRANSMISSION (Fig. 4.2)

During the resting phase, the interior of a peripheral nerve fibre has a potential difference of about −70 mV relative to the outside. When the nerve is stimulated, there is a rapid increase in the membrane potential to approximately +20 mV, followed by immediate restoration to the resting level. This depolarization/repolarization sequence lasts 1–2 ms and produces the familiar action potential associated with the passage of a nerve impulse.

The resting potential is the net result of several factors affecting the distribution of ions across the cell membrane. Electrochemical and concentration gradients modify ionic diffusion, which is adjusted further by the semipermeable nature of the membrane and the action of the sodium/potassium pump. The resulting balance of these factors is a slight excess of anions in intracellular fluid.

Depolarization of the fibre is the result of a sudden increase in membrane permeability to sodium, which may thus diffuse down both electrochemical and concentration gradients. Sodium ions enter the cell through large protein molecules in the membrane, known as channels. These are closed during the resting phase, but stimulation of the nerve changes the configuration of the protein molecules so that the channels open and allow positively charged sodium ions to enter the cell. The membrane potential increases to approximately +20 mV, when the electrochemical and concentration gradients for sodium balance each other and the channels close. Both concentration and electrochemical gradients then

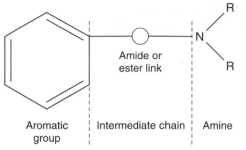

Fig. 4.1
General formula for local anaesthetic drugs.

favour movement of potassium out through the membrane until the resting potential is restored. This outward movement of potassium is also facilitated by the opening of specific channels in the membrane. Relative to the total amounts present, only small numbers of ions take part in this exchange and the sodium/potassium pump restores their distribution during the resting phase.

At sensory nerve endings, the initial opening of sodium channels is produced by the appropriate physiological stimulus, which may be mediated chemically in some instances. When these sodium channels open,

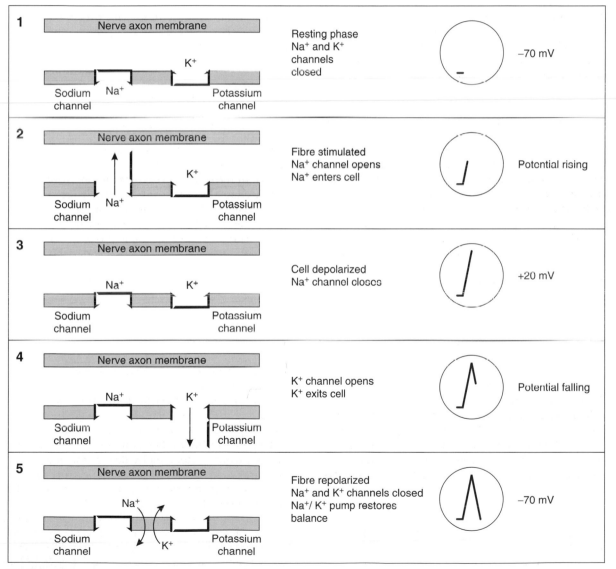

Fig. 4.2
Events occurring during transmission of a nerve impulse along an axon.

the potential at the nerve ending increases and results in a voltage gradient along the axon. This causes a current (known as a local current) to flow between the depolarized segment of nerve (which has a positive charge) and the next segment (which has a negative charge). The voltage change associated with this current causes the configurational change in the sodium channels in the next segment, so that the action potential is propagated along the nerve. A similar sequence is induced when transmitter substances act on specific receptors on the postjunctional membrane at synapses between nerves.

EFFECT OF LOCAL ANAESTHETIC DRUGS
(Fig. 4.3)

Local anaesthetics are usually injected in an acid solution as the hydrochloride salt (pH approximately 5). In such conditions, the tertiary amine group becomes quaternary and the molecules are thus soluble in water and suitable for injection. After injection, the pH increases as a result of buffering in the tissues and a proportion of the drug, determined by the pK_a, dissociates to release free base. Because it is lipid-soluble, the free base is able to pass through the lipid cell membrane to the interior of the axon, where re-ionization takes place. It is the re-ionized portion that enters and blocks the sodium channels, and prevents influx of sodium ions. As a result, no action potential is generated or transmitted, and conduction blockade occurs.

In addition to diffusing into nerves and surrounding tissues at the site of injection, the drug also enters capillaries and is removed by the circulation. Eventually, tissue concentration decreases below that in the nerve fibres and the drug diffuses out, so allowing restoration of normal function.

SYSTEMIC TOXICITY

If significant amounts of local anaesthetic drug reach the tissues of heart and brain, they exert the same membrane-stabilizing effect as on peripheral nerve, resulting in progressive depression of function. The earliest feature of systemic toxicity is numbness or tingling of the tongue and circumoral area; this is the result of a rich blood supply to these tissues depositing enough drug to have an effect on the nerve endings. The patient may become light-headed, anxious, drowsy and/or complain of tinnitus. If concentrations continue to increase, consciousness is lost and this may be preceded or followed by convulsions.

Coma and apnoea may develop subsequently. Cardiovascular collapse may result from direct myocardial depression and vasodilatation, but more commonly it is a result of hypoxaemia secondary to apnoea.

Factors affecting toxicity

The most common cause of life-threatening systemic toxicity is an inadvertent intravascular injection, but it may result also from absolute overdosage. The changes in plasma concentration of drug following injection (Fig. 4.4) are dependent on the total dose administered, the rate of absorption, the pattern of distribution to other tissues and the rate of metabolism.

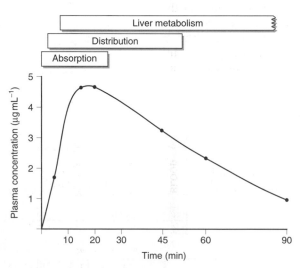

Fig. 4.4
Plasma concentration of lidocaine. Concentrations are shown after the injection into the lumbar epidural space of 400 mg of lidocaine without adrenaline (epinephrine). The injection was made at time zero and the phases of absorption, distribution and metabolism are indicated.

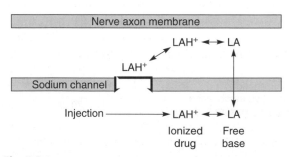

Fig. 4.3
Mode of action of a local anaesthetic (LA) drug. In order to penetrate the lipid cell membrane, the drug must be in free base form, while to effect a block, re-ionization must occur.

Absorption

Absorption from the site of injection depends on the blood flow; the higher the blood flow, the more rapid is the increase in plasma concentration, and the greater the resultant peak. Of the common sites of injection of large doses, the intercostal space has the highest blood supply, followed in turn by the epidural space, the brachial plexus and the sites of major lower limb nerve block. Absorption is slowest after infiltration anaesthesia.

Intravenous regional anaesthesia is a special case. If the tourniquet deflates immediately after drug injection, a large dose enters the circulation very rapidly. After 20 min of tourniquet application, sufficient drug has diffused out of the vessels into the tissues to result in the increase in systemic concentration being smaller than that following brachial plexus block.

Blood supply may be modified by the inherent vasoactive properties of the particular drug or by the addition of vasoconstrictors to the solution. Use of the latter permits the safe dose to be increased by 50–100%.

Distribution (Fig. 4.5)

After absorption, local anaesthetic drugs are distributed rapidly to, and taken up by, organs with a large blood supply and high affinity, e.g. brain, heart, liver and lungs. Muscle and fat, with low blood supplies, equilibrate more slowly, but the high affinity of fat for these drugs ensures that a large amount is taken up into adipose tissues. Local anaesthetic drugs are sequestered in (and possibly metabolized in) the lungs, thereby preventing a large proportion of the injected dose from reaching the coronary and cerebral circulations.

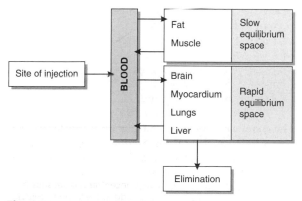

Fig. 4.5
Distribution of local anaesthetic drug after absorption from the site of injection.

Metabolism

In general, ester drugs are broken down so rapidly by plasma cholinesterase that systemic toxicity is unusual. Toxicity may occur with some of the slowly hydrolysed drugs or in patients with abnormal enzymes (cf. succinylcholine). The amides are metabolized by amidases located predominantly in the liver. Hepatocellular disease has to be severe before the rate of metabolism is slowed significantly, and in general the rate of disappearance of drug is dependent more upon liver blood flow. This has practical relevance to the use of lidocaine as an antiarrhythmic in cardiogenic shock, when liver blood flow is diminished.

Protein binding

Local anaesthetics are bound to plasma proteins to varying degrees. It is assumed sometimes that drugs with the greatest degrees of protein binding are less toxic because only a small fraction of the total amount in plasma is free to diffuse into the tissues and produce toxic effects. However, values for protein binding are obtained under laboratory conditions and probably bear little relationship to the dynamic situation that exists during the phase of rapid absorption. Furthermore, even if a drug is bound to protein, it is still available to diffuse into the tissues down a concentration gradient, because the bound portion is in equilibrium with that in solution in plasma. Thus, values for protein binding do not relate to acute toxicity of a drug.

Placental transfer

Much theoretical concern has been expressed about the mechanisms and effects of placental transfer of local anaesthetics administered to the mother during labour. Local anaesthetics cross the placenta as readily as other membranes, but their effects are of minimal significance when compared with those of conventional methods of analgesia and anaesthesia.

Fetal plasma protein may bind some drugs to a lesser extent than maternal protein so that *total* plasma concentration may be lower in the baby. It is claimed that such drugs are safer for the fetus. However, the concentration of *free* drug on each side of the placental membrane is the same, and as a result tissue concentrations are more similar in mother and fetus than total plasma concentrations. The neonatal liver metabolizes drugs slowly, but provided that delivery does not occur immediately after a toxic reaction, there should be little concern about effects on the baby.

Prevention of toxicity

The single most important factor in the prevention of toxicity is the avoidance of accidental intravascular injection. Careful aspiration tests are vital and should be repeated each time the needle is moved. However, a negative test is not an absolute guarantee, especially when a catheter technique is used. The initial injection of 2–3 mL of a solution that contains adrenaline (epinephrine) 1:200 000 has been advocated; an increase in heart rate during the succeeding 1–2 min should indicate intravascular injection. However, adrenaline is not the safest of drugs and this method is no guarantee against subsequent migration of needle or cannula into a vessel.

An alternative is to repeat the aspiration test after each 5–10 mL of solution and to inject slowly (about 5 mL per minute). The patient should be watched for early signs of toxicity so that the injection may be stopped before there are major sequelae. Particular care should be taken when performing head and neck blocks because a very small dose may produce a major reaction if injected into a carotid or vertebral artery.

Overdosage may be avoided by consideration of the behaviour of the various drugs after injection at the particular site. Most practical manuals indicate the appropriate drug and dosage for each block, and these recommendations should be followed. Maximum safe dosages (for use in any situation) are often quoted for local anaesthetics with and without vasoconstrictor, but such recommendations are not really helpful because they ignore variations caused by factors such as the site of injection, the patient's general condition and the concomitant use of a general anaesthetic. If the same total dose is used, variations in drug concentration have no effect on toxicity. In adults, body weight correlates poorly with the risk of toxicity and it is better to modify the dose on the basis of an informed assessment of the patient's general condition.

Treatment of toxicity

No matter how careful the anaesthetist is with regard to prevention, facilities for treatment must always be available. The airway is maintained and oxygen administered by face mask, using artificial ventilation if apnoea occurs. Convulsions may be controlled with small increments of either midazolam (2 mg) or thiopental (50 mg). The latter acts more rapidly. Excessive doses should not be given to control convulsions, because cardiorespiratory depression may be exacerbated. If cardiovascular collapse occurs despite adequate oxygenation (and this is rare), it should be treated with an adrenergic drug with α- and β-agonist properties, e.g. ephedrine in 3–5 mg increments.

ADDITIONAL SIDE-EFFECTS

Local anaesthetics are remarkably free from side-effects other than systemic toxicity which is an extension of pharmacological action. Complications of specific drugs are discussed later, but there are two general features – allergic reactions and drug interactions.

Allergic reactions

Allergy to the esters was relatively common, particularly with procaine, and was caused by p-aminobenzoic acid produced on hydrolysis. Most reactions were dermal in personnel handling the drugs, but fatal anaphylaxis has been recorded. Allergy to the amides is extremely rare and most reactions result from systemic toxicity, overdosage with vasoconstrictors, or are manifestations of anxiety. The occasional genuine allergic reaction is usually to a preservative in the solution rather than the drug itself.

Drug interactions

Interactions with other drugs do occur, although they rarely cause clinical problems. Therapy with anticholinesterases for myasthenia, or concomitant administration of other drugs hydrolysed by plasma cholinesterase, increases the toxicity of the ester drugs, and competition for plasma protein binding sites may occur with the amides. Of more practical importance is that heavy sedation with anticonvulsants (e.g. benzodiazepines) may mask the early signs of toxicity. These drugs may even prevent convulsions, so that if a severe reaction does occur the patient may suddenly become deeply unconscious.

LOCAL ANAESTHETIC DRUG CHEMISTRY

The chemical structures and physicochemical properties of individual local anaesthetic drugs are shown in Table 4.1. As indicated above (Fig. 4.1), all local anaesthetics have the same general structure of an aromatic group and an amine linked by either an ester or an amide bond. The important effects of the nature of this linkage on the route of metabolism and allergenicity of local anaesthetics have been discussed.

Table 4.1 The features of individual local anaesthetic drugs

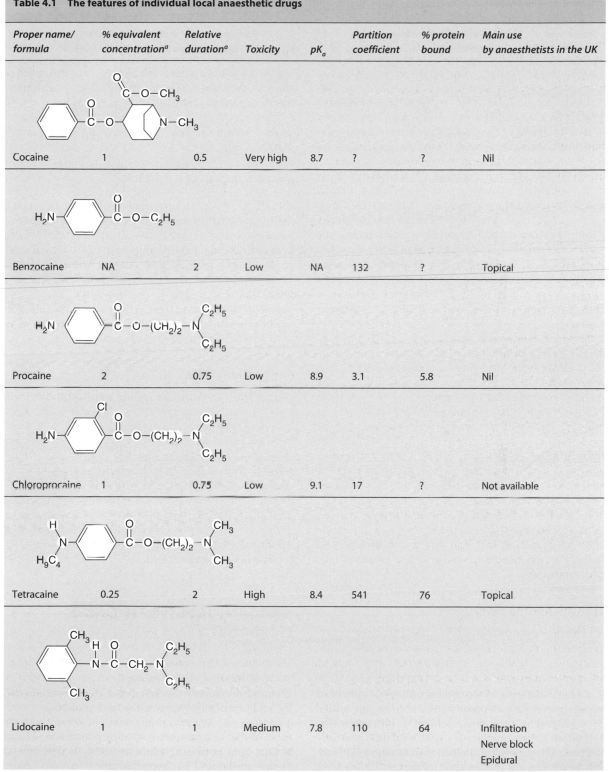

Proper name/ formula	% equivalent concentration[a]	Relative duration[a]	Toxicity	pK_a	Partition coefficient	% protein bound	Main use by anaesthetists in the UK
Cocaine	1	0.5	Very high	8.7	?	?	Nil
Benzocaine	NA	2	Low	NA	132	?	Topical
Procaine	2	0.75	Low	8.9	3.1	5.8	Nil
Chloroprocaine	1	0.75	Low	9.1	17	?	Not available
Tetracaine	0.25	2	High	8.4	541	76	Topical
Lidocaine	1	1	Medium	7.8	110	64	Infiltration Nerve block Epidural

Continued

Table 4.1   The features of individual local anaesthetic drugs — Cont'd

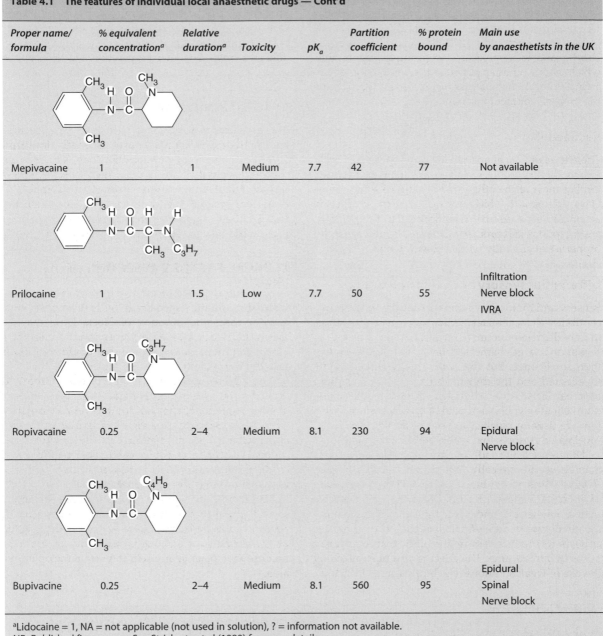

Proper name/ formula	% equivalent concentration[a]	Relative duration[a]	Toxicity	pK_a	Partition coefficient	% protein bound	Main use by anaesthetists in the UK
Mepivacaine	1	1	Medium	7.7	42	77	Not available
Prilocaine	1	1.5	Low	7.7	50	55	Infiltration Nerve block IVRA
Ropivacaine	0.25	2–4	Medium	8.1	230	94	Epidural Nerve block
Bupivacine	0.25	2–4	Medium	8.1	560	95	Epidural Spinal Nerve block

[a]Lidocaine = 1, NA = not applicable (not used in solution), ? = information not available.
NB: Published figures vary. See Strichartz et al (1990) for more details.

Other differences in the clinical profiles of individual agents (potency, onset, duration of action, etc.) are related to variations in their physicochemical properties. The important factors are the pK_a, lipid solubility (normally expressed as a partition coefficient) and degree of binding to protein. All of these are influenced by the basic chemical structure of the compound (ester or amide) and the addition of side chains to the basic molecule.

A low pK_a favours rapid onset of action because more of the drug is unionized at physiological pH and is thus lipid permeant. Lipid solubility is determined by the presence of hydrophobic side chains and more lipid-soluble drugs tend to be more potent. Duration of action relates to the degree of protein binding.

The effects of differences in molecular structure often interact in complex ways, but a simple example of a structure–activity relationship is the addition of a butyl group to mepivacaine to produce bupivacaine, which is four times as potent and significantly longer-acting. Alterations in structure also affect the rate and the products of metabolism.

Vasoactivity

The effects of a local anaesthetic drug on blood vessels also modify its profile. Cocaine is a potent vasoconstrictor, but most of the other agents produce some degree of vasodilatation, which tends to shorten duration of action and increase toxicity. Prilocaine and ropivacaine are exceptions and probably have slight vasoconstrictor properties at clinically used concentrations.

Differential sensory and motor blockade

Sensory and motor nerve fibres may differ in their susceptibility to local anaesthetics, because of differences in fibre diameter and myelination. In terms of absolute sensitivity, large-diameter fibres are more sensitive than small ones, but they are usually more heavily myelinated and the myelin sheath presents a significant barrier to drug diffusion. Therefore the small, unmyelinated C fibres of pain and temperature receptors are usually blocked more rapidly than the large, myelinated A fibres that innervate skeletal muscle.

Differential blockade of sensory and motor fibres may be useful clinically in producing analgesia with relatively little motor blockade: for example, provision of epidural analgesia for labour or the postoperative period. Higher pK_a and lower lipid solubility favour a greater degree of differential blockade and ropivacaine appears to produce less motor block than equivalent doses of bupivacaine. The effect is also maximized by the use of weak solutions (e.g. bupivacaine 0.125%).

Optical isomerism

Most local anaesthetics (lidocaine is an exception) exhibit optical isomerism because they contain an asymmetric carbon atom (i.e. a carbon atom which forms covalent bonds with four different chemical groups). Two possible spatial arrangements of the four groups around the carbon atom give rise to optical isomers, or enantiomers, which are mirror images of each other. These have identical physicochemical properties, but they differ in their stereoselective interactions with biological molecules.

Bupivacaine is usually presented as a racemic mixture of 'S' and 'R' enantiomers, but evidence that the R-isomer has greater cardiotoxicity has generated interest in the use of single enantiomeric forms. Ropivacaine was the first local anaesthetic to be commercially available as a single S-isomer preparation and levobupivacaine (S-bupivacaine) is also available now.

Stability and storage

The ester drugs have short shelf-lives because they tend to hydrolyse spontaneously, especially on warming. The amides may be stored for long periods without loss of potency and are not heat-sensitive unless mixed with glucose to produce hyperbaric spinal solutions. As a general rule, solutions of amides in glucose and solutions of any ester may be heat-sterilized once, and should be used soon after autoclaving.

CLINICAL FACTORS AFFECTING DRUG PROFILE

Increasing the dose of a drug shortens its onset time and increases the duration of block. Dose may be increased by using either a higher concentration or a larger volume; a large volume of a dilute solution is usually more effective.

The site of injection also affects onset time and duration (in addition to potential toxicity). Onset is almost immediate after infiltration and is progressively delayed with subarachnoid, peripheral nerve and epidural blocks, respectively. The slowest onset follows brachial plexus block. The dose required and the likely duration of action tend to increase in much the same order as for onset time.

Pregnancy and age are said to increase segmental spread of epidural blocks. For many blocks, young, healthy, tall patients seem to require more drug, as do obese, alcoholic or anxious patients, the last perhaps because they react to any sensation from the operative area.

PHARMACOLOGY OF INDIVIDUAL DRUGS

Only when all the above factors are taken into account may the properties of various drugs be compared. It is doubtful if, at equipotent concentrations, there are any significant differences in speed of onset, but there are certainly variations in potency, duration and toxicity. The features of individual drugs are described below and in Table 4.1. Appropriate volumes and concentrations of local anaesthetic agents used commonly for specific blocks are detailed in Chapter 17.

Cocaine

Cocaine has no role in modern anaesthetic practice, although it is used in ear, nose and throat surgery for its vasoconstrictor action. Because of its use as a drug of addiction, it is increasingly difficult to obtain cocaine legitimately at a reasonable price.

Benzocaine

This is an excellent topical agent of low toxicity. It does not ionize and therefore its use is limited to topical application. In addition, its mode of action cannot be explained according to the theory outlined above. Instead, it is thought that benzocaine diffuses into the cell membrane, but not into the cytoplasm, and either causes the membrane to expand in the same way as is suggested for general anaesthetics or enters the sodium channel from the lipid phase of the membrane. Whichever is the case, the mechanism may also be relevant to the action of the other agents.

Procaine

The incidence of allergic problems, its short shelf-life and brief duration of action of procaine have resulted in its infrequent clinical use at the present time.

Chloroprocaine

This is an ester, which is used widely in the USA. Its profile is very similar to that of procaine, from which it differs only by the addition of a chlorine atom (Table 4.1). As a result, it is hydrolysed four times more quickly by cholinesterase and seems to be less allergenic. It is claimed that it has a more rapid onset than any other agent, but this may relate to its very low toxicity, which permits the use of relatively larger doses. There has been some concern that chloroprocaine might be neurotoxic, because of several reports of paraplegia after accidental intrathecal injection. However, the evidence suggests that it was the preservative in the solution that caused the problems and not the drug itself.

Tetracaine

This drug is relatively toxic for an ester because it is hydrolysed very slowly by cholinesterase. It is also very potent and is the standard drug in North America for subarachnoid anaesthesia. It has a prolonged dura-

tion of action, but also a slow onset time. It may be used intrathecally in hyperbaric or isobaric solutions. In the UK its use is restricted to topical anaesthesia.

Lidocaine

Having been used safely and effectively for every type of local anaesthetic procedure, lidocaine is still the current standard agent. It has no unusual features and is also a standard antiarrhythmic. Lidocaine is used commonly for infiltration in concentrations of 0.5–1.0% and for peripheral nerve blocks if an intermediate duration is required. It may be used for intravenous regional anaesthesia, although prilocaine is preferred. Lidocaine 5% has been used for subarachnoid anaesthesia, although the degree of spread is unpredictable and the duration of action is relatively short. However, there have been concerns regarding transient neurological symptoms occurring after the use of such high concentrations. In a concentration of 1–2%, lidocaine produces epidural anaesthesia with a short onset time. Lidocaine 2–4% is used by many anaesthetists as a topical solution for anaesthesia of the upper airway before awake fibreoptic intubation.

Mepivacaine

This agent is very similar to lidocaine with neither advantages nor disadvantages in comparison.

Prilocaine

This is an underrated agent. It is equipotent with lidocaine, but in comparison it has virtually no vasodilator action, is either metabolized or sequestered to a greater degree by the lungs and is metabolized more rapidly by the liver. As a result, it is slightly shorter-acting, considerably less toxic and is the drug of choice when the risk of toxicity is high. Metabolism produces o-toluidine, which reduces haemoglobin; thus, methaemoglobinaemia may occur, but this complication is rare unless the dose exceeds 600 mg. Cyanosis appears when $1.5\,g\,dL^{-1}$ of haemoglobin is converted. Treatment with methylene blue ($1\,mg\,kg^{-1}$) is effective immediately. Fetal haemoglobin is more sensitive, and prilocaine should not be used for epidural block during labour. Prilocaine is used mostly for infiltration and for intravenous regional anaesthesia.

Bupivacaine

Bupivacaine is a potent local anaesthetic agent, with a long duration of action. Its introduction represented a significant advance in anaesthesia.

Relative to potency, the acute central nervous system toxicity of bupivacaine is slightly less than that of lidocaine and its longer duration of action reduces the need for repeated doses, and thus the risks of cumulative toxicity. However, several deaths have occurred after accidental intravenous administration of large doses of bupivacaine, and this drug appears to have a more toxic effect on the myocardium than other local anaesthetic agents. In addition, cardiovascular collapse may occur suddenly, without prior CNS symptoms, and resuscitation may be unsuccessful. There is evidence that myocardial toxicity is caused by the R-enantiomer (see above).

Bupivacaine may be used for infiltration, although only in small doses because of its toxicity. It is used frequently for peripheral nerve blockade and for subarachnoid and epidural anaesthesia because of its prolonged duration of action. Bupivacaine 0.5% is the most commonly used drug for subarachnoid anaesthesia in the UK. It may be used in a plain solution or in a hyperbaric formulation (see Ch. 17).

Ropivacaine

The cardiovascular toxicity of bupivacaine stimulated interest in the development of single enantiomeric preparations. Ropivacaine is similar chemically to bupivacaine (the butyl group attached to the amine is replaced by a propyl group), but it is presented as a single S-enantiomer. At equipotent concentrations it appears to be less toxic than bupivacaine. It is less likely to cause cardiac arrhythmias and collapse; resuscitation is more likely to be successful if toxicity occurs.

Ropivacaine is marginally less potent than bupivacaine, with a slightly shorter duration of action, but when used in dilute solutions it produces a greater degree of differential block. It is useful for peripheral nerve blockade and epidural anaesthesia, particularly when large doses of a long-acting local anaesthetic agent are required.

Levobupivacaine

The S-enantiomer of bupivacaine has the same chemical structure and physicochemical properties as racemic bupivacaine and produces the same block characteristics in clinical use. Volunteer studies have demonstrated that it is less toxic than the racemate, with higher plasma concentrations required to produce CNS symptoms, convulsions or cardiac arrhythmias. Thus the margin of safety between therapeutic and toxic doses is greater.

Levobupivacaine may be used for local infiltration, peripheral nerve blockade and epidural anaesthesia.

The concentrations and total doses required are the same as those for bupivacaine, with the advantage that the risks of toxicity are less.

ADDITIVES

Many substances are added to local anaesthetics for pharmaceutical purposes. Sodium hydroxide and hydrochloric acid are used to adjust the pH, sodium chloride the tonicity, and glucose and water the baricity of solutions. Preservatives, e.g. methyl hydroxybenzoate, are added to multidose bottles and manufacturers recommend that these should not be used for subarachnoid or epidural block. Other additions are made for pharmacological reasons.

Vasoconstrictors

The addition of a vasoconstrictor to a solution of local anaesthetic drug slows the rate of absorption, reduces toxicity, prolongs duration and may result in a more profound block. These are all desirable effects, but vasoconstrictors are not used universally for several reasons. They are absolutely contraindicated for injection close to end-arteries (ring blocks of digits and penis) and in intravenous regional anaesthesia because of the risk of ischaemia.

There is also a theoretical risk that the use of vasoconstrictors may increase the risk of permanent neurological deficit by rendering nerve tissue ischaemic. While evidence is inconclusive, many anaesthetists feel that vasoconstrictors should not be used unless there is no alternative method of prolonging duration or reducing toxicity in the specific clinical situation.

Adrenaline (epinephrine) is the most potent agent. It produces its own systemic toxicity and should be used with particular care, if at all, in patients with cardiac disease. Even in healthy patients, concentrations greater than 1:200 000 should not be used, and the maximum dose administered should not exceed 0.5 mg. Interactions with other sympathomimetic drugs, including tricyclic antidepressants, may occur, especially when adrenergic drugs are used systemically to treat hypotension.

Felypressin is a safer drug, although it causes pallor and may constrict the coronary circulation. It is usually available for dental use only.

Carbon dioxide

In order to speed the onset of blockade, some local anaesthetics have been produced as the carbonated salt, with carbon dioxide dissolved under pressure in the solution. The rationale for the use of these solutions is that after injection the carbon dioxide lowers intracellular pH and favours formation of more of the ionized active form of the drug. With blocks of slower onset, there is good evidence that a significant improvement is obtained.

Dextrans

There have been many attempts to prolong duration of action by mixing local anaesthetics with high-molecular-weight dextrans. The results are inconclusive, but the very large dextrans may be effective, especially in combination with adrenaline (epinephrine). 'Macromolecules' may be formed between dextran and local anaesthetic so that the latter is held in the tissues for longer periods.

Hyaluronidase

For many years, the enzyme hyaluronidase was added to local anaesthetics to aid spread by breaking down tissue barriers. There was little evidence that it had a significant effect and this practice has been abandoned, except perhaps in ophthalmic practice.

Mixtures

Some practitioners deliberately mix different local anaesthetics together in an attempt to obtain the advantages of both. One such combination (sometimes referred to as compounding) is lidocaine and bupivacaine; the aim is to achieve the rapid onset of the former and the long duration of the latter with a single injection. Another advantage claimed for compounding two drugs is a decrease in toxicity. However, local anaesthetic drug toxicity is additive, so that the use of 'half a dose' of each of two drugs is of no benefit. If an ester is combined with an amide, toxicity may increase because the amide slows hydrolysis of the ester by inhibiting plasma cholinesterase. It is more appropriate to use a catheter technique, to initiate the block with a dose of lidocaine and to maintain it with a dose of bupivacaine as the effect of lidocaine starts to regress.

A more effective combination is the eutectic mixture of local anaesthetics (EMLA). This is a mixture of the base (unionized) forms of lidocaine and prilocaine in a cream formulation. It is a local anaesthetic preparation which penetrates intact skin with some reliability. It takes up to 1 h to become effective but is very useful in paediatric practice, especially in children who need repeated venepuncture. It may also be of value for poor-risk patients undergoing skin grafting.

CHOICE OF LOCAL ANAESTHETIC AGENT

When using a local technique, the anaesthetist has to decide upon the concentration, volume and nature of the agent to be used. For lidocaine (the relative potencies of other agents are shown in Table 4.1), concentrations required are:

skin infiltration	0.5%
intravenous regional anaesthesia	0.5%
minor nerve block	1.0%
brachial plexus	1.0–1.5%
sciatic/femoral	1.0–1.5%
epidural	1.5–2.0%
subarachnoid	2.0–5.0%

Higher concentrations than these may be used to produce more profound peripheral blocks of faster onset. The volumes required for specific techniques are described in Chapter 17 and the interrelationships that exist between patient status and the required amount of drug are discussed above.

Ideally, several drugs of different potency, duration and toxicity should be available to permit a rational choice based upon the required dose, the particular risk of toxicity in that block and patient, and the likely duration of surgery. Often this is not possible, mainly for commercial reasons. For example, in the UK, lidocaine and bupivacaine are marketed in a full range of concentrations, but the range of solutions of other drugs is more restricted. The availability of spinal anaesthetic solutions is particularly poor. For more peripheral blocks, lidocaine and bupivacaine may be used safely unless the risk of toxicity is relatively high (e.g. intravenous regional anaesthesia when prilocaine is the drug of choice). When large volumes of more concentrated solutions are needed and the higher concentrations of prilocaine are not available, one of the other agents should probably be used in combination with adrenaline (epinephrine).

FURTHER READING

Covino B G, Wildsmith J A W 1998 Clinical pharmacology of local anesthetic agents. In: Cousins M J, Bridenbaugh P O (eds) Neural blockade in clinical anesthesia and management of pain, 3rd edn. Lippincott-Raven, Philadelphia, pp 97–128

Strichartz G R 1998 Neural physiology and local anesthetic action. In: Cousins M J, Bridenbaugh P O (eds) Neural blockade in clinical anesthesia and management of pain, 3rd edn. Lippincott-Raven, Philadelphia, pp 25–54

Tucker G T, Mather L E 1998 Properties, absorption, and disposition of local anesthetic agents. In: Cousins M J,

Bridenbaugh P O (eds) Neural blockade in clinical anesthesia and management of pain, 3rd edn. Lippincott-Raven, Philadelphia, pp 55–96

Wildsmith J A W, McClure J H, Armitage E N 2001 Principles and practice of regional anaesthesia, 3rd edn. Churchill Livingstone, Edinburgh

5   Analgesic drugs

The ideal analgesic should relieve pain with a minimum of side-effects. When formulating a management plan, it is worth considering what contributes to pain perception and associated distress. The International Association for the Study of Pain (IASP) defines pain as 'an unpleasant sensory and emotional experience associated with actual or potential tissue damage or described in terms of such damage'. It is clear from this definition that the degree of tissue damage and perception of pain are not necessarily correlated. Pain perception is a complex phenomenon, involving sensory, emotional and cognitive processes. Thus, while analgesic drugs can be effective in relieving both acute and chronic pain, other factors may also need to be addressed.

There is considerable evidence that patients continue to suffer pain, despite a wide range of available analgesic drugs. When devising a management plan for both acute and chronic settings, using 'balanced' or 'multimodal analgesia' may be helpful. These terms refer to the use of combinations of drugs acting by different mechanisms or at different sites within the pain pathway. Analgesic combinations may be additive or synergistic in their mode of action, with resultant dose-sparing effects and a reduction in side-effects. Effective and repeated assessment of patients is essential in determining optimal analgesic management.

OPIOIDS

Opioids are the most frequently used analgesics for the treatment of moderate to severe pain. Despite this, there are still major gaps in our knowledge of their clinical pharmacology; the choice of drug and dose is largely empirical. Although they may be highly effective, control of dynamic (pain on movement) or incident (breakthrough) pain may be poor and side-effects may be a significant problem. The term opioid refers to all drugs, both synthetic and natural, that act on opi-oid receptors. Opiates are naturally occurring opioids derived from the opium poppy *Papaver somniferum*. The most widely used opioid is morphine, although a variety of different opioids are available. Incomplete cross-tolerance occurs between them, so an alternative should be tried if morphine is poorly tolerated.

Table 5.1 shows the approximate equi-analgesic doses for some opioids.

MECHANISM OF ACTION

Opioid receptors belong to the G-protein coupled family of receptors with seven transmembrane domains, an extracellular N-terminal and intracellular C-terminal. Activation results in changes in enzyme activity such as adenylate cyclase or alterations in calcium and potassium ion channel permeability.

Opioid receptors were originally classified by pharmacological activity in animal preparations, and later by molecular sequence. The three main receptors were classified as μ (mu) or OP3, κ (kappa) or OP1 and δ (delta) or OP2. Another opioid-like receptor has been identified recently; it is termed the nociceptin orphanin FQ peptide receptor. Receptor nomenclature has changed several times in the last few years; the current International Union of Pharmacology (IUPHAR) classification is MOP (mu), KOP (kappa), DOP (delta) and NOP for the nociceptin orphanin FQ peptide receptor (Table 5.2).

Opioid receptors are distributed widely in both central and peripheral nervous systems. The different effects of currently available opioids are dependent on complex interactions at various receptors. There is a range of endogenous neuropeptide ligands active at these receptors (Table 5.2); they function as neurotransmitters, neuromodulators and neurohormones. The endogenous tetrapeptide endomorphins 1 and 2 are potent agonists acting specifically at the MOP receptor; they play a role in modulating inflammatory pain.

The analgesic action of morphine and most other opioids is related mainly to agonist activity at the

Table 5.1 Equi-analgesic doses of opioids

Opioid	~ Equi-analgesic dose	
	Parenteral	Oral
Morphine	10 mg	20–30 mg
Meperidine (pethidine)	100 mg	300 mg
Oxycodone	15 mg	20–30 mg
Fentanyl	100 μg	NA
Hydromorphone	1.5 mg	7.5 mg
Methadone	1–10 mg	20 mg
Codeine	NA	200 mg

MOP receptor. Unfortunately, many of the unwanted effects of opioids are also related to activity at this receptor. At a cellular level, MOP receptor activation has an overall inhibitory effect via: (i) inhibition of adenylate cyclase; (ii) increased opening of potassium channels (hyperpolarization of postsynaptic neurones, reduced synaptic transmission); and (iii) inhibition of calcium channels (decreases presynaptic neurotransmitter release).

PHARMACODYNAMIC EFFECTS OF OPIOIDS

The ubiquitous nature of opioid receptors implies that agents acting at them have wide-ranging effects, some of which may be problematic. Some opioids or their metabolites also have activity at other receptors, e.g. methadone acts at the N-methyl-D-aspartate (NMDA)

receptor. These particular actions are discussed for individual agents below. The more general effects of opioids are described in this section.

Analgesic action

Opioids with agonist activity mainly at the MOP receptor, and to a lesser extent at the KOP receptor, have analgesic effects. Analgesic effects have also been demonstrated for the spinal DOP receptor in certain situations.

Opioids should be titrated against pain; if higher than necessary doses are given, respiratory depression and excessive sedation may result. If the pain is incompletely opioid-responsive, as may occur with neuropathic pain, then care must be taken with dose titration and a detailed reassessment of analgesic response is essential. Opioids exert their analgesic effect by:

- a peripheral action in inflammatory states, where MOP receptors on cells of the immune system and nociceptors are important in regulating peripheral sensitization
- inhibitory effects within the dorsal horn of the spinal cord both pre- and postsynaptically
- supraspinal effects in the brainstem, thalamus and cortex, in addition to modulating descending systems in the midbrain periaqueductal grey matter, nucleus raphe magnus and the rostral ventral medulla.

Central nervous system

In addition to analgesia there are several potential central nervous system (CNS) effects of opioids:

Sedation and sleep. Opioids interfere with rapid-eye-movement sleep with changes in the EEG including

Table 5.2 Classification of opioid receptors as defined by the International Union of Pharmacology

Receptor	Previous classifications	Endogenous ligand	Site
MOP	Mu; OP3	Endomorphin 1 and 2; met-enkephalin; dynorphin A and B	Peripheral inflammation, pre- and postsynaptic neurones in spinal cord, periaqueduct grey matter, limbic system, caudate putamen, thalamus, cerebral cortex
KOP	Kappa; OP1	Dynorphin A and B; β-endorphin	Nucleus raphe magnus (midbrain), hypothalamus, spinal cord
DOP	Delta; OP2	Leu- and met-enkephalins; β-endorphin	Olfactory centres, cerebral cortex, nucleus accumbens, caudate putamen, spinal cord
NOP	Orphan; ORL-1	Orphanin FQ (nociceptin)	Nucleus raphe magnus, spinal cord, afferent neurones

a progressive decrease in EEG frequency and production of delta waves. However, burst suppression is not seen, even with large doses. Opioid-related ventilatory depression is more common during sleep. Opioid-induced sedation may be used therapeutically, e.g. critical care setting. There is a dose-related reduction in minimum alveolar concentration (MAC) for volatile anaesthetics

Mood. Significant euphoria is uncommon when opioids are used to treat pain but it occurs frequently when they are used inappropriately. Dysphoria (possibly via a KOP receptor action) and hallucinations can occur. Commonly, the hallucinations are visual in nature and may only affect part of the visual field.

Miosis. This is mediated via a KOP receptor effect on the Edinger–Westphal nucleus of the oculomotor nerve.

Tolerance (i.e. requirement of increasing doses to achieve the same effect) is important clinically because a significant number of patients are receiving long-term opioid therapy for malignant and chronic non-malignant pain; it is also relevant in illicit drug use. Additionally, tolerance may develop much more acutely e.g. when opioids are used for pain control before surgery or when given intrathecally. However, after the dose has been titrated initially, the majority of patients on long-term opioids are usually maintained on a stable dose.

At a cellular level, tolerance is caused by a progressive loss of active receptor sites combined with uncoupling of the receptor from the guanosine triphosphate (GTP)-binding subunit. There is also some evidence that the NMDA receptor may play a role in acute tolerance, via protein kinase C activity lifting the magnesium block at the NMDA site. There may therefore be a rationale for using ketamine in situations of acute tolerance, for example in the postoperative period. Interactions with the NOP receptor may also be important.

The incomplete cross-tolerance between different types of opioids may result from differential activity at opioid receptor subtypes. Withdrawal may occur if there is abrupt cessation of opioids or if an antagonist is given.

Addiction. This is defined as the compulsive use of opioids to the detriment of the patient in terms of physical, psychological or social function. Drug-seeking behaviour is not a problem if opioids are used appropriately for pain relief in both acute and chronic situations.

Respiratory

Opioids may cause respiratory depression, particularly in the elderly, neonates and when given without titrating effect to analgesic response. Tolerance does develop to this phenomenon, so it is less of a problem in chronic use. However, care must be taken if nociceptive input is reduced or removed, e.g. after a nerve block. Sensitivity to CO_2 is reduced, even with small doses of MOP agonists. This is caused by depression of sensitivity of neurones on the ventral surface of the medulla.

Opioids are effective at suppressing the stress response to laryngoscopy and airway manipulation. They may reduce the plasma concentrations of catecholamines, cortisol and other stress hormones by inhibiting the pituitary–adrenal axis, reducing central sympathetic outflow and influencing central neuroendocrine responses. Opioids also suppress cough activity and mucociliary function. This may cause inadequate clearing of secretions and hypostatic pneumonia, especially if there is associated sedation and respiratory depression. This antitussive activity is, at least in part, peripherally mediated.

Gastrointestinal

All opioids may cause nausea and vomiting, although tolerance develops. This may be mediated both centrally and peripherally, with a direct effect on the chemoreceptor trigger zone in addition to a delay in gastric emptying. Opioids increase gastrointestinal muscle tone and decrease motility. An increase in biliary pressure with gallbladder contraction may also occur. Constipation occurs commonly via a direct action on opioid receptors in the smooth muscle of the gut; many patients do not become tolerant to this when receiving long-term opioids.

Cardiovascular

In normovolaemic patients, the majority of opioids have no significant cardiovascular depressant effect. However, if histamine is released, then there may be tachycardia, decrease in systemic vascular resistance and a reduction in arterial pressure. Bradycardia may occur in response to some opioids. There is no direct action on baroreceptors but a minimal reduction in preload and afterload may occur. There is no effect on cerebral autoregulation. However, if respiratory depression is present, then the resultant increase in P_aCO_2 may increase cerebral blood flow.

Opioids decrease central sympathetic outflow. Therefore, in patients who are relying on increased sympathetic tone to maintain cardiovascular stability, opioids may lead to haemodynamic compromise. This may be severe, particularly if potent opioids are given by rapid intravenous bolus.

OPIOIDS **5**

Other effects

Myoclonic jerks may occur if there is opioid toxicity and may be associated with sedation and hallucinations. *Urinary retention* and urgency may occur, probably related to a centrally mediated mechanism as these problems are much more common when neuraxial opioids are used. *Pruritus* is relatively common after neuraxial administration. The nose, face and torso are particularly affected and this may be reversed by a low dose of a MOP antagonist. *Muscle rigidity* is a recognized complication, particularly after intravenous bolus administration of potent phenylpiperidines. This may cause significant problems with ventilation because of chest wall rigidity and decreased respiratory compliance. It may be minimized by co-administration with induction agents and benzodiazepines, reversed by naloxone or prevented by neuromuscular blocking agents. *Thermoregulation* is impaired to a similar extent as that seen with volatile agents. With long-term use, *depression of the immune system* may occur. *Endocrine problems* include impaired adrenal and sexual function, and infertility.

OPIOID STRUCTURE

The structures of opioid analgesics are diverse, although for most opioids it is usually the laevorotatory (*levo*) stereoisomer that is the active compound. The structures of some of the common agents are shown in Figures 5.1 and 5.2. Agents in current use include phenanthrenes (e.g. morphine – Fig. 5.1), phenylpiperidines (e.g. meperidine (pethidine), fentanyl – Fig. 5.2) and diphenylpropylamines (e.g. methadone, dextropropoxy-phene). Structural modification affects agonist activity and alters physicochemical properties such as lipid solubility.

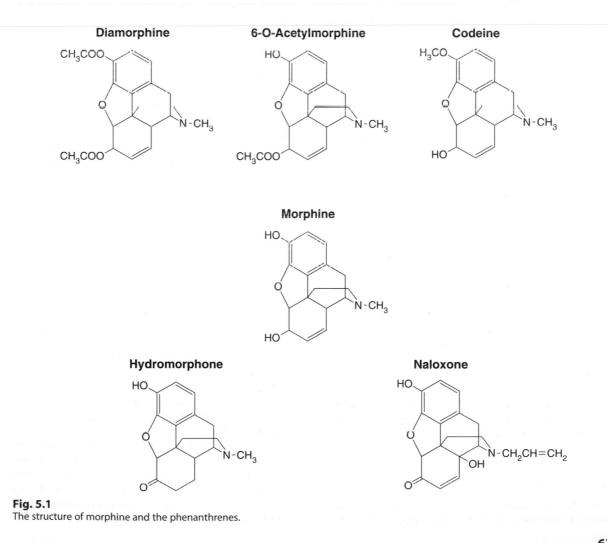

Fig. 5.1
The structure of morphine and the phenanthrenes.

Alfentanil

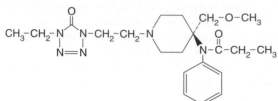

Fentanyl

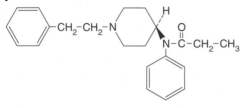

Sufentanil

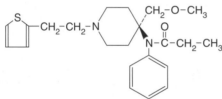

Remifentanil

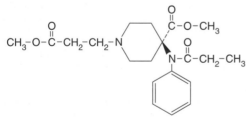

Fig. 5.2
The structures of phenylpiperidine opioids.

A tertiary nitrogen is necessary for activity, separated from a quaternary carbon by an ethylene chain. Chemical modifications that produce a quaternary nitrogen significantly reduce potency, as a result of decreased CNS penetration. If the methyl group on the nitrogen is changed, antagonism of analgesia may be produced.

Other important positions for activity and metabolism, as seen on the morphine molecule (Fig. 5.1), include the C-3 phenol group (the distance of this from the nitrogen affects activity) and the C-6 alcohol group. Potency may be increased by hydroxylation of the C-3 phenol; oxidation of C-6 (e.g. hydromorphone); double

acetylation at C-3 and C-6 (e.g. diamorphine); hydroxylation of C-14 and reducing the double bond at C-7/8. Further additions at the C-3 OH group reduce activity. A short-chain alkyl substitution is found in mixed agonist-antagonists, hydroxylation or bromination of C-14 produces full antagonists and removal or substitution of the methyl group reduces agonist activity.

PHARMACOKINETICS AND PHYSICOCHEMICAL PROPERTIES

Knowledge of the specific physicochemical properties and pharmacokinetics of individual agents is important in determining the optimal route of drug delivery in order to achieve an effective receptor site concentration for an appropriate duration of action. All opioids are weak bases. The relative proportion of free and ionized fractions is dependent on plasma pH and the pK_a of the particular opioid. The amount of opioid diffusing to the site of action (diffusible fraction) is dependent on lipid solubility, concentration gradient and degree of binding. Plasma concentrations of albumin and α_1-acid glycoprotein as well as tissue binding determine the availability of the unbound, unionized fraction. This diffusible fraction moves into tissue sites in the brain and elsewhere; the amount reaching receptors is dependent not only on lipophilicity but also on the amount of non-specific tissue binding, e.g. CNS lipids.

The ionized, protonated form is active at the receptor site. This has important implications for speed and duration of activity. For example, morphine is relatively hydrophobic and penetrates the blood–brain barrier slowly. However, a large mass of any given dose eventually reaches the receptor site because of low levels of non-specific tissue binding. This effect-site equilibration time $(t_{1/2}k_{eo})$ is measured by assessing the effect of opioids on the EEG. The offset time may also be prolonged, resulting in a longer duration of action than would be expected from the plasma half-life. Most opioids have a very steep dose–response curve. Therefore, if the dose is near the minimum effective analgesic concentration (MEAC), very small fluctuations in plasma or effect-site concentrations may lead to large changes in the level of analgesia.

Opioids tend to have a large volume of distribution (V_D) because of their high lipid solubility. A consequence of this can be that redistribution, particularly after a bolus dose or short infusion, can have significant effects on plasma concentrations. In addition, first-pass effects in the lung may remove significant amounts of drug from the circulation, reducing the initial peak plasma concentration. However, the drug re-enters the plasma several minutes later. Plasma concentrations of opioids such as fentanyl, sufentanil and meperidine (pethidine) are affected by this; the effect is negligible for remifentanil. Other lipophilic amines such as lidocaine and pro-pranolol are affected similarly and may reduce pulmonary uptake of co-administered opioids.

After prolonged infusion, significant sequestration in fat stores and other body tissues occurs for highly lipid-soluble opioids. This is reflected in the 'context-sensitive $t_\frac{1}{2}$', i.e. the time taken for the plasma concentration to reduce by 50% after the infusion has stopped (see Ch. 1). The context-sensitive $t_\frac{1}{2}$ is increased after prolonged infusion for most opioids apart from remifentanil. For example, the elimination $t_\frac{1}{2}$ for fentanyl after bolus administration is 3–5 h, but increases to 7–12 h after prolonged infusion.

Most opioid metabolism occurs in the liver (phase I and II reactions) with the hydrophilic metabolites predominantly excreted renally, although a small amount may be excreted in the bile or unchanged in the urine. As a result, hepatic blood flow is one of the major determinants of plasma clearance. Metabolism of individual drugs is shown in Table 5.3. Enterohepatic recirculation may occur when water-soluble metabolites excreted in the gut may be metabolized by gut flora to the parent opioid and then reabsorbed. Lipid-soluble opioids may diffuse into the stomach, become ionized because of the low pH and then be reabsorbed in the small intestine; this results in a secondary peak in plasma concentration.

A summary of physicochemical and pharmacokinetic properties of some opioids is shown in Table 5.4. Metabolism (including production of active metabolites), distribution between different tissues and elimination all interact within individual subjects to produce clinically important actions at receptor sites.

Factors affecting pharmacokinetics include:

* *Age.* Systemic dose is often calculated on body weight, although there is little evidence to support this in adult clinical practice. Age is often more important because of both pharmacokinetic and pharmacodynamic factors. Metabolism and volume of distribution are often reduced in the elderly, leading to increased free drug concentrations in the plasma. Hepatic blood flow may have declined by 40–50% by age 75 years, with reduced clearance of opioids. Increased CNS sensitivity to opioid effects is also found in the elderly.
* *Hepatic disease* has unpredictable effects, although there may be little clinical difference unless there is coexisting encephalopathy. Reductions in plasma

Table 5.3 Metabolism and excretion of some opioids

Drug	Metabolism	Faeces	Urine
Morphine	Glucuronidation, sulphation N-dealkylation	Trace	90% in 24 h (10% morphine; 70% glucuronides; 10% 3-sulphate; 1% normorphine; 3% normorphine glucuronide)
Codeine	O-demethylation, glucuronidation	Trace	86% in 24 h (5–10% codeine; 60% codeine glucuronide; 5–15% morphine (mainly conjugated); trace normorphine)
Diamorphine	O-deacetylation, glucuronidation	Trace	80% in 24 h (5–7% morphine; 90% morphine glucuronides; 1% 6-acetylmorphine; 0.1% diamorphine)
Buprenorphine	Glucuronidation, N-dealkylation	70% mainly unchanged	2–13% in 7 days; mainly N-dealkylbuprenorphine (and glucuronide); buprenorphine-3-glucuronide
Meperidine (pethidine)	N-demethylation, hydrolysis		70% in 24 h (10% meperidine; 10% normeperidine; 20% meperidinic acid; 16% meperidinic acid glucuronide; 8% normeperidinic acid; 10% normeperidinic acid glucuronide; plus small amounts of other metabolites)
Methadone	N-dealkylation	30%	60% in 24 h (33% methadone; 43% EDDP, 10% EMDP plus small amounts of other metabolites)
Fentanyl	N-dealkylation, hydroxylation	9%	70% in 4 days (5–25% fentanyl; 50% 4-N-(N-propionylanilino-piperidine) plus other metabolites)

EDDP; 2-ethylidine-1, 5-dimethyl-3, 3-diphenylpyrrolidine
EMDP; 2-ethyl-5-methyl-3, 3-diphenylpyraline

Table 5.4   Pharmacokinetic and physicochemical properties of some opioids

Opioid	pK_a	Protein binding (%)	Octanol:water partition coefficient	Terminal half-life (h)	Clearance (mL kg^{-1} min^{-1})	Volume of distribution (L kg^{-1})	Duration of action (h)
Morphine	7.9	30	6	1.7–3.0	15–20	3–5	3–5
Oxycodone	8.5	45		3–4	13	2–3	2–4
Codeine	8.2	20	0.6	2–4		2.5–3.5	
Meperidine (pethidine)	8.5	70	39	3–5	8–18	3–5	2–4
Fentanyl	8.4	90	813	2–4	10–20	3–5	1–1.5
Alfentanil	6.5	91	128	1–2	4–9	0.4–1	0.25–0.4
Remifentanil	7.3	70	18	0.1–0.2	40–60	0.3–0.4	2–5 min
Sufentanil	8.0	93	1778	2–3.5	10–15	2.5–3	0.8–1.3
Methadone	8.3	90	26–57	15–20	2	5	4–8

protein concentrations also have effects on plasma concentrations of free unbound drug.

- *Renal failure* may have significant effects for opioids with renally excreted active metabolites such as morphine, diamorphine and meperidine.
- *Obesity* will result in a larger V_D and prolonged elimination $t_{1/2}$. This may be a particular problem if infusions are being used.
- *Hypothermia, hypotension and hypovolaemia* may also result in variable absorption and altered distribution and metabolism.

ROUTES OF ADMINISTRATION

Opioids given parenterally have 100% bioavailability (see Ch. 1), although peak plasma concentrations may be affected by site of administration and haemodynamic status. Opioids may be given by many routes; variations between specific agents are discussed below. It is unclear how much cross-tolerance exists for different routes of administration, e.g. intravenous versus epidural.

The choice of route is dependent on the clinical situation and several factors may need to be considered:

- If there is delayed gastrointestinal transit time, the biological half-life may be prolonged with orally administered agents.
- Intrathecal administration is associated with fewer supraspinal effects, although both urinary retention

and pruritus may be more common. Highly lipid-soluble opioids (e.g. fentanyl) do not spread readily in cerebrospinal fluid (CSF). It is claimed that they are less likely than water-soluble opioids (e.g. morphine) to cause late respiratory depression due to rostral spread.

- Dural penetration from epidural administration is dependent on molecular size and lipophilicity. For example, only 3–5% of morphine crosses into the CSF, with a peak concentration after 60–240 min; fentanyl peaks at approximately 20 min.

MOP AGONISTS

Morphine is the standard opioid against which other agents are compared. Other MOP agonists have a similar pharmacodynamic profile but differ in relative potency, pharmacokinetics and biotransformation to other active metabolites.

Phenylpiperidine opioids (Fig. 5.2) are potent MOP receptor agonists with moderate (alfentanil) to high (sufentanil) lipid solubility and good diffusion through membranes. Both potency and time to reach the effect site vary considerably. In contrast to morphine, these agents do not cause histamine release. All except remifentanil may cause postoperative respiratory depression as a result of secondary peaks in plasma concentrations. This may be caused by release from body stores if large doses have been infused intraoperatively. Fentanyl, alfentanil and sufentanil are metabolized mainly in the liver to inactive metabolites. Very little is excreted unchanged in the urine (Table 5.3).

Morphine

Morphine is a relatively hydrophilic phenanthrene derivative. It may be given orally, rectally, topically, parenterally and via the neuraxial route. The standard parenteral dose for adults is 10 mg, although many factors affect this and the dose should be titrated to effect. Its oral bioavailability is dependent on first-pass hepatic metabolism and may be unpredictable (35–75%). Oral morphine is available either as immediate-release liquid, simple tablet or as a modified-release preparation. Single-dose studies of morphine bioavailability indicate that the relative potency of oral:intramuscular morphine is 1:6 although, with repeated regular administration, this ratio becomes approximately 1:3. The dose of short-acting morphine for breakthrough pain should be approximately one-sixth of the total daily dose. Morphine has a plasma half-life of approximately 3 h and a duration of analgesia of 4–6 h.

Morphine is metabolized, at least in part, by microsomal UDP glucuronyl transferases (UDPGT) found in the liver, kidney and intestines. Several of these metabolites may have clinically significant effects (see below). Although morphine conjugation occurs in the liver, there is evidence that extrahepatic sites may also be important, e.g. kidney, gastrointestinal tract. The site of conjugation on the molecule also varies, leading to a variety of metabolites (Table 5.3). After glucuronidation, metabolites are excreted in urine or bile, dependent on molecular weight and polarity, more than 90% of morphine metabolites are excreted in the urine. The main metabolite in humans is morphine-3-glucuronide (60–80%) and this may have an excitatory effect via CNS actions not related to opioid receptor activation. Morphine-6-glucuronide (M-6-G) is active at the MOP receptor, producing analgesia and other MOP-related effects. It is significantly more potent than morphine. Therefore, M-6-G produces significant clinical effects despite only 10% of morphine being metabolized in this way. As it is renally excreted, it may accumulate in patients with impaired renal function, causing respiratory depression. Current evidence indicates that accumulation of morphine metabolites, especially M-6-G, becomes significant when creatinine clearance declines to 50 mL min^{-1} or less.

Diamorphine

Diamorphine is a prodrug; it is inactive at opioid receptors. However, it is converted rapidly to the active metabolites 6-monoacetylmorphine, morphine and M-6-G. Further metabolism is similar to that of morphine (Table 5.3) and similar problems may arise if there is renal impairment.

It is available for parenteral and oral use. Diamorphine is more lipid soluble than morphine, affecting distribution and tissue penetration. One advantage over morphine is in settings where high concentrations are required in relatively low volumes, such as palliative care. Additionally, when lipid solubility is important in regulating site of action (e.g. epidural, intrathecal use), some practitioners believe that diamorphine has specific advantages over morphine.

Papaveretum

This naturally occurring opioid is used much less commonly now than previously. It is a mixture of morphine hydrochloride (253 parts), codeine hydrochloride (20 parts) and papaverine hydrochloride (23 parts). There is no oral preparation. A dose of 15.4 mg is approximately equivalent to 10 mg of anhydrous morphine.

Hydromorphone

This potent opioid is used mainly in the palliative care setting or in patients who are not opioid naive. Hydromorphone 1.3 mg is equi-analgesic to morphine 10 mg. Both immediate- and sustained-release preparations are available.

Meperidine (pethidine)

Meperidine (pethidine) is available as parenteral and oral preparations. There is no evidence that this opioid provides any advantage over morphine, e.g. treatment of colic-type pain. It is fairly short acting in terms of analgesia, and if repeated doses are given, the metabolite normeperidine can accumulate ($t_{1/2}$~15 h). This is a CNS stimulant and can cause seizures, especially if there is renal dysfunction. Its clearance is significantly reduced in hepatic disease. Chronic use may result in enzyme induction and an increase in normeperidine plasma concentrations. Its metabolism is decreased by the oral contraceptive pill.

Meperidine has other significant effects related to activity at non-opioid receptors. For example, its atropine-like action may cause a tachycardia, in addition to direct myocardial depression at high doses. It was used originally as a bronchodilator. It can also reduce shivering related to hypothermia or epidurals, although the mechanism for this is not fully understood. Meperidine also has a local anaesthetic-like membrane stabilizing action.

Fentanyl

Fentanyl is available in a variety of preparations for parenteral, transdermal and transmucosal administration. Due to high first-pass metabolism (~70%) it is not given orally. It is approx. 80–100 times more potent than morphine in the acute setting, although it is approx. 30–40 times as potent when given chronically, e.g. slow-release transdermal patches. With transdermal administration, the patch and underlying dermis act as a reservoir and plasma concentration does not reach steady state until approx 15 h after initial application. Plasma concentration also declines slowly after removal ($t_{1/2}$~ 15–20 h).

Fentanyl is very lipophilic with a relatively short duration of action. It has a large V_D with rapid peripheral tissue uptake limiting initial hepatic metabolism. This may result in significant variability in plasma concentrations and secondary plasma peaks. It binds to α_1-acid glycoprotein and albumin; 40% of the protein-bound fraction is taken up by erythrocytes. The lung may be important in exerting a first-pass effect on fentanyl (up to 75% of the dose), thus buffering the plasma from high peak drug concentrations.

Alfentanil

The low pK_a of alfentanil (6.9) results in it being largely unionized at plasma pH, allowing rapid diffusion to the effect site ($t_{1/2}k_{eo}$ ~ 1 min) and rapid onset of action. Although less lipid-soluble than some opioids, it has the most rapid onset time. It does not bind strongly to opioid receptors and the effect-site concentration also decreases rapidly as plasma concentrations decrease. It is metabolized by one of the most abundantly expressed isoforms of hepatic P450 (CYP3 A3/4). Genetic variability in the activity of this enzyme may result in two- to three-fold variations in pharmacokinetic values when given by infusion. Low, medium or high metabolizers have been identified; this has implications for duration of action when prolonged use is contemplated.

Sufentanil

Sufentanil is one of the most potent opioids; it has a rapid onset of action after intravenous administration and peak analgesic effect is at approximately 8 min. It is 625 times more potent than morphine and 12 times more potent than fentanyl. However, diffusion to tissues is slower than alfentanil because, although sufentanil is highly lipid soluble, it is also highly protein bound, resulting in low unbound plasma fractions at body pH. It has very low levels of non-specific binding that may increase potential effect-site concentrations. The speed of onset of a large dose is caused by saturation of receptors and non-specific sites, with potential for overdose. One of its metabolites (desmethylsufentanil) is active at the MOP receptor (10% of sufentanil's potency).

Remifentanil

Remifentanil is available for parenteral use as a lyophilized white crystalline powder containing glycine. It should not be administered epidurally or spinally. After being made up in solution, it is stable for 24 h. This MOP receptor agonist is ~25 times more potent than alfentanil. It differs from other opioids in that it has an ester linkage, resulting in degradation by tissue and non-specific plasma esterases. This process is non-saturable and clearance is significantly greater than hepatic blood flow. Plasma cholinesterase deficiency does not affect clearance. Hepatic and renal dysfunction have no effect on clearance also, although increased opioid sensitivity in hepatic disease may result in a lower dosage requirement. Other situations requiring a reduction in dose include haemorrhage or shock. Hydrolysis produces a carboxylic acid metabolite with limited action at the MOP receptor (~1000 times < remifentanil). It is not thought to be clinically significant, even in renal dysfunction.

Remifentanil has a rapid blood–brain equilibration time of just over 1 min, with a short context-sensitive half-time of 3–5 min which is unaffected by duration of infusion. This makes it ideally suited for infusion during anaesthesia and in the critical care setting. It may be titrated rapidly to achieve the desired effect. The high clearance and low V_D imply that the offset of effect is caused by metabolism rather then redistribution. Hypothermia, such as may occur in cardiac surgery, may reduce clearance by up to 20%.

There is some evidence that acute opioid tolerance and hyperalgesia may occur with intraoperative remifentanil infusions. If high doses are used without neuromuscular blockade, muscle rigidity may be a problem. It is unlikely to be a problem when using a concentration of $100\,\mu g\,mL^{-1}$ or less and an infusion rate of 0.2–$0.5\,\mu g\,kg^{-1}\,min^{-1}$. Bradycardia has also been reported.

Oxycodone

This potent semi-synthetic opioid has been in use for many years. In addition to actions at the MOP receptor, it may also have analgesic effects mediated via the

KOP receptor, resulting in incomplete cross-tolerance with morphine. It has a good oral bioavailability, and its plasma concentrations are more predictable than those of morphine after oral administration. It is available in both long- and short-acting oral preparations and, more recently, in a parenteral formulation.

Methadone

Methadone is a diphenylpropylamine. It has very good oral bioavailability (~85%) with an oral to parenteral ratio of 1:2. Its plasma half-life can be very variable (3–50 h, average 24 h) and its duration of action is relatively short. With repeated dosing, problems with accumulation can occur because of this discrepancy between half-life and analgesic effect. Careful monitoring is therefore required when converting patients to long-term methadone. Also, there is incomplete cross-tolerance with morphine. The racemic mixture in common use has agonist actions at the MOP receptor (mainly the *levo*-isomer) as well as antagonist activity at the NMDA receptor (*dextro*-isomer). Given the importance of this receptor in central sensitization in a variety of pain states, there may be cases where methadone offers particular advantages over and above other opioids, e.g. neuropathic pain.

Plasma concentrations of methadone can be reduced by carbamazepine and its metabolism is accelerated by phenytoin.

Codeine

Codeine is a constituent of opium and mainly metabolized in the liver to codeine conjugates, including norcodeine. It is considerably less potent than morphine. Up to 10% of it is metabolized by the hepatic microsomal enzyme CYP2D6 to morphine, which contributes significantly to its analgesic effect. Around 8% of Western Europeans are deficient in this enzyme due to genetic polymorphism and such individuals may not experience adequate analgesia with codeine. It can cause significant histamine release and its intravenous administration should be avoided. It has marked antitussive effects and also causes significant constipation. It is often combined with paracetamol.

Dextropropoxyphene

Dextropropoxyphene is a congener of methadone with limited analgesic effect. It has an active metabolite (norpropoxyphene) with a long half-life and excitatory effects including seizures.

Dihydrocodeine

Dihydrocodeine is a synthetic opioid developed in the early 1900s. Its structure and pharmacokinetics are similar to codeine and it is used for the treatment of postoperative and chronic pain. Both immediate- and sustained-release preparations are available. Despite its common use, there are very few clinical trials demonstrating efficacy. It has significant abuse potential.

Tramadol

Tramadol is thought to produce analgesia by two distinct actions. Firstly, it has agonist activity at the MOP and KOP receptors. Secondly, it enhances the descending inhibitory systems in the spinal cord by inhibiting noradrenaline (norepinephrine) reuptake and releasing serotonin from nerve endings. It is available in immediate- and sustained-release oral preparations and for parenteral administration. Its use is contraindicated in patients receiving MAOIs. Caution must also be exercised in hepatic impairment as its clearance is reduced to a much greater extent than morphine and related agents.

MIXED AGONIST-ANTAGONIST OPIOIDS

These agents have a ceiling effect for analgesia and possibly respiratory depression. They have agonist effects at the KOP receptor and weak antagonist effects at the MOP receptor. Dysphoria and hallucinations are relatively common and withdrawal effects may occur if given to patients taking MOP agonists. Pentazocine may be given orally or parenterally but is now rarely used. It may increase pulmonary and aortic blood pressure and myocardial oxygen demand. Hallucinations and dysphoria occur less commonly with nalbuphine.

PARTIAL AGONISTS

These agents have high affinity for the MOP receptor but limited efficacy (see Ch. 1). A ceiling effect is seen in the dose–response curve at less than the maximal analgesic effect of full MOP agonists. If given with a full MOP agonist, there may be a reduction in the maximal analgesic effect.

Buprenorphine

This is the only partial agonist in common use. It binds to the MOP receptor and dissociates very slowly from it. Consequently, although significant respiratory depression is less likely compared with morphine, it may be more difficult to reverse. It has poor oral bioavailability and parenteral, sublingual or transdermal formulations are used.

OPIOID ANTAGONISTS

Naloxone is a short-acting opioid antagonist that is relatively selective for the MOP receptor. It is structurally similar to morphine, with some modifications resulting in antagonist activity, including an OH group at C-14. It can reverse opioid-induced respiratory depression but repeated administration may be required because of its short duration of action; it can be given by continuous infusion. However, sudden and complete reversal of the analgesic effects of opioids may be accompanied by major cardiovascular and sympathetic responses. Naloxone has a very low oral bioavailability (~3%).

Naltrexone is a long-acting opioid antagonist used in the management of opioid dependence. It is available only in oral formulation.

PARACETAMOL

Paracetamol (acetaminophen) was first used in 1893 and is the only remaining *p*-aminophenol available in clinical practice. It is the active metabolite of the earlier, more toxic drugs acetanilide and phenacetin. Its structure is shown in Figure 5.3. Paracetamol is an effective analgesic and antipyretic but has no anti-inflammatory activity. In recommended doses, it is safe and has remarkably few side-effects.

MECHANISM OF ACTION

The mechanism of action of paracetamol is not well understood but it may act by inhibiting prostaglandin synthesis in the central nervous system with little effect on the peripheral nervous sys-

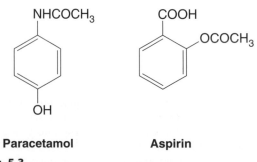

Paracetamol   **Aspirin**

Fig. 5.3
The structures of paracetamol and aspirin.

tem. Unlike morphine, paracetamol has no well-defined endogenous binding sites and, unlike NSAIDs, does not significantly inhibit cyclo-oxygenase (COX)-1 or COX-2. There is growing evidence of a central antinociceptive effect of paracetamol. It has also been shown to prevent prostaglandin production at cellular transcriptional level, independent of COX activity.

PHARMACOKINETICS

Paracetamol is absorbed rapidly from the small intestine after oral administration; peak plasma concentrations are reached after 30–60 min. It may also be given rectally and intravenously (either as paracetamol or the prodrug proparacetamol). It has good oral bioavailability (70–90%); rectal absorption is more variable (bioavailability ~ 50–80%) with a longer time to reach peak plasma concentration. The plasma half-life is approx. 2–3 h.

Paracetamol is metabolized by hepatic microsomal enzymes mainly to the glucuronide, sulphate and cysteine conjugates. None of these metabolites is pharmacologically active. A minimal amount of the metabolite *N*-acetyl-*p*-amino-benzquinoneimine is normally produced by cytochrome P450-mediated hydroxylation. This reactive toxic metabolite is rendered harmless by conjugation with liver glutathione, then renally excreted as mercapturic derivatives. With larger doses of paracetamol, the rate of formation of the reactive metabolite exceeds that of glutathione conjugation, and the reactive metabolite combines with hepatocellular macromolecules, resulting in cell death and potentially fatal hepatic failure. The formation of this metabolite is increased by drugs inducing cytochrome P450 enzymes, such as barbiturates or carbamazepine.

PHARMACODYNAMICS

Paracetamol has been shown to be effective in both acute and chronic settings. It is an effective postoperative analgesic but probably less effective than NSAIDs in many situations. It may reduce postoperative opioid requirements by up to 30%. The combination of paracetamol with an NSAID also improves efficacy. Paracetamol is also a very effective antipyretic. This is a centrally mediated effect.

OVERDOSE AND HEPATIC TOXICITY

In overdose, there is the potential for the toxic metabolite described above to cause centrilobular hepatocellular necrosis, occasionally with acute renal tubular necrosis. The threshold dose in adults is ~10–15 g.

Accidental overdosage can occur if combined preparations such as cocodamol are used together with paracetamol. Doses of more than 150 mg kg^{-1} taken within 24 h may result in severe liver damage, hypoglycaemia and acute tubular necrosis. Individuals taking enzyme-inducing agents are more likely to develop hepatotoxicity.

Early signs include nausea and vomiting, followed by right subcostal pain and tenderness. Hepatic damage is maximal 3–4 days after ingestion, and may lead to liver failure and death. Treatment consists of gastric emptying and the specific antidotes methionine and acetylcysteine. The former offers effective protection up to 10–12 h after ingestion. Acetylcysteine is effective within 24 h and perhaps beyond. The plasma paracetamol concentration related to time from ingestion indicates the risk of liver damage. Acetylcysteine is given if the plasma paracetamol concentration is >200 mg L^{-1} at 4 h and 6.25 mg L^{-1} at 24 h after ingestion

NON-STEROIDAL ANTI-INFLAMMATORY DRUGS

The analgesic, anti-inflammatory and antipyretic effects of salicylates, derived from the bark of the willow tree, were described as early as 1763. Acetylsalicylic acid (aspirin) was first produced in 1853 (Fig. 5.3). More recently, many other NSAIDs have been developed with actions similar to aspirin. Perioperative analgesia using NSAIDs is free from many of the adverse effects of opioids, such as respiratory depression, sedation, nausea and vomiting and gastrointestinal stasis. NSAIDs have been shown to be effective analgesics in acute and chronic conditions, although significant contraindications and adverse effects limit their use.

MECHANISM OF ACTION

The mechanism of action of aspirin was discovered in the 1970s. It was shown to irreversibly inhibit the production of prostanoids (i.e. prostaglandins and thromboxanes) from arachidonic acid released from phospholipids in cell membranes (Fig. 5.4). The basal rate of prostaglandin production is low and regulated by tissue stimuli or trauma that activate phospholipases to release arachidonic acid. Prostaglandins are then produced by the enzyme prostaglandin endoperoxide synthase which has both cyclo-oxygenase and hydroperoxidase sites. At least two subtypes of cyclo-oxygenase enzyme have been identified in humans: COX-1 and COX-2. The prostanoids produced by COX-1 are functionally active in many areas, including the gastrointestinal tract, kidney, lung and cardiovascular systems. By contrast, the functional COX-2

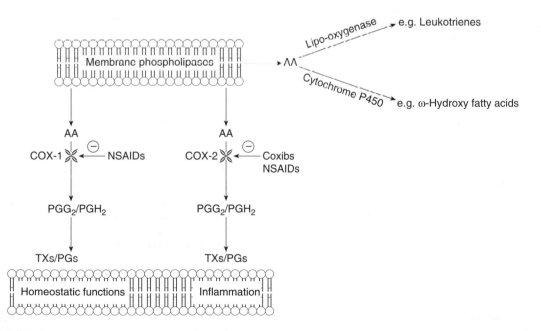

Fig. 5.4
Arachidonic acid metabolism. AA = arachidonic acid, COX = cyclo-oxygenase, PG = prostaglandin, TXs = thromboxanes.

enzyme is normally found less widely, e.g. brain, spinal cord, renal cortex, tracheal epithelium and vascular endothelium. However, COX-2 mRNA is widely distributed. In response to specific stimuli, especially those associated with inflammation, the expression of COX-2 isoenzyme is induced or upregulated, leading to increased local production of prostaglandins. A range of specific prostanoid receptors (e.g. EP1-4) are involved in peripheral sensitization associated with inflammation.

NSAIDs also have central effects as cyclo-oxygenases are widely distributed in both the peripheral and central nervous systems. NSAIDs may also have other mechanisms of action independent of any effect on prostaglandins, including effects on basic cellular and neuronal processes. NSAIDs are 'non-selective'; they inhibit both COX-1 and COX-2.

PHARMACOKINETICS

All NSAIDs are rapidly absorbed. They are weak acids and are therefore mainly unionized in the stomach where absorption can occur. When given orally, most absorption occurs in the small intestine because the absorptive area of the microvilli of the small intestine is much more extensive. Most have pK_a values lower than 5 and are therefore 99% ionized at a pH value greater than 7. Most are almost insoluble in water at body pH, although the sodium salt (diclofenac sodium, naproxen sodium) is more soluble. Ketorolac trometamol is the most soluble and can be given intravenously as a bolus and intramuscularly with less chance of significant irritation.

Most NSAIDs are highly protein bound (90–99%), with low volumes of distribution (approx. 0.1–0.2 L kg^{-1}). The unbound fraction is active. NSAIDs may potentiate the effects of other highly protein-bound drugs by displacing them from protein-binding sites (e.g. oral anticoagulants, oral hypoglycaemics, sulphonamides, anticonvulsants).

NSAIDs are mostly oxidized or hydroxylated and then conjugated and excreted in the urine. A few have active metabolites. For example, nabumetone is metabolized to 6-methoxy-2-naphthyl acetic acid, which is more active than the parent drug.

The interaction between NSAID and cyclo-oxygenase enzyme is often complex and plasma half-life may not reflect pharmacodynamic half-life. Diclofenac has a terminal half-life of 1–2 h. It is conjugated to glucuronides and sulphates, with 65% being excreted in the urine and 35% in the bile. The metabolites are less active than the parent compound. Ketorolac trometamol has a terminal half-life of 5 h and more than 90% is renally excreted. Naproxen has a terminal half-life of 12–15 h and is excreted almost entirely through the kidney as the conjugate. Tenoxicam is cleared mainly through the urine as the inactive hydroxypyridyl metabolite, although approximately 30% is via biliary excretion as the glucuronide.

PHARMACODYNAMICS

NSAIDs are very effective analgesics, although their use is limited by adverse effects due to their general effect on prostanoid synthesis and the ubiquitous nature of prostanoid. Generally, the risk and severity of NSAID-associated side-effects is increased in the elderly population or those with other significant co-morbidity.

Analgesia

NSAIDs have well-demonstrated efficacy both as post-operative analgesics and in chronic conditions such as rheumatoid and osteoarthritis. They can have significant opioid-sparing effects. NSAIDs are insufficient alone for severe pain after major surgery but are valuable as part of a multimodal analgesic regimen.

Gastrointestinal system

The gastric and duodenal epithelia have various protective mechanisms against acid and enzyme attack, and many of these involve prostaglandin production via a COX-1 pathway. Acute and particularly chronic NSAID administration can result in gastroduodenal ulceration and bleeding; the latter is exacerbated by the antiplatelet effect.

Platelet function

Platelet COX-1 is essential for the production of the cyclic endoperoxides and thromboxane A_2 that mediate the primary haemostatic response to vessel injury by producing vasoconstriction and platelet aggregation. Aspirin acetylates COX-1 irreversibly, whereas other NSAIDs do so in a reversible fashion. This can result in prolonged bleeding times and increased perioperative blood loss has been reported in some studies. The presence of a bleeding diathesis or co-administration of anticoagulants may increase the risk of significant surgical blood loss.

Renal function

Renal prostaglandins have many physiological roles, including the maintenance of renal blood flow and glomerular filtration rate in the presence of circulating vasoconstrictors, regulation of tubular electrolyte handling and modulation of the actions of renal hormones. NSAIDs can adversely affect renal function. High circulating concentrations of the vasoconstrictors renin, angiotensin, noradrenaline (norepinephrine) and vasopressin increase production of intrarenal vasodilators including prostacyclin, and renal function may be particularly sensitive to NSAIDs in these situations. Co-administration of other potential nephrotoxins, such as gentamicin, may increase the likelihood of renal toxicity.

Aspirin-induced asthma

Aspirin-induced asthma may affect up to 20% of asthmatics; it may be severe and there is often cross-sensitivity with other NSAID. Patients with coexisting chronic rhinitis and nasal polyps appear to be at most risk. A history of aspirin-induced asthma is a contraindication to NSAID use after surgery. There is no reason to avoid NSAIDs in other asthmatics if previous exposure has not been associated with bronchospasm. However, patients should be warned of potential problems and advised to stop taking them if their asthma worsens. The mechanism of this problem is unclear; it may be that cyclo-oxygenase inhibition increases arachidonic acid availability for production of inflammatory leukotrienes by lipo-oxygenase pathways.

CONTRAINDICATIONS

Specific contraindications to NSAID administration include a history of a bleeding diathesis, peptic ulceration, significant renal impairment or aspirin-induced asthma. Care should be taken in high-risk groups, such as the elderly, those with cardiovascular disease and the dehydrated.

COX-2-SPECIFIC INHIBITORS

These drugs are anti-inflammatory analgesics that reduce prostaglandin synthesis by specifically inhibiting COX-2 with little or no effect on COX-1 (relative specificity varies between drugs). They were developed as an alternative to traditional NSAIDs with the aim of avoiding COX-1-mediated side-effects, primarily gastric ulceration and platelet effects.

MECHANISM OF ACTION

The mechanism of action is similar to that of NSAIDs (Fig. 5.4). Both COX-1 and COX-2 enzymes have very similar active sites and catalytic properties, although COX-2 has a larger potential binding site because of a secondary internal pocket. This has allowed design of drugs to target predominantly COX-2. COX-2 is induced at sites of inflammation and trauma, producing prostaglandins, and these drugs, inhibit this process. However, COX-2 is an important constituitive enzyme in the CNS, including the spinal cord, and inhibition at this site is thought to be an important mechanism also.

PHARMACODYNAMICS

Analgesia

Systematic reviews and meta-analyses indicate similar efficacy to NSAIDs in both acute postoperative pain and for chronic conditions such as osteoarthritis. Agents are available orally (e.g. celecoxib, etoricoxib, valdecoxib) and parenterally (parecoxib).

Gastrointestinal

One of the commonest side-effects of NSAIDs is gastrointestinal toxicity. Approximately 1 in 1200 patients receiving chronic NSAID treatment (>2 months) die from related gastroduodenal complications. COX-1 isoenzyme is the predominant cyclo-oxygenase found in the gastric mucosa. The prostanoids produced here help to protect the gastric mucosa by reducing acid secretion, stimulating mucus secretion, increasing production of mucosal phospholipids and bicarbonate and regulating mucosal blood flow. Specific COX-2 inhibitors have less effect on these processes.

There is no doubt that short- to medium-term treatment with specific COX-2 inhibitors (up to 3 months) is associated with a significant reduction in the incidence of gastroduodenal ulceration. However, data have suggested that this effect is reduced during prolonged treatment and in patients taking low-dose aspirin. It is likely that the degree of COX-2 specificity is related to the efficacy of gastric protection.

Haematological

COX-2-specific agents have very little adverse effect on platelet function. This is potentially advantageous when compared with NSAIDs with respect to perioperative or gastrointestinal bleeding.

Cardiovascular

Some large long-term studies of COX-2 inhibitors have found an increased risk of cardiovascular events (e.g. myocardial infarction, stroke) compared with traditional NSAIDs and placebo. This has led to the recommendation that they should not be used in patients with ischaemic heart or cerebrovascular disease and that their use in others should be guided by individual risk assessments for each patient. Some drugs have been withdrawn. A similar phenomenon has been reported when some of these drugs have been used after coronary artery bypass surgery. An increased risk of myocardial events may not be confined to COX-2 inhibitors with some evidence for increased risk with general NSAIDs.

The mechanism of this adverse outcome is under investigation. However, it may be that COX-2 specificity itself is the cause. COX-2 is present in vessel endothelium where it produces prostacyclins which inhibit platelet function and cause vasodilatation. Inhibition of COX-2 at this site may increase the likelihood of thrombus formation and occlusion, and therefore myocardial infarction and stroke. NSAIDs inhibit COX-2 in addition but they also inhibit COX-1 which causes significant impairment of platelet function. Therefore, the combined effect of NSAIDs is such that the risk of adverse cardiovascular and cerebrovascular events is not increased; in fact, the incidence may be decreased (certainly true for low-dose aspirin).

Renal

COX-2 is normally found in the renal cortex and is therefore inhibited both by conventional NSAIDs and COX-2 inhibitors. There is the potential both for peripheral oedema and hypertension, as well as direct effects on renal excretory function with oliguria and decreased creatinine clearance.

KETAMINE

Ketamine (2-chlorophenyl-2-methylaminocyclohexanone hydrochloride) is an anaesthetic agent that has analgesic actions at low doses. It is structurally similar to phencyclidine. It is available in parenteral formulation in a variety of concentrations (10–100 mg mL^{-1}). It is normally presented as a racemic mixture, although the S(+) isomer is available in some countries and may have an improved therapeutic index. This isomer may be administered orally, but bioavailability is relatively low and unpredictable. If given epidurally, the preservative-free formulation must be used.

MECHANISM OF ACTION

The main analgesic effect of ketamine is likely to be mediated via antagonism at a specific glutamate receptor, the NMDA receptor. This receptor plays a role in central sensitization of the spinal cord, although its ubiquitous distribution in the CNS accounts for side-effects that often limit its use. The NMDA receptor is important in the mechanisms of neuropathic pain, both acutely and chronically, and may be involved in opioid tolerance.

PHARMACOKINETICS

Ketamine is water soluble, forming an acidic solution (pH = 3.5–5.5). It is ~45% unionized at body pH and rapidly distributed across the blood–brain barrier. It is mainly metabolized in the liver by mixed function oxidases, and has an elimination half-life of ~200 min. Its main metabolite is norketamine, which is renally excreted and has some limited activity. Other metabolites include hydroxynorketamine and hydroxyketamine glucuronide. Ketamine has a volume of distribution of 2.9–3.1 L kg^{-1} and clearance of ~20 mL kg^{-1} min^{-1}.

PHARMACODYNAMICS

Low-dose ketamine has analgesic effects in both acute and chronic pain. It appears to have an opioid-sparing effect in the postoperative setting, and there is evidence from systematic reviews of its efficacy for neuropathic pain. Unfortunately, its use is often limited by side-effects. It is unclear what the optimal route of administration is. Given parenterally, either intravenously or subcutaneously, bolus doses of 0.25–0.5 mg kg^{-1} or infusion rates of 0.125–0.25 mg kg^{-1} h^{-1} can provide analgesia.

Psychotomimetic effects can often limit use. Hallucinations and nightmares may be troublesome. In large doses, or in susceptible individuals, excess sedation can occur. Ketamine can cause hypertension, increased heart rate and cardiac output, and increased intracranial pressure.

FURTHER READING

Bernards C M 2002 Understanding the physiology and pharmacology of epidural and intrathecal opioids. Best Practice & Research. Clinical Anaesthesiology 16: 489–505

Christo P J 2003 Opioid effectiveness and side effects in chronic pain. Anesthesiology Clinics of North America 21: 699–713

Hocking G, Cousins M J 2003 Ketamine in chronic pain management: an evidence-based review. Anesthesia and Analgesia 97: 1730–1739

McDonald J, Lambert D G 2005 Opioid receptors. Continuing Education in Anaesthesia, Critical Care and Pain 5: 22–25

Mather L E 2001 Trends in the pharmacology of opioids: implications for the pharmacotherapy of pain. European Journal of Pain 5(suppl A): 49–57

Raffa R B, Clark-Vetri R, Tallarida R J, Wertheimer A I 2003 Combination strategies for pain management. Expert Opinion on Pharmacotherapy 4: 1697–1708

Yaksh T L 1997 Pharmacology and mechanisms of opioid analgesic activity. Acta Anaesthesiologica Scandinavica 41: 94–111

6 Muscle function and neuromuscular blockade

In the last 60 years, neuromuscular blocking drugs have become an established part of anaesthetic practice. They were first administered in 1942, when Griffith and Johnson in Montreal used Intocostrin, a biologically standardized mixture of the alkaloids of the plant *Chondrodendron tomentosum*, to facilitate relaxation during cyclopropane anaesthesia. Previously, only inhalational agents (nitrous oxide, ether, cyclopropane and chloroform) had been used during general anaesthesia, making surgical access for some procedures difficult because of lack of muscle relaxation. To achieve significant muscle relaxation, it was necessary to deepen anaesthesia, which often had adverse cardiac and respiratory effects. Local analgesia was the only alternative.

At first, muscle relaxants were used only occasionally, in small doses, as an adjuvant to aid in the management of a difficult case; they were not used routinely. A tracheal tube was not always used, the lungs were not ventilated artificially and residual block was not routinely reversed; all of these caused significant morbidity and mortality, as demonstrated in the famous retrospective study by Beecher & Todd (1954). By 1946, however, it was appreciated that using drugs such as curare in larger doses allowed the depth of anaesthesia to be lightened, and it was suggested that incremental doses should also be used during prolonged surgery, rather than deepening anaesthesia – an entirely new concept at that time. The use of routine tracheal intubation and artificial ventilation then evolved.

Gray & Halton (1946) in Liverpool reported their experience of using the pure alkaloid tubocurarine in more than 1000 patients receiving various anaesthetic agents. Over the following 6 years, they developed a concise description of the necessary ingredients of any anaesthetic technique; narcosis, analgesia and muscle relaxation were essential – the *triad* of anaesthesia. A fourth ingredient, controlled apnoea, was added at a later stage to emphasize the need for fully controlled ventilation, reducing the amount of relaxant required.

This concept is the basis of the use of neuromuscular blocking drugs in modern anaesthetic practice. In particular, it has allowed seriously ill patients undergoing complex surgery to be anaesthetized safely and to be cared for postoperatively in the intensive therapy unit.

PHYSIOLOGY OF NEUROMUSCULAR TRANSMISSION

Acetylcholine, the neurotransmitter at the neuromuscular junction, is released from presynaptic nerve endings on passage of a nerve impulse (an action potential) down the axon to the nerve terminal. The neurotransmitter is synthesized from choline and acetylcoenzyme A by the enzyme *choline acetyltransferase* and stored in vesicles in the nerve terminal. The action potential depolarizes the nerve terminal to release the neurotransmitter; entry of Ca^{2+} ions into the nerve terminal is a necessary part of this process. On the arrival of an action potential, the storage vesicles are transferred to the active zones on the edge of the axonal membrane, where they fuse with the terminal wall to release the acetylcholine (Fig. 6.1). There are about 1000 active sites at each nerve ending and any one nerve action potential leads to the release of 200–300 vesicles. In addition, small *quanta* of acetylcholine, presumably equivalent to the contents of one vesicle, are released at the neuromuscular junction spontaneously, causing miniature end-plate potentials (MEPPs) on the postsynaptic membrane, but these are insufficient to generate a muscle action potential.

The active sites of release are aligned directly opposite the acetylcholine receptors on the junctional folds of the postsynaptic membrane, lying on the muscle surface. The junctional cleft, the gap between the nerve terminal and the muscle membrane, has a width of only 60 nm. It contains the enzyme *acetylcholinesterase*, which is responsible for the ultimate breakdown of acetylcholine. This enzyme is also present, in higher

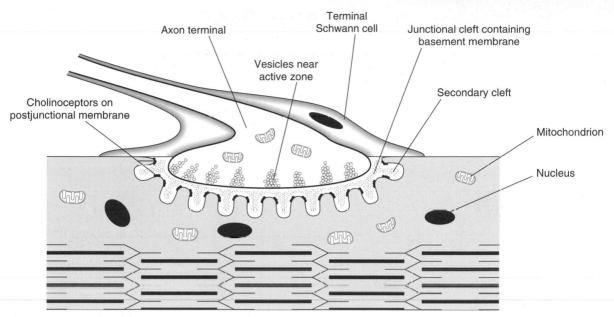

Fig. 6.1
The neuromuscular junction with an axon terminal, containing vesicles of acetylcholine. The neurotransmitter is released on arrival of an action potential and crosses the junctional cleft to stimulate the postjunctional receptors on the shoulders of the secondary clefts. (Reproduced with kind permission of Professor WC Bowman.)

concentrations, in the junctional folds in the postsynaptic membrane (Fig. 6.1). The choline produced by the breakdown of acetylcholine is taken up across the nerve membrane to be reused in the synthesis of the transmitter.

The nicotinic acetylcholine receptors on the postsynaptic membrane are organized in discrete clusters on the shoulders of the junctional folds (Fig. 6.1). Each cluster is about 0.1 µm in diameter and contains a few hundred receptors. Each receptor consists of five subunits, two of which, the alpha (α; MW = 40 000 Da), are identical. The other three, slightly larger subunits, are the beta (β), delta (δ) and epsilon (ε). In fetal muscle, the epsilon is replaced by a gamma (γ) subunit. Each subunit of the receptor is a glycosated protein – a chain of amino acids – coded by a different gene. The receptors are arranged as a cylinder which spans the membrane, with a central, normally closed, channel – the ionophore (Fig. 6.2). Each of the α subunits carries a single acetylcholine binding region on its extracellular surface. They also bind neuromuscular blocking drugs.

Activation of the receptor requires both α sites to be occupied, producing a structural change in the receptor complex that opens the central channel running between the receptors for a very short period, about 1 ms (Fig. 6.2). This allows movement of cations such as Na^+, K^+, Ca^{2+} and Mg^{2+} along their concentration gradients. The main change is influx of Na^+ ions, the *end-plate current*, followed by efflux of K^+ ions. The summation of this current through a large number of receptor channels lowers the transmembrane potential of the end-plate region sufficiently to depolarize it and generate a muscle action potential sufficient to allow muscle contraction.

At rest, the transmembrane potential is about –90 mV (inside negative). Under normal physiological conditions, a depolarization of about 40 mV occurs, lowering the potential from –90 to –50 mV. When the *end-plate potential* reaches this critical threshold, it triggers an *all-or-nothing* action potential that passes around the sarcolemma to activate muscle contraction via a mechanism involving Ca^{2+} release from the sarcoplasmic reticulum.

Each acetylcholine molecule is involved in opening one ion channel only before it is broken down rapidly by acetylcholinesterase; it does not interact with any of the other receptors. There is a large safety factor in the transmission process, in respect of both the amount of acetylcholine released and the number of postsynaptic receptors. Much more acetylcholine is released than is necessary to trigger the action potential. The end-plate region is depolarized for only a very short period (a few milliseconds) before it rapidly repolarizes and is ready to transmit another impulse.

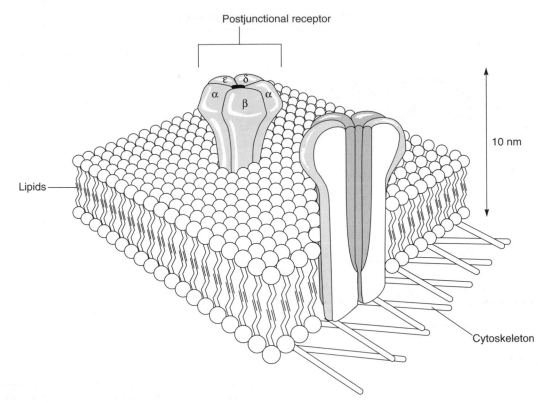

Fig. 6.2
Two postjunctional receptors, embedded in the lipid layer of the postsynaptic muscle membrane. The α, β, ε and δ subunits are demonstrated on the surface of one receptor and the ionophore is seen in cross-section on the other receptor. On stimulation of the two α subunits by two molecules of acetylcholine, the ionophore opens to allow the passage of the end-plate current. (Reproduced with kind permission of Professor WC Bowman.)

Acetylcholine receptors are also present on the presynaptic area of the nerve terminal. It is thought that a positive feedback mechanism exists for the further release of acetylcholine, such that some of the released molecules of acetylcholine stimulate these presynaptic receptors, producing further mobilization of the neurotransmitter to the readily releasable sites, ready for the arrival of the next nerve stimulus (Fig. 6.3).

In health, postsynaptic acetylcholine receptors are restricted to the neuromuscular junction by a mechanism involving the presence of an active nerve terminal. In many disease states affecting the neuromuscular junction, this control is lost and acetylcholine receptors develop on the adjacent muscle surface. The excessive release of K⁺ ions from diseased or swollen muscle on administration of succinylcholine is probably the result of stimulation of these *extrajunctional receptors*. They develop in many conditions, including polyneuropathies, severe burns and muscle disorders.

PHARMACOLOGY OF NEUROMUSCULAR TRANSMISSION

Neuromuscular blocking agents used regularly by anaesthetists are classified into *depolarizing* (or *non-competitive*) and *non-depolarizing* (or *competitive*) agents.

DEPOLARIZING NEUROMUSCULAR BLOCKING AGENTS

The only depolarizing relaxant now available in clinical practice is succinylcholine. Decamethonium was used clinically in the UK for many years, but it is now available only for research purposes.

Succinylcholine chloride (suxamethonium)

This quaternary ammonium compound is comparable to two molecules of acetylcholine linked together (Fig. 6.4). The two quaternary ammonium radicals,

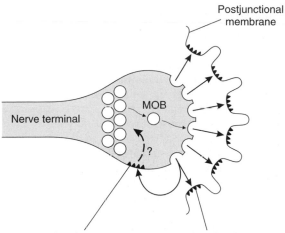

Fig. 6.3
Acetylcholine receptors are present on the shoulders of the axon terminal, as well as on the postjunctional membrane. Stimulation of the prejunctional receptors mobilizes (MOB) the vesicles of acetylcholine to move into the active zone, ready for release on arrival of another nerve impulse. The mechanism requires Ca^{2+} ions. (Reproduced with kind permission of Professor WC Bowman.)

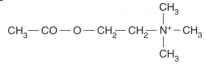

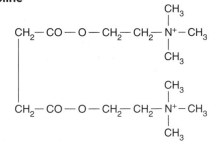

Fig. 6.4
The chemical structures of acetylcholine and succinylcholine. The similarity between the structure of succinylcholine and two molecules of acetylcholine can be seen. The structure of decamethonium is also shown. The quaternary ammonium radicals, $N^+(CH_3)_3$, cling to the α subunits of the postsynaptic receptor.

$N^+(CH_3)_3$ have the capacity to cling to each of the α units of the postsynaptic acetylcholine receptor, altering its structural conformation and opening the ion channel, but for a longer period than does a molecule of acetylcholine. Administration of succinylcholine therefore results in an initial depolarization and muscle contraction, termed *fasciculation*. As this effect persists, however, further action potentials cannot pass down the ion channels and the muscle becomes flaccid; repolarization does not occur (Appiah-Ankam & Hunter 2004).

The dose of succinylcholine necessary for tracheal intubation in adults is 1.0–1.5 mg kg^{-1}. This dose has the most rapid onset of action of any of the muscle relaxants presently available, producing profound block within 1 min. Succinylcholine is therefore of particular benefit when it is essential to achieve tracheal intubation rapidly, as in a patient with a full stomach or an obstetric patient. It is also indicated if tracheal intubation is expected to be difficult for anatomical reasons, as it produces optimal intubating conditions.

The drug is metabolized predominantly in the plasma by the enzyme *plasma cholinesterase*, at one time termed pseudocholinesterase, at a very rapid rate. Recovery from neuromuscular block may start to occur within 3 min and is complete within 12–15 min. The use of an anticholinesterase such as neostigmine,

which would inhibit such enzyme activity, is contraindicated (see below). About 10% of the drug is excreted in the urine; there is very little metabolism in the liver although some breakdown by non-specific esterases occurs in the plasma.

If plasma cholinesterase is structurally abnormal because of inherited factors, or if its concentration is reduced by acquired factors, then the duration of action of the drug may be altered significantly.

Inherited factors

The exact structure of plasma cholinesterase is determined genetically, by autosomal genes, and this has now been completely defined. Several abnormalities in the amino acid sequence of the normal enzyme, usually designated E_1^u, are recognized. The most common is produced by the atypical gene, E_1^a, which occurs in about 4% of the Caucasian population. Thus a patient who is a *heterozygote* for the atypical gene (E_1^u, E_1^a) demonstrates a longer effect from a standard dose of succinylcholine (about 30 min). If the individual is a *homozygote* for the atypical gene ($E_1{}^a$, $E_1{}^a$), the duration of action of succinylcholine may exceed 2 h. Other, rarer, abnormalities in the structure of plasma cholinesterase are also recognized, e.g. the fluoride ($E_1{}^f$) and silent ($E_1{}^s$) genes. The latter has very little capacity to metabolize succinylcholine and thus neuromuscular block in the homozygous state ($E_1{}^s$, $E_1{}^s$) lasts for at least 3 h. In such patients, non-specific esterases gradually clear the drug from plasma.

It has been suggested that a source of cholinesterase, such as fresh frozen plasma, should be administered in such cases, or an anticholinesterase such as neostigmine used to reverse what has usually developed into a *dual block* (see below). However, it is wiser to:

- Keep the patient anaesthetized and the lungs ventilated artificially.
- Monitor neuromuscular transmission accurately, until full recovery from residual neuromuscular block.

This condition is not life-threatening, but the risk of awareness is considerable, especially after the end of surgery, when the anaesthetist, who may not yet have made the diagnosis, is attempting to waken the patient. Anaesthesia must be continued until full recovery from neuromuscular block is demonstrable.

As plasma cholinesterase activity is reduced by the presence of succinylcholine, a plasma sample to measure the patient's cholinesterase activity should not be taken for several days after prolonged block has been experienced, by which time new enzyme has been synthesized. A patient who is found to have reduced enzyme activity and structurally abnormal enzyme should be given a warning card or alarm bracelet, detailing his or her genetic status. Examining the genetic status of the patient's immediate relatives should be considered.

Kalow & Genest (1957) first described a method for detecting structurally abnormal cholinesterase. If plasma from a patient of normal genotype is added to a water bath containing a substrate such as benzoylcholine, a chemical reaction occurs with plasma cholinesterase, emitting light of a given wavelength, which may be detected spectrophotometrically. If dibucaine is also added to the water bath, this reaction is inhibited; no light is produced. The percentage inhibition is referred to as the *dibucaine number*. A patient with normal plasma cholinesterase has a high dibucaine number of 77–83. A heterozygote for the atypical gene has a dibucaine number of 45–68; in a homozygote, the dibucaine number is less than 30.

If fluoride is added to the solution instead of dibucaine, the fluoride gene may be detected. If there is no reaction in the presence of the substrate only, the silent gene is present.

Acquired factors

In these instances, the structure of plasma cholinesterase is normal, but its activity is reduced. Thus, neuromuscular block is prolonged by only minutes, rather than hours. Causes of reduced plasma cholinesterase activity include the following:

- Liver disease, because of reduced enzyme synthesis.
- Carcinomatosis and starvation, also because of reduced enzyme synthesis.
- Pregnancy, for two reasons: an increased circulating volume (dilutional effect) and decreased enzyme synthesis.
- Anticholinesterases, including those used by the anaesthetist to reverse residual neuromuscular block after a non-depolarizing muscle relaxant (e.g. neostigmine or edrophonium); these drugs inhibit plasma cholinesterase in addition to acetylcholinesterase. The organophosphorus compound *ecothiopate*, once used topically as a miotic in ophthalmology, is also an anticholinesterase.
- Other drugs which are metabolized by plasma cholinesterase, and which therefore decrease its availability, include etomidate, propanidid, ester local analgesics, anti-cancer drugs such as methotrexate, monoamine oxidase inhibitors and esmolol (the short-acting β-blocker).
- Hypothyroidism.
- Cardiopulmonary bypass, plasmapheresis.
- Renal disease.

Side-effects of succinylcholine

Although succinylcholine is a very useful drug for achieving tracheal intubation rapidly, it has several undesirable side-effects which may limit its use.

Muscle pains

These occur especially in the patient who is ambulant soon after surgery, such as the day-case patient. The pains, thought possibly to be caused by the initial fasciculations, are more common in young, healthy patients with a large muscle mass. They occur in unusual sites, such as the diaphragm and between the scapulae, and are not relieved easily by conventional analgesics. They may be reduced by the use of a small dose of a non-depolarizing muscle relaxant given immediately before administration of succinylcholine, e.g. gallamine 10 mg (which is thought to be most efficacious in this respect), or atracurium 2.5 mg.

However, this technique, termed *pre-curarization* or *pretreatment*, reduces the potency of succinylcholine, necessitating administration of a larger dose to produce the same effect. Many other drugs have been used in an attempt to reduce the muscle pains, including lidocaine, calcium, magnesium and repeated doses of thiopental, but none is completely reliable.

Increased intraocular pressure

This is thought to be caused partly by the initial contraction of the external ocular muscles and contracture of the internal ocular muscles after administration of succinylcholine. It is not reduced by pre-curarization. The effect lasts for as long as the neuromuscular block and concern has been expressed that it may be sufficient to cause expulsion of the vitreal contents in the patient with an open eye injury. This is probably unlikely. Protection of the airway from gastric contents must take priority in the patient with a full stomach in addition to an eye injury, as inhalation of gastric contents may threaten life.

It is also possible that succinylcholine may increase intracranial pressure, although this is less certain.

Increased intragastric pressure

In the presence of a normal lower oesophageal sphincter, the increase in intragastric pressure produced by succinylcholine should be insufficient to produce regurgitation of gastric contents. However, in the patient with incompetence of this sphincter from, for example, hiatus hernia, regurgitation may occur.

Hyperkalaemia

It has long been recognized that administration of succinylcholine during halothane anaesthesia increases the serum potassium concentration by 0.5 mmol L^{-1}. This effect is thought to be caused by muscle fasciculation. It is probable that the effect is less marked with the newer potent inhalational agents, e.g. isoflurane, sevoflurane. A similar increase occurs in patients with renal failure, but as these patients may already have an elevated serum potassium concentration, such an increase may precipitate cardiac irregularities and even cardiac arrest.

In some conditions in which the muscle cells are swollen or damaged, or in which there is proliferation of extrajunctional receptors, this release of potassium may be exaggerated. This is most marked in the burned patient, in whom potassium concentrations up to 13 mmol L^{-1} have been reported. In such patients, pre-curarization is of no benefit. Succinylcholine should be avoided in this condition. In diseases of the muscle cell, or its nerve supply, hyperkalaemia after succinylcholine may also be exaggerated. These include the muscular dystrophies, dystrophia myotonica and paraplegia. Hyperkalaemia has been reported to cause death in such patients. Succinylcholine may also precipitate prolonged contracture of the masseter muscles in patients with these disorders, making tracheal intubation impossible. The drug should be avoided in any patient with a neuromuscular disorder, including the patient with *malignant hyperthermia*, in whom the drug is a recognized trigger factor (see p. 392).

Hyperkalaemia after succinylcholine has also been reported, albeit rarely, in patients with widespread intra-abdominal infection, severe trauma and closed head injury.

Cardiovascular effects

Succinylcholine has muscarinic in addition to nicotinic effects, as does acetylcholine. The direct vagal effect (muscarinic) produces sinus bradycardia, especially in patients with high vagal tone, such as children and the physically fit. It is also more common in the patient who has not received an anticholinergic agent (such as atropine) or who is given repeated increments of succinylcholine. It is advisable to use an anticholinergic routinely if it is planned to administer more than one dose of succinylcholine. Nodal or ventricular escape beats may develop in extreme circumstances.

Anaphylactic reactions

Anaphylactic reactions to succinylcholine are rare, but may occur, especially after repeated exposure to the drug. They are more common after succinylcholine than any other neuromuscular blocking agent.

Characteristics of depolarizing neuromuscular block

If neuromuscular block is monitored (see below), several differences between depolarizing and non-depolarizing block may be defined. In the presence of a small dose of succinylcholine:

- A decreased response to a single, low-voltage (1 Hz) twitch stimulus applied to a peripheral nerve is detected. Tetanic stimulation (e.g. at 50 Hz) produces a small, but sustained, response.
- If four twitch stimuli are applied at 2 Hz over 2 s (train-of-four stimulus), followed by a 10-s interval before the next train-of-four, no decrease in the height of successive stimuli is noted (Fig. 6.5).

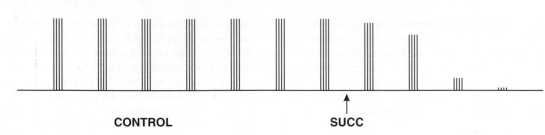

CONTROL   **SUCC**

Fig. 6.5
The train-of-four twitch response recorded before (CONTROL) and after a dose of succinylcholine. Before administration of succinylcholine 1 mg kg^{-1}, four twitches of equal height are visible. After giving the drug (SUCC), the height of all four twitches decreases equally; no 'fade' of the train-of-four is seen. Within 1 min, the trace has been ablated.

- The application of a 5-s burst of tetanic stimulation after the application of single twitch stimuli, followed 3 s later by a further run of twitch stimuli, produces no potentiation of the twitch height; there is no *post-tetanic potentiation* (sometimes termed *facilitation*).
- Neuromuscular block is *potentiated* by the administration of an anticholinesterase such as neostigmine or edrophonium.
- If repeated doses of succinylcholine are given, the characteristics of this depolarizing block alter; signs typical of a non-depolarizing block develop (see below). Initially, such changes are demonstrable only at fast rates of stimulation, but with further increments of succinylcholine they may occur at slower rates. This phenomenon is termed 'dual block'.
- Muscle fasciculation is typical of a depolarizing block.

Decamethonium

This depolarizing neuromuscular blocking agent has as rapid an onset of action as succinylcholine, but a longer duration of effect (about 20 min), as it is not metabolized by plasma cholinesterase, but mainly excreted unchanged through the kidney. It is prone to produce *tachyphylaxis* – a rapid increase in the dose required incrementally to produce the same effect – which, together with its route of excretion, limit its use. It is no longer available for clinical use.

NON-DEPOLARIZING NEUROMUSCULAR BLOCKING AGENTS

Unlike succinylcholine, these drugs do not alter the structural conformity of the postsynaptic acetylcholine receptor and therefore do not produce an initial contraction. Instead, they compete with the neurotransmitter at this site, binding reversibly to one or two of the α-recep-

tors, whenever these are not occupied by acetylcholine. The end-plate potential produced in the presence of a non-depolarizing agent is therefore smaller; it does not reach the threshold necessary to initiate a propagating action potential to activate the sarcolemma and produce an initial muscle contraction. More than 75% of the postsynaptic receptors have to be blocked in this way before there is failure of muscle contraction – a large safety factor. However, in large doses, non-depolarizing muscle relaxants impair neuromuscular transmission sufficiently to produce profound neuromuscular block.

Metabolism of neuromuscular blocking agents is not thought to occur at the neuromuscular junction. By the end of surgery, the end-plate concentration of the relaxant is decreasing as the drug diffuses down a concentration gradient into the plasma, from which it is cleared. Thus more receptors are stimulated by the neurotransmitter, allowing recovery from block. An anticholinesterase given at this time increases the half-life of acetylcholine at the neuromuscular junction, facilitating recovery.

Non-depolarizing muscle relaxants are highly ionized, water-soluble drugs, which are distributed mainly in plasma and extracellular fluid. Thus they have a relatively small volume of distribution. They are of two main types of chemical structure: either *benzylisoquinolinium compounds*, such as tubocurarine, alcuronium, atracurium, mivacurium and cisatracurium, or *aminosteroid compounds*, such as pancuronium, vecuronium, pipecuronium and rocuronium. All these drugs possess at least one quaternary ammonium group, $N^+(CH_3)_3$, to bind to an α subunit on the postsynaptic receptor. Their structural type determines many of their chemical properties. Some benzylisoquinolinium compounds consist of quaternary ammonium groups joined by a thin chain of methyl groups. They are therefore more liable to some breakdown in the plasma than are the aminosteroids. They are also more likely to release histamine.

Non-depolarizing muscle relaxants are administered usually in multiples of the effective dose (ED) required to produce 95% neuromuscular block (ED_{95}). A dose of at least $2 \times ED_{95}$ is required to produce adequate conditions for reliable tracheal intubation in all patients.

Benzylisoquinolinium compounds

Tubocurarine chloride

This is the only naturally occurring muscle relaxant. It is derived from the bark of the South American plant *Chondrodendron tomentosum* and has been used for centuries by South American Indians as an arrow poison. It was the first non-depolarizing neuromuscular blocking agent to be used in humans, by Griffith and Johnson in Montreal, in 1942. The intubating dose is of the order of 0.5–0.6 mg kg^{-1}. It has a long onset of action and a prolonged duration of effect (Table 6.1), and its effects are potentiated by inhalational agents and prior administration of succinylcholine. It has a marked propensity to produce histamine release and thus hypotension, with possibly a compensatory tachycardia. In large doses, it may also produce ganglion blockade, which potentiates these cardiovascular effects. It is excreted unchanged through the kidney, with some biliary excretion. It is no longer available in the UK.

Alcuronium chloride

This drug is a semi-synthetic derivative of toxiferin, an alkaloid of calabash curare. It has less histamine-releasing properties, and therefore cardiovascular effect, than tubocurarine, although it may have some vagolytic effect, producing a mild tachycardia. It also has a long onset time and nearly as long a duration of effect as tubocurarine (Table 6.1). It is almost entirely excreted unchanged through the kidney. The intubating dose is of the order of 0.2–0.25 mg kg^{-1}. Before the advent of atracurium and vecuronium, this inexpensive agent was used widely, but now its popularity has declined and it is no longer available commercially in the UK.

Gallamine triethiodide

This synthetic substance is a trisquaternary amine. It was first used in France in 1948. The intubating dose in adults is of the order of 160 mg. It has a similar onset to, but slightly shorter duration of action than, tubocurarine, and is excreted almost entirely by the kidney. Consequently, it should not be used in patients with renal impairment. Being more lipid-soluble than bisquaternary amines, it crosses the placenta to a significant degree and should not be used in obstetric practice. Gallamine has potent vagolytic properties and produces some direct sympathomimetic stimulation. Thus, it increases pulse rate and arterial pressure.

The only recent use of gallamine in the UK has been as a small pretreatment dose (10 mg) prior to succinylcholine, when it seems to be more efficacious than any other non-depolarizing muscle relaxant in minimizing muscle pains.

Atracurium besylate

This drug, introduced into clinical practice in 1982, was developed by Stenlake at Strathclyde University. He recognized that quaternary ammonium compounds break down spontaneously at varying temperature and pH, a phenomenon known for over 100 years as *Hofmann degradation*. Many such substances also have neuromuscular blocking properties, and

Table 6.1 Time to 95% depression of the twitch response, after a dose of $2 \times ED_{95}$ of a neuromuscular blocking drug (when tracheal intubation should be possible), and time to 20–25% recovery, when an anticholinesterase may be used reliably to reverse residual block produced by a non-depolarizing drug

	95% twitch depression (s)	20–25% recovery (min)
Succinylcholine	60	10
Tubocurarine	220	80+
Alcuronium	420	70
Gallamine	300	80
Atracurium	110	43
Cisatracurium	150	45
Doxacurium	250	83
Mivacurium	170	16
Pancuronium	220	75
Vecuronium	180	33
Pipecuronium	300	95
Rocuronium	75	33
Rapacuronium	<75	15

atracurium was developed in the search for such an agent that broke down at body temperature and pH. Hofmann degradation may be considered as a 'safety net' in the sick patient with impaired liver or renal function, as atracurium is still cleared from the body. Some renal excretion occurs in the healthy patient (10%), as does ester hydrolysis in the plasma; probably only about 45% of the drug is eliminated by Hofmann degradation in the normal patient.

Atracurium (and vecuronium) was developed in an attempt to obtain a non-depolarizing agent which had a more rapid onset, was shorter-acting and had less cardiovascular effects than the older agents. Atracurium $0.5 \, mg \, kg^{-1}$ does not produce neuromuscular block as rapidly as succinylcholine; the onset time is 2.0–2.5 min, depending on the dose used (Table 6.1). However, it produces more rapid recovery than the older non-depolarizing agents and may be reversed easily 20–25 min after administration of a dose of $2 \times ED_{95}$ ($0.45 \, mg \, kg^{-1}$). The drug does not have any direct cardiovascular effect, but may release histamine (about a third of that released by tubocurarine) and may therefore produce a local wheal and flare around the injection site, especially if a small vein is used. This may be accompanied by a slight reduction in arterial pressure.

A metabolite of Hofmann degradation, *laudanosine*, has epileptogenic properties, although fits have never been reported in humans. The plasma concentrations of laudanosine required to make animals convulse are much higher than those occurring during general anaesthesia, even if large doses of atracurium are given during a prolonged procedure, and there is little cause for concern about this metabolite in clinical practice. In patients in the ITU with multiple organ failure, who may receive atracurium for several days, laudanosine concentrations are higher, but as yet no reports of cerebral toxicity have occurred.

Cisatracurium

This is the most recently introduced benzylisoquinolinium neuromuscular blocker. It is of particular interest because it is an example of the development of a specific isomer of a drug to produce a 'clean' substance with the desired clinical actions but with reduced side-effects. Cisatracurium is the 1R-*cis* 1'R-*cis* isomer of atracurium, and one of the 10 possible isomers of the parent compound. It is three to four times more potent than atracurium ($ED_{95} = 0.05 \, mg \, kg^{-1}$) and has a slightly longer onset and duration of action. Its main advantage is that it does not release histamine and therefore is associated with greater cardiovascular stability. It undergoes even more Hofmann degradation than atracurium. As a lower dose of this more potent

drug is given, it produces less laudanosine than an equipotent dose of atracurium. It is therefore particularly useful in the critically ill patient requiring prolonged infusion of a neuromuscular blocking drug.

Doxacurium chloride

This bisquaternary ammonium compound is only available in the USA. It undergoes a small amount of metabolism in the plasma by cholinesterase (6%), but is excreted mainly through the kidney. It is the most potent non-depolarizing neuromuscular blocking agent available; an intubating dose is only $0.05 \, mg \, kg^{-1}$. It has a very long onset of action (Table 6.1) and a prolonged and unpredictable duration of effect. However, it has no cardiovascular effects and may therefore be of use during long surgical procedures in which cardiovascular stability is required, e.g. cardiac surgery.

Mivacurium chloride

This drug is metabolized by plasma cholinesterase at 88% of the rate of succinylcholine. An intubating dose ($2 \times ED_{95} = 0.15 \, mg \, kg^{-1}$) has a similar onset of action to an equipotent dose of atracurium, but in the presence of normal plasma cholinesterase, recovery after mivacurium is much faster (Table 6.1) and administration of an anticholinesterase may not be necessary (if neuromuscular function is being monitored and good recovery can be demonstrated). Full recovery in such circumstances takes about 20–25 min, but the drug may be antagonized easily within 15 min. Mivacurium is useful particularly for surgical procedures requiring muscle relaxation in which even atracurium and vecuronium seem too long-acting, and when it is desirable to avoid the side-effects of succinylcholine, e.g. for bronchoscopy, oesophagoscopy, laparoscopy or tonsillectomy. The drug produces a similar amount of histamine release as does atracurium.

In the presence of reduced plasma cholinesterase activity, because of either inherited or acquired factors, the duration of action of mivacurium may be increased. In patients heterozygous for the atypical cholinesterase gene, the duration of action of mivacurium is comparable to that of atracurium, negating its advantages. The action of the drug may also be prolonged in patients with hepatic and renal disease.

Aminosteroid compounds

These non-depolarizing neuromuscular blocking agents possess at least one quaternary ammonium group, attached to a steroid nucleus. They produce fewer adverse cardiovascular effects than do the benzylisoquinolinium compounds and do not stimulate histamine release from mast cells to the same degree. They are excreted unchanged through the kidney and also undergo deacetylation in the liver. The deacetylated metabolites may possess weak neuromuscular blocking properties. The parent compound may also be excreted unchanged in the bile.

Pancuronium bromide

This bisquaternary amine, the first steroid muscle relaxant used clinically, was developed by Savege and Hewitt and marketed in 1964. The intubating dose is 0.1 mg kg^{-1}, which takes 3–4 min to reach its maximum effect (Table 6.1). The clinical duration of action of the drug is long, especially in the presence of potent inhalational agents or renal dysfunction, as 60% of a dose of the drug is excreted unchanged through the kidney. It is also deacetylated in the liver; some of the metabolites have neuromuscular blocking properties.

Pancuronium does not stimulate histamine release and is therefore useful in patients with a history of allergy. However, it has direct vagolytic and sympathomimetic effects which may cause tachycardia and hypertension. It slightly inhibits plasma cholinesterase and therefore potentiates any drug metabolized by this enzyme, e.g. succinylcholine and mivacurium.

Vecuronium bromide

This steroidal agent was developed in an attempt to reduce the cardiovascular effects of pancuronium. It is similar in structure to the older drug, differing only in the loss of a methyl group from one quaternary ammonium radical. Thus it is a monoquaternary amine. An intubating dose of 0.1 mg kg^{-1} produces profound neuromuscular block within 3 min, which is slightly longer than the onset time of atracurium, but shorter than that of tubocurarine and pancuronium. This dose produces clinical block for about 30 min. Vecuronium rarely produces histamine release, nor does it have any direct cardiovascular effects, although it allows the cardiac effects of other anaesthetic agents, such as bradycardia produced by the opioids, to go unchallenged. Vecuronium is excreted through the kidney (30%), although to a lesser extent than pancuronium, and undergoes hepatic deacetylation; the deacetylated metabolites have neuromuscular blocking properties. Repeated doses should be used with care in patients with renal or hepatic disease.

Pipecuronium bromide

This analogue of pancuronium was developed in Hungary in 1980 and is marketed in Eastern Europe and the USA. The intubating dose is 0.07 mg kg^{-1}. The onset time and time to recovery from block are similar to those of pancuronium (Table 6.1), and excretion of the drug through the kidney is significant (66%). In contrast to pancuronium, pipecuronium possesses marked cardiovascular stability, having no vagolytic or sympathomimetic effects. It may therefore be useful during major surgery in patients with cardiac disease.

Rocuronium bromide

This monoquaternary amine has a very rapid onset of action for a non-depolarizing muscle relaxant. It is six to eight times less potent than vecuronium but has approximately the same molecular weight; consequently, a greater number of drug molecules may reach the postjunctional receptors within the first few circulations, enabling faster development of neuromuscular block. In a dose of 0.6 mg kg^{-1}, good or excellent intubating conditions are achieved usually within 60–90 s; this is only slightly slower than the onset time of succinylcholine. The clinical duration is 30–45 min.

In most other respects, rocuronium resembles vecuronium. The drug stimulates little histamine release or cardiovascular disturbance, although in high doses it has a mild vagolytic property which sometimes results in an increase in heart rate. The drug is excreted unchanged in the urine and in the bile, and thus the duration of action may be increased by severe renal or hepatic dysfunction. Rocuronium has no metabolites with significant neuromuscular blocking activity.

Anaphylactic reactions are more common after rocuronium than after any other aminosteroid neuromuscular blocking drug. They occur at a similar rate to anaphylactic reactions to atracurium and mivacurium.

Rapacuronium bromide

This was the last aminosteroid to become available. It is even less potent than rocuronium ($2 \times ED_{90} = 1.15$ mg kg^{-1}) and in equipotent doses may have an even more rapid onset of action (<75 s). It is cleared rapidly from the plasma by hepatic uptake and deacetylation and thus has a shorter duration of effect than rocuronium of 12–15 min (Table 6.1). As with the deacetylation of pancuronium and vecuronium, a metabolite of rapacuronium has neuromuscular blocking properties (Org 9488). This may prolong the effect of incremental doses of the drug.

Rapacuronium has similar cardiovascular effects to rocuronium but it may also produce bronchospasm, possibly because of the release of histamine or leukotrienes. After several reports to the US Food and Drug Administration of bronchospasm and hypoxaemia following administration of rapacuronium, especially in small children, the manufacturers voluntarily withdrew the drug from release in the USA in 2002. It has never been commercially available in the UK.

Factors affecting duration of non-depolarizing neuromuscular block

The duration of action of non-depolarizing muscle relaxants is affected by several factors. Effects are most marked with the longer-acting agents, such as tubocurarine and pancuronium. Prior administration of succinylcholine potentiates the effect and prolongs the duration of action of non-depolarizing drugs. Concomitant administration of a potent inhalational agent increases the duration of block. This is most marked with the ether anaesthetic agents such as isoflurane, enflurane and sevoflurane, but occurs to a lesser extent with halothane.

pH changes. Metabolic and, to a lesser extent, respiratory acidosis extend the duration of block. With monoquaternary amines such as tubocurarine and vecuronium, this effect is produced probably by the ionization, under acidic conditions, of a second nitrogen atom in the molecule, making the drug more potent.

Body temperature. Hypothermia potentiates block as impairment of organ function delays metabolism and excretion of these drugs. Enzyme activity is also reduced. This may occur in patients undergoing cardiac surgery; reduced doses of muscle relaxants are required during cardiopulmonary bypass.

Age. Non-depolarizing muscle relaxants which depend on organ metabolism and excretion may be expected to have a prolonged effect in old age, as organ function deteriorates. In healthy neonates, who have a higher extracellular volume than adults, resistance may occur, but if the baby is sick or immature then, because of underdevelopment of the neuromuscular junction and other organ function, increased sensitivity may be encountered. Children of school age tend to be relatively resistant to non-depolarizing muscle relaxants, when given on a weight basis.

Electrolyte changes. A low serum potassium concentration potentiates neuromuscular block by changing the value of the resting membrane potential of the postsynaptic membrane. A reduced ionized calcium concentration also potentiates block by impairing presynaptic acetylcholine release.

Myasthenia gravis. In this disease, the number and half-life of the postsynaptic receptors are reduced by autoantibodies produced in the thymus gland. Thus,

the patient is more sensitive to the effects of non-depolarizing muscle relaxants. Resistance to succinylcholine may be encountered.

Other disease states. Because of the altered pharmacokinetics of muscle relaxants in hepatic and renal disease, prolongation of action may be found in these conditions, especially if excretion of the drug is dependent upon these organs.

Characteristics of non-depolarizing neuromuscular block

If a small, subparalysing dose of a non-depolarizing neuromuscular blocking drug is administered, the following characteristics are recognized:

- Decreased response to a low-voltage twitch stimulus (e.g. 1 Hz) which, if repeated, decreases further in amplitude. This effect, which is in contrast to that produced by a depolarizing drug, also occurs to a greater degree when the train-of-four twitch response is applied, and even more so with higher, tetanic rates of stimulation. It is often referred to as 'fade' or decrement.
- Post-tetanic potentiation (PTP) or facilitation (PTF) of the twitch response may be demonstrated (Fig. 6.6).
- Neuromuscular block is reversed by administration of an anticholinesterase.
- No muscle fasciculation is visible.

ANTICHOLINESTERASES

These agents are used in clinical practice to inhibit the action of acetylcholinesterase at the neuromuscular junction, thus prolonging the half-life of acetylcholine and potentiating its effect, especially in the presence of residual amounts of non-depolarizing muscle relaxant at the end of surgery. The most commonly used anticholinesterase during anaesthesia is neostigmine, but edrophonium and pyridostigmine are also available. These carbamate esters are water-soluble, quaternary ammonium compounds which are absorbed poorly from the gastrointestinal tract. The more lipid-soluble tertiary amine, physostigmine, has a similar effect and is more suitable for oral administration, but crosses the blood–brain barrier. Organophosphorus compounds also inhibit acetylcholinesterase, but unlike other agents, their effect is irreversible; recovery occurs only on generation of more enzyme, which takes some weeks.

Anticholinesterases are also given orally to patients with *myasthenia gravis*. In this disease, the patient possesses antibodies to the postsynaptic nicotinic

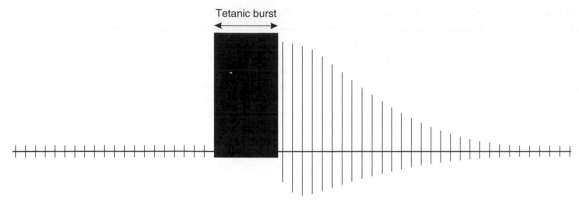

Fig. 6.6
A 5-s burst of tetanus (50 Hz), applied after a run of single twitch stimuli, causes a transient increase in the height of subsequent twitches, although they gradually decrease to their former height; this is post-tetanic potentiation (PTP) or facilitation (PTF).

receptor, reducing the efficacy of acetylcholine. The use of these drugs is thought to increase the amount and duration of action of acetylcholine at the neuro-muscular junction, thus enhancing neuromuscular transmission.

Neostigmine

This drug combines reversibly with acetyl-cholinesterase by formation of an ester linkage. Neostigmine is excreted largely unchanged through the kidney and has a half-life of about 45 min. It is pre-sented in brown vials, as it breaks down on exposure to light. Neostigmine potentiates the action of acetyl-choline wherever it is a neurotransmitter, including all cholinergic nerve endings; thus it produces bradycar-dia, salivation, sweating, bronchospasm, increased intestinal motility and blurred vision. These choliner-gic effects may be reduced by simultaneous adminis-tration of an anticholinergic agent such as atropine or glycopyrrolate. The usual dose of neostigmine is of the order of 0.035 mg kg^{-1}, in combination with either atropine 0.015 mg kg^{-1} or glycopyrrolate 0.01 mg kg^{-1}. Neostigmine takes at least 2 min to have an initial effect, and recovery from neuromuscular block is max-imally enhanced by 5–7 min.

Edrophonium

This anticholinesterase forms an ionic bond with the enzyme but does not undergo a chemical reaction with it. The effect is therefore more short-lived than with neostigmine, of the order of only a few minutes. Edrophonium has a quicker onset of action than neostigmine, producing signs of recovery within 1 min.

However, its effects are more evanescent; when edro-phonium is given in the presence of profound neuro-muscular block, the degree of neuromuscular block may *increase* after an initial period of recovery. The dose of edrophonium is 0.5–1.0 mg kg^{-1}.

Pyridostigmine

This drug has a longer onset time than neostigmine or edrophonium, and also a longer duration of action. It is used more frequently as oral therapy in patients with myasthenia gravis than in anaesthesia.

Physostigmine

This anticholinesterase, also known as *eserine*, is a ter-tiary amine and is more lipid-soluble than the other carbamate esters. It is therefore absorbed more easily from the gastrointestinal tract, and also crosses the blood–brain barrier.

Organophosphorus compounds

These substances are considered to be irreversible inhibitors of acetylcholinesterase; by phosphorylation of the enzyme they produce a very stable complex which is resistant to reactivation or hydrolysis. Synthesis of new enzyme must occur before recovery. These agents, which include di-isopropylfluorophos-phonate (DFP) and tetraethylpyrophosphate (TEPP), are used as insecticides and chemical warfare agents. They are absorbed readily through the lungs and skin. Poisoning is not uncommon among farm workers. Muscarinic effects, such as salivation, sweating and bronchospasm, are combined with nicotinic effects, such as muscle weakness. Central nervous effects such as tremor and convulsions may occur, as may unconsciousness and respiratory failure. Reactivators of acetylcholinesterase are used to treat this form of poisoning: they include *pralidoxime* and *obidoxime*. Atropine, anticonvulsants and artificial ventilation may be necessary. Chronic exposure may produce polyneuritis. Carbamates such as pyridostigmine are used prophylactically in those threatened by chemical warfare with these compounds.

Ecothiopate is an organophosphorus compound with a quaternary amine group; it was used as an eye drop preparation in ophthalmology to produce miosis in narrow-angle glaucoma. It inhibits cholinesterase by phosphorylation and thus potentiates all esters metabolized by this enzyme. It has now been withdrawn from the UK market.

A new generation of organophosphorus compounds may be beneficial in Alzheimer's disease, and clinical trials are in progress. Neuromuscular blockers must be used with caution if such patients require anaesthesia.

Org 25969 (Sugammadex)

Anticholinesterases, although used routinely in anaesthetic practice, are recognized to have disadvantages. The most important is that recovery from block must be established before they are given (see below). Their muscarinic effects may be disadvantageous in patients with a history of nausea and vomiting, or in the presence of cardiac arrhythmias or bronchospasm.

A novel approach to reversal of neuromuscular block is now undergoing clinical trials. Cyclodextrins are being used to *encapsulate* or *chelate* non-depolarizing neuromuscular blocking drugs in plasma, preventing their access to the nicotinic receptor and encouraging dissociation from it. Org 25969, a γ-cyclodextrin, is being used to chelate rocuronium and possibly vecuronium. It consists of eight oligosaccharides arranged in a cylindrical structure to encapsulate all four steroid rings of rocuronium completely. The complex is excreted in the urine and has no muscarinic effect. The use of anticholinergic agents is unnecessary. At this early stage of development, Org 25969 seems to be devoid of adverse cardiovascular effects, and to act about three times as rapidly as neostigmine in reversing neuromuscular block produced by rocuronium.

These chelating agents are drug specific, and would not be expected to reverse residual block produced by other muscle relaxants. For instance, Org 25969 does not antagonize neuromuscular block produced by atracurium.

NEUROMUSCULAR MONITORING

There is no clinical tool available to measure accurately neuromuscular transmission in a muscle group. Thus, neither the amount of acetylcholine released in response to a given stimulus nor the number of post-synaptic receptors blocked by a given non-depolarizing muscle relaxant may be assessed. However, it is possible to obtain a crude estimate of muscle contraction during anaesthesia using a variety of techniques. All require the application to a peripheral nerve of a current of up to 60 mA, for a fraction of a millisecond (often 0.2 ms), necessitating a voltage of up to 300 V. Usually, a nerve which is readily accessible to the anaesthetist, such as the ulnar, facial or lateral popliteal nerve, is used. The muscle response to the nerve stimulus may then be assessed by either *visual* or *tactile* means, or it may be recorded by more sophisticated methods.

Mechanomyography

A strain-gauge transducer may be used to measure the force of contraction of, for instance, the thumb, in response to stimulation of the ulnar nerve at the wrist. This measurement may then be charted using a recording device. Accurate measurements of the twitch or tetanic response may be made, although the hand must be splinted firmly for reproducible results. This technique is primarily a research tool.

Electromyography

The electromyographic response of a muscle is measured in response to the same electrical stimulus, using recording electrodes similar to ECG pads placed over the motor point of the stimulated muscle. For instance, if the ulnar nerve is stimulated, the recording electrodes are placed over the motor point of adductor pollicis in the thumb (Fig. 6.7). A compound muscle action potential may be recorded. Although primarily a research tool, there are now several simple clinical instruments, such as the Datex Relaxograph, which give a less accurate, but similar recording. Maintaining the exact position of the hand is not as essential with electromyography as with mechanomyography.

Accelerography

With this technique, the acceleration of the thumb is measured in response to the nerve stimulus and the force of contraction may be derived (force = mass × acceleration). Clinical equipment is available (e.g. the

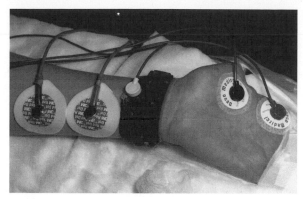

Fig. 6.7
Positioning of the hand necessary to obtain an electromyographic recording of the response of the adductor pollicis muscle to stimulation of the ulnar nerve is demonstrated. An earth electrode is placed round the wrist. Two recording electrodes are placed over the muscle on the hand; the distal one lies over the motor point.

TOF watch, which is an accelerograph) which provides a quantitative assessment of, for instance, the twitch height in comparison with a control reading.

MODES OF STIMULATION

Several different rates of stimulation can be applied to the nerve in an attempt to produce a sensitive index of neuromuscular function. It is considered essential always to apply a *supramaximal* stimulus to the nerve, i.e. the strength of the electrical stimulus (V) should be increased until the response no longer increases. It is then increased by an additional 25%.

Twitch

A square-wave stimulus of short duration (0.1–0.2 ms) is applied to a peripheral nerve. In isolation, such a stimulus is of limited value, although if applied repeatedly, before and after a dose of a muscle relaxant, it may be possible to assess crudely the effects of the drug. Such rates of stimulation have the benefit of being less painful, with no untoward effects after recovery from anaesthesia.

Train-of-four twitch response

In an attempt to assess the degree of neuromuscular block clinically, Ali et al (1971) described a development of the twitch response which, it was hoped, would be more sensitive than repeated single twitches. Four stimuli (at 2 Hz) are applied over 2 s, with at least a 10-s gap between each train-of-four. On administra-

tion of a small dose of a non-depolarizing muscle relaxant, *fade* of the amplitude of the train-of-four may be visible. The ratio of the amplitude of the fourth to the first twitch is called the *train-of-four ratio*. In the presence of a larger dose of such a drug, the fourth twitch disappears first, then the third, followed by the second and, finally, the first twitch (Fig. 6.8A). On recovery from neuromuscular block, the first twitch appears first, then the second (when the first twitch has recovered to about 20% control), then the third, and finally the fourth (Fig. 6.8B).

It is generally thought that at least three of the four twitches must be absent to obtain adequate surgical access for upper abdominal surgery. It is also preferable to reverse residual block with an anticholinesterase only when the second twitch is visible, if good recovery is to be relied upon. After reversal, good muscle tone – as assessed clinically by the patient being able to cough, raise his or her head from the pillow for at least 5 s, protrude the tongue and have good grip strength – may be anticipated when the train-of-four ratio has reached at least 0.7, and probably higher.

It is recognized that, although the number of twitches present in the train of four during profound neuromuscular block is easily counted by visual or tactile means, it is impossible, even for the expert, to assess the value of the train-of-four ratio accurately by these methods. In addition, visual or tactile evaluation fails to detect any fade of the train-of-four when the ratio is in excess of 50%. Thus, failure to detect fade with a nerve stimulator does not always guarantee adequate reversal. Recording of the response is preferable.

Tetanic stimulation

This is the most sensitive form of neuromuscular stimulation. Frequencies of 50–100 Hz are applied to a peripheral nerve to detect even minor degrees of residual neuromuscular block; thus, tetanic fade may be present when the twitch response is normal. Tetanic rates of stimulation may be applied under anaesthesia, but in the awake patient they are intolerable and painful. Indeed, on recovery from anaesthesia in which tetanic stimulation has been applied, the patient may be aware of some discomfort in the area of application.

Post-tetanic potentiation or facilitation

This method of monitoring was developed in an attempt to assess more profound degrees of neuromuscular block produced by non-depolarizing neuromuscular blocking agents. If a single twitch stimulus is applied to the nerve with little or no neuromuscular

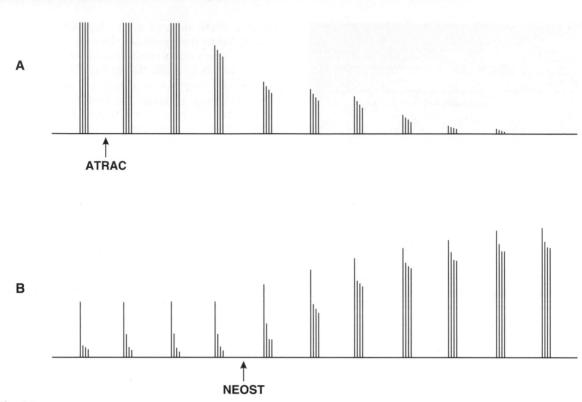

Fig. 6.8
(**A**) After administration of a non-depolarizing muscle relaxant (in this instance, atracurium (ATRAC) 0.5 mg kg^{-1}), the decrease in height of the fourth twitch of the train-of-four response is more marked than the decrease in height of the third twitch, which is more marked than the decrease in the second, which is greater than the decrease in the first. The effect is known as 'fade'. Within 2 min, the train-of-four response has been ablated completely. (**B**) On recovery, the first twitch response appears first, then the second, the third and finally the fourth. Marked fade is present, but after administration of an anticholinesterase (neostigmine (NEOST)) recovery of all four twitches occurs rapidly.

response, but after a 5 s delay a burst of 50-Hz tetanus is given for 5 s, the effect of a further twitch stimulus 3 s later produces an enhanced effect (Fig. 6.6). In the presence of profound block, repeated single twitches applied after the tetanus until the response disappears can be counted; this is termed the *post-tetanic count*. The augmentation of the twitch is thought to be caused by presynaptic mobilization of acetylcholine, as a result of the positive feedback effect of the run of tetanus.

Double-burst stimulation (DBS)

In an attempt to develop a clinical tool which would allow more accurate assessment by visual or tactile means of residual block than fade of the train-of-four response, Viby-Mogensen suggested the application of two or three short bursts of 50-Hz tetanus, each comprising two or three impulses separated by a 750-ms interval. Each square-wave impulse lasts for 0.2 ms

(Fig. 6.9). If records of the fade of the DBS and the train-of-four response are compared, they are very similar, but there is evidence to suggest that visual assessment of the DBS is more accurate.

INDICATIONS FOR NEUROMUSCULAR MONITORING

It is preferable always to monitor neuromuscular function when a muscle relaxant is used during anaesthesia, but it is especially indicated in the following circumstances:

- during prolonged anaesthesia, when repeated increments of neuromuscular blocking agents are required
- when infusions of muscle relaxants are given (including in the ITU)
- in the presence of renal or hepatic dysfunction
- in patients with neuromuscular disorders

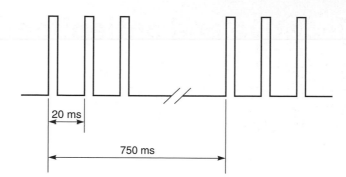

Fig. 6.9
The pattern of double-burst stimulation. Three bursts of 50-Hz tetanus, at 20-ms intervals, every 750 ms are shown.

- in patients with a history of sensitivity to a muscle relaxant or poor recovery from block
- when poor reversal of neuromuscular block is encountered unexpectedly.

FURTHER READING

Ali H H, Utting J E, Gray T C 1971 Quantitative assessment of residual antidepolarizing block. II. British Journal of Anaesthesia 43: 478–485

Appiah-Ankam J, Hunter J M 2004 Pharmacology of neuromuscular blocking drugs. British Journal of Anaesthesia CEPD Reviews 4: 2–7

King J M, Hunter J M 2002 Physiology of the neuromuscular junction. British Journal of Anaesthesia CEPD Reviews 2: 129–133

7 Sedative and antiepileptic drugs

Sedation may be defined as the use of pharmacological agents to produce depression of the level of consciousness sufficient to result in drowsiness and anxiolysis without loss of verbal communication.

The American Society of Anesthesiologists uses the following definitions for sedation:

Minimal sedation is a drug-induced state during which the patient responds normally to verbal commands. Although cognitive function and coordination may be impaired, ventilatory and cardiovascular functions are unaffected.

Moderate sedation (conscious sedation) is a drug-induced depression of consciousness during which the patient responds purposefully to verbal commands either alone or accompanied by light tactile stimulation. No interventions are required to maintain a patent airway and spontaneous ventilation is adequate. Cardiovascular function is usually maintained.

Deep sedation is a drug-induced depression of consciousness during which the patient cannot be easily aroused but will respond purposefully following repeated or painful stimulation. The ability to maintain ventilatory function independently may be impaired and patients may require assistance in maintaining a patent airway. Cardiovascular function is usually maintained.

There exists a seamless progression from minimal sedation to deep sedation where verbal contact and protective reflexes are lost. Deep sedation may progress easily to be indistinguishable from general anaesthesia, when the patient is not rousable, and a higher level of skill is needed to ensure safe management of the patient. The ability of the patient to maintain a patent airway independently is one characteristic of moderate or conscious sedation, but even at this level of sedation it cannot be assumed that protective reflexes are intact. The difference between sedative and anaesthetic drugs is largely one of usage. Many anaesthetic drugs may be used at reduced dosage to produce sedation. Drugs used more usually as sedatives produce a form of anaesthesia if given in high enough doses.

INDICATIONS FOR THE USE OF SEDATIVE DRUGS

Premedication

Sedative drugs may be given in the preoperative period to reduce the apprehension experienced before undergoing anaesthesia and surgery. Sedation may be particularly useful in young children, patients with learning difficulties and individuals who are very anxious. Sedative drugs given in this way augment the actions of anaesthetic agents. The choice of drug depends on the patient, the proposed surgery and the prevailing circumstances: e.g. requirements for patients undergoing ambulatory surgery are different from those scheduled for major surgery as an inpatient. The oral route of administration is preferred and benzodiazepines are the drugs used most commonly for this purpose.

Sedo-analgesia

This term describes the use of a combination of a sedative drug with local anaesthesia, e.g. during dental surgery or surgical procedures performed under regional block. The recent expansion in the development of minimally invasive surgery makes this technique more widely applicable.

Radiological procedures

Some patients, particularly children and anxious individuals, are unable to tolerate long and uncomfortable imaging procedures without sedation. Developments in the use and scope of interventional radiology have further increased the demand for sedation in the radiology department.

Endoscopy

Sedative drugs are used commonly to provide anxiolysis and sedation during endoscopic examinations and interventions. In gastrointestinal (GI) endoscopy, local analgesia is usually inappropriate, necessitating co-administration of sedative drugs and systemic opioids. The synergism between these groups of drugs significantly increases the risks of airway obstruction and ventilatory depression.

Intensive therapy

Most critically ill patients require sedation to facilitate mechanical ventilation and other therapeutic interventions in the intensive therapy unit (ITU). With the increasing sophistication of mechanical ventilators, the modern approach is to combine adequate analgesia with sufficient sedation to maintain the patient in a tranquil but rousable state. The pharmacokinetic profiles of individual drugs should be considered, as sedatives are inevitably given by infusion for prolonged periods in patients with potential organ dysfunction and impaired ability to metabolize or excrete drugs. Many different drugs and regimens have been used to provide short-term and long-term sedation in the ITU, including benzodiazepines, anaesthetic agents such as propofol, opioids, and most recently α_2-adrenergic agonists. There is a lack of high-quality randomized controlled trials to guide best practice in this field. The value of sedation scoring during critical care has been recognized for many years, but more attention has focused recently on the importance of daily sedation 'holds'; a strategy of daily interruption of the sedation regimen allows a more sensitive assessment of the requirements for sedation. This has been shown to decrease the incidence of some complications associated with mechanical ventilation during critical illness, and to reduce the length of stay.

Supplementation of general anaesthesia

Use is made of the synergy between sedative drugs and intravenous induction agents in the technique of co-induction. The administration of a small dose of sedative may result in a significant reduction in the dose of induction agent required, and therefore in the frequency and severity of side-effects.

TECHNIQUES FOR ADMINISTRATION

The administration of sedative drugs requires skill and vigilance, not least because of the seamless progression from light sedation to general anaesthesia. Traditionally, sedative drugs have been administered by intermittent intravenous bolus doses titrated to effect. There is considerable variability in the individual response to a given dose and there are many circumstances in which medical practitioners without anaesthetic training administer sedatives. Recent technological advances in microprocessor-controlled infusion pumps have improved the safety of administration of sedatives. Patient-controlled analgesia systems have been programmed for *patient-controlled sedation*, usually to maintain sedation after an initial bolus dose administered by the physician. When the system is wholly patient-controlled, the mean dose of sedative drug decreases while the range increases.

In *target-controlled infusion*, an adapted syringe pump is programmed with the pharmacokinetic model of a drug and designed to achieve a prescribed 'target' plasma concentration as rapidly as possible, based on the patient's weight. The patient's age should also be taken into consideration, as elderly patients have an increased sensitivity to the effects of sedative drugs on the CNS. To allow for variability in the pharmacodynamic effect of the drug, the operator may vary the target level.

Safe sedation practice

The practice of sedation has been under increasing scrutiny from regulatory agencies with the aim of making procedures safer and minimizing risk to the patient. When sedation is used in areas outside the operating theatre environment, there is a particular need to ensure adequate provision of facilities, equipment and competent personnel. Several practice guidelines have been published which address these issues. Guidelines relating to the provision of sedation for GI endoscopy, procedures in the emergency department, procedures in the dental surgery and the sedation of children have several common themes. Suitability of the patient to undergo a procedure under sedation should be evaluated in advance: e.g. excluding patients with potential airway problems. Facilities should be available to monitor physiological variables such as arterial oxygen saturation, and the individual who performs the procedure should not be responsible for monitoring the condition of the patient at the same time. Personnel should be trained to recognize, and competent to manage, cardiorespiratory complications, and resuscitation equipment must be comprehensive and immediately available. An assessment should be made of the patient's fitness for discharge, and the episode must be appropriately documented.

SEDATIVE DRUGS

Most sedative drugs may be categorized into one of three main groups: benzodiazepines, neuroleptics and α_2-adrenoceptor agonists. Drugs classified more usually as intravenous anaesthetic agents, particularly propofol and ketamine, are also used as sedatives in subanaesthetic doses; the pharmacology of these drugs is discussed in Chapter 3. Inhaled anaesthetics (see Ch. 2) are also used occasionally as sedatives, in subanaesthetic concentrations.

BENZODIAZEPINES

These drugs were developed initially for their anxiolytic and hypnotic properties and largely replaced oral barbiturates in the 1960s. As parenteral preparations became available, they rapidly became established in anaesthesia and intensive care. All benzodiazepines have similar pharmacological effects; their therapeutic use is determined largely by their potency and the available pharmaceutical preparations. Benzodiazepines are often classified by their duration of action as long-acting (e.g. diazepam), medium-acting (e.g. temazepam) or short-acting (e.g. midazolam).

Pharmacology

Mechanism of action

Benzodiazepines exert their actions by specific high-affinity binding to the benzodiazepine receptor, which is part of the γ-aminobutyric acid (GABA) receptor complex. GABA is the major inhibitory neurotransmitter in the central nervous system (CNS), with most neurones undergoing GABA-ergic modulation. The benzodiazepine receptor is an integral binding site on the $GABA_A$ receptor subtype. Binding of the agonist facilitates the entry of chloride ions into the cell, resulting in hyperpolarization of the postsynaptic membrane, which makes the neurone resistant to excitation. These drugs thereby facilitate the inhibitory effects of GABA. Benzodiazepine receptors are found throughout the brain and spinal cord, with the highest density in the cerebral cortex, cerebellum and hippocampus, and with a lower density in the medulla. The absence of $GABA_A$ receptors outside the CNS is consistent with the good cardiovascular safety profile of these drugs.

The clinical CNS effects of benzodiazepines have been shown to correlate with receptor occupancy (Table 7.1).

Table 7.1 Relationship between the effects seen with benzodiazepines and receptor occupancy

Midazolam dose	Effect	Receptor occupancy (%)	Flumazenil dose to reverse
Low dose	Antiepileptic	20–25	Low dose
	Anxiolysis	20–30	
	Slight sedation		
	Reduced attention	25–50	
	Amnesia		
	Intense sedation	60–90	
	Muscle relaxation		
High dose	Anaesthesia		High dose

The $GABA_A$ receptor is a large structure which also contains separate binding sites for other drugs including barbiturates, alcohol and propofol. The binding of other compounds to the benzodiazepine receptor explains the synergistic effects seen with some other drugs. This synergy may lead to dangerous depression of the CNS if drugs are used in combination and also results in pharmacological cross-tolerance, e.g. with alcohol. It is also consistent with the use of benzodiazepines to manage the symptoms associated with acute withdrawal or detoxification from alcohol or other drugs.

The benzodiazepine antagonist flumazenil occupies the receptor but produces no activity. Benzodiazepine compounds have been developed which are ligands at the receptor but have inverse agonist activity, resulting in cerebral excitement. These compounds are also antagonized by flumazenil. This mirrors the way in which paradoxical reactions to benzodiazepines in the elderly are reversed by flumazenil and exacerbated by increasing the dose of the original drug. Other more sinister causes of restlessness, such as hypoxaemia and local anaesthetic toxicity, should always be excluded first.

Chronic administration of benzodiazepines results in receptor downregulation, with decreased receptor binding and function, explaining, at least in part, the development of tolerance. Chronic administration also leads to physical and psychological dependence, although these drugs are less addictive than opioids and barbiturates. Abrupt withdrawal may lead to a clinical syndrome similar to that seen in acute alcohol withdrawal; consequently, doses of benzodiazepines should be reduced gradually after chronic administration.

Elderly patients are particularly sensitive to the effects of benzodiazepines and dosage should be reduced accordingly.

CNS effects

The characteristic CNS effects seen with all benzodiazepines are anxiolysis, sedation, amnesia and antiepileptic activity.

Anxiolysis occurs at low dosage and these drugs are used extensively for the treatment of acute and chronic anxiety states. Longer-acting oral drugs such as diazepam and chlordiazepoxide have a place in the management of acute alcohol withdrawal states. Anxiolysis is very useful in premedication and during unfamiliar or unpleasant procedures.

Sedation occurs as a dose-dependent depression of cerebral activity, with mild sedation at low receptor occupancy progressing to a state similar to general anaesthesia when most receptor sites are occupied. Midazolam is firmly established as a safe intravenous sedative. Benzodiazepines have a high therapeutic index (ratio of effective to lethal dose) because, in overdosage, differences in receptor density result in greater sensitivity to cortical than to medullary depression. However, upper airway obstruction and loss of protective reflexes occur before profound sedation ensues, and are a major hazard following inadvertent oversedation or self-poisoning.

Amnesia is a common sequel to intravenous administration of benzodiazepines and is useful for patients undergoing unpleasant or repeated procedures. Amnesia is anterograde, affecting the acquisition of new information; retrograde amnesia has not been demonstrated following administration of benzodiazepines. Prolonged periods of amnesia have been reported in association with the use of oral lorazepam, making it potentially dangerous in the day-case setting.

Antiepileptic activity is the result of prevention of the subcortical spread of seizure activity. Intravenous lorazepam and diazepam may be used to terminate seizures and clonazepam is used as an adjunct in chronic antiepileptic therapy. Benzodiazepines increase the threshold to seizure activity in local anaesthetic toxicity but may also mask the early signs.

Benzodiazepines have enjoyed wide use as a treatment for insomnia and are effective particularly for acute insomnia. However, chronic use is not recommended because of problems with tolerance and dependence, leading to difficulty in withdrawal of treatment. The use of benzodiazepines as hypnotics has now been partly superseded by more modern non-benzodiazepine hypnotics such as zopiclone, which also acts at the benzodiazepine receptor.

Benzodiazepines decrease cerebral metabolic oxygen requirement and cerebral blood flow, and the cerebrovascular response to carbon dioxide is preserved; consequently, they are suitable for use in some patients with intracranial pathology. However, it should be noted that midazolam does not prevent the increase in intracranial pressure associated with tracheal intubation. In addition, depression of ventilation caused by benzodiazepines in the spontaneously breathing patient results in an increase in arterial $Pa\text{CO}_2$, which is undesirable if intracranial compliance is reduced.

Unwanted CNS side-effects include drowsiness and impaired psychomotor performance. Even when residual sedative effects are minimal, there may be impaired cognitive function and motor coordination, which should be taken into consideration when assessing fitness for discharge in day-case patients.

Muscle relaxation

Benzodiazepines produce a mild reduction in muscle tone, which may be advantageous, e.g. during mechanical ventilation in the intensive care unit, when reducing articular dislocations or during endoscopy. However, muscle relaxation is partly responsible for the airway obstruction which may occur during intravenous sedation. The muscle relaxation is not related to any effect at the neuromuscular junction, but results from suppression of the internuncial neurones of the spinal cord and depression of polysynaptic transmission in the brain.

Respiratory effects

Benzodiazepines produce dose-related central depression of ventilation. The ventilatory response to carbon dioxide is impaired and hypoxic ventilatory responses are markedly depressed. It follows that patients with hypoventilation syndromes and type 2 respiratory failure are particularly sensitive to the respiratory depressant effects of benzodiazepines. Ventilatory depression is exacerbated by airway obstruction and is more common in the elderly. Synergism occurs when both opioids and benzodiazepines are administered. If both types of drug are to be given intravenously, the opioid should be given first and its effect assessed. A reduction of up to 75% in the dose requirement of the benzodiazepine should be anticipated. It should be standard practice to provide supplemental oxygen and to monitor oxygen saturation by pulse oximetry during intravenous sedation.

Cardiovascular effects

Benzodiazepines produce modest haemodynamic effects, with good preservation of homeostatic reflex mechanisms and a much wider margin of safety than intravenous anaesthetic agents. A decrease in systemic vascular resistance results in a small decrease in arterial pressure. Significant hypotension may occur in hypovolaemic or vasoconstricted patients.

Pharmacokinetics

Benzodiazepines are relatively small lipid-soluble molecules, which are readily absorbed orally and which pass rapidly into the CNS. Midazolam has a significant first-pass hepatic effect with only around 50% of an oral dose reaching the systemic circulation. After intravenous bolus administration, termination of action occurs largely by redistribution. Compared with drugs such as propofol, benzodiazepines have a slower effect-site equilibration time. This suggests that time should be allowed to assess the full clinical effect before administering a further intravenous incremental dose. There is extensive protein binding. Elimination takes place by hepatic metabolism followed by renal excretion of the metabolites. There are two main pathways of metabolism involving either microsomal oxidation or conjugation with glucuronide. The significance of this is that oxidation is much more likely to be affected by age, hepatic disease, drug interactions and other factors which alter the concentration of cytochrome P450. Some of the benzodiazepines, including diazepam, have active metabolites, which greatly prolong their clinical effects. Renal dysfunction results in the accumulation of metabolites, and this is an important factor in delayed recovery from prolonged sedation in the ITU.

Diazepam

Diazepam was the first benzodiazepine available for parenteral use. It is insoluble in water and was formulated initially in propylene glycol, which is very irritant to veins and which is associated with a high incidence of thrombophlebitis. A lipid emulsion (Diazemuls) was developed later. Both formulations are presented in 2-mL ampoules containing 5 mg mL^{-1}. Diazepam is also available orally as tablets or a syrup with a bioavailability of 100% and as a rectal solution and suppositories. The elimination half-life is 20–50 h, but active metabolites are produced, including desmethyldiazepam, which has a half-life of 36–200 h. Clearance is reduced in the presence of hepatic dysfunction.

Dosage

- *Premedication* – 10 mg orally 1–1.5 h preoperatively
- *Sedation* – 5–15 mg i.v. slowly; incremental boluses of 1–2 mg
- *Status epilepticus* – 2 mg, repeated every minute until seizure ends; maximum dose 20 mg
- *Intensive therapy* – not suitable for infusion; i.v. bolus dose 5–10 mg may be used 4-hourly.

Midazolam

Midazolam is an imidazobenzodiazepine derivative and it is the imidazole ring which imparts water solubility at pH less than 4. At blood pH, the drug becomes highly lipid-soluble and penetrates the brain rapidly with the onset of sedation in 90 s and peak effect at 2–5 min. It is available in 2-mL ampoules containing 5 mg mL^{-1} or 5-mL ampoules containing 2 mg mL^{-1} and, unlike diazepam, may be diluted. It is also available in 50-mL vials containing 1 mg mL^{-1}, and as a 15-mg tablet with a bioavailability of 44%. Midazolam undergoes hepatic oxidative metabolism and has an elimination half-life of 2 h. The major metabolite, hydroxy-midazolam, has a half-life of around 1 h, and although it is biologically active, it is clinically important only after prolonged infusion in patients with renal impairment. Midazolam is 1.5–2 times more potent than diazepam and has much more favourable pharmacokinetics for use as a short-term intravenous sedative.

Dosage

- *Premedication* – 15 mg orally or 5 mg i.m.; children over 6 months p.r. 70–100 µg kg^{-1}
- *Sedation* – 2–7 mg i.v. (elderly less than 4 mg); incremental boluses of 0.5–1 mg
- *Intensive therapy* – i.v. infusion 0.03–0.1 mg kg^{-1} h^{-1}.

Temazepam

This benzodiazepine is only available orally but is used widely as a premedicant because of its anxiolytic properties. Oral absorption is complete but it may take up to 2 h to reach peak plasma concentrations. Metabolism takes place in the liver by conjugation with glucuronide and there are no significant active metabolites. It has a relatively long elimination half-life of 8–15 h. A dose of 20 mg is effective within 1–2 h and lasts for a period of around 2 h, after which time there is little residual drowsiness. Tolerance and dependence are less likely to occur with chronic use of temazepam and it has been prescribed widely as a hypnotic.

Lorazepam

This drug is available for parenteral and oral administration but is not used routinely as an intravenous sedative as it is limited by a slow onset of action. Metabolism is by glucuronidation, with an elimination half-life of 15 h and much longer duration of action than temazepam. When used for premedication, a dose of 2–4 mg is given the night before or early on the day of surgery. Amnesia is a marked feature of this drug.

Intravenous lorazepam is currently the drug of choice in the management of major status epilepticus, because it has a longer duration of antiepileptic action than diazepam (see below). It can also be used in the management of severe acute panic attacks either intramuscularly or intravenously, in a dose of 25–30 μg kg⁻¹ (usual dose 1.5–2.5 mg). The intramuscular route should be used only when no other route is available.

Adverse reactions

Adverse reactions to benzodiazepines are dose-related and predictable from their pharmacodynamic effects. Oversedation, ventilatory depression, haemodynamic instability and airway obstruction may all follow inadvertent overdosage and are more likely in elderly and debilitated patients.

Flumazenil

Flumazenil is a very high-affinity competitive antagonist for all other ligands at the benzodiazepine receptor. It rapidly reverses all the CNS effects of benzodiazepines and also the other potentially dangerous adverse physiological effects, including respiratory and cardiovascular depression and airway obstruction.

Flumazenil has only very slight intrinsic activity at high dose and is very well tolerated, with minimal adverse effects.

Flumazenil is rapidly cleared from plasma and metabolized by the liver. It has a very short elimination half-life of less than 1 h. Its duration of action depends on the dose administered and the identity and dose of the agonist. It ranges from 20 min to 2 h and the potential exists for resedation if the agonist has a long half-life, necessitating a period of close observation. Repeated administration may be necessary.

Dosage and administration

Flumazenil is presented for intravenous use in 5-mL ampoules containing 100 μg mL⁻¹. The usual clinically effective dose is 0.2–1 mg given as 0.1–0.2 mg boluses and repeated at 1-min intervals. The dose in diagnosis of coma should not exceed 2 mg.

Indications

Reversal of sedation. It has been suggested that sedation be reversed electively to speed the through-put of day-case patients or to minimize the period of sedation in sick or debilitated patients. The risks of resedation make this undesirable as a routine. The reversal of inadvertent oversedation is uncontroversial and an important indication for the use of flumazenil.

In self-poisoning. Treatment of benzodiazepine overdosage in cases of unconsciousness and respiratory depression may avoid the need for artificial ventilation. Repeated doses or a continuous infusion are required until plasma concentrations of the agonist have decreased. In coma of unknown aetiology, flumazenil may be given as a diagnostic tool.

In the ITU. Prolonged sedation, resulting usually from the accumulation of midazolam in patients with renal failure, may be treated with an infusion of flumazenil. Occasionally, the drug is given as a bolus to reverse sedation and permit neurological assessment.

Precautions

Epileptic patients. There is a risk of seizures, especially if a benzodiazepine has been prescribed as antiepileptic therapy.

Benzodiazepine dependence. Withdrawal symptoms may be precipitated.

Anxiety reactions. These may occur after rapid reversal of heavy sedation.

Patients with severe head injury. Flumazenil may precipitate a sudden increase in intracranial pressure.

NEUROLEPTICS

This group of sedative drugs includes the phenothiazines and the butyrophenones; the drugs are also used as antipsychotics.

Neurolepsis describes a characteristic drug-induced change in behaviour. There is an altered state of awareness, with suppression of spontaneous movement and a placid compliant affect. Loss of consciousness does not occur, and spinal and central reflexes remain intact. The combination of a neuroleptic drug with an opioid, usually fentanyl, is termed neurolept-analgesia. This was a popular means of providing sedation before the advent of intravenous benzodiazepines. There is no amnesia and the patient may subsequently report unpleasant mental agitation despite a calm demeanour. The opioid obtunds the unpleasant mental experience but may result in respiratory depression. The addition of nitrous oxide may be used to produce neuroleptanaesthesia, in which consciousness is lost.

Mechanism of action

Neuroleptics interfere with dopaminergic transmission in the brain by blocking dopamine receptors. At some synapses, dopamine is the stimulatory transmitter and GABA the inhibitory transmitter, so in common with other sedatives, neuroleptics enhance the effects of GABA. Dopamine blockade results in useful antiemetic activity but also carries the inevitable potential for extrapyramidal side-effects. Neuroleptic drugs also have actions at cholinergic, α-adrenergic, histaminergic and serotinergic receptors, and these properties influence their side-effects and the degree of sedation produced.

Haloperidol

Haloperidol is a butyrophenone with a long duration of action. It has almost no α-adrenoceptor blocking activity. It is a potent antiemetic but has a high incidence of extrapyramidal side-effects. It has been reported as a cause of the *neuroleptic malignant syndrome*, a rare but potentially fatal reaction. The syndrome is characterized by hyperthermia, muscle hypertonicity, autonomic instability and fluctuating levels of consciousness and has some features in common with malignant hyperthermia associated with anaesthesia. Treatment includes supportive measures, dopamine agonists and dantrolene.

Haloperidol may be used in the short-term management of the acutely agitated patient, after sinister causes of confusion such as hypoxaemia and sepsis have been excluded. It may be given orally in a dose of 1.5–3 mg two to three times daily. It may also be administered by i.m. or i.v. injection in a dose of 2–5 mg. A dose of 1.25 mg is effective in prevention of postoperative nausea and vomiting.

Droperidol

Droperidol is a butyrophenone, a class of drug with structural similarities to the phenothiazines. It is a powerful antiemetic, acting at the chemoreceptor trigger zone. Large doses may produce dystonic reactions. Droperidol has mild α-adrenoceptor blocking actions, which may cause vasodilatation after intravenous administration, resulting in hypotension.

Droperidol has an onset time of 3–10 min after intravenous injection, with a duration of action of 12 h

or longer. It undergoes hepatic metabolism, but approximately 10% of the drug is excreted unchanged in the urine.

Droperidol is presently not available in the UK, but is still used in several other countries. Its uses include the following.

Premedication. Droperidol may be given orally or intramuscularly, and reliably produces sedation. It may result in delayed recovery, with sedation persisting well into the postoperative period because the effects of anaesthetic drugs are potentiated.

Antiemesis. The dose is often limited to 2.5 mg intravenously to provide antiemesis without unwanted sedation.

Neuroleptanalgesia/anaesthesia. Droperidol is administered intravenously in a dose of up to 10 mg in combination with an opioid, usually fentanyl, to produce neuroleptanalgesia; addition of nitrous oxide results in neuroleptanaesthesia.

Chlorpromazine

Chlorpromazine is a phenothiazine which is prescribed commonly as an antipsychotic but no longer used as an adjunct in anaesthesia. It may be used in the same way as haloperidol in the acutely confused or agitated patient. It has pronounced sedative properties and potentiates the actions of anaesthetic drugs. There is marked antiemetic activity. A mild anticholinergic action moderates the incidence of extrapyramidal effects. α-Adrenoceptor blockade produces vasodilatation and may result in hypotension which is exacerbated by direct cardiac depression and depression of vasomotor reflexes. Central temperature control mechanisms are affected by chlorpromazine, with a reduced shivering response. The neuroleptic malignant syndrome has been reported following its use. In elderly or debilitated patients the dose should be reduced by half.

The dose used to treat acute agitation is usually 25 mg i.m. or i.v. The drug must be diluted and given slowly when used intravenously.

α$_2$-ADRENOCEPTOR AGONISTS

α$_2$-Adrenoceptor agonists have been used widely in veterinary anaesthetic practice for many years. Their properties of sedation, anxiolysis and analgesia have been recognized as potentially beneficial in humans, but they have not found a place as sedatives in routine clinical practice. The main disadvantage is the risk of excessive cardiovascular depression. In anaesthetic practice, attention has turned to making use of the haemodynamic actions of these drugs to prevent perioperative cardiovascular complications. There is some evidence that they may be useful adjuncts in cardiac and vascular surgery.

Mechanism of action

α_2-Adrenergic receptors are involved in the regulation of the release of the neurotransmitter noradrenaline (norepinephrine). These receptors were initially classified anatomically as presynaptic, but α_2-adrenoceptors are also found postsynaptically and extrasynaptically. The more correct pharmacological classification is based on the predominantly α_2-selectivity of the antagonist yohimbine. α_2-Adrenoceptors are located peripherally and centrally, with the centrally mediated effects of particular relevance in anaesthesia.

The characteristic central effects of α_2-adrenoceptor agonists are sedation, anxiolysis and hypnosis. The locus caeruleus is a small neuronal nucleus in the upper brainstem that contains the major noradrenergic cell group in the brain. This nucleus is an important modulator of wakefulness. Activation of α_2-adrenoceptors results in inhibition of transmitter release. The locus caeruleus also has connections to the cortex, thalamus and vasomotor centre.

α_2-Adrenoceptor agonists have analgesic properties. Descending fibres from the locus caeruleus decrease nociceptive transmission at the spinal level. In addition, α_2-adrenoceptors occur in primary sensory neurones and the dorsal horn of the spinal cord.

Many ligands at α_2-adrenoceptors are substituted imidazoles. It has been demonstrated recently that in some tissues, including brain, non-adrenergic imidazole binding sites exist: the imidazoline (I) receptors. Imidazoline receptors are found in the medulla and are involved in the regulation of arterial pressure. First-generation, centrally acting antihypertensives such as clonidine were thought originally to act via α_2 actions alone, reducing sympathetic outflow. The main disadvantage of the perioperative use of clonidine is the potential for cardiovascular depression, with bradycardia and hypotension. Recent work suggests that the hypotensive effects are also mediated via I receptors. The new centrally acting antihypertensive moxonidine has activity primarily at I receptors and is much less sedative than clonidine. An α_2-adrenoceptor agonist sedative agent lacking adverse haemodynamic effects remains a hope for the future.

Clonidine

Clonidine is an imidazoline compound and a selective α_2-adrenoceptor agonist with an $\alpha_2 : \alpha_1$ ratio of 200:1. It is currently the only drug in this group available for use in anaesthetic practice. Clonidine has proved effec-

tive in the treatment of patients with severe hypertension but it is recognized that abrupt discontinuation of therapy can result in rebound hypertension. Clonidine is lipid-soluble and is absorbed rapidly and almost completely after oral administration, with peak plasma concentrations occurring in 60–90 min. It may be administered transdermally and is also available as a solution for intravenous, intramuscular, epidural, intrathecal and local use. The elimination half-life is 9–13 h; 50% is excreted unchanged by the kidneys and 50% is metabolized in the liver.

Pharmacological effects

Clonidine produces sedation and anxiolysis. It also results in a reduction in requirements for both intravenous and volatile anaesthetic agents. There is a ceiling to the reduction of MAC effect, because of the potential for activity at α_1-receptors at high dose. More selective α_2-adrenoceptor agonists reduce MAC to a much greater extent.

Clonidine is a potent analgesic, acting centrally and on the α_2-adrenoceptors of the dorsal horn. It may be administered intravenously, intrathecally or epidurally to produce an analgesic response. Synergism exists with opioids, and the actions of local anaesthetics are also potentiated. Clonidine is used to provide analgesia in the perioperative period and also in chronic pain syndromes.

The cardiovascular effects of clonidine probably involve both α_2-adrenoceptors and imidazoline receptors. Administration leads to a decrease in heart rate and arterial pressure. Clonidine is known to lower the 'set point' around which arterial pressure is regulated. The α_2-agonist effects are a reduction in sympathetic tone and an increase in parasympathetic tone. The resulting decreases in heart rate, myocardial contractility and systemic vascular resistance lead to a reduction in myocardial oxygen requirements. This may be used to advantage in attenuating stress-induced haemodynamic responses. However, undesirable cardiovascular depression has been the major limiting factor in developing the use of clonidine as a sedative.

Clonidine has minor respiratory effects, causing only a small reduction in minute ventilation.

Dosage and indications

Premedication. The oral dose is 200–300 µg given 1 h preoperatively.

Analgesia. Epidural clonidine is safe and effective in the management of acute postoperative pain. The epidural dose is 1–2 $\mu g\ kg^{-1}$.

Anaesthesia. Intravenous clonidine in a dose of 150–300 μg has been used as an adjunct to general anaesthesia and to attenuate haemodynamic responses. There may be a risk of awareness if haemodynamic variables alone are used to monitor the depth of anaesthesia. Prolonged duration of action and cardiovascular depression make clonidine unsuitable for use as a sedative for short procedures.

Withdrawal of drugs in dependence. Clonidine has been used to facilitate drug withdrawal in states of opioid, benzodiazepine and alcohol dependence.

Dexmedetomidine and medetomidine

Medetomidine is the prototype of the newer selective α_2-agonists. Its active ingredient, the D-stereoisomer dexmedetomidine, is used routinely as an adjunct in veterinary anaesthesia. It has much greater efficacy than clonidine and is shorter-acting. The $\alpha_2{:}\alpha_1$ selectivity ratio is 1600:1 and the lack of α_1 activity leads to a MAC-sparing effect of up to 90%. Dexmedetomidine is an imidazole and so also binds to I receptors. In common with clonidine, this drug produces sedation, anxiolysis, analgesia and haemodynamic depression. Dexmedetomidine is approved for sedating patients in the intensive care unit and recent evaluations have demonstrated that, given by infusion, it provides reliable and manageable sedation, although hypotension and bradycardia do occur more frequently than in control patients.

The selective α_2-adrenoreceptor antagonist atipamezole has been used in veterinary practice and reverses the sedation caused by dexmedetomidine.

ANTIEPILEPTICS

Epilepsy is a common condition, affecting 350 000 people in the UK. Most patients with recurrent seizures require antiepileptic therapy. Epilepsy is not a uniform condition but comprises a range of seizure types and epilepsy syndromes. In 30% of patients, there is an identifiable neurological or systemic disorder leading to epilepsy. In the event of seizures occurring unexpectedly, treatable causes should be excluded. In the perioperative period, precipitating factors such as hypoglycaemia, electrolyte abnormalities and metabolic disturbance must be considered. Antiepileptic drugs are increasingly establishing a place in the treatment of neuropathic pain.

General principles of antiepileptic therapy

An epileptic seizure is a sudden stereotypical episode with changes in motor activity, sensation, behaviour, emotion, memory or consciousness due to an abnormal electrochemical discharge in the brain. Epileptic seizures have many manifestations. Seizure classification is based on clinical description and EEG pattern and is important in selecting the most effective therapy. Monotherapy is preferred for most patients because combination therapy enhances toxicity and drug interactions may occur between antiepileptic drugs. The best drug for the specific seizure type and individual patient is selected and administered in a dose high enough to bring the plasma concentration into the therapeutic range without unacceptable side-effects. All antiepileptic drugs have significant dose-related side-effects and some are associated with serious idiosyncratic reactions. For most of the established antiepileptics, the complexity of their pharmacokinetic profiles makes therapeutic drug level monitoring necessary. Initial dosing schedules are complicated, because for many antiepileptic drugs it is important to increase the dose slowly to avoid toxic side-effects. If seizure control remains poor, a second drug is added or substituted while the original choice is withdrawn slowly. Up to 70% of patients may be managed successfully with a single drug, but a substantial minority report seizures despite combination therapy.

There are several problems associated with the established antiepileptics. These include sedation and cognitive impairment, long-term side-effects, pharmacokinetic interactions and teratogenesis. In the last decade, several new antiepileptics have become available. Some of these appear to offer greater efficacy with fewer disadvantages, although at a higher cost. In the UK, the use of newer drugs for the management of epilepsy in children and adults has been evaluated recently and national guidance has been issued. Use of the newer drugs is now recommended for patients who have not benefited from treatment with the older drugs and for those in whom the older drugs are unsuitable because of contraindications, drug interactions or child-bearing potential. Some of the newer drugs are recommended as first-line treatment in a number of childhood epilepsy syndromes.

Mechanisms of action

Antiepileptic drugs act by inhibiting the abnormal cerebral discharge leading to the seizure or inhibiting its propagation through the brain. There is no class action for this group of drugs; they act by several different single or multiple mechanisms. The most important of these include enhancement of the effects of GABA and limiting sustained repetitive neuronal firing through voltage- and use-dependent blockade of sodium channels. The indications for use, and the mechanisms of action, of new and established antiepileptics are shown in Table 7.2.

Pharmacokinetics

The pharmacokinetic profiles of many antiepileptic drugs determine dosing schedules and affect important drug interactions which can result in potential adverse effects. Some of the older drugs, including phenytoin and sodium valproate, have a high degree of protein binding. Bioactivity may be influenced by changes in the availability of binding sites. Factors which may decrease protein binding, such as competition with other drugs or a decrease in serum albumin concentration, may lead to toxicity.

Hepatic metabolism is important in the elimination of most antiepileptics. Plasma drug concentrations may be altered by changes in the activity of oxidative enzymes. Induction of microsomal enzymes accelerates the metabolism of both the inducer and other drugs. Some drugs inhibit metabolism and may interact with antiepileptics to produce higher serum drug concentrations. Hepatic dysfunction may also result in decreased metabolism. Significant renal excretion of phenobarbital and ethosuximide leads to accumulation of these drugs in patients with impairment of renal function.

INDIVIDUAL DRUGS

Phenytoin

Phenytoin is a hydantoin, similar in structure to barbiturates. The usual oral dose is 250–500 mg daily. It is also available for intravenous use and has an important place in the management of status epilepticus (see below). Phenytoin has membrane-stabilizing

Table 7.2   Antiepileptics: mechanisms of action and indications for use

Drug	Mechanism of action	Indications
Phenytoin	Voltage-dependent block of sodium channels	Partial and generalized tonic-clonic seizures
Pentobarbital	Increases chloride channel conductance and so enhances GABA-induced effects	Partial and generalized tonic-clonic seizures
Carbamazepine	Voltage-dependent block of sodium channels	Partial and generalized tonic-clonic seizures
Sodium valproate	Voltage-dependent block of sodium channels Increases calcium-dependent potassium conductance Other mechanisms also	All seizure types, especially idiopathic generalized epilepsy
Ethosuximide	Reduces slow calcium conductance in thalamic neurones	Uncomplicated absence seizures
Clonazepam, clobazam	Enhancement of GABA effects	All seizure types
Vigabatrin	Irreversible inhibition of the enzyme GABA transaminase	Add on for partial seizures ± secondary generalizations. Mono-infantile spasms
Lamotrigine	Prolongs inactivated state of voltage-dependent sodium channels	Adjunct or monotherapy for partial and tonic-clonic seizures
Gabapentin	Binds to calcium channels	Add on for partial seizures ± secondary generalizations
Topiramate	Blockade of sodium channels. Attenuation of neuronal excitation. Enhancement of GABA	Add on for refractory partial seizures ± secondary generalizations
Tiagabine	Inhibits uptake of GABA into neurones	Add on for partial seizures ± secondary generalizations

actions and as a result has the potential to cause profound cardiovascular depression when administered too rapidly by the intravenous route. As it is formulated in propylene glycol, it is very irritant, with a high incidence of thrombophlebitis after intravenous administration. It is unsuitable for admixture with concurrent infusions. A newer preparation, the prodrug fosphenytoin, is water-soluble and much less irritant, although more expensive. Fosphenytoin is rapidly converted by serum phosphatases to phenytoin when it is in the vascular compartment. Therapeutic concentrations may be obtained in less than 10 min after intravenous administration. Phenytoin is 90% protein-bound and undergoes hepatic metabolism. Phenytoin has several important interactions with other drugs. It is an enzyme inducer and so may accelerate the metabolism of other drugs. It is noteworthy that the elimination half-life of phenytoin is concentration-dependent. At high plasma concentrations, the metabolism changes from first-order to saturation (zero-order) kinetics, with the risk of a large increase in plasma concentration from a small increase in dose. Other drugs, including cimetidine and amiodarone, which inhibit the metabolism of phenytoin, are likely to lead to neurotoxic effects because of the saturatable metabolism.

Phenytoin has a range of dose-related and idiosyncratic adverse effects. Reversible cosmetic changes are a problem. Neurotoxic symptoms at high plasma concentrations include drowsiness, dysarthria, ataxia, tremor and cognitive difficulties.

Phenobarbital

Phenobarbital is a barbiturate with a long half-life of 70–140 h. The usual dose is 60–180 mg orally at night. It is 50% protein-bound and largely undergoes hepatic metabolism, with 25% excreted unchanged in the urine. Phenobarbital is an enzyme inducer and so accelerates the metabolism of other drugs. The main disadvantage of this drug is sedation and other CNS effects, including depression of mood, cognition and memory. Children may develop hyperactivity and aggression. As with all barbiturates, toxic levels may lead to respiratory depression and death. Phenobarbital also has a role in the management of status epilepticus.

Primidone

Primidone is essentially a prodrug and is metabolized to phenobarbital. It is tolerated less well than phenobarbital and is no longer recommended routinely in the management of epilepsy.

Carbamazepine

Carbamazepine is related structurally to tricyclic antidepressants. The usual daily dose is 0.8–1.2 g in divided doses. Carbamazepine is 70–80% protein-bound and undergoes hepatic metabolism. This produces an active metabolite, and with multiple doses the pharmacodynamic half-life is 8–24 h. Carbamazepine is an enzyme inducer and the eventual maintenance dose for each patient depends on the degree of autoinduction of its own metabolism. Carbamazepine accelerates hepatic oxidation and conjugation of other lipid-soluble drugs and has an important interaction with the oral contraceptive pill. Other drugs, including cimetidine, erythromycin and propoxyphene, inhibit the metabolism of carbamazepine and may lead to toxicity. Carbamazepine has a wider therapeutic index and fewer adverse effects than phenytoin or phenobarbital. The most common side-effects are diplopia, headache and nausea. A mild reversible leucopenia is not uncommon, but there have also been reports of agranulocytosis and aplastic anaemia following its use. At high doses, it has an ADH-like effect, with retention of water and the development of hyponatraemia.

Sodium valproate

Sodium valproate is a derivative of carboxylic acid. The usual maintenance dose is 1–2 g daily in divided doses. It is also available as an intravenous solution for use when oral administration is not possible.

Sodium valproate is approximately 90% protein-bound. It undergoes hepatic metabolism with production of active metabolites and has an elimination half-life of 7–17 h. Sodium valproate is an enzyme inhibitor and may inhibit the metabolism of other drugs, including other antiepileptics. Common side-effects include gastrointestinal disturbance, weight gain, menstrual irregularities and dose-related tremor. Mild hepatic dysfunction is common but there is also a risk of hepatotoxicity. Monitoring of liver function tests is recommended and administration of the drug should be discontinued if the prothrombin time is prolonged.

Ethosuximide

Ethosuximide is the drug of choice for simple absence seizures. The usual dose is 1–1.5 g daily in divided doses. Ethosuximide is not protein-bound. It undergoes hepatic metabolism, with 25% excreted unchanged. It has an elimination half-life of 20–60 h, with more rapid clearance in children. Enzyme inhibitors and inducers may affect its metabolism.

Common side-effects include gastrointestinal disturbance and adverse CNS effects, usually lethargy, dizziness and ataxia.

Clonazepam

Clonazepam is a benzodiazepine. The usual maintenance dose is 4–8 mg daily in divided doses. It is also available as an intravenous preparation which has a place in the management of status epilepticus.

Clonazepam is 90% protein-bound and undergoes hepatic metabolism with an elimination half-life of 30–40 h. The main disadvantage of clonazepam is its sedative effect. There is also a tendency to develop tolerance to its antiepileptic activity, with an unfortunate rebound increase in seizure frequency when it is withdrawn.

Vigabatrin

This is the first of the newer antiepileptics. The usual oral maintenance dose is 2–3 g daily. Vigabatrin is not protein bound and is excreted unchanged in the urine. It has a short elimination half-life but its duration of action is longer, as it takes several days for the enzyme GABA transaminase to regenerate after treatment is stopped. It has few interactions with other drugs. Vigabatrin is usually tolerated well but CNS side-effects, including sedation and dizziness, may occur. The drug should be avoided if there is a psychiatric history because depression and psychosis have been reported.

Lamotrigine

The usual maintenance dose is 150–200 mg daily. Lamotrigine is metabolized in the liver and has an elimination half-life of 22–36 h. Its metabolism is accelerated by enzyme-inducing antiepileptics such as phenytoin, and its action is prolonged by the enzyme inhibition of sodium valproate. Lamotrigine does not influence the metabolism of other drugs. Adverse effects are confined largely to the CNS, and include headache, diplopia, sedation, ataxia and tremor. These develop more commonly when lamotrigine is used in combination with carbamazepine.

Gabapentin

The usual maintenance dose is 1.2 g daily in three divided doses. Gabapentin is excreted unchanged by the kidneys and has a short half-life of 5–7 h. It does not interact significantly with other drugs. This drug is generally well tolerated, with a side-effect profile similar to that of lamotrigine.

Topiramate

The usual maintenance dose range is 100–400 mg daily in two doses. Topiramate undergoes hepatic metabolism which is accelerated by the enzyme inducers. Topiramate selectively reduces the clearance of phenytoin in some patients and may accelerate metabolism of the oral contraceptive pill. It has a wide range of adverse effects, the commonest being neurological symptoms, anorexia and weight loss. It also has the potential to cause nephrolithiasis as a result of inhibition of carbonic anhydrase; consequently, it is important to ensure adequate hydration throughout the perioperative period in surgical patients who are taking the drug. It is the only newer antiepileptic which shows evidence of possible teratogenicity. These disadvantages are offset by its high efficacy.

Tiagabine

The usual maintenance dose range is 15–30 mg daily in three divided doses. Tiagabine undergoes hepatic metabolism which is accelerated by enzyme inducers and consequently the dose should be increased when used with enzyme-inducing drugs. It has a short half-life of 5–9 h and does not affect the metabolism of other drugs. Side-effects include gastrointestinal upset and CNS effects, particularly dizziness.

ANAESTHETIC CONSIDERATIONS

Patients receiving long-term antiepileptic therapy should receive their usual treatment regimens as far as possible, with the aim of maintaining therapeutic drug concentrations. The propensity for adverse interactions with many different drugs is particularly high with the established antiepileptics. Changes in protein binding may result from disturbances of acid–base balance or hypoalbuminaemia. The development of renal or hepatic dysfunction in the perioperative period may reduce the elimination of antiepileptics, leading to toxicity.

STATUS EPILEPTICUS

Status epilepticus is an important medical emergency that is commonly seen in the emergency department and ITU. Failure to diagnose and treat status epilepticus may result in significant morbidity and mortality. Status epilepticus has been defined as continuous seizure activity lasting for 30 min, or intermittent activity of the same duration without recovery of consciousness between episodes. There should be a clear distinction between typical isolated seizure activity lasting for a few minutes and terminating spontaneously, and status epilepticus. It has been suggested that a much shorter duration of seizure activity (10–20 min) should trigger the diagnosis of status epilepticus and the instigation of appropriate intervention in order to reduce the progressive physiological and neurochemical changes associated with unremitting seizure activity. There is also evidence that the longer the seizure activity goes on, the more refractory to treatment it becomes. First-line therapy is effective in controlling seizures in 55% of patients and should be administered without delay.

The overall mortality of status epilepticus in adults is 25%, although most deaths are attributable to the underlying condition which causes the seizures. Individuals with a history of epilepsy are at particular risk of developing status epilepticus but these represent only 50% of patients with status. In known epileptics, a recent change in antiepileptic treatment may precipitate the seizures. In non-epileptics, many cases arise as a result of acute neurological problems including cerebrovascular accidents, cerebral trauma (including surgery), cerebral tumours, cerebral infections and cerebral anoxic/hypoxic damage. Acute systemic illness may also be a precipitating cause; seizures may occur as a result of sepsis, electrolyte imbalance, renal failure, drug toxicity and alcohol-related problems.

The clinical manifestations of status epilepticus vary according to the type of seizure activity; all seizure types may become prolonged. Seizures may be classified by the presence of motor convulsions and whether they affect the whole or part of the body. Accurate diagnosis, which is more difficult with non-convulsive seizures, may affect management. Generalized convulsive status epilepticus (GCSE) is the form most often seen and is a medical emergency requiring the most urgent control of seizures.

Pathophysiology

GCSE has both systemic and cerebral effects; systemic effects are much less marked with non-convulsive or partial status epilepticus. Cerebral effects are characterized by increased cerebral metabolic demand caused by abnormally discharging cells. This leads to an increase in cerebral blood flow initially. However, after about 30 min of seizure activity, autoregulation fails, cerebral blood flow decreases as systemic arterial pressure decreases and there is an increase in intracranial pressure. At this stage, cerebral oxygen delivery is insufficient to meet demand and clinically, although electrical seizure activity continues, it may be manifest as only minor twitching. Inhibition of GABA and excessive activity of the excitatory neurotransmitter glutamate are thought to play a role in cerebral cell damage.

During prolonged GCSE, systemic effects compound the inadequate cerebral oxygen supply. Increased minute ventilation occurs initially, but as seizure activity continues, ventilation becomes progressively inadequate, and apnoea may occur. Hypoxaemia may be exacerbated by pulmonary aspiration and pulmonary oedema. Cardiovascular changes follow a similar pattern, with an initial increase in cardiac output giving way to hypotension, which may progress to cardiogenic shock. Arrhythmias are common and ECG changes are usually a bad prognostic sign. Metabolic derangement also contributes to neuronal damage. Hyperthermia results from muscle activity and massive catecholamine release. In addition, anaerobic muscle metabolism results in a metabolic acidosis.

Treatment of status epilepticus

The aims of treatment are to terminate seizure activity, prevent seizure recurrence and to manage both the precipitating cause and the complications resulting from the seizures:

1. Basic life support: maintain the airway, ensure adequate ventilation and oxygenation and ensure adequate circulation. Tracheal intubation is usually required in status epilepticus to facilitate adequate ventilation and to secure and protect the airway. Neuromuscular blockade is required to permit tracheal intubation but should not be continued, as it interferes with monitoring of seizure activity.
2. A vein should be cannulated and blood samples should be taken to check the blood glucose concentration and for basic biochemical and haematological investigations. An immediate bedside measurement of blood glucose concentration is important, but glucose should not be given empirically as hyperglycaemia may exacerbate neuronal damage. Confirmed hypoglycaemia must be treated urgently.
3. First-line pharmacological therapy is i.v. lorazepam in a dose of up to 0.1 mg kg^{-1}, but with an initial dose of no more than 2–4 mg. Lorazepam is preferred to Diazemuls because it has a longer effective duration of action in the brain. Intravenous midazolam has also been used; it has a rapid onset of action but the disadvantage of a short duration of action. If it is impossible to obtain i.v. access, midazolam may be given by the buccal route in a dose of 10 mg or intranasally in a dose of 200 µg kg^{-1}; alternatively, diazepam may be given as a rectal solution (available as rectal tubes in a range of doses). Redistribution of diazepam may lead to seizure recurrence after about 20 min.

Respiratory depression may occur with standard clinical doses of benzodiazepines, and should be anticipated and managed accordingly.

4. If benzodiazepines fail to stop seizures within 10 min, second-line therapy should be used. Phenytoin (or fosphenytoin) is the second-line drug of choice and is indicated also to prevent recurrence of seizures, particularly following neurosurgery or head injury. An intravenous loading dose of 15 mg kg^{-1} is given at a rate not exceeding 50 mg min^{-1}. There is a risk of serious cardiovascular complications, particularly hypotension and arrhythmias; consequently, ECG and arterial pressure monitoring are mandatory. If phenytoin is administered via a vein distal to the antecubital fossa there is a 6% incidence of 'purple-glove' syndrome, a serious soft tissue reaction which may lead to tissue necrosis.

5. Refractory status. Phenobarbital 10–20 mg kg^{-1} is effective for refractory status epilepticus, but prolonged sedation is inevitable at this dosage, making neurological assessment difficult. Respiratory and cardiovascular depression are common. If seizure activity continues, the definitive treatment for refractory status epilepticus is general anaesthesia. This management should be undertaken only in an ITU. Artificial ventilation of the lungs is required because of the risk of profound respiratory depression. Paralysis with neuromuscular blocking agents facilitates ventilation and decreases oxygen consumption, but masks continued seizure activity; this is undesirable because, although no seizure activity is apparent externally, continuing electrical seizure activity in the brain results in a high cerebral metabolic rate for oxygen ($CMRo_2$), which may result in cerebral ischaemia. It is therefore necessary to monitor the EEG with a device such as the cerebral function analysing monitor. The electrophysiological goal for treatment remains a matter for debate, but the most commonly used end-point is burst suppression. Cardiovascular support may also be required. Thiopental has been used by infusion at a dose of 3–5 mg kg^{-1} h^{-1}. In adults, propofol has gained popularity as an alternative, given by infusion at a rate of 2–10 mg kg^{-1} h^{-1}. Barbiturates are immunosuppressive, and prolonged use increases the risk of infection. Metabolic acidosis and lipidaemia may occur with prolonged use of propofol. Long-acting antiepileptic therapy should be maintained during this period and drug concentrations must be monitored.

6. After seizures have been controlled, a precipitating cause should be sought. There may be diagnostic clues in the history or on examination, but urgent imaging of the brain is often indicated.

Clomethiazole

Clomethiazole is an antiepileptic with a limited place in the management of status epilepticus. It is a GABA agonist and was used extensively in the past to manage acute alcohol withdrawal states, a role for which benzodiazepines are now preferred.

In addition to its antiepileptic properties, it is a powerful sedative. Respiratory depression, airway obstruction and hypotension may follow rapid infusion. Prolonged infusion may be associated with a decreasing level of consciousness. Clomethiazole has a short half-life, but although the rate of infusion may theoretically be titrated against clinical effect, accumulation of the drug may lead to delayed recovery after prolonged administration. It should be avoided in patients who have impaired hepatic or renal function.

Dosage and administration. Clomethiazole is available as a 0.8% solution for intravenous infusion. This solution contains only 32 mmol L^{-1} of sodium and no other electrolytes. Administration of large volumes carries a risk of water intoxication and fluid overload. The solution is usually administered initially at a rate of 5–15 mL min^{-1} for about 6–8 min and the rate is then reduced to 0.5–1 mL min^{-1}. Clomethiazole is also available orally as capsules or a syrup.

FURTHER READING

American Society of Anesthesiologists Task Force 2002 Practice guidelines for sedation and analgesia by non-anesthesiologists. Anesthesiology 96: 1004–1017

Brodie M J, Dichter M A 1996 Antiepileptic drugs. New England Journal of Medicine 334: 168–175

Chapman M G, Smith M, Hirsch N P 2001 Status epilepticus. Anaesthesia 56: 648–659

Dichter M A, Brodie M J 1996 New antiepileptic drugs. New England Journal of Medicine 334: 1583–1590

Ostermann M E, Keenan S P, Seiferling R A, Sibbald W J 2000 Sedation in the intensive care unit: a systematic review. Journal of the American Medical Association 283: 1451–1459

UK Academy of Medical Royal Colleges and their Faculties, 2001. Implementing and ensuring safe sedation practice for healthcare procedures in adults.

Scottish Intercollegiate Guidelines Network 2004: sedation of children SIGN guidelines: www.sign.ac.uk

8 Drugs acting on the cardiovascular system

Many drugs have either primary or secondary effects on the cardiovascular and autonomic nervous systems. Several of the drugs discussed in this chapter have more than one clinical indication so drugs are considered according to their mechanism of action. An understanding of drugs acting on the cardiovascular and autonomic nervous systems requires an understanding of autonomic physiology and pharmacology.

THE AUTONOMIC NERVOUS SYSTEM

The term autonomic nervous system (ANS) refers to the nervous and humoral mechanisms which modify the function of the autonomous or automatic organs. These include heart rate and force of contraction, calibre of blood vessels, contraction and relaxation of smooth muscle in gut, bladder and bronchi, visual accommodation and pupillary size. Other functions include regulation of secretion from exocrine and other glands and aspects of metabolism (e.g. glycogenolysis and lipolysis) (Table 8.1). There is constant activity of both the sympathetic and parasympathetic nervous systems even at rest. This is termed sympathetic or parasympathetic tone and allows alterations in autonomic activity to produce rapid two-way regulation of physiological effect. The ANS is controlled by centres in the spinal cord, brainstem and hypothalamus, which are in turn influenced by higher centres in the cerebral and particularly the limbic cortex. The ANS is also influenced by visceral reflexes whereby afferent signals enter the autonomic ganglia, spinal cord, hypothalamus, or brainstem and directly elicit appropriate reflex responses via the visceral organs. The efferent autonomic signals are transmitted through the body to two major subdivisions (separated by anatomical, physiological and pharmacological criteria), the sympathetic and the parasympathetic nervous systems.

THE SYMPATHETIC NERVOUS SYSTEM

The sympathetic nervous system includes nerves that originate in the spinal cord between the first thoracic and second lumbar segments (T1 to L2). Fibres leave the spinal cord with the anterior nerve roots and then branch off as white rami communicantes to synapse in the bilateral paravertebral sympathetic ganglionic chains, though some preganglionic fibres synapse instead in the paravertebral ganglia (e.g. coeliac, mesenteric and hypogastric) in the abdomen before travelling to their effector organ with the relevant arteries. Postganglionic fibres travel from paravertebral ganglia in sympathetic nerves (to supply the internal viscera, including the heart) and spinal nerves (which innervate the peripheral vasculature and sweat glands). Sympathetic nerves throughout the circulation contain vasoconstrictor fibres, particularly in the kidneys, the spleen, the gut and the skin but in skeletal muscle, coronary and cerebral vessels, sympathetic vasodilator fibres predominate. Sympathetic stimulation therefore causes predominantly vasoconstriction but also a redistribution of blood flow to skeletal muscle; constriction of venous capacitance vessels may decrease their volume and thereby increase venous return. The effects of sympathetic stimulation at different receptors and effector organs is summarized in Table 8.1. The distribution of sympathetic nerve fibres to an organ or region may differ from the sensory or motor supply, according to its embryonic origin. For example, sympathetic fibres to the heart arise from T1 to T5 (but predominantly from T1 to T4), the neck is supplied by fibres from T2, the chest by fibres from T3 to T6 and the abdomen by fibres from T7 to T11.

Sympathetic neurotransmitters

The neurotransmitter present in preganglionic neurones is acetylcholine (ACh). These and other neurones containing ACh are termed *cholinergic*. However, the activity of preganglionic neurones is modulated by

Table 8.1 Effects of the sympathetic and parasympathetic nervous systems on peripheral effector organs, and receptor subtypes mediating these functions (where known). All postganglionic parasympathetic fibres are muscarinic (M), but in many sites the subtype has not been identified

| Organ | Sympathetic | | Parasympathetic | |
	Receptor subtype	Effect	Receptor subtype	Effect
Heart	β_1 also β_2, ? also α and DA_1	↑ Heart rate ↑ Force of contraction ↑ Conduction velocity ↑ Automaticity (β_2) ↑ Excitability	M_2	↓ Heart rate ↓ Force of contraction Slight ↓ conduction velocity
	α_1	↑ Force of contraction		
Arteries	β_1	Coronary vasodilatation	M^a	Vasodilatation in skin, skeletal muscle, pulmonary and coronary circulations
	β_2	Vasodilatation (skeletal muscle)		
	α_1, α_2	Vasoconstriction (coronary, pulmonary, renal and splanchnic circulations, skin and skeletal muscle)		
	DA_1, β_2	Splanchnic and renal vasodilatation		
Veins	α_1, also α_2 β_2	Vasoconstriction Vasodilatation		
Lung	β_2	Bronchodilatation Inhibition of secretions	M_3	Bronchoconstriction Stimulation of secretions
	α_1	Bronchoconstriction		
GI tract	$\alpha_1, \alpha_2, \beta_2$	Decreased motility	M	Increased motility Relaxation of sphincters Stimulation of secretions
	α_1, α_2	Contraction of sphincters Inhibition of secretions		
Pancreas	β_2 α_1, α_2	Increased insulin release Decreased insulin release		
Kidney	β	Renin secretion		
Liver	β_2, α $\beta_2, ?\alpha$	Glycogenolysis Gluconeogenesis	M	Glycogen synthesis
Bladder	β_2 α	Detrusor relaxation Sphincter contraction	M	Detrusor contraction Sphincter relaxation
Uterus	α_1 β_2	Myometrial contraction Myometrial relaxation		
Adipocytes	β_3	Lipolysis		
Eye	α_1	Mydriasis (radial muscle contraction) Ciliary muscle relaxation for far vision	M	Miosis Ciliary muscle contraction for near vision

Continued

111

Table 8.1 Effects of the sympathetic and parasympathetic nervous systems on peripheral effector organs, and receptor subtypes mediating these functions (where known). All postganglionic parasympathetic fibres are muscarinic (M), but in many sites the subtype has not been identified—Cont'd

| Organ | Sympathetic | | Parasympathetic | |
	Receptor subtype	Effect	Receptor subtype	Effect
Platelets	α_2	Promote platelet aggregation		
Sweat glands	M[b]	Sweating		

[a]Muscarinic receptors are present on vascular smooth muscle, but they are independent of parasympathetic innervation and have little or no physiological role in the control of vasomotor tone.
[b]Sympathetic cholinergic fibres supply sweat glands and arterioles in some sites.

several other neuropeptides including enkephalin, neurotensin, substance P, somatostatin, nitric oxide, serotonin and catecholamines. ACh is the transmitter at all preganglionic synapses, acting via nicotinic receptors. Postganglionic sympathetic neurones secrete noradrenaline and are termed *adrenergic* (except for postganglionic sympathetic nerve fibres to sweat glands, pilo-erector muscles and some blood vessels, which are cholinergic).

Activation of preganglionic nicotinic fibres to the adrenal medulla causes the release of adrenaline (epinephrine), which is released primarily as a circulating hormone and is only found in insignificant amounts in the nerve endings. Endogenous catecholamines (adrenaline, noradrenaline (norepinephrine) and dopamine) are synthesized from the essential amino acid phenylalanine. Their structure is based on a catechol ring (i.e. a benzene ring with -OH groups in the 3 and 4 positions), and an ethylamine side chain (Figs 8.1, 8.2); substitutions in the side chain produce the different compounds. Dopamine may act as a precursor for both adrenaline and noradrenaline when administered exogenously (see below).

The action of noradrenaline released from sympathetic nerve endings is terminated in one of three ways:

- re-uptake into the nerve terminal
- diffusion into the circulation
- enzymatic destruction.

Most noradrenaline released from sympathetic nerves is taken back into the presynaptic nerve ending for storage and subsequent reuse. Re-uptake is by active transport back into the nerve terminal cytoplasm and then into cytoplasmic vesicles. This mechanism of presynaptic re-uptake, termed *uptake*$_1$, is dependent on adenosine triphosphate (ATP) and Mg^{2+}, is enhanced by Li^+ and may be blocked by cocaine and tricyclic antidepressants. Endogenous catecholamines entering the circulation by diffusion from sympathetic nerve endings or by release from the adrenal gland are metabolized rapidly by the enzymes monamine oxidase (MAO) and catechol O-methyltransferase (COMT) in the liver, kidneys, gut and many other tissues. The metabolites are conjugated before being excreted in urine as 3-methoxy-4-hydroxymandelic acid, metanephrine (from adrenaline) and normetanephrine (from noradrenaline) (Fig. 8.3). Noradrenaline taken up into the nerve terminal may also be deaminated by cytoplasmic MAO.

Another mechanism for the postsynaptic cellular re-uptake of catecholamines, termed *uptake*$_2$, is present predominantly at the membrane of smooth muscle cells. It may be responsible for the termination of action of catecholamines released from the adrenal medulla.

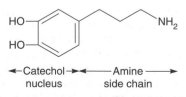

←Catechol→ ←—— Amine ——→
nucleus   side chain

Fig. 8.1
Standard molecular structure of catecholamines.

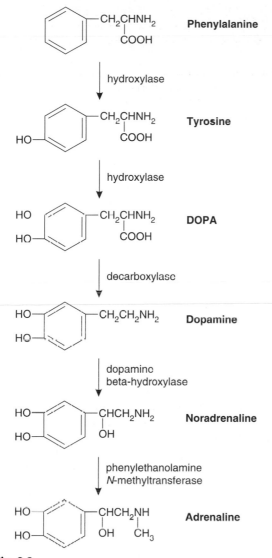

Fig. 8.2
Synthesis of endogenous catecholamines.

Adrenergic receptor pharmacology

The actions of catecholamines are mediated by specific postsynaptic cell surface receptors. The original classification of these receptors into α- and β-adrenergic receptors was based upon the effects of adrenaline at peripheral sympathetic sites, α-receptors being responsible for vasoconstriction and β-receptors mediating effects on the heart, bronchial and intestinal smooth muscle. However, several subtypes of α- and β-receptors exist in addition to receptors specific for dopamine (DA_1 and DA_2 subtypes). Two α- and β-receptor subtypes are well defined on functional,

anatomical and pharmacological grounds (α_1 and α_2, β_1 and β_2). A third β-receptor subtype, β_3, has been documented, and at least three further subtypes of both α_1- and α_2-receptors and five subtypes of DA receptor identified, although their precise functions are unclear. Differentiation of receptor subtypes is now based more directly on the effects of various catecholamine agonist compounds (including endogenous catecholamines). Adrenaline and noradrenaline are equipotent at β_1-receptors, but β_2-receptors are more sensitive to adrenaline. Noradrenaline and adrenaline are agonists at both α_1- and α_2-receptors. Although α_1-receptors are more sensitive in pharmacological terms to adrenaline, they mediate most of the physiological actions of noradrenaline.

Until recently it was thought that β_1-receptors predominated in the heart, mediating increases in force and rate of contraction, and β_2-receptors existed in bronchial, uterine and vascular smooth muscle, mediating relaxation. In fact, most organs and tissues contain both β_1- and β_2-receptors, which may even serve the same function. For example, up to 25% of cardiac β-receptors in the normal individual are of the β_2 subtype, and this proportion may be increased in patients with cardiac failure. It is now apparent that β_1-receptors in tissues are situated on the postsynaptic membrane of adrenergic neurones and respond to released noradrenaline. β_2-Receptors are presynaptic and when stimulated (principally by circulating catecholamines) they modulate autonomic activity by promoting neuronal noradrenaline release. β_3-Receptors are present on adipocytes and other tissues. Similarly, α_1-receptors are present on the postsynaptic membrane, whereas α_2-receptors are predominantly presynaptic, responding to circulating adrenaline but also mediating feedback inhibition of sympathetic nerve activity. Central α_2 stimulation causes decreases in arterial pressure, peripheral resistance, venous return, myocardial contractility, cardiac output and heart rate by inhibition of sympathetic outflow. Postsynaptic α_2-receptors present on platelets and in the CNS mediate platelet aggregation and membrane hyperpolarization, respectively.

Postsynaptic dopamine receptors (DA_1) are present in vascular smooth muscle of the renal, splanchnic, coronary and cerebral circulations, where they mediate vasodilatation. They are also situated on renal tubules, where they inhibit sodium reabsorption, causing natriuresis and diuresis. Postsynaptic DA_2-receptors are widespread in the CNS and occur on the presynaptic membrane of sympathetic nerves and in the adrenal gland. Stimulation of presynaptic DA_2-receptors inhibits dopamine release by negative feedback.

Postganglionic sympathetic fibres supplying sweat glands and arterioles in some areas of skin and skeletal

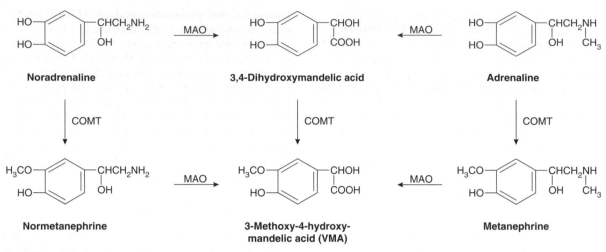

Fig. 8.3
Catecholamine metabolites. MAO=monoamine oxidase; COMT=catechol *O*-methyltransferase.

muscle are cholinergic. Vascular smooth muscle also contains non-innervated cholinergic receptors which mediate vasodilatation in response to circulating agonists. Cholinergic effects on vascular smooth muscle are usually minimal but may be involved in the mechanism of vasovagal attacks.

These subdivisions and the functions of the autonomic nervous system are summarized in Table 8.1.

Structure of adrenergic receptors

Both α- and β-adrenergic receptors are proteins with a similar basic structure, comprising seven hydrophobic transmembrane domains and an intracellular chain. Differences in amino acid sequences of the intracellular chain differentiate α- and β-receptors. Both are linked to guanine nucleotide binding proteins (G-proteins) in the cell membrane which mediate the generation of second messengers which activate intracellular events. These second messenger systems include enzymes (adenylate cyclase, phospholipases) and ion channels (for calcium and potassium).

Second and third messenger systems

In addition to functional differences, α- and β-receptors differ in the intracellular mechanisms by which they act. Stimulation of β_1- and β_2-receptors activates G_s-proteins, which activate adenylate cyclase and cause the generation of intracellular cyclic adenosine monophosphate (cAMP). cAMP activates intracellular enzyme pathways (the third messengers) to produce the associated alteration in cell function (e.g. increased force of cardiac muscle contraction, liver glycogenoly-

sis, bronchial smooth muscle relaxation). In cardiac myocytes, the intracellular pathway involves the activation of protein kinases to phosphorylate intracellular proteins and increase intracellular Ca^{2+} concentrations. Intracellular cAMP concentration is modulated by the enzyme phosphodiesterase, which breaks down cAMP to inactive 5′ AMP. This is the site of action of phosphodiesterase inhibitor drugs. The balance between production and degradation of cAMP is an important regulatory system for cell function. α_2-Receptors interact with G_i-proteins to *inhibit* adenylate cyclase and Ca^{2+} channels, but activate K^+ channels, phospholipase C and phospholipase A_2. Cholinergic M_2-receptors and somatostatin affect G_i-proteins in the same way.

In contrast, α_1-receptor stimulation does not directly affect intracellular cAMP levels, but causes coupling with another G-protein, G_q, to activate membrane-bound phospholipase C. This in turn hydrolyses phosphatidylinositol biphosphate (PIP_2) to inositol triphosphate (IP_3), which produces changes in intracellular Ca^{2+} concentration and binding. These lead, for example, to smooth muscle contraction.

THE PARASYMPATHETIC NERVOUS SYSTEM

The parasympathetic nervous system controls vegetative functions, e.g. the digestion and absorption of nutrients, excretion of waste products and the conservation and restoration of energy. Parasympathetic neurones arise from cell bodies of the motor nuclei of cranial nerves III, VII, IX and X in the brainstem, and from the sacral segments of the spinal cord ('the craniosacral outflow'). Preganglionic fibres run almost to the organ innervated and synapse in ganglia within the organ, giving rise to postganglionic fibres which then supply the relevant tissues. The ganglion cells may be well organized (e.g. the myenteric plexus of the intestine) or diffuse (e.g. in the bladder or vasculature). As the majority of all parasympathetic nerves are contained in branches of the vagus nerve, which innervates the viscera of the thorax and abdomen, increased parasympathetic activity is characterized by signs of vagal overactivity. Parasympathetic fibres also pass to the eye via the oculomotor (third cranial) nerve, and to the lacrimal, nasal and salivary glands via the facial (fifth) and glossopharyngeal (ninth) nerves. Fibres originating in the sacral portion of the spinal cord pass to the distal GI tract, bladder and reproductive organs. The effects of parasympathetic stimulation at different receptors and effector organs is summarized in Table 8.1

Parasympathetic neurotransmitters

The chemical neurotransmitter at both pre- and postganglionic synapses is ACh, although transmission at postganglionic synapses may be modulated by other substances, including GABA, serotonin and opioid peptides. ACh is synthesized in the cytoplasm of cholinergic nerve terminals by the combination of choline and acetate (in the form of acetyl-CoA, which is synthesized in the mitochondria as a product of normal cellular metabolism). ACh is stored in specific agranular vesicles and released from the presynaptic terminal in response to neuronal depolarization to act at specific receptor sites on the postsynaptic membrane. It is rapidly metabolized by the enzyme acetylcholinesterase (AChE) to produce acetate and choline. Choline is then taken up into the presynaptic nerve

ending for the regeneration of ACh. AChE is synthesized locally at cholinergic synapses, but is also present in erythrocytes and parts of the CNS. Butyryl cholinesterase (also termed plasma cholinesterase or pseudocholinesterase) is synthesized in the liver and is found in the plasma, skin, GI tract and parts of the CNS, but not at cholinergic synapses or the neuromuscular junction. It may metabolize ACh, in addition to some neuromuscular blockers (e.g. succinylcholine and mivacurium), but its physiological role probably involves the breakdown of other choline esters which may be present in the intestine.

Parasympathetic receptor pharmacology

Parasympathetic receptors have been classified according to the actions of the alkaloids muscarine and nicotine. The actions of ACh at the postganglionic membrane are mimicked by muscarine and are termed muscarinic, whereas preganglionic transmission is termed nicotinic. ACh is also the neurotransmitter at the neuromuscular junction, via nicotinic receptor sites. Five subtypes of muscarinic receptors (M_1–M_5) have been characterized and specific antagonists developed for M_1–M_3 receptors. All five subtypes exist in the CNS, but there are differences in their peripheral distribution and function (Table 8.2). M_1-receptors are found in the stomach where they mediate acid secretion, whereas M_2-receptors predominate in the myocardium, where they modulate heart rate and impulse conduction. Prejunctional M_2-receptors may also be involved in the regulation of synaptic noradrenaline and ACh release. M_3-receptors are present in classic postsynaptic sites in glandular tissue (of the GI and respiratory tract) and probably in bronchial smooth muscle. M_4-receptors have been isolated in cardiac and lung tissue in animal

Table 8.2   Properties of muscarinic (M_1–M_5) receptors

	M_1	M_2	M_3	M_4	M_5
Second messenger	IP_3	cAMP	IP_3	cAMP	IP_3
Location	CNS	Heart	CNS	CNS	CNS
	Stomach	CNS	Glands	Heart	?
Important clinical effects	Gastric acid production	Bradycardia	Secretion	?	?
Clinically selective agent	Pirenzepine	None	None	None	None

IP_3 stimulates inositol triphosphate production.
cAMP inhibits adenylate cyclase to decrease cAMP formation.

models and may have inhibitory effects, but the distribution and functions of M_5-receptors are not yet defined. In common with adrenergic receptors, muscarinic receptors are coupled to membrane-bound G-proteins though the subtypes differ in the second messenger system with which they interact. Currently available anticholinergics probably act at all muscarinic receptor subtypes but their clinical spectra differ, which suggests that they may have differential effects at different subtypes.

DRUGS ACTING ON THE SYMPATHETIC NERVOUS SYSTEM

SYMPATHOMIMETIC DRUGS

Sympathomimetic drugs partially or completely mimic the effects of sympathetic nerve stimulation or adrenal medullary discharge. They may act:

- directly on the adrenergic receptor, e.g. the catecholamines, phenylephrine, methoxamine
- indirectly, causing release of noradrenaline from the adrenergic nerve ending, e.g. amphetamine
- by both mechanisms, e.g. dopamine, ephedrine, metaraminol.

The drugs may be classified according to their structure (catecholamine/non-catecholamine), their origin (endogenous/synthetic) and their mechanism of action (via adrenergic receptors or a via a non-adrenergic mechanism) (Table 8.3). Drugs that affect myocardial contractility are termed inotropes, although this term is usually applied to those drugs that increase cardiac contractility (strictly 'positive inotropes'). Myocardial contractility may be increased by:

- increasing intracellular cAMP by activation of the adenylate cyclase system (e.g. catecholamines and other drugs acting via the adrenergic receptor)
- decreasing breakdown of cAMP (e.g. phosphodiesterase inhibitors)
- increasing intracellular calcium availability (e.g. digoxin, calcium salts, glucagon)
- increasing the response of contractile proteins to calcium (e.g. levosimendan) (Fig. 8.4).

Inotropes may also be classified into positive inotropic drugs that also produce systemic vasoconstriction ('inoconstrictors'), and those which also produce systemic vasodilatation ('inodilators'). Inoconstrictors include noradrenaline, adrenaline and ephedrine. Inodilators are dobutamine, dopexamine, isoprenaline and phosphodiesterase inhibitors. Dopamine is an inodilator at low dose, and an inoconstrictor at higher doses.

CATECHOLAMINES

Catecholamine drugs may be endogenous (adrenaline, noradrenaline and dopamine) or synthetic (dobutamine, dopexamine and isoprenaline). Several other drugs with a non-catecholamine structure produce sympathomimetic effects via adrenergic receptors, e.g. ephedrine and phenylephrine. All catecholamine drugs are inactivated in the gut by MAO and are usually only administered parenterally. They all have very short half-lifes in vivo, and so when given by intravenous infusion, their effects may be controlled by altering the infusion rate. The comparative effects of different inotropes and vasopressors are outlined below.

Endogenous catecholamines

Adrenaline

Adrenaline comprises 80–90% of adrenal medullary catecholamine content and is also an important CNS neurotransmitter. It is a powerful agonist at both α- and β-adrenergic receptors, being more potent than noradrenaline at α-receptors and more potent than isoprenaline at β-receptors. It is the treatment of choice in acute allergic (anaphylactic) reactions and is used in the management of cardiac arrest and shock, and occasionally as a bronchodilator. Except in emergency situations, i.v. injection is avoided because of the risk of inducing cardiac arrhythmias. Subcutaneous administration produces local vasoconstriction and so smoothes out its own effect by slowing absorption.

Table 8.3 Classification of sympathomimetic drugs

Catecholamines		Non-catecholamines	
Endogenous	*Synthetic*	*Acting via adrenergic receptors*	*Acting via non-adrenergic mechanisms*
Adrenaline	Isoprenaline	Ephedrine	Phosphodiesterase inhibitors
Noradrenaline	Dobutamine	Phenylephrine	Digoxin
Dopamine	Dopexamine	Methoxamine	Glucagon
		Metaraminol	Calcium salts

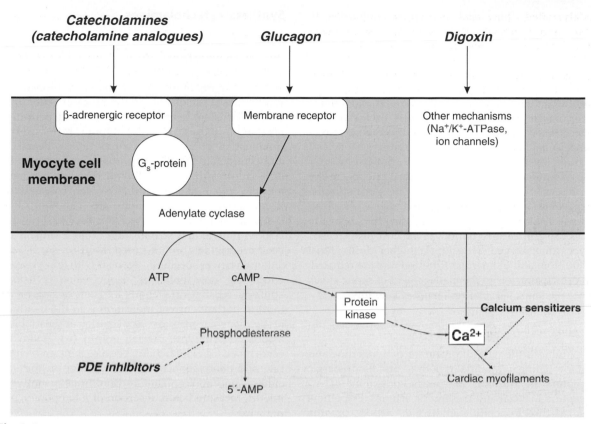

Fig. 8.4
Intracellular action of positive inotropic drugs. PDE; phosphodiesterase

The effects of adrenaline on arterial pressure and cardiac output are dependent on dose. Although both α- and β-receptors are stimulated, β_2 vasodilator effects are most sensitive. β_1-Effects cause increases in heart rate and contractility, cardiac output and systolic pressure. In low dosage, vasodilatation in skeletal muscle and splanchnic arterioles (β_2) is prominent; systemic vascular resistance and diastolic pressure may decrease, pulse pressure widens, but mean arterial pressure remains stable. At higher doses, α-mediated vasoconstriction occurs in the precapillary resistance vessels of skin, mucosa and kidney. Systolic pressure increases further, and cardiac output may decrease. Adrenaline causes marked decreases in renal blood flow, but coronary blood flow is increased. In contrast to other sympathomimetics, adrenaline has significant metabolic effects. Hepatic glycogenolysis and lipolysis in adipose tissue increase (β_1 and β_3 effects), and insulin secretion is inhibited (α_1 effect) so that hyperglycaemia occurs.

Adrenaline 0.5–1 mg i.m. (0.5–1.0 mL of 1:1000 solution) or 100 μg increments i.v. to a dose of 1 mg (1–10 mL of a 1:10 000 solution) is used to treat acute anaphylactic reactions. Adrenaline is important in the management of cardiac arrest (in doses of 1 mg i.v., repeated every 3 min), mostly because of its α effects: widespread systemic vasoconstriction occurs, increasing aortic diastolic pressure, and coronary and cerebral perfusion. Pure α-agonists are less effective than adrenaline in the management of cardiac arrest, and the β_2 effects of adrenaline may contribute to improved cerebral perfusion. In emergency situations, it may also be administered via the tracheal route, in doses of 2–3 mg diluted to a volume of 10 mL. It is effective by aerosol inhalation in bronchial asthma but has been superseded by selective β_2-agonists (see below). Unlike indirect-acting sympathomimetics that cause noradrenaline release, tachyphylaxis should not occur with adrenaline. Adrenaline is also used as a topical vasoconstrictor to aid haemostasis and is incorporated into local anaesthetic solutions to decrease systemic absorption and prolong the duration of local anaesthesia.

Noradrenaline

Noradrenaline acts as a potent arteriolar and venous vasoconstrictor, which acts almost exclusively at α-receptors, although it is less potent here than adrenaline. Infusions of noradrenaline increase systolic and diastolic systemic and pulmonary arterial pressures and central venous pressure. Heart rate decreases because of baroreflex activity. Despite some stimulatory effects on cardiac contraction, the widespread intense vasoconstriction leads either to no change or to a decrease in cardiac output at the cost of increased myocardial oxygen demand. At higher doses, renal blood flow and glomerular filtration rate are reduced. Its principal use is in the management of septic shock when systemic vascular resistance is very low.

Dopamine

Dopamine is the natural precursor of adrenaline and noradrenaline. It stimulates both α- and β-adrenergic receptors in addition to specific dopamine (DA_1) receptors in renal and mesenteric arteries. Dopamine has a direct positive inotropic action on the myocardium via β-receptors and also by release of noradrenaline from adrenergic nerve terminals. However, the overall effect of dopamine is related to dosage. In low dosage ($< 3 \mu g \ kg^{-1} \ min^{-1}$), renal and mesenteric vascular resistance is reduced by an action on DA_1-receptors, resulting in increased splanchnic and renal blood flows, glomerular filtration rate and sodium excretion. At doses of 5–10 $\mu g \ kg^{-1} \ min^{-1}$, the increasing direct β-mediated inotropic action predominates, increasing cardiac output and systolic pressure with little effect on diastolic pressure. Total peripheral resistance is usually unchanged. At doses $> 15 \mu g \ kg^{-1} \ min^{-1}$, α-receptor activity predominates, with direct vasoconstriction and increased cardiac stimulation (similar to noradrenaline). Renal and splanchnic blood flows decrease, and arrhythmias may occur. Dopamine receptors are widely present in the CNS, particularly in the basal ganglia, pituitary (where they mediate prolactin secretion) and the chemoreceptor trigger zone on the floor of the fourth ventricle where they mediate nausea and vomiting. Recently, dopamine infusions have been associated with decreased prolactin secretion, and the use of 'prophylactic' dopamine infusions in an attempt to preserve renal function in critically ill patients is declining.

Synthetic catecholamines

Isoprenaline

Isoprenaline is a β_1- and β_2-agonist, with virtually no activity at α-receptors. It acts via cardiac β_1-receptors, and β_2-receptors in the smooth muscle of bronchi, the vasculature of skeletal muscle and the gut. After intravenous infusion, heart rate increases and peripheral resistance is reduced. Cardiac output is increased by a combination of increased venous return, heart rate and contractility. Systolic pressure may increase, but diastolic pressure decreases and coronary perfusion may be impaired. Myocardial oxygen consumption is increased and arrhythmias are common. Other β_2-mediated effects include relaxation of bronchial smooth muscle and stabilization of mast cells. It has been used widely in the treatment of severe asthma, although newer specific β_2-agonists with fewer cardiac effects are now preferred. Isoprenaline is usually administered by intravenous infusion or aerosol. Its most important current indication is in the treatment of bradyarrhythmias or atrioventricular heart block associated with low cardiac output (e.g. following acute myocardial infarction), because it increases heart rate and conduction by a direct action on the subsidiary pacemaker. This indication is usually an interim measure before insertion of a temporary pacing wire.

Dobutamine

Dobutamine is primarily a β_1-agonist, with moderate β_2- and mild α_1-agonist activity, and no action at DA-receptors. Its primary effect is an increase in cardiac output via increased contractility (β_1 effect) augmented by a reduction in afterload. Heart rate also increases (β_2 effect). Systolic arterial pressure may increase, but peripheral resistance is reduced or unchanged. There is no direct effect on venous tone or renal blood flow, but preload may decrease and urine output and sodium excretion increase as a consequence of the increased cardiac output. Dobutamine increases SA node automaticity and conduction velocity in the atria, ventricles and AV node, but to a lesser extent than isoprenaline. Dobutamine infusion produces a progressive increase in cardiac output which is greater than with comparable doses of dopamine, although arterial pressure may initially remain unchanged. At higher doses, tachycardia and arrhythmias may occur, but dobutamine has less effect on myocardial oxygen consumption compared with other catecholamines. Dobutamine is considered the inotropic agent of choice for optimizing cardiac output (and therefore global organ blood flow) when cardiac output is low (measured or suspected) in septic shock; it is frequently combined with noradrenaline. Dobutamine is used alone or in combination with vasodilator drugs in cardiac failure when peripheral resistance is high.

Dopexamine

Dopexamine is a synthetic dopamine analogue which is an agonist at β_2- and DA_1-receptors. It is also a weak DA_2-agonist and it inhibits the neuronal re-uptake of noradrenaline (*uptake₁*), but has no direct effects at β_1-or α-receptors. Its principal effect is β_2-agonism, producing vasodilatation in skeletal muscle; it is less potent at DA_1-receptors, but a more potent β_2-agonist than dopamine. It produces mild increases in heart rate, contractility and cardiac output (effect on β_2-receptors and noradrenaline uptake), renal and mesenteric vasodilatation (β_2 and DA_1 effects), and natriuresis (DA_1 effect). Coronary and cerebral blood flows are also increased. Systemic vascular resistance decreases and arterial pressure may decrease if intravascular volume is not maintained. Dopexamine has theoretical advantages in maintaining splanchnic blood flow in patients with systemic sepsis, cardiac failure, or those who are undergoing major surgery, but definitive data are lacking. It also has anti-inflammatory effects (in common with other β-agonists) that are independent of its effects on gut mucosal perfusion. It is metabolized by hepatic methylation and conjugation and is eliminated mostly via the kidneys.

Fenoldopam is a dopamine (DA_1) agonist available in the USA that causes peripheral vasodilatation and increases renal blood flow and sodium and water excretion. It has been used in the treatment of hypertensive emergencies. Unlike some other vasodilators (e.g. sodium nitroprusside) it does not cause rebound hypertension after stopping the infusion.

Ibopamine is a non-selective DA_1- and DA_2-agonist with similar pharmacological effects to dopamine. Ibopamine is a prodrug, which is converted to epinine (*N*-methyldopamine) after oral administration, and produces a diuresis and natriuresis in patients with cardiac failure.

Non-catecholamine sympathomimetics

Synthetic sympathomimetic drugs may mimic the effect of adrenaline at adrenergic receptors (direct acting) or may produce effects by causing release of endogenous noradrenaline from postganglionic sympathetic nerve terminals (indirect acting). Some drugs have direct and indirect sympathomimetic effects (e.g. ephedrine, metaraminol). Direct-acting compounds

may affect α- or β-receptors selectively, whereas indirect-acting compounds have predominantly α- and β_1-agonist effects (as noradrenaline is only a weak β_2-agonist). Indirect-acting compounds are taken up into the nerve terminal via the noradrenaline re-uptake pathway, and so their effect is reduced by drugs which block noradrenaline re-uptake (e.g. tricyclic antidepressants). Conversely, the effect of direct-acting drugs is enhanced. In patients treated with drugs that decrease sympathetic nervous system activity (e.g. clonidine, reserpine), the cardiovascular response to indirect-acting drugs is diminished; however, upregulation of adrenergic receptors occurs and an increased response to direct-acting sympathomimetics is seen. Drugs with selective α-adrenergic receptor effects (e.g. phenylephrine, methoxamine) are potent vasoconstrictors.

Ephedrine

Ephedrine is a naturally occurring sympathomimetic amine which is now produced synthetically. It acts directly and indirectly as an agonist at α-, β_1- and β_2-receptors. The indirect actions are increased endogenous noradrenaline release and inhibition of MAO. Its cardiovascular effects are similar to those of adrenaline, but the duration of action is up to 10 times longer. It causes increases in heart rate, contractility, cardiac output and arterial pressure (systolic > diastolic). It may predispose to arrhythmias. Systemic vascular resistance is usually unchanged, as α-mediated vasoconstriction in some vascular beds is balanced by β-mediated vasodilatation in others, but renal and splanchnic blood flows decrease. It relaxes bronchial and other smooth muscle, and is occasionally used as a bronchodilator. It is active orally as it is not metabolized by MAO in the gut, and is useful by intramuscular injection as muscle blood flow is preserved. Ephedrine undergoes hepatic deamination and conjugation but significant amounts are excreted unchanged in urine. This accounts for its long duration of action and elimination half-life (3–6 h). Tachyphylaxis (a decreased response to repeated doses of the drug) occurs because of persistent occupation of adrenergic receptors and depletion of noradrenaline stores.

Ephedrine is often used to prevent or treat hypotension resulting from sympathetic blockade during regional anaesthesia or from the effects of general anaesthesia. It is particularly indicated during regional anaesthesia in obstetric patients, as uterine blood flow is maintained (whereas pure vasoconstrictors may restore systemic blood pressure at the expense of uterine blood flow). Oral or topical ephedrine is also useful as a nasal decongestant.

Phenylephrine

Phenylephrine is a potent synthetic direct-acting α_1-agonist, which has minimal agonist effects at α_2- and β-receptors. It has effects similar to those of noradrenaline, causing widespread vasoconstriction, increased arterial pressure, bradycardia (as a result of baroreflex activation) and a decrease in cardiac output. Venoconstriction predominates, and diastolic pressure increases more than systolic pressure, so that coronary blood flow may increase. It is also used topically as a nasal decongestant and mydriatic. Absorption of phenylephrine from mucous membranes may occasionally produce systemic side-effects.

Methoxamine

Methoxamine is a direct-acting α_1-agonist which also has a weak β-antagonist action. It produces vasoconstriction, increased diastolic arterial pressure and decreases in cardiac output and heart rate from baroreflex activation and the mild β-blocking effect. It is no longer available in the UK.

Metaraminol

Metaraminol is a direct- and indirect-acting α- and β-agonist, which acts partly by being taken up into sympathetic nerve terminals and acting as a false transmitter for noradrenaline. Its α effects predominate, causing pronounced vasoconstriction; arterial pressure increases and a reflex bradycardia may occur.

Vasopressin

Arginine-vasopressin (AVP) (formerly termed antidiuretic hormone) is a peptide hormone secreted by the hypothalamus. Its primary role is the regulation of body fluid balance. It is secreted in response to hypotension and promotes retention of water by action on specific cAMP-coupled V_2-receptors. It causes vasoconstriction by stimulating V_1-receptors in vascular smooth muscle and is particularly potent in hypotensive patients. It is occasionally used in the treatment of refractory vasodilatory shock that is resistant to catecholamines, although its role is uncertain because it can cause peripheral or splanchnic ischaemia.

Phosphodiesterase inhibitors

Phosphodiesterase inhibitors increase intracellular cAMP concentrations by inhibition of the enzyme responsible for cAMP breakdown (Fig. 8.4). Increased intracellular cAMP concentrations promote the activation of protein kinases, which lead to an increase in intracellular Ca^{2+}. In cardiac muscle cells, this causes a positive inotropic effect and also facilitates diastolic relaxation and cardiac filling (termed 'positive lusitropy'). In vascular smooth muscle, increased cAMP decreases intracellular Ca^{2+} and causes marked vasodilatation. Several subtypes of phosphodiesterase (PDE) isoenzyme exist in different tissues. Theophylline is a non-specific PDE inhibitor, but the newer drugs (e.g. enoximone and milrinone) are selective for the PDE type III isoenzyme present in the myocardium, vascular smooth muscle and platelets. PDE III inhibitors are positive inotropes and potent arterial, coronary and venodilators. They decrease preload, afterload, pulmonary vascular resistance and pulmonary capillary wedge pressure (PCWP), and increase cardiac index. Heart rate may increase or remain unchanged. In contrast to sympathomimetics, they improve myocardial function *without* increasing oxygen demand or causing tachyphylaxis. Their effects are augmented by the co-administration of β_1-agonists (i.e. increases in cAMP production are synergistic with decreased cAMP breakdown). They have particular advantages in patients with chronic cardiac failure, in whom downregulation of myocardial β-adrenergic receptors occurs, so that there is a decreased inotropic response to β-sympathomimetic drugs. A similar phenomenon occurs with advanced age, prolonged (> 72 h) catecholamine therapy and possibly with surgical stress.

PDE III inhibitors are indicated for acute refractory cardiac failure, e.g. cardiogenic shock, or pre- or postcardiac surgery. However, long-term oral treatment is associated with increased mortality in patients with congestive heart failure. All may cause hypotension, and tachyarrhythmias may occur. Other adverse effects include nausea, vomiting and fever. Their half-life is prolonged markedly in patients with heart or renal failure and they are commonly administered as an i.v. loading dose over 5 min with or without a subsequent i.v. infusion. *Milrinone* is a bipyridine derivative whereas *enoximone* is an imidazole derivative. Enoximone undergoes substantial first-pass metabolism, and is rapidly metabolized to an active sulphoxide metabolite which is excreted via the kidneys and which may accumulate in renal failure. The elimination $t_{\frac{1}{2}}$ of enoximone is 1–2 h in healthy individuals but up to 20 h in patients with heart failure.

Glucagon

Glucagon is a polypeptide secreted by the α cells of the pancreatic islets; its physiological actions include stimulation of hepatic gluconeogenesis in response to hypoglycaemia, amino acids and as part of the stress response. These effects are mediated by increasing adenylate cyclase activity and intracellular cAMP, by a mechanism independent of the β-adrenergic receptor (see Fig. 8.4). It increases cAMP in myocardial cells and so increases cardiac contractility. Glucagon causes nausea and vomiting, hyperglycaemia and hyper-kalaemia and is not used as an inotrope except in the management of β-blocker poisoning.

Calcium

Calcium ions are involved in cellular excitation, excitation–contraction coupling and muscle contraction in cardiac, skeletal and smooth muscle cells. Increased extracellular Ca^{2+} increases intracellular Ca^{2+} concentrations and consequently the force of contraction of cardiac myocytes and vascular smooth muscle cells. Massive blood loss and replacement with large volumes of calcium-free fluids or citrated blood (which chelates Ca^{2+}) may cause a decrease in serum Ca^{2+} concentration, especially in the critically ill. Therefore, Ca^{2+} salts (e.g. calcium chloride or gluconate) may be administered, particularly during and after cardiopulmonary bypass. Intravenous calcium 5 mg kg^{-1} may increase mean arterial pressure, but the effects on cardiac output and systemic vascular resistance are variable and there is little good evidence for the efficacy of Ca^{2+} salts. Moreover, high Ca^{2+} concentrations may cause cardiac arrhythmias and vasoconstriction, may be cytotoxic and may worsen the cellular effects of ischaemia. Calcium salts may be indicated for the treatment of hypocalcaemia (ionized Ca^{2+} < 0.8 mmol L^{-1}), hyperkalaemia and calcium channel blocker toxicity.

Levosimendan

Levosimendan belongs to a new group of positive inotropic drugs, the calcium sensitizers. These act by stabilizing the troponin molecule in cardiac myocytes (by a cAMP-independent mechanism) and so increase myocyte Ca^{2+} sensitivity without increasing Ca^{2+} influx. Contractility is increased without an increase in oxygen consumption or a tendency to arrhythmias. Levosimendan also causes vasodilatation by opening K^+ channels via an ATP-dependent mechanism and is a new alternative to dobutamine in acute heart failure. It is available in Europe.

Selective β$_2$-agonists

Selective β$_2$-receptor agonists (e.g. salbutamol, terbutaline, formoterol and salmeterol) relax bronchial, uterine and vascular smooth muscle whilst having much less effect on the heart than isoprenaline. These drugs are partial agonists (their maximal effect at β$_2$-receptors is less than that of isoprenaline) and are only partially selective for β$_2$-receptors. They are used widely in the treatment of bronchospasm (see Ch. 9). Although less cardiotoxic than isoprenaline, dose-related tremor, tachyarrhythmias, hyperglycaemia, hypokalaemia and hypomagnesaemia may occur. β$_2$-Agonists are resistant to metabolism by COMT and therefore have a prolonged duration of action (mostly 3–5 h). Salmeterol is highly lipophilic, has a strong affinity for the β$_2$-adrenergic receptor and is longer acting than the other β$_2$-agonists. β$_2$-Agonists are usually administered by the inhaled (metered dose inhaler or nebulizer) or intravenous routes because of unpredictable oral absorption and a high hepatic extraction ratio. When inhaled, only 10–20% of the administered dose reaches the lower airways; this proportion is reduced further when administered via a tracheal tube. Nevertheless, systemic absorption does occur, although adverse effects are less common during long term therapy.

Salbutamol

Salbutamol is the β$_2$-agonist used most commonly for the prevention and treatment of bronchospasm. When administered by metered dose inhaler (1–2 puffs, each delivering 100 μg), it acts within a few minutes, with a peak action at 30–60 min. In severe cases, it may be given by nebulizer (2.5–5.0 mg), repeated if required, or intravenously (either 250 μg by slow i.v. injection or as an infusion starting at 5 μg min^{-1} and titrated to response). It is metabolized in the liver and excreted in urine both as metabolites and as unchanged drug; the proportions are dependent on the route of administration.

Ritodrine

Ritodrine is a β$_2$-agonist used as a tocolytic to stop uterine contractions in premature labour. It is administered as an i.v. infusion until labour has stopped before continuing oral ritodrine therapy. Ritodrine infusions often cause tachycardia, which is mediated partly by β$_1$-agonism, and often limits its use. Other adverse effects include sodium and water retention, pulmonary oedema, hypokalaemia and hyperglycaemia, with the potential for reactive fetal hypoglycaemia. Careful monitoring of ECG, fluid balance, blood glucose and electrolytes is necessary. Ritodrine is contraindicated in patients with pre-eclampsia, antepartum haemorrhage requiring immediate delivery or maternal cardiac disease, and may be superseded by specific oxytocin antagonists.

SYMPATHOLYTIC DRUGS

Sympatholytic drugs antagonize the effects of the sympathetic nervous system either at central adrenergic neurones, peripheral autonomic ganglia or neurones, or at postsynaptic α- or β-receptors. Most are hypotensive drugs, although they have other effects and indications.

Centrally acting sympatholytic drugs

Centrally acting drugs act by stimulation of central α_2-receptors to decrease sympathetic tone. They were used as antihypertensive drugs, but have been superseded for this purpose by newer drugs with fewer adverse effects. They are also agonists at central imidazoline (I_1) receptors, which contributes to their hypotensive action. I_1 receptors are present in several peripheral tissues, including the kidney. Central α_2-stimulation causes decreases in arterial pressure, peripheral resistance, venous return, myocardial contractility, cardiac output and heart rate, but baroreceptor reflexes are preserved, and the pressor response to ephedrine or phenylephrine may be exaggerated. Stimulation of peripheral α_2-receptors on vascular smooth muscle causes direct arteriolar vasoconstriction, though the central effects of these drugs predominate overall. However, severe rebound hypertension may occur on stopping chronic oral therapy. α_2-Receptors in the dorsal horn of the spinal cord modulate upward transmission of nociceptive signals by modifying local release of substance P and CGRP. Centrally acting α_2-agonists produce analgesia by activation of descending spinal and supraspinal inhibitory pathways, and clonidine is now used mostly for its analgesic effects. These are greatest when administered by the epidural or spinal route. Other effects include dry mouth, sedation and anxiolysis.

Clonidine is a partial agonist at central and peripheral α_2-receptors, and a central imidazoline (I_1) receptor agonist. Clonidine has some effects at α_1-receptors ($\alpha_2{:}\alpha_1 >$ 200:1); dexmedetomidine and azepexole are more α_2-selective alternatives. Transient hypertension and bradycardia may occur after i.v. injection, caused by direct stimulation of peripheral vascular α_2-receptors though an α_1-agonist effect may also contribute. Clonidine potentiates the MAC of inhalational anaesthetic agents by up to 50%. It has a synergistic analgesic effect with opioids that may be partly pharmacokinetic, as the elimination half-life of opioids is also increased. Clonidine is well absorbed orally, with peak plasma concentrations after 60–90 min. It is highly lipid-soluble and

approximately 50% is metabolized in the liver to inactive metabolites; the rest is excreted unchanged via the kidneys, with an elimination half-life of 9–12 h. Clonidine 5 μg kg^{-1} as premedication attenuates reflex sympathetic responses and may improve cardiovascular stability during anaesthesia. It is also used in the treatment of opioid withdrawal and postoperative shivering. Epidural clonidine 1–2 μg kg^{-1} increases the duration and potency of analgesia provided by epidural opioid or local anaesthetic drugs. α_2-Agonists also have some antiarrhythmic effects, decreasing both the incidence of catecholamine-related arrhythmias and the toxicity of bupivacaine and cocaine.

Methyldopa crosses the blood–brain barrier easily and is converted to α-methyl noradrenaline, the active molecule, which is a full agonist at α_2-receptors ($\alpha_2{:}\alpha_1$ selectivity = 10:1). Adverse effects include peripheral oedema, hepatotoxicity, depression and a positive direct Coombs' test; some patients develop haemolytic anaemia. Its use is largely restricted to the management of pregnancy-associated hypertension.

Moxonidine is a moderately selective imidazoline I_1-receptor agonist ($I_1 > \alpha_2$) which reduces central sympathetic activity by stimulation of medullary I_1-receptors. It is used in the treatment of hypertension. Systemic vascular resistance is reduced, but heart rate and stroke volume are unchanged. Moxonidine has few α_2-related adverse effects but it may potentiate bradycardia and is contraindicated in sinoatrial, and second- or third-degree AV block.

Peripherally acting sympatholytic drugs

Ganglion blocking drugs

Nicotinic receptor antagonists (e.g. hexamethonium, pentolinium, trimetaphan) competitively inhibit the effects of ACh at autonomic ganglia and block both parasympathetic and sympathetic transmission. Sympathetic blockade produces venodilatation, decreased myocardial contractility and hypotension, but the effects vary depending on pre-existing sympathetic tone. Tachyphylaxis develops rapidly and these drugs have now been superseded.

Adrenergic neurone blocking drugs

Guanethidine decreases peripheral sympathetic nervous system activity by competitively binding to noradrenaline binding sites in storage vesicles in the cytoplasm of postganglionic sympathetic nerve terminals. Further uptake of noradrenaline into the vesicles is inhibited and it is metabolized by cytoplasmic monoamine oxidase, so the nerve terminals become depleted of noradrenaline. Guanethidine has local anaesthetic properties and does not cross the blood–brain barrier. It is sometimes used to produce intravenous regional sympathetic blockade in the treatment of chronic limb pain associated with excessive autonomic activity (reflex sympathetic dystrophy or complex regional pain syndromes). Bretylium has a similar mode of action; it is used in the treatment of resistant ventricular arrhythmias (see below).

α-Adrenergic receptor antagonists

α-Adrenergic antagonists (α blockers) selectively inhibit the action of catecholamines at α-adrenergic receptors. They are used mainly as vasodilators for the second-line treatment of hypertension or as urinary tract smooth muscle relaxants in patients with benign prostatic hyperplasia. They also have an important role in the preoperative management of phaeochromocytoma (see Ch. 37).

α-Blockers diminish vasoconstrictor tone, causing venous pooling and a decrease in peripheral vascular resistance. In common with other vasodilators, they may have indirect positive inotropic actions as a result of reductions in afterload and preload, so cardiac output may increase. They may be classified according to their relative selectivity for α_1- and α_2-receptors. Non-selective α-blockers commonly induce postural hypotension and reflex tachycardia, partly because α_2-blockade blocks the feedback inhibition of noradrenaline on its own release at presynaptic α_2-receptors, and neuronal noradrenaline concentrations increase. The action of noradrenaline at cardiac β-receptors then limits the hypotensive effects of non-selective α-blockers. In addition, the proportions of pre- and postsynaptic α_2-receptors in the arterial and venous smooth muscle may differ, so that α_1-selective drugs have a more balanced effect on venous and arterial circulations. The co-administration of a β-blocker may attenuate reflex tachycardia and produces a synergistic effect on arterial pressure.

α_1-Selective antagonists

Selective α_1-blockers include prazosin, doxazosin, indoramin, phenoxybenzamine and urapidil. *Doxazosin* has largely succeeded prazosin as it has a more prolonged duration of action. Reflex tachycardia and postural hypotension are less common than with direct-acting vasodilators (e.g. hydralazine) and the non-selective α-blockers, but may still occur on initiating therapy. Nasal congestion, sedation and inhibition of ejaculation may occur. *Phenoxybenzamine* binds covalently (i.e. irreversibly and non-competitively) to the receptor so that its effects last up to several days, and may be cumulative on repeated dosing. It is used for the preoperative preparation of patients with phaeochromocytoma (see Ch. 37).

Labetalol (see below) is a competitive α_1-, β_1- and β_2-antagonist, which is more active at β- than at α-receptors. At low doses (5–10 mg i.v.) it decreases arterial pressure without producing a tachycardia. At higher doses, the β effect becomes more prominent, with negative inotropic and chronotropic effects. *Carvedilol* is a α_1- and β-receptor antagonist which also has direct vasodilator effects (see below).

Urapidil is a peripheral postsynaptic α_1-selective antagonist, which is also an agonist at central serotonin 5-HT_{1A} receptors. It reduces blood pressure by arterial and venodilatation, with little effect on heart rate or cardiac output, because 5HT_{1A} receptor stimulation suppresses central autonomic activity and attenuates any reflex tachycardia. It has fewer adverse effects than other α_1-blockers. Intravenous urapidil as a bolus of 0.5–2 mg kg^{-1} may be useful in patients with pre-eclampsia, hypertensive crises or perioperative hypertension.

α_2-Selective antagonists

Drugs of this type, e.g. yohimbine, are not used because of the unacceptable incidence of adverse effects.

Non-selective α-antagonists

Non-selective α-blockers, e.g. phentolamine or tolazoline, block α_1- and α_2-receptors equally and produce more postural hypotension, reflex tachycardia and adverse gastrointestinal effects (e.g. abdominal cramps, diarrhoea) than α_1-selective drugs. Phentolamine 2–5 mg i.v. produces a rapid decrease in arterial pressure lasting 10–15 min and is used for the treatment of hypertensive crises.

β-Adrenergic receptor antagonists

β-adrenergic receptor antagonists (β-blockers) are structurally similar to the β-agonists, e.g. isoprenaline. Variations in the molecular structure (primarily of the catechol ring) have produced compounds that do not activate adenylate cyclase and the second messenger system despite binding avidly to the β-adrenergic receptor. Most are stereoisomers and the L-form is generally more potent (as an agonist or antagonist) than the D-form. β-blockers are competitive antagonists with high receptor affinity, although their effects are attenuated by high concentrations of endogenous or exogenous agonists. They may be classified according to:

- their relative affinity for β_1- or β_2-receptors
- agonist/antagonist activity
- membrane-stabilizing effect
- ancillary effects (e.g. action at other receptors).

β_1- or β_2-adrenergic receptor affinity

The relative potency of β-blockers is less important than their relative effects on the different β-receptor subtypes. Compounds are available which block preferentially either β_1- or β_2-receptors, although in clinical practice the β_1-selective drugs are more important. The first generation of β-blockers (e.g. propranolol, timolol) were non-selective; second-generation drugs (e.g. atenolol, metoprolol, bisoprolol) are selective for β_1-receptors but have no ancillary effects. The third generation of β-blockers are β_1-selective, but also have effects on other receptors (e.g. labetalol and carvedilol are antagonists at α_1-adrenergic receptors, and celiprolol produces vasodilatation by a mechanism involving endothelial nitric oxide). β_1-Selective (or 'cardioselective') drugs have theoretical advantages, as some of the adverse effects of β-blockers are related to β_2-antagonism, but the selectivity of both drugs and tissues is only relative: all β_1-selective drugs antagonize β_2-receptors at higher doses, and 25% of cardiac β-receptors are of the β_2 subtype. However β_1-selective drugs appear to have fewer adverse effects on blood glucose control in diabetics, less effect on serum lipids and less effect on bronchial tone in patients with chronic obstructive pulmonary disease.

Partial agonist activity

Some β-blockers have intrinsic sympathomimetic activity (ISA), i.e. they are partial agonists. This stimulant effect is apparent at low levels of sympathetic activity, but at high levels of sympathetic discharge, blockade of endogenously released catecholamines is the major clinical effect. Partial agonists may be advantageous in patients with a low resting heart rate as they reduce the risk of AV conduction disturbance, and have theoretical advantages in patients with peripheral vascular disease or hyperlipidaemia. However, only β-blockers *without* partial agonist activity have been shown to be beneficial after myocardial infarction.

Membrane-stabilizing effect

Some β-blockers have a quinidine-like action, inhibiting Na^+ transport in nerve and cardiac conducting tissue ('membrane-stabilizing effect'). This may be demonstrated in vivo as a stabilizing effect on the cardiac action potential, reducing the slope of phase 4 noticeably, thus decreasing excitability and automaticity of the myocardium (see below). However, the membrane-stabilizing activity probably has little clinical significance, as it occurs only at plasma concentrations above the therapeutic range, and the antiarrhythmic effect of β-blockade occurs via inhibition of the effects of catecholamines.

Ancillary effects

Some of the newer β-blockers drugs have additional effects, e.g. action at α-receptors, vasodilatation, antioxidant effects and other actions. The relevance of these properties is discussed below.

Pharmacological properties of β-blockers

The pharmacological properties of β-blockers are summarized in Table 8.4. All are weak bases and most are well absorbed to produce peak plasma concentrations 1–3 h after oral administration. The more lipid-soluble drugs are almost completely absorbed, but are metabolized to a greater extent and tend to have a marked first-pass effect through the liver. This reduces their bioavailability, but is offset by the fact that the 4-hydroxylated metabolites so formed are also active. These active metabolites are excreted via the kidneys and may accumulate in patients with renal failure. Propranolol decreases both the clearance of amide local anaesthetics (by decreasing hepatic blood flow and inhibiting metabolism) and the pulmonary first-pass uptake of fentanyl. The first-pass metabolic pathways may also become saturated, so that proportionately higher plasma concentrations of the parent drug occur at higher oral doses. The first-pass effect is also a source of wide inter-individual variation in plasma concentrations achieved from the same dose of primarily metabolized drugs, though β-blockers have a flat dose–response curve and large changes in plasma concentration may give rise to only a small change in degree of β-blockade. However, differences in individual plasma concentration–response relationships may occur, possibly as a result of variations in sympathetic tone or the formation of active metabolites. All β-blockers are distributed widely throughout the body and significant concentrations occur in the CNS, particularly for the more lipid-soluble drugs (e.g. propranolol).

The less lipid-soluble drugs (e.g. atenolol) are less well absorbed, are metabolized to a lesser extent, are excreted via the kidneys and tend to have longer half-lives. Atenolol, nadolol and sotalol are excreted largely unchanged in urine and so are little affected by impairment of liver function.

Table 8.4 Pharmacological properties of β-blockers

Drug	β₁ selectivity	Partial agonist activity	Membrane stabilizing effect	Lipid solubility	Absorption (%)	Bioavailability (%)	Protein binding (%)	Terminal half-life (h)	Significant active metabolites	Elimination
Acebutolol	±	+	+	Medium	90	50	20	8–10	Yes	Hepatic, renal
Atenolol	+	–	–	Low	50	40	5	6–8	No	Renal
Bisoprolol	++	–	–	Low	>90	90		10–12	No	Hepatic, renal
Carvedilol	–	–	?	High	>90	25	98	6–10	Yes	Hepatic
Celiprolol	+	+	?	Low	30	30			No	Plasma hydrolysis
Esmolol	+	–	–	High	70	30	55	0.15	No	Hepatic
Labetalol	–	±	+	High	90	50	50	4	No	Hepatic
Metoprolol	+	–	±	High	90	50	10–20	4	No	Renal
Nadolol	–	–	–	Low	30	30	20	20–24	No	Hepatic
Oxprenolol	–	+	+	High	80	50	80	2	No	Hepatic
Pindolol	–	++	±	Medium	90	90	50	4	No	Hepatic
Propranolol	–	–	++	High	90	30	90	5	Yes	Renal
Sotalol	–	+	+	Low	80	60		8–15	No	Hepatic, renal
Timolol	–	+	±	High	90	50	10	4	No	

Indications for β-blockade

See Tables 8.5 and 8.6 for indications of β-blockade.

Hypertension. β-Blockers are regarded as first-line therapy for the treatment of hypertension, either alone or in combination with other drugs (see below). They are of proven benefit in reducing the incidence of stroke and the morbidity and mortality from coronary heart disease in hypertensive patients. The antihypertensive effect results from a combination of factors:

- Reductions in heart rate, cardiac output and myocardial contractility.
- A reduction in central sympathetic nervous activity. The significance of this is uncertain, as different drugs vary widely in their CNS penetration, but have similar effects on arterial pressure.

Table 8.5   Clinical indications for β-blockade

Hypertension
Ischaemic heart disease
Secondary prevention of myocardial infarction
Obstructive cardiomyopathy
Congestive cardiac failure
Arrhythmias
Miscellaneous

Table 8.6   Specific perioperative indications for β-blockers

Prevention or treatment of intraoperative hypertension, tachycardia and supraventricular tachyarrhythmias associated with excessive sympathetic activity
Treatment of postoperative hypertension
Controlled hypotension
Prophylaxis or treatment of perioperative myocardial ischaemia
Pre- and perioperative management of phaeochromocytoma
Pre- and perioperative management of thyrotoxic patients

- *Decreased plasma renin concentration.* β-Blockers decrease resting and orthostatic release of renin to a variable extent. The non-selective drugs propranolol and timolol cause the greatest reduction, while partial agonists (oxprenolol, pindolol) or β_1-selective drugs are less effective. However, no correlation has been found between renin-lowering effect and antihypertensive activity or dosage of β-blocker used.
- *Effects on peripheral resistance.* β-Blockade does not reduce peripheral resistance directly and may even cause an increase by allowing unopposed α stimulation. As the vasodilating effect of catecholamines on skeletal muscle is β_2-mediated, unopposed α stimulation would be expected to be lower with cardioselective drugs or partial agonists. However, cardioselectivity decreases with dosage and, as hypertensive patients often require a large dose of β-blocker, little real advantage is offered. Drugs with partial agonist activity may not increase peripheral resistance as much as those without.

Arterial pressure reduction begins within an hour of β-blocker administration, but several days may elapse before the plateau is reached, and the full hypotensive effect of oral β-blockers takes about 2 weeks. This suggests the involvement of several mechanisms including readjustment of central and peripheral cardiovascular reflexes. During chronic administration, the hypotensive effects of β-blockers last longer than the pharmacological half-life, so that single daily dosage is adequate therapeutically. However, upregulation of receptors may occur, leading to adverse effects (tachycardia, hypertension, myocardial ischaemia) on abrupt withdrawal of β-blockers. This may be important in the perioperative period. All are equally effective as hypotensive drugs; patients unresponsive to one β-blocker are generally unresponsive to all.

Ischaemic heart disease. β-Blockers improve symptoms and decrease the frequency and severity of silent myocardial ischaemia in patients with ischaemic heart disease. The incidence of myocardial ischaemia in high-risk patients is reduced by perioperative β-blockade and long-term outcome may be improved. β-blockers reduce heart rate and contractility, with consequent decreases in wall tension and myocardial oxygen demand. A slower heart rate also permits longer diastolic filling time and hence potentially greater coronary perfusion. The perfusion of ischaemic regions may be improved by redistribution of myocardial blood flow, and other additional mechanisms may be involved.

β-Blockade also reduces exercise-induced increases in arterial pressure, velocity of cardiac contraction and oxygen consumption at any workload. Partial agonists have less effect on the resting heart rate and theoretically increase the metabolic demand of the myocardium; they may be less effective in patients with angina at rest or at very low levels of exercise. In contrast to effects on arterial pressure, there is a more direct relationship between plasma concentration and antianginal effect. To achieve effective plasma concentrations over a sustained period as a single daily dosage, either the long half-life drugs (e.g. atenolol, nadolol) or slow-release preparations (e.g. oxprenolol-SR, propranolol-LA, metoprolol-SR) are required.

Secondary prevention of myocardial infarction. Early i.v. administration after acute myocardial infarction can decrease infarct size, the incidence of ventricular and supraventricular arrhythmias and mortality in both lower- and higher-risk groups (e.g. elderly patients or those with left ventricular dysfunction). Mortality is reduced by 20–40%, and the risk of re-infarction is reduced if oral therapy is continued for 2–3 years.

Obstructive cardiomyopathy. β-Blockers improve exercise tolerance and alleviate symptoms in hypertrophic obstructive cardiomyopathy by decreasing heart rate, myocardial work, contractility and, thus, outflow tract obstruction. However, the incidence of sudden death in this condition is not affected. The incidence of cyanotic episodes caused by pulmonary outflow obstruction in patients with Fallot's tetralogy is reduced by a similar mechanism.

Congestive heart failure. Congestive heart failure is accompanied by a compensatory increase in sympathetic nervous stimulation with increased plasma and cardiac noradrenaline concentrations, leading to increases in cardiac output, systemic vascular resistance and afterload. Plasma renin concentration also increases. Whilst beneficial as an acute response in the short term, high circulating catecholamine concentrations are directly toxic to the myocardium. Desensitization of myocardial β_1 adrenergic receptors occurs via downregulation and altered signal transduction. In combination with chronically increased peripheral resistance, this leads to ventricular remodelling with progressively worsening myocardial function and a propensity to arrhythmias. Some second- and third-generation β-blockers (bisoprolol, metoprolol and carvedilol) have been shown to decrease morbidity and mortality in heart failure by improving ventricular function. The mechanism is primarily by upregulation of β-receptor density or function, though other factors may contribute, including slowing of heart rate or an antiarrhythmic effect. Bisoprolol and metoprolol are β_1-selective antagonists but carvedilol also has β_2- and α_1-antagonist and antioxidant effects which may contribute to its action. They must be introduced cautiously in heart failure as symptoms may initially worsen, and ventricular function improves only after 1 month of therapy.

Arrhythmias (see below). β-Blockers are effective in the treatment of arrhythmias caused by sympathetic nervous overactivity or after myocardial infarction. The mechanisms are related to β-blockade itself rather than any membrane-stabilizing effect, e.g. antagonism of catecholamine effects on the cardiac action potential and muscle contractility. The result is a slowing of rate of discharge from the sinus and any ectopic pacemaker, and slowing of conduction and increased refractoriness of the AV node. β-Blockers also slow conduction in anomalous pathways. They may be used i.v. to terminate an attack of supraventricular tachycardia, or decrease the ventricular rate in atrial fibrillation and flutter; conversion to sinus rhythm may also be achieved. If given within 30 min of i.v. verapamil, there is a danger of severe bradycardia or asystole. Most β-blockers have similar antiarrhythmic effects in adequate dosage, but esmolol has the advantage of a short half-life (see below) so that adverse effects are limited. They are also useful as second-line alternatives for the treatment of ventricular tachycardia. Sotalol has both class 2 and class 3 antiarrhythmic activity (see below), and is licensed for use only for its antiarrhythmic action, in particular for the treatment of supraventricular and ventricular tachycardias.

Miscellaneous. β-Blockers are prescribed for migraine prophylaxis, essential tremor and anxiety states. They are useful for glaucoma as they decrease intraocular pressure, probably by reducing the production of aqueous humour. Topical preparations (e.g. timolol, betaxolol, carteolol) are used in an attempt to decrease adverse effects, but significant systemic absorption may still take place; bradycardia, hypotension and bronchospasm may occur, particularly during anaesthesia. β-Blockers diminish the symptoms of thyrotoxicosis and are used as part of preoperative preparation before thyroidectomy. They also may be used as part of a hypotensive anaesthetic technique.

Adverse reactions to β-blockers

All available β-blockers have similar adverse effects, although their magnitude depends on β_1-selectivity and the presence or absence of partial agonist activity. The reactions may be classified as follows.

Reactions resulting from β-blockade

Cardiovascular effects. β-Blockers may precipitate heart failure in patients with poor LV function, and accentuate AV block. Their negative inotropic and chronotropic effects may be additive with other drugs affecting cardiac conduction or drugs used during anaesthesia. They prevent the compensatory tachycardia which accompanies hypovolaemia, so severe hypotension may occur if intravascular replacement is delayed. Bradycardia caused by excessive β-blockade may be treated by atropine, β-agonists (e.g. dobutamine or isoprenaline), glucagon or calcium chloride. Occasionally, cardiac pacing may be required.

Induction of bronchospasm. This occurs in patients with asthma or chronic bronchitis who rely on sympathetically (β_2) mediated bronchodilatation. Theoretically, β_1-selective drugs are less likely to aggravate bronchospasm in asthmatics, but as their selectivity is only relative, they should not be considered completely safe.

Raynaud's phenomenon. Raynaud's phenomenon and peripheral vascular disease are relative contraindications to the use of β-blockers, as symptoms of cold extremities may be exacerbated.

Diabetes mellitus. Cardiovascular (tachycardia-β_1) and metabolic (hepatic glycogenolysis-β_2) responses to insulin-induced hypoglycaemia are impaired. These effects may be more marked with non-selective drugs.

Other. Increased muscle fatigue, possibly resulting from blockade of β_2-mediated vasodilatation in muscles during exercise. A withdrawal phenomenon may occur after abrupt cessation of long-term therapy for angina, causing rebound tachycardia, worsening angina or precipitation of myocardial infarction. Impotence occurs commonly during chronic β-blocker therapy.

Idiosyncratic reactions

Central nervous system effects occur with some β-blockers, including nightmares, hallucinations, insomnia and depression. These effects are more common with the lipophilic drugs (e.g. propranolol, acebutolol, oxprenolol and metoprolol). Gastrointestinal reactions include nausea, vomiting, and diarrhoea.

Newer β-blockers

Recently introduced third-generation β-blockers (e.g. labetalol, bucindolol and carvedilol) are mostly non-selective ($\beta_1 > \beta_2$) antagonists which also produce vasodilatation by several mechanisms. Labetalol and carvedilol are also α_1-antagonists; bucindolol produces direct vasodilatation by a cAMP-dependent mechanism. The severity of some of the adverse effects of β-blockade may be less with those drugs with vasodilating properties.

Labetalol is a competitive α_1-, β_1- and β_2-antagonist, which is a partial agonist at β_2-receptors. It is four to seven times more potent at β- than at α-receptors and is useful for the prevention and treatment of perioperative hypertension, or to produce controlled hypotension (see Ch. 16). It is also available as an oral preparation for the treatment of chronic hypertension or the preoperative management of phaeochromocytoma (see Ch. 37). Intravenous labetalol in small increments (e.g. 5–10 mg) produces a controlled decrease in arterial pressure over 5–10 min with no change in cardiac output or reflex tachycardia, suggesting that at this dose the vasodilating action predominates. At higher doses, the β-effect becomes more prominent, with negative inotropic and chronotropic effects.

Carvedilol is an antagonist at α_1- and β-receptors (with relative β:α_1 selectivity of 10:1 and no partial agonist activity), but it has other effects including significant antioxidant activity, inhibition of endothelin synthesis and possibly calcium channel blockade in higher doses; these may account for some of its beneficial activity in patients with cardiac failure. Carvedilol is a stereoisomer which undergoes extensive first-pass metabolism with the production of active metabolites.

Nebivolol is a lipophilic β_1-selective blocker which is administered as a racemic mixture of equal proportions of D- and L-enantiomers. It has no membrane-stabilizing activity but has vasodilatory effects probably mediated by endothelial nitric oxide.

Bucindolol is a non-selective β-blocker which also produces vasodilatation by a cAMP-dependent mechanism. It also has β_3-agonist and α_1-antagonist actions.

Celiprolol is a β_1-selective blocker which is a weak β_2-agonist and has α_2-antagonist activity. It also has direct vasodilator effects which may be mediated by endothelial nitric oxide release. Celiprolol is excreted unchanged.

Esmolol is a rapid-onset, short-acting β_1-selective blocker with no membrane-stabilizing or partial agonist activity and is only available for i.v. use. It has an onset time of 1–2 min and is metabolized rapidly by red cell esterases (distinct from plasma cholinesterases); its elimination half-life is 9 min. The rapid onset and offset of effect are an advantage in the perioperative period, as any effects such as bradycardia or hypotension are short-lived. It is effective in preventing or controlling intraoperative tachycardia and hypertension, and is also useful for the treatment of supraventricular tachyarrhythmias, e.g. atrial fibrillation or flutter. It may be given as a slow i.v. bolus of 0.5–2.0 mg kg^{-1} or an infusion of 25–500 μg kg^{-1} min^{-1};

its effects terminate within 10–20 min of stopping the infusion.

DRUGS ACTING ON THE PARASYMPATHETIC NERVOUS SYSTEM

The major drugs in use which act on the parasympathetic nervous system are muscarinic antagonists (e.g. atropine, hyoscine and propantheline), and parasympathetic agonists (e.g. the anticholinesterases neostigmine and pyridostigmine). Neuromuscular blocking drugs act at nicotinic receptors, and are described in Chapter 6.

PARASYMPATHETIC ANTAGONISTS

Parasympathetic antagonists block muscarinic ACh receptors and are either tertiary or quaternary amine compounds. Tertiary amines, e.g. atropine and hyoscine, are more lipid- soluble and cross biological membranes, e.g. the blood–brain barrier, to affect central ACh receptors and produce sedative or stimulatory effects. Similar antimuscarinic drugs, e.g. benzatropine and procyclidine, are useful anti-parkinsonian agents because of their predominant central action; procyclidine is useful for the reversal of acute dystonic reactions to dopaminergic drugs (e.g. phenothiazines, droperidol). Other muscarinic antagonists used as gastrointestinal or urinary antispasmodics are quaternary amines; they are poorly absorbed after oral administration and produce minimal central effects.

Atropine

Atropine has widespread, dose-dependent antimuscarinic effects on parasympathetic functions. Salivary secretion, micturition, heart rate and visual accommodation are impaired sequentially. CNS effects (sedation or excitation, hallucinations and hyperthermia) may occur at high doses. Atropine is administered in doses of 0.6–3.0 mg i.v. to counteract bradycardia in the presence of hypotension and to prevent the bradycardia associated with vagal stimulation or the use of anticholinesterase drugs. Adverse cardiac effects of atropine include an increase in cardiac work and ventricular arrhythmias. Occasionally, atropine may produce an initial transient bradycardia, thought to be caused by increased ACh release mediated by M_2-receptor antagonism. In therapeutic dosage, effects mediated by M_3-receptors (tachycardia, bronchodilatation, dry mouth, mydriasis) predominate.

Hyoscine

Hyoscine hydrobromide has less effect on heart rate than atropine but crosses the blood–brain barrier more readily and may cause confusion, sedation and ataxia, particularly in the elderly. This may result in the 'central anticholinergic syndrome'. It has greater antisialagogue and mydriatic effects than atropine. It is also useful as an antiemetic, particularly for the prophylaxis of motion sickness, and is available as a transdermal patch for this purpose. Hyoscine butylbromide is used as a gastrointestinal or genitourinary antispasmodic.

Glycopyrronium bromide (glycopyrrolate)

This is a quaternary amine which has similar anticholinergic actions to those of atropine. It is used as an alternative to atropine during the reversal of neuromuscular blockade or for its antisecretory actions. Some other quaternary amines, e.g. propantheline and dicycloverine, have a mainly peripheral parasympathetic antagonist action and are used as gastrointestinal and urinary antispasmodics.

Ipratropium bromide is used as an inhaled anticholinergic bronchodilator.

Antimuscarinic drugs in premedication

Subcutaneous or oral atropine and hyoscine have long been used as premedicant drugs, usually in combination with an opioid or sedative, to decrease salivary and respiratory secretions and counteract vagal reflexes. Their use declined with the decreased use of ether, and many patients find the associated dry mouth and blurred vision unpleasant. However, if an antisialagogue is particularly indicated, glycopyrrolate is effective in a dose of 0.2 mg i.m. or i.v. with minimal central or cardiovascular effects.

PARASYMPATHETIC AGONISTS

Pilocarpine is a muscarinic agonist used as a topical miotic in the treatment of glaucoma. Other parasympathetic agonists used historically as gastrointestinal tract and bladder smooth muscle stimulants have been superseded.

Anticholinesterase drugs

Neostigmine and *pyridostigmine* antagonize acetylcholinesterase, thereby decreasing the breakdown of released ACh. They exert both nicotinic and muscarinic effects and are used in anaesthesia to reverse non-depolarizing neuromuscular blockade (see Ch. 6), accompanied by an antimuscarinic drug to minimize the adverse vagal effects. Other anticholinesterases include *edrophonium* (short-acting) and *pyridostigmine* (long-acting), used for the diagnosis and symptomatic management of myasthenia gravis, respectively.

VASODILATORS

Vasodilators dilate arteries or veins and may reduce afterload, preload or both. Acute and chronic heart failure are both associated with a reflex increase in sympathetic tone and an increase in systemic vascular resistance. By lowering this resistance (afterload), myocardial work and oxygen requirements are reduced. Vasodilators acting on the venous side of the circulation (e.g. nitrates) increase venous capacitance, reduce venous return to the heart and so decrease left ventricular filling pressure (preload), myocardial fibre length and myocardial oxygen consumption for the same degree of cardiac work performed. They have several clinical indications (Table 8.7).

Vasodilators may be classified into those acting directly on vascular smooth muscle (nitroprusside, nitrates, hydralazine, diazoxide, minoxidil, calcium channel blockers) and neurohumoral antagonists (α-blockers and ACE inhibitors). They may also be classified according to which side of the heart they act on preferentially. Hydralazine, calcium channel blockers, and minoxidil act mainly on afterload. Nitrates principally affect preload. Nitroprusside, α-blockers and ACE inhibitors have a balanced effect on arteries and veins.

Table 8.7 Indications for vasodilators
Acute and chronic left ventricular failure
Prophylaxis and treatment of unstable and stable angina
Treatment of acute myocardial ischaemia and infarction
Chronic hypertension
Acute hypertensive episodes
Elective controlled hypotensive anaesthesia

NITRATES

The organic nitrates (*glyceryl trinitrate* and *isosorbide mononitrate and dinitrate*) cause systemic and coronary vasodilatation. They act primarily on systemic veins, causing venodilatation, sequestration of blood in venous capacitance beds and a reduction in preload. Arteriolar dilatation occurs at higher doses and afterload is reduced; tachycardia, hypotension and headaches may occur. Systolic pressure decreases more than diastolic pressure, so coronary perfusion pressure is preserved. In left ventricular failure, venodilatation is beneficial, reducing pulmonary congestion; cardiac dynamics may be improved so that stroke volume and cardiac output increase. Nitrates are used widely for the prevention and treatment of angina and myocardial infarction as they cause vasodilatation in stenotic coronary arteries and redistribution of myocardial blood flow. Glyceryl trinitrate (GTN) is a powerful myometrial relaxant. Nitrates also inhibit platelet aggregation in vitro.

Nitrates are converted to the active compounds nitric oxide (NO) and nitrosothiols by a denitration mechanism involving reduced sulphydryl groups. NO and nitrosothiols activate guanylate cyclase in the cytoplasm of vascular smooth muscle cells to increase intracellular cGMP. This leads to protein kinase phosphorylation and decreased intracellular calcium, causing vascular smooth muscle relaxation and vasodilatation. Tolerance to nitrates develops rapidly during continuous therapy (within 24 h), caused by depletion of reduced sulphydryl groups or activation of neurohormonal counter-mechanisms, and a nitrate-free interval of 8–12 h is required. Nitrates may be administered by oral, buccal, transdermal and intravenous routes. Intravenous nitrates may be used for the treatment of perioperative hypertension or myocardial ischaemia or as part of a deliberate hypotensive anaesthetic technique. They are absorbed by rubber and plastics (especially PVC infusion bags), so are best administered by syringe pump.

SODIUM NITROPRUSSIDE

Sodium nitroprusside (SNP) is reduced to NO on exposure to reducing agents and in tissues, including vascular smooth muscle cell membranes. The process is non-enzymatic but SNP therefore has a similar ultimate mechanism of action to nitrates (increased intracellular cGMP). SNP produces similar effects on capacitance and resistance vessels so that preload and afterload are equally reduced, and it is useful in the management of acute left ventricular failure. Systolic and diastolic pressures decrease equally in a dose-dependent manner. In larger doses (as used for hypotensive anaesthesia), heart rate increases.

Release of NO from nitroprusside is accompanied by release of cyanide ions, which are detoxified by the liver and kidney to thiocyanate (requiring thiosulphate, vitamin B_{12} and the enzyme rhodanase), which is excreted slowly in urine. It has an immediate, short-lived effect (lasting only for a few minutes) so it must be given by intravenous infusion. SNP is photodegraded to cyanide ions, so infusion solutions should be protected from light and not used if they have turned dark brown or blue. Also, if the total dose of SNP exceeds 1.5 mg kg^{-1} or the infusion rate exceeds 1.5 µg kg^{-1} min^{-1}, cyanide and thiocyanate may accumulate, with the risk of metabolic acidosis; plasma bicarbonate concentration should be monitored. The risks of cyanide toxicity are increased in the presence of impaired renal or hepatic function, and symptoms may be delayed until after the SNP infusion has been discontinued. Plasma cyanide or thiocyanate concentrations may also be monitored if the drug is used for more than 2 days. Thiocyanate is potentially neurotoxic and may cause hypothyroidism. In cases of suspected cyanide toxicity, sodium thiosulphate (which promotes conversion to thiocyanate), dicobalt edetate (which chelates cyanide ions) and hydroxocobalamin (which combines with cyanide to form cyanocobalamin) may be given. In practice, nitroprusside is usually well tolerated and most symptoms are associated with too rapid a decrease in arterial pressure.

POTASSIUM CHANNEL ACTIVATORS

Hydralazine, minoxidil and diazoxide are direct-acting arteriolar vasodilators which have largely been superseded. Minoxidil and diazoxide activate ATP-sensitive K$^+$ channels in vascular smooth muscle cells, causing K$^+$ efflux and membrane hyperpolarization. This leads to closure of calcium channels, reduced intracellular calcium availability and consequently smooth muscle relaxation and arterial vasodilatation. Hydralazine may act via a similar mechanism. All these drugs reduce afterload, with little or no effect on preload. Their effects are limited by reflex tachycardia and a tendency to cause sodium and water retention (by activation of the renin–angiotensin system and a direct renal mechanism). Consequently, they are usually administered during long term therapy with a β-blocker and a diuretic.

Hydralazine is the most widely used of these drugs. Its half-life is short (approximately 2.5 h), but its antihypertensive effect is relatively prolonged. It may be given as a slow i.v. bolus of 5–10 mg, with appropriate monitoring, for the treatment of hypertensive emergencies.

Minoxidil is only available orally. It has a long duration of action (12–24 h) unrelated to its plasma half-life, and it causes hypertrichosis. T-wave abnormalities on ECG are observed in 60% of patients.

Diazoxide has a similar structure to thiazide diuretics. It causes sodium retention, increases plasma glucose concentration and may be used orally for the treatment of intractable hypoglycaemia. In hypertensive emergencies, diazoxide 1–3 mg kg^{-1} i.v. may be given rapidly (over 30 s) for effects lasting 4–24 h. However, it is difficult to control the action or duration of action of repeated doses, and it is rarely used.

Nicorandil

Nicorandil activates K$^+$ channels in vascular smooth muscle, but also causes NO release and increases intracellular cGMP in vascular endothelium, causing venous dilatation. It therefore reduces preload as well as afterload and is a potent coronary vasodilator with no effect on heart rate or contractility. It is metabolized in the liver, excreted via the kidneys and does not cause tolerance. Nicorandil is used for the treatment of angina, e.g. in nitrate-tolerant patients or those unresponsive to β-blockers. There is potential for an additive hypotensive effect with other vasodilators, although few data are available.

CALCIUM CHANNEL BLOCKERS

MECHANISM OF ACTION

The normal function of cardiac myocytes and conducting tissues, skeletal muscle, vascular and other smooth muscle, and neurones depends on the availability of intracellular calcium ions. Under physiological conditions, calcium entry into the cell induces further calcium release from the sarcoplasmic reticulum, which facilitates conduction of the cardiac action potential and excitation–contraction coupling by interaction with calmodulin (in smooth muscle) or troponin (within cardiac muscle). Calcium enters the cell via several ion channels situated on the plasma membrane, the most important being voltage-gated calcium channels, which are activated by nerve impulses or membrane depolarization. Other types of calcium channels are receptor-operated and stretch-activated channels. Calcium channel blockers (CCBs) are a diverse group of compounds which decrease calcium entry into cardiac and vascular smooth muscle cells through the L-subtype (long-lasting inward calcium current) of voltage-gated calcium channels. CCBs bind in several ways to the α_1 subunit of L-type channels to impede calcium entry. Phenylalkylamines (e.g. verapamil) bind to the intracellular portion of the channel and physically occlude it, whereas dihydropyridines modify the extracellular allosteric structure of the channel. Benzothiazepines (e.g. diltiazem) act on the α_1 subunit, although the mechanism has not been fully elucidated, and may have further actions on sodium–potassium exchange and calcium–calmodulin binding.

Cardiac cells in the SA and AV nodes are dependent on the slow inward calcium current for depolarization. CCBs which act here decrease calcium entry during phase 0 of the action potential of SA node and AV node cells, decreasing heart rate and AV node conduction. Calcium entry during phase 2 of the action potential of ventricular myocytes may be decreased (Fig. 8.5) and excitation–contraction coupling inhibited, causing decreased myocardial contractility. Some CCBs may also have favourable effects on endothelial function.

CLINICAL EFFECTS

CCBs differ in their selectivity for cardiac muscle cells, conducting tissue and vascular smooth muscle, but they all decrease myocardial contractility and produce coronary and systemic vasodilatation with a consequent decrease in arterial pressure. They have been used widely for the treatment of hypertension and angina, but have been partly superseded by newer

drugs. Other current indications include prevention of vasospasm in subarachnoid haemorrhage or Raynaud's disease. Verapamil and diltiazem also decrease SA node activity, AV node conduction and heart rate, and they are useful in the treatment of paroxysmal supraventricular tachyarrhythmias. CCBs may also inhibit platelet aggregation, protect against bronchospasm and improve lower oesophageal sphincter function. The non-dihydropyridines are contraindicated in the presence of second- or third-degree heart block and should not be combined with β-blockers as they may cause bradycardia or heart block. With the exception of amlodipine and felodipine, calcium channel blockers should not be used in patients with heart failure. In some patients, sudden cessation of CCBs may lead to an exacerbation of angina symptoms.

CLASSIFICATION

CCBs are a diverse group of compounds which have been classified in several ways, according to their structure, mechanism of action and specificity for slow calcium channels. They are classified here by their chemical structure, tissue selectivity and pharmacokinetic properties (Table 8.8).

First-generation calcium channel blockers

The first-generation CCBs (verapamil, diltiazem and nifedipine) have a rapid onset of action which may reduce arterial pressure acutely and produce reflex sympathetic activation. They have marked negative dromotropic and inotropic effects (especially verapamil and diltiazem). Their intrinsic duration of action is short, but slow-release formulations have been developed (see below). All are well absorbed but undergo a significant first-pass effect, leading to low bioavailability. They are highly protein-bound and metabolized extensively by hepatic demethylation and dealkylation, with wide individual pharmacokinetic variability (Table 8.9). Most CCBs possess one or more chiral centres, and the different enantiomeric forms have different pharmacokinetic and pharmacodynamic properties. For example, L-verapamil undergoes higher first-pass metabolism than the D-form, so plasma concentrations of L-verapamil are relatively higher after intravenous administration, producing more pronounced negative inotropic and chronotropic effects.

Nifedipine is a dihydropyridine derivative which is a systemic and coronary arterial vasodilator. It is effective in countering coronary artery spasm, thought to be an important component of all forms of angina, and it may bring symptomatic relief in patients with

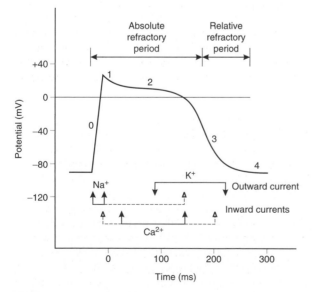

Fig 8.5
The cardiac action potential.

Table 8.8 Classification of calcium channel blockers

| Group | Prototype/ first-generation drugs | Second- and third-generation drugs | Effects on: | | | | |
			SA node	AV node conduction	Myocardial contractility	Peripheral arteries	Coronary arteries
Benzothiazepine	Diltiazem		−/+	+	+	+	++
Phenylalkylamine	Verapamil		++	++	+	+	+
Dihydropyridine	Nifedipine		−	−	+	++	++
		Nicardipine	−	−	+/−	++	+++
		Nimodipine	−	−	+/−	++	+/−
		Felodipine	−	−	−	+++	+
		Isradipine	−	−	−	+++	+
		Amlodipine[a]	−	−	−	+++	++
		Lacidipine[a]	−	−	−	++++	+/−
Phenylalkylamine/ benzimidazoyl	Mibefradil		−	−		+	++

[a]Third-generation calcium antagonists.

peripheral vasospastic (e.g. Raynaud's) disease. Its antianginal effect is additive with that of β-adrenergic blocking drugs and nitrates. Adverse effects include flushing, headaches, ankle oedema, dizziness, tiredness and palpitations. Nifedipine is absorbed rapidly, particularly when the stomach is empty, with an onset of action of 20 min. This may produce reflex tachycardia and increased myocardial contractility.

Verapamil is a phenylalkylamine which has more pronounced effects on the SA and AV nodes compared with other CCBs, and is used mainly as an antiarrhythmic (see below). It has vasodilator and negative inotropic properties and is also used for the treatment of angina, hypertension and hypertrophic obstructive cardiomyopathy. Verapamil has a marked negative inotropic action and may cause bradycardia, hypotension,

Table 8.9 Pharmacokinetic properties of some commonly used calcium channel blockers

Drug	Nifedipine	Verapamil	Diltiazem	Nicardipine	Felodipine	Amlodipine	Lacidipine
Bioavailability (%)	50	20	25–50	30	15	65–80	10
Elimination half-life (h)	3–5	5–8	2–6	3–8	25	35–50	13–19
Route of elimination	Renal, hepatic	Renal, hepatic,	Hepatic	Renal, hepatic	Renal, hepatic	Renal	Hepatic, renal
Time to peak plasma concentration (h)	1–2	4–8	3–4	1	12–24	6–12	1–3

AV block or heart failure when combined with β-blockers or other cardiodepressant drugs (including volatile anaesthetic agents). It may also potentiate the effects of neuromuscular blocking drugs. Both verapamil and diltiazem inhibit the hepatic metabolism of several drugs; plasma concentrations of digoxin, carbamazepine and theophyllines are increased by verapamil.

Diltiazem is a benzothiazepine whose predominant effect is on coronary arteries rather than conducting tissue, and is used mainly in the treatment of hypertension and angina. It can cause myocardial depression, especially when combined with β-blockers. It is metabolized in the liver, producing active metabolites, and is excreted via the kidneys.

Second- and third-generation CCBs

The second-generation CCBs are dihydropyridine derivatives (either sustained-release formulations or new compounds) which have a slower onset and longer duration of action, and greater vascular smooth muscle selectivity. The slow onset results in less sympathetic activation and reflex tachycardia. The new compounds (e.g. felodipine, nisoldipine, nicardipine) have less effect on AV conduction and less negative inotropic and chronotropic effects. All have little effect on lipid or glucose metabolism and may be used in patients with renal dysfunction. Some have special features.

Nimodipine is selective for cerebral vasculature and is used to prevent vasospasm after subarachnoid haemorrhage. *Nicardipine* causes less reduction in myocardial contractility than other CCBs. *Felodipine* acts predominantly on peripheral vascular smooth muscle and has negligible effects on myocardial contractility, although it does produce coronary vasodilatation. It also has a mild diuretic and natriuretic effect. It is indicated for the treatment of hypertension, but has been used in patients with impaired LV function.

The third generation of CCBs (lacidipine, amlodipine) bind to specific high-affinity sites in the calcium channel complex. They have a particularly slow onset and long duration of action, and so reflex sympathetic stimulation is not evident but adverse effects related to vasodilatation (headache, flushing, ankle oedema) do occur. Both are extensively metabolized in the liver to inactive metabolites which are excreted via the kidneys and liver. *Lacidipine* is highly lipophilic, so that it is sequestered in the lipid bilayer of vascular smooth muscle cells and may delay the development of atherosclerosis via effects on modulators of vascular smooth muscle and platelet function. Lacidipine may augment the action of endothelium-derived relaxing factors (e.g. NO – which has vasodilator, antiplatelet and antiproliferative effects) and antagonize endothelin-1, a potent vasoconstrictor which also stimulates endothelial proliferation.

ANAESTHESIA AND CALCIUM CHANNEL BLOCKERS

Both intravenous and volatile anaesthetic agents block conduction through L-type calcium channels in neuronal and cardiac tissues, and may therefore interact with CCBs through pharmacokinetic and pharmacodynamic mechanisms. In general, CCBs potentiate the hypotensive effects of volatile anaesthetics: verapamil (and to a lesser extent diltiazem) has additive effects with halothane on cardiac conduction and contractility, with the potential for bradycardia and myocardial depression. Verapamil decreases the MAC of halothane, and, in an animal model, nifedipine enhances the analgesic effects of morphine by stimulation of spinal 5-HT$_3$ receptors. Plasma concentrations of verapamil are increased during anaesthesia with volatile agents, possibly because of decreased hepatic blood flow.

CCBs also potentiate the effects of depolarizing and non-depolarizing neuromuscular blockers in experimental conditions, although the clinical relevance of this is uncertain.

DRUGS ACTING VIA THE RENIN–ANGIOTENSIN–ALDOSTERONE SYSTEM

The renin–angiotensin–aldosterone system (RAS) is intimately involved with cardiovascular and body fluid homeostasis. Angiotensin II (AT-II) is the major regulator of the renin–angiotensin system and is a potent vasoconstrictor with several renal and extrarenal effects. AT-II has an important role in the maintenance of circulating volume in response to several stressors, whilst direct renal effects are mostly responsible for long-term regulation of body fluid volume and blood pressure.

The production of AT-II from angiotensinogen occurs in the walls of small blood vessels in the lungs, kidneys, and other organs, and in the plasma. The rate-limiting step for this cascade is the plasma concentration of renin (Fig. 8.6). AT-II is metabolized by several peptidases to several breakdown products including angiotensin III (AT-III), which has some activity at angiotensin receptors. Four subtypes of angiotensin receptor have been defined (AT$_{1-4}$). AT$_1$ receptors are found principally in vascular smooth muscle, adrenal cortex, kidney, liver and some areas of the brain, and mediate all the known physiological functions of AT-II. AT_2 receptors are present in the kidney, adrenal medulla, uterus, ovary and the brain; they may play a role in cell growth and differentiation. The roles of AT_3 and AT_4 receptors are unclear.

AT_1 receptors are typical G-protein-coupled receptors that activate phospholipase C with the production of DAG and IP_3. IP_3 causes the release of intracellular Ca^{2+}, which activates enzymes to cause the phosphorylation of intracellular proteins. AT-II also increases Ca^{2+} entry through membrane channels.

AT-II (see Fig. 8.6) is a potent vasoconstrictor (by direct action on vascular smooth muscle of arterioles and veins) and it promotes sodium reabsorption both by direct action at the proximal tubules and by stimulating aldosterone secretion. AT-II produces preglomerular vasoconstriction and efferent arteriole vasoconstriction, and so maintains glomerular filtration rate in response to a decrease in renal blood flow. It also affects the local regulation of blood flow in other vascular beds, e.g. the splanchnic circulation, and stimulates the sympathetic nervous system via direct and indirect methods to increase noradrenaline and adrenaline release; it may also inhibit cardiac vagal activity. AT-II stimulates erythropoiesis and has direct trophic effects on vascular smooth muscle and cardiac muscle, promoting cellular proliferation, migration and hypertrophy. There is some evidence for relative downregulation of AT_1 receptors and

upregulation of AT_2 receptors in cardiac failure, with AT_2 receptors being responsible for some cardioprotective effects.

RAS activity tends to be low in the resting state, but renin production (the rate-limiting step in the production of AT-II) is activated by several stimuli, e.g. depletion of circulating volume, haemorrhage or sodium depletion. This increases AT-II production and causes vasoconstriction, increased sympathetic activity (with increased cardiac output and arterial pressure) and sodium retention. The RAS may be involved in the pathogenesis of hypertension, but the relationship is complex; RAS activity may be high (e.g. in renal artery stenosis), low (as in primary aldosteronism) or variable (essential hypertension).

DRUGS ACTING ON THE RENIN–ANGIOTENSIN SYSTEM

The activity of the RAS may be inhibited by several mechanisms:

- *Suppression of renin release or inhibition of renin activity.* Sympatholytic drugs (e.g. β-blockers or central α-antagonists) directly inhibit renin secretion. Renin inhibitors competitively inhibit the reaction between renin and angiotensinogen, preventing the production of AT-II. Because renin release still occurs, the consequent reduction of

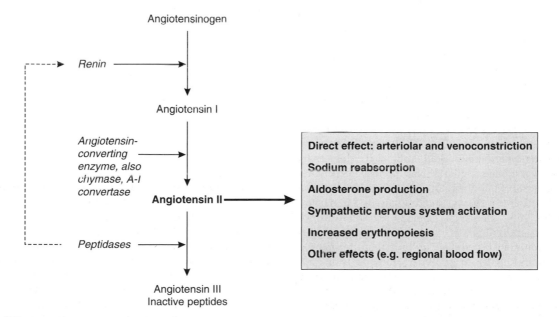

Fig. 8.6
The renin–angiotensin system.

plasma AT-II concentrations leads to a secondary increase in renin secretion, limiting the effect of such drugs.

- *Inhibition of angiotensin converting enzyme (ACE).* The primary mechanism of action of ACE inhibitors is to block the conversion of angiotensin I (AT-I) to AT-II, although effects on kinin and prostaglandin metabolism also contribute.
- *Blockade of AT-II receptors.* AT_1-receptor blockers non-competitively block AT_1 receptors and inhibit the RAS independently from the source of AT-II. They block any effects of AT-II resulting from compensatory stimulation of renin, such as reflex activation of the sympathetic nervous system.
- *Aldosterone antagonism.* Spironolactone and eplerenone are competitive antagonists of aldosterone at renal nuclear mineralocorticoid receptors (see Ch. 10).

ACE inhibitors

ACE inhibitors act principally by inhibition of AT-II formation, but effects on the kallikrein–kinin system are also important. All ACE inhibitors reduce arteriolar tone, peripheral resistance and arterial pressure by decreasing both AT-II-mediated vasoconstriction and sympathetic nervous system activity. Renal blood flow increases, further inhibiting aldosterone and antidiuretic hormone secretion and promoting sodium excretion. ACE inhibitors are useful in patients with heart failure, as preload and afterload decrease without an increase in heart rate, and cardiac output increases.

ACE is the same enzyme as kininase II and is involved in the metabolism of both kinins and prostaglandins. ACE inhibitors therefore block the degradation of kinins, substance P and endorphins, and increase prostaglandin concentrations. Bradykinin and other kinins are highly potent arterial and venous dilators which stimulate the production of arachidonic acid metabolites, NO and endothelial-derived hyperpolarization factor, via specific bradykinin B_2-receptors in vascular endothelium. Bradykinin also enhances the uptake of circulating glucose into skeletal muscle and has a protective effect on cardiac myocytes by a mechanism involving prostacyclin stimulation. Kinins have no major effect on arterial pressure regulation in normotensive individuals or those with low-renin hypertension, but they account for up to 30% of the effects of ACE inhibitors in renovascular hypertension. The adverse effects of dry cough and angioneurotic oedema sometimes associated with ACE inhibitors may be kinin-dependent. ACE is widely distributed in tissues and plasma; ACE inhibitors may differ in their affinity for ACE at different sites. Other tissue enzymes (AT-I convertase and chymase) may also produce AT-II, from AT-I or directly from angiotensinogen, so that the inhibition of the RAS by ACE inhibitors is incomplete.

Clinical applications of ACE inhibitors

ACE inhibitors are established in the treatment of hypertension and congestive heart failure. They improve left ventricular dysfunction after myocardial infarction, delay the progression of diabetic nephropathy and have a protective effect in non-diabetic chronic renal failure. ACE inhibitors improve vascular endothelial function by their effects on AT-II and bradykinin and improve long-term cardiovascular outcome in patients with established vascular disease. ACE inhibitors have a common mechanism of action, differing in the chemical structure of their active moieties, in potency, bioavailability, plasma half-life, route of elimination, distribution and affinity for tissue-bound ACE (Table 8.10). Most of the newer compounds are prodrugs, converted to an active metabolite by the liver, and have a prolonged duration of action. Most are excreted via the kidneys, and dosage should be reduced in the elderly and those with impaired renal or cardiac function. Enalapril is also available as the active drug, enalaprilat, and may be administered i.v. for the treatment of hypertensive emergencies.

ACE inhibitors are generally well tolerated, with no rebound hypertension after stopping therapy and few metabolic effects. Symptomatic first-dose hypotension may occur, particularly in hypovolaemic or sodium-depleted patients with high plasma renin concentrations. Symptomatic hypotension was more common with the higher doses originally used. ACE inhibitors have a synergistic effect with diuretics (which increase the activity of the renin–angiotensin system), but are less effective in patients taking NSAIDs.

Adverse effects of ACE inhibitors are classified into those that are class-specific (related to inhibition of ACE) and those that relate to specific drugs. Class-specific effects include hypotension, renal insufficiency, hyperkalaemia, cough (10%) and angioneurotic oedema (0.1–0.2%). ACE inhibitors may cause renal impairment, particularly if renal perfusion is decreased (e.g. because of renal artery stenosis, congestive heart failure or hypovolaemia) or if there is pre-existing renal disease. Renal impairment is also more likely in the elderly or those receiving NSAIDs, and renal function should be checked before starting ACE inhibitor therapy, and monitored subsequently. Hyperkalaemia (plasma K^+ concentration usually increases by 0.1–0.2 mmol L^{-1} because of decreased

Table 8.10 **Pharmacology of ACE inhibitors**

	Captopril	*Lisinopril*	*Enalapril*	*Perindopril*	*Quinapril*	*Trandolapril*	*Ramipril*	*Fosinopril*
Zinc ligand	Sulphydryl	Carboxyl	Carboxyl	Carboxyl	Carboxyl	Carboxyl	Carboxyl	Phosphinyl
Prodrug	No	No	Yes	Yes	Yes	Yes	Yes	Yes
Bioavailability (%)	75	25	60	65	40	70	50	35
t_{max} (h)[b]	0.8	6–8	3–4	3–4	2	4–6	2–3	3–6
$t_{1/2e}$ (h)	2	12	11	25[a]	20–25[a]	16–24[a]	4–50 [a]	12
Metabolism	Oxidation (50%)	Minimal	Minimal	Prodrug	Prodrug	Prodrug	Prodrug	Prodrug
Elimination	Renal	Renal	Renal	Renal	Renal	Renal, hepatic	Renal	Renal, hepatic

[a]These drugs have polyphasic pharmacokinetics, with a dose-dependent prolonged terminal elimination phase from plasma of over 24 hours.
[b]The prodrugs are metabolized in the gut mucosa and liver to active compounds. Pharmacokinetic data refer to the active compounds.

aldosterone concentrations) may be more marked in those with impaired renal function or in patients taking potassium supplements or potassium-sparing diuretics. The mechanism of cough is not known but is mediated by C fibres and may be related to bradykinin or substance P production. It is reversible on stopping the ACE inhibitor. Other adverse effects include upper respiratory congestion, rhinorrhoea, gastrointestinal disturbances, and increased insulin sensitivity and hyperglycaemia in diabetic patients.

Some adverse effects, e.g. skin rashes (1%), taste disturbances, proteinuria (1%) and neutropenia (0.05%), are related to the presence of a sulphydryl group (e.g. captopril). ACE inhibitors are contraindicated in pregnancy.

Although anaesthesia per se has no direct effect on the RAS or ACE inhibitors, the RAS is activated by several stimuli which may occur during the perioperative period. These include blood or fluid losses and the stress response to surgical stimulation. RAS activation contributes to the maintenance of arterial pressure after haemorrhage, or during anaesthesia. The incidence of hypotension during anaesthesia is increased in patients receiving long-term antihypertensive treatment with ACE inhibitors, and it has been argued that they should be stopped before surgery if significant blood loss or fluid shifts are likely. ACE inhibitors improve ventricular function in patients with heart failure or after myocardial infarction, but it is not known whether acute cessation before surgery is harmful. Conversely, they may have beneficial effects on regional blood flow and have been associated with improved renal function in patients undergoing aortic surgery.

AT_1 receptor blockers

These drugs specifically and non-competitively block the AT_1 receptor, inhibiting the RAS independently, and blocking any effects of AT-II resulting from compensatory stimulation of renin. Hence, they reduce afterload and increase cardiac output without causing tachycardia and are used in the treatment of hypertension, diabetic nephropathy and heart failure. As they have no effect on bradykinin metabolism or prostaglandin synthesis, AT_1 blockers do not produce the cough or rash associated with ACE inhibitors, though angio-oedema has been reported. However, plasma renin, AT-I and AT-II concentrations increase, and aldosterone concentrations decrease during long term therapy: hyperkalaemia may occur if potassium-sparing diuretics are also administered. Losartan is also uricosuric. All available AT_1 blockers are non-peptide imidazole compounds and are highly protein bound, with a prolonged duration of action exceeding their plasma half-life, and a maximum antihypertensive effect 2–4 weeks after starting therapy. In common with ACE inhibitors, they are contraindicated in pregnancy and are likely to have an adverse effect in patients with renal artery stenosis or those taking NSAIDs. The pharmacological properties of some AT_1-receptor blockers are shown in Table 8.11. There are few data describing the effects of AT_1 blockers in the perioperative period, but caution would be appropriate when large fluid or blood losses are expected.

ANTIARRHYTHMIC DRUGS

Cardiac arrhythmias are irregular or abnormal heart rhythms and include bradycardias or tachycardias outside the physiological range. Patients may present for surgery with a pre-existing arrhythmia; alternatively, arrhythmias may be precipitated or accentuated during anaesthesia by several surgical, pharmacological or physiological factors (Table 8.12). Although several drugs (including anaesthetic drugs) have effects on heart rate and rhythm, the term antiarrhythmic is applied to drugs that primarily affect ionic currents within myocardial conducting tissue. Therapy for long-term arrhythmias has changed during the last two decades with the development of non-pharmacological techniques, e.g. DC cardioversion, implantable cardioverter-defibrillator (ICD) devices or radiofrequency ablation of ectopic foci. Most forms of supraventricular tachycardia may be controlled by

radiofrequency ablation, and ICDs are increasingly used in patients who have suffered an episode of ventricular tachycardia. Long-term drug therapy has therefore declined and is now largely confined to patients with atrial fibrillation, or as an adjunct in patients with ICDs or benign arrhythmias resistant to catheter ablation. However, owing to the frequency of arrhythmias during anaesthesia, knowledge of the available drugs and their interactions is important for the anaesthetist. Antiarrhythmic drugs are classified according to their effects on the action potential (see below).

THE CARDIAC ACTION POTENTIAL

The cardiac action potential (AP) is generated by movement of charged ions across the cell membrane and comprises five phases (see Fig. 8.5). At rest, the cells are polarized and the resting membrane potential is negative (−50 to −60 mV in sinus node pacemaker cells and −80 to −90 mV in Purkinje, atrial and ventricular muscle fibres). The AP is triggered by a low intracellular leak of Na^+ ions (and Ca^{2+} ions at the AV node) until a threshold point is reached, when sudden rapid influx of Na^+ ions causes an increase in positive charge within the cell and generates an impulse (phase 0, depolarization). The AP starts to reverse (phase 1), but is sustained because of slower inward movement of Ca^{2+} ions (phase 2). Efflux of K^+ ions brings about repolarization (phase 3) and the gradual termination of the AP. Thereafter, re-equilibration of Na^+ and K^+ takes place and the resting membrane potential is restored

Table 8.11 Pharmacology of AT_1 antagonists

Drug	Losartan	Candesartan	Irbesartan	Valsartan	Eprosartan	Telmisartan
Prodrug	Yes	Yes	No	No	No	No
Bioavailability (%)	33	14–40	60–80	23	10–15	40
Peak effect (h)	1[a]	3–4	1.5–2	2–4	1–3	0.5–1
$t_{1/2e}$(h)	2[a]	9	11–15	9	5–9	24
Metabolism	Hepatic	Minimal	Hepatic	Minimal	Hepatic (most excreted unchanged)	Minimal
Elimination	Renal, hepatic	Renal, hepatic	Renal, hepatic	Bile, urine	Bile	Bile

[a]Undergoes significant first-pass metabolism, producing an active metabolite EXP 3174, which is 10–40 times more potent than the parent drug. Time to peak concentration, and elimination half-life of EXP 3174 are 3–4 h and 6–9 h, respectively.

Table 8.12   Precipitants of arrhythmias during anaesthesia

Myocardial ischaemia
Hypoxia
Hypercapnia
Halogenated hydrocarbons (volatile anaesthetic agents, e.g. trichloroethylene, cyclopropane, halothane)
Catecholamines (endogenous or exogenous)
Electrolyte abnormalities (hypo- or hyperkalaemia, hypocalcaemia, hypomagnesaemia)
Hypotension
Autonomic effects (e.g. reflex vagal stimulation, brain tumours or trauma)
Acid–base abnormalities
Mechanical stimuli (e.g. during CVP or PAFC line insertion)
Drugs (toxicity or adverse reactions)
Medical conditions (e.g. pneumonia, alcohol abuse)

(phase 4). The AP spreads between adjacent cells and is transmitted through the specialized conducting system from the AV node to the bundle of His and ventricular muscle fibres via the Purkinje fibres. The SA node pacemaker cells have the fastest spontaneous discharge rate and usually initiate the coordinated action potential. However, action potentials may also be generated by the AV node and other cells in the conducting system.

MECHANISMS OF ARRHYTHMIAS

Arrhythmias are caused by abnormalities of impulse generation or conduction, or both, via a number of mechanisms:

- *Altered automaticity.* Increased pacemaker activity in the SA node (e.g. caused by increased sympathetic tone) may cause sinus tachycardia, or atrial or ventricular tachyarrhythmias. Decreased SA node automaticity (e.g. as a result of enhanced vagal activity) may allow the emergence of latent pacemaker activity in distal conducting tissues, e.g. AV node or the bundle of His–Purkinje system, causing sinus bradycardia, AV nodal or

idioventricular escape rhythms. These rhythms are common during halothane anaesthesia.
- *Unidirectional conduction block.* Interruption of the normal conduction pathways caused by anatomical defects, alterations in refractory period or excitability may cause heart block and favours arrhythmias caused by abnormal re-entry or automaticity.
- *Ectopic foci.* Ectopic foci may give rise to arrhythmias in a variety of circumstances. In the presence of bradycardia or SA node block, pathological damage in cardiac muscle cells or conducting tissues may augment the generation of arrhythmias from ectopic foci, via:
  – increased automaticity
  – re-entry phenomena
  – pathological after-depolarizations.

Other factors may contribute. Increased automaticity in atrial, ventricular or conducting tissues caused by ischaemia or electrolyte disturbances (e.g. hypokalaemia) may trigger depolarization before the SA node and cause an arrhythmia. Re-entrant arrhythmias arise when forward conduction of impulses in a branch of the conduction pathway is blocked by disease and retrograde conduction occurs. If there is a discrepancy in the refractory periods of the two branches, retrograde conduction may occur in cells that have already discharged and repolarized, triggering a further AP which is both premature and ectopic. These premature APs become self-sustaining (circus movements), leading to atrial or ventricular tachycardia or fibrillation. Pathological after-depolarizations are spontaneous impulses arising just after the normal AP, and occur mostly in ischaemic myocardium (e.g. after myocardial infarction) especially in the presence of hypoxaemia, increased catecholamine concentrations, digoxin toxicity or electrolyte abnormalities.

ARRHYTHMIAS AND ANAESTHESIA

Arrhythmias are common during anaesthesia and in intensive care, especially in patients with preoperative arrhythmia, cardiomyopathy, ischaemia, or valvular or pericardial disease. They may be precipitated by several factors (see Table 8.13). Some arrhythmias are immediately life-threatening, but all warrant attention because they usually imply the presence of other disturbances, and the effects of specific therapy (e.g. drugs, electrical cardioversion or cardiac pacing) are enhanced by prior corrective measures. Specific antiarrhythmic treatment is usually reserved for those arrhythmias affecting cardiac output or that may progress to dangerous tachyarrhythmias.

In addition to volatile agents, several drugs used during anaesthesia may facilitate arrhythmias by direct toxicity (e.g. local anaesthetics), autonomic effects (e.g. succinylcholine, pancuronium), by enhancing the effects of catecholamines (e.g. nitrous oxide, thiopental, cocaine) or as a result of histamine release. Opioids potentiate central vagal activity, decrease sympathetic tone and have direct negative chronotropic effects on the SA node. They may therefore cause bradycardia but conversely decrease the incidence of ventricular arrhythmias.

MECHANISMS OF ACTION OF ANTIARRHYTHMIC DRUGS

An arrhythmia may be controlled either by slowing the primary mechanism or, in the case of supraventricular arrhythmias, by reducing the proportion of impulses transmitted through the AV node to the ventricular conducting system. The cardiac action potential may be pharmacologically manipulated in three ways:

- The *automaticity* (tendency to spontaneous discharge) of cells may be reduced. This result can be achieved by reducing the rate of leakage of sodium (reducing the slope of phase 4), by increasing the electronegativity of the resulting membrane potential or by decreasing the electronegativity of the threshold potential.
- The *speed of conduction* of the action potential may be suppressed as reflected by a lowering of the height and slope of the phase 0 discharge. A reduction in the electronegativity of the membrane potential at the onset of phase 0 reduces both the amplitude and the slope of the phase 0 depolarization. This situation occurs if the cell discharges before it has been completely repolarized.
- The *rate of repolarization* may be reduced, which prolongs the refractory period of the discharging cell.

All antiarrhythmic drugs may themselves induce arrhythmias. Many (particularly class 1 antiarrhythmics) have a narrow therapeutic index and some have been associated with an increase in mortality in large-scale studies. Antiarrhythmic agents may be classified empirically on the basis of their effectiveness in supraventricular tachycardias (e.g. digoxin, β-blockers and verapamil) or in ventricular arrhythmias (lidocaine, mexiletine, tocainide, phenytoin and bretylium). Many drugs (disopyramide, amiodarone, quinidine and procainamide) are effective in both supraventricular and ventricular arrhythmias (Table 8.13). The Vaughan Williams classification (Table 8.14) is based on electrophysiological mechanisms. This classification has limitations (some drugs belong to more than one class, some arrhythmias may be caused by several mechanisms, some drugs, e.g. digoxin, adenosine, do not fit into the classification) but it remains in use and is therefore described below.

Class 1 antiarrhythmic drugs (Table 8.15) inhibit the fast Na^+ influx during depolarization; they inhibit arrhythmias caused by abnormal automaticity or re-entry. All class 1 drugs decrease the maximum rate of rise of phase 0, and decrease conduction velocity, excitability and automaticity to varying degrees. In addition to these local anaesthetic properties, some have membrane-stabilizing effects. Class 1a drugs antagonize primarily the fast influx of Na^+ ions and so reduce conduction velocity through the AV node and His–Purkinje system, whilst prolonging the duration of the action potential and the refractory period. They also have varying antimuscarinic and sympathomimetic effects. Class 1b drugs have much less effect on conduction velocity in usual therapeutic doses and they shorten the refractory period. Agents in class 1c affect conduction profoundly without altering the refractory period.

β-Blockers (class 2) depress automaticity in the SA and AV nodes, and attenuate the effects of cate-

---

Table 8.13 Drug treatments for specific arrhythmias

Atrial fibrillation	Paroxysmal atrial fibrillation	Atrial flutter	Paroxysmal SVT	WPW	Ventricular arrhythmias
Digoxin β-blockers Verapamil Amiodarone	Amiodarone Disopyramide Quinidine	Digoxin Amiodarone	Adenosine Verapamil β-blockers	Amiodarone Disopyramide Flecainide β-blockers	Lidocaine Amiodarone Bretylium Mexiletine (Disopyramide) Magnesium

WPW; Wolff–Parkinson–White syndrome

Table 8.14 Vaughan Williams classification of antiarrhythmic drugs

Class	Examples	Mechanism	Effects	Indication
1a	Quinidine Disopyramide	Na$^+$ channel blockade (moderate) ↓ Conduction velocity Prolonged polarization	Moderate ↓ V$_{MAX}$ ↑ Action potential duration ↑ Refractory period QRS widened	Prevention of SVT, VT, atrial tachycardia WPW
1b	Lidocaine Mexiletine	Na$^+$ channel blockade (mild) ↓ Conduction velocity Shortened repolarization	Mild ↓ V$_{MAX}$ ↓ Action potential duration ↓ Refractory period QRS unchanged	Prevention of VT/VF during ischaemia
1c	Flecainide Propafenone	Na$^+$ channel blockade (marked) ↓ Conduction velocity No change in repolarization	Marked ↓ V$_{MAX}$ Minimal change in action potential duration and refractory period QRS widened	Conversion/prevention of SVT/VT/VF
2	β-Blockers	β-Adrenergic receptor blockade	Decreased automaticity (SA and AV nodes)	Prevention of sympathetic-induced tachy-arrhythmias, rate control in AF, 2° prevention after MI, prevention of AV node re-entrant tachycardia
3	Amiodarone Bretylium Sotalol	Inhibition of inward K$^+$ current	Markedly prolonged repolarization ↑ Action potential duration ↑ Refractory period QRS unchanged	Prevention of SVT/VT/VF
4	Diltiazem	Calcium channel blockade	↓ Depolarization and V$_{MAX}$ of slow response cells in SA and AV nodes ↓ Action potential duration ↓ Refractory period of AV node	Rate control in AF Prevention of AV node re-entrant tachycardias

cholamines on automaticity and conduction velocity in the sinus and AV nodes. Class 3 drugs prolong the AP and so lengthen the refractory period. Verapamil (class 4) also prolongs the AP, in addition to depressing automaticity (especially in the AV node).

Class 1 antiarrhythmics

Class 1a

These drugs (see Tables 8.14 and 8.15) are used for the treatment and prevention of ventricular and supraventricular arrhythmias. Their use in the prevention of atrial fibrillation has declined because of proarrhythmic effects causing increased mortality, especially in patients with ischaemic heart disease or poor LV func-

tion. They may induce torsades de pointes (a form of polymorphic ventricular tachycardia) even in patients without structural heart disease.

Quinidine is an isomer of quinine formerly used in the treatment of atrial and supraventricular tachycardias which has antimuscarinic and α-blocking properties. The latter causes vasodilatation and decreased myocardial contractility so that severe hypotension may occur after i.v. administration.

Disopyramide is useful in supraventricular tachycardias and as a second-line agent to lidocaine in ventricular arrhythmias. It has less action on the His–Purkinje system than quinidine, but greater antimuscarinic and negative inotropic effects.

Procainamide has similar effects to quinidine and may cause hypotension after i.v. administration. It

Table 8.15 Pharmacology of some class 1 antiarrhythmic drugs

Drug	Quinidine	Disopyramide	Procainamide	Mexiletine	Flecainide
Class	Ia	Ia	Ia	1b	Ic
Indications	Supraventricular tachyarrhythmias	Supraventricular and ventricular tachy-arrhythmias	Supraventricular tachyarrhythmias	Ventricular tachyarrhythmias	Supraventricular and ventricular tachyarrhythmias
Metabolism and elimination	80% metabolized in liver, 20% excreted unchanged via kidneys	Renal; 50–80% excreted unchanged	15–30% by hepatic acetylation, 40–70% excreted unchanged by kidneys	85% hepatic, 15% excreted unchanged by kidneys	Renal 80–90% excreted unchanged
Elimination $t_{1/2}$ (h)	5–8 h	4–6 h	3–5 h	6–10 h	7–15 h
Active metabolites?	Yes	one of metabolites has marked anti-cholinergic effects	Yes (N-acetyl procainamide)	No	Weakly active metabolites
Adverse effects	Ventricular arrhythmias; visual and auditory disturbances with vertigo; gastrointestinal symptoms; rashes, thrombo-cytopenia and agranulocytosis	Arrhythmias (ventricular tachycardia, AV block); hypotension; dry mouth, blurred vision, urinary retention, GI irritation	Nausea; myocardial depression; drug-induced systemic lupus erythe-matosus; agranulocytosis	Nausea, vomiting; cardiotoxicity (bradycardia, hypotension, conduction defects); CNS toxicity (confusion, dysarthria, paraesthesiae, dizziness and convulsions)	Arrhythmias (ventricular tachycardia, AV block); myocardial depression; nausea, vomiting
Notes	Additive with other cardiodepressant drugs (e.g. disopyramide, β-blockers and calcium channel blockers); potentiates non-depolarizing neuromuscular blockers; enhances digoxin toxicity by displacing digoxin from binding sites and reducing its clearance	Negative inotropic effects more marked in combination with β-blockers or verapamil	Metabolism to N-acetyl procainamide dependent on hepatic N-acetyl transferase; usually only administered i.v.	Elimination enhanced by hepatic enzyme induction (e.g. by rifampicin or phenytoin); elimination reduced in cardiac or hepatic disease	Polymorphic metabolism; elimination prolonged in renal or cardiac failure; increases digoxin and propranolol concentrations

may be used i.v. to terminate ventricular arrhythmias, or as an oral antiarrhythmic, although it has a short half-life and requires frequent administration or the use of a sustained-release oral preparation.

Ajmalin is a quinidine-like drug used for the treatment of Wolff-Parkinson-White (WPW) syndrome. It inhibits intraventricular conduction and prolongs AV conduction time, and is available in Europe.

Class 1b

Class 1b drugs are useful for the prevention and treatment of premature ventricular contractions, ventricular tachycardia and ventricular fibrillation, particularly associated with ischaemia.

Lidocaine is the first-choice drug for ventricular arrhythmias resistant to DC cardioversion. It decreases normal and abnormal automaticity and decreases action potential and refractory period duration. The threshold for ventricular fibrillation is raised, but it has minimal haemodynamic effects. The antiarrhythmic properties of lidocaine are enhanced by hypoxaemia, acidosis and hyperkalaemia, so it is particularly effective in ischaemic cells, e.g. after acute myocardial infarction, during cardiac surgery or in arrhythmias associated with digitalis toxicity. Lidocaine may cause CNS toxicity. Cardiotoxic effects (hypotension, bradycardia or heart block) occur at higher doses and are potentiated by hypoxaemia, acidosis and hypercapnia. Clearance is decreased if hepatic blood flow is decreased (e.g. in the elderly, those with congestive cardiac failure, after myocardial infarction), and also by β-blockers, cimetidine and liver disease. In these circumstances, the dose should be reduced by 50%. It is less effective in the presence of hypokalaemia.

Mexiletine is a lidocaine analogue which is well absorbed orally with high bioavailability. Adverse effects are similar to those of lidocaine; nausea and vomiting are also common during oral treatment.

Class 1c

Class 1c drugs are used for the prevention and treatment of supraventricular and ventricular tachyarrhythmias and junctional tachycardias with or without an accessory pathway. They are proarrhythmogenic, particularly in patients with myocardial ischaemia, poor left ventricular function or after myocardial infarction, and although effective in chronic atrial fibrillation, they are reserved for life-threatening arrhythmias.

Flecainide is a procainamide derivative with little effect on repolarization, the refractory period or AP duration, but unlike other drugs in this class, it decreases automaticity and produces dose-dependent widening of the QRS complex. In acute atrial fibrillation, intravenous flecainide usually restores sinus rhythm and is useful prophylaxis against further episodes of atrial fibrillation. However, it increases the risk of ventricular arrhythmias after myocardial infarction, especially in patients with structural cardiac disease.

Propafenone has a complex pharmacology including weak antimuscarinic, β-adrenergic receptor and calcium channel blocking effects. It should be used with caution in patients with reactive airways disease. Interaction with digoxin may increase plasma digoxin concentrations.

Class 2 antiarrhythmic drugs

β-Blockers are used mainly for the treatment of sinus and supraventricular tachycardias, especially those provoked by endogenous or exogenous catecholamines, emotion or exercise. Their antiarrhythmic effects are an intrinsic property of β-blockade, i.e. reduced automaticity in ectopic pacemakers, prolonged AV node conduction and refractory period, although some β-blockers have class 1 activity in high doses ('membrane-stabilizing activity'). Although beneficial in chronic heart failure, their negative inotropic effects may be disadvantageous in patients with acute left ventricular dysfunction.

Class 3 antiarrhythmic drugs

Class 3 antiarrhythmics prolong the AP in conducting tissues and myocardial muscle. They prolong repolarization by K^+ channel blockade, and decrease outward K^+ conduction in the bundle of His, atrial and ventricular muscle, and accessory pathways. They are used for the treatment of supraventricular and ventricular tachyarrhythmias, including those associated with accessory conduction pathways. Some drugs have other actions (e.g. sotalol also produces β-blockade, and disopyramide has class 1 effects). All may prolong the QT interval and precipitate torsades de pointes, especially in high doses or in the presence of electrolyte disturbance.

Sotalol is a non-selective β-blocker with class 3 antiarrhythmic effects. Action potential duration and refractory period are lengthened, and it is effective in the treatment of supraventricular tachyarrhythmias, especially atrial flutter and fibrillation, which may be converted to sinus rhythm. It also suppresses ventricular tachyarrhythmias and ventricular ectopic beats. However, sotalol may cause torsades de pointes and other life-threatening arrhythmias, particularly in the presence of hypokalaemia.

Amiodarone is primarily a class 3 drug; it acts by inhibition of inward K^+ current. It also blocks sodium and calcium channels, and has competitive inhibitory actions at α- and β-adrenoceptors, and may therefore be considered to have class 1, 2 and 4 antiarrhythmic activity. It prolongs AP duration, repolarization and refractory periods in the atria and ventricles. In addition, AV node conduction is markedly slowed and refractory period increased. Ventricular conduction velocity is slowed. Amiodarone is effective against a wide variety of supraventricular and ventricular arrhythmias, including WPW syndrome, and is preferred to other drugs in the presence of left ventricular dysfunction. Intravenous amiodarone is contraindicated in the presence of bradycardia or AV block, but is less likely than other agents to cause arrhythmias. Bradycardia unresponsive to atropine, and hypotension, have been reported during general anaesthesia in patients receiving amiodarone therapy. Long-term oral therapy may produce a number of adverse effects. Amiodarone is an iodinated compound, which explains its effects on the thyroid (Table 8.16).

Bretylium is a quaternary ammonium compound which prevents noradrenaline uptake into sympathetic nerve endings. It prolongs AP duration and refractory period with no effect on automaticity, and is used as second-line therapy to lidocaine for resistant life-threatening ventricular tachyarrhythmias. It may also facilitate electrical defibrillation to sinus rhythm and is useful for the treatment of ventricular arrhythmias associated with local anaesthetic toxicity. Catecholamine concentrations increase initially, causing transient increases in heart rate and arterial pressure. Bretylium is excreted unchanged in urine. Bradycardia or asystole occasionally occur and ventricular arrhythmias may be worsened, particularly those caused by digoxin. Bretylium is no longer avilable in the UK.

Ibutilide and *dofetilide* are new class 3 antiarrhythmics that selectively inhibit inward K^+ currents and so prolong repolarization, effective refractory period and the QT interval. Dofetilide has high bioavailability and is excreted mostly unchanged by the kidney. Both are used for long-term treatment of atrial fibrillation.

Class 4 antiarrhythmic drugs

Class 4 drugs (calcium channel blockers) prevent voltage-dependent calcium influx during depolarization, particularly in the SA and AV nodes. Verapamil is more selective for cardiac cells than other calcium channel blockers, but it is also a coronary and peripheral vasodilator, and decreases myocardial contractility. It depresses AV conduction, is effective in supraventricular or re-entrant tachycardia and controls the ventricular rate in atrial fibrillation. However, it is contraindicated in WPW syndrome, as conduction through the accessory pathway may be encouraged, leading to ventricular fibrillation. Intravenous administration may cause hypotension (by vasodilatation), and caution is necessary in low-output states and in patients treated with negative inotropic drugs, e.g. β-blockers, disopyramide, quinidine or procainamide. Verapamil and diltiazem are effective by both i.v. and oral routes.

Other antiarrhythmics

Adenosine is an endogenous purine nucleoside which mediates a variety of natural cellular functions via membrane-bound adenosine receptors, of which several subtypes (A_1–A_4) have been identified. Myocardial A_1 receptors activate potassium channels and decrease cAMP by activating inhibitory G_i-proteins; A_2 receptors mediate coronary vasodilatation by stimulating endothelial-derived relaxing factor and increasing intracellular cAMP. Increased potassium conductance induces membrane hyperpolarization in the SA and AV nodes, reducing automaticity, and blocking AV node conduction. Adenosine also has an antiadrenergic effect in calcium-dependent ventricular tissue. It effectively converts paroxysmal supraventricular tachyarrhythmias (including those associated with WPW syndrome) to sinus rhythm, is used in the diagnosis of broad complex tachycardias when the origin (ventricular or supraventricular) is uncertain, but is ineffective in the conversion of atrial flutter or fibrillation. In patients unable to exercise, adenosine is used as a coronary vasodilator in combination with myocardial perfusion scanning to diagnose coronary artery disease. Adenosine is metabolized to AMP or inosine by erythrocytes and vascular endothelial cells, so has a very short duration of action and is given as a rapid i.v. bolus.

Magnesium sulphate. Magnesium is a cofactor for many enzyme systems, including the myocardial Na^+/K^+ ATPase. It antagonizes atrial L and T type Ca^{2+} channels, so prolongs both atrial refractory periods and conduction, and also inhibits K^+ entry and suppresses ventricular after-depolarizations. Intravenous magnesium sulphate is the treatment of choice for torsades de pointes, a type of ventricular tachycardia occasionally induced by class 1a or class 3 antiarrhythmic drugs that prolong the QT interval. It is a second-line treatment for supraventricular and ventricular arrhythmias, particularly those associated with digoxin toxicity or hypokalaemia, and is used as an anticonvulsant in patients with pre-eclampsia. Magnesium is redistributed rapidly into bone (50%) and intracellular fluid (45%) with the remainder excreted via the kidneys. It is therefore administered as an i.v. infusion.

Cardiac glycosides

Digoxin and digitoxin are cardiac glycosides derived from plant sources, principally *Digitalis purpura* and *Digitalis lanata*. Their structure comprises a cyclopentanophenanthrene nucleus, an aglycone ring (responsible for the pharmacological activity) and a carbohydrate chain made up of sugar molecules (which aid solubility). Digitalis compounds have been used for over 200 years for the treatment of cardiac failure but have been largely superseded and are now principally indicated for the control of ventricu-

Table 8.16 Pharmacological properties of some commonly used intravenous antiarrhythmic drugs

Drug (class)	Lidocaine (1b)	Adenosine	Digoxin	Amiodarone (3)	Magnesium sulphate
Typical i.v. dose	50–100 mg, repeated after 5–10 min or followed by continuous infusion	3 mg, repeated up to 6 mg and 12 mg after 1–2 min	Loading dose 250–500 µg i.v. over 10–20 min, repeated after 6–12 h	5 mg kg^{-1} over at least 5–10 min, followed by infusion of 900 mg over 24 h	8 mmol over 10–15 min followed by continuous i.v. infusion of 4–72 mmol over 24 h
Metabolism and elimination	Extensive first-pass hepatic metabolism	Vascular endothelium	Mostly excreted unchanged via kidneys	Hepatic; drug and active metabolite accumulate in tissues	Redistributed or excreted unchanged via kidneys
Elimination $t_{(1/2)}$ (h)	< 2 h	< 10 s	36 h	35–40 days	< 1 h
Active metabolites?	Monoethylglycine-xylidide (MEGX), glycine xylidide (GX)	No	No	Desethylamiodarone	No
Adverse effects	CNS toxicity (confusion, dysarthria, tremor, paraesthesiae, dizziness and convulsions). Cardiotoxicity (bradycardia, hypotension, asystole)	Dyspnoea, flushing, bronchospasm, bradycardia and, occasionally, ventricular standstill or malignant tachyarrhythmias	Cardiac arrhythmias (especially ventricular arrhythmias, heart block), CNS toxicity (fatigue, agitation, nightmares, visual disturbances), anorexia and nausea or abdominal pain	Bradycardia, hypotension, thrombophlebitis. With long-term therapy, corneal microdeposits, cutaneous rash, hypothyroidism, confounding of thyroid function tests	Vasodilatation, hyporeflexia, neuromuscular blockade, cardiac conduction changes, cardiac arrest and electrolyte disturbances.
Notes			Toxicity increased by hypokalaemia; plasma concentrations increased by quinidine, amiodarone, verapamil; specific digoxin antibody available for treatment of toxicity. Plasma concentrations should be monitored	Avoid co-administration with other drugs which prolong QT interval (e.g. diltiazem, verapamil, phenothiazines, sotalol or class 1a antiarrhythmics; significant drug interactions, including increasing plasma digoxin concentrations and potentiation of warfarin and heparin	Plasma concentrations should be monitored

lar rate in supraventricular arrhythmias, particularly atrial fibrillation. They have several actions, including direct effects on the myocardium and both direct and indirect actions on the ANS. They increase myocardial contractility and decrease conduction in the AV node and bundle of His. Action potential and refractory period duration in atrial cells are reduced, and the rate of phase 4 depolarization in the SA node (automaticity) is decreased. The refractory periods of the AV node and bundle of His are increased, but in the ventricles, refractory period is decreased and spontaneous depolarization rate increases. This increased ventricular excitability is more marked in the presence of hypokalaemia and may lead to the appearance of ectopic pacemaker foci. The principal direct cardiac action is inhibition of membrane Na^+/K^+-ATPase activity. Intracellular Na^+ concentration and Na^+/Ca^{2+} exchange increase, leading to increased availability of intracellular Ca^{2+} and increased myocardial contractility. Increased local catecholamine concentrations as a result of decreased neuronal re-uptake and increased central sympathetic drive may also contribute to this positive inotropic action. In addition to direct cardiac actions, digitalis compounds have direct and indirect vagal effects. Central vagal tone, cardiac sensitivity to vagal stimulation, and local myocardial concentrations of acetylcholine are all increased, and these effects may be partly antagonized by atropine.

Digoxin has a large apparent volume of distribution and a long half-life, so effective plasma concentrations occur after approximately 5–7 days unless a loading dose is given. Doses should be reduced in renal impairment or elderly patients. The therapeutic index is low and toxicity is likely at plasma concentrations > 2.5 ng mL^{-1}. However, plasma concentrations are a poor guide to toxicity as the drugs are concentrated in cardiac and other tissues. Even at therapeutic plasma concentrations, digitalis affects the ECG, causing repolarization abnormalities. The classic 'digoxin effect' on ECG is of downsloping ('reverse tick') ST-segment depression with T wave inversion which may be wrongly interpreted as ischaemia. These changes are usually widespread, are not confined to the territory of one coronary artery and do not indicate toxicity. Digoxin toxicity usually causes cardiac, CNS, visual and gastrointestinal disturbances, including almost any arrhythmia, although ventricular arrhythmias (extrasystoles, bigeminy and trigeminy) and various degrees of heart block are commonest. Supraventricular arrhythmias also occur, often with some degree of conduction block. Digoxin should be avoided in the presence of second-degree heart block, ventricular tachycardia or aberrant conduction pathways (e.g. WPW syndrome), as arrhythmias may be precipitated, and used with caution after myocardial infarction. Sensitivity to digoxin is increased by hypokalaemia, hypomagnesaemia, hypercalcaemia, renal impairment, chronic pulmonary or heart disease, myxoedema and hypoxaemia. β-Blockers and verapamil have combined effects on the AV node, and digoxin should be administered cautiously. Treatment of serious arrhythmias involves careful administration of KCl under ECG monitoring (especially in the presence of heart block or renal impairment). Lidocaine and phenytoin are useful for ventricular arrhythmias, β-blockade for supraventricular arrhythmias, and bradyarrhythmias may be treated with atropine. Digoxin should be stopped for at least 48 h before elective DC cardioversion, otherwise ventricular fibrillation may be precipitated. If cardioversion is required, the initial energy level should be low (e.g. 10–25 J) and increased if necessary.

Digitoxin is metabolized by the liver, and is less dependent upon renal function for its elimination. It has a very long half-life (4–6 days), so maintenance doses may be required only on alternate days, but this is also a disadvantage as toxic effects are very persistent.

FURTHER READING

Calvey T N, Williams N E 2001 Principles and practice of pharmacology for anaesthetists, 4th edn. Blackwell Science, Oxford

Stoelting R K 2005 Pharmacology and physiology in anesthetic practice, 4th edn. Lippincott, Williams & Wilkins, Philadelphia

Sweetman S C (ed.) 2004 Martindale: the complete drug reference, 34th edn. Pharmaceutical Press, London

Drugs acting on the respiratory system

9

Many drugs used in anaesthetic practice have effects on the respiratory system. For example, opioids depress the respiratory centre, inhalational agents and anticholinergics dilate bronchi, and anticholinesterases cause bronchial constriction. These are the secondary effects of these drugs. This chapter describes the pharmacology of drugs used primarily for their effects on the respiratory system. These may be classified as:

- drugs acting on the respiratory centre
- drugs acting on airway calibre
- drugs acting on pulmonary vascular resistance
- drugs acting on mucociliary function
- surfactant replacement therapy.

DRUGS ACTING ON THE RESPIRATORY CENTRE

These drugs may either be true stimulants of ventilation or reverse respiratory depression caused by opioids or benzodiazepines.

RESPIRATORY STIMULANTS

Several classes of drug stimulate ventilation and may be used when ventilatory drive is inadequate. These agents increase respiratory drive through a variety of mechanisms. For example, strychnine blocks central inhibitory pathways, acetazolamide increases hydrogen ion concentration in the extracellular fluid around the respiratory centre, and nikethamide and doxapram stimulate the respiratory centre directly. Only doxapram is now used clinically.

In general, respiratory stimulants should not be used if respiratory failure is caused by muscle exhaustion. The suggested clinical indications for the use of respiratory stimulants include the following:

- overdose with sedatives
- postanaesthetic respiratory depression

- idiopathic hypoventilation
- opioid overdose
- acute exacerbation of chronic obstructive pulmonary disease (COPD).

It must be stressed that artificial ventilation is the best option for respiratory management in most of these circumstances and that respiratory stimulants should be used only as a short-term measure or when facilities for artificial ventilation are not immediately available. Respiratory stimulants are rarely indicated in the late stages of COPD because respiratory drive in these patients is already maximal.

Doxapram

At low doses ($0.5\,\text{mg kg}^{-1}$), doxapram stimulates carotid chemoreceptors. At high doses, it also stimulates medullary respiratory centres. However, the effect of a single dose is transient and a continuous intravenous infusion may be required for sustained action.

Uses

In addition to the indications listed above, it has been suggested that doxapram may be used in the following situations:

- prevention of postoperative atelectasis and thus maintenance of better oxygenation
- prevention of postoperative chest complications
- facilitation of blind nasal intubation
- treatment of apnoea in premature babies.

When it is used to reverse opioid-induced respiratory depression, doxapram has the advantage in comparison with opioid antagonists that it does not reverse the analgesic effect.

Dosage and administration

Doxapram is given intravenously as a slow bolus of $0.5\,\text{mg kg}^{-1}$. The effect lasts for 5–10 min. For sustained action, a continuous i.v. infusion of $1-2\,mg\,min^{-1}$ may be used.

Adverse effects

In common with other analeptics (such as nikethamide), doxapram has central excitatory effects, although it affects the respiratory centre preferentially. The main adverse effects are listed in Table 9.1. In extreme cases, convulsions may occur; hypoxaemia and hypercapnia are predisposing factors.

Doxapram is metabolized by the liver and should be used with caution if liver function is impaired.

OPIOID ANTAGONISTS

Naloxone

Naloxone is not a respiratory stimulant per se. It is an oxymorphone derivative and is an opioid antagonist without significant intrinsic agonist activity. It reverses opioid-induced respiratory depression, analgesia and sedation; however, careful titration allows reversal of respiratory depression without reversing analgesia.

Uses

The main indication for naloxone is reversal of opioid-induced respiratory depression. It does not reverse the depressant effects of other drugs or depression of ventilation caused by neurological disease.

Table 9.1 Adverse effects of doxapram

Restlessness
Sweating
Anxiety
Agitation
Confusion
Headache
Hallucinations
Tachycardia
Hypertension
Convulsions

Although artificial ventilation is usually a safer option for treatment of opioid-induced respiratory depression, administration of naloxone is indicated particularly under the following circumstances:

- neonatal respiratory depression caused by administration of an opioid to the mother during labour
- as a diagnostic test if the cause of sedation and respiratory depression is not clear.

Dosage and administration

Naloxone may be given either intravenously or intramuscularly. In adults, a bolus dose of up to 0.4 mg can be given initially. The action is apparent in 2–5 min and lasts for about 30–40 min. This duration of action is shorter than that of most opioid agonists. Consequently, repeated doses are often required, and the patient's condition must be monitored closely so that recurrence of respiratory depression is detected promptly. Alternatively, a continuous i.v. infusion may be used in adults at a rate of $0.4-2\,mg\,h^{-1}$. The rate of infusion should be adjusted according to the response.

Adverse effects

Adverse effects are rare but include arrhythmia, hypertension and pulmonary oedema. The main undesirable effect is reversal of the analgesic effect of the agonist.

BENZODIAZEPINE ANTAGONISTS

Flumazenil

In common with naloxone, flumazenil is not a direct respiratory stimulant. It is an imidazobenzodiazepine, which is a competitive binder to the benzodiazepine receptors. Its administration reverses all the central effects of benzodiazepines, including sedation and depression of ventilation.

Uses

- To reverse sedation and respiratory depression induced by benzodiazepines (e.g. diazepam and midazolam)
- As a diagnostic tool in patients with sedation and/or respiratory depression of unknown origin.

Dosage and administration

Flumazenil is usually administered intravenously. An initial dose of 0.2 mg is appropriate in adults. Additional doses of 0.1 mg can be given every 15 min.

The maximum recommended dose is 1.0 mg, although massive doses of up to 100 mg have been administered safely. The effect of each dose is short-lived (15–45 min) and unpredictable. The half-life is shorter than those of the benzodiazepine agonists, and sedation and depression of ventilation may recur, particularly if a large dose of agonist has been given; the patient must be monitored closely. For a longer duration of action, a continuous infusion of flumazenil at a rate of $0.1–1.0$ mg h^{-1} may be used.

Adverse effects

Flumazenil has no direct effect on the central nervous system. It is a relatively safe drug even in doses higher than recommended. However, the dose should be reduced in the presence of liver disease, because flumazenil is almost completely metabolized by the liver. Its use in patients with epilepsy is not recommended because it may precipitate convulsions by rapidly reversing the central effects of benzodiazepines.

DRUGS ACTING ON CALIBRE OF THE AIRWAYS

The normal tone of airway smooth muscles is the result of a balance between the opposing effects of sympathetic (mainly β_2) and parasympathetic influences (Fig. 9.1). At the cellular level, β_2-adrenergic drugs bind to the cell membrane receptor to activate adenylate cyclase. This catalyses the conversion of adenosine triphosphate (ATP) to cyclic adenosine monophosphate (cAMP) within the cell. Through different enzyme systems (kinases), cAMP relaxes bronchial smooth muscle. Cyclic AMP is inactivated by the enzyme phosphodiesterase to produce 5'-AMP. Thus, drugs which increase the concentration of cAMP relax the bronchi (β_2-agonists, phosphodiesterase inhibitors). Conversely, drugs which reduce the level of cAMP (β_2-antagonists) may cause bronchoconstriction.

Cholinergic drugs act on muscarinic receptors to activate guanylate cyclase, which converts guanosine triphosphate (GTP) into cyclic guanosine monophosphate (cGMP). Cyclic GMP, through kinases, causes bronchial constriction. Thus, cholinergic drugs increase cGMP and cause bronchoconstriction, while anticholinergic drugs reduce the production of cGMP and cause bronchial dilatation. The bronchial smooth muscle tone at any given time is determined by the balance between the concentrations of cAMP and cGMP (Fig. 9.1).

Histamine and other mediators also play an important role in promoting bronchial constriction

(H_1 receptors), especially during anaphylaxis, drug reactions, allergy, asthma and respiratory infections. Membrane stabilizers (sodium cromoglycate) and anti-inflammatory agents (steroids) may reduce or prevent bronchoconstriction in these conditions. Table 9.2 summarizes the factors that influence airway calibre.

BRONCHODILATORS

Bronchoconstriction leads to the following:

- increased difficulty in breathing
- inadequate ventilation
- $\dot{V}/\dot{Q}$ mismatch
- hypoxaemia
- impaired ability to cough.

The goal of bronchodilator therapy is to reverse these effects. Depending upon the condition of the patient, bronchodilators may be used either in isolation or as a part of respiratory support with other measures such as oxygen therapy, humidification of inspired gases, antibiotics, physiotherapy and mechanical ventilation. Three types of bronchodilator are in clinical use:

- β-adrenergic agonists
- methylxanthines
- anticholinergics.

Membrane stabilizers such as sodium cromoglycate may prevent bronchoconstriction, but do not have a direct bronchodilator action. Therefore, these drugs are ineffective when bronchoconstriction has already occurred.

β-Adrenergic agonists

Adrenaline (epinephrine) has been used in the treatment of asthma since the beginning of the twentieth century. In addition to increasing the intracellular concentration of cAMP, β-agonists have other complementary effects on the airways, the most notable being inhibition of mast cell mediator release. Table 9.3 summarizes the effects of β-agonists on the airways. These effects are mediated via subtype β_2-receptors, which are spread throughout the larger and smaller airways; β_2-selective agents are now used commonly as bronchodilators.

Uses

- Asthma
- COPD
- Hyperreactive airways in patients undergoing mechanical ventilation

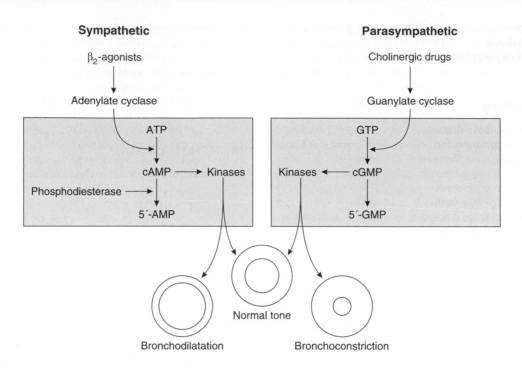

Fig. 9.1
Regulation of bronchomotor tone and mechanism of action of drugs. The relative quantities of cAMP and cGMP determine the state of bronchial tone; cAMP relaxes bronchial muscles and cGMP constricts them.

Table 9.2   Factors influencing airway calibre
Bronchodilatation
Sympathetic stimulation – increased intracellular cAMP
β_2-agonists
Methylxanthines
Anticholinergics
Bronchoconstriction
Parasympathetic stimulation – increased intracellular cGMP
Cholinergic drugs
β_2-antagonists
Inflammatory mediators
Allergy and anaphylaxis
Prevention of bronchoconstriction
Membrane stabilizers – sodium cromoglycate
Steroids

Table 9.3   Effects of β-agonists on the airways
Specific
Increase in intracellular cAMP and bronchodilatation
Non-specific but complementary
Inhibition of mast cell mediator release
Inhibition of plasma exudation and microvascular leakage
Prevention of airway oedema
Increased mucus secretion
Increased mucociliary clearance
Prevention of tissue damage mediated by oxygen free radicals
Decreased acetylcholine release in cholinergic nerves by an action on prejunctional β_2-receptors

- Bronchospasm caused by allergic reactions and anaphylaxis
- Bronchospasm following aspiration or inhalation of toxins.

Choice of drug

Epinephrine, ephedrine and isoproterenol have been used in the past for their bronchodilator effect. Their use has declined because of cardiovascular side-effects mediated by β_1-receptors; selective β_2-agonists are now preferred. However, epinephrine remains the drug of choice in anaphylaxis when a combination of β_1-, β_2- and α-agonist action is desirable. Some patients with acute asthma respond best to subcutaneous epinephrine, but in the large majority of patients, β_2-selective agonists such as salbutamol or terbutaline are the drugs of first choice because they are less likely to produce unwanted β_1 actions. However, it should be noted that the selectivity of β_2-agonists is only relative and that in high doses or in the presence of predisposing factors (hypoxaemia, hypercapnia), β_2-agonists may also produce β_1 effects (Table 9.4).

Dosage and administration

Inhalation is the method of choice because systemic side-effects are minimized. An inhaled drug may also be more effective because it reaches the surface cells (mast cells and epithelial cells) which are relatively inaccessible to a drug administered systemically. Salbutamol can be administered from a pressurized aerosol ($100\,\mu g$ per puff; dose 1–2 puffs). The effect lasts for 4–6 h. The drug may also be nebulized to be delivered with oxygen-enriched air using a face mask, or with inspiratory gases in patients undergoing mechanical ventilation. For this purpose, a dose of 2.5–5 mg ($1\,mg\,mL^{-1}$) every 4–6 h is used. In severe bronchospasm, up to 5–10 mg may be given as fre-quently as every 30 min initially. Side-effects are more likely when these drugs are used in nebulized form rather than a pressurized aerosol because aerosols deliver a smaller dose and a smaller proportion is absorbed systemically.

Oral administration has no advantage over inhalational and is associated with more side-effects. Intravenous administration is used occasionally as a last resort when bronchospasm is so severe that a nebulizer or aerosol is unlikely to deliver the drug to the target cells. Intravenous administration is associated with more frequent side-effects and should be used only when the patient is monitored intensively.

Adverse effects

In addition to those listed in Table 9.4, the adverse effects of β-agonists include the following:

- muscle tremor – resulting from a direct effect on β_2-receptors in skeletal muscle
- hypokalaemia caused by increased uptake of potassium ions by skeletal muscles (mediated by β_2-receptors)
- metabolic effects – increases in the plasma concentrations of free fatty acids, insulin, glucose, pyruvate and lactate.

In high doses, β_1-stimulants may cause dangerous arrhythmias, particularly in the presence of hypoxaemia and hypercapnia. Bronchodilatation may itself lead to hypoxaemia because of increased $\dot{V}/\dot{Q}$ mismatch; this hypoxaemia tends to be transient and may be readily overcome with supplementary oxygen. Thus, the therapy should not be withheld for this reason.

Methylxanthines

The bronchodilator effect of strong coffee was described in the nineteenth century. Methylxanthines, which are related to caffeine, have been used widely to control asthma since 1930. Theophylline is the most commonly used parent compound. Aminophylline is a water-soluble salt that contains over 75% theophylline and is used as the injectable form of theophylline. Methylxanthines have widespread effects involving various organ systems. With regard to their bronchodilator effects, the following mechanisms have been proposed:

- phosphodiesterase inhibition – this leads to an increased level of intracellular cAMP (Fig. 9.1)
- adenosine receptor antagonism – adenosine, especially in asthmatic subjects, causes mast cell histamine release which is prevented by theophylline

Table 9.4 Adverse β_1 effects of β-agonists
Anxiety
Nausea and vomiting
Tachycardia and other tachyarrhythmias
Hypertension
Headache
Dizziness

- endogenous catecholamine release
- prostaglandin inhibition
- interference with calcium mobilization
- potentiation of β_2-agonists.

All these mechanisms have therapeutic effects on the airways and respiratory muscles, which are summarized in Table 9.5.

The net effect is reduced airways resistance, reduced work of breathing and increased efficiency of the respiratory muscles. Other potentially beneficial effects include increases in cardiac output and diaphragmatic contractility. Many of the effects of methylxanthines contribute to their side-effects.

Central nervous system effects. Stimulation of the CNS may lead to nausea, restlessness, agitation, insomnia, tremor and seizures. Some CNS effects (e.g. tremor) may occur even with therapeutic plasma concentrations of the drug.

Cardiovascular effects. Methylxanthines have positive chronotropic and inotropic effects on the heart. They are potent vasodilators and may have a beneficial effect in left ventricular failure. Tachyarrhythmias occur with therapeutic doses.

Renal effects. Methylxanthines cause increased urine output which may be related to an effect on tubular function or may be an indirect effect of the increased cardiac output.

Miscellaneous effects. Methylxanthines are known to increase gastric acid secretion and promote gastro-oesophageal reflux.

Uses

Methylxanthines are the second line of bronchodilators if β_2-agonists alone are not effective or are only partly effective. They are particularly useful in COPD. Recently, they have been shown to improve exercise tolerance in intensive care patients who are on a weaning programme.

Dosage and administration

Aminophylline is a strong alkaline solution and should *never* be given intramuscularly or subcutaneously. Oral sustained-release tablets are available; the dosage is 225–450 mg (6–12 mg kg^{-1} in children) twice daily. For i.v. administration, the loading dose of aminophylline is 5 mg kg^{-1} (slow injection over 20 min) followed by an infusion of 0.5 mg kg^{-1} h^{-1}. If the patient is already taking theophylline, then half the loading dose should be given and the plasma concentration should be checked frequently.

There is a close relationship between the degree of bronchial dilatation and the plasma concentration of theophylline. A concentration of less than 10 mg L^{-1} is associated with a mild effect and a concentration of more than 25 mg L^{-1} is associated with frequent side-effects. Consequently, the therapeutic window is narrow and the plasma concentration should be maintained within the range 10–20 mg L^{-1}. Approximately 40% of the drug is protein-bound. Theophylline is metabolized mainly in the liver by cytochrome P450 and P448 microenzymes; 10% is excreted unchanged in urine. Factors which affect the activity of hepatic enzymes and thus the clearance of the drug are summarized in Table 9.6. The infusion rate of aminophylline should be adjusted accordingly (e.g. 1.6 times for smokers, 0.6 times for patients receiving cimetidine). Frequent estimation of plasma concentration is required to prevent undertreatment or toxicity.

Adverse effects

Adverse effects of methylxanthines are frequent (Table 9.7). They are more likely to occur in patients who are already receiving β-agonist bronchodilators or sympathomimetic drugs. Extreme care should be exercised in the presence of hypoxaemia, hypercapnia, dehydration, hypokalaemia or cardiac arrhythmias. Patients receiving intravenous aminophylline must be monitored closely. Death caused by gross hypokalaemia and cardiac arrhythmias has been reported.

If toxic symptoms develop, administration of the drug should be discontinued. Symptomatic treatment should be provided. The serum potassium concentration should be measured, and corrected if necessary. In some cases, haemodialysis may be required to hasten elimination of the drug.

Table 9.5 Respiratory effects of methylxanthines
Specific
Bronchodilatation by phosphodiesterase inhibition
Non-specific but complementary
Increased mucociliary clearance
Decreased mediator release
Decreased microvascular leakage
Decreased airway oedema
Increased contraction of fatigued respiratory muscles

Table 9.6 Factors affecting the plasma concentration of methylxanthines for a given dose

Factors which lower the plasma concentration

Children

Smoking

Enzyme induction – rifampicin, ethanol

Increased protein diet

Reduced carbohydrate diet

Factors which reduce clearance and thus increase plasma concentration

Old age

Congestive heart failure

Liver disease – cirrhosis

Pneumonia

Viral infection or vaccination

Increased carbohydrate diet

Enzyme inhibition – cimetidine, erythromycin

Table 9.7 Common adverse effects of methylxanthines

Nausea and vomiting

Gastrointestinal upset

Gastro-oesophageal reflux

Headache and restlessness

Diuresis

Arrhythmias

Seizures

Hypokalaemia

Anticholinergic drugs

The use of anticholinergic agents for their bronchodilator properties dates back two centuries when *Datura* plants were smoked for the relief of asthma. Atropine was used later but the side-effects, particularly dry secretions, made it unpopular. Less-soluble ammonia compounds such as ipratropium were then introduced. Ipratropium is active topically and there is little systemic absorption from the respiratory or gastrointestinal tract. It has been suggested that the cholinergic mechanism (increased intracellular cGMP) may be responsible for hyperreactive airways. Thus, ipratropium is effective in both prevention and treatment of reflex bronchoconstriction. Mast cell stabilization has also been proposed as a complementary mechanism of action. The maximum effect occurs 30–60 min after inhalation. The effect may persist for up to 8 h.

Uses

Ipratropium is a second-line bronchodilator which has an additive effect when used with β-agonists. Its safety profile is well proven and it may be used in both acute asthma and COPD. It is particularly effective in older patients with COPD.

Dosage and administration

Ipratropium is used as an aerosol, which delivers 20 µg per puff. The dose is 1–2 puffs three to four times daily. It may also be delivered in a nebulized form; 2–3 mL of a solution containing 250 µg mL^{-1} is used.

Adverse effects

These are uncommon, but include dry secretions, a bitter taste and exacerbation of glaucoma (caused by direct effects of the nebulized drug on the eye).

Magnesium sulphate

Magnesium is an important regulator of intracellular calcium and its effects. It is an effective bronchodilator and is being evaluated for its role in treating refractory severe asthma. Patients with asthma who have a high intake of magnesium tend to have better lung function. Intravenous infusion of magnesium sulphate produces rapid and marked bronchodilatation in both mild and severe asthma.

Uses

Magnesium sulphate has been used successfully in the treatment of refractory severe bronchospasm. Intravenous infusion may be started in patients who fail to respond to conventional therapy. Patients should be monitored regularly for serum concentration of magnesium. There is now enthusiasm to consider it as a first-line bronchodilator in acute asthma requiring hospital admission; however, clinical trials are in progress to define its role precisely.

Dosage and administration

Magnesium sulphate is administered intravenously. Several dose regimens have been described. In acute asthma, 16 mmol may be administerd intravenously over 30 min followed by an infusion of 4–8 mmol h^{-1}. Serum concentrations should be monitored regularly and the dose adjusted correspondingly. Normal serum concentration of magnesium is 0.7–1.0 mmol L^{-1}. The therapeutic range is 1.5–2.5 mmol L^{-1}.

Adverse effects

Minor side-effects include warmth, flushing, nausea, headache and dizziness. Use of magnesium sulphate is contraindicated in hypocalcaemia, heart block or renal failure. It should be given cautiously in patients with oliguria. It potentiates both depolarizing and non-depolarizing neuromuscular block. At serum concentrations greater than 4 mmol L^{-1}, somnolence, double vision, slurred speech and areflexia may occur. At concentrations greater than 6 mmol L^{-1}, profound muscle weakness, respiratory arrest, arrhythmias, bradycardia and hypotension may occur. In the short term, toxic effects may be treated with intravenous infusion of calcium gluconate. In the longer term, use of haemofiltration or dialysis may be required.

MEMBRANE STABILIZERS

Disodium cromoglycate

This is a derivative of khellin, an Egyptian herbal remedy which was found to protect bronchi against allergens. It has no intrinsic bronchodilator effect.

The main mechanism of action of disodium cromoglycate is the stabilization of the mast cell membrane, which in turn inhibits the release of mediators by allergens. It closes the calcium channels and thus prevents the entry of calcium ions, which trigger mast cell degranulation. Long-term treatment with this drug reduces hyperreactivity of the bronchial tree. Other possible mechanisms include an interaction with sensory nerves and effects on other inflammatory cells including macrophages and eosinophils.

Uses

Disodium cromoglycate reduces or prevents bronchospasm in children and adults who suffer from mild asthma, especially if it is exacerbated by fog or exercise.

It is also useful in allergic rhinitis and conjunctivitis. To be effective, it needs to be administered frequently (up to four times a day) even if the patient is symptom-free.

Dosage and administration

Disodium cromoglycate is not soluble and is not absorbed after oral administration. It is administered as an inhaled metered dose (50 μg per puff).

Adverse effects

These are rare, but include cough, wheeze (pre-treatment with a β$_2$-agonist prevents it), pharyngeal discomfort and a transient rash and urticaria in patients with pulmonary eosinophilia.

ANTI-INFLAMMATORY AGENTS

Steroids

Steroids remain the most effective anti-inflammatory agents for lung disease. A variety of mechanisms may be involved in achieving the anti-inflammatory effects (Table 9.8). There is growing evidence that hyperreactive airways are the result of an inflammatory process. Steroids reduce hyperreactivity of airways but have no direct bronchodilator effect. The anti-asthma property of an inhaled steroid is proportional to its anti-inflammatory potency. In addition to their anti-inflammatory actions, steroids sensitize β$_2$-adrenoceptors to the effects of agonists, increase the receptor population and prevent tachyphylaxis.

Uses

The main indications are

- asthma
- COPD
- sarcoidosis
- interstitial lung disease
- pulmonary eosinophilia.

Steroids are a second-line treatment in acute asthma. There is a delayed onset of action, with a peak effect about 6–12 h after intravenous administration. Steroids are of particular use in acute severe asthma (but not for an immediate effect) and in acute exacerbations of COPD. They are also effective in reducing the frequency and severity of acute episodes in chronic asthma. Intravenous hydrocortisone reduces the duration of hospital admission in patients with asthma. Some patients with COPD also benefit from the long-term use of inhaled steroids.

Table 9.8 Sites of action and mechanisms of anti-inflammatory effects of steroids

Intracellular steroid receptors. Steroid–receptor complex alters the transcription of genes leading to altered protein synthesis

Lipocortin. Increase in production of lipocortin which inhibits the release of arachidonic acid metabolites and platelet-activating factor from lung and macrophages

Eosinophils. Decrease in the number of eosinophils and inhibition of degranulation

T lymphocytes. Reduction in the number of T lymphocytes and the production of cytokines

Macrophages. Reduced secretion of leukotrienes and prostaglandin

Endothelial cells. Reduction of the leak around endothelial cells

Airway smooth muscle β_2-adrenoceptors. Increased sensitivity of β_2-adrenoceptors and therefore augmentation of the effect of agonists together with increase in receptor density and prevention of tachyphylaxis

Mucous glands. Reduced mucus secretions

Dosage and administration

Prednisolone may be administered orally in a dose of 30–40 mg daily, reducing later to 10–15 mg daily. Prednisolone is absorbed rapidly after oral administration. Ninety per cent of the drug is protein-bound and it is metabolized by the liver. Enzyme induction by ethanol or rifampicin reduces the half-life of prednisolone.

Hydrocortisone is the drug of choice for intravenous administration. The dose is 3–4 mg kg^{-1} 6-hourly.

Administration by inhalation is preferred for chronic use because it is associated with delivery of a lower dose and with a reduced incidence of systemic side-effects. Beclometasone is used in a dose of 400–500 μg daily. Inhaled steroids may be absorbed systemically either by surface absorption or by swallowed pharyngeal deposits.

Adverse effects

Steroids are well known for their widespread side-effects, which involve almost every system. Systemic effects are less likely with inhaled steroids, but the local effects may be troublesome. The high incidence of adverse effects is the main factor which limits the long-term use of steroids in clinical practice. If it is necessary to use steroids, the dose should be adjusted to achieve the optimal balance between clinical benefit and adverse effects. The adverse effects of steroids are summarized in Table 9.9.

Table 9.9 Common adverse effects of steroids

| **Local (inhaled steroids)** |
| Hoarseness |
| Oral pharyngeal candidiasis |
| Throat irritation and cough |
| **Systemic** |
| Adrenergic suppression |
| Fluid retention |
| Hypertension |
| Peptic ulceration |
| Diabetes mellitus |
| Increased appetite |
| Weight gain |
| Bruising and skin thinning |
| Increased bone metabolism, osteoporosis |
| Cataracts |
| Stunted growth in children |
| Psychosis |

DRUGS ACTING ON PULMONARY VESSELS

A rational approach to manipulating pulmonary vascular tone relies on an understanding of the complex physiological and pathophysiological control of pulmonary resistance vessels. The underlying mechanisms are not understood fully, but there are several broad principles which have been recognized recently:

- Lungs and pulmonary vessels produce and metabolize many vasoactive substances.
- The adrenergic nerves innervate pulmonary vessels; α-stimulation causes vasoconstriction and β-stimulation causes vasodilatation.
- Arachidonic acid metabolites may cause vasoconstriction (thromboxane) or vasodilatation (prostaglandins PGI_2 and PGD_2).
- Oxygen has a strong influence on the pulmonary blood vessels; hypoxia constricts the vessels and oxygen inhalation dilates them.
- Acetylcholine, ATP and bradykinin cause vasodilatation via a specific receptor to produce endothelium-derived relaxing factor (EDRF) and/or endothelium-derived nitric oxide (EDNO), which diffuses into muscle cells to increase the concentration of cyclic GMP, resulting in vasodilatation.

The therapeutic value of drugs acting on pulmonary vessels is mainly as a means of reducing pulmonary vascular resistance. Occasionally, increased pulmonary vascular resistance may be desirable in order to obtain temporary relief in some congenital heart diseases with a large left-to-right shunt. A decrease in pulmonary vascular resistance causes a reduction in right heart afterload. Usually, oxygen inhalation is sufficient to obtain a moderate decrease in pulmonary vascular resistance, but drugs may be needed if more profound vasodilatation is required. It is important to remember that these measures are helpful only if there is a reversible element to the increased pulmonary vascular resistance.

Drugs affecting the pulmonary vascular resistance are summarized in Table 9.10. They may be used either for initial diagnostic or therapeutic evaluation, or for long-term management of pulmonary hypertension, in a variety of clinical conditions:

- primary pulmonary hypertension
- congenital heart disease
- mitral valve disease
- COPD and cor pulmonale

Table 9.10   Factors affecting pulmonary vascular resistance

Factors increasing pulmonary vascular resistance
Hypoxia
Acidosis
α-Adrenergic agonists
β-Adrenergic antagonists
Protamine
Histamine
Serotonin
Angiotensin II
Thromboxane
Factors decreasing pulmonary vascular resistance
Oxygen
Alkalosis
α-Adrenergic antagonists
β-Adrenergic agonists
Prostaglandins PGI_2 and PGD_2
Calcium channel blockers
ACE inhibitors
Acetylcholine
Aminophylline
Nitrates and nitrites
Nitric oxide
Sodium nitroprusside
Hydralazine
Diazoxide

- acute respiratory distress syndrome (ARDS)
- acute respiratory failure
- acute pulmonary oedema.

Pulmonary vasodilators may be administered either by systemic vascular infusion or by inhalation (oxygen, nitric oxide). In patients with acute respiratory failure and/or ARDS, systemic pulmonary vasodilators may worsen the clinical situation, whilst inhaled pulmonary vasodilators may improve it.

INITIAL DIAGNOSTIC AND THERAPEUTIC EVALUATION

Initial evaluation aims to ascertain simply and safely whether significant and reversible pulmonary vasoconstriction is present. Accurate evaluation of pulmonary vascular reactivity requires direct measurement of pulmonary arterial pressure and pulmonary blood flow. Non-invasive approaches using Doppler techniques are not yet sufficiently accurate to obviate an invasive approach. However, an improvement in oxygenation is an indirect measure of the success of therapy. To evaluate vascular reactivity, the agents with the least side-effects and shortest duration of action should be used.

Inhalation of 100% oxygen for at least 10 min is sufficient to demonstrate a change in most cases. Tolazoline hydrochloride (an α-antagonist and a directly acting vasodilator) in a dose of 0.5–1.0 mg kg^{-1} given over 30 s into the right atrium or pulmonary artery is probably the most commonly used agent for evaluating the pulmonary vascular response in individuals with congenital heart disease. It has the disadvantage of significant systemic effects (hypotension, tachycardia) which limit the dose that can be given. Other agents that have been used and are being evaluated include acetylcholine, prostaglandin PGI$_2$, nitroprusside and ATP-magnesium chloride infusion.

LONG-TERM MANAGEMENT WITH VASODILATORS

Oxygen

In acute forms of specific hypoxic pulmonary vasoconstriction such as high-altitude pulmonary hypertension, increasing the inspired oxygen concentration immediately may be life-saving; descent to lower altitude is curative. In chronic forms of lung disease, particularly COPD, oxygen assists management by reducing pulmonary vascular resistance to varying degrees and therefore reducing the severity of cor pulmonale. In these patients, administration of oxygen should be as continuous as is feasible and should continue during sleep. In general, the beneficial effects are only modest and in most instances oxygen is supplemented by at least one other vasodilator.

Adrenergic agonists and antagonists

Tolazoline, phentolamine and prazosin have been used for their α-adrenergic blocking effect. Trials of long-term therapy have been inconclusive. β-Adrenergic stimulation by isoprenaline and terbutaline has also been used. These agents are not uniformly effective and are associated with significant side-effects including angina, tachycardia, arrhythmias and tremors. Children with congenital heart disease and pulmonary vascular disease often have hyperreactive pulmonary vessels and may develop a pulmonary hypertensive crisis postoperatively, especially during tracheal suction and weaning from the ventilator. These episodes may be managed with adequate sedation, intrathecal lidocaine before tracheal suction and systemic α-adrenergic blockade.

Calcium channel blockers

All three of the currently available agents (verapamil, diltiazem and nifedipine) prevent hypoxia-induced pulmonary vasoconstriction. Clinical trials of long-term oral treatment with diltiazem or nifedipine have shown some improvement in survival of a subset of patients with primary pulmonary hypertension.

Arachidonic acid metabolites

PGI$_2$ is a pulmonary vasodilator. Continuous infusion of PGI$_2$ has been used in pulmonary hypertension, but systemic hypotension may be a problem. Non-steroidal anti-inflammatory drugs such as indometacin or aspirin inhibit production of PGI$_2$; these agents may accentuate hypoxic pulmonary vasoconstriction.

Directly acting agents

Hydralazine and tolazoline are direct pulmonary vasodilators (tolazoline has an α-blocking effect as well). Only tolazoline has been used with success (see above). Inhaled nitric oxide has gained immense popularity recently. Its pharmacology and clinical role are discussed below.

Miscellaneous agents

Theophylline, used mainly as a bronchodilator, also has a direct dilator effect on the pulmonary vasculature. Angiotensin II increases pulmonary vascular resistance, and captopril, an angiotensin II inhibitor, reduces pulmonary vascular resistance. Long-term treatment with captopril has proved beneficial in some studies.

Nitric oxide

Nitric oxide is produced endogenously by vascular epithelium. The production is modulated by shear stress in the vessel wall; this ensures a constant basal production. In 1991, it was first used therapeutically in patients who had pulmonary hypertension and respiratory failure.

Organic nitrates and nitrites relax smooth muscle in both arteries and veins. They release nitric oxide, which results in cGMP-mediated smooth muscle relaxation. Studies have indicated that systemic administration of these agents results in significant relief of pulmonary hypertension. Intravenous glyceryl trinitrate is effective when relief is required immediately. On a long-term basis, sublingual isosorbide, in combination with another vasodilator, provides effective treatment. Intravenous sodium nitrite also appears to be an effective pulmonary vasodilator.

In some respiratory conditions, such as ARDS, a combination of hypoxaemia, hypercapnia and acidosis promotes excessive pulmonary vasoconstriction, particularly in hypoventilated areas of the lung. Other factors that may aggravate this disproportionate vasoconstriction include platelet aggregation, white cell aggregation and cytokine release. Pulmonary vasoconstriction in ARDS may be regarded either as an increased afterload on the right ventricle or as a locally protective mechanism which reduces ventilation-perfusion mismatch (i.e. hypoventilated areas receive less blood supply; Fig. 9.2). Intravenous systemic vasodilators act on pulmonary vasculature as a whole and induce vasodilatation simultaneously in well-ventilated and poorly ventilated alveolar units. Thus, the proportion of total pulmonary blood flow which perfuses the hypoventilated areas increases. This leads to an increase in shunt fraction and deterioration in the oxygenation of arterial blood.

By contrast, an inhaled vasodilator (nitric oxide) is delivered preferentially to the well-ventilated areas and thus causes vasodilatation primarily in those areas. Consequently, the proportion of total pulmonary blood flow that perfuses the hypoventilated areas decreases. This leads to a decrease in shunt fraction and an improvement in oxygenation of arterial blood (Fig. 9.2). The other main site of action of inhaled nitric oxide is the bronchial tree; there, it causes bronchodilatation. These advantages of inhaled nitric oxide in comparison with intravenous vasodilators have led to the surge in its popularity in recent years. Administration of other vasodilators such as PGI_2 and tolazoline by inhalation is currently under investigation.

Uses

In a dose of 40–80 ppm, nitric oxide has been used as a pulmonary vasodilator in a wide variety of condi-

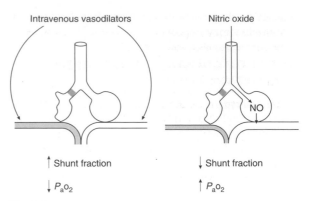

Fig. 9.2
Pulmonary vasodilators, on systemic administration, dilate the vessels supplying hypoventilated areas in addition to adequately ventilated areas; this may result in an increase in shunt fraction and deterioration in oxygenation of arterial blood. Inhaled vasodilators, such as nitric oxide, are delivered preferentially to the well-ventilated areas; this results in a decrease in shunt fraction and an improvement in oxygenation of arterial blood.

tions. The main indications for inhaled nitric oxide are shown in Table 9.11. In all these situations, inhaled nitric oxide has been shown to reduce pulmonary vascular resistance, reduce right ventricular wall stress, increase coronary artery blood flow, reduce the need for inotropic support, increase right ventricular output and increase systemic cardiac output.

In addition, bronchodilatation and reduction in shunt fraction result in an improvement in oxygenation in patients with ARDS. In neonates, nitric oxide also helps to keep the ductus arteriosus closed and has been shown to reduce the need for extracorporeal membrane oxygenation (ECMO).

Another advantage of inhaled nitric oxide is that it does not produce significant systemic effects. This is because inhaled nitric oxide first diffuses through the alveoli to reach vascular smooth muscle and then through the endothelial cells to reach the bloodstream, where it is inactivated rapidly by haemoglobin.

Dosage and administration

Nitric oxide is stored in concentrations of 1000 ppm in nitrogen (in oxygen it is converted into higher oxides). For clinical use, it is diluted in an air–oxygen mixture to produce concentrations of 20–100 ppm. It is delivered through a mechanical ventilator. In the pulmonary bloodstream, it is inactivated rapidly as it combines with haemoglobin to form mainly nitrosyl-haemoglobin (NOHb) but also some methaemoglobin

Table 9.11   The main clinical indications for administration of inhaled nitric oxide

Acute respiratory distress syndrome
Neonatal hypoxic respiratory failure
Lung transplantation
Increased right heart afterload and impaired right ventricular function after cardiac surgery
Mitral valve disease
Right ventricular infarction
Heart transplantation

and nitrates. Nitric oxide has an effective half-life of 0.5–1.0 s. NOHb is converted into nitrites and nitrates, which are excreted by the kidney.

The toxicity of nitric oxide is related to the total amount delivered and to its concentration. Consequently, the design of the delivery system is crucial for the safety of patients. Several delivery systems are now available. Monitoring the concentrations of nitric oxide and higher oxides (NO_2) is essential with all systems.

Adverse effects

Because of its single unpaired electron, nitric oxide is also a free radical and is potentially harmful. Both endogenous and exogenous nitric oxide react readily with oxygen, water, superoxide, nucleotides, metalloproteins, amines and lipids. Biochemical end-products of these reactions may lead to an array of toxic effects. The following have been demonstrated in experimental and/or clinical settings:

- lipid peroxidation
- impaired mitochondrial function
- mutagenesis
- prolonged bleeding time
- impaired surfactant function.

It is difficult to wean some patients from nitric oxide. This difficulty is related mainly to rebound pulmonary hypertension on withdrawal of nitric oxide. Underlying mechanisms include lack of endogenous nitric oxide and the exaggerated constrictive response of pulmonary vessels to hypoxia. In some patients, sudden withdrawal of nitric oxide may precipitate life-threatening pulmonary hypertension and deterioration in gas exchange.

DRUGS ACTING ON MUCOCILIARY FUNCTION

The effectiveness of the mucociliary system depends upon the integrity of the mucus 'blanket' and ciliary motility. The 'blanket' is a high-viscosity mucopolysaccharide gel floating over a low-viscosity serous layer. In health, secretions from goblet cells and bronchial glands maintain the composition of airway secretions. The goblet cells secrete mucopolysaccharides and are stimulated by irritant factors; their response is under local control. Bronchial gland secretions are serous in nature and are controlled by vagal stimulation in addition to local factors. Consequently, both stimulation and blockade of vagal tone affect bronchial gland secretions. The secretions are reduced by administration of opioid drugs.

Cilia are important in propelling the outer 'blanket' of mucus (with entrapped dust, soot or microorganisms) over the serous layer. They act in unison to set the flow of mucus from peripheral airways to central airways from which the mucus is expectorated. Several factors affect ciliary movement and thus mucociliary function. These are summarized in Table 9.12. It is also important to realize that impaired mucociliary function has an indirect effect on the viability of surfactant. Drugs used to improve mucokinetics may be classified as hydrating agents or mucolytics.

HYDRATING AGENTS

Aerosolized water and good systemic hydration help mucociliary clearance. Aerosolized saline may provoke bronchospasm. Hypertonic saline is administered if irritation is desired to provoke ciliary clearance. Hypotonic saline is used for hydration.

Humidification

In health, the upper airways warm and humidify the inspired gases. In disease or when the upper airway is bypassed (mouth-breathing, tracheal intubation), inspiration of dry, cold gases results in increased viscosity of mucus, depressed ciliary function, impaired surfactant function, airway obstruction by tenacious secretions, tracheal inflammation and mucosal ulceration. For these reasons, the inspired gases delivered via a tracheal tube should be saturated with water vapour at body temperature.

Table 9.12 Factors affecting mucociliary function

Factors that depress mucociliary function

Extremes of temperature

Acidic environment

Smoking

Dehydration

Alcohol

Atropine

Anaesthetics

Dry gases

Opioids

Factors that optimize mucociliary function

Temperature (airway) range 29–34°C

Hydration

Humidification

Sympathomimetics

Methylxanthines

Methods of humidification

A variety of methods may be used to achieve humidification of the inspired gases. These include condensers (heat and moisture exchangers), cold water bubble humidifiers, hot water bath humidifiers, and aerosol generators. The details of each method are beyond the scope of this chapter. Condensers are less efficient than heated humidifiers but are useful for short-term humidification. Cold water bubble humidifiers are inefficient and unnecessary; they also have an increased risk of microbial infection. Heated water bath humidifiers are commonly used in intensive care units; the disadvantages are condensation of water, risk of infection and thermostat malfunction. Aerosol generators are effective and may be used with a face mask or mechanical ventilator; the disadvantages include infection and overhydration.

MUCOLYTICS

Cysteine derivatives such as *N*-acetylcysteine may cause mucolysis. *N*-acetylcysteine may be given sys-temically or by inhalation. However, because of its unpleasant odour, irritation of the upper airway and bronchospasm, its use seems to be associated with more problems than benefits. The results of trials in patients with COPD have been disappointing.

SURFACTANT REPLACEMENT THERAPY

Natural surfactant is produced by type II cells in the alveolar epithelium. It is a lipoprotein of complex structure. It lines the alveoli and reduces the surface tension at the air–alveolar interface to prevent the alveoli from collapsing during expiration. An inadequate quantity or quality of endogenous surfactant causes reduced compliance and atelectasis of the lungs, increased pressure gradient between capillaries and pulmonary interstitial space (leading to interstitial oedema), increased work of breathing, increased shunt fraction and hypoxaemia.

In order to reduce surface tension during expiration, natural surfactant forms a mobile and flexible surface film that expands and collapses with the change in alveolar surface area that occurs throughout the respiratory cycle. In order to do so, it must be capable of adsorbing rapidly to the surface of the air–liquid interface, re-spreading rapidly at the onset of inspiration and forming a stable film that is capable of lowering surface tension to a very low value. No single synthetic substance exhibits all of these properties of functional surfactant; this is one of the difficulties in replacing natural surfactant with an artificial compound. The most surface-active phospholipid (85% of surfactant) in natural surfactant is dipalmitoylphosphatidyl choline. However, when administered alone, this phospholipid is ineffective because it does not spread and absorb effectively under physiological conditions. It is necessary to co-administer various other protein components to achieve adequate spread and adsorption.

In infants with respiratory distress syndrome (RDS) the production of natural surfactant is inadequate. In ARDS there is either inadequate production or poor quality of natural surfactant caused by endogenous (capillary leak, endothelial damage, sepsis) or exogenous (smoke inhalation, drowning, aspiration of gastric contents) factors. Administration of artificial surfactant has established its role in RDS in neonates, but in ARDS there is no convincing evidence that it offers benefit.

To date, the following substances have been investigated for their potential to replace exogenous surfactant:

- natural surfactants isolated from human amniotic fluid aspirated during caesarean section for term pregnancy
- natural preparations from minced calf or porcine lungs
- semi-synthetic mixtures of minced calf lung extract with surfactant phospholipid
- synthetic surfactant preparations containing a mixture of dipalmitoylphosphatidyl choline and dispersing and emulsifying agents.

Human surfactant from healthy subjects would be the ideal replacement, but practical difficulties in obtaining sufficient quantities and the risk of transmission of infections (cytomegalovirus, herpes, HIV) restrict its use. Bovine extracts have been used with some success in RDS of neonates, but the potential remains for infection and immunological reactions to the foreign protein content. Synthetic surfactants are protein-free and there is no threat of transmission of infection.

Exosurf

This is a sterile, protein free, synthetic preparation which is presented as lyophilized powder stored in a vacuum. It contains 80% dipalmitoylphosphatidyl choline mixed with hexadecanol and tyloxapol. The blend of these three components achieves the biophysical properties necessary for pulmonary surfactant to prevent alveolar collapse during expiration. Dipalmitoylphosphatidyl choline decreases the surface tension and the other two compounds facilitate its rapid spread and adsorption to the air–fluid interface during the respiratory cycle.

Uses

In RDS in infants who weigh more than 700 g, the use of Exosurf has shown promise:

- 66% reduction in mortality from RDS
- 44% reduction in 1-year mortality from any other cause
- improvement in survival without bronchopulmonary dysplasia
- reduction in incidences of pneumothorax and pulmonary interstitial oedema
- reduction in the number of days of mechanical ventilation
- reduction in the incidence of patent ductus arteriosus
- no change in the incidence of infection or sepsis.

In ARDS, no definite advantage has been shown to date.

Adverse effects

In neonates, the use of Exosurf is associated with an increased incidence of apnoea. Other adverse effects include episodes of transient oxygen desaturation (followed by improvement) and mucus plugging.

FURTHER READING

Berge K H, Warner D O 2006 Drugs that affect the respiratory system. In: Hemmings H, Hopkins P (eds) Foundations of anaesthesia 2nd edn. Mosby, London
Katzung BG 2003 Basic and clinical pharmacology, 9th edn. McGraw-Hill, New York

10 Drugs used in renal disease

DRUG CONSIDERATIONS IN PATIENTS WITH RENAL DYSFUNCTION

INFLUENCE OF RENAL DISEASE ON PHARMACOKINETICS

Renal disease may affect drug pharmacokinetics via several mechanisms. Acidic drugs bind mainly to albumin. In renal failure, a decrease in serum albumin concentration, an increase in serum urea concentration, and the competition between endogenous substrates and drug metabolites for plasma protein binding sites lead to a decrease in the plasma protein binding of drugs. Highly protein-bound drugs have an increased unbound, active, free fraction. Under these circumstances, there may be an increase in the volume of distribution. Drugs are metabolized in the liver to water-soluble, inactive metabolites. Although uraemia has an effect on the intermediary metabolism of the liver, it does not seem to affect hepatic drug metabolism in humans.

The duration of action of most drugs administered by bolus or short-term infusion is dependent on redistribution and not elimination. It is usually not necessary to decrease the initial loading dose in patients with renal dysfunction, but subsequent maintenance doses may cause drug accumulation and should be reduced appropriately. The inactive water-soluble metabolites of drugs are eliminated by passive filtration at the glomerulus. A reduction in glomerular filtration in renal disease may lead to the accumulation of these metabolites.

INFLUENCE OF DRUGS ON RENAL FUNCTION

All anaesthetic agents may cause generalized depression of renal function which is transient and clinically insignificant. However, nephrotoxic drugs can impair renal function permanently (Table 10.1). For example,

they may lead to severe sodium and water depletion, reduction in renal blood supply, direct renal damage or renal obstruction. Some drugs cause renal insufficiency by more than one mechanism.

Some of the fluorinated inhalational agents have well-recognized nephrotoxic effects, because they increase the serum inorganic fluoride concentration. Prolonged exposure of the renal tubules to fluoride ions causes polyuric renal dysfunction, leading to dehydration, hypernatraemia and increased plasma osmolarity. Experience with methoxyflurane (no longer in clinical use) has suggested that a plasma fluoride concentration of $50\,\mu mol\,L^{-1}$ is potentially nephrotoxic. Although halothane and isoflurane do not seem to have a significant effect, prolonged administration of enflurane may lead to nephrotoxic fluoride ion concentrations.

Sevoflurane undergoes approximately 5% metabolism and one of the primary metabolites is fluoride. There were initial concerns that sevoflurane may be similar to methoxyflurane and impair the ability of the kidneys to concentrate urine. However, after sevoflurane administration is stopped, there is a rapid decrease in plasma fluoride concentration because of its insolubility and rapid pulmonary elimination. The intrarenal metabolic production of fluoride is also much lower with sevoflurane than with methoxyflurane. Although after extensive use it appears that sevoflurane renal toxicity is not a problem in clinical practice, prolonged use is not recommended in patients with significantly impaired renal function.

Aprotinin is a serine-protease inhibitor and an antifibrinolytic agent administered occasionally during major surgery to improve haemostasis. It undergoes active reabsorption by the proximal tubules and is metabolized by enzymes in the kidney. There is some controversy about its effect on renal function. Although some studies have shown a low incidence of reversible renal dysfunction, others have shown changes in biochemical markers of tubular damage without evidence of renal impairment.

Table 10.1   Mechanisms of drug-induced renal damage

Sodium and water depletion
Reduced renal perfusion
Direct renal toxicity
Urinary obstruction

Other drugs with potential for impairing renal function include aminoglycosides and NSAIDs in the presence of sepsis, radiocontrast agents and various chemotherapeutic drugs.

VASOACTIVE DRUGS USED IN RENAL DYSFUNCTION

DOPAMINE

Dopamine is an important endogenous catecholamine, a precursor of noradrenaline (norepinephrine) and adrenaline (epinephrine), and a neurotransmitter in its own right. It may be administered pharmacologically and has complicated pharmacodynamic effects, including inotropy, chronotropy, vasoconstriction, and renal and splanchnic vasodilatation. Dopamine is inactive orally and has to be administered as an intravenous infusion, because it is metabolized within minutes by the enzymes dopamine β-hydroxylase and monoamine oxidase ($t_{1/2}$ < 2 min). Dopamine must be diluted before infusion.

Mechanism of action

In common with all catecholamines, dopamine acts on different receptors in a diverse dose-related fashion. Dopamine receptors are present in various sites in the body and have been classified into five subtypes. The two most important receptors in the peripheral cardiovascular and renal systems are DA_1 and DA_2.

The infusion of relatively low concentrations of dopamine activates postsynaptic DA_1 receptors in blood vessels and the renal tubules. Stimulation leads to vasodilatation and improves some measures of renal function, such as cortical renal blood flow, glomerular filtration rate (GFR), sodium excretion and urine output. There is also an increase in mesenteric flow. Activation of presynaptic DA_2 receptors decreases intrarenal noradrenaline release, which leads to vasodilatation. It also causes inhibition of aldos-

terone secretion from the adrenal glands and a consequent decrease in sodium reabsorption. Theoretically, this should decrease renal oxygen consumption and improve the renal oxygen supply/demand relationship.

Dopamine stimulates its receptors in the renal and splanchnic beds at low infusion rates (0.1–2 μg kg^{-1} min^{-1}). This effect is accompanied by little change in cardiac output or heart rate. A reduction in arterial pressure may occur because of inhibition of the sympathetic nervous system by stimulation of the DA_2 receptors, and by DA_1-induced vasodilatation.

Increased infusion (2–5 μg kg^{-1} min^{-1}) stimulates $β_1$- and $β_2$-adrenergic receptors, which causes increases in myocardial contractility, stroke volume and cardiac output. At this infusion rate, the heart rate usually does not change.

Higher doses of dopamine (>10 μg kg^{-1} min^{-1}) lead to stimulation of the α-adrenergic receptors, causing vasoconstriction, an increase in peripheral vascular resistance and a decrease in renal and splanchnic blood flow.

The dopamine infusion rates given above are guidelines and there is considerable intra- and interpatient variation. The maximum dose at which dopamine affects only dopamine receptors is debatable and must be individually determined. Because of the up- and downregulation of receptors, in any one patient, the appropriate dose for a required effect may vary from hour to hour.

Clinical uses

Dopamine is often used to preserve regional blood flow, but its perceived effectiveness is based largely on anecdotal reports and experimental data. Improved haemodynamics, renal vasodilatation and increase in renal blood flow do have diuretic and natriuretic effects. Because the urine output of the critically ill patient is considered a good marker of tissue perfusion by many clinicians, the diuretic properties of dopamine are valued. However, clinical studies have not demonstrated any benefit of 'low-dose' dopamine for renal protection or for the prevention and treatment of acute renal failure in critically ill patients. In fact, it induces regional redistribution of blood flow within the kidney by shunting blood away from the outer medulla to the cortex. This is potentially detrimental in acute renal failure given that the outer medulla is very susceptible to ischaemic injury.

The use of higher doses of dopamine as an inotrope during cardiac failure, or a vasopressor during hypotension, is well established. Under these circumstances, it has a beneficial effect on renal function, but it is important to ensure that there is an adequate circulating blood volume.

Side-effects

Side-effects of dopamine include tachyarrhythmias, vasoconstriction with acute hypertension, and nausea and vomiting because of a direct effect on receptors within the chemoreceptor trigger zone. Intravenous administration of dopamine does not result in central nervous system effects as dopamine does not cross the blood–brain barrier. Other potentially detrimental effects of low-dose dopamine in the critically ill patient include:

- a decrease in splanchnic oxygen consumption in septic patients despite an increase in splanchnic blood flow
- a possible decrease in gastric motility compromising enteral feeding and absorption
- impairment of regional ventilation–perfusion matching in the lung and the ventilatory drive in response to hypoxaemia and hypercapnia
- reduced output of anterior pituitary hormones including prolactin, growth hormone, TSH and thyroid hormones.

Ideally, dopamine should be administered through a central venous catheter because extravasation may cause sloughing and necrosis of local surrounding tissues.

DOPEXAMINE

Dopexamine is a synthetic catecholamine with structural and pharmacological similarities to dopamine, and is used for its increase in cardiac output and renal and splanchnic vasodilator effects. It is inactive orally and, because of its short half-life (~6 min), it is administered intravenously as an infusion. Infusion rate starts at $0.5\ \mu g\ kg^{-1}\ min^{-1}$ and is titrated to a therapeutic response (up to $6\ \mu g\ kg^{-1}\ min^{-1}$). Tolerance is associated usually with receptor downregulation. It is metabolized by the recognized pathways for all the catecholamines.

Dopexamine is an agonist at vascular and renal dopaminergic DA_1 and DA_2 receptors. It also stimulates cardiac and vascular β_2-receptors, and has a limited indirect β_1 effect. It therefore combines vasodilator, chronotropic and mild inotropic activity and is used in low cardiac output states where specific renal and hepatosplanchnic vasodilatation is considered beneficial. The heart rate is increased in a dose-related manner and it produces natriuresis and diuresis. The protective effect of dopexamine on the kidneys is theoretical and an effect on outcome still has to be proven.

The most common side-effects are a tachycardia and ventricular ectopic beats when higher doses are used. Nausea and vomiting, probably caused by stimulation of DA_2 receptors in the chemoreceptor trigger zone, have been reported.

FENOLDOPAM

Fenoldopam is a selective DA_1 agonist. It may be administered orally or intravenously and has been used for the management of congestive cardiac failure and hypertension.

ADENOSINE

Adenosine is a natural purine and is an important mediator in the control of renal blood flow and glomerular filtration. It causes peripheral vasodilatation and decreases arterial pressure when given intravenously. Adenosine-induced arterial hypotension inhibits renin release by the juxtaglomerular cells and has an interesting effect on the renal vasculature. It causes transient vasoconstriction of the afferent arterioles, combined with vasodilatation of the efferent arterioles. This results in decreases in renal blood flow and glomerular filtration pressure and rate. There have been suggestions that this temporary decrease in renal function may play a protective role against an ischaemic insult. A decrease in GFR is associated usually with decreases in ultrafiltrate volume, reabsorption and oxygen demand. Whether adenosine changes the outcome of an ischaemic insult and acute renal injury in clinical practice has not been confirmed.

Recently a novel A1 adenosine receptor antagonist, BG9719, has been described; this apparently promotes diuresis without worsening renal function.

Adenosine also slows the heart rate and impairs atrioventricular conduction and is used in the treatment of supraventricular tachycardias.

CALCIUM CHANNEL BLOCKERS

Calcium antagonists (see Ch. 8) act selectively on calcium channels in the cellular membrane of cardiac and vascular smooth muscle cells. Free calcium within the vascular smooth muscle enhances vascular tone and contributes to vasoconstriction. Calcium antagonists reduce the transmembrane calcium influx in these cells and via this mechanism are responsible for relaxation of the vascular smooth muscle and subsequent vasodilatation.

Apart from vasodilatation, these drugs have a direct diuretic effect that contributes to their long-term antihypertensive action. Nifedipine increases urine volume and sodium excretion, and may inhibit aldosterone release. This diuretic action is independent of any change in renal blood flow or GFR.

Because of the vasodilator effect on the vasculature, these drugs have been found to be useful in the management of conditions in which pathological vasoconstriction occurs, such as hypertension, Raynaud's disease, migraine and Prinzmetal angina.

Calcium antagonists are often used as renovascular vasodilators in selected situations, e.g. renal transplantation. In kidney recipients, diltiazem has been shown to cause vasodilatation within the kidney and to improve intrarenal circulation. Calcium antagonists also decrease calcium influx and production of oxygen free radicals on reperfusion after the ischaemic insult. In these patients, calcium antagonists significantly improve renal function and decrease the incidence of post-transplant acute tubular necrosis. Furthermore, they may reduce the vasoconstrictor action of ciclosporin. In spite of all the apparent beneficial effects, calcium antagonists have failed to improve graft survival.

Calcium antagonists may cause hypotension and thereby decrease renal perfusion. Therefore their use is not really justified in most cases of postischaemic acute renal failure. The effects of the depolarizing and non-depolarizing neuromuscular blocking agents might be enhanced by the calcium antagonists. Caution should always be exercised when this combination is used in patients with renal dysfunction.

ANGIOTENSIN-CONVERTING ENZYME (ACE) INHIBITORS

Many patients with hypertension or cardiac failure have an increased activity of the renin–angiotensin–aldosterone system. This leads to an elevated systemic vascular resistance, further decreases in cardiac output and renal perfusion, and more sodium and fluid retention. These patients are often receiving diuretic treatment, which in itself triggers renin activity. The ACE inhibitors (e.g. captopril, enalapril, lisinopril) are being used increasingly in this scenario, in place of, or in combination with, diuretics.

ACE inhibitors have a much greater affinity for the active site on ACE than the natural substrate, angiotensin I. Consequently, the conversion of angiotensin I to angiotensin II is blocked. ACE is also responsible for the breakdown of bradykinin, which is a potent vasodilator. Therefore, ACE inhibitors not

only lead to vasodilatation but, because of the decreases in aldosterone formation and sodium reuptake, also have an indirect potassium-retaining diuretic effect. The combination of ACE inhibitors and the potassium-saving diuretics should be avoided because of the risk of hyperkalaemia.

Angiotensin II is important for the maintenance of an adequate glomerular filtration pressure in patients with decreased renal perfusion. In the presence of renal artery stenosis, the use of ACE inhibitors may lead to an impairment of renal function by decreasing renal perfusion pressure, caused by the decrease in arterial pressure together with dilatation of the efferent arteriole of the glomerulus. Underlying renal impairment should therefore always be excluded before using ACE inhibitors, and patients receiving these agents should be monitored carefully.

NORADRENALINE (NOREPINEPHRINE)/ ADRENALINE (EPINEPHRINE)/ PHENYLEPHRINE

Although noradrenaline (norepinephrine) and adrenaline (epinephrine) also have β-receptor effects, all three of these drugs are very potent vasoconstrictors acting on the vascular α-receptors (see Ch. 8). Their use is often accompanied by fear of inducing decreases in renal blood flow, GFR and renal function.

The efferent arterioles are the major sites of flow resistance in the kidney and determine renal blood flow, perfusion pressure and GFR. In cases of hypotension or septic shock, restoring the perfusion pressure of the kidney is of the utmost importance. An infusion of one of these vasoconstrictors may improve renal perfusion pressure provided that fluid resuscitation has been adequate.

ANTIDIURETIC HORMONE/ VASOPRESSIN/DESMOPRESSIN/DDAVP

Antidiuretic hormone (ADH) is a naturally occurring hormone, produced in the hypothalamus, transported by nerve axons down to the posterior pituitary gland and, from there, secreted into the blood. The release of ADH is regulated by the osmolarity of the extracellular body fluids, changes in arterial pressure and intravascular volume, and the sympathetic nervous system. An increase in blood osmolarity and hypovolaemia stimulate the hypothalamic osmoreceptors and arterial baroreceptors as part of the stress response. ADH is released and acts primarily on receptors in the distal convoluted tubule and collecting ducts of the nephron, to increase free water reabsorption and restore the plasma volume. The presence or absence of ADH determines to a large extent whether the kidney excretes a dilute or a concentrated urine. ADH is also termed vasopressin, because it has a very potent vasoconstrictor effect, even more powerful than that of angiotensin.

Vasopressin decreases splanchnic and renal blood flow and is sometimes used to treat bleeding oesophageal varices. Desmopressin (DDAVP, 1-desamino-8-D-arginine vasopressin) is a synthetic form of vasopressin that does not cause vasoconstriction. It is used in cases of central diabetes insipidus (i.e. spontaneous diuresis with a urine osmolarity below 200 mosm L^{-1}).

DDAVP also has an influence on the coagulation system by increasing factor VIII von Willebrand (VIII:vWF), factor VIII coagulant (VIII:C), and factor VIII-related antigen (VIIIr:Ag) activity by stimulating release from the storage sites. A dose of 0.3 µg kg^{-1} is often used in the treatment of haemorrhage in haemophiliacs.

Platelet dysfunction often occurs in renal disease when a high urea concentration occurs. The increase in bleeding time (>15 min), despite a normal platelet count (>100×10^9 L^{-1}), may be corrected before major surgery. The most appropriate treatment currently is administration of DDAVP in the same dose as above. It has also been used prophylactically to reduce bleeding after cardiac surgery.

DDAVP cannot be used repeatedly because the endothelial storage sites of factor VIII:C become depleted, resulting in tachyphylaxis. Because it also seems to release tissue plasminogen activator, DDAVP enhances fibrinolysis and the simultaneous use of an antifibrinolytic agent should be considered. Although vasopressin is a vasoconstrictor, rapid injection of DDAVP may cause acute hypotension as a result of vasodilatation.

DIURETICS

Diuretics are probably among the most frequently prescribed groups of drugs in clinical practice. By definition, they cause a diuresis of water and sodium. When used on a long-term basis as antihypertensive agents, or for chronic cardiac failure, they not only change the body's sodium and fluid balance but also act as mild vascular dilators. In the more acute perioperative and critical care scenario when a major diuretic effect is required, diuretics are used in higher doses. In acute cardiac failure, these drugs are very valuable because of their high benefit–risk ratio. Diuretics are often used to 'protect' the kidneys dur-

ing ischaemic episodes such as aortic cross-clamping and cardiopulmonary bypass. However, human studies have failed to show the effectiveness of these agents in the prevention of ischaemic acute renal failure. There is also no clear evidence that polyuric renal dysfunction has a better outcome than oliguric renal failure, but it is generally accepted that the intensive care management of a critically ill patient is easier if there is a urine output.

Diuretics are classified according to their mechanism and site of action on the nephron (Fig. 10.1):

- glomerulus and proximal renal tubule, e.g. osmotic diuretics, carbonic anhydrase inhibitors
- ascending limb of the loop of Henle, e.g. loop diuretics
- distal tubule, e.g. thiazides, potassium-sparing diuretics
- collecting ducts, e.g. aldosterone antagonists.

CARBONIC ANHYDRASE INHIBITORS

Acetazolamide

Acetazolamide is well absorbed, not metabolized, but excreted almost unchanged by the kidney within 24 h. Toxicity is very rare.

Acetazolamide is a carbonic anhydrase inhibitor and acts in the proximal convoluted tubule of the nephron. Under normal physiological conditions, this enzyme is responsible for reabsorption of sodium and excretion of hydrogen ions in this part of the kidney. Inhibition of the carbonic anhydrase enzyme decreases the excretion of hydrogen ions, and therefore sodium and bicarbonate ions stay in the renal tubule. This results in the production of an alkaline urine with a high sodium bicarbonate content. This increased sodium excretion leads to a modest diuresis. Chloride ions are retained instead of bicarbonate to maintain an ionic balance. All these changes result in a hyperchloraemic metabolic acidosis.

Carbonic anhydrase inhibitors are seldom used as primary diuretics because of their weak diuretic effect. In the management of salicylate overdose, they may be used to start an alkaline diuresis to eliminate the weak organic acid. The most common use of acetazolamide is to reduce the intraocular pressure of patients with glaucoma. The inhibition of carbonic anhydrase results in decreased formation of ocular aqueous humour and cerebrospinal fluid. It is valuable in the prevention and management of acute mountain sickness. When used in patients with familial periodic paralysis, the metabolic acidosis increases the potassium concentration in skeletal muscles and improves symptoms.

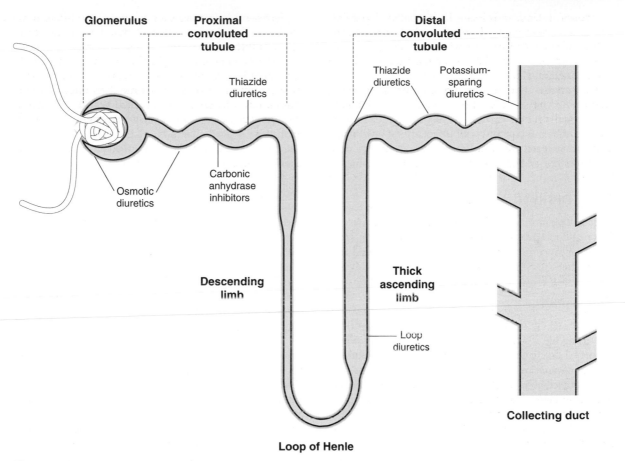

Fig. 10.1
Sites of action of diuretics.

OSMOTIC DIURETICS

Mannitol

Mannitol is absorbed unreliably from the gastrointestinal tract and therefore has to be given by intravenous injection; doses of $0.25–1 \text{ g kg}^{-1}$ are used. Initially it stays within the intravascular space but is then redistributed slowly into the extravascular compartment. Mannitol does not undergo metabolism and is excreted unchanged through the kidneys.

Mannitol expands the intravascular volume and then undergoes free glomerular filtration with almost no reabsorption in the proximal tubule. It also decreases the energy-consuming process of sodium and water reabsorption in the proximal tubule. This leads to an osmotic force that retains water and sodium in the tubule with a consequent osmotic diuresis, i.e. increased urinary excretion of sodium, water, bicarbonate and chloride. Mannitol does not alter urinary pH. The raised renal blood flow reduces the rate of renin secretion, which decreases the urine-concentrating effect of the kidney.

Mannitol is often used prophylactically to protect the kidneys against an ischaemic incident (e.g. cardiopulmonary bypass, aortic cross-clamping or hypotensive episodes) and subsequent acute renal failure. It has been suggested that decreasing the oxygen demand in the proximal tubular cells preserves oxygen balance. By increasing tubular flow, it might also provide a flushing effect to remove necrotic cellular debris from the renal tubules after ischaemic injury. The hyperosmotic and oxygen radical scavenging effects of this drug might also reduce tubular endothelial cell swelling. However, although mannitol has been shown to be effective in animal experiments, studies have failed to show a renal protective effect in clinical practice. There is also little evidence that conversion from an oliguric to non-oliguric renal failure decreases the mortality rate in critically ill patients. Nevertheless, mannitol is used regularly during renal transplantation to help 'preserve' the donor kidney.

Anaesthetists often administer mannitol to reduce intracranial and intraocular pressure.

In patients with compromised cardiac function, mannitol may precipitate pulmonary oedema. Occasionally it may cause hypersensitivity reactions. If the blood–brain barrier is not intact after a head injury or neurosurgery, mannitol may enter the brain, draw water with it and cause rebound cerebral swelling.

LOOP DIURETICS

Furosemide, bumetanide and ethacrynic acid are classified as loop diuretics because of their common site of action. Furosemide is the most commonly used loop diuretic.

Furosemide

Furosemide is usually administered intravenously $(0.1–1 \text{ mg kg}^{-1})$ or orally $(0.75–3 \text{ mg kg}^{-1})$. It is well absorbed orally and about 60% of the dose reaches the central circulation within a short period, with the peak effect after 1–1.5 h. Intravenous furosemide is usually started as a slow 20–40 mg injection in adults, but higher doses or even an infusion may be required in the case of elderly patients with renal failure or severe congestive cardiac failure. Approximately 90% of the drug is bound to plasma proteins and its volume of distribution is relatively low. Metabolism and excretion into the gastrointestinal tract contribute to about 30% of the elimination of a dose of furosemide. The remainder is excreted unchanged through glomerular filtration and tubular secretion. Impaired renal function affects the elimination process, but liver disease does not seem to influence this. The elimination half-life of furosemide is 1–1.5 h.

Loop diuretics act primarily on the medullary part of the ascending limb of the loop of Henle. After initial glomerular filtration and proximal tubular secretion, furosemide inhibits the active reabsorption of chloride in the thick portion of the ascending limb. This leads to chloride, sodium, potassium and hydrogen ions remaining in the tubule to maintain electrical neutrality, and their increased excretion in the urine. The extent of the following diuresis is determined by the concentration of furosemide active in this part of the tubule. Because the ascending limb plays an important role in the reabsorption of sodium chloride in the kidney, furosemide results in a marked diuretic response. The decrease in sodium chloride reabsorption leads to a reduced urine-concentrating ability of the normally hypertonic medullary interstitium.

Furosemide increases renal artery blood flow if the intravascular fluid volume is maintained. It causes redistribution so that flow to the outer part of the cortex remains unchanged while flow to the inner cortex and medulla is increased. It leads to an improved renal tissue oxygen tension. This effect, together with the increased release of renin and activation of the angiotensin–aldosterone axis, is mediated via prostaglandins. A particular advantage of loop diuretics is the high ceiling effect (i.e. increasing doses lead to increasing diuresis).

Furosemide is the diuretic of choice in acute pulmonary oedema or other oedematous states of fluid overload due to cardiac, renal or liver failure. It reduces the intravascular fluid volume by promoting a rapid, powerful diuresis even in the presence of a low GFR. The pulmonary vascular bed and capacitance vessels are dilated by furosemide, and often relief of dyspnoea and a reduction in pulmonary pressures may take place before the diuretic effect has occurred. In hypertensive patients, the vasodilatation and preload reduction lead to a decrease in arterial pressure.

The use of furosemide for prophylactic protection of the kidney against ischaemic injury and in the treatment of acute renal failure is controversial. In common with mannitol, furosemide has been shown in animal studies to help protect the kidney against ischaemic damage. Human studies, however, failed to support this. Loop diuretics, if administered early in the course of ischaemic acute renal failure, may change an oliguric into a non-oliguric state. Although non-oliguric acute renal failure is generally associated with a lower mortality rate, there is little evidence that conversion produced by furosemide changes the outcome. Furosemide should never be used, however, to treat oliguria caused by a decreased intravascular fluid volume or dehydration, because the following diuresis could exaggerate hypovolaemia and renal ischaemic injury. It is important to restore the intravascular volume status first before any pharmacological intervention.

A raised intracranial pressure is often treated with furosemide. It mobilizes the oedema fluid, decreases cerebrospinal fluid production and lowers the intracranial pressure without changing the plasma osmolarity. In contrast to mannitol, a disrupted blood–brain barrier does not influence the effect of furosemide on the intracranial pressure.

Excessive doses of furosemide often lead to fluid or electrolyte abnormalities. Severe hypokalaemia may precipitate dangerous cardiac arrhythmias, especially in the presence of high concentrations of digitalis. It may also enhance the effect of non-depolarizing muscle relaxants. Hypovolaemia, dehydration and the consequent haemoconcentration may lead to changes in blood viscosity. Hyperuricaemia and prerenal uraemia may develop and may precipitate an acute gout attack in a patient with pre-existing gout.

Furosemide may cause high concentrations of aminoglycosides and cephalosporins in the kidneys and this may enhance their nephrotoxic effect. Prolonged high blood concentrations of furosemide may have a detrimental effect on renal function through a direct toxic action resulting in interstitial nephritis. It may also cause transient or permanent deafness because of changes in the endolymph electrolyte composition. Patients allergic to other sulphonamide drugs may have a cross-sensitivity, although idiosyncratic reactions are rare.

Bumetanide

The mechanism of action of bumetanide and its effects are similar to those of furosemide. The difference between these two drugs is the greater potency and bioavailability of bumetanide; therefore, smaller doses are needed. The normal adult dose is 0.5–3 mg i.v. over 1–2 min. The onset of diuresis is within 30 min and usually lasts for about 4 h. The pharmacokinetics are similar to those of furosemide, with the exception that bumetanide is absorbed completely after oral administration and its rate of elimination is less dependent on renal function. Potassium loss is also a problem with bumetanide. Ototoxicity may be slightly less frequent than with furosemide, but renal toxicity is more of a problem. In clinical practice, there is no clear advantage or disadvantage over furosemide, providing that equivalent doses are administered.

Ethacrynic acid

Although the molecular structure of ethacrynic acid is very different from that of furosemide, it has almost identical pharmacological properties. After intravenous administration, it binds strongly to plasma proteins and the majority of the drug is eliminated by active secretion into the renal tubule. Almost one-third is excreted in the bile. The risk of toxicity and side-effects is probably equivalent to that of furosemide.

THIAZIDE DIURETICS

Although thiazide diuretics are seldom used by anaesthetists, many patients scheduled for surgery are receiving these drugs for chronic hypertension or cardiac failure. There is a large number of thiazides available, all with a similar dose–response curve and diuretic effect. Bendroflumethiazide, chlorothiazide, hydrochlorothiazide and chlortalidone are a few examples of the better-known thiazide diuretics. The majority have a duration of action of 6–12 h. In comparison with loop diuretics, thiazides have a longer duration of action, act at a different site, have a low 'ceiling' effect and are less effective in renal failure.

Thiazide diuretics are administered orally, absorbed rapidly from the gastrointestinal tract and initiate a diuresis within 1–2 h. The major distinction between the available thiazides is their difference in elimination rate. They are distributed in the extracellular space and eliminated in the proximal tubule of the nephron by active secretion.

Thiazides inhibit the active pump for sodium and chloride reabsorption in the cortical ascending part of the loop of Henle and the distal convoluted tubule. Therefore, the urine-concentrating ability of the kidney is not impaired, as normally this area is responsible for less than 5% of sodium reabsorption. The diuresis achieved by the thiazides is therefore never as effective as that of the loop diuretics. It is mild but sustained. In contrast with loop diuretics, the excretion of calcium is decreased and hypercalcaemia may become a problem. In the presence of aldosterone activity, the increase in sodium delivery to the distal renal tubules is associated with increased potassium loss, similar to that of the loop diuretics. The reduced clearance of uric acid by thiazides may cause hyperuricaemia.

Thiazides are used extensively in low doses, and often combined with a low-sodium diet, for the management of essential hypertension. A reduction in extracellular fluid volume and mild peripheral vasodilatation are responsible for the sustained antihypertensive effect. The full antihypertensive effect may take up to 12 weeks to become established. Higher doses of thiazides are used for the management of congestive cardiac failure and other oedematous conditions such as nephrotic syndrome and liver cirrhosis.

The most common side-effects of the thiazides are probably dehydration and hypovolaemia. This may present as orthostatic hypotension. When administered chronically, these drugs lead typically to a diuretic-induced hypokalaemic, hypochloraemic, metabolic alkalosis. In combination with magnesium depletion, the hypokalaemia may trigger serious cardiac arrhythmias, in addition to digitalis toxicity, muscle weakness and the potentiation of non-depolarizing muscle relaxants.

Thiazides decrease the tubular secretion of urate, which may lead to hyperuricaemia and gout. They are sulphonamide derivatives and may therefore cause inhibition of insulin release from the pancreas and blockade of peripheral glucose utilization. This may precipitate hyperglycaemia or an increase in insulin requirements in a patient with diabetes mellitus. They also lead to an increase in total blood cholesterol concentration.

POTASSIUM-SPARING DIURETICS

Only a small part of sodium reabsorption into the renal cells takes place via the sodium–potassium exchange mechanism in the distal tubules. The potassium-retaining diuretics act on the distal convoluted tubules and the collecting ducts and therefore cause only a limited diuresis. There are two subgroups in this category: drugs acting independently of the aldosterone mechanism (e.g. triamterene and amiloride) and aldosterone antagonists (e.g. spironolactone).

These drugs increase the urinary excretion of sodium, chloride and bicarbonate and lead to an increase in urinary pH. They prevent excessive loss of potassium that occurs with the loop and thiazide diuretics by reducing sodium–potassium exchange. Potassium-sparing drugs do, however, augment the diuretic response of these drugs when given in combination.

Amiloride and triamterene

Amiloride acts directly on the distal tubule and collecting duct. It causes potassium retention and an increase in sodium loss. After oral intake, up to 25% is absorbed, the onset of its peak effect is within 6 h, and it is then excreted unchanged in the urine. Amiloride is almost always used in combination with a thiazide or loop diuretic. It then has a synergistic action in terms of diuresis, although it opposes the potassium loss. Amiloride has few side-effects. Hyperkalaemia and acidosis may occur, and it is therefore contraindicated in patients with renal failure.

Triamterene has characteristics similar to those of amiloride.

Spironolactone

Aldosterone causes sodium reabsorption and potassium loss in the distal convoluted tubule. Spironolactone has a steroid molecular structure, acts as a competitive antagonist on the aldosterone receptors and inhibits sodium reabsorption and potassium loss. In the absence of aldosterone, it has no effect.

After oral absorption, spironolactone is immediately metabolized to several metabolites. Some of these are active and act for up to 15 h.

Spironolactone is the logical choice of diuretic in the management of cirrhosis of the liver, ascites and secondary hyperaldosteronism. Cardiac failure or hypertension in the presence of high mineralocorticoid levels (Conn's syndrome or prednisone therapy) is another indication. It is often combined with a thiazide to maximize the diuretic effect and prevent potassium loss.

Hyperkalaemia may develop if spironolactone is used in the presence of renal dysfunction. If it is used in high doses, it may cause gynaecomastia and impotence.

When diuretics are prescribed in a patient with fluid retention and oedema, three important principles have to be kept in mind. First, although a dramatic diuretic response may be required in pulmonary oedema and acute cardiac failure, a mild sustained diuresis is more appropriate in the majority of patients with a need for diuretics. This approach reduces the extent of side-effects. Secondly, plasma potassium concentration and hydration status must always be monitored when a diuretic is being used. Thirdly, diuretic therapy only treats the symptoms and does not influence the underlying cause or change the outcome of a patient with oedema.

ACUTE RENAL FAILURE, SEPSIS AND THE INTENSIVE CARE UNIT

Acute renal failure is a common complication of sepsis and septic shock; the combination is associated with a 70% mortality. The arterial vasodilatation that accompanies sepsis is mediated in part by cytokines that upregulate inducible nitric oxide synthase with a subsequent increased release of nitric oxide. The potent vasodilatory effect of nitric oxide is partly responsible for the vascular resistance to the pressor response to noradrenaline (norepinephrine) and angiotensin II. Early in sepsis-related acute renal failure, cytokines such as tumour necrosis factor alpha (TNF-α) cause vasoconstriction of the renal vasculature. However, the use of monoclonal antibody against TNF-α did not result in any improvement in patient survival. Although this early vasoconstrictor phase is potentially reversible, clinical studies to optimize haemodynamics with goal-directed therapy did not show any benefit and in some cases even showed increased mortality. There is evidence that administration of vasopressin (see earlier) in patients with septic shock may help maintain arterial pressure despite the relative ineffectiveness of other vasopressors such as noradrenaline (norepinephrine) and angiotensin II. Vasopressin constricts the glomerular efferent arteriole and therefore increases the filtration pressure and glomerular filtration rate.

ACUTE RENAL FAILURE FOLLOWING CARDIAC SURGERY

The incidence of acute renal failure after cardiac surgery is approximately 10% and it is associated with a high morbidity and mortality. Clinical evidence suggests that preoperative renal insufficiency, diabetes mellitus, prolonged cardiopulmonary bypass time and postoperative hypotension are all independent risk factors for acute renal failure in the cardiac surgical patient. Prevention of renal damage by adequate hydration and perfusion pressure during cardiopulmonary bypass (CPB), and the maintenance of cardiac output in the postoperative period, is the most effective way to combat this problem. Hypothermia during CPB, pulsatile CPB flow or avoiding CPB altogether through off-pump cardiac surgical techniques, have not been consistently associated with a reduced incidence of acute renal failure.

Many drugs have been studied for renal protection during CPB but none has been conclusively proven to be effective. As explained earlier, low-dose dopamine offers no renal protection and may even be harmful. Although mannitol is used in routine CPB pump prime in many cardiac units and furosemide potentially reduces renal medullary oxygen consumption, both seem to be ineffective in preventing acute renal failure in this setting. There is currently no pharmacological strategy known to reduce its incidence reliably.

DRUGS AND RENAL TRANSPLANTATION

The optimal treatment for end-stage renal failure is renal transplantation. Apart from optimizing the recipient's general health (e.g. correction of anaemia, preoperative dialysis, etc.), immunosuppression plays an extremely important role in graft survival.

ERYTHROPOIETIN

Erythropoietin is a circulating hormone secreted by the kidneys. It stimulates the bone marrow to produce red blood cells. The ability of the kidney to secrete erythropoietin deteriorates as excretory function decreases. Patients with severe chronic renal failure are unable to produce adequate quantities of erythropoietin, which leads to diminished red blood cell production. The retention of toxic substances also contributes to bone marrow depression. In addition, red cell survival is reduced by 50% in advanced renal failure. Therefore these patients almost always develop chronic anaemia.

Long-term administration of recombinant human erythropoietin (rHUEPO) in chronic renal failure patients results in global stimulation of the bone marrow, increasing red blood cell differentiation and maintaining cell viability, thereby improving anaemia. It also decreases bleeding by increasing platelet adhesion in haemodialysed uraemic patients. A side-effect of rHUEPO is the development of hypertension or exacerbation of existing hypertension.

IMMUNOSUPPRESSION

Prednisolone and azathioprine

Corticosteroids were the first drugs to be used as immunosuppressive agents. Initially, very high doses were used, producing the typical steroid side-effects, e.g. cushingoid appearance, hypertension, hyperglycaemia and osteoporosis. Experience and research showed that large doses were not necessary and that better results and fewer side-effects were possible with lower doses.

The 'modern era' of immunosuppression started with the discovery of azathioprine. For a long period of time, the combination of azathioprine and corticosteroids was the 'gold standard' in transplant surgery. Azathioprine is a derivative of 6-mercaptopurine and is metabolized to its active form in the liver. It affects the synthesis of DNA and RNA and is broken down by the enzyme xanthine oxidase. Co-administration of allopurinol (xanthine oxidase inhibitor) is contraindicated because it may result in bone marrow suppression, agranulocytosis and leucopenia. Patients receiving azathioprine are prone to develop viral warts or malignancies of the skin and hepatic dysfunction.

Ciclosporin A and ciclosporin (Neoral)

The next major advance in transplant surgery was the discovery of ciclosporin A. This fungal peptide prevents the proliferation and clonal expansion of T lymphocytes. The chance of acute rejection is reduced significantly by administration of this drug. In spite of the large number of side-effects of ciclosporin A, it has been accepted as the new standard against which all other immunosuppressants are judged. Ciclosporin A is lipophilic and incompletely absorbed in the small bowel. Serious side-effects such as gingival hypertrophy, hepatotoxicity and nephrotoxicity make this a less than perfect drug. For a long time, classic triple therapy consisted of prednisolone, azathioprine and ciclosporin A.

Recently, ciclosporin has been released in a new form under the trade name Neoral. This form is a microemulsion that enhances the bioavailability of ciclosporin through improved absorption. Ciclosporin (Neoral) is equipotent to the parent drug and most renal transplant patients are presently receiving this agent.

Rapamycin

Rapamycin is a macrolide with antifungal and potent immunosuppressant effects. It prevents proliferation of T cells and antagonizes the action of interleukin-2 on its receptor. This agent is 100 times more potent than ciclosporin A. It has no adverse effects on liver or renal function, but has the potential to enhance the nephrotoxicity and hepatotoxicity of ciclosporin.

FK506 (Tacrolimus)

FK506 is a new macrolide antibiotic with a similar structure to rapamycin. It is a very potent immunosuppressant drug that inhibits the activation of T cells and interleukin-2 generation. The principal side-effects are nephrotoxicity and neurotoxicity.

Mycophenolate mofetil

Mycophenolate mofetil (MMF) is the newest immunosuppressant licensed for use in renal transplantation. It inhibits a key enzyme in the purine synthesis pathway and therefore has a specific effect on B and T lymphocytes. The synthesis of adhesion molecules is also inhibited by MMF. It seems as though MMF effectively prevents chronic rejection in renal transplant patients. MMF is neither nephrotoxic nor hepatotoxic.

There is a variety of substances with potent immunosuppressant properties which are usually used in combination with each other. This allows individualized therapy according to the patient's comorbidity and immunological risk. A typical perioperative regimen for renal transplantation is shown in Table 10.2.

Despite their powerful immunosuppressant effects, it is unlikely that any of the new or existing drugs may be used as monotherapy. The role of drugs inhibiting antigen presentation and the use of monoclonal antibodies are still being defined.

Table 10.2   A typical perioperative regimen for renal transplantation

Preoperative
Induction immunosuppression (ciclosporin (Neoral), FK506, rapamycin)
Heparin 5000 units subcutaneously
Ranitidine 150 mg orally (stress ulcer prophylaxis)
Nifedipine 20 mg orally (vasodilator, free radical scavenger)
At induction
Antibiotic prophylaxis – co-amoxiclav (Augmentin) 1.2 g intravenous methylprednisolone 0.5 g i.v.
During vascular anastomosis
Mannitol 0.5 g kg^{-1} intravenously ± dopamine 3–5 µg kg^{-1} min^{-1}
Postoperative
Antibiotic prophylaxis
Heparin 5000 units subcutaneously, twice daily
Aspirin 150 mg orally
Ranitidine 150 mg orally, twice daily
Co-trimoxazole 480 mg orally, daily (protection against *Pneumocystis carinii*)
Immunosuppression ('triple therapy')

Guyton A C, Hall J E 1997 The body fluids and the kidneys. In: Guyton A C, Hall J E (eds) Human physiology and mechanisms of disease, 6th edn. WB Saunders, Philadelphia, pp 201–254

Schrier RW, Wang W 2004 Acute renal failure and sepsis. New England Journal of Medicine 351: 159–169

FURTHER READING

Debaveye Y A, Van den Berghe G H 2004 Is there still a place for dopamine in the modern intensive care unit? Anesthesia and Analgesia 98: 461–468

Fischereder M, Kretzler M 2004 New immunosuppressive strategies in renal transplant recipients. Journal of Nephrology 17: 9–18

Basic physics for the anaesthetist

THE APPLICATION OF PHYSICS IN ANAESTHESIA

Knowledge of simple physics is required in order to understand fully the function of many items of anaesthetic apparatus. This chapter is designed to emphasize the more elementary aspects of physical principles and it is hoped that the reader may be stimulated to read some of the excellent books which are designed for anaesthetists and examine this topic in greater detail (see 'Further reading'). Sophisticated measurement techniques may be required for more complex types of anaesthesia, in the intensive therapy unit and during anaesthesia for severely ill patients, and an understanding of the principles involved in performing such measurements is required in the later stages of the anaesthetist's training.

This chapter does not describe all the physical principles which may be encountered in the early stages of anaesthetic training, but concentrates on the more common applications, including pressure and flow in gases and liquids, electricity and electrical safety. However, it is necessary first to consider some basic definitions.

BASIC DEFINITIONS

It is now customary in medical practice to employ the International System (Système Internationale; SI) of units. Common exceptions to the use of the SI system include measurement of arterial pressure and, to a lesser extent, gas pressure. The mercury column is commonly used to calibrate electronic arterial pressure measuring devices and so 'mmHg' is retained. Pressures in gas cylinders are also referred to frequently in terms of the 'normal' atmospheric pressure of 760 mmHg; this is equal to 1.01 bar (or approximately 1 bar). Low pressures are expressed usually in the SI units of kPa whilst higher pressures are referred to in bar (100 kPa = 1 bar). The basic and derived units of the SI system are shown in Table 11.1.

The fundamental quantities in physics are mass, length and time.

Mass (m) is defined as the amount of matter in a body. The unit of mass is the kilogram (kg), for which the standard is a block of platinum held in a Physics Reference Laboratory.

Length (l) is defined as the distance between two points. The SI unit is the metre (m), which is defined as the distance occupied by a specified number of wavelengths of light.

Time (t) is measured in seconds. The reference standard for time is based on the frequency of resonation of the caesium atom.

From these basic definitions, several units of measurement may be derived:

Velocity is defined as the distance travelled per unit time:

$$\text{velocity } (v) = \frac{\text{distance}}{\text{time}} \quad \text{m s}^{-1}$$

Acceleration is defined as the rate of change of velocity:

$$\text{acceleration } (a) = \frac{\text{velocity}}{\text{time}} \quad \text{m s}^{-2}$$

Force is that which is required to give a mass acceleration:

$$\text{force} = \text{mass} \times \text{acceleration}$$
$$= ma$$

The SI unit of force is the newton (N). One newton is the force required to give a mass of 1 kg an acceleration of 1 m s^{-1}:

$$1\,\text{N} = 1\,\text{kg m s}^{-2}$$

Weight is the force of the earth's attraction for a body. When a body falls freely under the influence of gravity, it accelerates at a rate of 9.81 m s^{-2}:

$$\text{weight} = \text{mass} \times g$$
$$= m \times g$$
$$= m \times 9.81 \text{ kg m s}^{-2}$$

Table 11.1   Physical quantities

Quantity	Definition	Symbol	SI unit
Length	Unit of distance	l	metre (m)
Mass	Amount of matter	m	kilogram (kg)
Density	Mass per unit volume (m/V)	ρ	$kg\ m^{-3}$
Time		t	second (s)
Velocity	Distance per unit time (l/t)	v	$m\ s^{-1}$
Acceleration	Rate of change of velocity (v/t)	a	$m\ s^{-2}$
Force	Gives acceleration to a mass (ma)	F	newton (N) ($kg\ m\ s^{-2}$)
Weight	Force exerted by gravity on a mass (mg)	W	$kg \times 9.81\ m\ s^{-2}$
Pressure	Force per unit area (F/A)	P	$N\ m^{-2}$
Temperature	Tendency to gain or lose heat	T	kelvin (K) or degree Celsius (°C)
Work	Performed when a force moves an object (force × distance)	U	joule (J) (N m)
Energy	Capacity for doing work (force × distance)	U	joule (J) (N m)
Power	Rate of performing work (joules per second)	P	watt (W) ($J\ s^{-1}$)

Momentum is defined as mass multiplied by velocity:

$$momentum = m \times v$$

Work is undertaken when a force moves an object:

$$work = force \times distance$$
$$= F \times l$$
$$= N\ m\ (or\ joules,\ J)$$

Energy is the capacity for undertaking work. Thus it has the same units as those of work.

Power is the rate of doing work. The SI unit of power is the watt, which is equal to $1\ J\ s^{-1}$:

$$power = work\ per\ unit\ time$$
$$= joules\ per\ second$$
$$= watt\ (W)$$

Pressure is defined as force per unit area:

$$pressure\ (P) = \frac{force}{area}$$
$$= N\ m^{-2}$$
$$= pascal\ (Pa)$$

As 1 Pa is a rather small unit, it is more common in medical practice to use the kilopascal (kPa).

FLUIDS

Substances may exist in solid, liquid or gaseous form. These forms or phases differ from each other according to the random movement of their constituent atoms or molecules. In solids, molecules oscillate about a fixed point, whereas in liquids the molecules possess higher velocities and move more freely and thus do not bear a constant relationship in space to other molecules. The molecules of gases also move freely, but to an even greater extent.

Both gases and liquids are termed fluids. Liquids are incompressible and at constant temperature occupy a fixed volume, conforming to the shape of a container; gases have no fixed volume but expand to occupy the total space of a container.

Heating a liquid increases the kinetic energy of its molecules, permitting some to escape from the surface into the vapour phase. Random loss of molecules with higher kinetic energies from a liquid occurs in the process of vaporization. As these molecules possess higher kinetic states, this leads to a reduction in the energy state and cooling of the liquid.

Collision of randomly moving molecules in the gaseous phase with the walls of a container is responsible for the pressure exerted by a gas.

GAS PRESSURES

There are three important laws which determine the behaviour of gases and which are important to anaesthetists.

Boyle's law states that, at constant temperature, the volume (V) of a given mass of gas varies inversely with its absolute pressure (P):

$$PV = k_1$$

Charles' law states that, at constant pressure, the volume of a given mass of gas varies directly with its absolute temperature (T):

$$V = k_2 T$$

The third gas law states that, at constant volume, the absolute pressure of a given mass of gas varies directly with its absolute temperature:

$$P = k_3 T$$

Combining these three gas laws:

$$PV = kT$$

or

$$\frac{P_1 V_1}{T_1} = \frac{P_2 V_2}{T_2}$$

The behaviour of a mixture of gases in a container is described by *Dalton's law of partial pressures*. This states that, in a mixture of gases, the pressure exerted by each gas is the same as that which it would exert if it alone occupied the container.

Thus, in a cylinder of compressed air at a pressure of 100 bar, the pressure exerted by nitrogen is equal to 79 bar (as the fractional concentration of nitrogen is 0.79).

Avogadro's hypothesis

Avogadro's hypothesis states that equal volumes of gases at the same temperature and pressure contain equal numbers of molecules.

Avogadro's number is the number of molecules in 1 g molecular weight of a substance and is equal to 6.022×10^{23}.

Under conditions of standard temperature and pressure, 1 g molecular weight of any gas occupies a volume of 22.4 litres (L).

These data are useful in calculating, for example, the quantity of gas produced from liquid nitrous oxide. The molecular weight of nitrous oxide is 44. Thus, 44 g of N_2O occupy a volume of 22.4 L at standard temperature and pressure (STP). If a full cylinder of N_2O contains 3.0 kg of liquid, then vaporization of all the liquid would yield:

$$\frac{22.4 \times 3.0 \times 1000 \, L}{44}$$

$$= 1527 \, L \text{ at STP}$$

Critical temperature

The critical temperature of a substance is the temperature above which that substance cannot be liquefied by pressure, irrespective of its magnitude.

The critical temperature of oxygen is $-118°C$, that of nitrogen is $-147°C$, and that of air is $-141°C$. Thus, at room temperature, cylinders of these substances contain gases. By contrast, the critical temperature of carbon dioxide is $31°C$ and that of nitrous oxide is $36.4°C$. The critical pressures are 73.8 and 72.5 bar, respectively; at higher pressures, cylinders of these substances at room temperature contain a mixture of gas and liquid.

Clinical application of the gas laws

A 'full' cylinder of oxygen on an anaesthetic machine contains compressed gaseous oxygen at a pressure of 137 bar (2000 lb in^{-2}). If the cylinder of oxygen empties at constant temperature, the volume of gas contained is related linearly to its pressure (by Boyle's law). In practice, linearity is not followed because temperature falls as a result of adiabatic expansion of the compressed gas; the term adiabatic implies a change in the state of a gas without exchange of heat energy with its surroundings.

By contrast, the pressure in a cylinder of nitrous oxide remains relatively constant as the cylinder empties to the point at which liquid has totally vaporized. Subsequently, there is a linear decline in pressure proportional to the volume of gas remaining within the cylinder.

Filling ratio

The degree of filling of a nitrous oxide cylinder is expressed as the mass of nitrous oxide in the cylinder divided by the mass of water that the cylinder could hold. Normally, a cylinder of nitrous oxide is filled to a ratio of 0.67. This should not be confused with the volume of liquid nitrous oxide in a cylinder. A 'full' cylinder of nitrous oxide at room temperature is filled to the point at which approximately 90% of the interior of the cylinder is occupied by liquid, the remaining 10% being occupied by gaseous nitrous oxide. Incomplete filling of a cylinder is necessary because thermally induced expansion of the liquid in a totally full cylinder may cause an explosion.

Entonox

Entonox is the trade name for a compressed gas mixture containing 50% oxygen and 50% nitrous oxide. The mixture is compressed into cylinders containing gas at a pressure of 137 bar (2000 lb in^{-2}). The nitrous oxide does not liquefy because the two gases in this mixture 'dissolve' in each other at high pressure. In other words, the presence of oxygen reduces the critical temperature of nitrous oxide. The critical temperature of the mixture is $-7°C$. Cooling of a cylinder of Entonox to a temperature below −7°C results in separation of liquid nitrous oxide. Use of such a cylinder results in oxygen-rich gas being released initially, followed by a hypoxic nitrous oxide-rich gas. Consequently, it is recommended that when an Entonox cylinder may have been exposed to low temperatures, it should be stored horizontally for a period of not less than 24 h at a temperature of 5°C or above. In addition, the cylinder should be inverted several times before use.

Pressure notation in anaesthesia

Although the use of SI units of measurement is generally accepted in medicine, a variety of ways of expressing pressure is still used, reflecting custom and practice. Arterial pressure is still referred to universally in terms of mmHg because a column of mercury is still used occasionally to measure arterial pressure and also to calibrate electronic devices.

Measurement of central venous pressure is sometimes referred to in cmH_2O because it can be measured using a manometer filled with saline, but it is more commonly described in mmHg when measured using an electronic transducer system.

Atmospheric pressure (P_B) exerts a pressure sufficient to support a column of mercury of height 760 mm (Fig. 11.1).

$$
\begin{aligned}
1 \text{ atmospheric pressure} \quad &= 760 \text{ mmHg} \\
&= 1.01325 \text{ bar} \\
&= 760 \text{ torr} \\
&= 1 \text{ atmosphere absolute (ata)} \\
&= 14.7 \text{ lb in}^{-2} \\
&= 101.325 \text{ kPa} \\
&= 10.33 \text{ mH}_2\text{O}
\end{aligned}
$$

In considering pressure, it is necessary to indicate whether or not atmospheric pressure is taken into account. Thus, a diver working 10 m below the surface of the sea may be described as compressed to a depth of 1 atmosphere or working at a pressure of 2 atmospheres absolute (2 ata).

In order to avoid confusion when discussing compressed cylinders of gases, the term gauge pressure is used. This refers to the difference between the pressure of the contents of the cylinder and the ambient pressure. Thus, a full cylinder of oxygen has a gauge pressure of 137 bar, but the contents are at a pressure of 138 bar absolute.

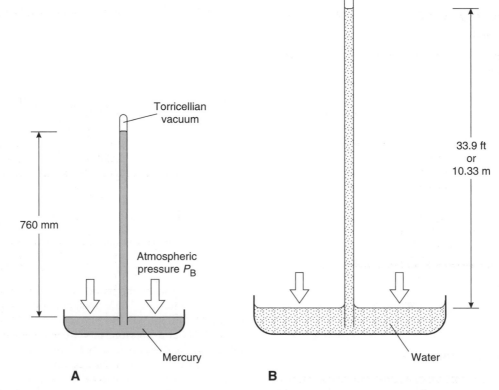

Fig. 11.1
The simple barometer described by Torricelli (not to scale). (**A**) Filled with mercury. (**B**) Filled with water.

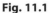

PRESSURE RELIEF VALVES

The Heidbrink valve is a common component of many anaesthesia breathing systems. In the Magill breathing system, the anaesthetist may vary the force in the spring(s), thereby controlling the pressure within the breathing system (Fig. 11.2). At equilibrium, the force exerted by the spring is equal to the force exerted by gas within the system:

$$\text{force } (F) = \text{gas pressure } (P) \times \text{disc area } (A)$$

Modern anaesthesia systems contain a variety of pressure relief valves, in each of which the force is fixed so as to provide a gas escape mechanism when pressure reaches a preset level. Thus, an anaesthetic machine may contain a pressure relief valve operating at 35 kPa, situated on the back bar of the machine between the vaporizers and the breathing system to protect the flowmeters and vaporizers from excessive pressures. Modern ventilators contain a pressure relief valve set at 7 kPa to protect the patient from barotrauma. A much lower pressure is set in relief valves which form part of anaesthetic scavenging systems and these may operate at pressures of 0.2–0.3 kPa to protect the patient from negative pressure applied to the lungs.

PRESSURE-REDUCING VALVES (PRESSURE REGULATORS)

Pressure regulators have two important functions in anaesthetic machines:

- They reduce high pressures of compressed gases to manageable levels (acting as pressure-reducing valves).
- They minimize fluctuations in the pressure within an anaesthetic machine, which would necessitate frequent manipulations of flowmeter controls.

Modern anaesthetic machines are designed to operate with an inlet gas supply at a pressure of 3–4 bar (usually 4 bar in the UK). Hospital pipeline supplies also operate at a pressure of 4 bar and therefore pressure regulators are not required between a hospital pipeline supply and an anaesthetic machine. By contrast, the contents of cylinders of all medical gases (i.e. oxygen, nitrous oxide, air and Entonox) are at much higher pressures. Thus, cylinders of these gases require a pressure-reducing valve between the cylinder and the flowmeter.

The principle on which the simplest type of pressure-reducing valve operates is shown in Figure 11.3. High pressure gas enters through the valve and forces the flexible diaphragm upwards, tending to close the valve and prevent further ingress of gas from the high-pressure source.

If there is no tension in the spring, the relationship between the reduced pressure (p) and the high pressure (P) is very approximately equal to the ratio of the areas of the valve seating (a) and the diaphragm (A):

$$\frac{P}{P} = \frac{a}{A}$$

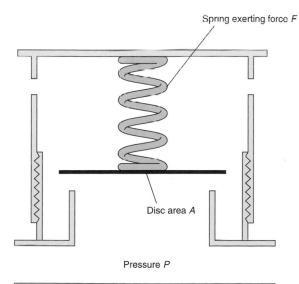

Fig. 11.2
A pressure relief valve.

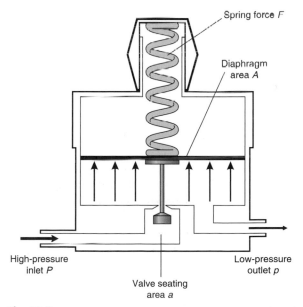

Fig. 11.3
A simple pressure-reducing valve.

By tensing the spring, a force F is produced which offsets the closing effect of the valve. Thus, p may be increased by increasing the force in the spring.

Without the spring, the simple pressure regulator has the disadvantage that reduced pressure decreases proportionally with the decrease in cylinder pressure. The addition of a force from the spring considerably reduces but does not eliminate this problem, and in order to overcome it, newer pressure regulators contain an extra closing spring. During high flows, the input to the valve may not be able to keep pace with the output. This can cause the regulated pressure to fall. A two-stage regulator can be employed in order to overcome this. Simple one-stage regulators are often designed for use with a specific gas. A universal regulator in which the body is used for all gases but has different seatings and springs fitted for each particular gas is now available.

PRESSURE DEMAND REGULATORS

These are regulators in which gas flow occurs when an inspiratory effort is applied to the outlet port. The Entonox valve is a two-stage regulator and its mode of action is demonstrated in Figure 11.4. The first stage is identical to the reducing valve described above. The second-stage valve contains a diaphragm. Movement of this diaphragm tilts a rod, which controls the flow of gas from the first-stage valve. The second stage is adjusted so that gas flows only when pressure is below atmospheric.

FLOW OF FLUIDS

Viscosity is defined as that property of a fluid that causes it to resist flow. The coefficient of viscosity (η) is defined as:

$$\eta = \frac{\text{force} \times \text{velocity gradient}}{\text{area}}$$

In this context, velocity gradient is equal to the difference between velocities of different fluid molecules divided by the distance between molecules (Fig. 11.5B). The units of the coefficient of viscosity are Pascal seconds (Pa s).

Fluids that obey this formula are referred to as Newtonian fluids and η is a constant for each fluid. However, some biological fluids are non-Newtonian. A prime example is blood; viscosity changes with the rate of flow of blood (as a result of change in distribution of cells) and, in stored blood, with time (blood thickens on storage).

Viscosity of liquids diminishes with increase in temperature, whereas viscosity of a gas increases with increase in temperature.

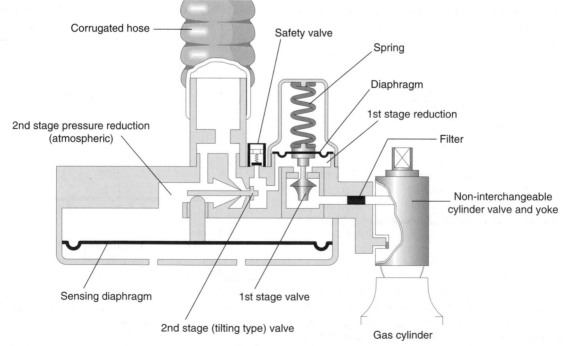

Fig. 11.4
The Entonox two-stage pressure demand regulator.

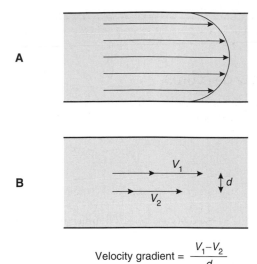

A

B

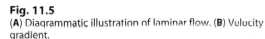

$$\text{Velocity gradient} = \frac{V_1 - V_2}{d}$$

Fig. 11.5
(**A**) Diagrammatic illustration of laminar flow. (**B**) Velocity gradient.

Laminar flow

Laminar flow through a tube is illustrated in Figure 11.5A. In this situation, there is a smooth, orderly flow of fluid such that molecules travel with the greatest velocity in the axial stream, whilst the velocity of those in contact with the wall of the tube may be virtually zero. The linear velocity of axial flow may be twice the average linear velocity of flow.

In a tube, the factors determining flow are given by the Hagen–Poiseuille formula:

$$\dot{Q} = \frac{\pi \Delta P r^4}{8 \eta l}$$

where $\dot{Q}$ is the flow, ΔP is the pressure gradient along the tube, r is the radius of the tube, η is the viscosity of fluid and l is the length of the tube.

The Hagen–Poiseuille formula applies only to Newtonian fluids. In non-Newtonian fluids such as blood, increase in velocity of flow may alter viscosity because of variation in the dispersion of cells within plasma.

Turbulent flow

In turbulent flow, fluid no longer moves in orderly planes but swirls and eddies around in a haphazard manner as illustrated in Figure 11.6. Although viscosity affects laminar flow, it should be noted that this does not apply to turbulent flow, which is affected by changes in density.

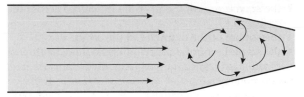

Fig. 11.6
Diagrammatic illustration of turbulent flow.

It may be seen from Figure 11.7 that the relationship between pressure and flow is linear within certain limits. However, as velocity increases, a point is reached (the critical point or critical velocity) at which the characteristics of flow change from laminar to turbulent. The critical point is dependent upon several factors, which were investigated by the physicist Reynolds. The factors are related by the formula used for calculation of Reynolds' number:

$$\text{Reynold's number} = v \rho r / \eta$$

where v is the linear velocity, r is the radius of the tube, ρ is the density and η is the viscosity.

Studies with cylindrical tubes have shown that if Reynolds' number exceeds 2000, flow is likely to be turbulent, whereas a Reynolds' number of less than 2000 is usually associated with laminar flow.

Flow of fluids through orifices

In an orifice, the diameter of the fluid pathway exceeds the length. The flow rate of a fluid through an orifice is partly turbulent and it is dependent upon:

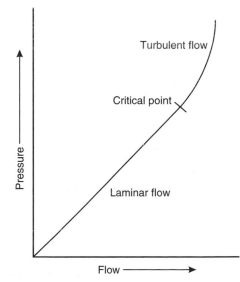

Fig. 11.7
The relationship between pressure and flow in a fluid is linear up to the critical point, above which flow becomes turbulent.

- the square root of the pressure difference across the orifice
- the square of the diameter of the orifice
- the square root of density (ρ) of the fluid, as flow through an orifice inevitably involves some degree of turbulence.

Flow through an orifice:

$$= \frac{\alpha \sqrt{\Delta P} \times (R^2)}{\sqrt{\rho}}$$

Applications in anaesthetic practice

- In upper respiratory tract obstruction of any severity, flow is inevitably turbulent; thus for the same respiratory effort, a lower tidal volume is achieved than when flow is laminar. The extent of turbulent flow may be reduced by reducing gas density; clinically it is common practice to administer oxygen-enriched helium rather than oxygen alone (the density of oxygen is 1.3 and that of helium is 0.16).
- In anaesthetic breathing systems, a sudden change in diameter of tubing or irregularity of the wall may be responsible for a change from laminar to turbulent flow. Thus, tracheal and other breathing tubes should possess smooth internal surfaces, gradual bends and no constrictions, and should be of as large a diameter and as short a length as possible.
- Resistance to breathing is much greater when a tracheal tube of small diameter is used (Fig. 11.8).

In a variable orifice flowmeter, gas flow at low flow rates is predominantly laminar. Flow depends on viscosity. At higher flow rates, because the flowmeter behaves as an orifice, turbulent flow dominates and density is more important than viscosity.

THE INJECTOR

The injector is frequently termed a Venturi, although the principles governing such an apparatus were formulated by Bernoulli in 1778, some 60 years earlier than Venturi. The relationship between pressure (P) and velocity (v) at any point in a fluid is illustrated in the following equation:

$$\tfrac{1}{2} \rho v^2 \; (KE) + P \; (PE) = constant$$

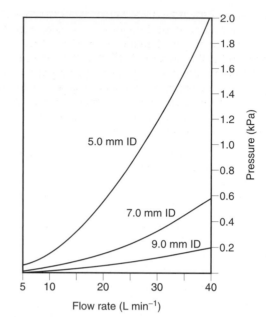

Fig. 11.8
Resistance to gas flow through tracheal tubes of different internal diameter (ID).

Bernoulli's principle shows that as fluid passes through a constriction, there is an increase in velocity of the fluid (increase in kinetic energy) and a reduction in pressure (decrease in potential energy); beyond the constriction, velocity decreases to the initial value. The principle is illustrated in Figure 11.9. At point A, the energy in the fluid is both potential and kinetic, but at point B the amount of kinetic energy is much greater because of the increased velocity. As the total energy state must remain constant, potential energy is reduced at point B and this is reflected by a reduction in pressure. Venturi's contribution to the injector lay in

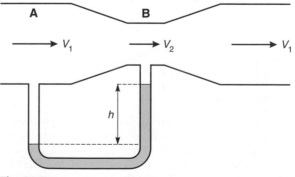

Fig. 11.9
The Bernoulli principle. See text for full details.

the design of the tube distal to the site of the constriction. For optimum performance, it is necessary for fluid flow to remain laminar in such a tube. In the Venturi tube, the pressure is least at the site of maximum constriction and, by gradual opening of the tube beyond the constriction, a subatmospheric pressure may be induced distal to the constriction (Fig. 11.10).

The injector principle may be seen in anaesthetic practice in the following situations:

- *Oxygen therapy.* Several types of Venturi oxygen masks are available which provide oxygen-enriched air. With an appropriate flow of oxygen (usually exceeding $4\,L\,min^{-1}$), there is a large degree of entrainment of air. This results in a total gas flow that exceeds the patient's peak inspiratory flow rate, thus ensuring that the inspired oxygen concentration remains constant, and it prevents an increase in apparatus dead space which always accompanies the use of low-flow oxygen devices.
- *Nebulizers.* These are used to entrain water from a reservoir. If the water inlet is suitably positioned, the entrained water may be broken up into a fine mist by the high gas velocity.
- *Portable suction apparatus.*
- *Oxygen tents.*
- *As a driving gas in a ventilator* (Fig. 11.11).

The Coanda effect

The Coanda effect describes a phenomenon whereby when gas flows through a tube and enters a Y junction, gas tends to cling either to one side of the tube or to the other. The gas is not divided equally between the two outlets. The principle has been used in anaesthetic ventilators (termed fluidic ventilators), as the applica-

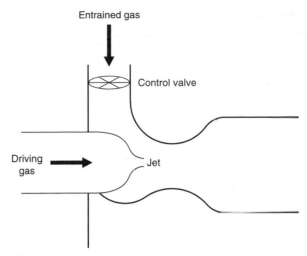

Fig. 11.11
A simple injector.

tion of a small pressure distal to the restriction may enable gas flow to be switched from one side to another (Fig. 11.12).

HEAT AND TEMPERATURE

Temperature is a measure of the tendency of an object to gain or lose heat. Heat is the energy which may be transferred from a body at a hotter temperature to one at a colder temperature.

THERMOMETRY

In the SI system, the unit of temperature is the kelvin (K). The zero reference point on this scale is absolute zero (0K or −273.15°C) and the upper point is the triple point of water (the temperature at which water exists simultaneously in solid, liquid and gaseous states); this corresponds to 273.16 K or 0.01°C. The Celsius

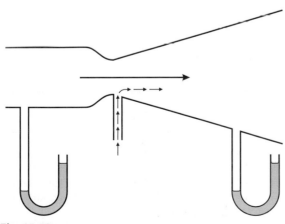

Fig. 11.10
Fluid entrainment by a Venturi injector.

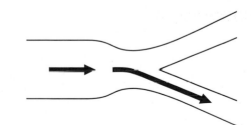

Fig. 11.12
The Coanda effect.

scale is also widely used. The intervals on this scale are identical to those on the kelvin scale (K) and the relationship between the two scales is as follows:

temperature (K) = temperature (°C) + 273.15

Temperature is measured in clinical practice by one of the following techniques:

- *Liquid expansion thermometer*. Mercury and alcohol are the more commonly used liquids.
- *Thermistor*. This is a semiconductor, which exhibits a reduction in electrical resistance with increase in temperature.
- *Thermocouple*. This relies on the Seebeck effect. When two metal conductors are joined together to form a circuit, a potential difference is produced which is proportional to the difference in temperatures of the two junctions. In order to measure temperature, one junction has to be kept at a constant temperature.
- *Chemical thermometers*. These thermometers are described in more detail in Chapter 12.

HEAT CAPACITY

The heat capacity of a body is the amount of heat required to raise the temperature of the body by 1°C; in the SI nomenclature, heat capacity is measured in units of joules per kelvin ($J\,K^{-1}$).

Specific heat capacity

The specific heat capacity of a substance is the energy required to raise the temperature of 1 kg of a substance by 1 K. Thus:

heat capacity = mass × specific heat capacity

The specific heat capacity of different substances is of interest because anaesthetists are frequently concerned with maintenance of body temperature in unconscious patients.

Heat is lost from patients by the processes of:

- conduction
- convection
- radiation
- evaporation.

The specific heat capacity of gases is up to 1000 times smaller than that of liquids. Consequently, humidification of inspired gases is a more important method of conserving heat than warming dry gases; in addition, the use of humidified gases minimizes the very large energy loss produced by evaporation of fluid from the respiratory tract.

The skin acts as an almost perfect radiator; radiant losses in susceptible patients may be reduced by the use of reflective aluminium foil ('space blanket').

VAPORIZATION AND VAPORIZERS

In a liquid, molecules are in a state of continuous motion because of mutual attraction by Van der Waal's forces. Some molecules may develop velocities sufficient to escape from these forces, and if they are close to the surface of a liquid these molecules may escape to enter the vapour phase. Increasing the temperature of a liquid increases its kinetic energy and a greater number of molecules escape. As the faster moving molecules escape into the vapour phase, the net velocity of the remaining molecules reduces; thus the energy state and therefore temperature of the liquid phase are reduced. The amount of heat required to convert a unit mass of liquid into a vapour without a change in temperature of the liquid is termed the heat of vaporization.

In a closed vessel containing liquid and gas, a state of equilibrium is reached when the number of molecules escaping from the liquid is equal to the number of molecules re-entering the liquid phase. The vapour concentration is then said to be saturated at the specified temperature. Saturated vapour pressure of liquids is independent of the ambient pressure, but increases with increasing temperature.

The boiling point of a liquid is the temperature at which its saturated vapour pressure becomes equal to the ambient pressure. Thus, on the graph in Figure 11.13, the boiling point of each liquid at 1 atmosphere is the temperature at which its saturated vapour pressure is 101.3 kPa.

VAPORIZERS

Vaporizers may be classified into two types:

- drawover vaporizers
- plenum vaporizers.

In the former type, gas is pulled through the vaporizer when the patient inspires, creating a subatmospheric pressure. In the latter type, gas is forced through the vaporizer by the pressure of the fresh gas supply. Consequently, the resistance to gas flow through a drawover vaporizer must be extremely small; the resistance of a plenum vaporizer may be high enough to prevent its use as a drawover vaporizer, although this is not necessarily so.

The principles of both devices are similar. If we consider the simplest form of vaporizer (Fig. 11.14), the

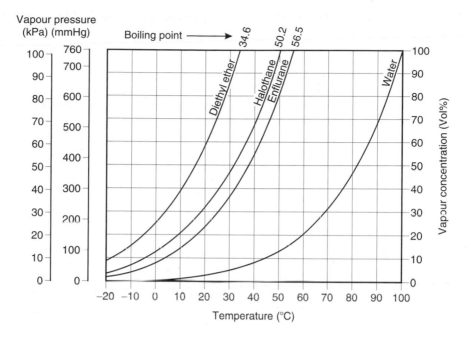

Fig. 11.13
Relationship between vapour pressure and temperature for different anaesthetic agents.

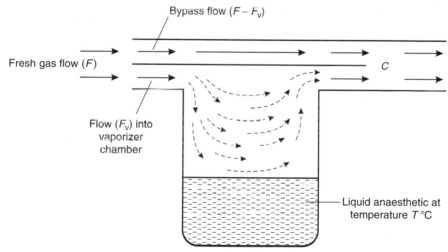

Fig. 11.14
A simple type of vaporizer.

concentration (C) of anaesthetic in the gas mixture emerging from the outlet port is dependent upon:

- *The saturated vapour pressure* of the anaesthetic liquid in the vaporizer. Thus, a highly volatile agent such as diethyl ether is present in a much higher concentration than a less volatile agent (i.e. with a lower saturated vapour pressure) such as halothane.

- *The temperature* of the liquid anaesthetic agent, as this determines its saturated vapour pressure.
- *The splitting ratio*, i.e. the flow rate of gas through the vaporizing chamber (F_v) in comparison with that through the bypass ($F - F_v$). Regulation of the splitting ratio is the usual mechanism whereby the anaesthetist controls the output concentration from a vaporizer.

- *The surface area* of the anaesthetic agent in the vaporizer. If the surface area is relatively small during use, the flow of gas through the vaporizing chamber may be too rapid to achieve complete saturation with anaesthetic molecules of the gas above the liquid.
- *Duration of use*. As the liquid in the vaporizing chamber evaporates, its temperature, and thus its saturated vapour pressure, decreases. This leads to a reduction in concentration of anaesthetic in the mixture leaving the exit port.
- *The flow characteristics* through the vaporizing chamber. In the simple vaporizer illustrated, gas passing through the vaporizing chamber may fail to mix completely with vapour as a result of streaming because of poor design. This lack of mixing is flow-dependent.

Modern anaesthetic vaporizers overcome many of the problems described above. Maintenance of full saturation may be achieved by making available a large surface area for vaporization. In the TEC series of vaporizers, this is achieved by the use of wicks which draw up liquid anaesthetic and provide a very large surface area. Efficient vaporization and prevention of streaming of gas through the vaporizing chamber are achieved by ensuring that gas travels through a concentric helix, which is bounded by the fabric wicks. Another method of ensuring full saturation is to bubble gas through liquid anaesthetic via a sintered disc; the final concentration is determined by mixing a known flow of fresh gas with a measured flow of fully saturated vapour.

Temperature compensation

Temperature-compensated vaporizers possess a mechanism which produces an increase in flow through the vaporizing chamber (i.e. an increased splitting ratio) as the temperature of liquid anaesthetic decreases. In the TEC vaporizers, a bimetallic strip controls (by bending) a valve which alters flow through the exit port of the vaporizing chamber. In the EMO and Ohio vaporizers, a bellows mechanism is used to regulate the valve (by shortening with decreased temperature), whilst in the Drager Vapor 19 vaporizers, a metal rod acts in a similar fashion.

Back pressure (pumping effect)

Some gas-driven mechanical ventilators (e.g. Manley) produce a considerable increase in pressure in the outlet port and back bar of the anaesthetic machine. This pressure is highest during the inspiratory phase of ventilation. If the simple vaporizer shown in Figure 11.14 is attached to the back bar, the increased pressure during inspiration compresses the gas in the vaporizer; some gas in the region of the outlet port of the vaporizer is forced back into the vaporizing chamber, where more vapour is added to it. Subsequently, there is a temporary surge in anaesthetic concentration when the pressure decreases at the end of the inspiratory cycle.

This effect is minimal with efficient vaporizers (i.e. those which saturate gas fully in the vaporization chamber) because gas in the outlet port is already saturated with vapour. However, when pressure reduces at the end of inspiration, some saturated gas passes retrogradely out of the inspiratory port and mixes with the bypass gas. Thus, a temporary increase in total vapour concentration may still occur in the gas supplied to the patient. Methods of overcoming this problem include:

- incorporation of a one-way valve in the outlet port
- construction of a bypass chamber and vaporizing chamber which are of equal volumes so that the gas in each is compressed or expanded equally
- construction of a long inlet tube to the vaporizing chamber so that retrograde flow from the vaporizing chamber does not reach the bypass channel (as in the Mark 3 TEC vaporizers).

HUMIDITY AND HUMIDIFICATION

Absolute humidity (g m^{-3}) is the mass of water vapour present in a given volume of gas. Relative humidity is the ratio of mass of water vapour in a given volume of gas to the mass required to saturate that volume of gas at the same temperature.

Relative humidity (RH) may be expressed as:

$$RH = \frac{\text{actual vapour pressure}}{\text{saturated vapour pressure}}$$

In normal practice, relative humidity may be measured using:

- *The hair hygrometer*. This operates on the principle that a hair elongates if humidity increases; the hair length controls a pointer. This simple device may be mounted on a wall. It is reasonably accurate only in the range 15–85% relative humidity.
- *The wet and dry bulb hygrometer*. The dry bulb measures the actual temperature, whereas the wet bulb measures a lower temperature as a result of the cooling effect of evaporation of water. The rate

of vaporization is related to the humidity of the ambient gas and the difference between the two temperatures is a measure of ambient humidity; the relative humidity is obtained from a set of tables.

- *Regnault's hygrometer*. This consists of a thin silver tube containing ether and a thermometer to show the temperature of the ether. Air is pumped through the ether to produce evaporation, thereby cooling the silver tube. When gas in contact with the tube is saturated with water vapour, it condenses as a mist on the bright silver. The temperature at which this takes place is known as the *dew point*, from which relative humidity is obtained from tables.

HUMIDIFICATION IN THE RESPIRATORY TRACT

Air drawn into the respiratory tract becomes fully saturated in the trachea at a temperature of 37°C. Under these conditions, the SVP of water is 6.3 kPa (47 mmHg); this represents a fractional concentration of 6.2%. The concentration of water is $44\,mg\,L^{-1}$. At 21°C, saturated water vapour contains 2.4% water vapour or $18\,mg\,L^{-1}$. Thus, there is a considerable capacity for patients to lose both water and heat when the lungs are ventilated with dry gases.

There are three means of humidifying inspired gas:

- heated humidifier (water vaporizer)
- nebulizer
- condenser humidifier (also known as heat and moisture exchanging humidifier).

The hot water bath humidifier is a simple device for heating water to 45–60°C. These devices have several potential problems, including infection if the water temperature decreases below 45°C, scalding the patient if the temperature exceeds 60°C (these high temperatures may be used to prevent growth of bacteria) and condensation of water in the inspiratory anaesthetic tubing. These devices are approximately 80% efficient.

Some nebulizers are based upon a Venturi system; a gas supply entrains water, which is broken up into a large number of droplets. The ultrasonic nebulizer operates by dropping water onto a surface, which is vibrated at a frequency of 2 MHz. This breaks up the water particles into extremely small droplets. The main problem with these nebulizers is the possibility that supersaturation of inspired gas may occur and the patient may be overloaded with water.

The condenser humidifier (or artificial nose) may consist of a simple wire mesh, which is inserted between the tracheal tube and the anaesthetic breathing system. More recently, humidifiers constructed of rolled corrugated paper have been introduced. These devices are approximately 70% efficient.

SOLUTION OF GASES

Henry's law states that, at a given temperature, the amount of a gas which dissolves in a liquid is directly proportional to the partial pressure of the gas in equilibrium with the liquid. If a liquid is heated and its temperature rises, the partial pressure of its vapour increases. As the total ambient pressure remains constant, the partial pressure of any dissolved gas must decrease.

It is customary to confine the term 'tension' to the partial pressure of a gas exerted by gas molecules in solution.

SOLUBILITY COEFFICIENTS

The Bunsen solubility coefficient is the volume of gas which dissolves in a unit volume of liquid at a given temperature when the gas in equilibrium with the liquid is at a pressure of 1 atmosphere.

The Ostwald solubility coefficient is the volume of gas which dissolves in a unit volume of liquid at a given temperature. Thus, the Ostwald solubility coefficient is independent of pressure.

The partition coefficient is the ratio of the amount of substance in one phase compared with a second phase, each phase being of equal volume and in equilibrium. As with the Ostwald coefficient, it is necessary to define the temperature but not the pressure. The partition coefficient may be applied to two liquids, but the Ostwald coefficient applies to partition between gas and liquid.

DIFFUSION AND OSMOSIS

If two different gases or liquids are separated in a container by an impermeable partition which is then removed, gradual mixing of the two different substances occurs as a result of the kinetic activity of each molecule. This is illustrated in Figure 11.15. The principle governing this process is described by Fick's law of diffusion, which states that the rate of diffusion of a substance across unit area is proportional to the concentration gradient. Graham's law (which applies to gases only) states that the rate of diffusion of a gas is inversely proportional to the square root of its molecular weight.

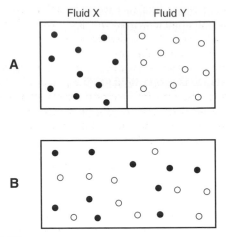

Fig. 11.15
Illustration of diffusion in fluids. (**A**) Fluids X and Y separated by partition. (**B**) Mixing of fluids after removal of partition.

In the example shown in Figure 11.15B, the interface between fluids X and Y after removal of the partition would be the surface of the fluid. In biology, however, there is normally a membrane separating gases or separating gas and liquids.

The rate of diffusion of gases may be affected by the nature of the membrane. In the lungs, the alveolar membrane is moist and may be regarded as a water film. Thus, diffusion of gases through the alveolar membrane is dependent not only on the properties of diffusion described above but also on the solubility of gas in the water film. As carbon dioxide is highly soluble compared with oxygen, it diffuses more rapidly across the alveolar membrane, despite the larger partial pressure gradient for oxygen.

OSMOSIS

In the examples given above, the membranes are permeable to all substances. However, in biology, membranes are frequently semipermeable, i.e. they allow the passage of some substances but are impermeable to others. This is illustrated in Figure 11.16. In Figure 11.16A, initially equal volumes of water and glucose solution are separated by a semipermeable membrane. Water molecules pass freely through the membrane to dilute the glucose solution (Fig. 11.16B). By application of a hydrostatic pressure (Fig. 11.16C), the process of transfer of water molecules can be prevented; this pressure (P) is equal to the osmotic pressure exerted by the glucose solution.

Substances in dilute solution behave in accordance with the gas laws. Thus, 1 g molecular weight of a dissolved substance occupying 22.4 L of solvent exerts an osmotic pressure of 1 bar at 273 K. Dalton's law also applies; the total osmotic pressure of a mixture of solutes is equal to the sum of osmotic pressures exerted independently by each substance.

The osmotic pressure of a solution depends on the number of dissolved particles per litre. Thus, a molar solution of a substance which ionizes into two particles exerts twice the osmotic pressure exerted by a molar solution of a non-ionizing substance.

The term osmolarity refers to the osmotic pressure produced by all substances in a fluid. Thus, it is the sum of the individual molarities of each particle.

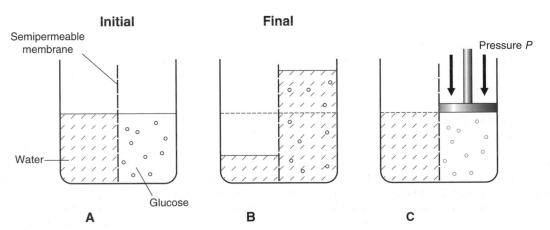

Fig. 11.16
Diagram to illustrate osmotic pressure. (**A**) Water and glucose placed into two compartments separated by a semipermeable membrane. (**B**) At equilibrium, water has passed into the glucose compartment to balance the pressure. (**C**) The magnitude of osmotic pressure of the glucose is denoted by a hydraulic pressure P applied to the glucose to prevent any movement of water into the glucose compartment.

The term osmolality refers to the number of osmoles per kilogram of water or other solvent (whilst osmolarity refers to osmoles per litre of solution). Thus, osmolarity may vary slightly from osmolality as a result of changes in density due to the effect of temperature on volume, although in biological terms the difference is extremely small.

In the circulation, water and the majority of ions are freely permeable across the endothelial membrane, but plasma proteins do not traverse into the interstitial fluid. The term oncotic pressure is used to describe the osmotic pressure exerted by the plasma proteins alone. Plasma oncotic pressure is relatively small (approximately $1 \, mosmol \, L^{-1}$ equivalent to 25 mmHg) in relation to total osmotic pressure exerted by plasma (approximately $300 \, mosmol \, L^{-1}$ equivalent to 6.5 bar).

ELECTRICAL SAFETY

Basic quantities and units

An ampere (A) is the unit of electric current in the SI system. It represents the flow of 6.24×10^{18} electrons and it is defined by means of the electromagnetic force which is associated with an electric current. The ampere is defined as the current which, if flowing in two parallel wires of infinite length, placed 1 m apart in a vacuum, produces a force of 2×10^{-7} newtons/metre $(N \, m^{-1})$ on each of the wires.

Electric charge is the measure of the amount of electricity and its SI unit is the coulomb (C). The coulomb is the quantity of electric charge that passes some point when a current of 1 ampere (A) flows for a period of 1 s:

$$coulombs \ (C) = amperes \ (A) \times seconds \ (s)$$

Electrical potential exists when one point in an electric circuit has more positive charge than another. Electrical potential is analogous to height in a gravitational field where a mass possesses potential energy due to its height. The electrical potential of the earth is regarded as the reference point for zero potential and is referred to as 'earth'. When a potential difference is applied across a conductor, it produces an electric current and current flows from an area of higher potential to one of lower.

The unit for potential difference is the volt. One volt is defined as the potential difference which produces a current of 1 ampere in a substance when the rate of energy dissipation is 1 watt, as demonstrated in the equation:

$$potential \ difference \ (volts) = \frac{power \ (watts)}{current \ (amperes)}$$

A volt can also be defined as a potential difference producing a change in energy of 1 joule when 1 coulomb is moved across it. This definition is often used in connection with defibrillators.

Ohm's law states that the current flowing through a resistance is proportional to the potential difference across it. The unit for electrical resistance is the ohm (Ω). The ohm is that resistance which will allow 1 ampere of current to flow under the influence of a potential difference of 1 volt.

$$resistance \ (\Omega) = \frac{potential \ (V)}{current \ (I)}$$

The anaesthetist is in daily contact with a large amount of equipment which is powered by mains supply electricity; this includes monitoring equipment, some ventilators, suction apparatus, defibrillators and diathermy equipment.

Whilst a total understanding of this equipment and its mode of action may depend upon a detailed knowledge of electronics, the equipment can usually be used safely as a type of 'black box', i.e. the inside of the box may be a mystery, but the anaesthetist must be familiar with the operating controls and the ways in which the apparatus may malfunction or, if a recording instrument, give rise to artefacts.

It is not possible in this brief chapter to provide a full synopsis of the basic principles of electricity and electronics, but it is essential to stress some elements which have a bearing on the safety of both the patient and the anaesthetist in the operating theatre.

In the UK, the mains electricity is supplied at a voltage of 240 V with a frequency of 50 Hz, and in the USA at a voltage of 110 V and a frequency of 60 Hz. These voltages are potentially dangerous, although the danger is related predominantly to the current which flows through the patient as governed by Ohm's law.

When dealing with alternating current, it is necessary to use the term impedance in place of resistance, as impedance takes into account the presence of capacitors and resistors. Direct current cannot pass through capacitors; the resistance of a capacitor is inversely proportional to the frequency of an alternating current.

If an increasing electrical current at 50 Hz passes through the body, there is initially a tingling sensation at a current of 1 mA. Increase in the current produces increasing pain and muscle spasm until, at 80–100 mA, arrhythmias and ventricular fibrillation may occur.

The damage to tissue by alternating current is related also to the current density; a current passing through a small area is more dangerous than the same current passing through a much larger area. Other factors relating to the likelihood of ventricular fibrillation are the duration of passage of the current and its frequency. Radio frequencies (such as those used in diathermy) have no potential for fibrillating the heart.

It is clear from Ohm's law that the size of the current is dependent upon the size of the impedance to current flow. A common way of reducing the risk of a large current injuring the anaesthetist in the operating theatre is to wear antistatic shoes and to stand on the antistatic floor. This provides a high impedance (see below).

There are three classes of electrical insulation which are designed to minimize the risk of a patient or anaesthetist forming part of an electrical circuit between the live conductor of a piece of equipment and ground:

- *Class I equipment* (fully earthed). The main supply lead has three cores (live, neutral and earth). The earth is connected to all exposed conductive parts, and in the event of a fault developing which short circuits current to the casing of the equipment, current flows from the case to earth and blows a fuse.
- *Class II equipment* (double-insulated). This has no protective earth. The power cable has only live and neutral conductors and these are 'double-insulated'. The casing is normally made of non-conductive material.
- *Class III equipment* (low voltage). This relies on a power supply at a very low voltage produced from a secondary transformer situated some distance away from the device. Potentials do not exceed 24 V (AC) or 50 V (DC). Electric heating blankets, for example, are rendered safer in this way.

ISOLATION CIRCUITS

All modern patient-monitoring equipment uses an isolation transformer so that the patient is connected only to the secondary circuit of the transformer, which is not earthed. Thus, even if the patient makes contact between the live circuit of the secondary transformer and ground, no current is transmitted to ground.

MICROSHOCK

Mains electricity supplies may induce currents in other circuits or on cases of instruments. The resulting induced currents are termed leakage currents and may pass through either the patient or anaesthetist to ground. Although the currents are very small, they may present problems to patients with an intracardiac pacemaker or a saline-filled intracardiac monitoring catheter.

The International Electrotechnical Commission has produced recommendations (adopted by the British Standards Institute) defining the levels of permitted leakage currents and patient currents from different types of electromedical equipment. Whenever new equipment is bought for a hospital, it should be subjected to tests, which verify that the leakage currents and other electrical safety characteristics are within the allowed specifications. Regular servicing of equipment should be carried out to ensure that these safe characteristics are maintained.

THE DEFIBRILLATOR

Capacitance is the ability to store electric charge. The defibrillator is an instrument in which electric charge is stored in a capacitor and then released in a controlled fashion. Direct current (DC) rather than alternating current (AC) energy is used. DC energy is more effective, causes less myocardial damage and is less arrhythmogenic than AC energy. Defibrillators are set according to the amount of energy stored and this depends on both the stored charge and the potential:

available energy (J) = stored charge (C) × potential (V)

To defibrillate a heart, two electrodes are placed on the patient's chest; one is placed just to one side of the sternum and the other over the apex of the heart. When it is discharged, the energy stored in the capacitor is released as a current pulse through the patient's chest and heart. This current pulse gives a synchronous contraction of the myocardium after which a refractory period and normal or near-normal beats may follow. The voltage may be up to 5000 V with a stored energy of up to 400 J. In practice, an inductor is included in the output circuit to ensure that the electric pulse has an optimum shape and duration. The inductor absorbs some of the energy which is discharged by the capacitor.

DIATHERMY

The effect of passing electric current through the body varies from slight physical sensation, through muscle contraction to ventricular fibrillation. The severity of these effects depends on the amount and the frequency of the current. These effects become less as the frequency of the current increases, being small above 1 kHz and negligible above 1 MHz. However, the heating and burning effects of electric current can occur at all frequencies.

A diathermy machine is used to pass electric current of high frequency (about 1 MHz) through the body in order to cause cutting and/or coagulation by burning local tissue where the current density is high. In the electrical circuit involving diathermy equipment, there are two connections with the patient. In unipolar diathermy, these are the patient plate and the active electrode used by the surgeon (Fig. 11.17A). The current travels from the active electrode, through the patient and exits through the patient plate. The current density is high at the active end where burning or cutting occurs, but it is low at the plate end where no injury occurs. If for any reason (e.g. a faulty plate) the current flows from the patient through a small area of contact between the patient and earth, then a burn may occur at the point of contact.

In bipolar diathermy, there is no patient plate, but the current travels down one side of the diathermy forceps and out through the other side (Fig. 11.17B). This type of diathermy uses low power and, because the current does not travel through the patient, it is advisable to use this in patients with a cardiac pacemaker.

ISOTOPES AND RADIATION

An atom consists of electrons which are negatively charged and these orbit around a nucleus which contains protons (positive charge) and neutrons (no charge) (Fig. 11.18). Isotopes are variations of similar atoms but with different numbers of neutrons. Isotopes with unstable nuclei are known as radioisotopes and are radioactive.

The process of change from one unstable isotope to another is known as radioactive decay. The rate of decay is measured by the half-life. The half-life of an isotope is the time required for half of the radioactive atoms present to disintegrate. When one atom changes from one unstable state to another, it emits gamma rays, or alpha or beta particles. Gamma rays, and alpha and beta particles all cause damage to or death of cells.

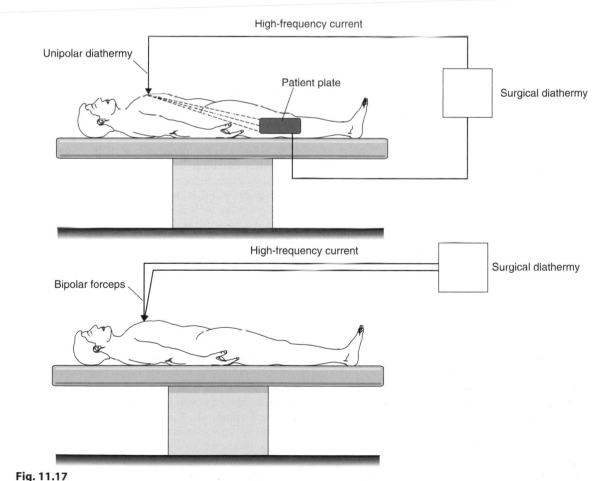

Fig. 11.17
Principle of the surgical diathermy system. (**A**) Unipolar diathermy. (**B**) Bipolar diathermy.

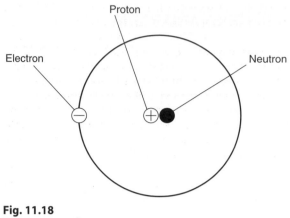

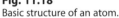

Fig. 11.18
Basic structure of an atom.

Because of this, radioisotopes are used for the treatment of cancer (e.g. cobalt-60 and caesium-137) and for conditions such as thyrotoxicosis (iodine-131). They may also be used for diagnostic purposes. Technetium-99m, krypton-81m and xenon-133 are used in imaging techniques such as scanning. Chromium-51 is used in non-imaging techniques such as labelling of red blood cells in order to measure red cell volume.

Radiation may be detected using a scintillation counter. The SI unit for radioactivity is the becquerel.

X-RAYS

X-rays are electromagnetic radiation produced when a beam of electrons is accelerated from a cathode to strike an anode (often made of tungsten). They are used for imaging purposes.

RADIATION SAFETY

Exposure to radioisotopes and X-rays should be kept to a minimum because of the risk of tissue damage and chromosomal changes that they can cause. Guidelines regarding the use of ionizing radiation were issued in the UK by the Department of Health in May 2000 in a document called Ionising Radiation (Medical Exposure) Regulations 2000 (IRMER 2000). The aims of this document are to protect patients against unnecessary exposure to radiation and to set standards for practitioners using ionizing radiation. The request of non-essential X-rays by clinicians is strongly discouraged. In the UK a doctor requires a certificate of authorization before he or she can administer radiation compounds to patients or use X-ray equipment. Lead absorbs X-rays and so it is incorporated into aprons worn by staff who are exposed to radiation. Staff who are exposed regularly to radiation should wear film badges. The film badge contains a piece of photographic film which permits estimation of the energy and dose of radiation received.

MAGNETIC RESONANCE IMAGING

Nuclear magnetic resonance (NMR) is a phenomenon that was first described by Bloch and Purcell in 1945 and has been used widely in chemistry and biochemistry. The more recent application of NMR to imaging came to be known as magnetic resonance imaging (MRI). The word nuclear was removed in order to emphasize that this technique was not associated with any radiation risk.

PHYSICAL PRINCIPLES OF MRI

Because of the presence of protons, all atomic nuclei possess a charge. In addition, the nuclei of some atoms spin. The combination of the spinning and the charge results in a local magnetic field. When some nuclei are placed in a powerful static magnetic field, they tend to align themselves longitudinally with the field. Approximately one-half of the nuclei are aligned parallel to the field and the other half antiparallel to it. However, there is an excess of nuclei which are parallel to the field and it is this population of nuclei which are of interest in the principles of MRI. When such a population of nuclei is intermittently subjected to a second magnetic field which is oscillating at the resonant frequency of the nucleus and at right angles to the static field, they tend to precess (i.e. they rotate about an axis different from the one about which they are spinning). The precession of the nuclei produces a rotating magnetic field and this is measured from the magnitude of the electrical signal induced in a set of coils within the MRI unit. The atoms then revert to their normal alignment. As they do so, images are made at different phases of relaxation known as T1, T2 and other sequences. These sequences are recorded. From the timings of these sequences, referred to as different weightings, the recorded images are compared with each other. The detected signals are then used to form an image of the body.

The hydrogen ion is commonly used for imaging because it is abundant in the body and has a strong response to an external magnetic field. Phosphorus may also be used.

The SI unit for magnetic flux density is the tesla (T) and magnets that are used in most MRI units have a magnetic flux density of 0.1–4 T. The powerful magnetic field may be created by either a permanent magnet (which cannot be switched on and off and tends to be heavy) or an electromagnet.

The presence of a strong magnetic field and restricted access to the patient imply that anaesthesia for patients undergoing an MRI scan presents unique problems which should be taken into account when planning MRI services. MRI-compatible anaesthetic equipment is essential. The hazards associated with using incorrect equipment include the projectile effect, burns and malfunction. Significant levels of acoustic noise are produced during MRI imaging because of vibrations within the scanner. Ear protectors should be provided to staff who may remain within the examination room during the scan and to the patients. The noise level may also make audible alarms inappropriate.

LASERS

A laser produces an intense beam of light that results from stimulation of atoms (the laser medium) by electrical or thermal energy. Laser light has three defining characteristics: coherence (all waves are in phase both in time and in space), collimation (all waves travel in parallel directions) and monochromaticity (all waves have the same wavelength). The term laser is an acronym for Light Amplification by Stimulated Emission of Radiation.

PHYSICAL PRINCIPLES OF LASERS

When atoms of the lasing medium are excited from a normal ground state into a high-energy state by a 'pumping' source, this is known as the excited state. When the atoms return from the excited state to the normal state, the energy is often dissipated as light or radiation of a specific wavelength characteristic of the atom (spontaneous emission). In normal circumstances, when this change from higher to lower energy state occurs, the light emitted is likely to be absorbed by an atom in the lower energy state rather than meet an atom in a higher energy state and cause more light emission. In a laser, the number of excited atoms is raised significantly so that the light emitted strikes another high-energy atom and, as a result, two light particles with the same phase and frequency are emitted (stimulated emission). These stages are summarized below:

- *Excitation*: stable atom + energy → high-energy atom
- *Spontaneous emission*: high-energy atom → stable atom + a photon of light
- *Stimulated emission*: photon of light + high-energy atom → stable atom + 2 photons of light.

The light emitted is reflected back and forth many times between mirrored surfaces, giving rise to further stimulation. This amplification continues as long as there are more atoms in the excited state than in the normal state.

A laser system has four components (Fig. 11.19):

- *The laser medium* may be gas, liquid or solid. Common surgical lasers are CO_2, argon gas and neodymium-yttrium-aluminium-garnet (Nd-YAG) crystal. This determines the wavelength of the radiation emitted. The Nd-YAG and CO_2 lasers emit invisible infrared radiation and argon gives blue-green radiation.

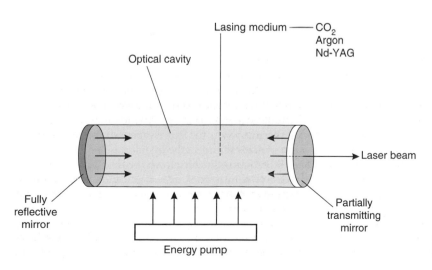

Fig. 11.19
Principle of a laser system.

- *The pumping source* supplies energy to the laser medium and this may be either an intense flash of light or electric discharge.
- *An optical cavity* is the container in which the laser medium is encased. It also contains mirrors used to reflect light in order to increase the energy of the stimulated emission. One of the mirrors is a partially transmitting mirror, which allows the laser beam to escape.
- *The light guide* directs the laser light to the surgical site. This may be in the form of a hollow tube or a flexible fibreoptic guide.

The longer the wavelength of the laser light, the more strongly it is absorbed, and the power of the light is converted to heat in shallower tissues, e.g. CO_2. The shorter the wavelength, the more scattered is the light, and the light energy is converted to heat in deeper tissues, e.g. Nd-YAG.

Lasers are categorized according to the degree of hazard they afford into four classes: class 1 is the least dangerous and class 4 the most dangerous. Surgical lasers which are specifically designed to damage tissue are class 4.

OPTICAL FIBRES

Optical fibres are used in the design of endoscopes and bronchoscopes in order to be able to see around corners. Optical fibres use the principle that when light passes from one medium to another, it is refracted (i.e. bent). If the direction of the light is altered, the light may be totally reflected instead and this allows transmission of the light along the optical fibres (Fig. 11.20). As a result, if light passes into one end of a fibre of glass or other transparent material, it may pass along the fibre by being continually reflected from the glass/air boundary. Endoscopes and bronchoscopes contain bundles of flexible transparent fibres.

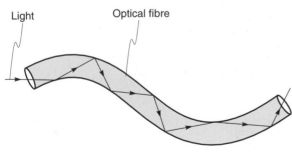

Light   Optical fibre

Fig. 11.20
Principle of the optical fibre.

FIRES AND EXPLOSIONS

Although the use of inflammable anaesthetic agents has declined greatly over the last two to three decades, ether is still used in some countries. In addition, other inflammable agents may be utilized in the operating theatre, e.g. alcohol for skin sterilization. Thus the anaesthetist should have some understanding of the problems and risks of fire occurring in the operating theatre.

Fires are produced when fuels undergo combustion. A conflagration differs from a fire in having a more rapid and more violent rate of combustion. A fire becomes an explosion if the combustion is sufficiently rapid to cause pressure waves that, in turn, cause sound waves. If these pressure waves possess sufficient energy to ignite adjacent fuels, the combustion is extremely violent and termed a detonation.

Fires require three ingredients:

- fuel
- oxygen or other substance capable of supporting combustion
- source of ignition, i.e. a source of heat sufficient to raise the fuel temperature to its ignition temperature. This quantity of heat is termed the activation energy.

FUELS

The modern volatile anaesthetic agents are non-flammable and non-explosive at room temperature in either air or oxygen.

Oils and greases are petroleum-based and form excellent fuels. In the presence of high pressures of oxygen, nitrous oxide or compressed air, these fuels may ignite spontaneously, an event termed dieseling (an analogy with the diesel engine). Thus oil or grease must not be used in compressed air, nitrous oxide or oxygen supplies.

Surgical spirit burns readily in air and the risk is increased in the presence of oxygen or nitrous oxide. Other non-anaesthetic inflammable substances include methane in the gut (which may be ignited by diathermy when the gut is opened), paper dressings and plastics found in the operating theatre suite.

Ether burns in air slowly with a blue flame, but mixtures of nitrous oxide, oxygen and ether are always explosive. It has been suggested that if administration of ether is discontinued 5 min before exposure to a source of ignition, the patient's expired gas is unlikely to burn provided that an open circuit has been used after discontinuation of ether.

The stoichiometric concentration of a fuel and oxidizing agent is the concentration at which all combustible vapour and agent are completely utilized. Thus the most violent reactions take place in stoichiometric mixtures, and as the concentration of the fuel moves away from the stoichiometric range, the reaction gradually declines until a point is reached (the flammability limit) at which ignition does not occur.

The inflammability range for ether is 2–82% in oxygen, 2–36% in air and 1.5–24% in nitrous oxide. The stoichiometric concentration of ether in oxygen is 14% and there is a risk of explosion with ether concentrations of approximately 12–40% in oxygen. In air, the stoichiometric concentration of ether is 3.4% and explosions do not occur.

SUPPORT OF COMBUSTION

It should always be remembered that as the concentration of oxygen increases, so does the likelihood of ignition of a fuel and the conversion of the reaction from fire to explosion.

Nitrous oxide supports combustion. During laparoscopy, there is a risk of perforation of the bowel and escape of methane or hydrogen into the peritoneal cavity. Consequently, the use of nitrous oxide to produce a pneumoperitoneum for this procedure is not recommended; carbon dioxide is to be preferred, as it does not support combustion (and, in addition, has a much greater solubility in blood than nitrous oxide, thereby diminishing the risk of gas embolism).

SOURCES OF IGNITION

The two main sources of ignition in the operating theatre are static electricity and diathermy.

Static electricity

Electrostatic charge occurs when two substances are rubbed together and one of the substances has an excess of electrons while the other has a deficit. Electrostatic charges are produced on non-conductive material, such as rubber mattresses, plastic pillow cases and sheets, woollen blankets, nylon, terylene, hosiery garments, rubber tops of stools and non-conducting parts of anaesthetic machines and breathing systems. Static electricity may be a source of ignition.

Diathermy

Diathermy equipment has now become an essential element of most surgical practice. However, it should not be used in the presence of inflammable agents.

Other sources of ignition

- Faulty electrical equipment.
- Heat from endoscopes, thermocautery, lasers, etc.
- Electric sparks from switches, X-ray machines, etc.

Prevention of static charges

Where possible, antistatic conducting material should be used in place of non conductors. The resistance of antistatic material should be between $50\,k\Omega\,cm^{-1}$ and $10\,M\Omega\,cm^{-1}$.

All material should be allowed to leak static charges through the floor of the operating theatre. However, if the conductivity of the floor is too high, there is a risk of electrocution if an individual forms a contact between mains voltage and ground. Consequently, the floor of the operating theatre is designed to have a resistance of $25–50\,k\Omega$ when measured between two electrodes placed 1 m apart. This allows the gradual discharge of static electricity to earth. Personnel should wear conducting shoes, each with a resistance of between 0.1 and $1\,\Omega$.

Moisture encourages the leakage of static charges along surfaces to the floor. The risk of sparks from accumulated static electricity charges is reduced if the relative humidity of the atmosphere is kept above 50%.

FURTHER READING

Association of Anaesthetists of Great Britain and Ireland 2002 Provision of anaesthetic services in magnetic resonance units. May 2002

Davis P D, Kenny G N C 2003 Basic physics and measurement in anaesthesia, 5th edn. Heinemann, London

Davey A, Diba A 2005 Ward's anaesthetic equipment, 5th edn. WB Saunders, London

12 Clinical measurement

Modern anaesthetic practice depends on the reliable measurement of the physiological and pharmacological state of the patient and the physical functioning of supportive anaesthetic equipment. The anaesthetist is responsible for the correct use of sophisticated instruments for clinical measurement which extend clinical observations beyond the human senses and enhance patient care. This requires vigilance and awareness of the limitations of the processes of measurement and the many causes of error. Uncritical acceptance of the recordings of monitoring equipment in the face of contradictory evidence is a common mistake. Unreliable measurements that are taken at face value and used to change patient management compromise the safety and effectiveness of care.

Clinical measurement is limited by four major constraints:

- *Feasibility of measurement*. The sensitivity and inherent variability of a clinical measurement depend on complex interactions and technical difficulties at the biological interface between the patient and the instrument.
- *Reliability* of measurements is determined by the properties of the measurement system. This is influenced by the calibration and correct use of the instrument. Simple examples include the correct placement of ECG electrodes, or the appropriate size of cuff for non-invasive measurement of arterial pressure. Delicate equipment, e.g. a blood gas analyser, requires regular maintenance and calibration.
- *Interpretation* depends on the critical faculties of the anaesthetist who interprets the significance of measurements in the context of complex physiological systems. Arterial pressure may be within the normal range despite severe hypovolaemia or derangement of cardiovascular function within the limits of physiological compensation. Global measurements of end-tidal CO_2 or pulse oximetry are influenced by many factors in a highly complex system. More information is required to deduce the cause of a change in the measurement.
- *Value* of clinical measurements in patient care is defined by the role of a measurement in improving patient care. This includes the ease, convenience, continuity and usefulness of a clinical measurement, and evidence of improvement in patient safety and clinical outcome.

This chapter describes the feasibility and reliability of clinical measurements relevant to anaesthetic practice. The correct interpretation of measurements and appropriate actions in the context of the condition of the patient, and the value of an instrument to the process of anaesthesia and outcomes for the patient are important but separate issues.

PROCESS OF CLINICAL MEASUREMENT

STAGES OF CLINICAL MEASUREMENT

There are four stages of clinical measurement:

- detection of the biological signal, by a sensing device which responds to a characteristic signal in the form of electrical, mechanical, electromagnetic, chemical or thermal energy
- transduction in which the output from the sensor is converted into another form of energy, usually to a continuous electrical signal
- amplification and signal processing to extract and magnify the relevant features of the signal and reduce unwanted noise
- display and storage – the output from the instrument is presented to the operator. Storage for future use may be achieved using mechanical markers, printed copy or computer memory.

Mechanical instruments use the signal energy to drive a display, with minimal intermediate processing. The height of a fluid-column manometer provides a visible index of pressure. The expansion of mercury within the confines of a thin glass column is a measure of temperature. Mechanical springs and gearing translate the rotation of a vane into the recording of expired volume on a dial. However, the overwhelming trend is for non-electrical signals to be converted by a transducer to an electrical signal suitable for electronic processing by digital computers.

THE MICROPROCESSOR REVOLUTION

The development of digital microprocessors over the last 25 years has revolutionized anaesthetic practice. Beautifully engineered mechanical instruments, e.g. the von Recklinghausen oscillotonometer, are now obsolete in developed countries.

Advantages of digital signal processing include:

- continuous real-time detection, processing and recording of measurements
- increased range of measurements possible
- miniaturization of complicated and powerful instruments
- sophisticated artefact rejection and noise reduction algorithms
- complex on-line mathematical and statistical signal processing in upgradeable software, e.g. Fourier analysis of the EEG
- automated control of the apparatus and the timing and process of measurement, and integration of alarms
- storage in memory, permitting trend analysis, future display and further analysis
- user-friendly audiovisual display of recordings, integrating many simultaneous clinical measurements, and able to be customized by the user
- less maintenance than analogue instruments.

There are a few important disadvantages:

- dependence on electrically powered equipment
- degradation of clinical skills and alternative manual measurements through disuse
- impoverished understanding of the principles of complex measuring equipment and the requirements for correct use
- illusion of the unquestionable accuracy of measurements produced by expensive computer-controlled equipment and presented on an impressive display or typed copy.

ESSENTIAL REQUIREMENTS FOR CLINICAL MEASUREMENT

All clinical measurement systems detect a biological signal and reproduce this input signal in the form of a display or record that is presented to the operator. The degree to which a discrete measurement is a true reflection of the underlying signal is defined by its accuracy and precision.

Accuracy is the difference between the measurements and the real biological signal, or in practice, a different and superior 'gold standard' measurement. Calibration against predetermined signals is used to test and optimally adjust measuring instruments. For absolute measurements, e.g. arterial pressure, one point must be a fixed reference or 'zero'.

Precision describes the reproducibility of repeated measurements of the same biological signal. This dispersion is usually described by summary statistics, standard deviation for normally distributed measurements, or the range for non-normal distributions. A single recording is unreliable when the measurement is imprecise. This is especially true of tests which require patient cooperation, practised skill or effort, e.g. peak expiratory flow rate. Repeated measurements demonstrate the variability in response.

The importance of repeated measurements

Differences in repeated clinical measurements arise from three causes:

- change in the clinical condition of the patient
- variability inherent in the biological signal or measuring instrument
- confounding errors – the recorded measurement does not reflect the signal.

The anaesthetist must be satisfied with the accuracy and precision of any clinical measurement used in patient management. Repeated measurements that are consistent ensure that the measurement is representative, i.e. precise, but do not ensure accuracy. For example, repeated recordings of invasive arterial pressure may be extremely consistent but erroneous if the transducer is not calibrated against the correct zero point. Defences against the uncritical acceptance of inaccurate measurements include meticulous care in calibrating instruments and recording of clinical measurements, and reflection on clinical measurements that do not fit the clinical state of the patient or other related measurements. A discrepant result should be rechecked, using a different measurement technique if possible, before it is used to change patient management. This is especially true of complex, operator-dependent techniques such as measurement of cardiac output.

MEASUREMENT OF CONTINUOUS SIGNALS OVER TIME

Continuous signals, which include the majority of modern clinical measurements such as biological electrical signals and the electrical output of signal transducers, introduce the complication of the response of the measuring instrument to a changing signal over time. The reliability with which a continuous signal is reproduced is defined by the relationship between input and output of the measurement system over the clinical range of signal magnitude and frequency. The input–output function of an accurate clinical measurement system would demonstrate good zero and gain stability, minimal amplitude non-linearity and hysteresis, and an adequate frequency response. This cannot be taken for granted, particularly with older equipment or with variations in environmental temperature or humidity.

Zero stability

The ability of a measurement to maintain a zero reading on the display or record when the input signal is zero defines the zero stability. The importance of zero instability depends on the magnitude relative to the signal; e.g. a zero drift of a few millimetres of mercury is much less important for the recording of arterial pressure than it is for intracranial pressure.

Gain stability

The majority of biological signals are amplified before reproduction. This 'gain' may be fixed or controlled by the user. When set, this should remain constant over the period of recording.

Amplitude linearity

The degree of amplification of the signal should be constant over the whole range of signal amplitudes. Manufacturers usually specify the degree of linearity of electronic components over a certain amplitude range. The amplitude linearity of a complete clinical system may be confirmed easily in an electronics laboratory by comparing the output to known, standardized test signals.

Hysteresis

Certain instruments such as thermistors and humidity sensors may display hysteresis. This is a special case of non-linearity, in which the output differs depending on whether the input signal is increasing or decreasing.

Frequency response

Many biological signals vary in a complicated and rapidly changing pattern. Accurate reproduction of a complex waveform requires that all of the component frequencies that make up the waveform are processed in an identical manner. This requires more than equal amplification irrespective of frequency, i.e. no amplitude distortion. It also implies that the relative positions of the various frequency components of the waveform are not shifted, i.e. no phase distortion. In practice, accurate reproduction up to the 10th harmonic of the fundamental frequency is sufficient for clinical purposes, e.g. 30 Hz for an arterial pressure waveform associated with heart rates up to 180 beats min^{-1} (3 Hz).

Signal-to-noise ratio

Biological signals are obscured to a variable degree by unwanted or extraneous signals which have similar physical characteristics and are described as noise, e.g. heart sounds become difficult to detect in the presence of continuous, noisy breath sounds. The efficiency of isolation of the signal from unwanted biological signals and electronic noise sources in the equipment is defined by the signal-to-noise ratio. The variability of the amplitudes of signal and noise is enormous and the signal-to-noise ratio is described using a logarithmic scale of decibels. Microvolt EEG measurements are particularly susceptible to noise from many sources. Biological noise includes contaminating ECG and EMG potentials, particularly from the scalp muscles, and interference from electrochemical activity at the skin–electrode interface. Electrostatic and electromagnetic linkage between the recording wires and nearby sources of mains electricity generates noise that is predominantly 50 Hz frequency and harmonics. Radiofrequency noise from diathermy or transmitters may also be picked up at this stage. Physical disturbance of the recording wires causes tiny changes in capacitative potentials and may add low-frequency noise, called microphony. Thermal noise is added during amplification, particularly at the input stage when the signal is in the microvolt range. Good amplifier design, electronic filtering of unwanted frequencies and modern techniques of digital signal processing may extract small signals from considerable background noise, but this inevitably introduces some distortion of the signal. Prevention of contamination of the signal by minimizing sources of noise before the signal is amplified is always preferable. The operator is responsible for correctly using measuring instruments to optimize the signal and for applying knowledge of the physical principles of the measurement to minimize contamination by noise.

ANALOGUE AND DIGITAL PROCESSING

Following signal detection and appropriate transduction, the continuously variable analogue signal is amplified, processed and displayed for the attention of the clinician.

Mechanical measuring instruments

Measuring instruments based on mechanical principles lack the flexibility and automated control of computerized devices, but use ingenious methods for processing and displaying analogue measurements. For example, mechanical spirometers use precision-engineered gears to translate the movement of a piston or vane into the rotation of a calibrated dial.

Analogue computers

Analogue computers use hardware comprising electronic circuits and operational amplifiers. Signals are processed in the form of continuously variable electric potentials. Analogue hardware components continuously perform a wide variety of mathematical functions on a rapidly changing input waveform. Integration and differentiation are formidable mathematical tasks for a digital computer, which can be solved simply and cheaply using analogue circuits comprising capacitors and resistors. Integration of the flow signal from a pneumotachograph produces a volume waveform.

Microcomputers and digital signal processing

Digital signal processing offers a powerful alternative to mechanical processing and analogue computation. A fundamental step in this process is the conversion of a continuous analogue electrical signal into a discrete digital form. This analogue-to-digital conversion is achieved by measuring or 'sampling' the continuous input signal at regular intervals, to produce a series of discrete measurements over time which are in a suitable format for digital computation. The overwhelming advantage of digital processing is that the manipulation of the digitized signal is performed by a flexible and unlimited series of software calculations which range from mathematical functions to the analysis of statistical properties and trends.

Analogue-to-digital conversion

The core processing units of digital computers assume one of two stable states, i.e. a binary, rather than decimal, code. This imposes a limit on the resolving power of the digital processor. A binary number of eight digits (called 8 bits) may represent a range of integer decimal numbers, from binary 00000000 = decimal 0 to binary 11111111 = decimal 255. In short, an 8-bit converter can resolve an analogue signal with an accuracy of one part in 255, i.e. with an amplitude resolution of 0.4% of full scale. A 12-bit converter is more accurate, with a resolving power of one part in 4095 or 0.02% of full scale. The cost of this improvement in resolution is more expensive hardware to digitize, process and store considerably more digital information.

Amplitude resolution is not the only determinant of the accuracy of analogue-to-digital conversion. Resolution over time, determined by the sampling frequency, is also important. A relatively low sampling frequency may provide a representative sample of values for a slowly changing waveform; it may inadequately represent high-frequency components and introduce aliasing error. The Nyquist theorem suggests that the minimum sampling frequency to maintain the integrity of the waveform is at least twice the highest frequency component with significant amplitude in the input signal waveform; e.g. a sampling frequency of 100 Hz would adequately capture the fastest rate of change in a physiological pressure signal.

The immensely powerful and complicated hardware and software programming instructions responsible for performing the tasks of digitizing, processing, storing and displaying the input signal are hidden from view in the commercial 'black box'.

DATA DISPLAY

Useful instruments communicate measurements in an appropriate and user-friendly manner.

Analogue displays

A continuously variable signal, such as pressure or temperature, is represented by an analogue display in terms of the amplitude of a physical quantity on a calibrated scale, dial, electrical meter or printed record. The glass thermometer incorporates a wedge-shaped lens which magnifies the appearance of the mercury column against the calibrated background scale. The height of a water column manometer is a linear, visual scale of pressure. Simple mechanical displays are accurate and easily understood, but are inconvenient to read and most suitable for intermittent discrete measurements.

Mechanical spirometers and flowmeters record flow on a dial driven by gears. Electrical moving coil meters use a coil of wire suspended in a magnetic field which rotates in proportion to the applied current and moves a pointer on a calibrated dial. Alternatively, the amplified and filtered electrical signal could drive a chart recorder which produces a continuous printed record of the amplitude of measurements against time. Limitations common to these mechanical devices include fragile moving parts, and inertia which impairs the frequency response to rapidly changing signals.

The cathode ray oscilloscope is an effective screen-based display for continuous analogue electrical signals. A heated cathode generates a stream of electrons which are focused and accelerated onto phosphorescent coating which lines the flat surface of the tube to generate a bright spot. The position of the electron beam in both x- and y-axes is controlled by electrostatic plates. The continuously varying input signal is applied to the y-plates so that deflection in the vertical y-axis is proportional to the amplitude of the signal. The absence of mechanical parts results in a high-frequency response. An electronic time-base circuit delivers a saw-tooth voltage to the x-plates which drives the electron beam across the x-axis at a constant rate and returns the beam to the left-hand side at the start of each sweep. This produces a dynamic image of signal amplitude against time. Alternatively, a second input signal may be applied to the x-plates to produce an x–y graphical plot, e.g. pressure–volume loop. Cathode ray oscilloscopes are widely used in electronic engineering and signal processing, but have been replaced in clinical practice by microprocessor-controlled displays.

Microprocessor-controlled displays

Digital signal processing has revolutionized clinical measurement. However, digital information in the form of a list of numbers is extremely difficult to interpret quickly and easily. Digital records are appropriate for discrete measurements such as drug concentrations or blood gas tensions, but a digital time series of a continuously varying signal, such as pressure in the form of a list of numbers, would be incomprehensible. The human brain is accustomed to continuous analogue sensory input and modern microprocessor-controlled measuring instruments convert the discrete digital record back into continuous analogue waveforms for display on a monitor in a manner familiar to anaesthetists.

This paradox illustrates the real power of digital signal processing to manipulate and present information in a relevant and user-friendly manner. Continuous waveforms, e.g. invasive pressure, may be displayed alongside discrete numerical measurements of amplitude or frequency and a graphical display of trends over time. These can be recreated or processed in other ways from the original digital signal, which is stored in a digital computer record without degradation of the quality of the signal.

BIOLOGICAL ELECTRICAL SIGNALS

The detection and recording of biological electrical potentials are important clinical measurements which incorporate many of the key principles of clinical measurement.

Depolarization of the cell membrane of excitable cells is fundamental to the action of these cells and generates a transient potential difference between the active cell and surrounding tissues. The summation of synchronous extracellular potentials from a large number of excitable cells generates a widespread electric field which can be detected by electrodes on the body surface.

The electrocardiogram is a well-established measure of myocardial electrical activity. The synchronous depolarization and prolonged action potentials in cardiac muscle summate to generate a potential field of high amplitude. Body surface ECG recordings are approximately 1 mV in amplitude, with a frequency content in the range 0.05–100 Hz.

The electroencephalogram is a smaller and more complex signal, with an amplitude of 50–200 µV and a frequency content that is classified conventionally into four categories:

- delta waves: 0–4 Hz
- theta waves: 4–8 Hz
- alpha waves: 8–13 Hz
- beta waves: 13 Hz and above.

The spiking, transient depolarization, then repolarization, of action potentials in neurones in the brain is sufficiently asynchronous and transient to be unrecordable from the scalp or surface of the brain. It is believed that the EEG is generated by the summation of synchronous postsynaptic potentials on the dendrites of sheets of large and symmetrically arranged pyramidal cells in cortical layers III and IV. Recording of these microvolt signals with acceptable levels of artefact and interference is difficult. Visual analysis of EEG recordings is subjective and requires experience.

Statistical processing can produce summary data at several levels of complexity. The power spectrum derived from Fourier analysis of the EEG signal represents the amplitudes of the different frequency components represented in the original EEG signal. Median and spectral edge frequencies represent the frequencies below which is contained 50% and 95% of the total EEG power respectively.

Bispectral analysis is a higher-order statistical process that estimates phase coupling between different frequency components in the EEG signal. The bispectral index (BIS) is derived from complex EEG analysis incorporating weighted information derived from the degree of burst suppression, spectral power and the bispectrum. The BIS number decreases with increasing hypnosis.

Evoked potentials are small, specific changes in the EEG in response to a series of auditory, visual or somatosensory stimuli. These tiny evoked potentials are overwhelmed by the larger background EEG. They are, however, time-locked to the stimulus and may be extracted from the asynchronous background EEG by the digital signal processing technique of signal-averaging of several hundred responses.

DETECTION OF BIOLOGICAL ELECTRICAL SIGNALS: ELECTRODES

Modern electrodes are constructed of silver, electrolytically coated with silver chloride. Low, stable impedances minimize mains interference. Symmetrical electrode impedance and insignificant polarization control drift. However, care is still required to achieve optimum results. The silver chloride layer is very thin, prone to deterioration and only suitable for single use. Movement artefacts which alter the electrode potential and impedance are greatly reduced if the electrode surface is separated from the skin by a foam pad impregnated with electrolyte gel. It is no longer necessary to abrade the skin to achieve ultra-low impedance, but de-greasing with alcohol before applying the electrode helps to reduce skin impedance and ensures satisfactory adhesion.

Needle electrodes deliver poor electrical performance, are sensitive to movement and increase the risk of diathermy burns.

AMPLIFIERS FOR BIOLOGICAL SIGNALS

The amplitude of tiny bioelectrical signals must be increased by amplification, and unwanted noise and interference minimized. Calibration voltages may be incorporated for correct adjustment of the gain of the amplifier.

Input impedance and common mode rejection

Amplifiers for biological signals require high common mode rejection and high input impedance. The input and electrode impedances act as a potential divider: high electrode impedance and low amplifier input impedance attenuate the electrical signal across the amplifier. The input impedance of modern amplifiers exceeds $5\,M\Omega$ to avoid problems, and careful attention must be paid to minimizing electrode impedance, particularly for EEG recordings.

Differential amplification is a powerful method of reducing unwanted noise. The potential difference between two input signals is amplified, but electrical signals common to both are attenuated. This feature is termed 'common mode rejection' and very effectively reduces mains interference in all biological signals and electrocardiographic contamination of much smaller electroencephalographic signals. The common mode rejection ratio (CMRR) for a typical differential amplifier exceeds 10 000:1. In other words, a signal applied equally to both input terminals would need to be 10 000 times larger than a signal applied between them for the same change in output.

Frequency response

The bandwidth of the amplifier must cover the range of frequencies that are important in the signal. In practice, amplifiers require a flat frequency response for ECG from 0.14 to 50 Hz, for EEG from 0.5 to 100 Hz and for EMG from 20 Hz to at least 2 kHz.

Low-frequency interference, largely caused by slow fluctuating potentials generated in the electrodes, produces baseline instability and drift. This is removed by incorporating a network of resistors and capacitors which function as a simple high-pass filter allowing biological signals to pass, but attenuating low-frequency noise. This introduces a compromise in amplifier design between signal trace fidelity and stability of recording. For example, amplifiers designed for diagnostic electrocardiography have long time constants with optimal reproduction of the waveform at the expense of baseline instability, especially to movement. In comparison, continuity of recording is more important when the electrocardiogram is used for monitoring during anaesthesia; high-pass filtering produces a short time constant and good baseline stability at the expense of waveform reproduction. Low-frequency elements of the ECG, such as the T wave, may become differentiated by phase shift in the high-pass filter and appear distorted or biphasic.

Other filters can attenuate particular frequencies. Highly selective band reject filters attenuate 50 Hz interference from the signal. Low-pass filters are used to eliminate higher-frequency artefacts from an EEG signal. The purpose of filtering is to reduce unwanted noise relative to the signal. When the frequency range of signal and noise overlap, some degree of signal degradation is inevitable.

Noise and interference

Electrical noise arising from the patient, the patient–electrode interface or the surroundings may seriously interfere with accurate recording of biological potentials.

Noise originating from the patient

Millivolt ECG potentials on the body surface are hundreds of times larger than microvolt EEG signals on the scalp. EMG signals may be even larger, and muscular activity, especially shivering, causes severe interference. Two features of electronic amplifier design substantially improve the EEG signal-to-noise ratio. ECG potentials are essentially the same across the scalp and are ignored by amplifiers with a high common mode rejection. EMG activity has a higher frequency content than the EEG signal, and may be minimized by a low-pass filter which attenuates the higher-frequency response of the amplifier to a level which attenuates the EMG signals and does not interfere with the characteristics of the EEG.

Noise originating from the patient–electrode interface

Recording electrodes do not behave as passive conductors. All skin–metal electrode systems employ a metal surface in contact with an electrolyte solution. Polarization describes the interaction between metal and electrolyte which generates a small electrical gradient. Electrodes comprising metal plated with one of its own salts, e.g. silver–silver chloride, avoid this problem because current in each direction does not significantly change the electrolyte composition. Mechanical movement of recording electrodes may also cause significant potential gradients – alteration in the physical dimensions of the electrode changes the cell potential and skin–electrode impedance. Differences in potential between two electrodes connected to a differential amplifier are amplified and asymmetry of electrode impedance seriously impairs the common mode rejection ratio of the recording amplifier.

Noise originating outside the patient

Electrical interference. Mains frequency interference with the recording of biological potentials may be troublesome, particularly in electromagnetically noisy clinical environments. Patients function physically as large unscreened conductors and interact with nearby electrical sources through the processes of capacitative coupling and electromagnetic induction.

Capacitance permits alternating current to pass across an air gap. A live mains conductor and nearby patient behave as the two plates of a capacitor. The very small mains frequency current that flows through the patient is of no clinical significance but confounds the detection and amplification of biological potentials, creating unwanted interference in the recording. Capacitatively coupled interference is minimized by reducing the capacitance and the alternating potential difference. This is achieved by moving the patient away from the source of interference and by screening mains-powered equipment with a conductive surround which is maintained at earth potential by a low-resistance earth connection and by surrounding leads with a braided copper screen – stray capacitances couple with the screen instead of the lead.

Alternating currents in a conductor generate a magnetic flux. This induces voltages in any nearby conductors which lie in the changing magnetic flux, including the patient or signal leads to the amplifier, which function as inefficient secondary transformers. This source of interference is minimized by keeping patients as far as possible from powerful sources of electromagnetic flux, especially mains transformers. Electromagnetic inductance may be minimized by ensuring that all patient leads are the same length, closely bound or twisted together until very close to the electrodes. This ensures that the induced signals are identical in all leads and therefore susceptible to common mode rejection.

The importance of low electrode impedance. Low electrode impedance may exaggerate the effects of surrounding electrical interference. Capacitive and inductive coupling produce very small currents in the recording leads. If the electrode impedance is low, the potential at the amplifier input must remain close to the potential at the skin surface, so that minimal interference results. If electrode impedance is high, the small induced currents may create a significant potential difference across that impedance, leading to severe 50 Hz interference.

Radiofrequency interference from diathermy is a severe problem for the recording of biological potentials. ECG amplifiers may be provided with some protection by filtering the signal before it enters the isolated input circuit, filtering the power supply to block mains-borne radiofrequencies and enclosing the electronic components in a double screen: the outer earthed and the inner at amplifier potential.

MECHANICAL SIGNALS: MEASUREMENT OF ARTERIAL PRESSURE

Several physical principles and a wide range of instruments are used to measure pressure. Liquid column manometers display pressure according to the height of a column of fluid relative to a predefined zero-point, and the density of the fluid. Mechanical pressure gauges are used widely, particularly in high-pressure gas supplies; pressure dependent mechanical movement is amplified by a gearing mechanism which drives a pointer across a scale.

For most physiological pressure measurements, diaphragm gauges are used – a flexible diaphragm moves according to the applied pressure. Mechanical display of diaphragm movement is limited by poor sensitivity to small pressures, inertia to changing pressure and a narrow range of linear response. In modern diaphragm gauges used for sensing dynamic pressures, movement of the diaphragm is sensed by a device which converts the mechanical energy imparted to the diaphragm into electrical energy.

ELECTROMECHANICAL TRANSDUCERS

The first step in transduction is movement of the diaphragm caused by the relationship to applied pressure. This depends on the stiffness of the diaphragm and substantially determines the operating characteristics of the transducer. Linearity of amplitude and frequency response are improved by using small stiff diaphragms which require a more sensitive mechanism for sensing diaphragm movement.

Wire strain gauges are based on the principle that stretching or compression of a wire changes the electrical resistance. Changes in capacitance or inductance have also been coupled to movement of a diaphragm. Silicon strain gauges use the changes in resistance in a thin slice of silicon crystal that occur when it is compressed or expanded. They are very sensitive and suitable for incorporation into a small stiff diaphragm with excellent frequency response, but non-linearity and temperature dependence are difficult technical problems.

Optical transduction senses movement of the diaphragm by reflecting light from the silvered back of the convex diaphragm onto a photocell. Applied pressure causes the silvered surface to become more convex. This causes the reflected light beam to diverge, reducing the intensity of reflected light sensed by the photoelectric cell. This design is used in a fibreoptic cardiac catheter for intravascular pressure measurement. These miniature pressure transducers are expensive but have a high-frequency response and fibreoptic light sources eliminate the risk of microshock.

DIRECT MEASUREMENT OF INTRAVASCULAR PRESSURE

Liquid manometers remain a simple, cheap and useful method of measuring central venous pressure. However, electromechanical transducers are commonly used for the invasive measurement of intravascular pressures; cost and complexity are compensated by convenience, accuracy, continuity of measurement and an electrical output which may be processed, stored and displayed according to the requirements.

Fourier showed that all complex waveforms may be described as a mixture of simple sine waves of varying amplitude, frequency and phase. These consist of a fundamental wave, in this case at the pulse frequency, and a series of harmonics. The lower harmonics tend to have the greatest amplitude and a reasonable approximation to the arterial pressure waveform may be obtained by accurate reproduction of the fundamental and first 10 harmonics. In other words, to reproduce an arterial waveform at 120 beats min^{-1} accurately would require transduction with a linear frequency response up to a frequency of at least $120 \times 10/60 = 20$ Hz. Accurate reproduction of a waveform requires that both the amplitude and phase difference of each harmonic are faithfully reproduced. This requires a transduction system with a natural frequency higher than the significant frequency components of the system, and the correct amount of damping.

The commonest method for the direct measurement of intravascular pressure uses a pressure transducer connected to the lumen of the vessel by a fluid-filled catheter. The fluid and diaphragm of the transducer constitute a mechanical system which oscillates in simple harmonic motion at the natural resonant frequency. This determines the frequency response of the measurement system (Fig. 12.1). The resonant frequency of a catheter–transducer measuring system is highest and the frictional resistance to fluid flow which dampens the frequency response is

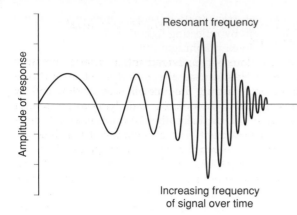

Fig. 12.1
Simulation of the output of a catheter–transducer system with increasing frequency of a constant amplitude input signal. The linearity of response is lost as the frequency approaches the resonant frequency of the system.

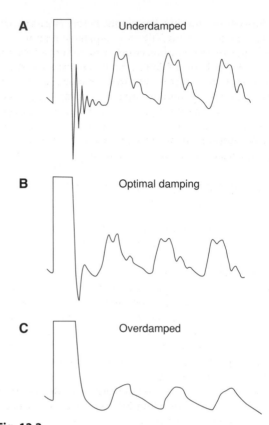

Fig. 12.2
Damping of arterial pressure waves and the response to a square wave signal from the fast flush device.

lowest when the velocity of movement of fluid in the catheter is minimized. This is achieved with a stiff, low-volume displacement diaphragm and a short, wide, rigid catheter.

Transduced vascular pressures should always be displayed. Inspection of the arterial waveform provides a qualitative assessment of the adequacy of the frequency response and damping. Modern instruments calculate mean arterial pressure automatically by integrating the area under the pressure waveform. This measurement is affected less by non-linear characteristics of the catheter–transducer system and is more accurate and precise than the peak systolic and trough diastolic pressures. It is also more relevant to the physiology of organ perfusion.

DETERMINATION OF THE RESONANT FREQUENCY AND DAMPING

The resonant frequency and the effects of damping may be estimated by applying a step change in pressure to the catheter–transducer system and recording the response (Fig. 12.2). The underdamped system responds rapidly but overshoots and oscillates close to the natural resonant frequency of the system; frequency components of the pressure wave close to the resonant frequency are exaggerated. By contrast, the overdamped system responds slowly and the recorded signal decreases slowly to reach the baseline with no overshoot. High-frequency oscillations are damped, underestimating the true pressure changes. These extremes are undesirable.

Optimal damping

Optimal damping maximizes the frequency response of the system, minimizes resonance and represents the best compromise between speed of response and accuracy of transduction. A small overshoot represents approximately 7% of the step change in pressure, with the pressure then following the arterial waveform (Fig. 12.2).

Damping is relatively unimportant when the frequencies being recorded are less than two-thirds of the natural frequency of the catheter–transducer system. Modern transducer systems using small compliance transducers connected to a short, stiff catheter, with a minimum of constrictions or connections, approximate to this ideal. Air bubbles in the system, clotting or kinking in the vascular catheter and arterial spasm lower the natural resonant frequency and increase the damping.

In clinical practice, the resonant frequency of the whole system is uncomfortably close to the frequency content of the signal, and accurate measurements require optimal damping. However, damping is difficult to measure and control, and is poor compensation for an inadequate frequency response in the pressure recording system. Adjustment of damping is difficult to achieve and mechanical methods which include inserting constrictions or a compliant tube into the system to increase damping further reduce the resonant frequency. Electronic damping of the electrical output from the transducer cannot correct for non-linear amplification and attenuation of frequencies in the pressure wave before transduction.

INDIRECT METHODS FOR MEASURING ARTERIAL PRESSURE

Indirect methods of measuring arterial pressure do not depend on contact between arterial blood and the system for signal recognition and transduction. The majority depend on signals generated by the occlusion of a major artery using a cuff, known as the Riva–Rocci method. Clinical methods of signal detection include palpation to estimate the systolic pressure at the return of a palpable distal pulse, and auscultation of the Korotkoff sounds for systolic and diastolic pressures. Measuring devices depend on the detection of movement of the arterial wall using changes in pressure or sound below audible frequencies and detection of blood flow using the Doppler shift of an ultrasound signal or plethysmography.

Accuracy of pressure measurements

The accuracy of pressure measurements, particularly using indirect methods, needs to be considered. Invasive direct measurement of arterial pressure is the usual standard for comparison. However, the catheter–transducer system must be carefully set up and tested for optimal performance and this is hard to achieve in clinical practice. Arterial pressure varies throughout the arterial tree and the measured pressure depends on the site of measurement. As the pulse wave travels from the ventricle to peripheral arteries, changes in vessel diameter and elasticity affect the pressure waveform which becomes narrower with increased amplitude. Differences in arterial pressure between limbs are common, particularly in patients with arterial disease.

Indirect methods using an occluding cuff make intermittent measurements, with the systolic and diastolic readings reflecting the conditions in the artery at two instants at which the end-points are detected. By contrast, direct pressure measurements are the average of a number of cycles, more precisely reflecting mean pressures. Indirect measurements may be compromised by taking a small number of infrequent samples from a variable signal.

Oscillometric measurement of arterial pressure

The oscillometric measurement of arterial pressure estimates arterial pressure by analysis of the pressure oscillations that are produced in an occluding cuff by pulsatile blood flow in the underlying artery during deflation of the cuff (Fig. 12.3). Mechanical oscillotonometers use a second sensing cuff which drives rotation of a mechanical dial. Automated oscillometers sense transient pressure fluctuations with an electromechanical pressure transducer. In common with other instruments for indirect measurement of arterial pressure, accurate estimation of the systolic pressure requires slow cuff deflation and estimates of diastolic pressure are unreliable. During slow deflation, each pulse wave produces a pressure transient in the cuff which may be distinguished from the slowly decreasing ambient pressure in the cuff. Above systolic pressure, the transients are small, but suddenly increase in magnitude when the cuff pressure reaches the systolic point. As the cuff pressure decreases further, the amplitude reaches a peak and then starts to diminish. The mean arterial pressure correlates closely with the lowest cuff pressure at which the maximum amplitude is maintained. As the cuff pressure reaches diastolic pressure, the transients abruptly diminish in amplitude.

Commercial instruments incorporate mechanisms for improving the reliability of the measurement. For example, at each successive plateau pressure during the controlled deflation, successive pressure fluctuations are compared and accepted only if they are similar. All automatic oscillometric instruments require a regular cardiac cycle with no great differences between successive pulses. Accurate and consistent readings may be impossible to record in patients with an irregular rhythm, particularly atrial fibrillation.

Clinical studies comparing automatic oscillometric instruments with direct arterial pressure have demonstrated good correlation for systolic pressure with a tendency to overestimate at low pressures and underestimate at high pressures. Mean and diastolic pressures were less reliable. The 95% confidence interval for all three indices exceeded 15 mmHg.

MEASUREMENT OF BLOOD FLOW: CARDIAC OUTPUT

Three different approaches are discussed for the measurement of cardiac output based on different and contrasting principles:

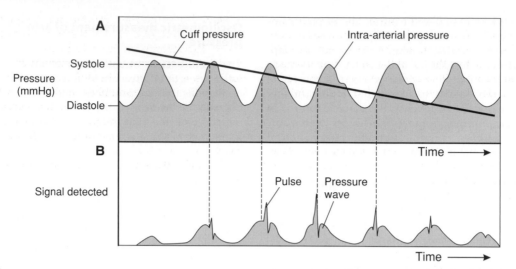

Fig. 12.3
Diagram showing: (**A**) relationship between cuff pressure and intra-arterial pressure as cuff pressure decreases during oscillometry; (**B**) the signal created by the relative pressure changes in **A**. The sharp spikes of pressure in **B** are created by the walls of the artery opening and closing. These spikes are detected by a transducer first when the cuff pressure is just below systolic arterial pressure; their amplitude reaches a peak at mean arterial pressure and they cease when the cuff pressure is below diastolic pressure.

- indicator dilution, and other techniques based on the Fick principle
- Doppler ultrasonography
- thoracic electrical bioimpedance.

More detail concerning these and other techniques of measuring blood flow are described in the further reading.

THE FICK PRINCIPLE

The Fick principle defines flow by the ratio of the uptake or clearance of a tracer within an organ to measurements of the arteriovenous difference in concentration. It may be used to measure cardiac output, notably when applied to oxygen uptake or indicator dilution, and also regional blood flow, e.g. cerebral blood flow using the uptake of nitrous oxide, and renal blood flow from the excretion of compounds cleared totally by the kidney, such as *para*-aminohippuric acid.

In subjects with minimal cardiac shunt and reasonable pulmonary function, pulmonary blood flow may be calculated from the ratio of the oxygen consumption and the difference in oxygen content between arterial and mixed venous blood, as follows:

$$\text{Pulmonary blood flow} = \frac{\text{oxygen consumption}}{\text{arteriovenous oxygen content difference}}$$

Oxygen consumption from a reservoir is measured using an accurate spirometer, and oxygen content of blood requires a co-oximeter. The patient should be at steady state when the measurements are made, with constant inspired oxygen concentration and blood samples obtained slowly whilst the oxygen consumption is being determined. True mixed venous blood samples must be obtained from a pulmonary artery catheter, in which case alternative indicator dilution techniques described below are less demanding. The effects of ventilation and beat-to-beat variation in cardiac output are averaged over the long period of measurement of oxygen consumption. Errors in measurement of oxygen consumption limit the accuracy of this technique ($\pm 10\%$).

INDICATOR DILUTION

An indicator is injected as a bolus into the right heart and the concentration reaching the systemic side of the circulation is plotted against time (Fig. 12.4). The average concentration is calculated from the area under the concentration–time curve divided by the duration of the curve. The cardiac output during the period of this measurement is the ratio of the dose of indicator to average concentration.

The general formula is:

$$\begin{array}{l}\text{Cardiac output} \\ \text{(L min}^{-1}\text{)}\end{array} = \frac{\text{indicator dose (units)} \times 60}{\text{average concentration (units L}^{-1}\text{)} \times \text{time (s)}}$$

Recirculation of the indicator before the downslope is complete is a problem (Fig. 12.4). This may be circumvented by extrapolation of the early exponential downslope to define the tail of the curve which would have been recorded if recirculation had not occurred. The area under the curve is calculated by integration.

Chemical indicator dilution

Indocyanine green is the commonest chemical indicator. It is non-toxic and has a relatively short half-life so that repeated measurements may be made. It also has a peak spectral absorption at 800 nm, which is the wavelength at which absorption of oxygenated haemoglobin is identical to that of reduced haemoglobin. The measurement is therefore not affected by arterial saturation.

Chemical indicator dilution techniques have been overtaken by the use of pulmonary flotation catheters and heat energy as the signal indicator.

Thermal indicator dilution

This technique is used commonly in the intensive care patient where a pulmonary artery catheter is required frequently for monitoring of cardiac output and left-sided pressures. The principle of the method is similar to other indicator dilution methods, but the injection and sampling are performed on the right side of the heart. A bolus of 10 mL of saline at room temperature

is injected into the right atrium and the temperature change is recorded by a thermistor in the pulmonary artery. The recorded temperatures generate an exponential dilution curve with no recirculation. The 'heat dose' is the product of the difference in temperature between the injectate and blood multiplied by the density, specific heat and volume of the injectate. The average change in heat content is the area under the temperature–time graph multiplied by the density and specific heat of blood.

Thermal dilution techniques offer many advantages:

- the indicator is cheap and non-toxic
- repeated measurements may be made without accumulation of the indicator
- arterial puncture and blood sampling are not required
- absence of recirculation greatly facilitates measurement of the area under the curve, particularly in low output states.

Disadvantages of thermal dilution include the following:

- invasive and expensive pulmonary artery catheterization is required
- the thermistor probe must be matched to the cardiac output processor
- mixing of the large bolus with venous blood may be incomplete

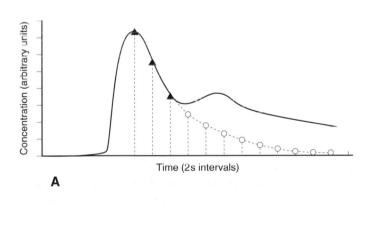

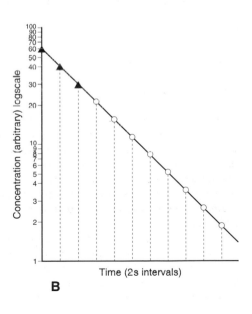

Fig. 12.4
(A) Single injection indicator dilution curve showing distortion of downslope produced by recirculation. (B) Re-plot on semi-logarithmic paper. ▲ = points taken from the downslope in **A** to establish the slope of the re-plot in **B**; ○ = points taken from **B** to plot tail of curve in **A**. Reproduced from Fig. 16.13, page 216, in Principles of measurement and monitoring in anaesthesia and intensive care, by Sykes MK, Vickers MD, Hull CJ, third edition, published 1991. Permission from Blackwell Scientific Publications.

- pulmonary artery flow varies more with respiration than does systemic flow
- corrections are required, e.g. for changes in injectate temperature during injection through the catheter.

The measurement of cardiac output using both dye and thermodilution is now automated with computer-controlled sampling, calculation of indicator dilution curves, rejection algorithms for artefacts or curves which are not exponential, and on-line calculation of cardiac output.

Instruments with rapidly responding thermistors and a heating element incorporated in the pulmonary flotation catheter can measure the stoke volume of a single right ventricular contraction, and derive a continuous estimate of cardiac output.

Pulse contour analysis

The area under the systolic part of the arterial pressure waveform correlates directly with left ventricular stroke volume and inversely with aortic impedance. Multiplication by heart rate provides an estimate of cardiac output. Aortic impedance is estimated from arterial pressure and cardiac output, usually measured by a thermodilution technique. Ongoing pulse contour analysis provides a continuous estimate of cardiac output. This measurement is sensitive to changes in systemic vascular resistance and requires intermittent recalibration by thermodilution.

DOPPLER ULTRASONOGRAPHY

Ultrasound techniques can detect the shape, size and movement of tissue interfaces, especially soft tissues and blood, including the echocardiographic measurement of blood flow and the structure and function of the heart. Sound waves are transmitted by the oscillation of particles in the direction of wave transmission and are defined by the amplitude of oscillation (the difference between ambient and peak pressures) and the wavelength (distance between successive peaks) or frequency (inversely proportional to wavelength, the number of cycles per second). These characteristics are measured by a pressure transducer placed in the path of an oncoming wave. The human ear detects frequencies within the range of 20–20 000 Hz. Diagnostic ultrasound uses frequencies in the range of 1–10 MHz. Short-term diagnostic use of ultrasound appears to be free from hazard.

Generation and detection of ultrasound

Generation and sensing of ultrasound are performed by transducers which are manufactured from ceramic materials containing lead zirconate and lead titanate which display the piezoelectric effect. These substances are cheap, easily shaped and very efficiently transform mechanical to electrical energy and vice versa. Pressure on the surface of these materials generates a related and measurable electric charge. Conversely, applying a high-frequency alternating potential difference across the transducer changes the thickness and generates ultrasound of the same frequency as the applied voltage.

Properties of ultrasound

Shorter wavelengths and higher frequencies improve the resolution of distance, but tissue penetration is simultaneously reduced. Amplitude determines the intensity of the ultrasound beam, the number and size of echoes recorded and therefore the sensitivity of the instrument. Ultrasound is absorbed by tissues and reflected at tissue interfaces. The intensity of the beam decreases exponentially as it passes through tissue. Attenuation depends on the nature and temperature of the tissue, and is related linearly to the frequency of the ultrasound.

The reflection of the ultrasound beam from the junction between two tissues or from tissue–fluid or tissue–air interfaces forms the basis of the majority of diagnostic techniques. Reflections at most soft-tissue interfaces are therefore weak, but bone–fat and tissue–air interfaces reflect the majority of incident energy. Structures lying behind a bone or air interface cannot be studied using ultrasound.

Ultrasound scanning techniques have been developed which are suited to different applications and which have extremely sophisticated two-dimensional, real-time, brightness- and colour-modulated displays under microprocessor control.

Detection of motion by the Doppler effect: cardiac output

The frequency of ultrasound waves reflected from a stationary object is the same as that of the transmitted waves. However, if the reflector is moving towards the transmitter, it encounters more oscillations in a given time than a stationary reflector, so that the frequency of the waves impinging on the reflector is apparently increased. This physical phenomenon is termed the Doppler effect. The apparent increase in frequency is directly proportional to the velocity of the reflecting object relative to the source and two constants, the frequency of the transmitted ultrasound and the velocity of ultrasound in the medium. This difference in frequency lies within the range of hearing and provides a vivid audible description of pulsatile blood flow. A Doppler signal proportional to blood flow may be obtained from the ascending aorta via the suprasternal notch or the aortic root from a transoesophageal probe which provides a non-invasive index of cardiac output.

The blood flow velocity curve is integrated to calculate the average velocity over each cardiac cycle. The stroke volume is calculated by multiplying the average velocity per cycle by an echocardiographic estimation of the cross-sectional area of the aorta. Multiplication of the stroke volume by heart rate yields cardiac output.

There are three major problems with Doppler measurements of cardiac output:

- Aortic diameter must be measured accurately. This may be done reasonably accurately by echocardiography, but errors also arise because the aorta is not completely circular, it expands by up to 12% during systole, and the sites of measurement of diameter and velocity may differ.
- The shape of the velocity profile is not uniform, with central streaming in the large-diameter aorta. Low and unrepresentative velocities may be recorded if the ultrasound beam is not aligned exactly along the central core of the aorta.
- The Doppler shift depends on the direction of the ultrasound beam relative to the axis. Provided that the angle is less than 20°, the error in cardiac output is only about 6%.

Unacceptable variation in measurements, operator dependence and poor correlation with thermal dilution for absolute measurements of cardiac output have limited the application of Doppler ultrasonography in clinical practice. However, it is less invasive with fewer serious complications, records a continuous measurement and provides a useful indication of trends in cardiac output.

THORACIC ELECTRICAL BIOIMPEDANCE

Tissue impedance depends on blood volume. Measurement of thoracic impedance provides an index of stroke volume. Two circumferential electrodes are placed around the neck and two around the upper abdomen. A small (<1 mA) constant, high-frequency (>1 kHz) alternating current is passed between the outer electrodes and the resulting potential difference is detected by the inner pair. This potential is rectified, smoothed and filtered to record voltage fluctuations which reflect changes in impedance due to respiration and cardiac activity. The cardiac activity is extracted by signal-averaging relative to the ECG R wave. This represents changes in thoracic blood volume and clearly resembles the pulse waveform.

Modern instruments show a modest agreement with invasive measurements of cardiac output, although trends and rapid changes in cardiac output are reliably demonstrated. This method is inaccurate when there are intracardiac shunts or arrhythmias, and underestimates cardiac output in a vasodilated circulation.

MEASUREMENT OF GAS FLOW AND VOLUME

The relationships between volume, flow and velocity are central to understanding gas flow and volume. Flow rate is defined as the volume passing a fixed point in unit time, i.e. volume per second. Integration of a continuous flow signal is the volume that has flowed over a defined period. Velocity is the distance moved by gas molecules in unit time. These are related directly and depend upon the cross-sectional area of flow:

$$Velocity = flow\ rate/area$$

The concept of velocity is important in flow measurement because several instruments measure the velocity of flow and not the flow rate. The velocities of all molecules in a gas or liquid are not the same. Axial streaming is characteristic of laminar flow (Fig. 12.5).

Methods of measuring gas volume and flow are considered in three groups:

- volume measurements
- steady gas flow rates
- unsteady gas flow rates.

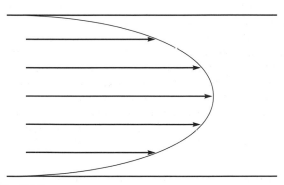

Fig. 12.5
Velocity profile during laminar flow. Velocity is zero at the walls of the containing tube and maximal in the axial stream.

VOLUME MEASUREMENTS

Measurements of gas volume depend on collecting the gases in a calibrated spirometer or passing the gases through some type of gas meter.

Spirometers

Wet spirometers consist of a rigid cylinder suspended over an underwater seal and counterbalanced. Gas entering the bell causes it to rise. This linear displacement is proportional to the volume of gas. Wet spirometers are accurate at steady state and have been used to calibrate other volume-measuring devices. However, they are bulky and inconvenient to use, and the frequency response is damped by friction between the moving parts, causing the instrument to under-read with rapidly changing rates of flow.

Dry spirometers are more convenient for clinical work. Gas displaces a rolling diaphragm or bellows and the expansion is recorded and related to gas volume. The 'Vitalograph' is a specialized type of bellows spirometer used for lung function testing. The patient makes a maximal forced exhalation into the spirometer through a wide-bore tube. The expansion of the wedge-shaped bellows is recorded by a stylus on a pressure-sensitive chart. The stylus moves across the x-axis (time) at a constant rate. The resultant plot represents the volume–time plot of the patient's expiration (Fig. 12.6). The FVC is the maximal volume expired. Understanding of technique and active cooperation of the patient are essential for accurate and precise recordings. The patient must make an airtight seal with the mouthpiece and the nose is occluded with a nose clip. Expiration should be as forcible and rapid as possible. Several attempts are recorded. The highest value measured is recorded because the technique is dependent on voluntary effort, which usually improves with practice.

Gas meters

Dry gas meters are widely used in the gas industry and are used also in medicine, e.g. in some mechanical ventilators, to measure large volumes of gas. Displacement of bellows controls valves which alternately direct gas flow to fill and empty the bellows, and also drives the pointer on a calibrated recording dial. Irregularities within each cycle disappear when the meter has returned to the same position in the cycle; hence, accuracy of measurements improves with increasing multiples of meter volume.

The Dräger volumeter

The volume of gas that flows through the Dräger volumeter is related to the rotation of two light, interlocking, dumbbell-shaped rotors. It is a simple meter and accurate when dry, but is affected by moisture.

The Wright respirometer

This device contains a light mica vane which rotates within a small cylinder (Fig. 12.7). Inflowing air is directed on to the vane by tangential slits. Rotation of the vane drives a gear chain and pointer on a dial. This mechanism is described as inferential because it does not measure either the volume or the flow of all of the gas flowing through the device. It is calibrated for normal tidal volumes and breathing rates by a sine wave pump. However, the meter seriously over-reads at high tidal volumes and under-reads at low tidal volumes because of the inertia of the moving parts.

Integration of the flow signal

The flow signal from a rapidly responding flowmeter may be integrated electronically over time to calculate volume. However, the process of integration exaggerates the effect of baseline drift; a small and insignificant change in the baseline of the flow signal may produce substantial and increasing error in the volume signal over time. This effect is minimized by limiting the duration of integration, e.g. to a single tidal volume by resetting the integrator to zero at the end of each inspiration.

Indirect methods of measuring tidal volume

Methods which depend on measuring inspired or expired gases require a leak-free connection. This is feasible with tracheal intubation. A physiological

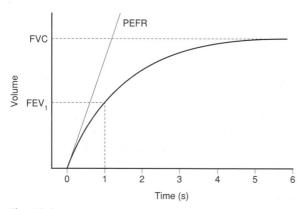

Fig. 12.6
Forced vital capacity (FVC), forced expiratory volume in 1 second (FEV$_1$) and peak expiratory flow rate can all be derived from the volume–time plot (Sykes et al 1991).

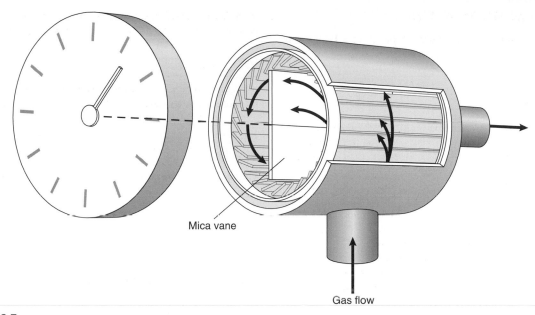

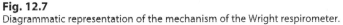

Mica vane

Gas flow

Fig. 12.7
Diagrammatic representation of the mechanism of the Wright respirometer.

mouthpiece and connection to the measuring apparatus may change the pattern of breathing and is suitable only for short-term use. Several indirect methods have been developed which enable tidal volume to be derived from measurements of chest wall movement.

Pneumography

Pneumographs sense changes in chest and abdominal circumference. Non-elastic tapes are placed around the chest and abdomen and the ends are connected to a displacement sensor. The output may be calibrated to provide a tidal volume signal. However, these devices are sensitive to position and require frequent calibration.

Respiratory inductance plethysmography

Respiratory inductance plethysmography uses a wire coil sewn into an elasticated strap. Expansion of the chest or abdomen increases the space between the coils and so alters the inductance generated by a high-frequency alternating (AC) current. The change in inductance depends on the cross-sectional area enclosed by the coil, which is closely related to change in volume. Inductance plethysmography has been used in various physiological studies to monitor postoperative respiratory depression and to detect apnoea.

MEASUREMENT OF GAS FLOW RATE

Volume–time methods

Flow rate may be calculated from spirometric measurements of volume of gas per unit time. These methods are accurate when corrected for temperature and pressure and are used widely to calibrate other flowmeters, but are slow, cumbersome and have limited clinical application.

Most clinical methods are based on the relationship between pressure decrease and flow across a resistance – either a fixed pressure decrease across a variable orifice or a variable pressure change across a fixed orifice.

Variable orifice (constant pressure change) flowmeters

The orifice through which gas flows enlarges with the flow rate so that the pressure difference across the orifice remains constant. This is the physical principle of the Rotameter.

Rotameter

The Rotameter consists of a vertical glass tube inside which rotates a light metal alloy bobbin (Fig. 12.8). The flow of gas is controlled by the fine-adjustment flow

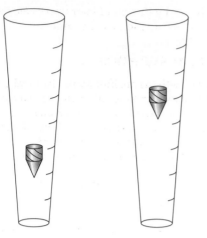

Fig. 12.8
Physical principle of the Rotameter flowmeter. The weight of the bobbin is exactly opposed by the pressure drop across the cross-sectional area of the annular space around the bobbin.

control valve at the bottom of the Rotameter, and when this is opened the pressure of the gas forces the bobbin up the tube. The inside of the tube is shaped like an inverted cone, so that the cross-sectional area of the annular space exactly opposes the downward pressure resulting from the weight of the bobbin. The pressure decrease remains constant throughout the range of flows for which the tube is calibrated and the bobbin rotates freely in the steady stream of gas. Each Rotameter must be calibrated for a specific gas. Laminar flow predominates at low flow rates and depends on the viscosity of gas. Turbulent flow increases at higher flow rates and the density of the gas becomes an important factor. Both density and viscosity of a gas vary with temperature and pressure, and each Rotameter must be calibrated for one specific gas in appropriate conditions.

The peak flowmeter

This useful clinical instrument is capable of measuring flow rates up to $1000\,L\,min^{-1}$. Air flow causes a vane to rotate or a piston to move against the constant force of a light spring. This opens orifices which permit air to escape. The position adopted by the vane or piston depends primarily on the flow rate and on the area of the orifice which must be exposed to the air flow to maintain a constant pressure. The light moving vane or piston rapidly attains a maximum position in response to the peak expiratory flow. It is held in this position by a ratchet. The reading is obtained from a mechanical pointer which is attached to the vane or piston.

Accurate results demand good technique. These devices must be held horizontally to minimize the effects of gravity on the position of the moving parts. The patient must be encouraged to exhale as rapidly as possible. Consistency of repeated recordings suggests maximal effort and the peak expiratory flow rate is the maximum reading recorded.

Variable pressure change (fixed orifice) flowmeters

The resistance is maintained constant so that changes of flow are accompanied by changes in pressure across the resistance element.

Bourdon gauge flowmeter

A Bourdon gauge is used to sense the pressure change across an orifice and is calibrated to the gas flow rate. These rugged meters are not affected by changes in position and are useful for metering the flow from gas cylinders at high ambient pressure. Back-pressure causes over-reading of the actual flow rate.

Pneumotachograph

The pneumotachograph measures flow rate by sensing the pressure change across a small but laminar resistance. Careful design ensures that the differential manometer senses the true lateral pressure exerted by the gas on each side of the resistance element (Fig. 12.9). The differential manometer needs to be very sensitive to record the tiny changes in pressure across the resistance

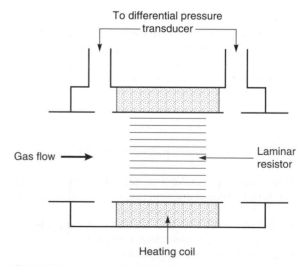

Fig. 12.9
The Fleisch pneumotachograph.

and transduce them to a continuous electrical output. This signal may be integrated to give volume and the manometer must have good zero and gain stability.

Pneumotachographs are sensitive instruments with a rapid response to changing gas flow and are used widely for clinical measurement of gas flows in respiratory and anaesthetic practice. The principles are easy to understand and they are used widely in the clinical measurement of respired gases. However, practical application requires frequent calibration and correction or compensation for differences in temperature, humidity, gas composition and pressure changes during mechanical ventilation.

Other devices for measuring gas flow

Measurements other than pressure change across an orifice have been used to measure flow.

Hot wire flowmeters

These employ the rate of cooling of a heated wire which depends on the gas flow rate and is measured by sensing the change in temperature. It also depends on the thermal conductivity of the gas, which is affected by changes in the gas composition and the presence of water vapour.

Ultrasonic flowmeters

These flowmeters use the vortex-shedding technique. Gas is passed through a tube containing a rod 1–2 mm in diameter, mounted at right angles to the direction of gas flow. Vortices form downstream of the rod, the number of vortices formed being directly related to the flow rate. The vortices are detected using ultrasound and integrated to give a volume signal. Measurement is not affected greatly by temperature, humidity or changes in gas composition. A critical flow rate is required for the formation of vortices and the flowmeter is most accurate when the tidal volume is large.

GAS AND VAPOUR ANALYSIS

Three main applications of gas and vapour analysis are used in anaesthetic practice:

- to establish identity and concentrations of gases and vapours delivered to the patient
- to detect atmospheric pollution
- to assess metabolic or cardiorespiratory function either by analysis of the respired gases (O_2, CO_2

and N_2) or by the use of inert tracer gases such as helium, carbon monoxide or argon.

CHEMICAL METHODS

Chemical methods are important historically for measurement of oxygen and carbon dioxide concentrations. They involve the removal of fractional volumes from the gas phase by chemical reactions to non-gaseous compounds, the fractional concentration being determined by the reduction in volume that occurs:

$$\text{Fractional concentration} = \frac{\text{reduction in gas volume}}{\text{original volume}}$$

Several types of apparatus have been described, e.g. the Haldane. Carbon dioxide is absorbed in a strongly alkaline potassium hydroxide solution. Subsequently, oxygen is absorbed in alkaline pyrogallol or sodium anthraquinone.

PHYSICAL METHODS

In contrast with chemical methods, instruments based on the physical properties of a gas or vapour are convenient, responsive and more suitable for continuous operation.

Speed of response of the system is determined by two components:

- *Transit time* required for the sample to flow along the sampling catheter usually accounts for the greater part of the total delay. It is minimized by using a narrow and short sampling catheter with a rapid sampling flow rate.
- *Response time* required for the instrument to react to the change in gas concentration. It consists of the time required to wash out the analysis cell and delays imposed by the sensing mechanism.

Zero drift and variations in gain are common problems and most gas analysers have to be calibrated frequently, ideally against gas mixtures of known composition.

NON-SPECIFIC METHODS

Non-specific methods use a property of the gas which is common to all gases, but which is possessed by each gas to a differing degree.

Thermal conductivity

A gas with a high thermal conductivity conducts heat more readily than one with a low conductivity. In the katharometer, gas is passed over a heated wire and the degree of cooling of the wire depends on the temperature of the gas, the rate of gas flow and the thermal conductivity of the gas. The reduction in temperature of the wire reduces its resistance and produces an electrical signal related to the gas concentration. In clinical practice, katharometers are usually used for the measurement of CO_2 and He, and as detectors in gas chromatography systems.

Refractive index: interference refractometers

The speed of light slows through transparent materials to a degree determined by the refractive index of that substance. The delay caused by the passage of light through the gas depends on the number of gas molecules present; hence the refractive index also depends on the pressure and temperature of the gas. This extremely small delay is measured using the phase lag by the principle of interference. When light waves from a common source are passed through two linear slits in an opaque sheet and focused onto a screen, an interference pattern is produced. Bright areas where light from the two sources in phase is reinforced alternate with dark bands where the light paths differ in length by half a wavelength, i.e. they are out of phase and attenuating each other. When a gas is introduced into one light path, it delays transmission of the light waves with a reduction in wavelength and an alteration in the position of the dark bands. If the refractive index of the gas is known, the change in position may be related to the number of gas molecules in the light path and hence to the partial pressure of the gas. Interference refractometers are calibrated using known concentrations of gas or vapour. The response is essentially linear and after calibration remains stable.

This method of analysis is used to calibrate flowmeters and vaporizers accurately. Portable devices are useful for monitoring pollution by anaesthetic gases and vapours.

SPECIFIC METHODS

Specific methods identify and measure a gas using some unique property and are particularly suitable for complex mixtures of gases.

Magnetic susceptibility

Most gases are repelled by a magnetic field and are termed diamagnetic. Two unpaired electrons spinning in the same direction in the outer electron shell of the oxygen atom make the molecules strongly paramagnetic, i.e. attracted into a magnetic field.

The first paramagnetic analyser consisted of a cell containing the pole pieces of a permanent magnet. Two small spheres filled with a weakly diamagnetic gas such as nitrogen were connected by a short bridge and suspended by a taut wire in the strongest part of a non-homogeneous magnetic field. Molecules of a paramagnetic gas such as oxygen were attracted to the centre of the magnetic field and displaced the glass spheres with a force related to the concentration of oxygen molecules. This rotational force was detected by a reflected light spot or by the current required by an opposing induction coil to maintain the sensing element in the zero position. Accuracy was high but the mechanism was delicate and the response time slow.

Alternative designs of oxygen analyser are based on the paramagnetic property of oxygen. A fast differential paramagnetic oxygen sensor has been designed on the pneumatic bridge principle. The sample and reference gas are drawn by a common pump through two tubes surrounded by an electromagnet alternating at 110 Hz. Pressure differences between the two tubes are related to the paramagnetic properties of the sample and reference gases. The phasic changes in pressure are extremely small and measured with a miniature microphone. The output of the device is linear, very stable and has a fast response time of less than 150 ms.

Absorption of radiation

All gases absorb electromagnetic radiation in either the infrared or ultraviolet regions of the spectrum. The wavelengths are specific for each gas and depend on the molecular configuration.

Infrared gas analysers

Infrared radiation (1–15 μm) is absorbed by all gases with two or more dissimilar atoms in the molecule. The infrared spectrophotometer uses infrared light dispersed through a prism or diffraction grating into a spectrum of different wavelengths, which is absorbed to different degrees by the gas to be analysed, in a concentration-dependent manner, and the resulting absorption spectrum is specific to the gas. Modern infrared analysers use special photocells to detect and transduce the infrared radiation to a continuous electrical output.

There are several sources of error with infrared analysis:

- The absorption wavebands of different gases may be coincident. For instance, the peak absorption bands for carbon dioxide, nitrous oxide and carbon monoxide are at 4.3, 4.5 and 4.7 μm, respectively, and the absorption spectra inevitably overlap. Error is minimized by narrowing the band of infrared light.

- The phenomenon of 'collision broadening' describes the apparent widening of the absorption spectrum of CO_2 by the physical presence of certain other gases, notably N_2 and N_2O. Correction factors have been described, but the error may be minimized by calibrating the instrument with similar background gas mixtures as the gas to be analysed.
- Absorption is related to the number of molecules in the absorbent gas in the cuvette, i.e. partial pressure. The reading is affected by changes in atmospheric pressure, pressurization of a breathing system or variation in the resistance of the sampling flow line.

Modern CO_2 analysers for clinical use are very stable but require regular calibration of the zero point and scale. Accuracy at normal breathing frequencies also requires a satisfactory response time, typically a 90% or 95% rise time less than 150 ms. Slow response is usually caused by blockage of the sampling line with condensation or sputum, or failure of the suction pump.

Mass spectrometry

Mass spectrometers are capable of separating the components of complex gas mixtures according to their mass and charge by deflecting the charged ions in a magnetic field. Molecules of sample gas are drawn into an evacuated ionization chamber where they are bombarded by a transverse beam of electrons. The positively charged ions then diffuse out of a slit in the chamber wall and are accelerated by a plate to which a negative voltage is applied. A magnetic field from plates or parallel cylindrical rods deflects the ions according to their mass:charge ratio. The ions impinge on a detector in proportion to the partial pressure of the sample gas. Streams of ions of different masses are detected by varying the accelerating and focusing voltages. A mass spectrum is produced by relating the detector output on the y-axis (calibrated to concentration of gas) to the accelerating voltage on the x-axis (calibrated to molecular weight).

Mass spectrometers are bulky and expensive, but have a very short response time (approx. 100 ms for a 95% response) and require very small sample flow rates (approx. $20\,mL\,min^{-1}$). All mass spectrometers operate under conditions of a very high vacuum, which takes time to achieve and must be maintained.

Some molecules may lose two electrons and become doubly charged – they behave like ions with half the mass. Some fragmentation of molecules also occurs in the ionization process, resulting in the production of a mass spectrum rather than a single peak for each molecule. These secondary peaks may be used to advantage, e.g. in the identification and quantification of CO_2 and N_2O, both of which share a parent peak at 44 Da, but produce secondary peaks at 12 and 30 Da, respectively.

Gas–liquid chromatography

Gas–liquid chromatographs achieve separation of the components of a mixture using the principle of partition chromatography. The molecules of a solute partition between two solvents in a way that reflects the balance of attractive and repulsive forces between solute and solvent. One solvent is absorbed onto an inert material such as firebrick granules or a diatomaceous earth. This 'stationary phase' is packed into a narrow, stainless steel or glass tube (up to 2 m long) to form the chromatographic column. The second solvent is a moving stream of gas which flows through the column. The mixture to be analysed is injected as a bolus into this stream of carrier gas and its constituents then partition between the two solvents as the mixture is carried down the column. Components which have a high volatility or low solubility in the stationary phase are eluted before the less volatile or more soluble compounds and are the first to appear at the outlet of the column. Increasing temperature also pushes the partition in favour of the gaseous phase. This speeds the elution of the compound from the column. Careful control of temperature is used to separate two substances which have a similar solubility in the liquid phase, but different volatility.

The various components of the mixture thus emerge at varying intervals after injection and pass to a non-specific detector unit which yields an electronic signal proportional to the quantity of each substance present. Commonly used detectors include katharometers, flame ionization and electron capture detectors. Identification of the source of a deflection produced by a non-specific detector remains a problem in normal practice. Identification of known mixtures may be determined by the retention time for each constituent in the chromatograph column. The combination of a gas chromatograph and mass spectrometer is a particularly powerful analytical tool – the mass spectrometer identifies the molecular fragments present in any component eluted from a chromatograph column.

In addition to gas analysis, the gas–liquid chromatograph may be used to analyse blood samples containing volatile or local anaesthetic agents, anticonvulsants and intravenous anaesthetic drugs.

BLOOD GAS ANALYSIS

THE GLASS pH ELECTRODE

A potential difference is generated across hydrogen ion-sensitive glass depending on the gradient of hydrogen ions. The hydrogen ion concentration within the pH electrode is fixed by a buffer solution, so that the potential across the glass is dependent on the hydrogen ion concentration in the sample (Fig. 12.10).

Measurement of this potential gradient is complicated by the difficulty in making stable electrical contact with the sample and buffer solutions. Two silver:silver chloride electrodes generate an electrode potential, but this is constant at a fixed temperature and provides a stable electrical connection with the buffer solution in the pH electrode, and with a potassium chloride solution in the reference electrode separated from the test sample by a semi-permeable membrane. The potential difference between the electrodes is determined by the pH of the test solution and the temperature, and is calibrated using two phosphate buffers of known and fixed pH. Careful daily calibration is required to maintain accuracy and the electrodes must be regularly cleaned of protein deposits. Reliable measurement of blood pH also depends on the quality of the blood sample, which must be free from air bubbles, heparinized and analysed promptly.

Dissociation of acids and bases is temperature-dependent and the electrodes and blood sampling channel are maintained at 37°C. The measured pH is then corrected to indicate the pH at the temperature of the patient.

THE CO$_2$ ELECTRODE

The main methods of measuring CO$_2$ tension in liquids are based on pH measurement: CO$_2$ equilibrates in solution with hydrogen and bicarbonate ions. A glass pH electrode is in contact with a thin layer of bicarbonate buffer. The buffer is trapped in a nylon mesh spacer and separated by a thin Teflon or silicone membrane which is permeable to CO$_2$ but not to blood cells, plasma or charged ions.

The whole unit is maintained at 37°C. Carbon dioxide diffuses from the blood into the buffer, and so changes the hydrogen ion concentration. The electrode is calibrated by equilibrating the buffer with two known CO$_2$ concentrations to establish the relationship between pH and $P\text{CO}_2$.

OXYGENATION

Oxygenation may be assessed by measuring the tension, saturation or content of oxygen, the relationship between these three measurements being determined by the shape and position of the oxyhaemoglobin dissociation curve. There are many causes of variations in both the shape and position of the curve and it is usually necessary to measure the oxygen tension or saturation directly. Tension measurements are required for most respiratory problems, although saturation or content may be required for calculation of the percentage shunt.

Oxygen tension is usually measured using an oxygen electrode.

Content is measured by vacuum extraction and chemical absorption, by driving the O$_2$ into solution and measuring the increase in $P\text{O}_2$ or by a galvanic cell analyser.

Saturation is determined by photometric techniques, involving the transmission or reflection of light at certain wavelengths.

Oxygen tension

Oxygen electrode: the polarographic method

The oxygen electrode (Clark) consists of a platinum wire, nominally 2 nm in diameter, embedded in a rough-surfaced glass rod. This is immersed in a phosphate buffer which is stabilized with KCl and contained in an outer jacket which incorporates an oxygen-permeable polyethylene or polypropylene membrane (Fig. 12.11). A polarizing voltage of between 600 and 800 mV is applied to the platinum wire and as oxygen diffuses

The pH electrode

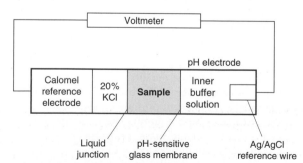

Fig. 12.10
Component parts of the pH electrode. Reproduced from the Radiometer Reference Manual. Permission from Radiometer A/S, Åkandevej 21, DK-2700 Brønshøj, Denmark.

The pO₂ electrode

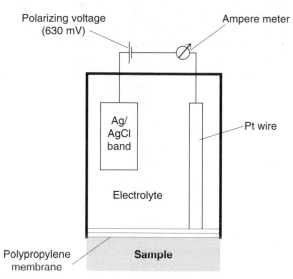

Fig. 12.11
The oxygen electrode. Reproduced from the Radiometer Reference Manual. Permission from Radiometer A/S, Åkandevej 21, DK-2700 Brønshøj, Denmark.

through the membrane electro-oxidoreduction occurs at the cathode:

$$O_2 + 2H_2O + 2e^- = H_2O_2 + 2OH^-$$

Corresponding oxidation occurs at the Ag:AgCl anode:

$$4Ag \rightarrow 4Ag^+ + 4e^-$$

$$4Ag^+ + 4Cl^- \rightarrow 4AgCl$$

Thus a half cell is set up and a tiny current is generated dependent on the oxygen tension at the platinum cathode. The change in current is measured as a change in voltage using the same potentiometric circuit as the pH and $P\text{CO}_2$ measurement systems. The oxygen electrode may be used with gas mixtures or blood. Two-point calibration includes zero with an oxygen-free reference gas or an electronic zero with no electrode output, and the second point with 12% O_2. Temperature control is important and the electrode is maintained at 37°C. Accuracy is compromised by protein deposits or perforation of the delicate plastic membrane which must be regularly inspected. Oxygen continues to be consumed in blood samples which should be taken anaerobically, heparinized and analysed promptly.

Galvanic or fuel cell

Galvanic cells convert energy from an oxidation–reduction chemical process into electrical energy. The potential generated is dependent on the oxygen concentration.

A gold mesh cathode catalyses the reduction of oxygen by reaction with water to hydroxyl ions, while lead is oxidized at the anode. Unlike the oxygen electrode, no battery is required. The reaction in the fuel cell generates a potential gradient. The chemical reaction uses up the components of the cell, so that its life depends on the concentration of oxygen to which it is exposed and on the duration of exposure: in practice, 6–12 months. Fuel cells are widely used in reliable and portable oxygen analysers which incorporate a digital readout and audible alarms. These are cheap and require little maintenance. Inaccurate responses to calibration with oxygen and air suggest that the fuel cell is exhausted and should be replaced.

Transcutaneous electrodes

Transcutaneous electrodes are non-invasive and used extensively for monitoring neonatal blood gas tensions. The electrodes are based on principles similar to those used in blood gas analysers but also incorporate a heating element. The electrode is attached to the skin to form an airtight seal using a contact liquid and the area is heated to 43°C. At this temperature, the blood flow to the skin increases and the capillary oxygen diffuses through the skin, allowing measurement of the diffused gases by the attached electrode. The values obtained from the transcutaneous electrode are lower than those from a simultaneous arterial specimen. Many factors affect the transcutaneous measurement of oxygen tension, including the skin site and thickness. Most importantly, the electrode depends on local capillary blood flow and reads low with hypotension and microcirculatory perfusion failure. Problems occur with surgical diathermy; the heating current circuit provides a return path for the cutting current which may cause the transcutaneous electrode to overheat.

Other methods of measuring oxygen tension in blood include mass spectrometry and optodes, which employ the quenching of fluorescence from illuminated dye.

Oxygen content

The total amount of oxygen in blood may be measured directly, but this is technically demanding and rarely used. The van Slyke technique uses a chemical and volumetric or manometric analysis of oxygen content.

Oxygen is driven from a small sample by denaturing the haemoglobin with acid. The volume of gas at atmospheric pressure, or the pressure at constant volume, is recorded before and after the chemical absorption of oxygen. The change is related directly to the oxygen content of the fixed volume of blood. Alternative detectors have been used to measure oxygen displaced from haemoglobin, e.g. a galvanic cell.

These time-consuming and operator-dependent laboratory techniques have been replaced by calculation of oxygen content from measurements of the oxygen saturation of haemoglobin, haemoglobin concentration and the tension of oxygen in blood:

Oxygen content of blood (mL dL^{-1})

$$= [So_2 (\%) \times Hb (g\,dL^{-1}) \times 1.34] + [0.0225 \times Po_2 (kPa)]$$

Accurate estimates require that the oxygen saturation of haemoglobin is measured directly, and not calculated from oxygen tension and an arbitrary but unmeasured oxyhaemoglobin dissociation curve.

Oximetry: measurement of oxygen saturation

In vitro oximetry

Oximetry relies on the differing absorption of light at different wavelengths by the various states of haemoglobin. The absorption of radiation passing through a sample is measured. The degree of absorption of light, defined by the ratio of incident to emergent light intensities on a logarithmic scale, is proportional to the concentration of the molecules absorbing light (Beer's law) and the thickness of the absorbing layer (Lambert's law).

Oxyhaemoglobin and deoxyhaemoglobin differ at both the red and infrared portions of the spectrum (Fig. 12.12). The differential absorption of two wavelengths of red and infrared light permits the calculation of the ratio of the concentration of oxygenated and reduced haemoglobins. Additional wavelengths are added in co-oximeters for the calculation of the proportions of other species of haemoglobin, such as carboxyhaemoglobin and methaemoglobin, and the absolute absorbance is used to estimate total haemoglobin concentration from the sum of the various haemoglobins. This is important in measurements of oxyhaemoglobin for use in the calculation of oxygen content.

Commercial co-oximeters draw a small blood sample which is haemolysed before entering a cuvette. Light is filtered to produce monochromatic beams, shone through the cuvette and detected by a photocell. The absorption by the sample is the difference in the intensity of both incident and transmitted light and both must be measured. Spectrophotometers apply a double-beam technique which improves the accuracy and precision. Light from the monochromator is split into two beams, which pass through the test sample or a reference sample. Photocells generate two signals corresponding to the sample and the reference light intensities. Electronic processing compares the two signals and generates an output proportional to the difference. This greatly improves the signal-to-noise ratio because any variation which affects both the sample and reference beams equally is ignored and the difference remains constant.

The saturation of mixed venous blood may be measured using an oximeter incorporated into a pulmonary

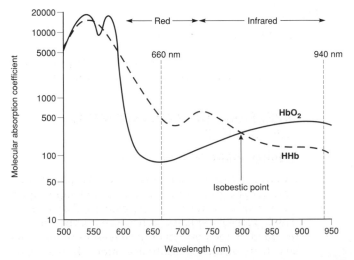

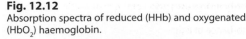

Fig. 12.12
Absorption spectra of reduced (HHb) and oxygenated (HbO$_2$) haemoglobin.

artery catheter. Fibreoptic cables transmit incident light of at least two wavelengths, and reflected light from red blood cells back to a detector.

The same spectrophotometric principles used by co-oximeters in vitro on haemolysed blood samples have been applied to patients in vivo.

Pulse oximetry

Light transmitted through tissues is absorbed not only by arterial blood but also by other tissue pigments and venous blood. However, the variation in light absorption with each pulse beat results almost entirely from pulsatile arterial blood flow. Two light-emitting diodes – red (660 nm) and infrared (940 nm) – shine light through a finger or earlobe and a photocell detects the transmitted light. The output of the sensor is processed to display a pulse waveform and the arterial oxygen saturation.

To identify the absorption at each wavelength, the light emitting diodes are switched on and off at 30 Hz to detect the cyclical changes in the signal due to pulsatile arterial blood flow. The electrical output from the photodetector consists of a steady (DC) signal which depends on the strength of the light source and absorption by the tissues and by the arterial, venous and capillary blood. On this is superimposed a pulsatile (AC) signal resulting from absorbance associated with the greater volume of blood in the light path with each pulse wave (Fig. 12.13). These raw signals require complex processing. The AC level is scaled relative to the DC component so that it is no longer a function of the incident light intensity. The ratio of the amplitude of the red and infrared pulsatile signals is related to

arterial saturation using an algorithm which is non-linear and derived from empirical measurements.

Several important sources of error are common in the measurement of pulse oximetry:

- The AC signal sensed by the pulse oximeter is less than 5% of the DC signal when the pulse volume is normal. Inadequate signals are caused by vasoconstriction or poor perfusion from whatever cause. Modern instruments display a continuous waveform and include algorithms which warn of inadequate pulsation or probe misplacement.
- Errors in measurement are underestimated. Calibration points in the range 80–100% are derived from volunteer studies and values below this are extrapolated and unreliable. Accuracy within the working range is ±3%, and the variability between different instruments is significantly higher.
- The response time is slow and includes two separate components: instrument delay and circulatory delay. Instrument delay is caused by averaging times of 10–15 s which are designed to improve reliability. Circulatory delay depends on the distribution of blood from the lungs to the tissues. Response time at the fingertip may exceed 1 min in normal subjects, and is exaggerated by low cardiac output or vasoconstriction.
- Having only two transmitted wavelengths does not permit pulse oximeters to differentiate oxyhaemoglobin from other species of haemoglobin, especially carboxyhaemoglobin and methaemoglobin. Dyes, including methylene blue and bilirubin, may also cause interference.

THERMOMETRY

Several temperature-dependent phenomena have been incorporated in commercial thermometers.

DIRECT READING NON-ELECTRICAL THERMOMETERS

Liquid expansion thermometers

Liquid expansion thermometers are simple, reliable instruments. A glass bulb is filled with a liquid (generally alcohol or mercury) and connected to an evacuated, closed capillary tube. The temperature is recorded by the position of the meniscus in the capillary tube against a calibrated scale. If the cross-

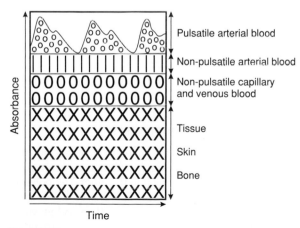

Fig. 12.13
Schematic representation of the contribution of pulsatile arterial blood, non-pulsatile blood and tissues to the absorbance of light.

sectional area of the capillary tube is constant, movement of the meniscus with changing temperature is linear.

Several simple and elegant design features improve usability. A large bulb and very narrow capillary increase the sensitivity. Visibility of the narrow capillary is improved by shaping the thermometer so that the glass forms a lens and by incorporating a strip of white glass behind the capillary. A constriction in the capillary tube permits the mercury to expand but hinders its return to the bulb so that the reading is preserved until the mercury is shaken down. However, glass thermometers are fragile. A large thermal capacity results in a slow response. The instrument is hand-held, awkward to read and reset, and cannot be used for remote measurement or recording.

Dial thermometers

Dial thermometers exploit the increase in pressure caused by the temperature-dependent expansion of a liquid or gas in an enclosed cavity. This is sensed by a Bourdon pressure gauge and recorded on a dial. Although cheap and robust, they are relatively inaccurate, slow to respond and are only suitable for large temperature changes in heated equipment, e.g. autoclaves.

Bimetallic strip thermometers

If strips of two metals with different coefficients of expansion are fastened together throughout their length, the combined strip will bend when heated. Sensitivity is improved by using a long strip which is usually bent in a spiral or coil, with one end fixed and the other connected to a recording pointer. This technique is used for temperature compensation in some anaesthetic vaporizers, and in cheap mechanical thermometers for measuring air temperature.

CHEMICAL THERMOMETERS

Thermometers based on temperature-dependent changes in chemical mixtures have been marketed. Reversible chemical thermometers contain several cells filled with liquid crystals, each of slightly different composition. At a critical temperature, the optical properties change because of realignment of the molecules, causing reflection instead of absorption of the incident light. An alternative technique consists of rows of cells filled with chemical mixtures which melt at specific temperatures releasing a dye; this single-use, disposable design prevents cross-infection but is relatively expensive.

INFRARED THERMOMETERS

The amount of infrared radiation emitted by the tympanic membrane depends on its temperature, emissivity compared to a black body at the same temperature and the Stefan–Boltzmann constant. Infrared tympanic membrane thermometers based on this principle are in common clinical use.

REMOTE READING INSTRUMENTS

Temperature-dependent electrical properties may be incorporated into thermometers suitable for automation.

Resistance-wire thermometers

Resistance-wire thermometers are based on the principle that the resistance of certain metal wires increases as their temperature increases. Platinum resistance thermometers have a large temperature coefficient of resistance and are very sensitive to small changes in temperature, but are fragile and slow to respond. Single-use probes which incorporate a tiny copper element have been marketed with an acceptable clinical accuracy and response time.

Thermistor thermometers

Thermistors are semiconductors made from the fused oxides of heavy metals such as cobalt, manganese and nickel. They demonstrate marked and non-linear variation in resistance with temperature, which is usually compensated by electronic processing. Disadvantages include inconsistent variation between individual thermistors, change in resistance over time, and hysteresis during rapid heating and cooling. However, the large temperature coefficient permits the detection of small temperature changes and the tiny 'pin-head' size results in a rapid response. They are used widely in invasive temperature monitoring, e.g. in pulmonary artery catheters.

Thermocouple thermometers

If two dissimilar metals are joined to create an electrical circuit and the junctions are at different temperatures, a current flows from one metal to the other. The potential difference that is generated is a function of the temperature difference between the two junctions. All junctions made from the same metals have identical properties. The reference junction must be kept at a constant temperature, or incorporate temperature compensation into the measurement. Common combinations of metals include copper–constantan or platinum–rhodium. The output is small (about 40 mV per °C temperature difference between the junctions), but this is sufficient to be sensed by a galvanometer.

FURTHER READING

Cruikshank S 1998 Mathematics and statistics in anaesthesia. Oxford Medical Publications, Oxford

Kenny G, Davis PD 2003 Basic physics and measurement in anaesthesia, 5th edn. Butterworth-Heinemann, Oxford

Sykes M K, Vickers M D, Hull C J 1991 Principles of clinical measurement, 3rd edn. Blackwell Scientific Publications, Oxford

13 Anaesthetic apparatus

Anaesthetists must have a sound understanding and firm knowledge of the functioning of all anaesthetic equipment in common use. Although primary malfunction of equipment has not featured highly in surveys of anaesthetic-related morbidity and mortality, failure to understand the use of equipment and failure to check equipment prior to use feature in these reports as a cause of morbidity and mortality. This is true especially of ventilators, where lack of knowledge regarding the function of equipment may result in a patient being subjected to the dangers of hypoxaemia and/or hypercapnia.

It is essential that anaesthetists check that all equipment is functioning correctly before they proceed to anaesthetize patients (see Ch. 14). In some respects, the routine of testing anaesthetic equipment resembles the airline pilot's checklist, which is an essential preliminary to aircraft flight.

The purpose of this chapter is to describe briefly apparatus which is used in delivery of gases, from the sources of supply to the patient's lungs. Clearly, it is not possible to describe in detail equivalent models produced by all manufacturers. Consequently, this chapter concentrates only on principles and some equipment which is used commonly.

It is convenient to describe anaesthetic apparatus sequentially from the supply of gases to point of delivery to the patient. This sequence is shown in Table 13.1.

GAS SUPPLIES

BULK SUPPLY OF ANAESTHETIC GASES

In the majority of modern hospitals, piped medical gases and vacuum (PMGV) systems have been installed. These obviate the necessity for holding large numbers of cylinders in the operating theatre suite. Normally, only a few cylinders are kept in reserve, attached usually to the anaesthetic machine.

The advantages of the PMGV system are reductions in cost, in the necessity to transport cylinders and in accidents caused by cylinders becoming exhausted. However, there have been several well-publicized incidents in which anaesthetic morbidity or mortality has resulted from incorrect connections in piped medical gas supplies.

The PMGV services comprise five sections:

- bulk store
- distribution pipelines in the hospital
- terminal outlets, situated usually on the walls or ceilings of the operating theatre suite and other sites
- flexible hoses connecting the terminal outlets to the anaesthetic machine
- connections between flexible hoses and anaesthetic machines.

Responsibility for the first three items lies with the engineering and pharmacy departments. Within the operating theatre, it is partly the anaesthetist's responsibility to check the correct functioning of the last two items.

BULK STORE

Oxygen

In small hospitals, oxygen may be supplied to the PMGV from a bank of several oxygen cylinders attached to a manifold.

Oxygen cylinder manifolds consist of two groups of large cylinders (size J). The two groups alternate in supplying oxygen to the pipelines. In both groups, all cylinder valves are open so that they empty simultaneously. All cylinders have non-return valves. The supply automatically changes from one group to the other when the first group of cylinders is nearly empty. The changeover also activates an electrical signalling system which alerts staff to change the empty cylinders.

However, in larger hospitals, pipeline oxygen originates from a liquid oxygen store. Liquid oxygen is stored at a temperature of approximately −165°C at 10.5 bar in a giant Thermos flask – a vacuum insulated evaporator (VIE). Some heat passes from the environ-

Table 13.1   Classification of anaesthetic equipment described in this chapter

Supply of gases:
   From outside the operating theatre
   From cylinders within the operating theatre, together with the connections involved

The anaesthetic machine:
   Unions
   Cylinders
   Reducing valves
   Flowmeters
   Vaporizers

Safety features of the anaesthetic machine

Anaesthetic breathing systems

Ventilators

Apparatus used in scavenging waste anaesthetic gases

Apparatus used in interfacing the patient to the anaesthetic breathing system:
   Laryngoscopes
   Tracheal tubes
   Catheter mounts and connectors

Accessory apparatus for the airway:
   Anaesthetic masks and airways
   Forceps
   Laryngeal sprays
   Bougies
   Mouth gags
   Stilettes
   Suction apparatus

ment through the insulating layer between the two shells of the flask, increasing the tendency to evaporation and pressure increase within the chamber. Pressure is maintained constant by transfer of gaseous oxygen into the pipeline system (via a warming device). However, if the pressure increases above 17 bar (1700 kPa), a safety valve opens and oxygen runs to waste. When the supply of oxygen resulting from the slow evaporation from the surface in the VIE is inadequate, the pressure decreases and a valve opens to allow liquid oxygen to pass into an evaporator, from which gas passes into the pipeline system.

Liquid oxygen plants are housed some distance away from hospital buildings because of the risk of fire. Even when a hospital possesses a liquid oxygen plant, it is still necessary to hold reserve banks of oxygen cylinders in case of supply failure.

Oxygen concentrators

Recently, oxygen concentrators have been used to supply hospitals and it is likely that the use of these devices will increase in future. The oxygen concentrator depends upon the ability of an artificial zeolight to entrap molecules of nitrogen. These devices cannot produce pure oxygen, but the concentration usually exceeds 90%; the remainder comprises nitrogen, argon and other inert gases. Small oxygen concentrators are provided for domiciliary use.

Nitrous oxide

Nitrous oxide and Entonox may be supplied from banks of cylinders connected to manifolds similar to those used for oxygen.

Medical compressed air

Compressed air is supplied from a bank of cylinders into the PMGV system. Air of medical quality is required, as industrial compressed air may contain fine particles of oil.

Piped medical vacuum

Piped medical vacuum is provided by large vacuum pumps which discharge via a filter and silencer to a suitable point, usually at roof level, where gases are vented to atmosphere. Although concern has been expressed regarding the possibility of volatile anaesthetic agents dissolving in the lubricating oil of vacuum pumps and causing malfunction, this fear has not been substantiated.

TERMINAL OUTLETS

There has been standardization of terminal outlets in the UK since 1978, but there is no universal standard.

Six types of terminal outlet are found commonly in the operating theatre. The terminals are colour-coded and also have non-interchangeable connections specific to each gas:

- Vacuum (coloured yellow) – a vacuum of at least 53 kPa (400 mmHg) should be maintained at the outlet, which should be able to take a free flow of air of at least 40 L min^{-1}.

- Compressed air (coloured white/black) at 4 bar – this is used for anaesthetic breathing systems and ventilators.
- Air (coloured white/black) at 7 bar – this is to be used only for powering compressed air tools and is confined usually to the orthopaedic operating theatre.
- Nitrous oxide (coloured blue) at 4 bar.
- Oxygen (coloured white) at 4 bar.
- Scavenging – there is a variety of scavenging outlets from the operating theatre. The passive systems are designed to accept a standard 30-mm connection.

Whenever a new pipeline system has been installed or servicing of an existing pipeline system has been undertaken, a designated member of the pharmacy staff should test the gas obtained from the sockets, using an oxygen analyser. Malfunction of an oxygen/air mixing device may result in entry of compressed air into the oxygen pipeline, rendering an anaesthetic mixture hypoxic. Because of this and other potential mishaps, it has been advocated that oxygen analysers be used routinely during anaesthesia.

GAS SUPPLIES

Gas supplies to the anaesthetic machine should be checked at the beginning of each session to ensure that the gas which issues from the pipeline or cylinder is the same as that which passes through the appropriate flowmeter. This ensures that pipelines are not connected incorrectly. Both the machine in the operating theatre and that in the anaesthetic room should be checked. Checking of anaesthetic machine and medical gas supplies is discussed fully in Chapter 14.

CYLINDERS

Modern cylinders are constructed from molybdenum steel. They are checked at intervals by the manufacturer to ensure that they can withstand hydraulic pressures considerably in excess of those to which they are subjected in normal use. One cylinder in every 100 is cut into strips to test the metal for tensile strength, flattening impact and bend tests. Medical gas cylinders are tested hydraulically every 5 years and the tests recorded by a mark stamped on the neck of the cylinder.

The cylinders are provided in a variety of sizes, and colour-coded according to the gas supplied. The cylinders comprise a body and a shoulder containing threads into which are fitted a pin index valve block, a bull-nosed valve or a handwheel valve.

The pin index system was devised to prevent interchangeability of cylinders of different gases. Pin index valves are provided for the smaller cylinders of oxygen and nitrous oxide (and also carbon dioxide) which may be attached to anaesthetic machines. The pegs on the inlet connection slot into corresponding holes on the cylinder valve.

Full cylinders are supplied usually with a plastic dust cover in order to prevent contamination by dirt. This cover should not be removed until immediately before the cylinder is fitted to the anaesthetic machine. When fitting the cylinder to a machine, the yoke is positioned and tightened with the handle of the yoke spindle. After fitting, the cylinder should be opened to make sure that it is full and that there are no leaks at the gland nut or the pin index valve junction, caused, for example, by absence of or damage to the washer. The washer used is normally a Bodok seal which has a metal periphery designed to keep the seal in good condition for a long period.

Cylinder valves should be opened slowly to prevent sudden surges of pressure and should be closed with no more force than is necessary, otherwise the valve seating may be damaged.

The sealing material between the valve and the neck of the cylinder may be constructed from a fusable material which melts in the event of fire and allows the contents of the cylinder to escape around the threads of the joint.

The colour codes used for medical gas cylinders in the United Kingdom are shown in Table 13.2 and cylinder sizes and capacities are shown in Table 13.3.

THE ANAESTHETIC MACHINE

The anaesthetic machine comprises:

- a means of supplying gases either from attached cylinders or from piped medical supplies via appropriate unions on the machine
- methods of measuring flow rate of gases
- apparatus for vaporizing volatile anaesthetic agents
- breathing systems and a ventilator for delivery of gases and vapours from the machine to the patient
- apparatus for scavenging anaesthetic gases in order to minimize environmental pollution.

SUPPLY OF GASES

In the UK, gases are supplied at a pipeline pressure of 4 bar (400 kPa, 60 lb in^{-2}) and this pressure is transferred directly to the bank of flowmeters and back bar

Table 13.2 Medical gas cylinders used in the UK

	Colour		Pressure at 15°C		
	Body	Shoulder	lb in^{-2}	kPa	bar
Oxygen	Black	White	1987	13700	137
Nitrous oxide	Blue	Blue	638	4400	44
CO$_2$	Grey	Grey	725	5000	50
Helium	Brown	Brown	1987	13700	137
Air	Grey	White/black quarters	1987	13700	137
O$_2$/helium	Black	White/brown quarters	1987	13700	137
N$_2$O/O$_2$ (Entonox)	Blue	White/blue quarters	1987	13700	137

Table 13.3 Medical gas cylinder sizes and capacities by cylinder size (A–J) and height (inches)

	Capacities (L)							
	A/10 in	B/10 in	C/14 in	D/18 in	E/31 in	F/34 in	G/49 in	J/57 in
Oxygen			170	340	680	1360	3400	6800
Nitrous oxide			450	900	1800	3600	9000	
CO$_2$			450	900	1800			
Helium				300		1200		
Air							3200	6400
O$_2$/helium					600	1200		
O$_2$/CO$_2$						1360	3400	
Entonox							3200	6400

of the anaesthetic machine. The flexible colour-coded hoses connect the pipeline outlets to the anaesthetic machine. The anaesthetic machine end of the hoses should be permanently fixed using a nut and liner union where the thread is gas-specific and non-interchangeable. The non-interchangeable screw thread (NIST) is the British Standard.

The gas issuing from other medical gas cylinders is at a much higher pressure, necessitating the interposition of a pressure regulator between the cylinder and the bank of flowmeters. In some older anaesthetic machines (and in some other countries), the pressure in the pipelines of the anaesthetic machine may be 3 bar (300 kPa, 45 lb in^{-2}).

PRESSURE GAUGES

Pressure gauges measure the pressure in the cylinders or pipeline. The anaesthetic machines have pressure gauges for oxygen, air and nitrous oxide. These are mounted usually on the front panel of the anaesthetic machine.

PRESSURE REGULATORS

Pressure regulators are used on anaesthetic machines for three purposes:

- to reduce the high pressure of gas in a cylinder to a safe working level
- to prevent damage to equipment on the anaesthetic machine, e.g. flow control valves
- as the contents of the cylinder are used, the pressure within the cylinder decreases and the regulating mechanism maintains a constant outlet pressure, obviating the necessity to make continuous adjustments to the flowmeter controls.

The principles underlying the operation of flowmeters are described in detail in Chapters 11 and 12.

Flow restrictors

Pressure regulators are omitted usually when anaesthetic machines are supplied directly from a pipeline at a pressure of 4 bar. Changes in pipeline pressure would cause changes in flow rate, necessitating adjustment of the flow control valves. This is prevented by the use of a flow restrictor upstream of the flowmeter (flow restrictors are simply constrictions in the low-pressure circuit).

A different type of flow restrictor may be fitted also to the downstream end of the vaporizers to prevent back-pressure effects (see Ch. 11). The absence of such a flow restrictor may be detected if a ventilator such as the Manley is used, as this leads to fluctuations in the positions of the flowmeter bobbins during the respiratory cycle.

Pressure relief valves on regulators

Pressure relief valves are often fitted on the downstream side of regulators to allow escape of gas if the regulators were to fail (thereby causing a high output pressure). Relief valves are set usually at approximately 7 bar for regulators designed to give an output pressure of 4 bar.

FLOWMETERS

The principles of flowmeters are described in detail in Chapters 11 and 12.

Problems with flowmeters

- *Non-vertical tube.* This causes a change in shape of the annulus and therefore variation in flow. If the

bobbin touches the side of the tube, resulting friction causes an even more inaccurate reading.
- *Static electricity.* This may cause inaccuracy (by as much as 35%) and sticking of the bobbin, especially at low flows. This may be reduced by coating the inside of the tube with a transparent film of gold or tin.
- *Dirt* on the bobbin may cause sticking or alteration in size of the annulus and therefore inaccuracies.
- *Back-pressure.* Changes in accuracy may be produced by back-pressure. For example, the Manley ventilator may exert a back-pressure and depress the bobbin; there may be as much as 10% more gas flow than that indicated on the flowmeter. Similar problems may be produced by the insertion of any equipment which restricts flow downstream, e.g. Selectatec head, vaporizer.
- *Leakage.* This results usually from defects in the top sealing washer of a flowmeter.

It is unfortunate that in the UK the standard position of the oxygen flowmeters is on the left followed by either nitrous oxide or air (if all three gases are supplied). On several recorded occasions, patients have suffered damage from hypoxia because of leakage from a broken flowmeter tube in this type of arrangement, as oxygen, being at the upstream end, passes out to the atmosphere through any leak. This problem is reduced if the oxygen flowmeter is placed downstream (i.e. on the right-hand side of the bank of flowmeters) as is standard practice in the USA. In the UK, this problem is now avoided by designing the outlet from the oxygen flowmeter to enter the back bar downstream from the outlets of other flowmeters (Fig. 13.1). Most modern anaesthetic machines do not have a flowmeter for carbon dioxide.

The emergency oxygen flush is a non-locking button which, when pressed, delivers pure oxygen from the anaesthetic outlet. On modern anaesthetic machines, the emergency oxygen flush lever is situated downstream from the flowmeters and vaporizers. A flow of about 35–45 L min^{-1} at pipeline pressure is delivered. This may lead to dilution of the anaesthetic mixture with excess oxygen if the emergency oxygen tap is opened partially by mistake and may result in awareness. There is also a risk of barotrauma should the high pressure be accidentally delivered directly to the patient's lungs.

Quantiflex

The Quantiflex mixer flowmeter (Fig. 13.2) eliminates the possibility of reducing the oxygen supply inadvertently. One dial is set to the desired percentage of

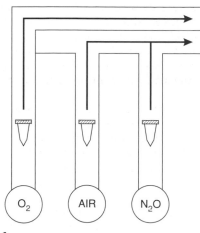

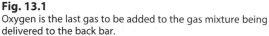

Fig. 13.1
Oxygen is the last gas to be added to the gas mixture being delivered to the back bar.

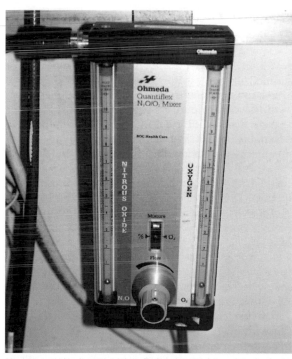

Fig. 13.2
A Quantiflex flowmeter. The required oxygen percentage is selected using the dial, and total flow of the oxygen/nitrous oxide mixture is adjusted using the grey knob.

oxygen and the total flow rate is adjusted independently. The oxygen passes through a flowmeter to provide evidence of correct functioning of the linked valves. Both gases arrive via linked pressure-reducing regulators. The Quantiflex is useful in particular for varying the volume of fresh gas flow (FGF) from

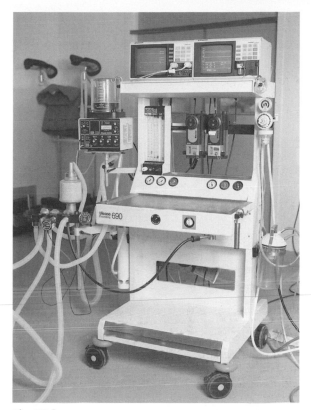

Fig. 13.3
A Blease Frontline anaesthetic machine.

moment to moment whilst keeping the proportions constant. In addition, the oxygen flowmeter is situated downstream of the nitrous oxide flowmeter.

Linked flowmeters

The majority of modern anaesthetic machines such as that shown in Figure 13.3 possess a mechanical linkage between the N_2O and O_2 flowmeters. This causes the N_2O flow to decrease if the oxygen flowmeter is adjusted to give less than 25–30% O_2 (Fig. 13.4).

VAPORIZERS

The principles of vaporizers are described in detail in Chapter 11.

Modern vaporizers may be classified as:

- *Drawover vaporizers.* These have a very low resistance to gas flow and may be used for emergency use in the field (e.g. Oxford miniature vaporizer) or in developing countries (e.g. EMO vaporizer) (Figs 13.5–13.7).

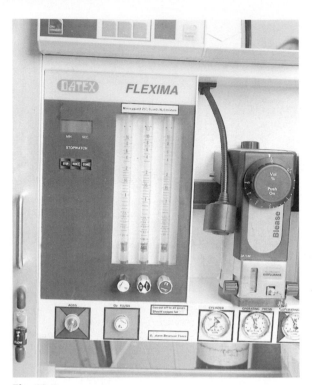

Fig. 13.4
Flowmeters with mechanical linkage between nitrous oxide and oxygen.

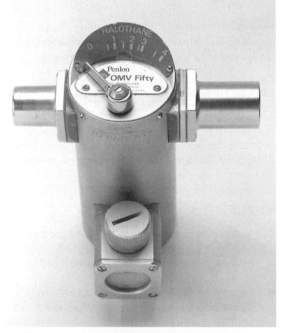

Fig. 13.5
Oxford miniature vaporizer (OMV).

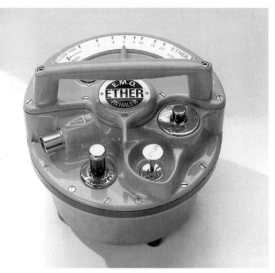

Fig. 13.6
The EMO (Epstein and Macintosh of Oxford) drawover ether vaporizer. A cutaway diagram is shown in Figure 13.7.

- *Plenum vaporizers.* These are intended for unidirectional gas flow, have a relatively high resistance to flow and are unsuitable for use either as drawover vaporizers or in a circle system. Examples include the 'TEC' type in which there is a variable bypass flow. Commonly used types of equipment are shown in Figures 13.8 and 13.9.

Methods of temperature regulation include a bimetallic strip (TEC) and bellows (EMO).

There has been more than one model of the 'TEC' type of vaporizer. The TEC Mark 2 vaporizer is now obsolete. The TEC Mark 3 had characteristics which were an improvement on the Mark 2. These included improved vaporization as a result of increased area of the wicks, reduced pumping effect by having a long tube through which the vaporized gas leaves the vaporizing chamber, improved accuracy at low gas flows and a bimetallic strip which is situated in the bypass channel and not the vaporizing chamber. In the Mark 4 the improvements were as follows: no spillage into the bypass channel if the vaporizer is accidentally inverted and the inability to turn two vaporizers on at the same time when they are on the back bar of the anaesthetic machine. The TEC Mark 5 vaporizer (Fig. 13.9) has improved surface area for vaporization in the chamber, improved key-filling action and an easier mechanism for switching on the rotary valve and lock with one hand.

Desflurane presents a particular challenge as it has a saturated vapour pressure of 664 mmHg at 20°C and

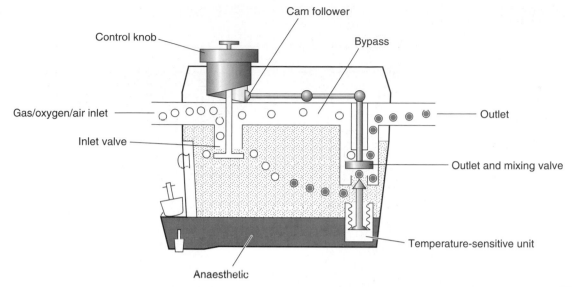

Fig. 13.7
Working principles of the EMO vaporizer. The water jacket provides a heat sink to reduce the decrease in temperature during vaporization. Temperature compensation is provided by a valve operated by bellows, filled with ether vapour. When the control lever is moved to the 'closed' position, the ether chamber is sealed to prevent spillage during transit.

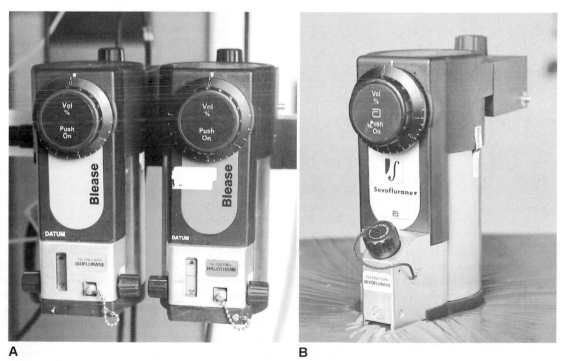

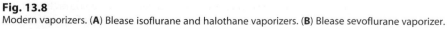

Fig. 13.8
Modern vaporizers. (**A**) Blease isoflurane and halothane vaporizers. (**B**) Blease sevoflurane vaporizer.

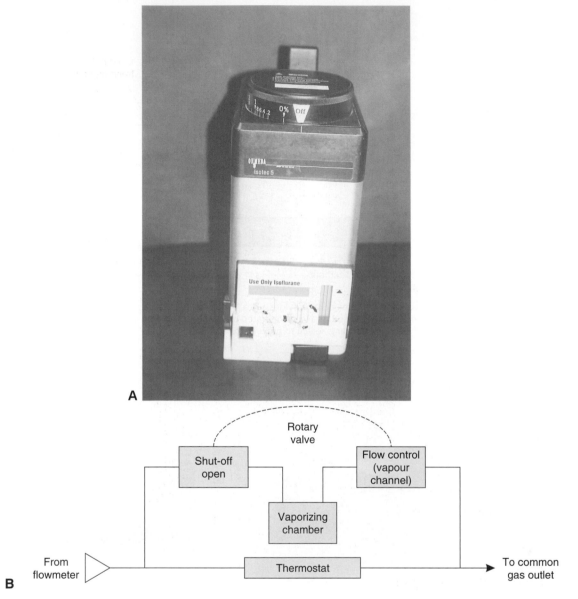

Fig. 13.9
(**A**) A Mark 5 TEC vaporizer. (**B**) Schematic diagram of the TEC Mark 5 vaporizer.

Continued

a boiling point of 23.5°C. In order to combat this problem, a new vaporizer, the TEC 6, was developed (Fig. 13.10). It is heated electrically to 39°C with a pressure of 1550 mmHg (approx. 2 atmospheres). The vaporizer has electronic monitors of vaporizer function and alarms. The FGF does not enter the vaporization chamber. Instead, desflurane vapour enters into the path of the FGF. A percentage control dial regulates the flow of desflurane vapour into the FGF. The dial calibration is from 1% to 18%. The vaporizer has a

back-up 9 volt battery should there be a mains failure. The functioning of the vaporizer is shown diagrammatically in Figure 13.11.

Anaesthetic-specific connections are available to link the supply bottle (container of liquid anaesthetic agent) to the appropriate vaporizer (Fig. 13.12). These connections reduce the extent of spillage (and thus atmospheric pollution) and also the likelihood of filling the vaporizer with an inappropriate liquid. In addition to being designed specifically for each liquid,

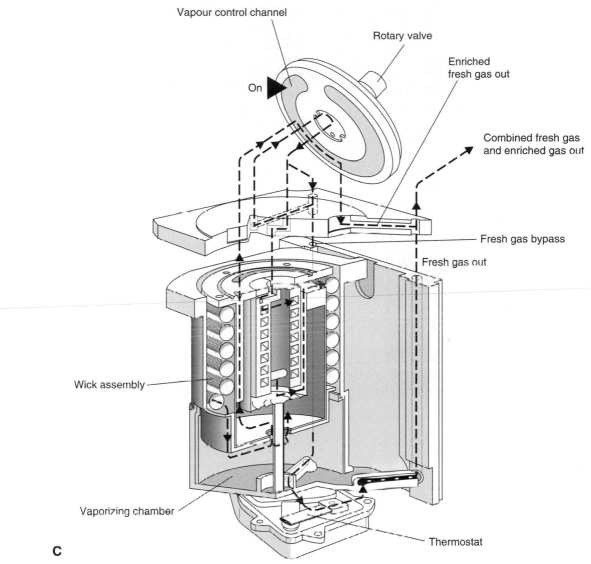

Vapour control channel

Rotary valve

Enriched
fresh gas out

On

Combined fresh gas
and enriched gas out

Fresh gas bypass

Fresh gas out

Wick assembly

Vaporizing chamber

Thermostat

C

Fig. 13.9 — Cont'd
(**C**) Diagram of the TEC Mark 5 vaporizer.

the connections themselves may be colour-coded (e.g. purple for isoflurane, yellow for sevoflurane, orange for enflurane, red for halothane).

Halothane contains a non-volatile stabilizing agent (0.01% thymol) to prevent breakdown of the halothane by heat and ultraviolet light. Thymol is less volatile than halothane and its concentration in the vaporizer increases as halothane is vaporized. If the vaporizer is used and refilled regularly, the concentration of thymol may become sufficiently high to impair vaporization of halothane. In addition, very high concentrations may result in a significant degree of thymol vaporization, which may be harmful to the patient. Consequently, it is

recommended that halothane vaporizers are drained once every 2 weeks. Enflurane and isoflurane vaporizers require to be emptied at much less frequent intervals.

SAFETY FEATURES OF MODERN ANAESTHETIC MACHINES

- Specificity of probes on flexible hoses between terminal outlets and connections with the anaesthetic machine. The flexible hoses are colour-coded.

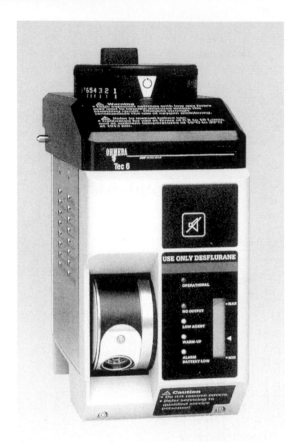

Fig. 13.10
The TEC 6 desflurane vaporizer.

- Pin index system to prevent incorrect attachment of gas cylinders to anaesthetic machine. Cylinders are colour-coded and they are labelled with the name of the gas that they contain.
- Pressure relief valves on the downstream side of pressure regulators.
- Flow restrictors on the upstream side of flowmeters.
- Arrangement of the bank of flowmeters such that the oxygen flowmeter is on the right (i.e. downstream side) or oxygen is the last gas to be added to the gas mixture being delivered to the back bar (Fig. 13.1).
- Non-return valves. Sometimes a single regulator and contents meter is used both for cylinders in use and for the reserve cylinder. When one cylinder runs out, the presence of a non-return valve prevents the empty cylinder from being refilled by the reserve cylinder and also enables the empty

cylinder to be removed and replaced without interrupting the supply of gas to the patient.
- Pressure gauges indicate the pressures in the pipelines and the cylinders.
- An oxygen bypass valve (emergency oxygen) delivers oxygen directly to a point downstream of the vaporizers. When operated, the oxygen bypass should give a flow rate of at least 35 L min^{-1}.
- Mounting of vaporizers on the back bar. There is concern about contamination of vaporizers if two vaporizers are turned on at the same time. Temperature-compensated vaporizers contain wicks and these can absorb a considerable amount of anaesthetic agent. If two vaporizers are mounted in series, the downstream vaporizer could become contaminated to a dangerous degree with the agent from the upstream vaporizer. However, the newer TEC Mark 4 and 5 vaporizers have the interlocking Selectatec system (Fig. 13.13) which has locking rods to prevent more than one vaporizer being used at the same time. When a vaporizer is mounted on the back bar, the locking lever needs to be engaged (Mark 4 and 5). If this is not done, the control dial cannot be moved.
- Pressure-linked flow controls. Some anaesthetic machines possess a device which switches off the supply of nitrous oxide automatically in the event of failure of the oxygen supply.
- A non-return valve situated downstream of the vaporizers prevents back-pressure (e.g. when using a Manley ventilator) which might otherwise cause output of high concentrations of vapour.
- A pressure relief valve may be situated downstream of the vaporizer, opening at 34 kPa to prevent damage to the flowmeters or vaporizers if the gas outlet from the anaesthetic machine is obstructed.
- A pressure relief valve set to blow off at a low pressure of 5 kPa may be fitted to prevent the patient's lungs from being damaged by high pressure. The presence of such a valve prevents the use of the machine with minute volume divider ventilators, such as the Manley.
- Oxygen failure warning devices. There is a variety of oxygen failure warning devices. The ideal warning device:
  – does not depend on the pressure of any gas other than the oxygen itself
  – does not use a battery or mains power
  – gives a signal which is audible, of sufficient duration and volume, and of distinctive character
  – should give a warning of impending failure and a further warning that failure has occurred
  – should interrupt the flow of all other gases when it comes into operation.

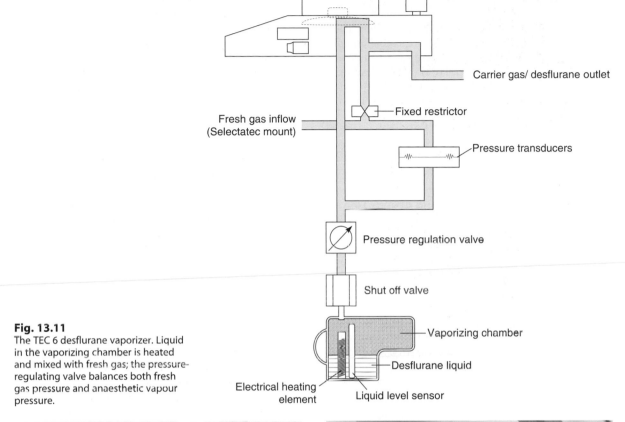

Concentration selection dial

Carrier gas/ desflurane outlet

Fixed restrictor

Fresh gas inflow
(Selectatec mount)

Pressure transducers

Pressure regulation valve

Shut off valve

Vaporizing chamber

Desflurane liquid

Electrical heating
element

Liquid level sensor

Fig. 13.11
The TEC 6 desflurane vaporizer. Liquid in the vaporizing chamber is heated and mixed with fresh gas; the pressure-regulating valve balances both fresh gas pressure and anaesthetic vapour pressure.

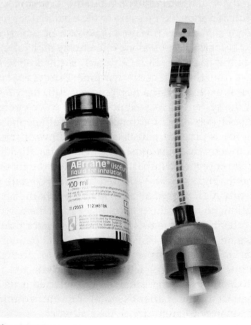

Fig. 13.12
An agent-specific connector for filling a vaporizer.

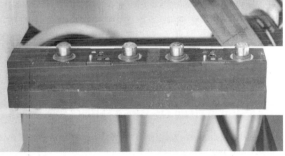

Fig. 13.13
A Selectatec block on the back bar of an anaesthetic machine. This permits the vaporizer to be changed rapidly without interrupting the flow of carrier gas to the patient.

The breathing system should open to the atmosphere, the inspired oxygen concentration should be at least equal to that of air, and accumulation of carbon dioxide should not occur. In addition, it should be impossible to resume anaesthesia until the oxygen supply has been restored.

- The reservoir bag in an anaesthetic breathing system is highly distensible and seldom reaches pressures exceeding 5 kPa.

BREATHING SYSTEMS

The delivery system which conducts anaesthetic gases from the machine to the patient is termed colloquially a 'circuit' but is described more accurately as a breathing system. Terms such as 'open circuits', 'semi-open circuits' or 'semi-closed circuits' should be avoided. The 'closed circuit' or circle system is the only true circuit, as anaesthetic gases are recycled.

Adjustable pressure-limiting valve

Most breathing systems incorporate an adjustable pressure-limiting valve (APL valve, spill valve, 'pop-off' valve, expiratory valve) which is designed to vent gas when there is a positive pressure within the system. During spontaneous ventilation, the valve opens when the patient generates a positive pressure within the system during expiration; during positive pressure ventilation, the valve is adjusted to produce a controlled leak during the inspiratory phase.

Several valves of this type are available. They comprise a lightweight disc (Fig. 13.14) which rests on a 'knife edge' seating to minimize the area of contact and reduce the risk of adhesion resulting from surface tension of condensed water. The disc has a stem which acts as a guide to position it correctly. A light spring is incorporated in the valve so that the pressure required to open it may be adjusted. During spontaneous breathing, the tension of the spring is low so that the resistance to expiration is minimized. During controlled ventilation, the valve top is screwed down to increase the tension in the spring so that gas leaves the system at a higher pressure than during spontaneous ventilation.

CLASSIFICATION OF BREATHING SYSTEMS

In 1954, Mapleson classified anaesthetic breathing systems into five types (Fig. 13.15); the Mapleson E system was modified subsequently by Rees, but is classified as the Mapleson F system. The systems differ considerably in their 'efficiency', which is measured in terms of the fresh gas flow (FGF) rate required to prevent rebreathing of alveolar gas during ventilation.

Mapleson A systems

The most commonly used version is the Magill attachment. The corrugated hose should be of adequate length (usually approximately 110 cm). It is the most efficient system during spontaneous ventilation, but one of the least efficient when ventilation is controlled.

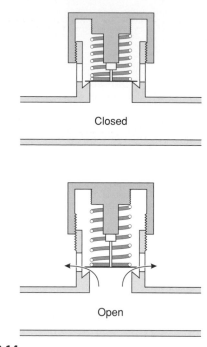

Fig. 13.14
Diagram of a spill valve. See text for details.

During spontaneous ventilation (Fig. 13.16), there are three phases in the ventilatory cycle: inspiratory, expiratory and the expiratory pause. Gas is inhaled from the system during inspiration (Fig. 13.16B). During the initial part of expiration, the reservoir bag is not full and thus the pressure in the system does not increase; exhaled gas (the initial portion of which is dead space gas) passes along the corrugated tubing towards the bag (Fig. 13.16C), which is filled also by fresh gas from the anaesthetic machine. During the latter part of expiration, the bag becomes full, the pressure in the system increases and the spill valve opens, venting all subsequent exhaled gas to atmosphere. During the expiratory pause, continued flow of fresh gas from the machine pushes exhaled gas distally along the corrugated tube to be vented through the spill valve (Fig. 13.16D). Provided that the FGF rate is sufficiently high to vent all *alveolar* gas before the next inspiration, no rebreathing takes place from the corrugated tube. If the system is functioning correctly and no leaks are present, a FGF rate equal to the patient's alveolar minute ventilation is sufficient to prevent rebreathing. In practice, a higher FGF is selected in order to compensate for leaks; the rate selected is usually equal to the patient's total minute volume (approximately $6\,L\,min^{-1}$ for a 70-kg adult).

The system increases dead space to the extent of the volume of the anaesthetic face mask and angle piece to

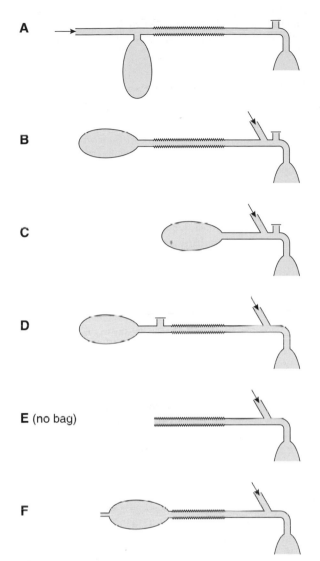

A

B

C

D

E (no bag)

F

Fig. 13.15
Mapleson classification of anaesthetic breathing systems. The arrow indicates entry of fresh gas to the system.

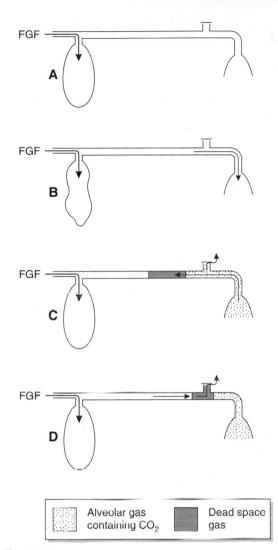

FGF

A

FGF

B

FGF

C

FGF

D

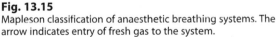

| | Alveolar gas containing CO_2 | | Dead space gas |

Fig. 13.16
Mode of action of Magill attachment during spontaneous ventilation. See text for details. FGF = fresh gas flow.

the spill valve. The volume of this dead space may amount to 100 mL or more for an adult face mask. Paediatric face masks reduce the extent of dead space, but it remains too high to allow use of the system in infants or small children (<4 years old).

The characteristics of the Mapleson A system are different during controlled ventilation (Fig. 13.17). At the end of inspiration (produced by the anaesthetist squeezing the reservoir bag), the bag is usually less than half full (see below). During expiration, dead space and alveolar gas pass along the corrugated tube and are likely to reach the reservoir bag, which therefore contains some carbon dioxide (Fig. 13.17A).

During inspiration, the valve does not open initially because its opening pressure has been increased by the anaesthetist in order to generate a sufficient pressure within the system to inflate the lungs. Thus, alveolar gas re-enters the patient's lungs and is followed by a mixture of fresh, dead space and alveolar gases (Fig. 13.17B). When the valve does open, it is this mixture which is vented (Fig. 13.17C). Consequently, the FGF rate must be very high (at least three times alveolar minute volume) to prevent rebreathing. The volume of gas squeezed from the reservoir bag must be sufficient both to inflate the lungs and to vent gas from the system.

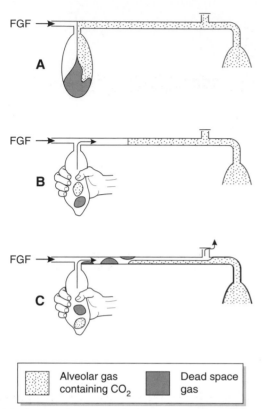

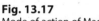

Fig. 13.17
Mode of action of Magill attachment during controlled ventilation. See text for details. FGF = fresh gas flow.

The major disadvantage of the Magill attachment during surgery is that the spill valve is attached close to the mask. This makes the system heavy, particularly when a scavenging system is used, and it is inconvenient if the valve is in this position during surgery of the head or neck. The Lack system (Fig. 13.18B) is a modification of the Mapleson A system with a coaxial arrangement of tubing. This permits positioning of the spill valve at the proximal end of the system. The inner tube must be of sufficiently wide bore to allow the patient to exhale with minimal resistance. The Lack system is not quite as efficient as the Magill attachment.

Mapleson B and C systems

These systems cause mixing of alveolar and fresh gas during spontaneous or controlled ventilation. Very high FGF rates are required to prevent rebreathing. There is no clinical role for the Mapleson B system. The Mapleson C system is used in some hospitals to venti-

late the lungs with oxygen during transport, but a self-inflating bag with a non-rebreathing valve is preferable.

Mapleson D system

The Mapleson D arrangement is inefficient during spontaneous breathing (Fig. 13.19). During expiration, exhaled gas and fresh gas mix in the corrugated tube and travel towards the reservoir bag (Fig. 13.19B). When the reservoir bag is full, the pressure in the system increases, the spill valve opens and a mixture of fresh and exhaled gas is vented; this includes the dead space gas, which reaches the reservoir bag first (Fig. 13.19C). Although fresh gas pushes alveolar gas towards the valve during the expiratory pause, a mixture of alveolar and fresh gases is inhaled from the corrugated tube unless the FGF rate is at least twice as great as the patient's minute volume (i.e. at least $12 \, L \, min^{-1}$ in the adult); in some patients, a FGF rate of $250 \, mL \, kg^{-1} \, min^{-1}$ is required to prevent rebreathing.

However, the Mapleson D system is more efficient than the Mapleson A during controlled ventilation (Fig. 13.20), especially if an expiratory pause is incorporated into the ventilatory cycle. During expiration, the corrugated tubing and reservoir bag fill with a mixture of fresh and alveolar gas (Fig. 13.20A). Fresh gas fills the distal part of the corrugated tube during the expiratory pause (Fig. 13.20B). When the reservoir bag is squeezed, this fresh gas enters the lungs, and when the spill valve opens a mixture of fresh and alveolar gas is vented. The degree of rebreathing may thus be controlled by adjustment of the FGF rate, but this should always exceed the patient's minute volume.

The Bain coaxial system (Fig. 13.18A) is the most commonly used version of the Mapleson D system. FGF is supplied through a narrow inner tube. This tube may become disconnected, resulting in hypoxaemia and hypercapnia. Before use, the system should be tested by occluding the distal end of the inner tube transiently with a finger or the plunger of a 2-mL syringe; there should be a reduction in the flowmeter bobbin reading during occlusion and an audible release of pressure when occlusion is discontinued. Movement of the reservoir bag during anaesthesia does not necessarily indicate that fresh gas is being delivered to the patient.

The Bain system may be used to ventilate the patient's lungs with some types of automatic ventilator (e.g. Penlon Nuffield 200; Fig. 13.21). A 1-m length of corrugated tubing is interposed between the patient valve of the ventilator and the reservoir bag mount (Fig. 13.22); the spill valve *must* be closed completely. An appropriate tidal volume and ventilatory rate are

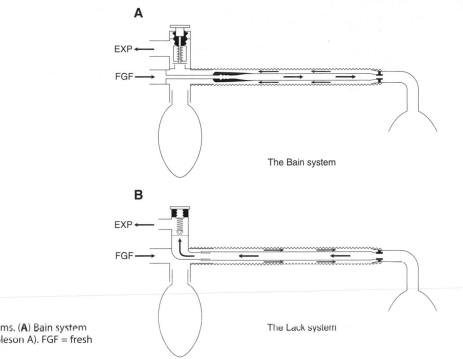

A

EXP ←

FGF →

The Bain system

B

EXP ←

FGF →

The Lack system

Fig. 13.18
Coaxial anaesthetic breathing systems. (**A**) Bain system
(Mapleson D). (**B**) Lack system (Mapleson A). FGF = fresh
gas flow; EXP = expired gas

selected on the ventilator and anaesthetic gases are supplied to the Bain system. During inspiration, the gas from the ventilator pushes a mixture of anaesthetic and alveolar gas from the corrugated outer tube into the patient's lungs; during expiration, the ventilator gas and some of the alveolar gas are vented through the exhaust valve of the ventilator. The degree of rebreathing is regulated by the anaesthetic gas flow rate; a flow of 70–80 mL kg^{-1} min^{-1} should result in normocapnia and a flow of 100 mL kg^{-1} min^{-1} in moderate hypocapnia. A secure connection between the Bain system and the anaesthetic machine must be assured. If this connection is loose, a leak of fresh gas occurs; this causes rebreathing of ventilator gas and results in awareness, hypoxaemia and hypercapnia.

Mapleson E and F systems

The Mapleson E system, or Ayre's T-piece, has virtually no resistance to expiration and was used extensively in paediatric anaesthesia before the advantages of continuous positive airways pressure (CPAP) were recognized. It functions in a manner similar to the Mapleson D system in that the corrugated tube fills with a mixture of exhaled and fresh gas during expiration and with fresh gas during the expiratory pause. Rebreathing is prevented if the FGF rate is 2.5–3 times the patient's minute volume. If the volume of the cor-

rugated tube is less than the patient's tidal volume, some air may be inhaled at the end of inspiration; consequently, an FGF rate of at least 4L min^{-1} is recommended with a paediatric Mapleson E system.

During spontaneous ventilation, there is no indication of the presence, or the adequacy, of ventilation. It is possible to attach a visual indicator, such as a piece of tissue paper or a feather, at the end of the corrugated tube, but this is not very satisfactory.

Intermittent positive pressure ventilation (IPPV) may be applied by occluding the end of the corrugated tube with a finger. However, there is no way of assessing the pressure in the system and there is a possibility of exposing the patient's lungs to excessive volumes and pressures.

The Mapleson F system, or Rees' modification of the Ayre's T-piece, includes an open-ended bag attached to the end of the corrugated tube. This confers several advantages:

- It provides visual evidence of breathing during spontaneous ventilation.
- By occluding the open end of the bag temporarily, it is possible to confirm that fresh gas is entering the system.
- It provides a degree of CPAP during spontaneous ventilation and positive end-expiratory pressure (PEEP) during IPPV.

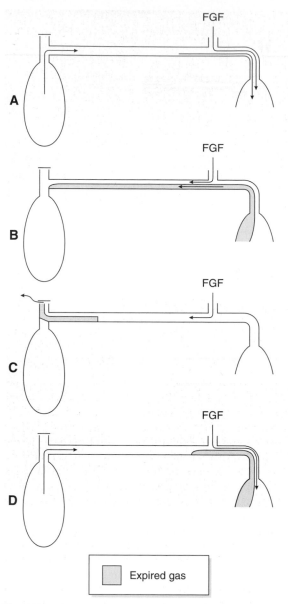

Fig. 13.19
Mode of action of Mapleson D breathing system during spontaneous ventilation. See text for details. FGF = fresh gas flow.

- It provides a convenient method of assisting or controlling ventilation. The open end of the reservoir bag is occluded between the fourth and fifth fingers and the bag is squeezed between the thumb and index finger; the fourth and fifth fingers are relaxed during expiration to allow gas to escape from the bag. It is possible with experience to assess (approximately) the inflation pressure and to detect changes in lung and chest wall compliance.

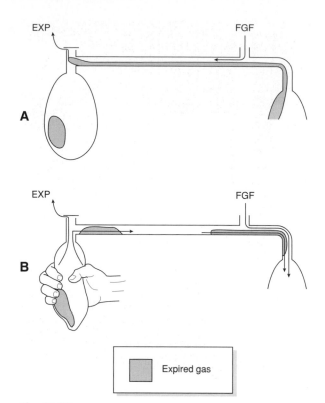

Fig. 13.20
Mode of action of Mapleson D breathing system during controlled ventilation. See text for details. FGF = fresh gas flow.

However, one main disadvantage of the Mapleson F system is that efficient scavenging is unsatisfactory and is non-standard.

Mapleson ADE system

This system provides the advantages of the Mapleson A, D and E systems. It can be used efficiently for spontaneous and controlled ventilation in both children and adults.

It consists of two parallel lengths of 15-mm bore tubing; one delivers fresh gas and the other carries exhaled gas. One end of the tubing connects to the patient via a Y-connection and the other end contains the Humphrey block (Fig. 13.23). The Humphrey block (Fig. 13.24) consists of an APL valve, a lever to select spontaneous or controlled ventilation, a reservoir bag, a port to connect a ventilator and a safety pressure relief valve which opens at a pressure above 6-kPa.

When the lever is in the A mode (up), the reservoir bag is connected to the breathing system as it would be in the Mapleson A system. The breathing hose connecting the bag to the patient is the inspiratory limb.

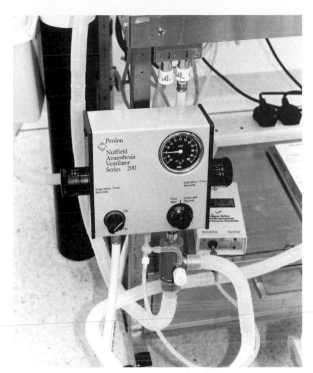

Fig. 13.21
The Penlon Nuffield 200 ventilator.

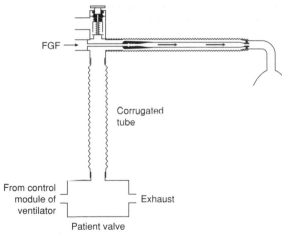

Fig. 13.22
The Bain system for controlled ventilation by a mechanical ventilator (e.g. Penlon Nuffield 200). A 1-m length of corrugated tubing with a capacity of at least 500 mL is required to prevent gas from the ventilator reaching the patient's lungs. P_aCO_2 is controlled by varying the fresh gas flow (FGF) rate.

The expired gases travel along the other tubing back to the APL valve, which is connected to the scavenging system.

With the lever in the D/E mode (down), the reservoir bag and the APL valve are isolated from the

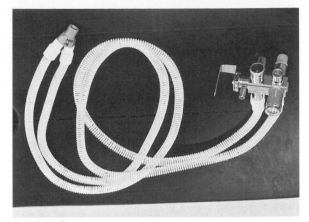

Fig. 13.23
The ADE system.

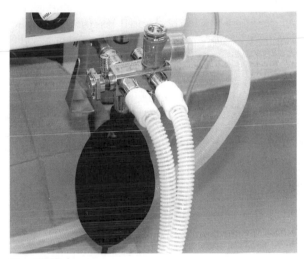

Fig. 13.24
The Humphrey block. This consists of an APL valve, a lever to select spontaneous or controlled ventilation, a reservoir bag, a port to connect to the ventilator and a safety pressure relief valve.

breathing system. What was the inspiratory limb in the A mode now delivers gas to the patient. The hose returning gas to the Humphrey block now functions as a reservoir to the T-piece. This hose would open to atmosphere via a port adjacent to the bag mount, but in practice this port is connected to a ventilator such as the Penlon Nuffield .

In adults, an appropriate FGF is 50–60 mL kg^{-1} min^{-1} in spontaneously breathing patients and 70 mL kg^{-1} min^{-1} in ventilated patients.

Drawover systems

Occasionally, it is necessary to administer anaesthesia at the scene of a major accident. If inhalation anaesthesia is required, it is necessary to use simple, portable equipment. The Triservice apparatus has been designed by the British armed forces for use in battle conditions (Fig. 13.25). It comprises a self-inflating bag, a non-rebreathing valve (e.g. Ambu E, Rubens) which vents all expired gases to atmosphere, one or two Oxford miniature vaporizers (which have a low internal resistance), an oxygen supply and a length of corrugated tubing which serves as an oxygen reservoir. Either spontaneous or controlled ventilation may be employed using this apparatus.

REBREATHING SYSTEMS

Anaesthetic breathing systems in which some gas is rebreathed by the patient were designed originally to economize in the use of cyclopropane. In addition, they reduce the risk of atmospheric pollution and increase the humidity of inspired gases, thereby reducing heat loss from the patient. Rebreathing systems may be used as 'closed' systems, in which fresh gas is introduced only to replace oxygen and anaesthetic agents absorbed by the patient. More commonly, the system is used with a small leak through a spill valve, and the fresh gas supply exceeds basal oxygen requirements. Because rebreathing occurs, these systems must incorporate a means of absorbing carbon dioxide from exhaled alveolar gas.

Soda lime

Soda lime is the substance used most commonly for absorption of carbon dioxide in rebreathing systems. The composition of soda lime is shown in Table 13.4. The major constituent is calcium hydroxide, but sodium and potassium hydroxides may also be pres-

Table 13.4 Composition of soda lime

$Ca(OH)_2$	94%
NaOH	5%
KOH	<1% or nil
Silica	0.2%
Moisture content	14–19%

ent. Absorption of carbon dioxide occurs by the following chemical reactions:

$$CO_2 + 2NaOH \rightarrow Na_2CO_3 + H_2O + heat$$
$$Na_2CO_3 + Ca(OH)_2 \rightarrow 2NaOH + CaCO_3$$

Water is required for efficient absorption. There is some water in soda lime and more is added from the patient's expired gas and from the chemical reaction. The reaction generates heat and the temperature in the centre of a soda lime canister may exceed 60°C. Trichloroethylene degenerates at high temperatures, forming toxic substances including the neurotoxin dichloroacetylene; consequently, trichloroethylene must never be used in rebreathing systems which contain soda lime. Sevoflurane has been shown to interact with soda lime to produce substances that are toxic in animals. However, this does not appear to impose any significant risk in humans (see Ch. 2). There is new evidence suggesting that the presence of strong alkalis such as sodium and potassium hydroxides could be the trigger of the interaction between volatile agents

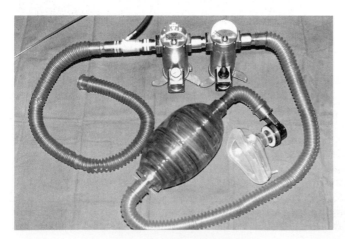

Fig. 13.25
The Triservice apparatus. Courtesy of Dr S. Kidd.

and soda lime. New carbon dioxide absorbers are now being manufactured without these hydroxides in order to reduce this interaction.

The size of soda lime granules is important. If granules are too large, the surface area for absorption is insufficient; if they are too small, the narrow space between granules results in a high resistance to breathing. Granule size is measured by a mesh number. Soda lime consists of granules in the range of 4–8 mesh. (A 4-mesh strainer has four openings per inch and an 8-mesh strainer has eight openings.) Silica is added to soda lime to reduce the tendency of the granules to disintegrate into powder. In addition, soda lime contains an indicator which changes colour as the active constituents become exhausted. The rate at which soda lime becomes exhausted depends on the capacity of the canister, the FGF rate and the rate of carbon dioxide production. In a completely closed system, a standard 450-g canister becomes inefficient after approximately 2 h.

Baralyme

Baralyme is another carbon dioxide absorber. It is a mixture of approximately 20% barium hydroxide and 80% calcium hydroxide. It may also contain some potassium hydroxide, an indicator and moisture. Barium hydroxide contains eight molecules of water of crystallization, which help to fuse the mixture so that it retains the granular structure under various conditions of heat and moisture. The granules of Baralyme are similar to those of soda lime.

'To-and-fro' (Waters') system

This breathing system comprises a Mapleson C breathing system with a canister of soda lime interposed between the spill valve and the reservoir bag (Fig. 13.26). The soda lime granules nearest the patient become exhausted first, increasing the dead space of the system; in addition, the canister is positioned horizontally and gas may be channelled above the soda lime unless the canister is packed tightly. The system is cumbersome and there is a risk that patients may inhale soda lime dust from the canister.

Circle system

This system has replaced the 'to-and-fro' system. The soda lime canister is mounted on the anaesthetic machine, and inspiratory and expiratory corrugated tubing conducts gas to and from the patient (Fig. 13.27). The system incorporates a reservoir bag and spill valve and two low-resistance one-way valves to ensure unidi-

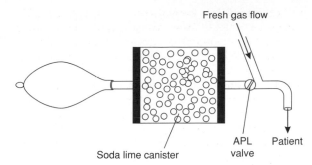

Fig. 13.26
Waters' anaesthetic breathing system, incorporating a canister of soda lime.

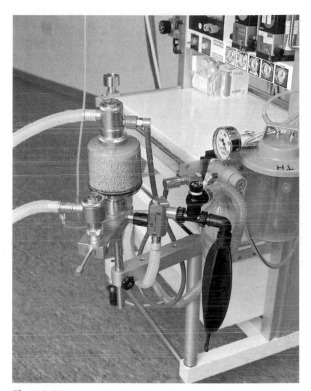

Fig. 13.27
The circle breathing system mounted on an anaesthetic machine.

rectional movement of gas (Fig. 13.28). These valves are normally mounted in glass domes so that they may be observed to be functioning correctly. The spill valve may be mounted close to the patient or beside the absorber; during surgery to the head or neck, it is more convenient to use a valve near the absorber. Fresh gas enters the system between the absorber and the inspiratory tubing.

The soda lime canister is mounted vertically and thus channelling of gas through unfilled areas is not

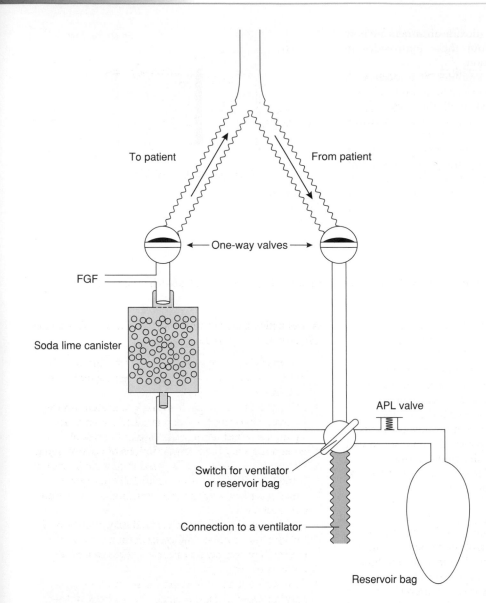

To patient

From patient

← One-way valves →

FGF

Soda lime canister

APL valve

Switch for ventilator
or reservoir bag

Connection to a ventilator

Reservoir bag

Fig. 13.28
Mechanism of the circle system.
The direction of gas flow is
controlled via the unidirectional
valves. A lever allows the
ventilation to be either
spontaneous through the
reservoir bag and APL valve or
controlled by a ventilator.

possible. The canister cannot contribute to dead space; consequently, a large canister may be used and the soda lime needs to be changed less often.

The major disadvantage of the circle system arises from its volume. If the system is filled with air initially, low flow rates of anaesthetic gases are diluted substantially and adequate concentrations cannot be achieved. Even if the system is primed with a mixture of anaesthetic gases, the initial rapid uptake by the patient results in a marked decrease in concentrations of anaesthetic agents in the system, resulting in light anaesthesia. Consequently, it is necessary usually to provide a total FGF rate of 3–4 L min⁻¹ to the system

initially. This flow rate may be reduced subsequently, but it must be remembered that dilution of fresh gas continues at low flow rates and that rapid changes in depth of anaesthesia cannot be achieved.

Volatile anaesthetic agents may be delivered to a circle system in two ways:

- *Vaporizer outside the circle (VOC)* (Fig. 13.29A). If a standard vaporizer (e.g. TEC series) is used, it must be placed on the back bar of the anaesthetic machine because of its high internal resistance. If low FGF rates (<1 L min⁻¹) are used, the change in concentration of volatile anaesthetic agent achieved

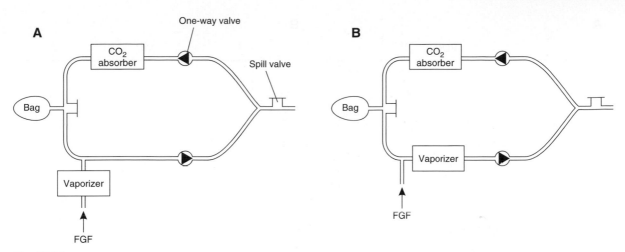

Fig. 13.29
Diagrammatic representation of circle system. (**A**) Vaporizer outside the circle (VOC). (**B**) Vaporizer inside the circle (VIC).

in the circle system is very small because of dilution, even if the vaporizer is set to deliver a high concentration (Fig. 13.30A). It may be necessary to change FGF rate rather than the vaporizer setting in order to achieve a rapid change in depth of anaesthesia. The concentration of volatile agent in the system depends on the patient's expired concentration (which is recycled), the rate of uptake by the patient (which decreases with time and is lower with agents of low blood/gas solubility coefficient), the concentration of agent supplied and the FGF rate.

- *Vaporizer inside the circle (VIC)* (Fig. 13.29B). Drawover vaporizers with a low internal resistance (e.g. Goldman) may be placed within the circle system. During each inspiration, vapour is added to the inspired gas mixture. In contrast to a VOC system, the inspired concentration is higher at low FGF rates because the expired concentration is diluted to a lesser extent (Fig. 13.30B) and the vaporizer *adds* to the concentration present in the expired gas. Very high concentrations of volatile agent may be inspired if minute volume is large; this risk is greatest if IPPV is employed.

If FGF rate is low, the use of the circle system by the inexperienced anaesthetist may result either in inadequate anaesthesia or in severe cardiovascular and respiratory depression. In addition, a hypoxic gas mixture may be delivered if low flow rates of a nitrous oxide/oxygen mixture are supplied, because after 10–15 min oxygen is taken up in larger volumes than nitrous oxide. These difficulties may be overcome by monitoring the inspired concentrations of oxygen, carbon dioxide and volatile

anaesthetic agent continuously (see Ch. 18). The trainee anaesthetist *must* be aware that:

- It is inadvisable to use a VIC system unless inspired concentrations of anaesthetic agents are monitored continuously.
- IPPV must *never* be used with a VIC system unless inspired concentrations of anaesthetic agents are monitored continuously, because of the risk of generating very high concentrations of volatile agent.
- Nitrous oxide must *not* be used in any circle system if the total FGF rate is less than 1000 mL min^{-1}, unless inspired oxygen concentration is measured continuously.
- It is essential to monitor inspired concentration of oxygen and inhalational anaesthetic agent and expired concentration of carbon dioxide when using the circle system.
- One-way valves may stick. These should be checked both at the pre-anaesthetic check of the machine and during anaesthesia.
- Because the circle system has many connections, the anaesthetist should be vigilant about checking for any leak or disconnection.

The advantages and disadvantages of the circle system are summarized in Table 13.5.

VENTILATORS

Mechanical ventilation of the lung may be achieved by several mechanisms, including the generation of a negative pressure around the whole of the patient's

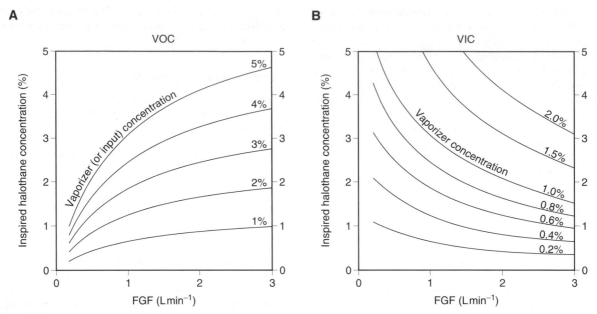

Fig. 13.30
Variation of inspired concentration of halothane with fresh gas flow (FGF) rate. Total minute ventilation is 5 L min⁻¹. (**A**) Vaporizer outside the circle (VOC); note that dilution of the fresh gas results in much lower concentrations in the circle system than the concentration set on the vaporizer unless FGF rate approaches 3 L min⁻¹. (**B**) Vaporizer inside the circle (VIC); at low flow rates, lack of dilution of expired halothane concentration, with additional halothane vaporized during each inspiration, results in inspired concentrations much higher than those set on the vaporizer. Even at an FGF rate of 3 L min⁻¹, inspired concentration is approximately 50% higher than the vaporizer setting.

body except the head and neck (cabinet ventilator or 'iron lung'), a negative pressure over the thorax and abdomen (cuirass ventilators) or a positive pressure over the thorax and abdomen (inflatable cuirass ventilators). However, during anaesthesia, and in the majority of patients who require mechanical ventilation in the intensive care unit, ventilation is achieved by the application of positive pressure to the lungs through a tracheal tube. Only this mode of ventilation is described here.

An enormous selection of ventilators exists and it is possible in this section to discuss only the principles involved in their use. Before using any ventilator, it is *essential* that the trainee understands its functions fully; failure to do so may result in the delivery of a hypoxic gas mixture, rebreathing of carbon dioxide and/or delivery of a mixture that contains no anaesthetic gases. If an unfamiliar ventilator is encountered, it may be helpful to use a 'dummy lung' (a small reservoir bag on the patient connection) and to discuss the capabilities and limitations of the machine with a senior colleague. In addition, the manufacturer's 'user handbook' may be consulted or details may be obtained from a specialist book.

Table 13.5 Disadvantages and advantages of the circle system	
Disadvantages	*Advantages*
Cumbersome equipment	Inspired gases are humidified and warmed
Risk of delivering hypoxic mixture	Economical
Increased resistance to breathing	Minimal pollution
Slow change in the depth of anaesthesia	
Risk of awareness	
Risk of a rise in end-tidal CO_2	
Risk of unidirectional valves sticking	
Not ideal for paediatric patients breathing spontaneously	
Some inhalational agents may interact with soda lime	

Continuous clinical monitoring is essential when any ventilator is used, even those which incorporate sophisticated monitoring and warning devices. In addition to standard clinical monitoring systems attached to the patient (see Ch. 18), the minimum acceptable monitoring of ventilator function includes measurement of expired tidal volume, airway pressure and inspired oxygen concentration; in addition, a ventilator disconnection alarm should be incorporated in the system. Continuous monitoring of end-tidal carbon dioxide, oxygen saturation and inspired anaesthetic gas concentrations is essential.

The incorporation of a humidifier in the inspiratory limb, or of a condenser humidifier at the connection with the tracheal tube, is essential in long-term ventilation in the ICU. Bacterial filters (Fig. 13.31) are now recommended for all patients undergoing anaesthesia.

The principles of operation of ventilators are described best by considering each phase of the ventilatory cycle: inspiration; change from inspiration to expiration; expiration; and change from expiration to inspiration.

Inspiration

The pattern of volume change in the lung is determined by the characteristics of the ventilator. Ventilators may deliver a predetermined flow rate of gas (*constant flow generators*) or exert a predetermined pressure (*constant pressure generators*), although some machines produce a pattern which does not conform to either category. Most flow generators produce a constant flow of gas during inspiration, although a few generate a sinusoidal flow pattern if the ventilator

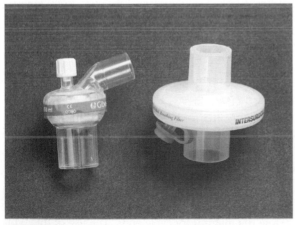

Fig. 13.31
Bacterial filters and humidifiers which are used in breathing systems: *left*, a paediatric filter incorporated into an angle piece; *right*, an adult filter.

bellows is driven via a crank. The characteristics of constant flow and constant pressure generators are shown in Figure 13.32.

Constant pressure generator

The ventilator produces inspiration by generating a constant, predetermined pressure. However, if airway resistance increases or if compliance decreases these ventilators deliver reduced tidal volume at the preset cycling pressure (Fig. 13.33). Therefore their perfomance is variable.

Constant flow generator

These ventilators produce inspiration by delivering a predetermined flow of gas. Changes in resistance or compliance make little difference to the volume delivered (unless the ventilator is pressure-cycled; see below), although airway and alveolar pressures may change (Fig. 13.34). For example, decreased compliance results in delivery of a normal tidal volume; however, the rate of increase of alveolar pressure is greater than normal (i.e. the slope is greater) and airway pressure is correspondingly higher to maintain a gradient between the tracheal tube and the alveoli. If airway resistance increases, the pressure at the tracheal tube (and the gradient between tracheal tube and alveolar pressures) is higher than normal throughout inspiration, but alveolar pressure and the slopes of both pressure curves are normal. Constant flow generators do not compensate for leaks; the tidal volume delivered to the lungs decreases.

Some ventilators generate a pressure rather higher than that required to inflate the lungs but not high enough to maintain constant flow throughout inspiration. The flow, volume and pressure changes within the lung are shown in Figure 13.35.

Change from inspiration to expiration

This is termed 'cycling' and may be achieved in one of three ways:

Volume-cycling. The ventilator cycles into expiration whenever a predetermined tidal volume has been delivered. The duration of inspiration is determined by the inspiratory flow rate.

Pressure-cycling. The ventilator cycles into expiration when a preset *airway* pressure is achieved. This allows compensation for small leaks but, in common with a constant pressure generator, a pressure-cycled ventilator delivers a different tidal volume if compliance or resistance changes. In addition, inspiratory time varies with changes in compliance and resistance.

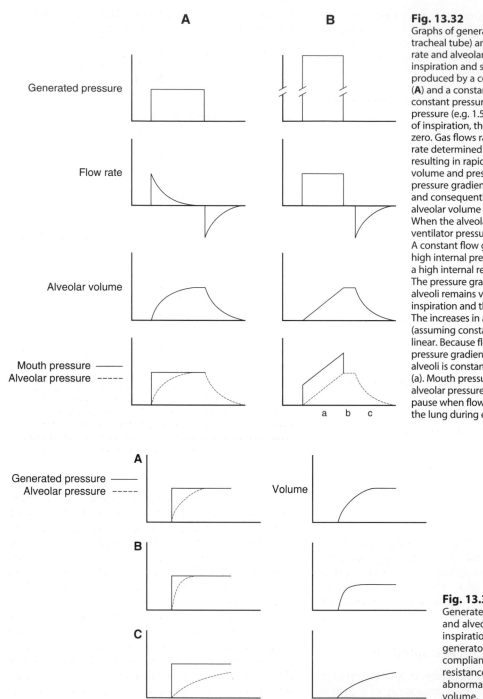

Fig. 13.32
Graphs of generated pressure, mouth (or tracheal tube) and alveolar pressures, flow rate and alveolar volume changes during inspiration and subsequent expiration produced by a constant pressure generator (**A**) and a constant flow generator (**B**). A constant pressure generator exerts a low pressure (e.g. 1.5 kPa, 15 cmH$_2$O). At the start of inspiration, the pressure in the alveoli is zero. Gas flows rapidly into the alveoli at a rate determined by airways resistance, resulting in rapid increases in alveolar volume and pressure. The mouth–alveolar pressure gradient decreases and flow rate, and consequently the rate of increase of alveolar volume and pressure, decrease also. When the alveolar pressure equals the ventilator pressure, flow ceases.
A constant flow generator generates a very high internal pressure (e.g. 400 kPa) but has a high internal resistance to limit flow rate. The pressure gradient between machine and alveoli remains virtually constant throughout inspiration and thus flow rate is constant. The increases in alveolar volume and (assuming constant compliance) pressure are linear. Because flow rate is constant, the pressure gradient between mouth and alveoli is constant throughout inspiration (a). Mouth pressure decreases to equal alveolar pressure during the inspiratory pause when flow ceases (b). Gas flow out of the lung during expiration (c) is passive.

Fig. 13.33
Generated and alveolar pressures, and alveolar volume, during inspiration with a constant pressure generator. (**A**) Normal. (**B**) Decreased compliance. (**C**) Increased airway resistance. Note that both abnormalities reduce alveolar volume.

Time-cycling. This is the method used most commonly by modern ventilators. The duration of inspiration is predetermined. With a constant flow generator, it may be desirable to preset a tidal volume; when this has been delivered, there is a short inspiratory pause (which improves gas distribution within the lung) before the inspiratory cycle ends. The use of this 'volume-preset' mechanism must be differentiated from volume-cycling. When a constant pressure generator is time-cycled, the tidal volume delivered depends on

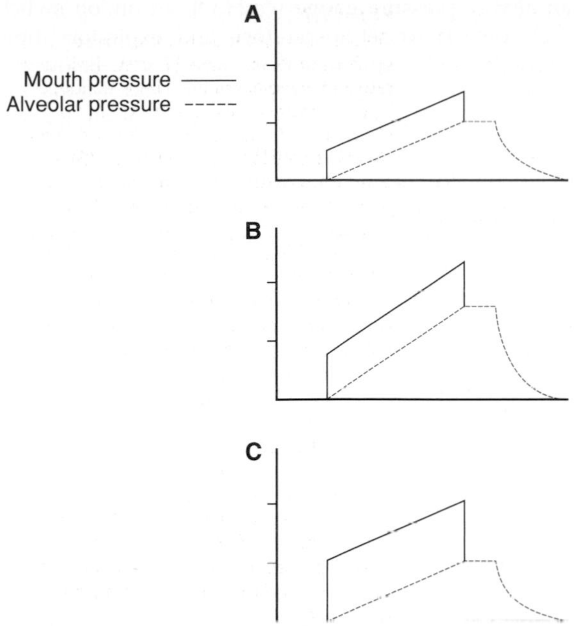

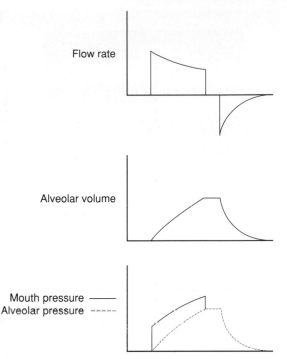

Fig. 13.34
Mouth and alveolar pressures during inspiration with a constant flow generator. (**A**) Normal. (**B**) Decreased compliance. (**C**) Increased airway resistance. Alveolar volume remains constant because flow rate is constant. Decreased compliance results in an increased rate of increase of alveolar pressure; mouth pressure also increases more steeply, but the gradient between mouth and alveolar pressures remains normal. Increased airway resistance increases the mouth–alveolar pressure gradient.

Fig. 13.35
Pressure, flow and alveolar volume characteristics during inspiration with a ventilator with a moderately high internal pressure. At higher bellows pressures, and in a patient with normal compliance and airway resistance, the characteristics approximate to those of a constant flow generator (Fig. 13.34). At low bellows pressures, if compliance decreases or if airway resistance increases, the pattern is similar to that of a constant pressure generator.

the compliance and resistance of the lungs and on the pressure within the bellows.

Expiration

Usually, the patient is allowed to exhale to atmospheric pressure; flow rate decreases exponentially. Subatmospheric pressure should not be used during expiration as it induces small airways' closure and air trapping. PEEP may be applied in some circumstances (see Ch. 41).

Change from expiration to inspiration

On most ventilators, this is achieved by time-cycling. However, it may be desirable occasionally to use pressure-cycling in response to a subatmospheric pressure generated by the patient's inspiratory effort.

Delivery of anaesthetic gas

Some ventilators deliver a minute volume determined by a preset tidal volume and rate. When used in anaes-

thesia, these machines must be supplied with a flow rate of anaesthetic gases which equals or exceeds the minute volume delivered, otherwise air, or gas used to drive the ventilator, is entrained and delivered to the patient. Several ventilators such as the Blease Manley ventilator (Fig. 13.36) are driven by the anaesthetic gas supply, can deliver only that gas, and divide it into predetermined tidal volumes (*minute volume dividers*).

Ventilators may be used to compress bellows in a separate system which contains anaesthetic gases ('bag-in-a-bottle'); it is possible to provide IPPV in a circle system in this way. The bag-in-a-bottle ventilator (Fig. 13.37) consists of a chamber with a tidal volume range of 0–1500 mL (adult mode) or 0–400 mL (paediatric mode) and ascending bellows which accommodate FGF. The control unit has controls, displays and alarms and these may include tidal volume, respiratory rate, I:E ratio, airway pressure and an on/off/standby switch. Compressed air or oxygen is used as the driving gas. On entering the chamber, the compressed gas forces the bellows down, delivering

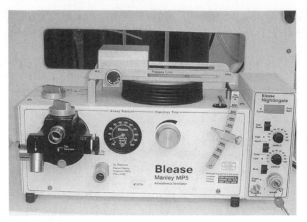

Fig. 13.36
The Blease Manley MP5 ventilator with ventilator alarm.

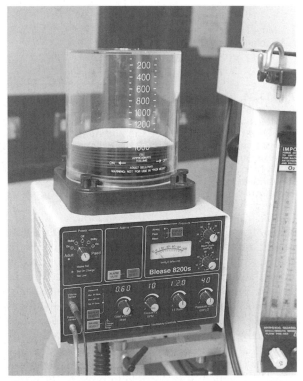

Fig. 13.37
Blease bag-in-a-bottle ventilator.

the FGF within the bellows to the patient. The driving gas in the chamber and the FGF in the bellows remain separate.

The Penlon Nuffield 200 ventilator (Fig. 13.21) is an intermittent blower. It is a very versatile ventilator which may be used in different age groups and using different breathing systems. The control unit consists of

an airway pressure gauge (cmH_2O), an on/off switch and controls to set inspiratory and expiratory time (seconds) and inspiratory flow rate ($L\,s^{-1}$). Below the control unit, there is a connection for the driving gas (oxygen or air) and the valve block. A small tubing connects the valve block to an airway pressure monitor and to a ventilator alarm. The valve block consists of a port for tubing to connect to the breathing system reservoir bag mount (Bain system) or the ventilator port (ADE system), an exhaust port which can be connected to the scavenging system and a pressure relief valve which opens at 6–7 kPa. With this standard valve, the ventilator is a time-cycled flow generator. The valve block can be changed to a paediatric Newton valve and this then converts the ventilator to a time-cycled pressure generator.

The Servo 900C ventilator is a sophisticated ventilator which is used mainly in the intensive care setting but may also be used to ventilate anaesthetized patients in the operating theatre. It is a time-cycled flow generator which can either be driven by anaesthetic gases or pipeline gases. It has electronically controlled inspiration and expiration valves. Although it is electrically powered, it requires gas to operate. Fresh gas from either the anaesthetic machine or pipeline gas is fed into spring-loaded bellows. The spring load can be varied with the front panel dial which alters the working pressure. The ventilator provides alternate modes of ventilation which include intermittent mandatory ventilation (IMV), synchronized intermittent ventilation (SIMV) and pressure support.

The characteristics of several common ventilators are summarized in Table 13.6.

HIGH-FREQUENCY VENTILATION

High-frequency ventilation (HFV) may be defined as ventilation at a respiratory rate of greater than four times the resting respiratory rate of the subject. The different modes of HFV are shown in Table 13.7.

Of the three types of HFV, high-frequency jet ventilation (HFJV) is the most commonly used. The tidal volume used in HFJV is small compared with conventional ventilation. This is delivered at high pressure (up to 5 bar) through a cannula or catheter placed in the trachea. Inspiratory flow rates of up to $100\,L\,min^{-1}$ may be required. The inspiratory time is adjustable from 20% to 50% of the cycle. The mechanism by which HFV is able to maintain gas exchange is not clear. Typical values for adult ventilation are:

- ventilation rate 100–150 cycles min^{-1}
- driving pressure 100–200 kPa
- inspiratory cycle of 20–40%.

Table 13.6 Classification of some common ventilators used during anaesthesia

Ventilator	Driven by	Cycling to expiration	Cycling to inspiration	Pressure/flow generator	Minute volume divider	Volume preset
Manley MP3, MP5	Anaesthetic gases	Time/volume	Time	Pressure	Yes	Yes
Manley Pulmovent	Anaesthetic gases	Volume	Time	Flow	Yes	Yes
Manley Servovent	Compressed air or oxygen	Volume	Time	Flow	No	Yes
Nuffield 200	Compressed air or oxygen	Time	Time	Flow	No	No
Servo 900	Anaesthetic gases	Time (electrically operated valves)	Time (electrically operated valves)	Flow (usually)	No	Yes
Bag-in-bottle	Compressed air or oxygen	Time	Time	Flow	No	Yes

HFJV is used during some operations on the larynx, trachea or lung and in a small number of patients in the ICU. Gases should be humidified when using HFJV. Gas exchange may be unpredictable and the technique should not be used by the trainee without supervision. Figure 13.38 illustrates a type of ventilator used for HFJV.

VENTURI INJECTOR DEVICE

The Venturi injector consists of a high-pressure oxygen source (at about 400 kPa from either the anaesthetic machine or direct from a pipeline), an on/off trigger and connection tubing that can withstand high pressure. The Manujet (Fig. 13.39) is a newer design of a Venturi injector device. It has a dial to alter the driving pressure to suit the size of patient from a neonate to an adult. This is connected to the side of a rigid broncho-scope, to a transtracheal catheter or to a cannula through the cricothyroid membrane. The injector is controlled manually. A 14G cannula or a specially designed cannula (Fig. 13.40) inserted through the cricothyroid membrane may be used to ventilate using the Venturi injector device. A Venturi effect is created which entrains atmospheric air and allows intermittent insufflation of the lungs with oxygen-enriched air at airway pressures of 2.5–3.0 kPa. It is used in operations on the larynx, trachea or lung. Possible complications include barotrauma, gastric distension and awareness if inadequate intravenous anaesthetic drugs are administered. When Venturi injector devices are employed, it is essential to ensure that gas is able to leave the lungs though the upper airway during expiration.

SCAVENGING

The possible adverse effects of pollution on staff in the operating theatre environment are discussed in Chapter 14. The principal sources of pollution by anaesthetic gases and vapours include:

- discharge of anaesthetic gases from ventilators
- expired gas vented from the spill valve of anaesthetic breathing systems
- leaks from equipment, e.g. from an ill-fitting face mask
- gas exhaled by the patient after anaesthesia. This may occur in the operating theatre, corridors and recovery room
- spillage during filling of vaporizers.

Although most attention has centred on removing gas from the expiratory ports of breathing systems and

Table 13.7 Types of high-frequency ventilation

Type of ventilation	Rate of ventilation (cycles min^{-1})
High-frequency positive pressure ventilation (HFPPV)	60–100
High-frequency jet ventilation (HFJV)	100–400
High-frequency oscillation ventilation (HFOV)	400–2400

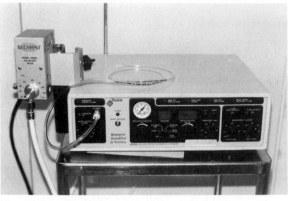

Fig. 13.38
Penlon Bromsgrove jet ventilator.

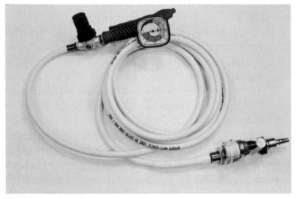

Fig. 13.39
Manually controlled Venturi injector.

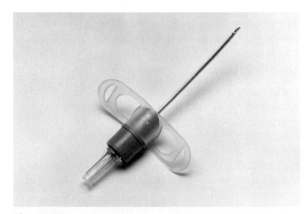

Fig. 13.40
A cricothyroid cannula to use with a Venturi injector device.

ventilators, other methods of reducing pollution should also be considered:

Reduced use of anaesthetic gases and vapours. The use of the circle system reduces the potential for atmospheric pollution. The use of inhalation anaesthetics may be obviated totally by using total intravenous anaesthesia or local anaesthetic techniques.

Air conditioning. Air conditioning units which produce a rapid change of air in the operating theatre reduce pollution substantially. However, some systems recycle air, and older operating theatres, dental surgeries and obstetric delivery suites may not be equipped with air conditioning.

Care in filling vaporizers. Great care should be taken not to spill volatile anaesthetic agent when a vaporizer is filled. The use of agent-specific connections (Fig. 13.12) reduces the risk of spillage. In some countries, vaporizers may be filled only in a portable fume cupboard.

SCAVENGING APPARATUS

Anaesthetic gases vented from the breathing system are removed by a collecting system. A variety of purpose-built scavenging spill valves is available; an example of an adjustable pressure-limiting (APL) valve is shown in Figure 13.41. Waste gases from ventilators are collected by attaching the scavenging system to the expiratory port of the ventilator. Connectors on scavenging systems have a diameter of 30 mm to ensure that inappropriate connections with anaesthetic apparatus cannot be made.

Disposal systems may be active, semi-active or passive.

Active systems

These employ apparatus to generate a negative pressure within the scavenging system to propel waste gases to the outside atmosphere. The system may be powered by a vacuum pump (Fig. 13.42) or a Venturi system (Fig. 13.43). The exhaust should be capable of accommodating 75 L min^{-1} continuous flow with a peak of 130 L min^{-1}. Usually, a reservoir system is used to permit high peak flow rates to be accommodated. In addition, there must be a pressure-limiting device within the system to prevent the application of negative pressure to the patient's lungs.

Semi-active systems

The waste gases may be conducted to the extraction side of the air-conditioning system, which generates a small negative pressure within the scavenging tubing.

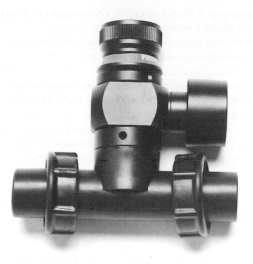

Fig. 13.41
An APL (adjustable pressure-limiting) valve with scavenging attachment.

These systems have variable performance and efficiency.

Passive systems

These systems vent the expired gas to the outside atmosphere (Fig. 13.44). Gas movement is generated by the patient. Consequently, the total length of tubing must not be excessive or resistance to expiration is high. The pressure within the system may be altered by wind conditions at the external terminal; on occasions, these may generate a negative pressure, but may also generate high positive pressures. Each scavenging location should have a separate external terminal to prevent gases being vented into adjacent locations. Relief valves must be incorporated to prevent negative or high positive pressures within the system.

Irrespective of the type of disposal system, tubing used for scavenging must not be allowed to lie on the floor of the operating theatre, as compression (e.g. by

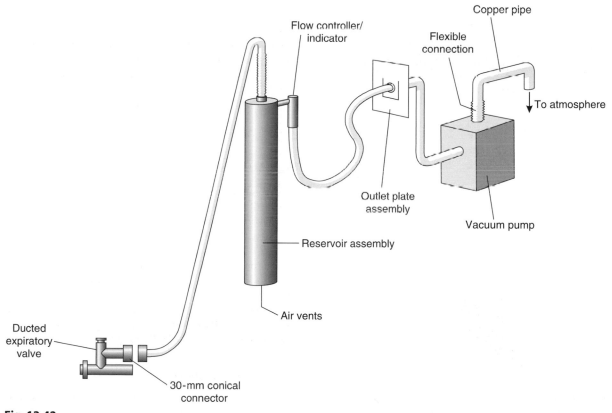

Fig. 13.42
An active scavenging system.

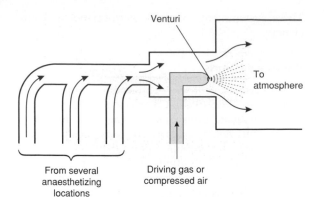

Fig. 13.43
A Venturi system for active scavenging of anaesthetic gases.

feet or by items of equipment) results in increased resistance to expiration and may generate dangerously high pressure within the patient's lungs.

RESERVOIR BAGS

Reservoir bags are used in breathing systems. Their functions include:

- serving as a reservoir of inspired gases
- providing a means of manual ventilation of the lungs

- serving as a visual or tactile observation to monitor the patient's spontaneous respiration
- protecting the patient from excessive pressure in the breathing system.

The reservoir bag may accommodate an increase in pressure in the breathing system to a maximum of approximately 50 cmH$_2$O (5 kPa).

The standard adult size is 2 L and the paediatric size is 0.5 L. However, the size of reservoir bags may vary from 0.5 to 6 L.

LARYNGOSCOPES

A laryngoscope consists of a blade which elevates the lower jaw and tongue, a light source near the tip of the blade to illuminate the larynx, and a handle to apply leverage to the blade. There are many forms of blade and handle.

Curved blade

The most commonly used adult laryngoscope blade is the Macintosh curved blade, which is manufactured in several sizes (Figs 13.45, 13.46).

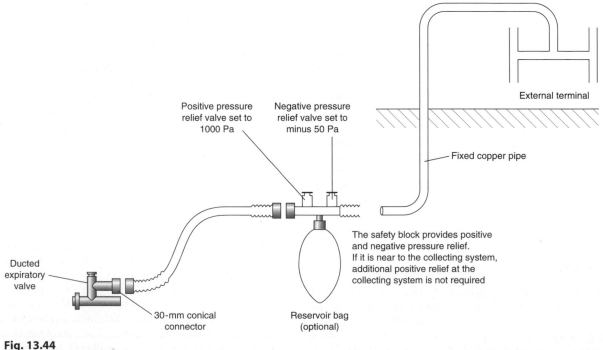

Fig. 13.44
A passive scavenging system.

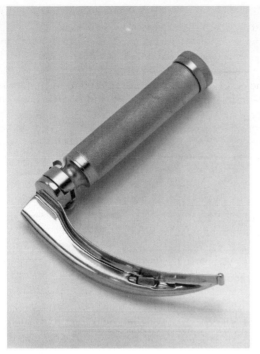

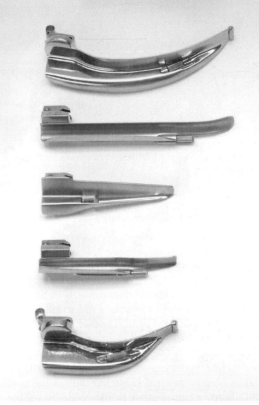

Fig. 13.45
A laryngoscope with the Macintosh adult blade.

The tip of the laryngoscope blade is advanced carefully over the surface of the tongue until it reaches the vallecula (Fig. 16.3). The tip of the blade is rotated upwards and the laryngoscope lifted along the axis of the handle to lift the larynx; the incisor teeth must not be used as a fulcrum to lever the tip of the blade upwards. When the arytenoids and posterior part of the cords are seen, gentle pressure on the larynx using the right thumb, or provided by an assistant, may help to improve the view. Concerns have been raised about the possibility that multiple-use laryngoscopes may transfer between patients the prions thought to be responsible for causing variant Creutzfeldt–Jakob disease (vCJD), especially if used during surgery for tonsillectomy or adenoidectomy. Therefore disposable laryngoscope blades with a plastic sheath over the handle (Fig. 13.47) are now available. The quality of disposable laryngoscopes has improved enormously and is now indistinguishable from that of non-disposable devices.

Straight blade

Straight-bladed laryngoscopes are useful adjuncts in safe airway management. However, they are not always as easy to use as curved blades. The technique of laryngoscopy is slightly different when a straight-bladed laryngoscope is used (see Fig. 16.3).

Fig. 13.46
A selection of laryngoscope blades. From the top downwards: Macintosh adult blade, Miller adult blade, Soper infant blade, Wisconsin infant blade and Macintosh infant blade.

Instead of placing the tip of the blade in the vallecula, it is advanced over the posterior border of the epiglottis, which is then lifted directly by the blade to provide a view of the larynx. This technique is useful particularly in babies, in whom the epiglottis is rather floppy and may obscure the view of the larynx if a curved blade is used. However, bruising of the epiglottis is more likely with a straight blade. The straight-bladed laryngoscopes available include the Miller, Magill, Soper and Wisconsin laryngoscopes.

Light source

Most laryngoscopes are powered by batteries contained within the handle; these must be replaced regularly to prevent failure during laryngoscopy. On many older models of laryngoscope, the light source is a bulb which screws into a socket on the blade; a tight connection should be ensured before laryngoscopy is attempted. It is usual for the electrical circuit between the batteries and the bulb to be closed by a switch

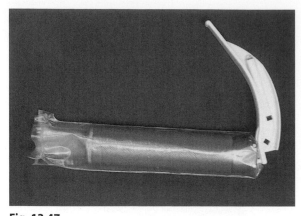

Fig. 13.47
A disposable laryngoscope blade with a plastic sheath over the handle.

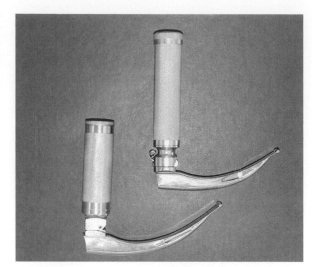

Fig. 13.48
Short and standard laryngoscope handles.

which operates automatically when the blade is opened. However, the electrical contacts of the switch may become corroded, causing a reduction in power or total failure. Because of these potential problems, it is important that the function of the laryngoscope is checked carefully before use. It is also wise to have a spare functioning laryngoscope and a variety of blades available. Newer designs place the bulb in the handle and the light is transmitted to the blade by means of fibreoptics.

Laryngoscope handle

The standard handle may result in difficult laryngoscopy in obese patients, and in women with large breasts. Short handles are available for use in these situations (Fig. 13.48). The short handle has almost replaced the use of the Polio blade (Fig. 13.49) in obstetric practice.

The McCoy laryngoscope (Fig. 13.50A) is based on the standard Macintosh blade but has a hinged tip. This is operated by a lever mechanism attached to the handle. When the lever is pressed (Fig. 13.50B), the tip of the blade bends forward and this improves the view of the larynx.

FIBREOPTIC LARYNGO/BRONCHOSCOPE

The fibreoptic scope (Fig. 13.51) is an endoscope which is used to view the upper and lower airway through either the nose or the mouth. The principle of the fibreoptic system is that light from a powerful external light source is transmitted through a flexible instrument and an image of the area is returned to an eyepiece or camera. The fibres which transmit the light

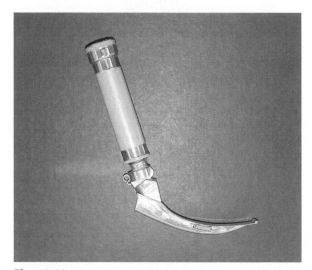

Fig. 13.49
The Polio blade

have a diameter of approximately 20 μm and are made up of a central glass core coated with a thin layer of glass material with a lower refractive index. The light passing down the fibre is repeatedly reflected down the inner glass.

The fibreoptic scope consists of a light source, a universal cord and light guide connector, a control unit, an eyepiece and an insertion tube. The light source (Fig. 13.52) is usually powered by mains electrical supply and contains either a xenon or a halogen lamp. The universal cord and light guide connector contain the light guide fibre bundle and transmit light from a light source to the fibreoptic bundle in the insertion tube.

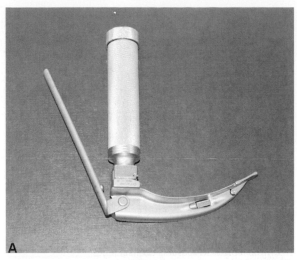

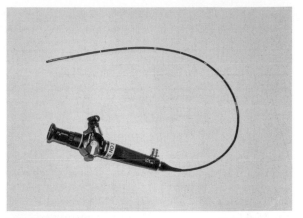

Fig. 13.51
The fibreoptic intubating laryngoscope which consists of a
control unit, insertion cord and a connector for a light guide.

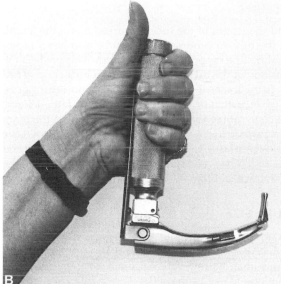

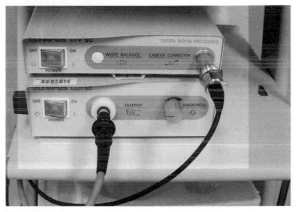

Fig. 13.52
The light source and a camera system for the fibreoptic
intubating laryngoscope.

Fig. 13.50
(**A**) The McCoy laryngoscope. (**B**) The McCoy laryngoscope,
demonstrating the hinged blade tip.

In some newer models, light is powered by a battery
and this enables these scopes to be easily portable and
be used in remote places like Accident and Emergency
departments.

The control unit consists of an angulation control
lever, suction port and a biopsy port. The angulation
lever controls the deflection of the tip of the scope. The
suction port is for connecting to a suction pump but it
can also be used for insufflation of oxygen. The biopsy
channel can be used for taking biopsy specimens but it
can also be used to attach a syringe to instil local
anaesthetic into the airway.

The eyepiece consists of the viewing lens and the
dioptre adjustment ring. A camera can be attached to
the eyepiece either to take photographs or to transmit
the pictures to a television monitor (Figs 13.52, 13.53).

The insertion tube contains two optical fibre bundles: the light guide and the image guide. The fibres
transmitting light (light guide) are arranged in a random fashion but those returning the image (image
guide) are precisely located relative to each other. The
insertion tube also contains the suction channel and
the biopsy channel. At the distal end of each optical
fibre, there is a lens. The size of the insertion tube
varies from 1.8 to 6.4 mm to fit inside tracheal tubes of
internal diameter 3.0–7.0 mm.

Most anaesthetists who use the fibreoptic scope
now attach a camera to the eyepiece and view the airway on the television monitor. The use of a camera

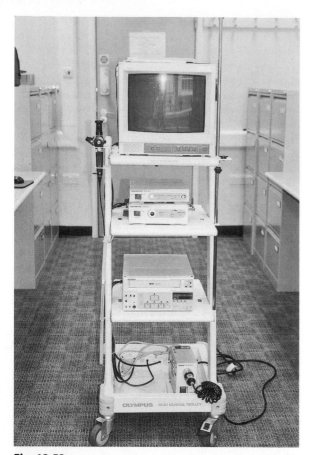

Fig. 13.53
The television monitor, camera system and light source used with the intubating fibreoptic scope.

and TV monitor have been demonstrated to enhance the speed with which anaesthetists can be taught fibreoptic endoscopy skills.

TRACHEAL TUBES

Most tracheal tubes are constructed of red rubber, silicone rubber or plastic. Red rubber tubes are re-usable, although they may start to show signs of deterioration after 2–3 years. Today, disposable plastic tubes are the preferred choice (Fig. 13.54) as they eliminate the need to collect, clean, sterilize and check tubes after use. Plastic tubes are presented in a sterile pack and should be cut to an appropriate length before use. The plastic disposable tubes have a cuff and a pilot balloon with a self-sealing valve. The cuff may be inflated with air, nitrous oxide or saline. The internal diameter of the tube is marked on the side of the tube in millimetres

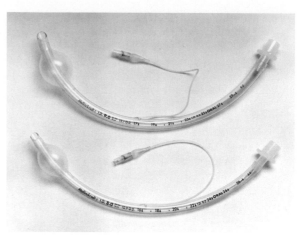

Fig. 13.54
Size 8 and 9 plastic disposable tracheal tubes.

and the length of the tube is marked along the length of the tube in centimetres. The tube also has a radio-opaque line running along its length. This enables the position of the tube to be determined on a chest X-ray.

Some tracheal tubes contain latex and must not be used in patients who have a history of latex allergy. Silicone rubber is increasingly being used in the manufacture of tracheal tubes. These are more expensive than the plastic tubes but they may be sterilized and re-used. They are softer than red rubber or plastic endotracheal tubes and they are non-irritant.

TUBE SIZE

In adults, there is little to be gained in the way of reduced resistance to breathing by selecting a tube larger than 8.0 mm internal diameter. However, it is common to use a tube of 9.0–9.5 mm internal diameter for male and 8.0–8.5 mm for female adults. Tubes of wide diameter may exert pressure on the laryngeal cords after insertion. Appropriate sizes of tracheal tubes for children are shown in Appendix B IX.

PLAIN TUBES

Uncuffed tubes are used in children (Fig. 13.55). A cuff is unnecessary to secure an airtight fit if the correct diameter of tube is selected, because the narrowest part of the airway is in the trachea at the level of the cricoid cartilage. However, the larynx is the narrowest part of the airway in the adult and a leak occurs if an uncuffed tube is used; in addition, there is a risk of aspiration of fluid from the pharynx into the trachea. Nasotracheal intubation is less traumatic if an uncuffed tube is used. The incidence of sore throat is

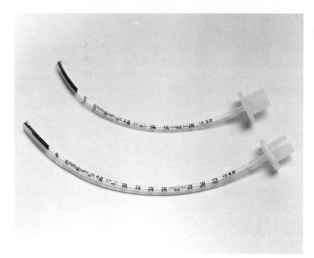

Fig. 13.55
Paediatric uncuffed plastic endotracheal tubes.

not influenced by the presence of a cuff on the tracheal tube.

CUFFED TUBES

It is usual to use a cuffed tube whenever tracheal intubation is required in the adult. It is mandatory if IPPV is to be used or if there is a risk of blood, pus or gastric fluid entering the pharynx. Tracheal tubes with a streamlined cuff are available and are suitable for nasotracheal intubation.

Cuff volume

Tracheal tube cuffs may be either low-volume/high-pressure or high-volume/low-pressure. A tube with a low-volume cuff may require inflation to a high pressure to effect a seal within the trachea. The pressure within a low-volume cuff does not necessarily relate to the pressure exerted by the cuff on the tracheal mucosa. However, a high pressure may be exerted on the mucosa if the cuff is overinflated. This may occur inadvertently during anaesthesia because nitrous oxide diffuses through some types of plastic. Some anaesthetists inflate the cuff with an oxygen/nitrous oxide mixture to obviate this problem. Alternatively, the cuff volume may be readjusted after 10–15 min of anaesthesia.

High-volume/low-pressure ('floppy') cuffs cover a larger area of tracheal wall and may effect a seal with less pressure exerted on the mucosa. However, they may cause more trauma during insertion and may become puckered in a relatively small trachea.

Herniation of an overinflated cuff may occlude the distal end of the tracheal tube and cause partial or total airway obstruction.

SHAPE OF TUBE

In most centres, a curved tracheal tube is used. These should be cut to the correct length as there is a risk of accidental intubation of a bronchus (usually the right main bronchus) if the tip is inserted too far. The Oxford tube is L-shaped and the angle of the tube lies in the pharynx; the distal end is of a fixed length. It is claimed that the use of an Oxford tube reduces the risk of bronchial intubation. There may be less risk of an Oxford tube kinking if the head is flexed during surgery. However, an introducer is required to pass an Oxford tube through the larynx.

Some plastic tracheal tubes are pre-formed in shapes which either fit the pharyngeal contour or carry the proximal end of the tube away from the mouth (Fig. 13.56); the latter design is useful when surgery on the face or head is planned. The RAE (Ring, Adair and Elwyn) tubes have pre-formed curves and they can be used either orally or nasally (Fig. 13.57). RAE tubes may be cuffed or non-cuffed. Care should be taken not to insert these pre-formed tubes too far as there is a risk of bronchial intubation.

SPECIALIZED TUBES

An armoured latex tube is useful if there is a danger of the tube kinking during surgery; a nylon spiral is incorporated in the wall of the tube and prevents obliteration of the lumen. Alternatively, a flexometallic tube, with a metal spiral in the wall, may be used. These tubes are very floppy and a wire stilette is required for their insertion.

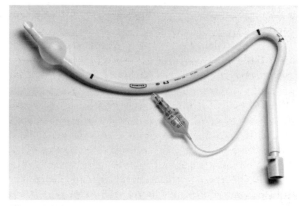

Fig. 13.56
Pre-formed north-facing nasotracheal tube.

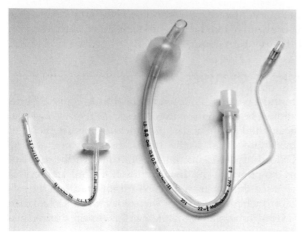

Fig. 13.57
Pre-formed RAE disposable plastic tracheal tubes. The cuffed adult tube and the uncuffed paediatric tube.

The flexometallic tubes are available in either uncuffed paediatric sizes or cuffed adult sizes (Fig. 13.58). These tracheal tubes are long and cannot be shortened because they have a fixed tracheal tube connector. Therefore, when inserting them into the trachea, care should be taken to avoid bronchial intubation. The adult cuffed tubes have two black rings and the paediatric uncuffed tubes have a black line at the distal end. These give guidance as to where the vocal cords should be, in order to avoid bronchial intubation.

A flexible metal tube (Fig. 13.59) may be used during procedures that require the use of lasers in the airway; plastic tubes may ignite if struck by the laser

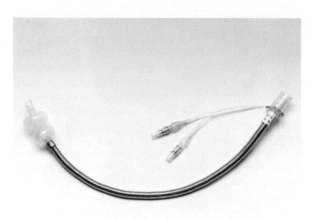

Fig. 13.59
Flexible metal tube suitable for use during laser surgery to the airway.

beam. Some designs have two cuffs. This ensures a tracheal seal should the upper cuff be damaged by laser. An air-filled cuff may ignite if it is hit by a laser beam. Therefore it is recommended that the cuffs are filled with saline instead of air.

The Parker tube (Fig. 13.60) has a curved bevel on the inner curvature of the tube. The bevel therefore lies on the anterior aspect of the tube during insertion. The manufacturer claims that it is less likely than the conventional tube to cause trauma to the larynx or trachea, particularly during insertion over a bougie or fibreoptic laryngoscope.

Double-lumen endobronchial tubes are used during thoracic surgery when there is a need for one lung to be

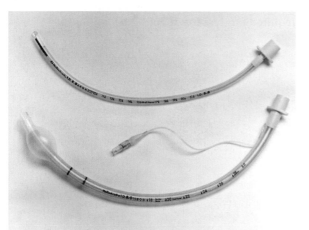

Fig. 13.58
The reinforced tracheal tube – the adult cuffed and paediatric uncuffed tubes.

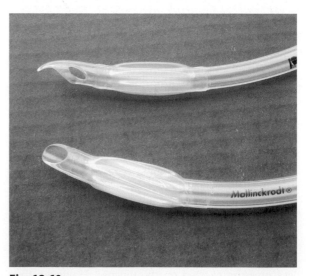

Fig. 13.60
The distal ends of a Parker (upper) and a conventional bevelled tracheal tube.

deflated. They allow selective deflation of one lung whilst maintaining ventilation of the other lung. The older Robertshaw double-lumen tubes are made of red rubber and are therefore re-usable. The disposable Bronchocath double-lumen tubes (Fig. 13.61), which are made of plastic, are used more commonly now.

Laryngectomy tubes (Fig. 13.62) are designed to be inserted through a tracheostomy into the trachea to maintain the airway during surgery for laryngectomy. Because of its shape, the connection to the breathing system is some distance away from the surgical field and this gives the surgeon a relatively clear field in which to operate.

A microlaryngeal tube is a small tube (usually 5 mm internal diameter) with an adult-sized cuff which is used during surgery on the larynx. It allows better surgical access to the larynx.

TRACHEOSTOMY TUBES

There are many types of tracheostomy tube. They may be cuffed or non-cuffed. The proximal end of a

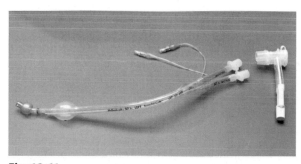

Fig. 13.61
Bronchocath double-lumen endobronchial tube with catheter mount.

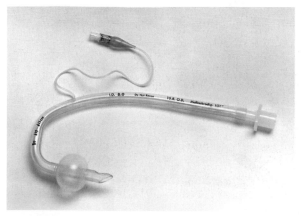

Fig. 13.62
Laryngectomy tube.

tracheostomy tube has a standard 15-mm connector and there are two wings with slots to which the securing tape is attached (Fig. 13.63). Tracheostomy tubes have a replaceable inner cannula which facilitates insertion and is removed once the tracheostomy tube is in place.

The fenestrated tracheostomy tube has a hole (fenestration) along its greater curvature. This allows the patient to speak by directing some of the air past the vocal cords.

Silver tracheostomy tubes are used in many patients who require long-term intubation. They have an inner tube which may be removed for cleaning. Some designs have a one-way flap valve to allow the patient to speak. Silver is non-irritant and bactericidal.

CONNECTIONS

Catheter mount

This is a flexible link between the breathing system and a tracheal tube, laryngeal mask airway, face mask or tracheostomy tube (Fig. 13.64). It may be made of rubber or plastic and some have a gas sampling port. The proximal end, which attaches to the breathing system, has a standard 22-mm connection and the distal end is a 15-mm connector. The length of catheter mounts varies from 45 to 170 mm.

Tracheal tube connectors

Disposable 15-mm-diameter connectors are provided with plastic disposable tubes; the diameter of the distal end is of an appropriate size to fit the internal diameter of the tube. Several other connections (Fig. 13.65)

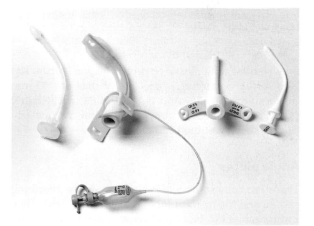

Fig. 13.63
Tracheostomy tubes. Adult cuffed (size 7) and paediatric Shiley uncuffed tube with the replaceable inner cannulae.

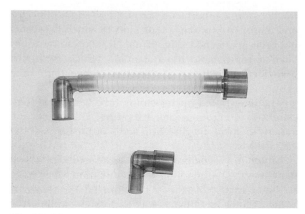

Fig. 13.64
A disposable catheter mount to connect the tracheal tube to the breathing system (top). A disposable angle piece to connect a face mask or tracheal tube to the breathing system (bottom).

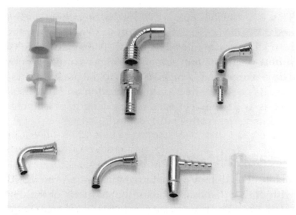

Fig. 13.65
A variety of tracheal tube connectors. From top left in clockwise rotation: Portex with 15-mm tracheal tube connector, Nosworthy, Knight's paediatric connector, Cobbs, Rowbotham, Magill oral, Magill nasal.

may be used with plastic or rubber tracheal tubes. The Nosworthy connector is less bulky than the 15-mm disposable connector and is used often in paediatric practice. The Magill connector is useful, particularly during surgery of the head or neck.

Angle pieces

These are connectors which fit between the breathing system and the tracheal tube or mask (Fig. 13.64). They incorporate a 90° bend and have either 15- or 22-mm connectors at each end. Some angle pieces have a condenser humidifier, bacterial filter and a port for gas sampling incorporated into them (Fig. 13.31).

PROTECTING THE BREATHING CIRCUIT IN ANAESTHESIA

Following recent fatal incidents in which anaesthetic tubing became blocked, the UK Department of Health has made recommendations to minimise the risk of recurrence. The recommendations include training and increasing awareness of the potential problem of anaesthetic tubing becoming blocked accidentally, and protecting vulnerable components of the breathing system by keeping the components individually wrapped until use. The Department of Health recommends the use of the Association of Anaesthetists of Great Britain and Ireland (AAGBI) document 'Checking anaesthetic equipment' and that all trainees should be trained in the correct procedure for checking anaesthetic equipment.

SUPRAGLOTTIC DEVICES

THE LARYNGEAL MASK AIRWAY (LMA)

This device consists of a shortened conventional silicone tube with an elliptical cuff, inflated through a pilot tube, attached to the distal end (Fig. 13.66). The cuff, which resembles a miniature face mask, has been designed to form a relatively airtight seal around the posterior perimeter of the larynx (Fig. 13.67). A variety of sizes of cuff are available, ranging from size 1 which is used in the neonate to size 5 which is used in large adults. The mask is inserted and the cuff inflated until no air leak is detected. It is important to ensure that the maximum inflation volume is not exceeded (Table 13.8).

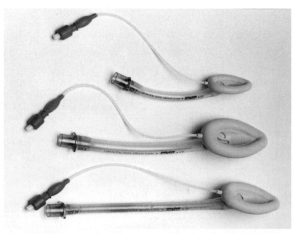

Fig. 13.66
Laryngeal masks. A paediatric size 2 mask, an adult size 4 mask and a size 3 reinforced LMA.

longer and narrower and therefore offers more resistance to breathing (Fig. 13.66). Because of the wire in the tube, it is unsuitable for use in the MRI unit. The classic LMA is re-usable up to 40 times. However, disposable LMAs are now available.

THE INTUBATING LMA

The intubating LMA (ILMA) is an advanced form of the standard LMA (Fig. 13.68). It has a shorter tube and a metal handle. The handle permits single-handed insertion without moving the head and neck and without placing fingers in the mouth. It may be passed through an interdental gap as narrow as 20 mm. The mask floor has an elevating bar which replaces the two bars in the standard LMA. The caudal end of the bar is not fixed to the mask floor and this allows a tracheal tube to be passed in order to intubate the trachea. The ILMA is available in sizes 3, 4 and 5. The recommended cuff volumes are similar to the corresponding sizes of the standard LMA. The rigid curved airway has a standard 15-mm connector at the proximal end. The tube is wide enough to allow passage of a cuffed 8-mm tracheal tube. The ILMA is a re-usable device which may be cleaned and sterilized up to 40 times.

THE LMA PRO-SEAL

The LMA Pro-seal is another advanced form of the classic LMA and it is designed to have additional benefits over the ordinary LMA (Fig. 13.69). It has a double lumen. The drain tube passes lateral to the airway tube and traverses the floor of the mask to open in the mask tip opposite the upper oesophageal sphincter. It may permit drainage of gastric contents or allow

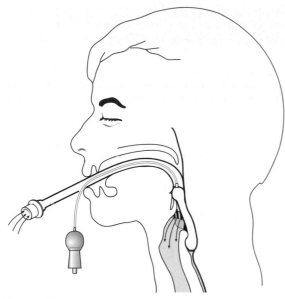

Fig. 13.67
A laryngeal mask in situ.

The device is very effective in maintaining a patent airway in the spontaneously breathing patient. Positive pressure ventilation may be applied if necessary. The mask is not suitable for patients who are at risk from regurgitation of gastric contents (emergency surgery, hiatus hernia or history of reflux, and obesity) and should be used with caution if pharyngeal soiling is anticipated.

The flexible LMA differs from the standard LMA in that it has a flexible, wire reinforced tube. It is available in sizes 2, 2.5, 3, 4 and 5. The size of the cuff is similar to that of the standard LMA but the tube is

	Length of		Volume of	Largest size of tracheal tube
Size of LMA	LMA	Size of patient	cuff (mL)	that fits into the LMA
1	8	Neonates and infants up to 6.5 kg	Up to 4	3.5
1.5	10	Infants 5–10 kg	Up to 7	4.0
2	11	Infants and children 10–20 kg	Up to 10	4.5
2.5	12.5	Children 20–30 kg	Up to 14	5.0
3	16	Children and small adults 30–50 kg	Up to 20	6.0
4	16	Normal adults 50–70 kg	Up to 30	6.0
5	18	Large adults >70 kg	Up to 40	7.0

Table 13.8 Characteristics of laryngeal mask airways (LMAs)

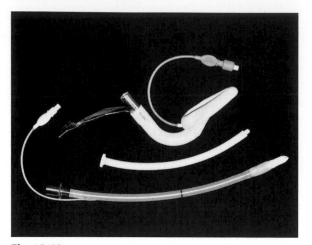

Fig. 13.68
An intubating laryngeal mask with the silicone tracheal tube and the introducer.

passage of an orogastric tube. The drainage tube is also intended to prevent gastric insufflation. The airway tube is wire reinforced to prevent collapse and it ends with a standard 15-mm connector. The cuff arrangement allows a higher seal than the LMA for a given intracuff pressure, which permits more effective ventilation of the lungs. It has a built-in bite-block to reduce the danger of airway obstruction from the patient biting on the LMA. The Pro-seal LMA is re-usable up to 40 times and all its components are latex free. It can be mounted on an introducer which facilitates the insertion of the LMA Pro-seal into the patient's mouth (Fig. 13.69B).

THE COMBITUBE

The Combitube (Fig. 13.70) is a double-lumen airway which is designed to be inserted blindly in difficult and emergency situations. When inserted, it allows establishment of an effective airway whether it is placed into the oesophagus or the trachea. It combines the function of an oesophageal obturator and conventional tracheal tube and it protects the airway against aspiration of gastric contents. The tube has two cuffs, a proximal larger pharyngeal cuff (85–100 mL) and the smaller distal cuff (10–15 mL). The distal cuff may be placed in either the oesophagus or the trachea. Between 94% and 98% of blind insertions usually result in oesophageal placement. In this situation, the breathing system is attached to the longer blue connecting tube and the Combitube acts as a pharyngeal airway (Fig. 13.71A). If the tube enters the trachea, ventilation of the lungs should be carried out using the shorter connecting tube and it acts as an ordinary tracheal tube (Fig. 13.71B).

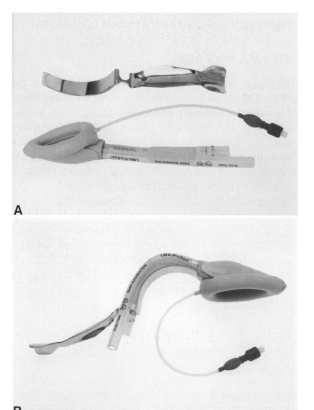

A

B

Fig. 13.69
(**A**) The LMA Pro-seal. (**B**) The LMA Pro-seal mounted on the LMA Pro-seal introducer.

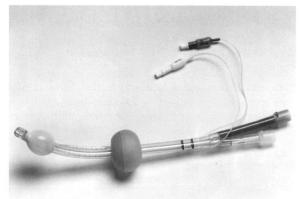

Fig. 13.70
The Combitube, showing the larger proximal pharyngeal cuff and smaller distal cuff.

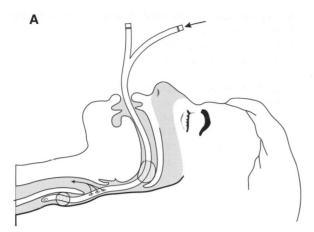

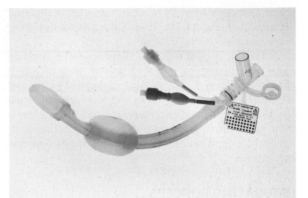

Fig. 13.72
The airway management device (AMD).

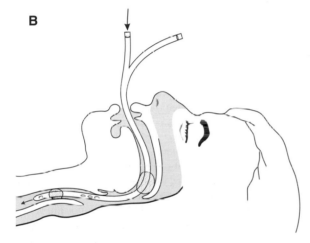

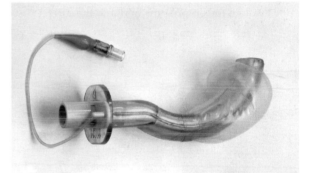

Fig. 13.73
The cuffed oropharyngeal airway (COPA).

Fig. 13.71
The two possible positions of the Combitube. (**A**) Combitube inserted in the oesophagus. (**B**) Combitube inserted in the trachea.

THE AIRWAY MANAGEMENT DEVICE (AMD)

The AMD is a another supraglottic device which is inserted blindly (Fig. 13.72). It has a single lumen, a double cuff and two pilot balloons. An oesophageal aperture becomes patent when the distal cuff is deflated. Its role in airway management is yet to be fully established as it does not offer many further benefits over other devices already available.

THE CUFFED OROPHARYNGEAL AIRWAY (COPA)

The cuffed oropharyngeal airway (COPA, Fig. 13.73) is essentially a Guedel airway with an extended pharyngeal section in which an inflatable cuff is embedded.

Inflation of the cuff is designed to produce an airtight seal in the oropharynx and lift the tongue. It may be attached to the anaesthetic breathing system. It is designed to avoid tracheal intubation and is easier to place than the LMA. The advantages and disadvantages of this device are similar to those of the LMA, although it possibly does not form a sealed airway as well as the LMA. Four sizes are available (8, 9, 10, and 11), each colour-coded and representing the length of the COPA in centimetres.

OTHER APPARATUS

FACE MASKS

These are designed to fit the face perfectly so that no leak of gas occurs, but without applying excessive pressure to the skin. An appropriate size of face mask must be selected to ensure a proper fit, but the smallest size possible should be used to minimize dead space. Disposable masks made of transparent material are available (Fig. 13.74). These allow the detection of vomitus or secretions.

A harness system (e.g. Clausen harness) is used by some anaesthetists to hold the mask on the face during surgery. However, airway obstruction may occur at any time and the excursion of the reservoir bag must be observed constantly. In many countries, the LMA is now used during maintenance of anaesthesia in almost all situations in which a face mask was formerly used.

INTUBATING FORCEPS

The most commonly used intubating forceps is that designed by Magill (Fig. 13.75). The instrument is employed to manipulate a nasotracheal or nasogastric tube through the oropharynx and into the correct posi-

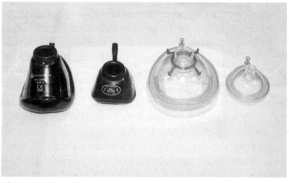

Fig. 13.74
Sizes 1 and 5 disposable and re-usable face masks.

tion. A laryngoscope is used to obtain a view of the oropharynx.

LARYNGEAL SPRAY

This is used to deposit a fine mist of local anaesthetic solution (usually lidocaine 4% or 10%) on the mucosa of the larynx and upper trachea (Fig. 13.76). These sprays are particularly useful in applying local anaesthetic to the upper airway during awake fibreoptic intubation.

MOUTH GAG

A mouth gag (Fig. 13.75) may be used during dental anaesthesia and is required occasionally to open the mouth in patients with trismus, or if masseter spasm is present. It is positioned between the molar teeth and must be used with great care to avoid dental trauma.

BOUGIE

If the larynx cannot be seen adequately during laryngoscopy, or if the tracheal tube cannot be manoeuvred into the laryngeal inlet, a bougie may be used as an aid to tracheal intubation. The lubricated bougie is inserted into the trachea to act as a guide for the tracheal tube. The tube should be rotated so that the bevel does not become lodged against the aryepiglottic fold. In a difficult intubation scenario, the correct type of bougie should be used (Fig. 13.77). The bougie with a curved tip at the end is designed to assist in this situation whereas the straight-ended bougie is intended for endotracheal tube exchange only. Disposable bougies are now available but their efficacy over the re-usable ones is yet to be demonstrated. The Eschmann multiple-use bougie has the

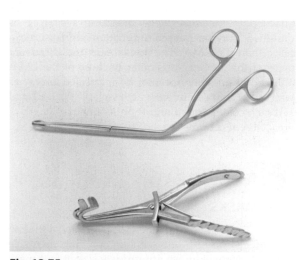

Fig. 13.75
Magill intubating forceps (above). The Ferguson mouth gag (below).

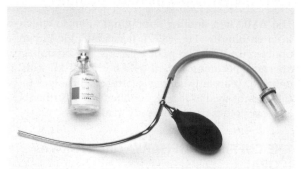

Fig. 13.76
Laryngeal sprays. Forrester spray and the 10% lidocaine pre-filled laryngeal spray.

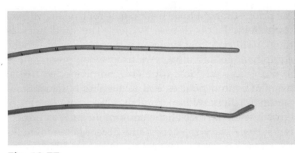

Fig. 13.77
The straight-ended multiple-use bougie (above) and the angled-end multiple-use bougie (below).

highest success rate, least likelihood of causing trauma and has reliable and clinically tested signs of confirmation of tracheal placement when compared with either the Frova, single-use intubation introducer or the Portex single-use introducer.

STILETTES

A malleable metal stilette may be used to adjust the degree of curvature of a tracheal tube as an aid to its insertion. The stilette must not protrude from the distal end of the tube.

AIRWAYS

An *oropharyngeal* airway (Guedel airway, Fig. 13.78) may be required to prevent obstruction caused by the tongue or collapse of the pharynx in the patient without a tracheal tube. A *nasopharyngeal* airway (Fig. 13.78) is tolerated better during light anaesthesia and may also be used if it is difficult to insert an oropharyngeal airway, e.g. trismus. However, the use of nasopharyngeal airways may be associated with significant bleeding from the nose.

SUCTION APPARATUS

Suction apparatus is vital during anaesthesia and resuscitation to clear the airway of any mucus, blood or debris. It is also used during surgery to clear the operating field of either blood or fluid.

Suction apparatus consists of a source of vacuum, a suction unit and suction tubing. The source of vacuum can be either piped vacuum or electrically or manually operated units. Piped vacuum is the most commonly used source in many operating theatres.

The suction unit consists of a reservoir jar, bacterial filter, vacuum control regulator and a vacuum gauge (Fig. 13.79). The reservoir jar is graduated so that the volume of aspirate may be estimated. It contains a cut-off valve. The cut-off valve has a float that rises as the fluid level increases and shuts off the valve when the reservoir jar is full. This prevents liquid from the suction jar entering the suction system. There is a bacterial filter between the cut-off valve and the suction control unit to prevent air that has been contaminated during passage through the apparatus infecting the atmosphere when it is blown out. The filter also traps any particulate or nebulized matter. Filters should be changed at regular intervals.

The vacuum regulator adjusts the degree of vacuum. The vacuum is indicated on the pressure gauge. This is normally marked in mmHg or kPa. The needle on the gauge goes in an anticlockwise direction as the vacuum increases. Suction units can achieve flows of

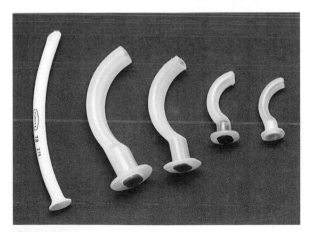

Fig. 13.78
Guedel airways and a nasopharyngeal airway.

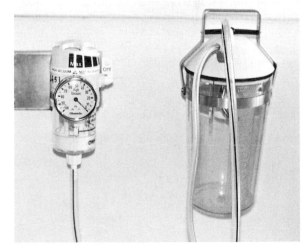

Fig. 13.79
Suction apparatus.

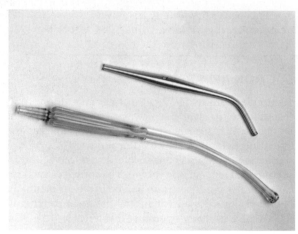

Fig. 13.80
Yankauer suction connectors. Adult and paediatric apparatus.

greater than $25\,L\,min^{-1}$ and a vacuum of greater than 67 kPa. However, flows and vacuum as high as these are seldom necessary and can cause harm if used inappropriately, particularly in children.

The suction reservoir jar is connected to the patient via a suction tubing and either a Yankauer handpiece (Fig. 13.80) or suction catheters.

DECONTAMINATION OF ANAESTHETIC EQUIPMENT

Anaesthetic equipment is a potential vector for transmission of diseases between patients. Concerns have been raised about the possibility that multiple-use devices may transfer blood-borne infections between patients and there is also the possibility of transfer of the prions thought to be responsible for causing variant Creutzfeldt–Jakob disease (vCJD). The guidelines of the AAGBI state that single-use, disposable anaesthetic equipment should always be used when possible. For re-usable anaesthetic equipment, compliance with local hospital control policies and awareness of decontamination practices are important in minimizing the risk of cross-infection. Anaesthetic equipment such as breathing systems, laryngoscopes and fibreoptic endoscopes are classified as semi-critical items because they come in contact with mucous membranes and non-intact skin but do not ordinarily break the blood barrier. They present an intermediate risk of transmitting infection. It is therefore recommended that these should have a high level of disinfection. High levels of disinfectants such as gluteraldehyde, stabilized hydrogen peroxide, peracetic acid, chlorine and chlorine-releasing compounds should be used.

FURTHER READING

Al-Shaikh B, Stacey S 2002 Essentials of anaesthetic equipment, 2nd edn. Churchill Livingstone, London

Association of Anaesthetists of Great Britain and Ireland 2002 Infection control in anaesthesia. AAGBI, London

Association of Anaesthetists of Great Britain and Ireland 2004 Checking anaesthetic equipment 3. AAGBI, London

Dorsch J A, Dorsch S E 1999 Understanding anaesthetic equipment, 4th edn. Williams and Wilkins, London

Gabbott B M 2001 Recent advances in airway technology. BJA CEPD Reviews 1: 76–80

Davey A, Diba A 2005 Anaesthetic equipment, 5th edn. WB Saunders, London

Murray J M, Bedi A 2000 Carbon dioxide absorption during anaesthesia. RCA Newsletter 50: 287–299

Sabir N, Ramachandra V 2004 Decontamination of anaesthetic equipment. Continuing Education in Anaesthesia, Critical Care and Pain 4: 103–106

The operating theatre environment

14

Until the middle of the nineteenth century, surgery was carried out in any convenient room, frequently one which was used for other purposes. Although the introduction of antisepsis resulted in the washing of instruments and the operating table, the operating room itself was ignored as a source of infection. Operating rooms were designed with tiers of wooden benches around the operating table for spectators; thus the term operating *theatre* was introduced. During the early part of the twentieth century, large windows were incorporated, as artificial light was relatively ineffective, and high ceilings were introduced to improve ventilation. Additional facilities became necessary for preparing and anaesthetizing the patient, for sterilization of instruments and for the surgeon and other theatre staff to change clothes and scrub up. In addition, the design of operating theatres changed, and smaller theatres were introduced to facilitate frequent cleaning.

A modern operating theatre incorporates the following design features:

- environmental controls of varying degrees of complexity, to reduce the risk of airborne infection
- services for surgical and anaesthetic equipment
- an operating table on which the patient may be placed in the position required for surgery
- artificial lighting appropriate for the requirements of both surgeon and anaesthetist
- measures to ensure the safety of patient and staff.

In addition, provision should be made immediately adjacent to the operating theatre for anaesthetizing the patient, preparing instruments, cleaning dirty instruments and for the surgeon to scrub up. There should also be separate areas for reception and recovery of patients. It is the usual practice for each hospital to have a suite of theatres, rather than operating theatres close to each of the surgical wards, which was formerly a common feature. The use of theatre suites permits more flexible and efficient use of staff and resources.

THE OPERATING THEATRE SUITE

The number of operating theatres required is difficult to calculate, but approximates in most British cities to one for every 40 000 of the population served. Ideally, the operating theatre suite should be close to the surgical wards, and adjacent to, and on the same floor as, the accident and emergency department, intensive care unit, X-ray department, day-case ward and sterile supplies unit. It is logical for the anaesthetic department to be immediately adjacent to, or an integral part of, the operating theatre suite, although this seldom occurs in practice.

The main purpose of the operating theatre environment is to minimize the risk of transmission of infection to the patient from the air, the building or the staff. The operating theatre suite contains four zones of increasing degree of cleanliness (Table 14.1).

TRANSFER OF PATIENT

There is some evidence that anxiety in the surgical patient peaks as transfer from the ward to the operating theatre begins, and it is important that facilities for transfer minimize stress. A nurse from the ward usually accompanies the patient, but it is customary for the ward nurse to leave adult patients before anaesthesia has been induced. In paediatric practice, it is now the normal routine that a ward nurse and parent remain with the child during induction of anaesthesia.

On arrival at the reception area, the patient's identity and surgical procedure are checked. In a theatre suite, it may be necessary for patients to wait for some time in the reception area to prevent delays in the operating schedules. Consequently, adequate space should be provided for several beds, and there should be screens for patients who wish for privacy. The staff in the reception area should include nurses. The décor should be cheerful, and the lighting subdued.

Transport should involve the minimum number of changes of trolley. A trolley is used commonly to

Table 14.1 Zones of cleanliness in the operating theatre suite

Outer zone – hospital areas up to and including the reception area

Clean zone – the circulation area used by staff after they have changed, and the route taken by patients from the transfer bay to the anaesthetic room

Aseptic zone – scrub-up and gowning area, anaesthetic room, theatre preparation room, operation room, exit bay

Disposal zone – disposal area for waste products and soiled or used equipment and supplies

transfer the patient to the operating theatre suite, but changes of trolley may be required to enter the clean area and also for transfer to the operating table after anaesthesia has been induced.

Alternatively, the patient's own bed may be taken to the operating theatre suite. If the patient is infirm or in severe pain, the bed may be taken to the anaesthetic room, and transfer delayed until after induction of anaesthesia, but this is appropriate only if the bed has the facility to be tipped head-down if necessary. In some hospitals, a single transfer is effected by transporting the patient to the theatre suite in bed, where the patient is moved on to the operating theatre table-top, which is mounted on a wheeled frame. After induction of anaesthesia, the table-top is wheeled into the theatre and the top attached to a fixed base, which allows it to be positioned for surgery.

There is no universal method of transferring patients from one trolley to another. This may be achieved by the use of canvas and poles, rollers or other 'sliding' devices, or lifting the patient bodily. There is increasing awareness of the risk of injury to operating theatre personnel as a result of lifting patients, and thus an increasing tendency to install transfer systems which do not require great physical effort. There are also risks to patients arising from transfer to and from trolleys, operating tables and beds, including physical injury, disconnection of intravenous infusions or intravascular catheters, displacement of a tracheal tube and disconnection of monitoring apparatus.

All trolleys in the operating theatre suite should be equipped with oxygen, and this should be administered routinely to patients during transfer from theatre to the recovery room at the end of the procedure if general anaesthesia has been used or if there is any other clinical indication.

ANAESTHETIC ROOM

In several countries, the anaesthetic room has developed from a small annexe to the theatre to an integral part of the operating theatre suite. However, this is not universal, and in many parts of the world anaesthesia is induced in the operating theatre after the patient has been transferred onto the operating table. The main advantages of the anaesthetic room are:

- The patient's anxiety may be reduced by avoiding the sights and sounds of the operating theatre. This is of special importance in children.
- The equipment which may be necessary during induction of anaesthesia can be stored in an uncluttered manner, with each item readily available and its location obvious, in contrast to the cramped 'cart' which is usually employed to provide equipment and drugs when anaesthesia is induced in the operating theatre.
- Time is saved by inducing anaesthesia while surgery is being completed on another patient. This is useful particularly if preparation is prolonged, e.g. performance of local anaesthetic blocks or establishment of invasive cardiovascular monitoring, but is safe only if at least two anaesthetists and two trained assistants are present.

However, there are several disadvantages:

- Anaesthetic and monitoring equipment must be duplicated, or moved to the operating theatre with the patient; this usually necessitates temporary disconnection from electrical or gas supplies.
- Hazards are involved in transferring an unconscious patient from a trolley to the operating table.
- Construction and maintenance of anaesthetic rooms are expensive.

Even in countries where anaesthetic rooms are used, it is customary to induce anaesthesia in the high-risk patient on the operating table, as the delay between onset of unconsciousness and the start of surgery must be kept to a minimum, e.g. for emergency caesarean section or severe haemorrhage.

The design of the anaesthetic room should allow easy access all round the patient's trolley, and should provide space for anaesthetic and monitoring equipment, and storage cupboards and shelves. The minimum floor area recommended by the Department of Health in the UK is 17 m², but this is inadequate. A floor area of 21 m² is more appropriate. Piped gases and suction, and electrical sockets, are required near the head of the trolley. An anaesthetic machine, mechanical ventilator and monitoring system are also necessary. Cupboards must be available to store equipment and drugs, and worktops must be of sufficient size to allow syringes, needles, cannulae and drugs to be prepared. There should be a clock with a second hand.

OPERATING ROOM

The operating room is designed around its centrally situated operating table with overhead lighting and ventilation systems. The ideal shape for the operating room is circular, but this is inefficient and most operating rooms are square or nearly square. The Royal College of Surgeons of England has suggested that the floor should be $625 \, ft^2$ (approximately $58 \, m^2$) in area, and no smaller than $484 \, ft^2$ (approximately $45 \, m^2$). Theatres for specialized surgery may require a larger area to accommodate bulky equipment.

Outlets for piped gases and electrical sockets must be positioned close to the head of the operating table; they are provided most conveniently by a boom or stalactite system. Electrical cables should not lie across the floor. The operating room should be of sufficient size to allow all types of surgery without moving the position of the head of the table; this location should be reached easily and without complex manoeuvres as the patient enters the theatre from the anaesthetic room.

Temperature, humidity and ventilation

The temperature in the operating theatre and anaesthetic room should be sufficiently high to minimize the risk of inducing hypothermia in the patient, but must be comfortable for theatre staff. The patient may develop hypothermia at an ambient temperature of less than $21°C$. Temperatures of $22-24°C$ are usually acceptable in the operating room, with a relative humidity of 50–60%; a higher environmental temperature is required during surgery in the neonate or infant. Slightly lower temperature and humidity are acceptable in other parts of the theatre suite. Controls for temperature and humidity should be located within the operating theatre so that adjustments can be made by theatre staff.

Heating and humidity are controlled usually by an air-conditioning and ventilation system, which provides an ambient pressure inside the operating room slightly higher than atmospheric. In general, air is introduced directly over the operating table, and leaves at the periphery through ducts positioned near floor level. In the area of the table, 400 air changes per hour are required to minimize the risk of airborne transmission of infection. More effective systems of ventilation, involving radial exponential air flow away from the operating table, or laminar flow, are used in some centres for some types of surgery, e.g. joint replacement, in which infection is especially undesirable. High-flow systems may accelerate cooling of the patient (and staff).

Light

Daylight is not necessary in the operating theatre, although it is more pleasant for staff if there are windows in the theatre suite, e.g. in corridors and common rooms. A high level of illumination is required over the operating table, and ceiling-mounted lamps are standard; it is preferable if they can be positioned directly by the surgeon.

The intensity and colour temperature of general lighting are very important to the anaesthetist, as appreciation of skin colour is affected by the spectrum of the source of illumination. The spectrum provided by lighting tubes should be similar to that of daylight, with an emission temperature of $4000-5000 \, K$. The colour of the décor should be neutral and uniform. The intensity of general illumination should be up to $325 \, lm \, m^{-2}$ in the operating theatre, and it should be diffuse to avoid glare. In the anaesthetic room and recovery area, a light intensity of approximately $220 \, lm \, m^{-2}$ is acceptable, but a spotlight should be available if increased illumination is required for specific procedures.

SAFETY IN THE OPERATING THEATRE

Trailing electrical wires, gas supply hoses, ventilator tubing, intravenous tubing and monitoring cables represent a hazard to both staff and patients in the operating theatre. Staff may trip and suffer injury, and it is easy to disconnect the electrical supply to vital equipment. If the power to modern anaesthetic machines is disconnected, monitoring, ventilation and gas supplies fail simultaneously. In addition, there may be a risk to staff from pollution of the atmosphere with anaesthetic gases and vapours, and of contracting infection, particularly human immunodeficiency virus (HIV) or hepatitis, from infected patients. Potential hazards in the operating theatre are shown in Table 14.2.

Electrical safety

Although some mention is made of electrical hazards in the operating theatre in Chapter 11, a detailed description is beyond the scope of this book, and the reader is referred to the article by Hull (1978) in the further reading list. The electrical supply to the

Table 14.2   Potential hazards in the operating theatre
Electricity
Liquids
Gases and vapours
Temperature
Humidity
Fire
Cables and tubes

operating theatre and all electrical equipment connected to the patient incorporate design features which minimize the risk of electrical currents being transmitted through the patient to earth.

Explosions

Explosive anaesthetic gases and vapours (diethyl ether, cyclopropane, ethyl chloride) are no longer used in developed countries. However, diethyl ether is still used occasionally in some countries. Ether burns in air, but forms an explosive mixture with oxygen. An explosion may be initiated by a spark of very low energy (<1 μJ) or by contact with a temperature of 300°C or higher. The risk of explosion is highest within and close to the anaesthetic breathing system because of the presence of a high oxygen concentration. Beyond a distance of 10 cm from the breathing system, the oxygen concentration diminishes and the risk is reduced. Ethyl chloride is used in some centres to generate a cold stimulus when testing the extent of regional or local anaesthetic blocks, and the risk of fire or explosion should not be forgotten.

The construction of anaesthetic apparatus is designed to minimize explosion hazards from generation of sparks caused by cumulation of static electricity. All rubber is conductive, so that electrical charges leak to earth, and non-conductive substances are treated with antistatic material. In most operating theatres more than 15–20 years old, the floor has a high but finite resistance, so that static charges leak to earth but electrocution risks are minimized. Until recently, theatre footwear was also designed to earth static charges. Sparks may be generated by clothing made of synthetic materials such as nylon. The risk of accumulation of static electricity on walls and equipment is reduced if the environment humidity exceeds 70%.

Diathermy must not be used if flammable or explosive anaesthetics are employed. However, because the use of these agents has ceased in developed countries, many of the precautions against generation of sparks, and the use of expensive antistatic flooring, have become unnecessary.

Fire is still a hazard if alcohol-based solutions are used by the surgeon to sterilize the skin; the usual ignition source is a spark from the diathermy probe.

Atmospheric pollution

There has been considerable controversy regarding the risk to theatre staff from atmospheric pollution by anaesthetic gases and vapours. Earlier investigations suggested that theatre staff are more likely than other hospital personnel to suffer from hepatic and renal disease, to have non-specific neurological symptoms and for their children to have an increased risk of congenital abnormality. However, none of these problems has been substantiated.

There was more convincing evidence from some studies that female staff who worked in the operating theatre during the early months of pregnancy suffered an increased incidence of spontaneous abortion, and there is experimental evidence to suggest that constant exposure of rats to a concentration of more than 1000 ppm of nitrous oxide produces adverse results on their reproduction. However, the most recent, comprehensive and only randomized prospective investigation of operating theatre staff failed to demonstrate any increased health risk.

Trace concentrations of anaesthetic gases have been implicated in another area of concern – impairment of professional performance. Motor and intellectual performance were shown in an early laboratory study in volunteers to deteriorate in the presence of concentrations of nitrous oxide of 500 ppm, with or without halothane 15 ppm. However, subsequent studies failed to confirm these findings, and the consensus of several studies is that concentrations of 8–12% nitrous oxide are required before significant impairment of performance occurs. Such concentrations might be inhaled if the anaesthetist is close to an unscavenged expiratory valve, or during inhalation induction of anaesthesia, but exceed those present in other areas of an adequately ventilated operating theatre.

Nevertheless, it is sensible to minimize atmospheric pollution in the operating theatre, and hospital regulations in both western Europe and North America require the installation of anaesthetic gas-scavenging systems in all areas where anaesthesia is administered. In the USA, the National Institute of Occupational Safety and Hygiene (a federal regulatory body) dictates that environmental concentrations of anaesthetic gases should not exceed a value of 25 ppm of nitrous oxide and 2 ppm of volatile agent. In the UK, the Health and Safety Executive introduced maximum limits of exposure to anaesthetic agents in January 1996; these are shown in Table 14.3. Scavenging systems are described in Chapter 13.

Anaesthetic gases are not the only source of environmental pollution in the operating theatre; volatile skin-cleaning fluids and aerosol sprays, e.g. iodine or plastic skin dressing, should be used sensibly, and inhalation of vapours should be avoided.

Infection

The most serious types of acquired infection in operating theatre staff are HIV and hepatitis, which may be contracted by contact with blood or body fluids from an infected patient. Several healthcare workers have been infected in this way, either by a needlestick injury or through cuts and abrasions. The risk of percutaneous transmission of HIV is believed to be extremely low; the incidence of seroconversion after occupational exposure to HIV is 0.39%. However, the risk is 5–30% after an occupational inoculation injury.

Two thousand cases of hepatitis B are reported each year in the UK, although the true incidence is probably very much higher. Hepatitis B surface antigen persists for at least 6 months in 5–10% of infected individuals. The virus is highly infectious, and minute amounts of blood may transmit the disease. The Association of Anaesthetists of Great Britain and Ireland (AAGBI) recommends that all anaesthetists should receive active immunization against hepatitis B and most hospitals in the UK insist that evidence of immunity to the virus is present in an anaesthetist's serum before allowing employment to start. A single dose of hepatitis B immunoglobulin combined with active immunization is required immediately if an unprotected individual is inoculated with infected material.

Hepatitis C and D viruses are also blood-borne. Up to 50% of people infected with the hepatitis C virus develop chronic liver disease. Occupational transmission of this virus has been reported.

The incidence of acquired immunodeficiency syndrome (AIDS) continues to increase. For every patient with fully developed AIDS, there are estimated to be five with a less severe form of the disease, and up to 50 asymptomatic carriers. At present, it is unclear what proportion of these develop AIDS, but it may approach 100%. Thus, anaesthetists are likely to be exposed to an increasing number of patients who may transmit HIV. At present, compulsory screening of hospital patients for HIV is regarded as unacceptable. Consequently, precautions must be taken in patients who are believed to be at high risk of being HIV-positive; these include homosexual or bisexual men, haemophiliacs and sexual partners of high-risk patients. In some locations, it has been recommended that precautions should be taken with all patients.

Human T-cell leukaemia virus (HTLV-1) is also of potential importance.

The following precautions are recommended to reduce the risks of transmission of HIV; these are also applicable when patients infected with other blood-borne viruses are anaesthetized.

- Gloves must be worn during induction of anaesthesia, performance of venepuncture or insertion of any intravascular cannula, and during insertion or removal of airways and tracheal tubes; this should be a routine when dealing with any patient. A plastic apron, mask and eye protection should be worn if substantial spillage of blood is anticipated, e.g. during insertion of an arterial cannula. Gloves should normally be discarded on taking the patient into the operating theatre and a fresh pair donned when any of these procedures is carried out during or at the end of anaesthesia. Equipment, notes and other articles must not be handled with contaminated gloves.
- Needles which have been in contact with the patient must not be resheathed or handed from one person to another.
- All needles and other sharp objects should be disposed of in an appropriate tough disposal bin; cardboard bins are unsatisfactory.

Table 14.3 Maximum levels of exposure to anaesthetic agents in the operating theatre suite over an 8 h time-weighted average reference period, as laid down in the UK by the Health and Safety Executive

Agent	Maximum concentration (ppm)
Nitrous oxide	100
Halothane	10
Enflurane	50
Isoflurane	50
Sevoflurane	20[*]

[*]Manufacturer's recommendation.

- Cuts or abrasions on the anaesthetist's hands should be covered with a waterproof dressing. An anaesthetist with considerable skin lesions, such as eczema, chapping or several scratches, is particularly at risk of being infected.
- If a needlestick injury or contamination of a cut or abrasion occurs, bleeding should be encouraged and the skin washed thoroughly with soap and water.
- Advice should be obtained immediately from the hospital's occupational health department if there is reason to believe that contamination has occurred.
- Disposable equipment should be used where possible. Non-disposable equipment should be decontaminated with 2% glutaraldehyde, washed with soap and water and left in glutaraldehyde for a further 3 h. Contaminated floors and surfaces should be washed with 1% hypochlorite solution. Gloves must be worn.

There have been a number of instances in which items of disposable equipment, e.g. angle-pieces and catheter mounts, have been re-used, but in which the lumen has become obstructed, probably accidentally, by other items of equipment kept in the anaesthetic room. Equipment intended for single use should be discarded after use; re-usable equipment should be checked carefully to ensure that it is functioning correctly.

It is standard practice that a bacterial filter should be placed between the tracheal tube or airway and the anaesthetic breathing system in all patients to prevent cross-infection from a patient with undiagnosed infection.

In some countries, and particularly the UK, there has been increasing concern in recent years about the possibility of transmission of the prion responsible for the development of variant Creutzfeldt–Jakob disease (vCJD), attributed to infection from cows affected by bovine spongiform encephalitis (BSE). In infected patients, the prion is believed to be present in high concentrations in the tonsils. It is resistant to conventional methods of cleaning or sterilizing equipment. Consequently, many hospitals in the UK have taken steps to stop the use of non-disposable items of equipment which could come in contact with structures in the pharynx. These items include laryngoscopes, bougies and laryngeal mask airways, and single-use devices are being introduced. Although they eliminate the risk of transmission of vCJD, the currently available single-use devices are not always as successful in achieving their primary aim as their re-usable counterparts.

Noise

Noise in the operating theatre should be kept to a minimum. Patients in the anaesthetic room before induction of anaesthesia may be made more anxious by boisterous laughter or loud conversation coming from the operating theatre. Similarly, as patients recover consciousness after the operation, undue noise is undesirable.

Surgeons and operating theatre staff may enjoy listening to music during surgery, and it is not uncommon for hi-fi systems to be installed in operating theatres. The anaesthetist must ensure that sounds from the monitoring system, e.g. the tone indicating arterial oxygen saturation and the sounds of alarms, can be heard, either by turning up the volume of tones from the monitoring system or turning down the volume of the hi-fi system.

EQUIPMENT CHECKS

Anaesthetic equipment should be up to date, maintained regularly and the instruction manuals should be available and accessible. Monitoring apparatus should be in accordance with existing guidelines. Appropriate alarm limits must be set, and alarms must not be disabled. An equipment check must be performed before an operating theatre session begins because a frequent cause of misadventure is the use of a machine which has not been checked properly, and which malfunctions. An adequate check of anaesthetic apparatus is an integral part of good practice; failure to check the anaesthetic equipment properly may amount to malpractice.

Operating theatre staff usually carry out checks when setting up an operating theatre for use, or after apparatus has been serviced or repaired, but the ultimate responsibility for ensuring that the apparatus is safe for its intended use rests with the anaesthetist. Sophisticated tests may have been performed after major servicing, but key control settings may have been altered and it is essential that the anaesthetist checks that the equipment is in proper working order and ready for clinical use. The final pre-use check is the sole responsibility of the anaesthetist who is to use the machine. It cannot be delegated to any other person. The necessary checks can be carried out in a few minutes and must be undertaken before any operating theatre session is started.

It is strongly recommended that a record of the checks is kept and this is best achieved by the use of a specific logbook attached to the anaesthetic machine, in which should be recorded the date and time that the equipment was checked, the name of the individual carrying out the check and any faults encountered, however minor. There is no justification for proceeding with an anaesthetic when faults have been identified in the equipment. If there is no record of an adequate preoperative check of equipment and a problem occurs as a result of equipment failure, it is very difficult to defend an allegation of negligence.

Checking the anaesthetic machine

At its most basic, the function of an anaesthetic machine is to enable the anaesthetist to administer to a patient oxygen under pressure without leaks. If all else fails, this allows the anaesthetist to preserve life.

Anaesthetic apparatus should be checked in a logical sequence as recommended in the AAGBI checklist shown in Table 14.4. The primary intention of the check of the anaesthetic machine is to ensure that it is safe to use and to deliver gases under pressure without leaks. The presence of an oxygen analyser is essential to check and use an anaesthetic machine.

In most industries in which complex equipment is used, full training is provided for users. It is not

Table 14.4   Checklist for anaesthetic apparatus. (Reproduced with permission from AAGBI 2004)

The following checks should be made prior to each operating session:

Check that the anaesthetic machine and relevant ancillary equipment are connected to the mains electrical supply (if appropriate) and switched on. Switch on the gas supply master switch (if one is fitted). Check that the system clock (if fitted) is set correctly

Check that all monitoring devices are functioning and that appropriate parameters have been set, including the cycling times, or frequency of recordings, of automatic non-invasive blood pressure monitors

Check that gas sampling lines are properly attached and free from obstruction or kinks. Check that the oxygen analyser, pulse oximeter and capnograph are functioning correctly and that appropriate alarm limits are set

Perform a 'tug test' to ensure that each gas pipeline is correctly inserted

Check that the anaesthetic apparatus is connected to a supply of oxygen and that an adequate reserve supply of oxygen is available from a spare cylinder

Check that adequate supplies of any other gases intended for use are available and connected

Check that all pressure gauges for pipelines connected to the anaesthetic machine indicate 400–500 kPa

Check the operation of flowmeters, ensuring that each control valve operates smoothly and that the bobbin moves freely throughout its range

Operate the emergency oxygen bypass control and ensure that flow occurs without a significant decrease in the pipeline supply pressure

Check that vaporizers are fitted correctly to the anaesthetic machine, with the back bar locking mechanism fully engaged. Check that the vaporizers are adequately filled and that the filling port is tightly closed

Check the breathing system visually and manually

Check that the ventilator is configured correctly and that the ventilator tubing is securely attached

Check that the anaesthetic scavenging system is switched on and functioning, and that the tubing is attached to the appropriate exhaust port

Check that all ancillary equipment (e.g. face masks, laryngeal mask airways, tracheal tubes, connectors, laryngoscopes, intubation aids) which may be needed is present and in working order. Check that all tubes and connectors are patent

Check that the suction apparatus is functioning correctly

Check that the trolley or bed can be tilted head-down rapidly

Ensure that an alternative oxygen supply and means of ventilation are readily available in case the anaesthetic machine fails

Document the fact that the anaesthetic machine and equipment have been checked acceptable for anaesthetists to assume that they intuitively understand an anaesthetic machine which they have not used before. Those new to the speciality require detailed instruction and training in the use of anaesthetic equipment, but even experienced anaesthetists need tuition in the use of new equipment.

Anaesthetic machine

The anaesthetic machine and associated ancillary equipment should be connected to the mains electrical supply (if appropriate) and switched on. Microprocessor-based machines may start self-check routines, and these should be observed and responded to as appropriate. A visual check of the apparatus should confirm that all essential equipment is present and assembled correctly. If the oxygen analyser is not functioning correctly, then it is not safe to use the anaesthetic machine.

Medical gas supplies

Pipelines

It is essential to know which gases are being supplied by pipeline from a central supply and to confirm that the connections between the anaesthetic machine and the pipelines are secure and correct. The anaesthetist should check the connections visually and then perform a 'tug test' on each pipeline connection to confirm that the connections are secure. The Schrader sockets and probes are manufactured to ensure that misconnection is almost impossible, but there have been instances in which the wrong gas has been supplied through pipeline systems. Consequently, it is important to ensure that the oxygen analyser confirms that oxygen is being supplied through the oxygen pipeline.

Having confirmed that the correct gas is being delivered and that the pipeline connections are secure, the anaesthetist should check that the pipeline pressure gauges on the anaesthetic machine indicate a pressure of 400–500 kPa.

Cylinders

Machine-mounted cylinders provide reserve gas supplies, although in some situations they may provide the sole gas supply. The anaesthetist should ensure that cylinders are installed in the correct position. The pin-index system (see Ch. 13) is designed to prevent incorrect installation, but no system is foolproof. Leaks caused by faulty connections or a missing Bodok seal should be evident because of the high pressures involved. The pressure of the gas in the cylinders should be checked, and a cylinder should be replaced if the pressure of gas is low, indicating that it contains little gas. If a pipeline system is the primary source of gas supply, all cylinders should be turned off after they have been checked.

An adequate reserve supply of oxygen should be available from a spare cylinder, and the pressure in the cylinder should be checked. There is debate about the need for a reserve supply of nitrous oxide, and in many hospitals, nitrous oxide cylinders are no longer present on anaesthetic machines because of the economic consequences in conjunction with the fact that they are very rarely used. Carbon dioxide is not required in modern anaesthetic practice, and a carbon dioxide cylinder should not normally be present on an anaesthetic machine.

A blanking plug should be fitted to all unused cylinder yokes.

Oxygen failure alarm

When the primary oxygen supply is by pipeline, it is no longer considered necessary to check the oxygen failure warning device as part of the daily routine. Unscheduled oxygen pipeline failure is extremely rare. Routinely checking the oxygen failure alarm requires the pipelines to be disconnected and reconnected, with a potential for damage and error. However, if the primary oxygen supply is from cylinders, then a test of the oxygen failure alarm is essential.

Although the oxygen failure alarm is not tested routinely, all anaesthetists must be aware of the presence and warning tone of such an alarm.

Flowmeters

The operation of all flowmeters should be checked. Flowmeter tubes should be inspected visually to ensure that they are seated correctly and devoid of cracks, and should be operated through their full range. Flowmeter tubes are calibrated for specific gases, and inspection should confirm that the correct tubes are in position. This is particularly important after servicing.

At this stage, the purity of the oxygen supply should be verified by closing all but the oxygen flowmeter, setting the flowmeter to deliver 2–3 L min^{-1} and checking that the oxygen analyser display approaches 100%. Close the flowmeter, and then operate the emergency oxygen bypass control. There should be no significant decrease in the oxygen pipeline supply pressure during this manoeuvre, and the oxygen analyser display should still approach 100%. When the emergency oxygen bypass control is released, check that it has ceased to operate; some older machines allow the emergency oxygen bypass control to be locked in the open position, and failure to ensure its release can result in barotrauma to a patient's lungs or awareness during anaesthesia.

The remainder of the anaesthetic machine should now be checked to ensure that there are no leaks.

Vaporizers

Vaporizers and their mountings are a common source of leaks within an anaesthetic machine. These leaks lead primarily to inadequate delivery of vapour to the breathing system, resulting in awareness. Large leaks may result in total failure to deliver any fresh gas to the breathing system. Careful checking and care in the use of vaporizers prevent these problems. The commonest cause of leaks is a missing or defective 'O'-ring on the mounting port, and the presence and integrity of these 'O'-rings must be verified before a vaporizer is installed on the anaesthetic machine. Failure to ensure that a vaporizer is properly mounted on the anaesthetic machine is also a cause of leaks. When a vaporizer is fitted to an anaesthetic machine, ensure that it is correctly seated, with the back bar locking mechanism fully engaged. If more than one vaporizer is fitted, each should be turned on in sequence and checked for leaks by occluding the common gas outlet, when there should be no audible gas leak or leak of liquid from the vaporizer. Ensure that all vaporizers are turned off again after the check is completed.

There are several types of vaporizer in use, some of which are fitted with interlock devices which ensure that only one vaporizer can be operated at a time, to avoid the inadvertent delivery of mixtures of vapours, and contamination of the liquid in the 'downstream' vaporizer. If vaporizers with no interlock device are used, then it is very important to ensure that all are turned off after checking, and that only one is turned on during anaesthesia.

It is sometimes necessary to change a vaporizer during the course of an operating list. If this is necessary, then it is essential that the new vaporizer is fitted carefully, and that the system is rechecked for leaks. Failure to do this is a common cause of critical incidents.

Breathing systems

Breathing systems are considered in detail in Chapter 13. The general principle of checking breathing systems is the same for all types. The breathing system should be inspected visually for correct configuration and assembly. All connections within the breathing system, and between the breathing system and anaes-thetic machine, should be checked carefully. It is important that all connections have been completed with a 'push and twist' action in order to make a firm connection, the slight twisting action being very important to the security of the connection. A pressure leak test should be performed on the breathing system. It is particularly important to perform an occlusion test on the inner tube of a Bain coaxial breathing system, as a fault on the inner tube results in failure to deliver fresh gas to the patient. The pressure relief valve on the breathing system should be tested.

Even if it is not proposed to use a mechanical ventilator during an operating list, the ventilator tubing should be checked in case its use is required unexpectedly.

Ventilators

The advice for checking of ventilators is the same for all types. In particular, mechanical ventilators should be checked for their ability to generate an adequate inspiratory pressure. The anaesthetist must ensure that the ventilator is configured correctly and that the controls are set appropriately for each patient. The ventilator tubing should already have been checked for leaks. It is essential to ensure that the pressure relief valve functions correctly, at the desired pressure, in order to minimize the risk of barotrauma. There must be a pressure disconnection alarm within the system; its presence must be sought and correct function confirmed. The settings of the high-pressure alarm should also be checked.

Whenever anaesthesia is undertaken, there must always be available, reasonably close to hand, an alternative means of ventilating the patient's lungs in the event of malfunction of the anaesthetic machine or ventilator. All anaesthetists should ensure that they know where to find a self-inflating resuscitation bag if necessary.

Scavenging

The scavenging system should be checked. The tubing should be attached correctly to the appropriate expiratory ports of the breathing system and ventilator. If an active system is present, then the anaesthetist should ensure that it is switched on and that it is functioning correctly.

Monitoring

Monitoring is considered in detail in Chapter 18. Before each session in an operating theatre, the oxygen analyser should be switched on and calibrated according to the manufacturer's instructions. The alarm settings on all monitoring equipment should be reviewed and the upper and lower limits set appropriately. The manufacturer's default settings are often inappropriate.

Failure to set alarm variables correctly has been identified by the medical defence organizations in the UK as a major risk factor for adverse outcomes. Incorrect settings of alarms, disabling alarms or ignoring alarms may be considered to amount to dangerous practice.

Ancillary equipment

The preoperative check is completed by ensuring that all items of ancillary equipment which may be needed (e.g. laryngoscopes, intubation aids) are available and close at hand in the anaesthetic room. Appropriate face masks, airways, tracheal tubes and connectors must be available. Tracheal tubes should be ready for use, cut to the correct length, with the cuff checked and with all connections secured. The patency of all tubes and connectors must be ensured.

Consideration should be given to the need for a blood warmer, warm air blower or warming blanket.

Suction apparatus should be functional and all connections should be secure. It should be tested before anaesthesia starts to ensure that an adequate negative pressure develops rapidly. The patient's trolley, bed or operating table must be capable of being placed rapidly into a head-down position; as with all equipment, the anaesthetist must be familiar with the operating mechanism before anaesthesia starts.

Emergencies

Some eventualities are unpredictable. There are many action plans available to guide anaesthetists during emergency situations, and these protocols, guidelines and action plans should be displayed prominently in the operating theatre suite. Rare emergencies such as malignant hyperthermia call for prompt action and the availability of large quantities of ice and dantrolene; the anaesthetist should know where these are located. It is also essential that the anaesthetist knows where emergency equipment, and particularly the defibrillator, is situated.

RECOVERY ROOM

A recovery room or ward is an essential requirement in the operating theatre. All patients require close surveillance in the immediate postoperative period and, after major surgery or in vulnerable patients, for up to 24 h after major surgery.

The recovery room should be an integral part of the operating theatre suite and should be located within the clean area. Department of Health guidelines suggest that there should be 1.5 places in the recovery area for each operating theatre, although a greater number may be required if surgery with a high turnover, e.g. gynaecology or day-case surgery. Each place requires a minimum floor area of approximately $10 \, m^2$, and there must be sufficient space to move a patient without disturbing the remainder.

It is appropriate for many patients to lie on a trolley in the recovery room, but beds should be available for those who are likely to stay for more than 30–45 min, e.g. patients who have undergone major surgery, or ASA (American Society of Anesthesiologists) grade III or IV patients who may require prolonged observation even after minor surgery. Each place should have piped oxygen and suction outlets on the wall, with an oxygen flowmeter and suction apparatus attached to a wall rail. Lighting should conform to the same standards as apply to the operating theatre, and additional spotlights should be provided. It is not common practice in the UK to monitor the electrocardiogram in all patients in the recovery ward, but oxygen saturation and blood pressure should be monitored routinely and the facility to monitor ECG should be available. Most large recovery areas have two or three places which are fully equipped with piped nitrous oxide, a mechanical ventilator and complete cardiovascular monitoring facilities.

An anaesthetic machine, a defibrillator, and equipment and drugs for resuscitation must be available in the recovery room. Oxygen is usually administered by disposable face mask, but each place should have a self-inflating resuscitation bag and anaesthetic mask.

Drug cupboards and storage space for equipment should be provided and, in a large recovery area, special telephones are required. Nursing staff spend most of their time with the patient, but require a nursing station at which notes may be written and from which wards can be contacted by telephone. At least one nurse is required for each three bed spaces. At present there is no specific training course in the UK for recovery room nurses. Student nurses may receive as little as 1 week of training in this area.

In many hospitals, it is possible to provide supervision of patients in the recovery ward for up to 24 h after major surgery, although it is now usual for patients who require close supervision for more than a few hours to be transferred to a high-dependency unit.

Clinical aspects of recovery room care are discussed in Chapter 24.

HIGH-DEPENDENCY UNIT

A high-dependency unit is an area for patients who require more invasive observation, treatment and nursing care than can be provided on a general ward. It would not normally accept patients requiring mechanical ventilation, but could manage those who require invasive monitoring. A survey conducted by the AAGBI in the 1990s indicated that many intensive care units admitted patients who could have been managed appropriately in a high-dependency unit. An unknown number of patients return from the recovery area to a general ward requiring monitoring or an intensity of nursing or medical care which cannot be provided safely in that location.

The facilities required to provide high-dependency care vary. Essential features are a high nurse-to-patient ratio, provision of piped oxygen and suction at every bed, and appropriate monitoring equipment. Protocols must be in place for admission and discharge criteria, and medical staffing must be clearly defined. In large hospitals, several units may be desirable, each dedicated to the care of specific groups of patients; in smaller hospitals, a single, multi-user unit may be more appropriate.

OTHER ACCOMMODATION

Storage space is required for large items of equipment. In most modern operating theatre suites, instruments are sterilized in a separate department, which should be situated in close proximity. Access to a facility for blood gas analysis and measurement of serum electrolyte concentrations is essential, especially if major surgery is to be undertaken, and large operating theatre suites usually contain a small laboratory or are adjacent to an ITU with these facilities.

Staff accommodation includes changing rooms and rest rooms. There should be facilities for beverages and snacks. Offices are provided for the theatre supervisor and senior operating department practitioners, and there should be a tutorial or seminar room for staff training. Some theatre suites incorporate an office for the anaesthetic department.

OTHER ANAESTHETIZING LOCATIONS

The anaesthetist is often required to work in areas outside the operating theatre suite. Many hospitals have peripheral theatres for some types of surgery, e.g. a self-contained day-case unit or treatment centre. In addition, patients may require anaesthesia in the accident and emergency unit, the radiology and radiotherapy departments or, in some instances (e.g. paediatric oncology), the side room of a ward. In these circumstances, where conditions are frequently not ideal, it is essential that the same precautions are taken as in the operating theatre suite to ensure that the identity of the patient and the nature of the proposed procedure are checked, that equipment is functioning correctly, that skilled help for the anaesthetist is available and that recovery facilities and staff are satisfactory. It is wise to avoid sending junior and inexperienced anaesthetists to these remote locations without direct senior supervision.

ANCILLARY STAFF

Skilled and dedicated help should be available to the anaesthetist at all times. In the majority of hospitals in the UK, this is provided by operating department practitioners (ODPs), who undergo a 2-year training programme in recognized institutions and are required to sit examinations. In some hospitals, anaesthetic nurses assist the anaesthetist. It is important to differentiate between anaesthetic nurses and the nurse anaesthetists who are trained to deliver anaesthesia in some countries (e.g. CRNAs in the USA). The anaesthetic nurse performs essentially the same functions as the ODP. These include:

- Preparation and preliminary checking of equipment. It should be stressed that this does not absolve the anaesthetist from the responsibility of checking the equipment fully before an operating list is started.
- Alleviation of anxiety by reassurance and constant communication with the patient while awaiting anaesthesia.
- Checking the correct identity of the patient. It is the responsibility of the surgeon to ensure that the appropriate procedure is undertaken on the correct patient, but the anaesthetist must also confirm the identity of the patient and, as far as is possible, confirm that the surgeon is performing the correct operation. This is one of the many reasons why the anaesthetist must see every patient preoperatively.
- Preparation of intravenous infusions, cardiovascular monitoring transducers, etc.
- Assistance during anaesthesia, particularly during induction, when special manoeuvres such as cricoid pressure may be required, and after transfer to the operating theatre to assist in re-establishment of monitoring.
- Assistance in positioning the patient for local or regional blocks.
- Assistance in obtaining drugs or equipment if complications arise during anaesthesia.
- Assistance in the immediate postoperative period before the patient is transferred to the recovery room.

The ODP or anaesthetic nurse should never be left alone with an anaesthetized patient unless a dire emergency requires the anaesthetist's presence elsewhere.

THE MEDICOLEGAL ENVIRONMENT

The increasing volume of litigation instituted by patients in respect of alleged or actual injury arising from treatment is causing great concern within the medical profession. Insurance premiums for medical practice have escalated rapidly. Anaesthesia represents a high insurance risk, because anaesthetists manipulate the physiology of the cardiovascular and respiratory systems to administer potentially lethal drugs for reasons which are not primarily therapeutic; consequently, when a serious accident occurs, it may cause a very rapid and profound reduction in delivery of oxygen to the major organs, and result in death or permanent neurological damage. In addition, even minor morbidity caused by anaesthesia or the anaesthetist may be regarded by the patient as unacceptable when it does not appear to be related to the primary illness.

MORTALITY ASSOCIATED WITH ANAESTHESIA

The overwhelming majority of anaesthetics are uneventful. However, both surgery and anaesthesia carry a finite risk. Mortality is usually related to the extent of surgery and the preoperative condition of the patient (see Ch. 15). However, avoidable deaths occur. In 1982, Lunn & Mushin estimated that the risk of death attributable to anaesthesia alone was approximately 1 in 10 000. In a subsequent study of more than half a million operations (Confidential Enquiry into Perioperative Deaths; CEPOD), the overall death rate after anaesthesia and surgery was 0.7% (Buck et al 1987). Anaesthesia alone was responsible for death in approximately 1 in 180 000 operations, but *contributed* to 14% of all deaths; in almost one-fifth of these deaths, avoidable errors occurred. Factors which contributed to death in these instances are listed in Table 14.5.

MORBIDITY ASSOCIATED WITH ANAESTHESIA

The incidence of major morbidity (causing permanent disability) related to anaesthesia is difficult to assess. Its causes are often similar to those associated with mortality. Table 14.6 lists the causes of death or cerebral damage reported to the Medical Defence Union between 1970 and 1982. Table 14.7 shows the detailed causes of the incidents resulting from errors in technique. Permanent disability may result also from spinal cord damage. Although these figures are old, they reflect the largest study of its type, and there is

Table 14.5   Factors involved in deaths attributable in part to anaesthesia, in decreasing order of frequency (CEPOD report)

Failure to apply knowledge
Lack of care
Failure of organization
Lack of experience
Lack of knowledge
Drug effect
Failure of equipment
Fatigue

evidence that the pattern of causes of death and serious morbidity associated with anaesthesia remain similar today.

Other, albeit less serious, incidents may result in distress or physical injury to patients. Table 14.8 lists untoward events, other than death and cerebral damage, which result commonly in litigation against anaesthetists.

CRITICAL INCIDENTS

These are incidents that could or do lead to death, permanent disability or prolongation of hospital stay. Most critical incidents in anaesthesia are detected before damage occurs; their incidence is 400–500 times greater than those of death or serious injury attributable to anaesthesia. It has been estimated that a critical incident occurs on average once in every 80 anaesthetics. Analysis of the causes of critical incidents is valuable in indicating the potential causes of anaesthetic-related mortality and major morbidity. Human error is responsible for approximately 70% of critical incidents in anaesthesia; the commonest errors are shown in Table 14.9. Factors associated with critical incidents are shown in Table 14.10.

MINIMIZING THE RISK

The most effective means of reducing the risk of an anaesthetic accident is to ensure that every aspect of anaesthetic management is conducted competently (Table 14.11). Preoperative assessment (see Ch. 15) is essential. In the anaesthetic room, the anaesthetist must check the identity of the patient and the intended

Table 14.6 Causes of anaesthetic-related death or cerebral damage reported to the Medical Defence Union between 1970 and 1982

Mainly misadventure	%	Mainly error	%
Coexisting disease	14	Faulty technique	43
Unknown	6	Failure of postoperative care	9
Drug sensitivity	5	Drug overdosage	5
Hypotension/blood loss	4	Inadequate preoperative assessment	3
Halothane-associated hepatic failure	3	Drug error	1
Hyperpyrexia	2	Anaesthetist's failure	1
Embolism	2		

Table 14.7 Causes of anaesthetic-related death or cerebral damage reported to the Medical Defence Union and thought to be the result of errors in technique

Cause	% of total
Errors associated with tracheal intubation	31
Misuse of apparatus	23
Inhalation of gastric contents	14
Errors associated with induced hypotension	8
Hypoxia	4
Obstructed airway	4
Accidental pneumothorax/haemopericardium	4
Errors associated with extradural analgesia	3
Use of nitrous oxide instead of oxygen	2
Use of carbon dioxide instead of oxygen	2
Errors associated with Bier's block	2
Underventilation	1
Use of halothane with adrenaline (epinephrine)	1
Mismatched blood transfusion	<1
Vasovagal attack	<1

Table 14.8 Less serious injuries which are common sources of litigation against anaesthetists

Damage to teeth
Awareness: During general anaesthesia   During regional or local anaesthesia
Peripheral nerve damage: Pressure   Related to nerve block
Spinal cord damage: Direct injury during spinal/epidural block   Epidural haematoma   Epidural abscess
Perioperative myocardial infarction
Pneumothorax
Extravasation of injected drugs
Intra-arterial injection of drugs
Lacerations, falls from table
Superficial thrombophlebitis and minor injuries (e.g. abrasions)
Burns

Table 14.9   Types of human error contributing to critical incidents during anaesthesia

Type of error	% of total
Wrong drug administered	24
Misuse of anaesthetic machine	22
Problem with airway management	16
Problem with breathing system	11
Fluid therapy mismanagement	5
Intravenous infusion disconnection	6
Failure of monitoring	4
Others	12

Table 14.10   Associated factors producing critical incidents during anaesthesia, in decreasing order of frequency

Failure to check
First experience of procedure
Inadequate experience
Inattention/carelessness
Haste
Unfamiliarity
Visual restriction
Fatigue

operation before proceeding. The information contained in Tables 14.6–14.10 indicates areas of particular concern regarding intraoperative management. All anaesthetic equipment must be checked before use. The anaesthetist must understand the principles of all the equipment used, especially mechanical ventilators. Drug doses must be calculated carefully and syringes labelled. After induction of anaesthesia, the correct placement of the tracheal tube must be confirmed on every occasion.

Studies of critical incidents indicate that the time of highest risk is during maintenance of anaesthesia. For this reason, appropriate clinical and instrumental monitoring (see Ch. 18) must be used throughout anaesthesia. After operation, the anaesthetist is responsible for the patient until consciousness has

Table 14.11   Summary of important factors which should minimize the risk of accidents during anaesthesia and the risk of litigation against the anaesthetist

- Careful preoperative assessment should be undertaken to identify risk factors such as concurrent disease, chronic medication history of allergy or other untoward reactions to anaesthesia, and potential difficulties in tracheal intubation

- Anaesthetic equipment must be maintained according to the manufacturers' recommendations, and checked thoroughly before every operating theatre session, or when the equipment is changed during an operating session

- The anaesthetic technique should be recognized as appropriate for the individual patient and for the proposed type of surgery

- The anaesthetist must be present at all times during anaesthesia

- Appropriate monitoring, in accordance with national recommendations, should be used at all times during anaesthesia and in the immediate recovery period. Alarms should be set at appropriate levels and must not be disabled

- At the end of anaesthesia, the anaesthetist should transfer the care of the patient only to an appropriately experienced recovery room nurse

- All anaesthetists should be taught how to manage uncommon emergencies, such as failed intubation, anaphylaxis or malignant hyperthermia. It is advisable to have protocols available in every anaesthetizing location to act as an *aide-mémoire* for uncommon emergencies, and anaesthetists and operating theatre staff should rehearse emergency management on a regular basis

- The anaesthetist should keep careful records

returned and until the cardiovascular and respiratory systems are stable. He or she may be required to defend a decision to delegate the care of the patient to a nurse in the recovery room.

The following factors should also be considered:

Awareness. Patients may recall intraoperative events, and may experience pain and discomfort, if the doses or concentrations of anaesthetic drugs are insufficient (see p. 389). In high-risk groups, it may be advisable to warn the patient of the possibility of awareness.

Anaesthetic record. A legible and comprehensive record must be made of every anaesthetic. The record should include details of preoperative findings, the doses and timing of all drugs administered during anaesthesia, frequent and regular recordings of cardiovascular and respiratory measurements, and notes regarding any untoward intraoperative event. This is an important document because it provides information which may assist other anaesthetists in the future and because a comprehensive record is essential in the event of medicolegal proceedings.

Communication. If a mishap occurs, failure on the part of the anaesthetist to communicate with the patient or relatives may arouse feelings of anger and suspicion. While no admission (or accusations) of liability should be made, an explanation should be offered. An interview with a patient or relatives in these circumstances requires skill and tact; the trainee should discuss the event with a consultant, and, if possible, the consultant should be present at the interview.

Each anaesthetic department should ensure that the channels of communication between trainees and consultants are clear, especially with regard to emergency procedures.

Audit. Standards of anaesthetic practice may be improved by identifying areas in which patient care has been suboptimal. Although case reports published in anaesthetic journals form a useful source of information, local audit, meetings to discuss morbidity and mortality related to anaesthesia and surgery and critical incident analysis should be undertaken regularly.

Risk management strategies. There is much to commend adoption of a system in which there is identification of adverse events, investigation at an early stage, assessment of the risk of complaint or litigation, and identification of areas in which care could be improved in future.

FURTHER READING

Aitkenhead A R 2005. Injuries associated with anaesthesia. A global perspective. British Journal of Anaesthesia 95: 95

Association of Anaesthetists of Great Britain and Ireland 2002 Immediate postanaesthetic recovery. AAGBI, London

Association of Anaesthetists of Great Britain and Ireland 2002 Infection control and anaesthesia. AAGBI, London

Association of Anaesthetists of Great Britain and Ireland 2004 Checking anaesthetic equipment 3. AAGBI, London

Boumphrey S, Langton JA, 2003. Electrical safety in the operating theatre. BJA CEPD Reviews 3: 10

Buck N, Devlin H B, Lunn J N 1987 The report of a confidential enquiry into perioperative deaths. Nuffield Provincial Hospitals Trust, London

Johnston I D A, Hunter A R (eds) 1984 The design and utilization of operating theatres. Edward Arnold, London

Runciman W B, Sellen A, Webb R K, Williamson J A, Currie M, Morgan C A, Russell W J 1993 Errors, incidents and accidents in anaesthetic practice. Anaesthesia and Intensive Care 21: 506

Spence A A 1987 Environmental pollution by inhalation of anaesthetics. British Journal of Anaesthesia 59: 96

Taylor T H, Major E (eds) 1994 Hazards and complications of anaesthesia, 2nd edn. Churchill Livingstone, Edinburgh

15 Preoperative assessment and premedication

All patients scheduled to undergo surgery should be assessed in advance with a view to planning optimal preparation and perioperative management. This is one mechanism by which the standard and quality of care provided by an individual anaesthetist or an anaesthetic department may be measured. Failure to undertake this activity places the patient at increased risk of perioperative morbidity or mortality.

The overall aims of preoperative assessment should include the following:

- Confirm that the surgery proposed is realistic when comparing the likely benefit to the patient with the possible risks involved.
- Anticipate potential problems and ensure that adequate facilities and appropriately trained staff are available to provide satisfactory perioperative care.
- Ensure that the patient is prepared correctly for the operation, improving where feasible any existing factors which may increase the risk of an adverse outcome.
- Provide appropriate information to the patient and obtain consent for the planned anaesthetic technique.
- Prescribe premedication and/or other specific prophylactic measures if required.
- Ensure that proper documentation is made of the assessment process, that specific plans are considered, and that, if indicated, communication is made with other relevant professionals.

It is implicit that the anaesthetist has sufficient knowledge and experience of both the proposed surgery and necessary anaesthetic management to predict the potential progress of an individual patient during the perioperative period. Appropriate skills must be achieved and maintained by an ongoing commitment to education, both individually and within the profession overall. There are organizational issues to be considered within any hospital in order that preoperative assessment and preparation of patients can be accomplished successfully. Increasingly, this makes use of a nurse-led assessment process combined with gaining an anaesthetic opinion when appropriate, guided and supported by the use of evidence-based protocols.

THE PROCESS OF PREOPERATIVE ASSESSMENT

WHO, WHEN AND WHERE?

The decision regarding the need for an operation is normally made by an experienced surgeon on the basis of the patient's presenting pathology. The patient subsequently undergoes a more extensive assessment of general health closer to the time of admission for surgery. This is undertaken usually by the least experienced member of the surgical team, and in some circumstances is delegated (in part) to an experienced nurse practitioner. Identification of potential problems by these individuals relies upon their application of general medical knowledge and common sense, often assisted by the use of screening protocols developed either nationally, or locally by the anaesthetic department. When a patient is recognized to be at special risk, referral to an appropriate anaesthetist should be made. This need not be the anaesthetist ultimately responsible for the patient's care if surgery is not urgent, provided that decisions made regarding preoperative preparation are communicated and recorded clearly in the medical notes. If surgery is more imminent then it becomes relevant to involve the anaesthetist who will be responsible for the patient's perioperative care.

The need to improve efficiency of hospital bed occupancy has led to the increasing use of pre-admission clerking appointments, arranged to allow completion of the majority of the necessary administrative details. This is an ideal opportunity for anaesthetic assessment to take place, but in reality it is often not feasible to guarantee the availability of an experienced anaesthetist for these sessions. One direct consequence of this change is that patients are subsequently admitted onto the ward close to the time of surgery, allowing significantly less time for the anaesthetist to organize perioperative management. In order to optimize preparation for surgery within this system, many hospitals now use preoperative questionnaires which are completed by the patient in advance of clerking and are designed specifically to identify key features in the medical history which need further clarification. In addition, guidelines may be provided by the anaesthetic department for the surgical team or nurse practitioner to ensure that appropriate investigations are undertaken and suitable action taken if problems are identified.

Regardless of the timing and the individual personnel involved in clerking patients before surgery, the fundamental process of taking a detailed history and performing a systematic clinical examination remains the foundation on which preoperative assessment relies, backed up by ordering appropriate investigations where indicated. This allows the anaesthetist to concentrate on areas of particular relevance to perioperative care.

HISTORY

Direct questions should be asked about the following items of specific relevance to anaesthesia.

Presenting condition and concurrent medical history

The indication for surgery determines its urgency and thus influences aspects of anaesthetic management. There are many surgical conditions which have systemic effects and these must be sought and quantified, e.g. bowel cancer may be associated with malnourishment, anaemia and electrolyte imbalance. The presence of coexisting medical disease must also be identified, together with an assessment of the extent of any associated limitations to normal activity. The most relevant tend to be related to cardiovascular and respiratory diseases because of their potential effect on perioperative management. Specific questioning should ascertain the degree of exertional dyspnoea, paroxysmal nocturnal dyspnoea, orthopnoea, angina of effort, etc. Limitations to exercise because of other factors should be identified, e.g. intermittent claudication, arthritis, etc., so that effort-related symptoms such as dyspnoea and angina may be interpreted correctly.

Anaesthetic history

Details of the administration and outcome of previous anaesthetic episodes should be documented, espe-

cially if problems were encountered. Some sequelae such as sore throat, headache or postoperative nausea may not seem of great significance to the anaesthetist but may form the basis of considerable preoperative anxiety for the patient. The patient may be unaware of anaesthetic problems in the past if managed uneventfully and hence the anaesthetic records should be examined if they are available. More serious problems such as difficulty maintaining a patent airway, performing tracheal intubation or some other specific procedure (e.g. insertion of an epidural catheter) should have been documented. Other serious problems such as unexpected admission to the intensive care unit following surgery should be explored carefully in order to identify contributing factors which might be encountered once again. Because of the risk of postoperative hepatotoxicity, the Medicine Healthcare Products Regulatory Agency (MHRA) recommends that repeated exposure to halothane should be avoided within a 3-month period unless specifically indicated.

Family history

There are several hereditary conditions which influence planned anaesthetic management, such as malignant hyperthermia, cholinesterase abnormalities, porphyria, some haemoglobinopathies and dystrophia myotonica. Some of these disorders may not limit the patient's normal activities, but their presence is usually confirmed by asking about details of anaesthetic problems encountered by immediate family members and any subsequent investigations required; the family history is particularly important in patients who have not undergone surgery and anaesthesia previously.

Drug history

A complete history of concurrent medication must be documented carefully. Many drugs interact with agents or techniques used during anaesthesia, but problems may occur if drugs are withdrawn suddenly during the perioperative period (Table 15.1). Knowledge of pharmacology is essential to permit the anaesthetist to adjust the doses of anaesthetic agents appropriately and to avoid possibly dangerous interactions. In addition, the anaesthetist must maintain up-to-date knowledge of pharmacological advances as new drugs continue to emerge on the market. Any potential interactions observed with new drugs must always be reported to the MHRA.

In general terms, administration of most drugs should be continued up to and including the morning of the operation, although some adjustment in dose

Table 15.1   Drugs with potential anaesthetic interaction during anaesthesia

Drug group	Comments
Cardiovascular	

Angiotensin-converting enzyme inhibitors
  Captopril
  Enalapril
  Lisinopril
	Hypotensive effects may be potentiated by anaesthetic agents. Sudden withdrawal tends not to produce haemodynamic effects, perhaps because of relatively long duration of action

Angiotensin II receptor antagonists
  Losartan
  Valsartan
	May be associated with severe hypotension at induction or during maintenance of anaesthesia; consideration should be given to stopping treatment 24 h preoperatively

Antihypertensives
  Clonidine
  Guanethidine
  Methyldopa
  Reserpine
	Hypotension with all anaesthetic agents, requiring extreme care with dosage and administration. *Clonidine* (or *dexmedetomidine*) allows reduction in dosage of anaesthetic agents and opioids. Acute withdrawal of long-term treatment may result in a hypertensive crisis. *Guanethidine* potentiates effect of sympathomimetics. *Reserpine* depletes noradrenaline (norepinephrine) stores, so attenuating the action of pressor agents acting via noradrenaline release

β-blockers	Negative inotropic effects additive with anaesthetic agents to cause exaggerated hypotension. Mask compensatory tachycardia. Caution with concomitant use of any cardiovascular depressant drugs. Acute withdrawal may result in angina, ventricular extrasystoles, or even precipitate myocardial infarction
Ca²⁺ channel blockers Verapamil	Depresses AV conduction and excitability. Interacts with volatile anaesthetic agents leading to bradyarrhythmias and decreased cardiac output
Diltiazem Nifedipine	Negative inotropic effect and vasodilatation. Interact with volatile anaesthetic agents to cause hypotension. May augment action of competitive muscle relaxants. Acute withdrawal may exacerbate angina
Others Digoxin	Arryhthmias enhanced by calcium. Toxicity is enhanced by hypokalaemia, which must be corrected preoperatively. Succinylcholine enhances toxicity, and should therefore be used with caution. Beware of bradyarrhythmias
Diuretics	Can cause hypokalaemia, which may potentiate the effect of competitive muscle relaxants
Magnesium	Potentiates action of muscle relaxants, the dosage of which may need to be reduced
Quinidine	Intravenous administration can produce neuromuscular blockade, notable particularly following succinylcholine
Central nervous system	
Anticonvulsants	Cause liver enzyme induction. May increase requirements for sedative or anaesthetic agents. Recommended to avoid enflurane. Caution with propofol. Sudden withdrawal may produce rebound convulsive activity
Benzodiazepines	Additive effect with many CNS-depressant drugs. Caution with dosage of intravenous anaesthetic agents and opioids. Additive effect with competitive muscle relaxants, causing potentiation of their action. Action of succinylcholine may be antagonized

Continued

Table 15.1   Drugs with potential anaesthetic interaction during anaesthesia—Cont'd

Drug group	Comments
Central nervous system — Contd.	
Monoamine oxidase inhibitors (MAOIs)	React with opioids causing coma or CNS excitement. Severe hypertensive response to pressor agents. Treatment of regional anaesthetic-induced hypotension may be difficult, especially as indirect sympathomimetics (e.g. ephedrine) are contraindicated due to unpredictable and exaggerated release of noradrenaline (norepinephrine). Adverse effects do not always occur, but recommended to withdraw drugs 2–3 weeks before surgery and use alternative medication
Tricyclic antidepressants	Inhibit the metabolism of catecholamines, increasing the likelihood of arrhythmias. Imipramine potentiates the cardiovascular effects of adrenaline (epinephrine). Delay gastric emptying
Phenothiazines Butyrophenones	Interact with other hypotensive agents, necessitating care with administration of all agents with potential cardiovascular effect
Others	
Lithium	Potentiates non-depolarizing muscle relaxants. Consider changing to alternative treatment 48–72 h prior to anaesthesia
L-Dopa	Risks of tachycardia and arrhythmias with halothane. Actions antagonized by droperidol. Augments hyperglycaemia in diabetes. Some suggest discontinuing on day of surgery, but this must be balanced against possible detrimental effects as a result
Antibiotics	
Aminoglycosides	Potentiation of neuromuscular block. Caution with the use of muscle relaxants. Effect may be partially antagonized with Ca^{2+}
Sulphonamides	Potentiation of thiopental
Non-steroidal anti-inflammatory drugs	Interfere with platelet function to varying degrees by inhibition of platelet cyclooxygenase. Possible effect on coagulation mechanism makes use of regional anaesthesia controversial
Steroids	Potential adrenocorticoid suppression. Additional steroid cover may be required for the perioperative period
Anticoagulants	Problems with minor trauma resulting from cannulation, laryngoscopy and intubation (especially nasotracheal), intramuscular injections and the use of local anaesthetic blocks. Full anticoagulation is an absolute contraindication to the use of regional anaesthetic techniques. Surgical haemorrhage more likely. Preoperative management of anticoagulant therapy is discussed elsewhere
Anticholinesterases	
Ecothiopate eye drops Organophosphorus insecticides	Rarely encountered nowadays. Inhibition of plasma cholinesterase. Caution should be exercised with the use of succinylcholine
Oral contraceptive pill	Increased risk of thromboembolic complications with oestrogen-containing formulations. Recommended that OCP is stopped 4 weeks before elective surgery or that some form of prophylactic therapy is provided
Antimitotic agents	Inhibition of plasma cholinesterase. Caution should be exercised with the use of succinylcholine

may be required (e.g. antihypertensives, insulin). Consideration must also be given to possible perioperative events that influence subsequent drug administration (e.g. postoperative ileus), and appropriate plans made to use an alternative route or an alternative product with similar action. It is advised that some drugs should be discontinued several weeks before surgery if feasible (e.g. oestrogen-containing oral contraceptive pill, long-acting monoamine oxidase inhibitors), because of the potential severity of perioperative complications with which they are associated. Consideration must be given to the potential consequences of stopping drugs preoperatively, and appropriate advice or alternative treatment provided to the patient.

There are occasions when patients with an illicit drug habit present for surgery. The patterns of abuse geographically are prone to frequent change, as are the specific drugs taken. Abuse of opioids and cocaine is not uncommon and there is significant information available about potential perioperative problems related to acute or chronic toxicity; however, the same is not true for the increasing number of 'designer drugs' available.

History of allergy

A history of allergy to specific substances must be sought, whether it is a drug, foods or adhesives, and the exact nature of the symptoms and signs should be elicited in order to distinguish true allergy from some other predictable adverse reaction. Latex allergy is becoming an increasing problem and requires specific equipment to be used perioperatively. Atopic individuals do not have an increased risk of anaphylaxis, but may demonstrate increased cardiovascular or respiratory reactivity to any vasoactive mediators (e.g. histamine) released following administration of some drugs.

A small number of patients describe an allergic reaction to previous anaesthetic exposure. A careful history and examination of the relevant medical notes should clarify the details of the problem, together with the documentation of any postoperative investigations.

Smoking

Long-term deleterious effects of smoking include vascular disease of the peripheral, coronary and cerebral circulations, carcinoma of the lung and chronic bronchitis. It has been suggested that there are good theoretical reasons for advising all patients to cease cigarette smoking for at least 12 h prior to surgery, although there is little evidence to suggest that this influences patients' behaviour in this period.

There are several potential mechanisms by which cigarette smoking can contribute to an adverse perioperative outcome. The cardiovascular effects of smoking are caused by the action of nicotine on the sympathetic nervous system, producing tachycardia and hypertension. Furthermore, smoking causes an increase in coronary vascular resistance; cessation of smoking improves the symptoms of angina. Cigarette smoke contains carbon monoxide, which converts haemoglobin to carboxyhaemoglobin. In heavy smok-

ers, this may result in a reduction in available oxygen by as much as 25%. The half-life of carboxyhaemoglobin is short and therefore abstinence for 12 h leads to an increase in arterial oxygen content. Finally, the effect of smoking on the respiratory tract leads to a sixfold increase in postoperative respiratory morbidity. It has been suggested that abstinence for 6 weeks results in reduced bronchoconstriction and mucus secretion in the tracheobronchial tree.

Alcohol

Patients may present with acute intoxication from alcohol or sequelae of chronic consumption. The latter are mainly non-specific features of secondary organ damage such as cardiomyopathy, pancreatitis and gastritis. Establishing the diagnosis may be far from straightforward, and needs to be complemented by a decision about whether to allow continued alcohol consumption during the hospital admission or risk the development of a withdrawal syndrome.

PHYSICAL EXAMINATION

A physical examination should be performed on every patient admitted for surgery and the findings documented in the medical notes. It might be argued that this is unnecessary in young healthy patients undergoing short or minor procedures. However, the exercise is a simple and safe method for confirming good health or otherwise, and provides important information in case unexpected morbidity arises postoperatively, e.g. foot drop as a result of incorrect positioning on the operating theatre table, prolonged sensory anaesthesia following local anaesthetic techniques, etc. The information obtained from clinical examination should complement the patient's history and allows the anaesthetist to focus further on features of relevance (Table 15.2).

In addition, the anaesthetist must predict any potential difficulty in maintaining the patient's airway during general anaesthesia. The teeth should be inspected closely for the presence of caries, caps, loose teeth and particularly protruding upper incisors. The extent of mouth opening is assessed, together with the degree of flexion of the cervical spine and extension of the atlanto-occipital joint. The thyromental distance should also be documented. Specific features associated with difficulty in performing tracheal intubation are described elsewhere (Ch. 16).

SPECIAL INVESTIGATIONS

In general, the results of many investigations may be predicted if a detailed history and examination have

Table 15.2 Features of the clinical examination relevant to the anaesthetist

System	Features of interest
General	Nutritional state, fluid balance
	Condition of the skin and mucous membranes (anaemia, perfusion, jaundice)
	Temperature
Cardiovascular	Peripheral pulse (rate, rhythm, volume)
	Jugular venous pressure and pulsation
	Arterial pressure
	Heart sounds
	Carotid bruits
	Dependent oedema
Respiratory	Central vs. peripheral cyanosis
	Observation of dyspnoea
	Auscultation of lung fields
Airway	Mouth opening
	Neck movements
	Thyromental distance
	Dentition
Nervous	Any dysfunction of the special senses, other cranial nerves, or peripheral motor and sensory nerves

Table 15.3 Guidelines for preoperative investigations

Urinalysis	All patients
Full blood count	Males over 50 years of age
	All female adults
	Before surgery which is likely to result in significant blood loss
	When indicated clinically, e.g. history of blood loss, previous anaemia or haemopoietic disease, cardiovascular disease, malnutrition, etc.
Urea, creatinine and electrolytes	All patients over 65 years, or with a positive urinalysis result
	Any patient with cardiopulmonary disease, or taking cardiovascular active medication, diuretics or corticosteroids
	Patients with renal or liver disease, diabetes or abnormal nutritional status
	Patients with a history of diarrhoea, vomiting or metabolic disorder
	Patients receiving intravenous fluid therapy for greater than 24 h
Blood glucose	Fasting sample in patients with diabetes mellitus, vascular disease or taking corticosteroids
Liver function tests	Any history of liver disease, alcoholism, previous hepatitis or an abnormal nutritional state
Coagulation screen	Any history of a coagulation disorder, drug abuse, significant chronic alcohol abuse, acute or chronic liver disease or anticoagulant medication
ECG	Male smokers older than 45 years; all others older than 50 years
	Any history (actual or suspected) of heart disease or hypertension
	Any patient taking medication active on the cardiovascular system or a diuretic
	Patients with chronic or acute-on-chronic pulmonary disease
Chest X-ray	History suggesting a possible abnormality, e.g. cardiovascular disease, pulmonary disease with localizing signs, possible lung tumour (primary or secondary), thyroid enlargement (combined with a thoracic inlet view)
	Previous abnormal chest X-ray

been performed. Routine laboratory tests in patients who are apparently healthy on the basis of the history and clinical examination are invariably of little use and a waste of resources. Before ordering extensive investigations, the following questions should be considered:

- Will this investigation yield information not revealed by clinical assessment?
- Will the results of the investigation alter the management of the patient?

In order to reduce the volume of routine preoperative investigations, the following suggestions are made. It should be noted that these are guidelines only and should be modified according to the assessment obtained from the history and clinical examination (Table 15.3). Attention should be paid to ensuring that the results of any investigations requested are seen by the surgical team and properly documented, and that this process is undertaken in a timely manner to allow any necessary intervention with the patient's management to be considered and implemented.

Urine analysis

This should be performed in every patient. It is inexpensive and may occasionally reveal undiagnosed diabetes mellitus or the presence of urinary tract infection. Positive results should be confirmed by seeking further evidence of pathology.

Full blood count

This provides information about the haemoglobin concentration, white blood cell count and platelet count, together with details of red cell morphology. Haemoglobin concentration tends to be of greatest interest to the anaesthetist. Patients whose ethnic origin or family history suggests that a haemoglobinopathy may be present should have their haemoglobin concentration measured and haemoglobin electrophoresis undertaken if it has not been performed previously or if the result is not available. If such patients are scheduled for emergency surgery, a Sickledex test should be performed; if this is positive, haemoglobin electrophoresis should be undertaken as soon as possible but should not delay emergency surgery.

Blood chemistry

The measurements available include the serum concentrations of urea, creatinine and electrolytes, blood glucose concentration and liver function tests. There are specific conditions in which knowledge of preoperative values is important (e.g. diuretic therapy, impaired renal function, chronic alcohol abuse). Beyond these situations, the value of preoperative screening is less clear, and detection of an unexpected abnormality seldom alters anaesthetic management. Blood sugar measurement is informative in patients receiving corticosteroid drugs and in those who have diabetes mellitus or vascular disease; a fasting sample is usually required.

Chest X-ray

This investigation should be reserved for an older population (e.g. over 60 years of age) and patients with a clear indication. It probably has little value as a preoperative baseline because postoperative abnormalities are treated predominantly on the basis of their clinical relevance.

Other X-rays

Cervical spine X-rays should be considered in any patient in whom there is a possibility of vertebral instability, e.g. in the presence of rheumatoid arthritis. Thoracic inlet X-rays are required in patients with thyroid enlargement.

ECG

A 12-lead electrocardiogram can demonstrate many acute or longstanding pathological conditions affecting the heart, particularly changes in rhythm or the occurrence of myocardial ischaemia or infarction. It has some value as a preoperative baseline in patients with known or potential cardiovascular disease, although in the resting state the trace may appear normal despite the presence of clinically significant coronary artery disease. More extensive investigations are available in many departments to supplement the 12-lead ECG and these are discussed elsewhere (see Chs 23 and 40).

Pulmonary function tests

Peak expiratory flow rate, forced vital capacity (FVC) and forced expiratory volume in 1 s (FEV_1) should be measured in all patients with significant dyspnoea on mild or moderate exertion. This acts as a valuable preoperative baseline reference in assessing the effects of postoperative complications, although the results may not be predictive of such problems. Arterial blood gas analysis is required in all patients with dyspnoea at rest and in patients scheduled for elective thoracotomy; the information is a useful supplement to spirometry values. In patients with progressive disease, these investigations serve as a useful reference for future admissions.

Coagulation studies

Coagulation tests (PTTK and INR) are required in patients who give a history of bleeding disorders, in patients receiving anticoagulant therapy and in those with liver disease. Assessment of platelet function is worth considering in patients with potential inherited or acquired disturbances, especially if a regional anaesthetic technique is being proposed; however, this involves measurement of the bleeding time or thromboelastography.

PREDICTION OF PERIOPERATIVE MORBIDITY OR MORTALITY

After the patient's history, examination and relevant investigations have been collated the anaesthetist must answer two questions:

- Is the patient in optimum physical condition for anaesthesia and surgery?
- Are the anticipated benefits of surgery greater than the combined risks of undergoing anaesthesia and surgery, taking into account any concurrent disease?

In principle, if there is any medical condition that may be improved (e.g. pulmonary disease, hypertension, cardiac failure, chronic bronchitis, renal disease), surgery should be postponed and appropriate therapy instituted. The reasoning behind such a decision must be recorded clearly in the patient's medical notes, with the anticipated time required to achieve reasonable improvement. At this stage, the patient should be reassessed and the decision about when or whether to proceed with surgery reviewed.

There is continued interest in quantifying factors preoperatively which correlate with the occurrence of postoperative morbidity and mortality. Some accuracy is possible for populations of patients, but precision does not extend to accurate prediction of risk for an individual patient. Frequently, the decision to proceed may be made only by discussion between surgeon and anaesthetist.

Scoring systems for determining the likelihood of adverse outcome may be divided into two main groups:

- general scoring systems designed to predict non-specific undesirable events
- systems which focus on prediction of specific morbidity or technical difficulty, e.g. adverse cardiac events, difficulty with tracheal intubation.

PREDICTION OF NON-SPECIFIC ADVERSE OUTCOME

Over a broad range of operations and age, the overall mortality rate from surgery is of the order of 0.6%. This is many times greater than the incidence of deaths in which anaesthesia has made a significant contribution or has been the sole cause (approximately 1 in 10 000). In many large studies of mortality, e.g. NCEPOD reports, common factors which have emerged as contributing to anaesthetic mortality include inadequate assessment of patients in the preoperative period, inadequate supervision and monitoring in the intraoperative period and inadequate postoperative supervision and management. However, it remains difficult to evaluate formally whether it is the patient's characteristics, the surgical features or the anaesthetic technique that is the most influential in terms of final outcome. This is primarily a result of the high standards of practice which exist, the relative infrequency with which

significant perioperative morbidity or mortality occurs and the multifactorial background for many adverse events.

Any prospective studies intended to evaluate predictive factors of perioperative risk rely upon the incorporation of large numbers of patients and scrupulous design. Those that have been published tend to agree on several factors identified from physiological, demographic and laboratory data which can combine to indicate the likelihood of adverse outcome (Table 15.4).

ASA (American Society of Anesthesiologists) grading

The ASA grading system (Table 15.5) was introduced in the 1960s as a simple description of the physical state of a patient, along with an indication of whether surgery is elective or emergency. Despite its apparent simplicity, it remains one of the few prospective descriptions of the patient that correlates with the risks of anaesthesia and surgery. However, it does not embrace all aspects of anaesthetic risk, as there is no allowance for inclusion of many criteria such as age or difficulty in intubation. In addition, it does not take into account the severity of either the presenting disease or the surgery proposed, nor does it identify factors which can be improved preoperatively in order to influence outcome. Nevertheless, it is extremely useful and should be applied to all patients who present for anaesthesia.

POSSUM

This stands for 'Physiological and Operative Severity Score for the enUmeration of Mortality and morbidity'. First reported in 1991, this tool was developed to compare mortality and morbidity over a wide range of general surgical procedures, and takes into account 12 physiological and six operative factors that are either readily available or predictable in the immediate preoperative period (Table 15.6). These factors are weighted according to their value, and a logistic regression formula applied to calculate 'risk' of mortality or morbidity. Some groups have modified the formula (P-POSSUM) after suggestions that the original overestimated the risk of death in low-risk patient groups, and others have produced speciality-specific variants (e.g. V-POSSUM for elective vascular surgery). It should be emphasized that the POSSUM scoring system was designed to compare observed with expected death rates among populations rather than to predict mortality for an individual, and should be applied only in this way.

Table 15.4   Typical preoperative features which may increase the likelihood of significant perioperative complications or mortality

Demographic/surgical	Physiological	Laboratory
Age > 70 years	Dyspnoea at rest or on minimal exertion	Plasma urea >20 mmol L^{-1}
Major thoracic, abdominal or cardiovascular surgery	Myocardial infarction < 6 months previously	Serum albumin <30 g L^{-1}
Perforated viscus (excluding appendix), pancreatitis or intraperitoneal abscess	Cardiac symptoms requiring medical treatment	Haemoglobin <10 g dL^{-1}
Intestinal obstruction	Confusional state	
Palliative surgery	Clinical jaundice	
Smoking	Significant weight loss (>10%) in 1 month	
Cytotoxic or corticosteroid treatment	Productive cough with sputum, especially if persistent	
Controlled diabetes	Haemorrhage or anaemia requiring transfusion	

Table 15.5   ASA classification of physical status and the associated mortality rates (for elective and emergency cases)

ASA rating	Description of patient	Mortality rate (%)
Class I	A normally healthy individual	0.1
Class II	A patient with mild systemic disease	0.2
Class III	A patient with severe systemic disease that is not incapacitating	1.8
Class IV	A patient with incapacitating systemic disease that is a constant threat to life	7.8
Class V	A moribund patient who is not expected to survive 24 h with or without operation	9.4
Class E	Added as a suffix for emergency operation	

PREDICTION OF SPECIFIC ADVERSE EVENTS

The difficult airway

There are specific medical or surgical conditions which are associated with potential airway problems during anaesthesia, such as obesity, the later stages of pregnancy, a large neck, mediastinal tumours and some faciomaxillary deformities. Apart from these, it requires an experienced anaesthetist to collate various physical features which can predict likely difficulty. Several classifications or scoring systems have been designed for this purpose, although none is entirely reliable; they are discussed elsewhere (see Ch. 16).

Adverse cardiac events

Over 25 years ago, Goldman and colleagues published a retrospective analysis of preoperative risk factors which were associated with an adverse cardiac event following non-cardiac surgery. This topic has been re-evaluated extensively in the intervening years, with many studies agreeing broadly with Goldman's conclusions. However, conflicting opinions exist regarding identification of the most accurate predictors, probably as a result of the diversity of methods used in these studies, together with the significant and continued advances made in the understanding and

Table 15.6 Factors contributing to the POSSUM score for risk of perioperative mortality and morbidity. A higher score is awarded for increasing deviation from the 'normal' value or range

Physiological factors	Operative factors
Age (years)	Operative complexity
Cardiac status	Single vs. multiple procedures
Respiratory status	Expected blood loss
Systolic blood pressure	Peritoneal contamination (blood, pus, bowel content)
Pulse rate	Extent of any malignant spread
Glasgow Coma Score	Urgency of surgery
Haemoglobin concentration	
White cell count	
Serum urea concentration	
Serum sodium concentration	
Serum potassium concentration	
ECG rhythm	

management of cardiovascular pathophysiology. The Detsky risk calculation tool is one such modification which introduced a simplified points allocation and added limiting angina as an independent risk factor (Table 15.7).

Respiratory complications

Patients at risk of developing postoperative pulmonary complications include smokers, those with pre-existing lung disease, the obese and those undergoing thoracic or abdominal surgery. Unfortunately, predicting the likelihood and severity of such adverse events remains difficult. Sophisticated tests of pulmonary function (e.g. functional residual capacity, closing capacity, pulmonary diffusing capacity, etc.) are no more valuable in assessment of lung disease than simple spirometric tests, particularly vital capacity, FVC and FEV_1. Blood gas analysis should be performed preoperatively if there is concern about postoperative lung function; the presence of a preop-erative arterial oxygen tension of less than 9 kPa, together with the presence of dyspnoea at rest, is the most sensitive method of predicting the need for mechanical ventilation in the postoperative period.

PREOPERATIVE PREPARATION

Having taken a full clinical history, performed a physical examination and reviewed the relevant investigations, the anaesthetist should decide if further measures are required to prepare the patient satisfactorily before proceeding to anaesthesia and surgery. This is the time to address any factors which place the patient at increased risk of adverse outcome and which could be improved to the patient's benefit before surgery. It is also appropriate to consider factors such as preoperative fasting; providing information to the patient and obtaining consent to proceed; ensuring blood products are available during the perioperative period if this is thought necessary; and organizing appropriate staff and equipment within the operating theatre suite.

POSTPONING SURGERY FOR CLINICAL REASONS

There are several common reasons for postponing surgery, some of which are mentioned below. One key issue relates to communication; the reason(s) for the decision to postpone surgery must be clear to the patient, the surgical team and any other staff who have been contacted to review the patient (e.g. cardiologists, physiotherapists). This helps to ensure that the time course for any improvement remains realistic and apparent to everyone involved, and that it can be balanced against the possible detriment of delaying surgery.

Acute upper respiratory tract infection

Although many patients may admit to the presence of a cold, clarification of such an admission should be made. In general, the presence of nasal secretions, pyrexia or the unexpected presence of physical signs on clinical examination of the chest suggest that non-urgent surgery should be postponed for a few weeks until the patient has recovered.

Coexisting medical disease and drug therapy

If the patient has coexisting medical disease which may affect outcome adversely if not under optimum

Table 15.7 Cardiac risk factors in non-cardiac procedures: the Goldman and Detsky systems. Within each system a higher total score indicates increased risk of severe or significant cardiac complications (i.e. cardiac death, perioperative myocardial infarction, pulmonary oedema, life-threatening tachyarrhythmia or significant coronary insufficiency)

Risk factor	Points	
	Goldman	Detsky
History and examination		
Age > 70 years	5	5
Myocardial infarction:		
<6 months/>6 months	10/0	10/5
Angina (Canadian Heart Association classification):		
Class 3/Class 4	n/a	10/20
Unstable angina within 3 months	n/a	10
Alveolar pulmonary oedema <1 week/ever	n/a	10/5
Signs of congestive heart failure	11	n/a
Aortic stenosis (significant or critical)	3	20
Investigations		
12-lead ECG:		
Arrhythmia other than sinus or premature atrial beats	7	5
5 or more premature ventricular ectopics per minute	7	5
Poor general medical condition (any one from those listed below):	3	5
P_aO_2 <8 kPa, P_aCO_2 >6.5 kPa, K^+ <3.0 mmol L^{-1}, HCO_3 <20 mmol L^{-1}, urea >7.5 mmol L^{-1}, creatinine >270 μmol L^{-1}, SGOT (ALT) abnormal, chronic liver disease		
Specific type of surgery		
Emergency procedure	4	10
Intraperitoneal or intrathoracic	3	n/a
Vascular – aortic surgery	3	n/a

control, there is a strong argument to postpone non-urgent surgery until further specialized advice has been sought.

Emergency surgery for which the patient has not been resuscitated adequately

Postponement may be necessary for only 1–2 h to permit restoration of circulating blood volume. This important principle may be breached if haemorrhage is extensive and continuous.

Recent ingestion of food

In general, anaesthesia for elective surgery should not be undertaken within 6 h of ingestion of food, although clear fluids may be taken up to 2 h before surgery (see below).

Failure to obtain consent

Consent for surgery should be obtained from all adult patients unless the patient is incapable of providing consent and the treatment proposed is clearly in his or her best interests (see below). If there is any doubt regarding the validity of the consent, surgery should be postponed where feasible until appropriate advice has been obtained.

PREOPERATIVE FASTING

The time of last oral intake of solid and fluid must be established. One of the commonest causes of anaesthetic-related mortality and morbidity is aspiration of gastric contents.

Many anaesthetic departments have re-evaluated their standing orders on the issue of preoperative fasting for clear fluids in light of clinical studies which have demonstrated the speed of gastric emptying in healthy adults. Several important points need to be emphasized on this topic.

- There are many factors which can increase the likelihood of significant gastric content regardless of the period of starvation (e.g. pain, anxiety, some drugs and premedication including opioid analgesics, paralytic ileus, later stages of pregnancy, etc.).
- The normal daily secretion of gastric fluid can approach 2000 mL in adults; consequently, the stomach is never truly 'empty'.
- Clinical studies which encourage changes in practice should be scrutinized carefully to ensure that the results are not extrapolated beyond the sample of the population upon which they were based.

PROVIDING INFORMATION TO THE PATIENT AND OBTAINING CONSENT

Consent for anaesthesia is a vital part of preoperative preparation. It must be obtained by an individual with sufficient knowledge of the procedure and the risks involved. In order for consent to be valid, it must encompass three elements:

- The patient must have the capacity to consent to the treatment offered.
- The patient must have sufficient information to enable him/her to make a balanced decision to consent.
- The consent must be voluntary.

Capacity to consent refers to the patient's ability to comprehend the information provided, come to a decision on what is involved and communicate that decision. There is no fixed age limit below which a minor cannot consent to treatment, although caution should

be exercised when dealing with patients less than 16 years old; if in doubt, consent should also be sought from a person with parental responsibility. Capacity may also be invalidated by a patient's confusion, pain, shock or fatigue, and administration of some drugs such as opioid analgesics or benzodiazepine premedication. Appropriate advice should be sought if there is any concern.

Patients are confronted by a barrage of information on arrival in hospital, in addition to having to comply with an often alien environment with its own routines and practices. It is common for surgical consent forms to include consent to anaesthesia, despite the fact that the surgical team rarely has the knowledge to inform the patient fully on this subject. During the preoperative visit, the anaesthetist must ensure that the patient has been given an adequate amount of information about the proposed anaesthetic technique, and in particular its nature and consequences. The amount of information provided should be determined by an assessment of the needs of the patient to receive detailed information and the likelihood of adverse events:

- All patients should be told of common complications associated with the proposed anaesthetic technique (e.g. succinylcholine pains, postdural puncture headache).
- All patients should be told what they may experience in the perioperative period, including temporary numbness and weakness in the postoperative period if a local or regional technique is to be used.
- If a technique of a sensitive nature (e.g. insertion of an analgesic suppository) is to be used during anaesthesia, the patient should be informed.
- Patients should be informed of any increased risk related to their preoperative condition (e.g. damage to loose or crowned teeth, or cardiac complications in the presence of severe coronary artery disease).
- All patients should be given the opportunity to ask questions, and specific questions relating to anaesthesia must be answered honestly; if the questions relate to surgery, then the anaesthetist should ensure that a surgeon speaks to the patient before anaesthesia is induced.
- A summary of the matters discussed, the risks explained and the techniques agreed should be documented on the anaesthetic record.

In many hospitals, patients receive information leaflets which describe anaesthesia and its associated risks.

BLOOD TRANSFUSION REQUESTS

Blood products are an expensive commodity and blood transfusion carries small but finite risks of incompatibility reactions and transmission of infection. In addition, there is the potential for supplies to be short, and the need for transfusion should be considered very carefully. The object of transfusion is to ensure that adequate oxygen delivery to the tissues can be maintained throughout the perioperative period. The amount of blood ordered from the blood transfusion service depends upon both the patient's preoperative haemoglobin concentration and the anticipated extent of surgery. Consideration should also be given to the use of anaesthetic techniques which reduce intraoperative blood loss, the use of cell salvage techniques perioperatively if available, preoperative red cell donation immediately before surgery, or acute normovolaemic haemodilution.

PREOPERATIVE ORGANIZATION OF THE OPERATING THEATRE AND THE POSTOPERATIVE PERIOD

The process of preoperative assessment provides the anaesthetist with a wealth of information about the patient and the proposed surgery. This allows the anaesthetist to plan various aspects of perioperative management. Some aspects must be conveyed to staff in the operating theatre suite in advance. Examples include the planned use of invasive monitoring, issues related to patient positioning, and any special needs the patient might have, such as an interpreter. If senior anaesthetic assistance is needed, this should be arranged in advance, and organization of appropriate postoperative care should also be initiated.

PREMEDICATION AND OTHER PROPHYLACTIC MEASURES

Premedication refers to the administration of drugs in the period 1–2 h before induction of anaesthesia. It is no longer a routine part of preoperative preparation, but the need for premedication must be considered after all of the relevant factors have been identified. The objectives of premedication are to:

- allay anxiety and fear
- reduce secretions
- enhance the hypnotic effect of general anaesthetic agents

- reduce postoperative nausea and vomiting
- produce amnesia
- reduce the volume and increase the pH of gastric contents
- attenuate vagal reflexes
- attenuate sympathoadrenal responses.

Relief from anxiety

Surgical patients have a high incidence of anxiety and there is a significant inverse relationship between anxiety and smoothness of induction of anaesthesia. Relief from anxiety is accomplished most effectively by non-pharmacological means, which may be termed psychotherapy. This is effected at the preoperative visit by establishment of rapport, explanation of events which occur in the perioperative period and reassurance regarding the patient's anxieties and fears. There is good evidence that this approach has a significant calming effect.

In some patients, reassurance and explanation may be insufficient to allay anxiety. In these patients, it is appropriate to offer anxiolytic medication; the benzodiazepine drugs are the most effective for this purpose.

Reduction in secretions

Ether stimulated the production of secretions from pharyngeal and bronchial glands and premedication with an anticholinergic agent was common. This problem occurs rarely with modern anaesthetic agents, and anticholinergic premedication is no longer used as a routine. However, premedication with an anticholinergic drug is advisable for patients in whom an awake fibre-optic intubation is planned (when excessive salivation can create extra difficulty), or before using ketamine.

Sedation

Sedation is not synonymous with anxiolysis. Some drugs, e.g. the barbiturates and to a lesser extent the opioids, provide sedation but have no anxiolytic properties. In general, it is unnecessary to use a sedative preoperatively. An exception to this may be in paediatric practice. It is unwise to administer any sedative medication if the patient is in a critical condition, particularly if the airway and/or respiratory function are at risk of compromise.

Postoperative antiemesis

Nausea and vomiting are extremely common after anaesthesia. Opioid drugs administered during and after operation are often responsible. Occasionally, antiemetics may be given with the premedication, but they are more effective if administered intravenously during anaesthesia.

Amnesia

Under some circumstances, it may be desirable for patients, especially children, to be amnesic throughout the perioperative period in case unpleasant memories cause difficulties if subsequent operations are required. Some anaesthetists believe that amnesia should not be induced in children, lest they associate natural sleep with awakening to find a surgical incision. Although claims have been made for retrograde amnesia, it is unlikely that this can be achieved by pharmacological means. However, anterograde amnesia (loss of memory of events after administration of a drug) is produced commonly by the benzodiazepines; in this respect, lorazepam is two to five times more potent than diazepam. It is inappropriate to prescribe an amnesic drug with the object of reducing the risks of awareness during general anaesthesia.

Reduction in gastric volume and elevation of gastric pH

In patients who are at risk of vomiting or regurgitation (e.g. emergency patients with a full stomach or elective patients with hiatus hernia), it may be desirable to promote gastric emptying and elevate the pH of residual gastric contents. Gastric emptying may be enhanced by the administration of metoclopramide, which also possesses some antiemetic properties, whilst elevation of the pH of gastric contents may be produced by administration of sodium citrate. This topic is described in greater detail in Chapter 28.

Reduction in vagal reflexes

Premedication with an anticholinergic drug may be considered in specific situations in which vagal bradycardia may occur:

- Traction of the eye muscles, particularly the rectus medialis, during squint surgery may result in bradycardia and/or arrhythmias (the oculocardiac reflex). Premedication with atropine protects against this, but it is not as effective as the intravenous administration of atropine at induction of anaesthesia or in anticipation of traction of the muscles.
- Repeated administration of succinylcholine often results in bradycardia, which sometimes proceeds to asystole. Administration of atropine should always precede the administration of a second dose of succinylcholine.
- Induction of anaesthesia with halothane, particularly in children, may be associated with bradycardia.
- Surgical stimulation during a balanced anaesthetic technique may be associated with bradycardia.
- The administration of propofol to patients with a slow heart rate may result in dangerous degrees of bradycardia.

Limitation of sympathoadrenal responses

Induction of anaesthesia and tracheal intubation may be associated with marked sympathoadrenal activity, manifest by tachycardia, hypertension and elevation of plasma catecholamine concentrations. These responses are undesirable in the healthy individual and may be harmful in patients with hypertension or ischaemic heart disease. A β-blocker drug or clonidine may be given as premedication in order to attenuate these responses.

DRUGS USED FOR PREMEDICATION

Some of the objectives listed above may be achieved by administration of drugs at induction or during maintenance of anaesthesia. The ability to achieve all objectives by administration of a variety of drugs either preoperatively or at induction is responsible for the wide variation in prescribing habits among anaesthetists.

Benzodiazepines

The benzodiazepines possess several properties which are useful for premedication, including anxiolysis, sedation and amnesia. The extent of each of these effects differs among individual drugs. Diazepam was the first drug of this group to be used commonly, although temazepam (10–30 mg) is now often preferred because of its shorter duration of action. Lorazepam (1–5 mg) produces a greater degree of amnesia than the other drugs in this group. Benzodiazepines produce anxiolysis in doses that do not produce excessive sedation, and this is advantageous if respiratory function is compromised; however, great caution should be exercised in these patients because depression of ventilation may be precipitated even by small doses. Some benzodiazepines may be administered by intramuscular injection, but evidence suggests that oral administration gives better results. There is a very wide variation in response to benzodiazepines and effects may be unpredictable. A specific antagonist (flumazenil) is available.

Opioid analgesics

It is necessary to prescribe opioid analgesic drugs for premedication only when patients are in pain preoperatively. This is uncommon except in some patients who require surgery as an emergency. Opioid drugs were used commonly for premedication in the past. The opioids cause sedation, but are not good anxiolytic agents. Although they produce euphoria in the presence of pain, they tend to cause dysphoria in its absence. They contribute to a smoother intraoperative course, and premedication with an opioid with a long half-life may provide some analgesia in the early postoperative period. Tachypnoea, which occurs during spontaneous breathing of volatile agents, is reduced and a lower concentration of anaesthetic agent is required for maintenance of anaesthesia. However, it is more logical to administer an opioid intravenously at or after induction of anaesthesia rather than intramuscularly for premedication.

There are several important side-effects of the opioids:

- Depression of ventilation and delayed resumption of spontaneous ventilation at the end of anaesthesia in which a muscle relaxant has been used.
- Nausea and vomiting, produced by stimulation of the chemoreceptor trigger zone in the medulla, are extremely common. Opioids should always be used in combination with an antiemetic agent.
- Morphine causes spasm of the sphincter of Oddi and this may result in right upper quadrant pain in patients presenting for surgery on the biliary tract.

Phenothiazines

These have been regarded as useful agents for premedication because they produce the following effects:

- central antiemetic action
- sedation
- anxiolysis
- H_2-receptor antagonism
- α-adrenergic antagonism
- anticholinergic properties
- potentiation of opioid analgesia.

Disadvantages include extrapyramidal side-effects, synergism with opioids which may delay postoperative recovery, and potentiation of the hypotensive effects of anaesthetic agents. Postoperatively, particularly in children given alimemazine (trimeprazine), the patient may exhibit pallor with mild tachycardia and hypotension, mimicking the signs of hypovolaemia.

Anticholinergic agents

The three anticholinergic agents used commonly in anaesthesia are atropine, hyoscine and glycopyrronium. Atropine and hyoscine are tertiary amines that cross the blood–brain barrier; glycopyrronium is a quaternary amine which does not cross the blood–brain barrier and which is not absorbed from the gastrointestinal tract. Although atropine is absorbed from the gastrointestinal tract, this occurs in an unpredictable manner and is dependent upon gastric content, pH and motility.

These three drugs differ in respect of their dose–response effects at various cholinergic receptors. In standard clinical doses, hyoscine 0.4 mg produces a greater antisialagogue effect than atropine 0.6 mg and has little action on cardiac vagal receptors. Hyoscine possesses sedative and amnesic actions and, in contrast to atropine, does not cause stimulation of higher centres. Hyoscine should be avoided in the elderly (over 60 years of age) as it can produce dysphoria and restlessness. Glycopyrronium has no central effects, a much longer duration of action and, in a standard clinical dose of 0.4 mg, causes less change in heart rate than atropine 0.6 mg.

Anticholinergic drugs are used clinically to produce the following effects:

- *Antisialagogue effects.* Glycopyrronium and hyoscine are more potent than atropine in this respect. These drugs block secretions when irritant anaesthetic gases are used and reduce excessive secretions and bradycardia associated with succinylcholine when it is given either repeatedly or as an infusion.
- *Sedative and amnesic effects.* In combination with morphine, hyoscine produces powerful sedative and amnesic effects.
- *Prevention of reflex bradycardia.* Anticholinergics are given for both prophylaxis and treatment of bradycardia. Atropine is used commonly as premedication in ophthalmic surgery to block the oculocardiac reflex in patients undergoing squint surgery and has been used also in small children to reduce the bradycardia which may occur in association with halothane anaesthesia.

Side-effects of anticholinergic drugs include the following:

- *CNS toxicity.* The central anticholinergic syndrome is produced by stimulation of the CNS (usually by atropine). Symptoms include restlessness, agitation and somnolence and, in extreme cases, convulsions and coma. With hyoscine there is more commonly prolonged somnolence. Physostigmine 1–2 mg i.v. has been recommended to reverse the central anticholinergic syndrome, but is no longer available in the UK. Diazepam has been reported to have a beneficial effect, but the patient must be observed closely and steps taken if necessary to deal with depression of ventilation or upper airway obstruction.

- *Reduction in lower oesophageal sphincter tone.* Theoretically, a reduction in tone may lead to an increased risk of gastro-oesophageal reflux, although in clinical practice there is no suggestion that the use of anticholinergics for premedication is associated with an increased incidence of regurgitation and aspiration.
- *Tachycardia*, which should be avoided in patients with cardiac disease (e.g. obstructive cardiomyopathy, valvular stenosis or ischaemic heart disease) or when a hypotensive anaesthetic technique is planned.

- *Mydriasis and cycloplegia*, which lead to visual impairment. This may be troublesome, but is not a serious side-effect. Theoretically, mydriasis may be associated with reduced drainage of aqueous humour from the anterior chamber of the eye, thereby increasing intraocular pressure in patients with glaucoma. However, this effect is not important in practice and atropine may be prescribed safely to patients with glaucoma provided that appropriate therapy is maintained.
- *Pyrexia.* By suppressing secretion of sweat, anticholinergics predispose to an increase in body temperature. These drugs should therefore be avoided in the presence of pyrexia, particularly in children.
- *Excessive drying.* Although anticholinergics are given for the specific purpose of producing antisialagogue effects, this may be most unpleasant for the patient.
- *Increased physiological dead space.* Atropine and hyoscine increase physiological dead space by 20–25%, but this is compensated for by an increase in ventilation.

Table 15.8 Prophylactic measures against specific complications

Complication	Methods of prophylaxis
Deep vein thrombosis	Early postoperative mobilization
	Leg exercises (active/passive)
	Pneumatic compression of limbs
	Electrical stimulation of calf muscles
	Graduated stockings
	Low-dose subcutaneous heparin
	Warfarin anticoagulation
	Dextran-70
	(Regional anaesthetic techniques, especially for orthopaedic lower-limb procedures)
Aspiration of gastric contents	Nil by mouth
	Antacids: sodium citrate
	H_2-antagonists
	Omeprazole
	Metoclopramide
Infection	
Surgical procedure	Directed by local or national practice with advice of microbiologists
Infective endocarditis	Follow guidelines of the Endocarditis Working Party
Adrenocortical suppression – suggested for patients who have received exogenous systemic steroids during the 2 months preceding surgery	Hydrocortisone 50 mg 4-hourly or 80 mg 6-hourly, or continue usual steroids if this is in excess of the current requirements (i.e. >300 mg hydrocortisone equivalent, which is the maximum daily production in response to stress)

β-Blockers

The use of β-blockers (e.g. atenolol) during the perioperative period limits the haemodynamic response to nociceptive stimuli, such as tracheal intubation and surgical stimulation, and inhibits the neuroendocrine stress response. Recent studies suggest that the use of β-blockers in patients at risk of coronary artery disease may be associated with improved outcome. However, their use incurs a limitation on appropriate increases in cardiac output during the perioperative period, and their administration to patients with impairment of left ventricular function should be considered very cautiously.

Clonidine and dexmedetomidine

These are α_2-agonists which potentiate anaesthetics by decreasing central noradrenergic activity. Dexmedetomidine is more specific for the α_2-receptor and probably has greater potential as a premedicant. Administration results in decreased intraoperative requirements for inhaled anaesthetic agents or propofol, although recovery times may be prolonged. These agents may also have a role in attenuating sympathoadrenal responses at induction of anaesthesia.

OTHER PROPHYLACTIC MEASURES

Thought should be given to the value of giving prophylactic treatment for the specific situations summarized in Table 15.8.

FURTHER READING

Association of Anaesthetists of Great Britain and Ireland 2001 Pre-operative assessment: the role of the anaesthetist. www.aagbi.org

Auerbach A, Goldman L 2002 Beta-blockers and reduction of cardiac events in non-cardiac surgery. Journal of the American Medical Association 287: 1435–1444

Janke E, Chalk V, Kinley H 2002 Pre-operative assessment: setting a standard through learning. University of Southampton, 2002

National Institute for Clinical Excellence 2003 CG3 – pre-operative testing, the use of routine pre-operative tests for elective surgery. www.nice.org.uk

Stoelting R K, Diedrorf S F 2002 Handbook of anesthesia and co-existing disease, 4th edn. Elsevier Health Sciences, Edinburgh

The practical conduct of anaesthesia 16

Planning the conduct of anaesthesia starts normally after details concerning the surgical procedure and the medical condition of the patient have been ascertained at the preoperative visit. Preoperative assessment and selection of appropriate premedication are discussed in Chapter 15.

PREPARATION FOR ANAESTHESIA

Before starting, consideration should be given to the induction and maintenance of anaesthesia, the position of the patient on the operating table, the equipment necessary for monitoring, the use of intravenous (i.v.) fluids or blood for infusion and the postoperative care and recovery facilities that will be required.

The anaesthetic machine to be used must be tested for leaks, misconnections and proper function. A checklist, e.g. that published by the Association of Anaesthetists of Great Britain and Ireland (AAGBI), is recommended. This is discussed in Chapter 14. The breathing system to be used should be new for each patient, or a filter of appropriate size should be placed between the patient and the system and a new filter used for each patient according to the recommendations of the Blood Borne Advisory Group of the AAGBI, 1996.

The availability and function of all anaesthetic equipment should be checked before starting (see Table 16.1). After the patient's arrival in the anaesthetic room, the anaesthetist should be satisfied that the correct operation is being performed upon the correct patient and that consent has been given. The patient must be on a tilting bed or trolley and the anaesthetist should have a competent assistant.

INDUCTION OF ANAESTHESIA

Anaesthesia is induced using one of the following techniques.

INHALATIONAL INDUCTION

The most common indications for induction of anaesthesia by an inhalational technique are listed in Table 16.2.

The proposed procedure should be explained to the patient before starting. A 'no-mask' technique using a cupped hand around the fresh gas delivery tube may be preferred for young children. When an Ayre's T-piece is used for inhalational induction in young children, it is recommended that a filter is not used as its presence provides excessive resistance to gas flow, diverting fresh gas flow to the efferent limb and slowing induction. The mask or hand is introduced *gradually* to the face from the side, as the sight of a mask descending onto the face may be disturbing. However, the use of a transparent perfumed mask can render the procedure less unpleasant. While talking to the patient and encouraging him/her to breathe normally, the anaesthetist adjusts the mixture of the fresh gas flow and observes the patient's reactions. Initially, nitrous oxide 70% in oxygen is used and anaesthesia is deepened by the gradual introduction of increments of a volatile agent, e.g. sevoflurane. This may also be used starting at an inspired concentration of 8% which achieves more rapid induction than its use incrementally. Maintenance concentrations of isoflurane (1–2%) or sevoflurane (2–3%) are used when anaesthesia has been established.

A single-breath technique of inhalational induction has been advocated for patients who are able to cooperate. One vital capacity breath from a prefilled 4 L reservoir bag containing a high concentration of volatile agent (e.g. sevoflurane 8%) in oxygen (or nitrous oxide 50% in oxygen) results in smooth induction of anaesthesia within 20–30 s.

Observation of the colour of the patient's skin and pattern of ventilation, palpation of the peripheral pulse, ECG and S_pO_2 monitoring and measurement of arterial pressure are important accompaniments to the technique of inhalational induction.

Table 16.1 Equipment required for tracheal intubation

Correct size of laryngoscope and spare (in case of light failure)
Tracheal tube of correct size + an alternative smaller size
Tracheal tube connector
Wire stilette
Gum elastic bougies
Magill forceps
Cuff-inflating syringe
Artery forceps
Securing tape or bandage
Catheter mount(s)
Local anaesthetic spray – 4% lidocaine
Cocaine spray/gel for nasal intubation
Tracheal tube lubricant
Throat packs
Anaesthetic breathing system and face masks – tested with O_2 to ensure no leaks present

Table 16.2 Indications for inhalational induction

Young children
Upper airway obstruction, e.g. epiglottitis
Lower airway obstruction with foreign body
Bronchopleural fistula or empyema
No accessible veins

If spontaneous ventilation is to be maintained throughout the procedure, the mask is applied more firmly as consciousness is lost and the airway is supported manually. Insertion of an oropharyngeal airway, a laryngeal mask airway or a tracheal tube may be considered when anaesthesia has been established.

Complications and difficulties

- slower induction of anaesthesia
- problems particularly during stage 2 (see below)

- airway obstruction, bronchospasm
- laryngeal spasm, hiccups
- environmental pollution.

INTRAVENOUS INDUCTION

Induction of anaesthesia with an i.v. agent is suitable for most routine purposes and avoids many of the complications associated with the inhalational technique. It is the most appropriate method of rapid induction for the patient undergoing emergency surgery, in whom there is a risk of regurgitation of gastric contents during induction. All drugs which may be required at induction should be prepared and a cannula inserted into a suitable vein before starting. The anaesthetist should wear rubber gloves for this and other procedures during induction of anaesthesia and during airway manipulations such as insertion of an airway or tracheal tube.

If an existing i.v. cannula is to be used, its function must be checked. Cannulae with a side injection port ('Venflon' type) are useful; large cannulae (e.g. 16G, 14G) are necessary for transfusion of fluids or blood. A vein in the forearm or on the back of the hand is preferable; veins in the antecubital fossa should be avoided because of the risks of intra-arterial injection and problems with elbow flexion. After selection of a suitable vein, skin preparation is performed using iodine or alcohol. Subcutaneous local anaesthetic should be used for large cannulae. Alternatively, local anaesthetic cream (EMLA or Ametop (tetracaine)) may have been applied preoperatively. Intravenous entry is confirmed with blood aspiration and the device is secured firmly with tape. 'Opsite' dressings may be used when long-term use is anticipated.

Monitoring should be commenced before induction of anaesthesia, including S_pO_2, ECG and arterial pressure measurement. Preoxygenation may be started, using a close-fitting face mask, and 100% oxygen delivered, for example, by a Magill breathing system for 5 min. Alternatively, three to four large (vital capacity) breaths may be used. Preoxygenation before routine elective induction of anaesthesia avoids transient hypoxaemia before establishment of effective lung ventilation.

Doses of the common i.v. agents are shown in Table 16.3. The induction dose varies with the patient's weight, age, state of nutrition, circulatory status, premedication and any concurrent medication. A small test dose is commonly administered and its effects are observed. Slow injection is recommended in the aged and in those with a slow circulation time (e.g. shock, hypovolaemia, cardiovascular disease) while the effects of the drug on the cardiovascular and respiratory systems are assessed.

Table 16.3 Intravenous induction agents

Agent	Induction dose (mg kg^{-1})
Thiopental	3–5
Etomidate	0.3
Propofol	1.5–2.5
Ketamine	2

A rapid-sequence induction technique is indicated for patients undergoing emergency surgery and for those in whom vomiting or regurgitation is a potential problem. After i.v. induction, a rapid transition to stage 3 anaesthesia (see below) is achieved; this is maintained by the introduction of an inhalational agent or by repeated bolus injections or a continuous infusion of an i.v. anaesthetic agent. Emergency anaesthesia is discussed fully in Chapter 28.

Complications and difficulties

Regurgitation and vomiting. If regurgitation occurs, the patient should be placed immediately into the Trendelenburg position and material aspirated with suction apparatus. Should inhalation of gastric contents occur, treatment is with 100% oxygen, bronchodilators and tracheal suction. Steroids and antibiotics may be considered. Continued IPPV may be required if the resultant pneumonitis is severe.

Intra-arterial injection of thiopental. This rare complication should be avoided by the appropriate choice of venous site, use of a 'plastic' cannula and checking its function before injection. Pain and blanching in the hand and fingers occurs as a result of crystal formation in the capillaries. The needle should be left in the artery and 5 mL 0.5% procaine and 40 mg papaverine injected. Further treatment includes stellate ganglion block, brachial plexus block or sympathetic block with i.v. guanethidine.

Perivenous injection. This causes blanching and pain and may result in a small degree of tissue necrosis. Propofol produces less tissue damage than thiopental. Hyaluronidase may be used to speed dispersal of the drug.

Cardiovascular depression. This is likely to occur particularly in the elderly, the hypovolaemic or the untreated hypertensive patient. Reducing the dose and speed of injection is recommended in these patients. Infusion of i.v. fluid (e.g. 500 mL colloid or 1000 mL crystalloid solution) is usually successful in restoring arterial pressure.

Respiratory depression. Slow injection of an induction agent may reduce the extent of respiratory depression. Respiratory adequacy must be assessed carefully and the anaesthetist should be ready to assist ventilation of the lungs if necessary.

Histamine release. Thiopental in particular may cause release of histamine with subsequent formation of typical wheals. Severe reactions may occur to individual agents, and appropriate drugs and fluids should be available in the anaesthetic room for treatment. Guidelines for emergency management of acute major anaphylaxis are available (AAGBI) and may be displayed in the anaesthetic room. This is discussed further in Chapter 19.

Porphyria. An acute porphyric episode may be precipitated in susceptible individuals by barbiturates.

Other complications. Pain on injection (especially with etomidate or propofol), hiccup or muscular movements may occur. The use of lidocaine mixed with propofol reduces the incidence of pain on injection.

POSITION OF PATIENT FOR SURGERY

After induction of anaesthesia, the patient is placed on the operating table in a position appropriate for the proposed surgery. When positioning the patient, the anaesthetist should take into account surgical access, patient safety, anaesthetic technique, monitoring and position of i.v. cannulae, etc.

Some commonly used positions are shown in Figure 16.1. Each may have adverse effects in terms of skeletal, neurological, ventilatory and circulatory effects.

The lithotomy position may result in nerve damage on the medial or lateral side of the leg from pressure exerted by the stirrups, which must be well padded. Care must be taken to elevate both legs simultaneously so that pelvic asymmetry and resultant backache are avoided. The sacrum should be supported on the operating table and not allowed to slip off the end.

The lateral position may result in asymmetrical lung ventilation. Care is required with arm position and i.v. infusions. The pelvis and shoulders must be supported to prevent the patient from rolling either backwards (with a risk of falling from the table) or forwards into the recovery position.

The prone position may cause abdominal compression which may result in ventilatory and circulatory embarrassment. To prevent this, support must be

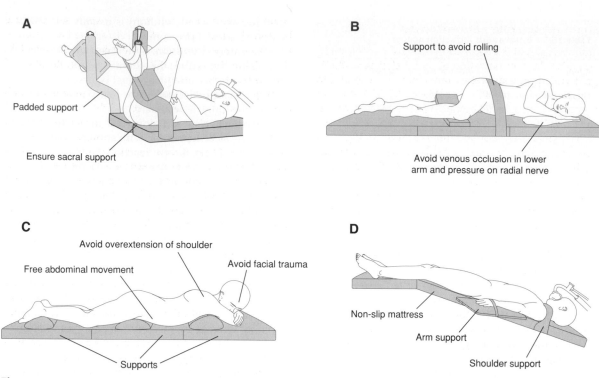

Fig. 16.1
Positions on the operating table. **(A)** Lithotomy position. **(B)** Lateral position. **(C)** Prone position. **(D)** Trendelenburg position.

provided beneath the shoulders and iliac crests. Excessive extension of the shoulders should be avoided. The face, and particularly the eyes, must be protected from trauma. The tracheal tube must be secured firmly in place as it is almost impossible to reinsert it with the patient in this position.

The Trendelenburg position may produce upward pressure on the diaphragm because of the weight of the abdominal contents. Damage to the brachial plexus may occur as a result of pressure from shoulder supports, especially if the arms are abducted.

The sitting position requires careful support of the head. In addition, venous pooling and resultant cardiovascular instability may occur.

The supine position carries the risk of the supine hypotensive syndrome during pregnancy (see Ch. 35) or in patients with a large abdominal mass.

Positioning during anaesthesia is discussed extensively by Martin & Warner (1997).

MAINTENANCE OF ANAESTHESIA

Anaesthesia may be continued using inhalational agents, i.v. anaesthetic agents or i.v. opioids either alone or in combination. Tracheal intubation with or without muscle relaxants may be used. Regional anaesthesia may be used to supplement any of these techniques to achieve the components of the familiar anaesthetic triad of sleep, muscular relaxation and analgesia.

INHALATIONAL ANAESTHESIA WITH SPONTANEOUS VENTILATION

This is an appropriate form of maintenance for superficial operations, minor procedures which produce little reflex or painful stimulation and operations for which profound muscle relaxation is not required.

Conduct

After induction of anaesthesia, nitrous oxide and/or a volatile agent may be used in the spontaneously breathing patient. Depending on the nature of surgery, the provision of analgesia in premedication (if used), and the patient's response (assessed by observation of ventilation, circulation and heart rate and rhythm), isoflurane 1–2% inspired concentration may be used in a mixture with nitrous oxide 70% in oxygen; sevoflurane 2–3% is an alternative.

Minimum alveolar concentration

Minimum alveolar concentration (MAC) is the minimum alveolar concentration of an inhaled anaesthetic agent which prevents reflex movement in response to surgical incision in 50% of subjects. MAC values of commonly used inhalational agents are shown in Appendix BII. MAC varies little with metabolic factors but is reduced by opioid premedication and in the presence of hypothermia. MAC is higher in neonates and is reduced in the elderly (see Ch. 2). The effects of inhalational anaesthetics are additive; thus, 1 MAC-equivalent could be achieved by producing an alveolar concentration of 70% nitrous oxide (0.67 MAC) and 0.4% isoflurane (0.33 MAC).

The rate at which MAC is attained may be increased by raising the inspired concentration and by avoidance of airway obstruction. Increasing ventilation at a constant inspired concentration produces more rapid equilibration between inspired and alveolar concentrations. The time taken for equilibration increases with the blood/gas solubility coefficient of the agent; those with a high blood/gas solubility coefficient (e.g. halothane) do not reach equilibrium for several hours (see Ch. 2). It follows, therefore, that the inspired concentration must be considerably higher than MAC to produce an adequate alveolar concentration when such agents are used.

Control of depth of anaesthesia by varying the inspired concentration of volatile agent requires constant assessment of the patient's reaction to anaesthesia and surgery to produce adequate anaesthesia, while avoiding overdosage and excessively 'deep' anaesthesia. This rapid control is one of the main advantages of inhalational anaesthesia. The signs of inadequate depth of anaesthesia include tachypnoea, tachycardia, hypertension and sweating.

Signs of anaesthesia

Guedel's classic signs of anaesthesia are those seen in patients premedicated with morphine and atropine and breathing ether in air. The clinical signs associated with anaesthesia produced by other inhalational agents follow a similar course, but the divisions between the stages and planes are less precise (Fig. 16.2).

Stage 1: the stage of analgesia. This is the stage attained when using nitrous oxide 50% in oxygen, as used in the technique of relative analgesia (see Ch. 33).

Stage 2: stage of excitement. This is seen with inhalational induction, but is passed rapidly during i.v. induction. Respiration is erratic, breath-holding may occur, laryngeal and pharyngeal reflexes are active and stimulation of pharynx or larynx, e.g. by insertion of a Guedel or laryngeal mask airway, may produce laryngeal spasm. The eyelash reflex (used as a sign of unconsciousness with i.v. induction) is abolished in stage 2, but the eyelid reflex (resistance to elevation of eyelid) remains present.

Stage 3: surgical anaesthesia. This deepens through four planes (in practice, three – light, medium, deep) with increasing concentration of anaesthetic drug. Respiration assumes a rhythmic pattern and the thoracic component diminishes with depth of anaesthesia. Respiratory reflexes become suppressed but the carinal reflex is abolished only at plane IV (therefore, a tracheal tube which is too long may produce carinal stimulation at an otherwise adequate depth). The pupils are central and gradually enlarge with depth of anaesthesia. Lacrimation is active in light planes but absent in planes III and IV – a useful sign in a patient not premedicated with an anticholinergic.

Stage 4: stage of impending respiratory and circulatory failure. Brainstem reflexes are depressed by the high anaesthetic concentration. Pupils are enlarged and unreactive. The patient should not be permitted to reach this stage. Withdrawal of the anaesthetic agents and administration of 100% oxygen lightens anaesthesia.

Observation of other reflexes provides a guide to depth of anaesthesia. Swallowing occurs in the light plane of stage 3. The gag reflex is abolished in upper stage 3. Stretching of the anal sphincter produces reflex laryngospasm even at plane III of stage 3.

Complications and difficulties

Airway obstruction. This is relieved by appropriate positioning and equipment (see below).

Laryngeal spasm. This may occur above light–medium stage 3 as a result of stimulation. Treatment is to stop the stimulation and gently deepen anaesthesia. If spasm is severe, 100% oxygen is applied with the face mask held tightly, while the airway is maintained by hand and pressure is applied to the reservoir bag. Attempts to ventilate the patient's lungs usually result only in gastric inflation. However, as the larynx partially opens, 100% oxygen flows through under pressure. Further gentle deepening of anaesthesia may then take place. In severe laryngeal spasm, i.v. succinylcholine may be required, and after the lungs have been inflated with oxygen it is advisable to intubate the trachea.

Bronchospasm. This may occur if volatile anaesthetic agents are introduced rapidly, particularly in smokers with excessive bronchial secretions. Humidification and warming of gases may minimize the problem. Bronchospasm may accompany laryngospasm. Administration of bronchodilators may be required. These respiratory reflexes are induced more readily

STAGE	RESPIRATION	PUPILS	EYE REFLEXES	URT & RESPIRATORY REFLEXES
1 Analgesia	Regular Small volume	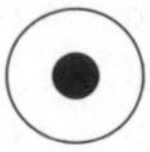		
2 Excitement	Irregular	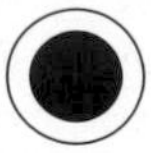	Eyelash absent	
3 Anaesthesia Plane I	Regular Large volume	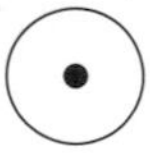	Eyelid absent Conjunctival depressed	Pharyngeal & vomiting depressed
Plane II	Regular Large volume		Corneal depressed	
Plane III	Regular Becoming diaphragmatic Small volume			Laryngeal depressed
Plane IV	Irregular Diaphragmatic Small volume	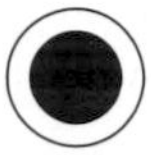		Carinal depressed
4 Overdose	Apnoea	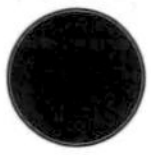		

Fig. 16.2
Stages of anaesthesia (modified from Guedel).

in the presence of or shortly after a respiratory tract infection.

Malignant hyperthermia. Volatile agents, succinylcholine or amide-type local anaesthetic agents may trigger this syndrome in susceptible individuals (see Ch. 19).

Raised intracranial pressure (ICP). All volatile agents may produce an increase in ICP and this is accentuated by retention of CO_2 which accompanies the use of volatile agents in the spontaneously breathing patient. A spontaneous ventilation technique is therefore contraindicated in patients with an intracranial space-occupying lesion or cerebral oedema.

Atmospheric pollution. The use of the appropriate scavenging apparatus helps to reduce levels of theatre pollution by volatile and gaseous agents (see Ch. 14).

Delivery of inhalational agents – airway maintenance

Maintenance of the airway is one of the most important of the anaesthetist's tasks. Inhalational agents may be delivered via a face mask, a laryngeal mask airway (LMA) or a tracheal tube. Insufflation techniques, although once popular, are now rarely used.

Use of the face mask

Inhalational anaesthesia usually involves the use of a face mask. The face mask has many variants of type and size, and selection of the correct fit is important to provide a gas-tight seal.

For children, a mask with excessive dead space should be avoided. Nasal masks may be used during dental anaesthesia. The patient's head position during mask anaesthesia is important; the mandible is held 'into' the mask by the anaesthetist using a boney contact point rather than pressing into the soft tissues, which may result in airway obstruction (especially in children). The mandible is held forward, helping to prevent posterior movement of the tongue and obstruction of the airway.

The importance of observation of the airway during mask anaesthesia cannot be overemphasized. Soft tissue indrawing in the suprasternal and supraclavicular areas is evidence of obstruction of the upper airway. Noisy ventilation or inspiratory stridor provides further evidence that airway obstruction requires correction. Maintenance of the airway may be assisted further by the use of an oropharyngeal (Guedel) airway. An appropriate stage of anaesthesia must be reached before insertion of the airway, as stimulation of the pharynx at stage 2 or at light stage 3 produces coughing, laryngospasm or breath-holding. The use of local anaesthetic spray or jelly to coat the airway may permit its insertion at an earlier stage. A nasopharyngeal airway may be tolerated better.

The face mask is used in current practice only before tracheal intubation or insertion of the laryngeal mask or during short non-invasive procedures, e.g. dental anaesthesia and orthopaedic manipulations. To ensure patency of the airway, other airway adjuncts such as an oropharyngeal or a nasopharyngeal airway may be used.

Use of the laryngeal mask airway

Indications

- To provide a clear airway without the need for the anaesthetist's hands to support a mask.
- To avoid the use of tracheal intubation during spontaneous ventilation.
- In a case of difficult intubation, to facilitate subsequent insertion of a tracheal tube via the intubating LMA.

Contraindications

- A patient with a 'full stomach' or with any condition leading to delayed gastric emptying.
- A patient in whom regurgitation of gastric contents into the oesophagus is likely (e.g. hiatus hernia).
- Where surgical access (e.g. to the pharynx) is impeded by the cuff of the LMA.

Conduct of LMA insertion. An appropriate depth of anaesthesia is required for successful insertion of the LMA. Fewer difficulties are encountered after i.v. induction of anaesthesia with propofol than with thiopental because of the greater tendency of the former to suppress pharyngeal reflexes. The appropriate size of LMA is chosen according to the weight of the patient (Table 16.4). In general, the largest size possible is used to create a seal with a cuff inflation less than the maximum. In adults, the larger sizes are used according to inspection. The patient's head is extended, the mouth is opened and, if necessary, the mandible can be held down by an assistant. The LMA cuff is evacuated and the LMA is inserted into the

Table 16.4 Laryngeal mask airway sizes

Mask size	Patient weight (kg)	Cuff volume (mL)
1	<5	2–5
1.5	5–10	5–7
2	10–20	7–10
2.5	20–30	12–14
3	>30	15–20
4	n/a	25–30
5	n/a	35–40

After Brimacombe et al. 1996

pharynx in a direction along the axis of the hard palate so that the cuff encounters the posterior pharyngeal wall and is swept distally into the laryngopharynx. This may be assisted by use of the gloved fingers in the 'classic' technique. The cuff then lies posterior to the larynx. Air is injected into the cuff and the breathing system is attached via a catheter mount to the 22-mm proximal connector. The LMA is secured in place with tape or a bandage after confirmation of correct placement by observation of movement of the reservoir bag, or of the chest after a gentle manual inflation of the lungs. The reinforced LMA may be useful when the standard LMA may hinder surgical access or be prone to kinking. Traditionally, the LMA has been re-used after autoclaving but disposable versions are now available.

TRACHEAL INTUBATION

Indications

- Provision of a clear airway, e.g. anticipated difficulty in using mask anaesthesia in the edentulous patient.
- An 'unusual' position, e.g. prone or sitting. A reinforced non-kinking tube may be necessary.
- Operations on the head and neck, e.g. ENT, dental. A nasotracheal tube may be required.
- Protection of the respiratory tract, e.g. from blood during upper respiratory tract or oral surgery and from inhalation of gastric contents in emergency surgery or patients with oesophageal obstruction. The use of a cuffed tube for adults is mandatory in these circumstances.

- During anaesthesia using IPPV and muscle relaxants.
- To facilitate suction of the respiratory tract.
- During thoracic operations.

    Contraindications. There are few contraindications. In emergency situations, hypoxaemia must be relieved if at all possible before insertion of a tracheal tube.

Preparation

Before starting, the anaesthetist must check the availability and function of the necessary equipment. He or she should have a 'dedicated' and experienced assistant. Laryngoscopes of the correct size are chosen and the function of bulb and batteries checked, the patency of the tracheal tube is checked and the integrity of the cuff ensured. Various aids to intubation must also be present (see Table 16.1).

Choice of equipment

Laryngoscopes

Laryngoscopes are manufactured in many shapes and sizes. There are two basic types of blade – straight or curved. Straight-blade laryngoscopes (e.g. Magill) are favoured for children, in whom the epiglottis is floppy, and are designed to pass posterior to the epiglottis and to lift it anteriorly, exposing the larynx. The curved blade (e.g. Macintosh) is designed so that the tip lies anterior to the epiglottis in the vallecula, pressing on the hyoepiglottic ligament and moving it anteriorly to expose the larynx and vocal cords (Fig. 16.3). The McCoy blade incorporates a movable distal tip to facilitate a view of the glottis in appropriate patients.

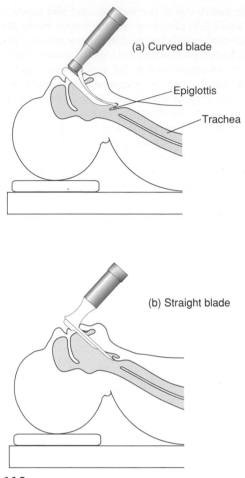

Fig. 16.3
Use of the laryngoscope.

Tracheal tubes

Modern tracheal tubes are disposable and made from PVC which is 'implant tested' for its inert effect upon the tissues. In some circumstances, e.g. head and neck or throat surgery, the tracheal tube may be subject to direct or indirect pressure and standard tubes may kink or become compressed. It may be appropriate to use a tube which is reinforced with a nylon or steel spiral in such cases. Tracheal tubes are introduced usually through the mouth, although it may be preferable to pass the tube through the nose, particularly for oral surgery. The supplied length of disposable tubes exceeds that required normally for oral intubation and the tube should be cut to the appropriate length before use. During thoracic surgery, it may be necessary to ventilate the lungs independently and a bronchial or double-lumen tube is required (see Ch. 39).

In order to seal the airway, most tracheal tubes are manufactured with an inflatable cuff at the distal end. The cuff may be of low or high volume; low-volume cuffs produce a seal over a smaller area of tracheal mucosa and tend to exert a high pressure on the mucosal cells, reducing the capillary blood supply and rendering the cells potentially ischaemic. High-volume cuffs cover a wide area of mucosa; the pressure exerted varies during the respiratory cycle, but on average is lower than that produced by a low-volume cuff. A medium-volume, low-profile cuffed tube represents a compromise and has some practical advantages.

Tracheal tubes of different sizes are required. The size quoted is the internal diameter (ID). Adult males normally require a tube of 9–9.5 mm ID and females

8–8.5 mm. For oral intubation, the tube should normally be 20–23 cm in length. The appropriate internal diameter of tube for paediatric use may be calculated from the following formula: (age/4) + 4 mm. This is an approximation and a tube 0.5 mm smaller and 0.5 mm larger should also be prepared. The length of tube required for oral intubation in children is approximately equal to (age/2) + 12 cm. A tube of slightly smaller internal diameter may be required for nasal intubation and its length may be calculated from the formula (age/2) + 15 cm.

An appropriate connector is required between the tracheal tube and the anaesthetic breathing system, e.g. curved connector for nasal tube, lightweight plastic with low dead space for children or a connector with a suction port for thoracic surgery. It is important before use to ensure the patency of breathing system connectors and the absence of foreign material occluding the lumen; vulnerable components of the breathing system should remain wrapped until use.

Anaesthesia for tracheal intubation

Tracheal intubation may be performed under local anaesthesia (using topical spray, transtracheal spray and superior laryngeal nerve block) or under general anaesthesia (either i.v. or inhalation, with or without the use of muscle relaxation). The usual approach is to provide general anaesthesia and muscle relaxation, to perform laryngoscopy and direct vision intubation and then to maintain anaesthesia via the tracheal tube with spontaneous or controlled ventilation.

Inhalational technique for intubation

Adequate depth of anaesthesia is necessary to depress the laryngeal reflexes and provide a degree of relaxation of the laryngeal and pharyngeal muscles. Halothane in concentrations up to 4% or sevoflurane 8% provides rapid attainment of the necessary depth, which can be judged from the pattern of respiration with predominance of diaphragmatic breathing (a useful sign in children is the 'dissociation' of the thoracic and abdominal excursion). The mask is removed and laryngoscopy and intubation performed. The anaesthetic circuit is then connected to the tracheal tube and anaesthesia maintained at a depth appropriate for surgery.

Relaxant anaesthesia for intubation

After i.v. or inhalational induction of anaesthesia, the short-acting depolarizing muscle relaxant succinylcholine may be used to provide relaxation for tracheal intubation. After loss of consciousness, the patient breathes 100% oxygen or 50% nitrous oxide in oxygen and succinylcholine is administered in a dose of 1–1.5 mg kg^{-1}. Assisted ventilation is maintained via the face mask until muscle relaxation occurs (except in emergency patients and those likely to regurgitate) and laryngoscopy and intubation are performed. Inhalational anaesthesia may be continued with manual ventilation until the effects of the relaxant have ceased, whereupon spontaneous ventilation is resumed. Alternatively, non-depolarizing neuromuscular blockade is produced and ventilation controlled.

Conduct of laryngoscopy

The position of the patient's head and neck is important. The neck should be flexed and the head extended with the support of a pillow; thus, the oral, pharyngeal and tracheal axes are brought into alignment (Fig. 16.4). The laryngoscope is designed for left-hand use and is introduced into the right side of the mouth while the right hand opens the mouth, parting the lips to avoid interposing them between laryngoscope and teeth. The teeth may be protected from blade trauma with the fingers or the use of a plastic 'guard'. The laryngoscope blade deflects the tongue to the left and the length of the blade is passed over the contour of the tongue. The laryngoscope is lifted upwards and forwards, avoiding a levering movement which can damage the upper anterior teeth. Using a straight blade, the tip is passed posterior to the epiglottis, which is lifted anteriorly, and the vocal cords are seen. With a curved blade, the tip is inserted into the vallecula and pressure on the hyoepiglottic ligament moves the epiglottis to expose the vocal cords. External pressure on the thyroid cartilage by an assistant may aid laryngeal vision at this stage. Alternatively, using the McCoy adaptation of the Macintosh blade, the distal

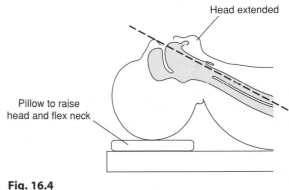

Fig. 16.4
Head position for laryngoscopy.

lever may be used to elevate the epiglottis to assist in viewing the larynx.

Conduct of intubation

After laryngeal visualization, the supraglottic area and cords may be sprayed, if required, with local anaesthetic solution (lidocaine 4%). The tracheal tube is passed from the right side of the mouth (which may be held open by the assistant's finger if necessary, permitting a clear view of the midline) and between the vocal cords into the trachea until the cuff is below the vocal cords. A semirigid stilette may be used during intubation to provide the correct degree of curvature of the tracheal tube to facilitate intubation. This is useful particularly with reinforced tubes.

The tube cuff is inflated sufficiently to abolish audible gas leaks on inflation of the lungs. The correct position of the tube must now be confirmed. If the tube has been seen clearly at laryngoscopy to pass through the vocal cords into the trachea, then equal movement of both sides of the chest during ventilation should be confirmed and auscultation in each axilla for breath sounds should be performed to ensure that the tip of the tracheal tube has not passed too far distally to enter, or occlude, one of the main bronchi (see Ch. 19); if there is unilateral air entry, the tube should be withdrawn slowly and carefully until air entry is equal in both lungs. If the tube has not been seen clearly to enter the trachea, or if there is any reason to suspect that its distal end is not in the trachea, then the steps outlined in Chapter 19 must be undertaken immediately to identify possible oesophageal intubation.

After its correct position has been determined, the tube is secured with cotton tape, bandage or sticking plaster strips. Correct fixation of the tube is important, particularly if the head is inaccessible during surgery, e.g. when the patient is in the prone position. On such occasions, extra security is gained using broad 'elastoplast' strapping over the primary fixing tape on the patient's face.

Nasal intubation

Nasal intubation may be used for dental operations, ENT operations, etc., and may be preferred for long-term intubation because it provides easier tube fixation, easier oral toilet and greater patient comfort.

A slightly smaller tube is used and is introduced preferentially into the right nostril, as the left-facing bevel of the tube favours this approach. The tube is passed along the floor of the nose and advanced *gently* into the pharynx, avoiding excessive force. Laryngoscopy takes place and the tube is advanced into the trachea by manipulation of the proximal end or by grasping the distal tip with Magill's intubating forceps to pass it between the cords.

Packing of the throat may be used after intubation, especially for oropharyngeal operations. The moist gauze pack is introduced using the laryngoscope and Magill forceps. The pharynx should be packed on each side of the tracheal tube. The pack should be applied gently to avoid abrasion of the mucosa. A 'tail' of the pack is left protruding from the mouth and the anaesthetist must accept responsibility for removal of the pack before extubation. A latex 'foam' pack may be used as an alternative to cotton gauze.

Difficult intubation

The reported incidence of difficult intubation is one in 65 patients. In practice, most cases represent difficulty with laryngoscopy. Poor management of difficult intubation is a significant cause of anaesthetic morbidity and mortality. Sequelae include dental and airway trauma, pulmonary aspiration and hypoxaemia.

Aetiology

Table 16.5 shows the common causes of difficult intubation. The single most important cause is an inexperienced or inadequately prepared anaesthetist, often complicated by equipment malfunction. There are numerous causes of difficult laryngoscopy related to patient factors. The anatomical features associated with difficult laryngoscopy are listed in Table 16.6 . Of these, the atlanto-occipital distance is the best predictor of difficulty but requires an X-ray examination. Many of these factors are normal anatomical variations; they may also be congenital or acquired.

Congenital. Many syndromes are associated with multiple anatomical abnormalities such as a small mouth, large tongue and cleft palate. Patients with encephalocele, cystic hygroma and hydrocephalus may have restricted head or jaw movement. Morquio and Down syndromes are associated with cervical spine instability.

Acquired. Acquired factors may affect jaw opening, neck movement or the airway itself. Reduced jaw movement is a common cause of difficult laryngoscopy. Trauma and infection may cause reflex spasm of the masseter and medial pterygoid muscles (trismus). This occurs typically with dental abscess or mandibular fractures and is usually relaxed by anaesthetic agents. In contrast, the reduced jaw movement associated with temporomandibular joint fibrosis is usually fixed. This may complicate chronic infection, rheumatoid arthritis, ankylosing spondylitis and radiotherapy. Any local soft tissue swelling or mass may also reduce jaw movement.

Table 16.5 Common causes of difficult intubation

Anaesthetist
Inadequate preoperative assessment
Inadequate equipment preparation
Inexperience
Poor technique

Equipment
Malfunction
Unavailability
No trained assistant

Patient

Congenital	Syndromes (Down, Pierre Robin, Treacher Collins, Marfan's)	
	Achondroplasia	
	Cystic hygroma	
	Encephalocele	
Acquired	Reduced jaw movement	Trismus (abscess/infection, fracture, tetanus)
		Fibrosis (postinfection/radiotherapy/trauma)
		Rheumatoid arthritis, ankylosing spondylitis
		Tumours
		Jaw wiring
	Reduced neck movement	Rheumatoid/osteoarthritis
		Ankylosing spondylitis
		Cervical fracture/instability/fusion
	Airway	Oedema (abscess/infection, trauma, angio-oedema, burns)
		Compression (goitre, surgical haemorrhage)
		Scarring (radiotherapy, infection, burns)
		Tumours/polyps
		Foreign body
		Nerve palsy
	Others	Morbid obesity
		Pregnancy
		Acromegaly

Reduced head and neck movement is an important cause of difficult laryngoscopy. Optimal positioning for laryngoscopy requires extension of the head at the atlanto-occipital joint; this joint may be damaged in patients with rheumatoid arthritis, osteoarthritis and ankylosing spondylitis. Cervical spine movement may be reduced by surgical fusion, fibrosis and soft tissue swellings of the head and neck. Cervical spine instability (e.g. fractures, tumours, rheumatoid arthritis) makes neck movement undesirable.

Disorders of the airway itself may pose a serious threat to ventilation in addition to preventing normal laryngoscopy. Soft tissue oedema of the face/upper airway from dental abscess, other infections, drug hypersensitivity, burns and trauma may cause considerable anatomical distortion with life-threatening airway obstruction. Foreign bodies, tumours and scarring after infection, burns and radiotherapy may also cause difficult laryngoscopy. Vocal cord apposition from recurrent laryngeal nerve palsy can hinder

Table 16.6   Anatomical factors associated with difficult laryngoscopy

Short, muscular neck
Protruding incisors (buck teeth)
Long, high arched palate
Receding lower jaw
Poor mobility of mandible
Increased anterior depth of mandible
Increased posterior depth of mandible (reduces jaw opening, requires X-ray)
Decreased atlanto-occipital distance (reduces neck extension, requires X-ray)

Table 16.7   Preoperative assessment of the airway

General appearance of neck, face, maxilla and mandible
Jaw movement
Head extension and neck movement
Teeth and oropharynx
Soft tissue of neck
Recent chest and cervical spine X-rays
Previous anaesthetic records

passage of the tracheal tube through the larynx. Positioning of the tracheal tube in the trachea may be difficult if there is compression or deviation caused by thyroid tumours, haematoma (traumatic, surgical) and thymic or lymph node tumours. Other rare disorders include vascular rings and laryngotracheomalacia. In clinical practice, the cause of difficult laryngoscopy is often multifactorial, for example in patients with morbid obesity, pregnancy and rheumatoid arthritis.

Management

Preoperative assessment. Preoperative examination of the airway (Table 16.7) is essential. Identifying patients with a potentially difficult airway (see Tables 16.5 and 16.6) allows time for planning an appropriate anaesthetic technique. Previous anaesthetic records should always be consulted. However, a past record of normal tracheal intubation is no guarantee for future anaesthesia as airway anatomy may be altered. Pregnancy is a common example. The presence of stridor or a hoarse voice is a warning sign for the anaesthetist. As it is impossible to identify all patients with a difficult airway during preoperative assessment, the anaesthetist must be prepared to manage the unexpected difficult laryngoscopy.

Many additional clinical tests to predict difficult laryngoscopy have been described. None of these tests is totally reliable, but their use may complement routine examination of the airway. The 'Mallampati' test is a widely used and simple classification of the pharyngeal view obtained during maximal mouth opening and tongue protrusion (Fig. 16.5). In practice, this test suggests a higher incidence of difficult laryngoscopy if the posterior pharyngeal wall is not seen. The predictive

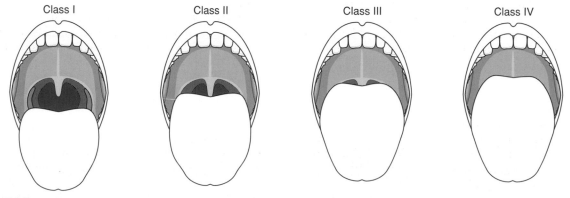

Class I   Class II   Class III   Class IV

Fig 16.5
Classification of the pharyngeal view when performing the Mallampati test. The patient must fully extend the tongue during maximal mouth opening. Class I: pharyngeal pillars, soft palate, uvula visible. Class II: only soft palate, uvula visible. Class III: only soft palate visible. Class IV: soft palate not visible.

value of this test may be strengthened if the thyromental distance (thyroid cartilage prominence to the bony point of the chin during full head extension) is less than 6.5 cm. The Mallampati classification correlates with the view obtained at laryngoscopy (Fig. 16.6). The difficulty associated with a 'grade 3' laryngoscopy may usually be overcome by posterior laryngeal displacement and/or the use of a suitable bougie. A patient whose epiglottis is not visible at laryngoscopy ('grade 4') usually has obvious preoperative anatomical abnormalities. Management of these patients requires the use of special techniques such as fibreoptic laryngoscopy.

Preoperative preparation. Premedication with an antisialagogue reduces airway secretions. This is advantageous before inhalational induction and essential for awake fibreoptic laryngoscopy to maximize the effectiveness of topical local anaesthesia. An anxiolytic may also be given but is contraindicated in patients with airway obstruction. The presence of a trained assistant is essential and the availability of an experienced anaesthetist and a special 'difficult intubation' trolley with a range of equipment such as bougies, laryngoscopes and tracheal tubes is desirable.

Regional anaesthesia. This should be used wherever possible in patients with a difficult airway, although the patient, anaesthetist and equipment must be prepared for general anaesthesia should a complication arise.

General anaesthesia. Unless tracheal intubation is essential for airway protection or to facilitate muscle relaxation and ventilation, the use of an artificial airway such as the laryngeal mask with spontaneous ventilation is a safe technique. If intubation is essential, the appropriate anaesthetic technique depends on the anticipated degree of difficulty, the presence of airway obstruction and the risk of regurgitation and aspiration. There is no place for the use of a long-acting muscle relaxant to facilitate intubation where difficulty is anticipated. Correct positioning of the head and neck is essential and the lungs should be preoxygenated after cannulation of a vein and appropriate

monitoring. The safest anaesthetic technique may usually be chosen from the following clinical examples:

1. *Patients with an increased risk of regurgitation and aspiration (e.g. full stomach, intra-abdominal pathology, pregnancy).* An inhalational induction is inappropriate in these patients. Regional anaesthesia is preferable in the parturient (see Ch. 35). Preoxygenation and a rapid sequence induction with succinylcholine can be used if there is little anticipated difficulty. If intubation is unsuccessful, no further doses of muscle relaxant should be used, the patient allowed to wake and further assistance sought. If there is a high degree of anticipated difficulty, an awake technique is recommended (see below).

2. *Patients with little anticipated difficulty and no airway obstruction (e.g. mild reduction of jaw or neck movement).* After a sleep dose of intravenous induction agent and confirmation of the ability to ventilate the lungs manually by mask, succinylcholine may be given to provide the best conditions for tracheal intubation. If difficulty is encountered, the patient is allowed to wake up and the procedure replanned. Where appropriate, anaesthesia is deepened by spontaneous ventilation using a volatile agent and alternative techniques to facilitate tracheal intubation used (see below).

3. *Patients with severe anticipated difficulty and no airway obstruction (e.g. severe reduction of jaw or neck movement).* Appropriate techniques include inhalational induction with sevoflurane or the use of fibreoptic laryngoscopy either in the awake patient or after inhalational induction. A muscle relaxant must not be used until the ability to ventilate the lungs manually and view the vocal cords is confirmed.

4. *Patients with airway obstruction (e.g. burns, infection, trauma).* An inhalational induction may be used; otherwise an awake technique should be

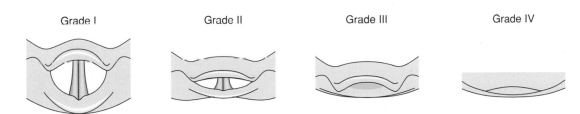

Grade I	Grade II	Grade III	Grade IV

Fig 16.6
Grading of the laryngoscopic view. Grade I: vocal cords visible. Grade II: arytenoid cartilages and posterior part of vocal cords visible. Grade III: epiglottis visible. Grade IV: epiglottis not visible. Note: the pharyngeal view (Fig. 16.5) is a clinical guide to the likely laryngoscopic view.

considered. Muscle relaxants should not be used until tracheal intubation is confirmed.

5. *Extreme clinical situations*. Tracheostomy performed under local anaesthesia may be the safest technique.

Inhalational induction

Premedication with an antisialagogue is desirable. Depth of anaesthesia is increased carefully by spontaneous ventilation of increasing concentrations of a volatile agent in 100% oxygen until laryngoscopy may be performed safely. Halothane may still be the agent of choice for this purpose. If the larynx is viewed easily, intubation may be performed with or without succinylcholine. If the view is limited, the use of a suitable bougie assists passage of the tracheal tube through the larynx. This is confirmed by detecting tracheal rings or resistance when the smaller bronchi are encountered. The tracheal tube is then 'railroaded' over the bougie into the trachea, often made easier by rotating the tracheal tube through 90° in an anticlockwise direction to align the bevel as it passes through the larynx. If this is unsuccessful, anaesthesia may be maintained and the use of fibre-optic laryngoscopy can be considered.

Awake intubation

Fibreoptic laryngoscopy and intubation require special equipment, skill and time. The procedure may be performed by the nasal or oral route after topical anaesthesia is achieved by spraying the nasal and oropharyngeal mucosa and/or gargling viscous preparations. The injection of 3–5 mL of lidocaine 2% through the cricothyroid membrane induces coughing and anaesthetizes the tracheal and laryngeal mucosa. Conventional laryngoscopy may also be performed in awake patients. After cricothyroid injection of lidocaine, laryngoscopy is performed in stages. The oropharynx is anaesthetized progressively with lidocaine spray until the patient tolerates deep insertion of the laryngoscope, enabling the larynx to be viewed.

Complications of tracheal intubation

Complications may be mechanical, respiratory or cardiovascular and may occur early or late.

Early complications

Trauma may occur to lips and teeth or dental crowns. Jaw dislocation and dislocation of arytenoids may be produced. Trauma during intubation may result in damage to larynx and vocal cords. Nasal intubation may produce epistaxis, trauma to the pharyngeal wall or dislodgement of adenoid tissue. Obstruction or kink-ing of the tube may occur and carinal stimulation or bronchial intubation may take place if the tube is too long. Laryngeal trauma may produce postoperative croup, bronchospasm or laryngospasm, especially in children. Mechanical complications may be avoided with a careful technique. Broken teeth must be retrieved and the event documented. Immediate postoperative respiratory complications may be minimized by humidification of inspired gases. Cardiovascular complications of intubation include arrhythmias and hypertension, especially in untreated hypertensive patients.

Late complications

These are more common after long-term intubation. Tracheal stenosis is rare, but damage to tracheal mucosa from a cuffed tube may be related to its design; high-volume, low-pressure cuffs may be preferred for long-term intubation. Trauma to vocal cords may result in ulceration or granulomata which may require surgical removal. Cord trauma may be more common in the presence of an upper respiratory tract infection.

ANAESTHESIA USING NEUROMUSCULAR BLOCKING AGENTS

Indications

As an alternative to deep anaesthesia with spontaneous ventilation and volatile agents leading to multisystem depression, the triad of sleep, suppression of reflexes and muscle relaxation may be provided separately with specific agents. The use of a neuromuscular blocking agent provides muscle relaxation, permitting lighter anaesthesia with less risk of cardiovascular depression. Thus, the technique is appropriate for major abdominal, intraperitoneal, thoracic or intracranial operations, prolonged operations in which spontaneous ventilation would lead to respiratory depression, and operations in a position in which ventilation is impaired mechanically.

Conduct of relaxant anaesthesia

After induction of anaesthesia, relaxation is produced by using either (a) a depolarizing muscle relaxant (succinylcholine) followed, after its action has subsided, by a non-depolarizing relaxant, or (b) in the case of an elective fasting patient with normal gastric emptying and no history of hiatus hernia or regurgitation, an intubating dose of a non-depolarizing muscle relaxant (see Table 6.1) The choice of agent depends upon operative indications or the patient's condition (e.g. vecuronium and rocuronium produce little cardiovascular depression). The airway is then secured with a tracheal tube.

Controlled ventilation is commenced, first manually by compression of the reservoir bag and then by a mechanical ventilator delivering the appropriate tidal and minute volumes (see Appendix B). Anaesthesia and analgesia are provided by nitrous oxide/oxygen or air/oxygen, together with a volatile agent and i.v. analgesic. The inspired and end-expired concentrations of volatile agents should be monitored. Analgesia may also be supplemented by opioid premedication or by use of regional or local anaesthetic techniques.

Assessment of relaxant anaesthesia

Light anaesthesia with preservation of reflexes permits the use of physical signs for the continued assessment of the adequacy of anaesthesia.

Adequacy of anaesthesia. Autonomic reflex activity with lacrimation, sweating, tachycardia, hypertension or reflex movement in response to surgery indicate 'light' anaesthesia and response to surgical stimulation, and warn that the depth of anaesthesia should be increased or further increments of i.v. analgesic given.

Awareness during anaesthesia. The possibility of conscious or unconscious awareness exists in a patient who is under the influence of a neuromuscular blocking drug if nitrous oxide/oxygen anaesthesia is unsupplemented or is supplemented by an opioid with little or no volatile agent. The anaesthetist should ensure that this possibility is avoided by constant observation of the patient for clinical signs of light anaesthesia and by use of small concentrations of a volatile agent. Up to 1% of patients may recall intraoperative events spontaneously if a mixture of nitrous oxide 67% in oxygen is administered, even with an i.v. opioid, and a proportion of these patients experience pain. Awareness during anaesthesia is now a common source of litigation. An appropriate concentration of volatile anaesthetic agent should be used routinely during elective surgery. The BIS monitor has been shown to decrease the incidence of awareness.

Adequacy of muscle relaxation Clinical signs of return of muscle tone include retraction of the wound edges during abdominal operations and abdominal muscle, diaphragmatic or facial movement. An increase in airway pressure (with a time- or volume-cycled ventilator) may indicate a return of muscle tone. Quantitative estimation of neuromuscular status may be obtained with a peripheral nerve stimulator (see Ch. 6). Small increments (e.g. 25–35% of the original dose) of muscle relaxant may be given to maintain relaxation; alternatively, an i.v. infusion may be a more convenient method of administration, but the use of a peripheral nerve stimulator is mandatory with this technique.

Adequacy of ventilation. Clinical signs of inadequate ventilation and an increase in P_aCO_2 include venous dilatation, wound oozing, tachycardia, hypertension and attempts at spontaneous ventilation by the patient.

Measurement of airway pressure and end-expired PCO_2 with a capnograph are mandatory during anaesthesia. Monitoring expired gas volume provides useful information to adjust the degree of mechanical ventilation, and occasionally arterial PCO_2 measurement may be used.

Reversal of relaxation

At the end of surgery, residual neuromuscular block is antagonized and spontaneous ventilation should begin before the tracheal tube is removed and the patient awakened. Residual neuromuscular block is antagonized with neostigmine 2.5–5 mg (0.05–0.08 mg kg^{-1} in children). Atropine 1.2 mg or glycopyrronium 0.5 mg (in adults) counteracts the muscarinic side-effects of the anticholinesterase and may be given before, or with, neostigmine. Care should be exercised in the use of an anticholinergic agent in the presence of existing tachycardia, pyrexia, carbon dioxide retention or ischaemic heart disease.

Resumption of spontaneous ventilation should occur if normocapnic ventilation has been used and assured by monitoring the end-expired PCO_2. Tracheobronchial suction (see below) has the beneficial side-effect of stimulating respiration if used at this stage.

OTHER TECHNIQUES

TOTAL INTRAVENOUS ANAESTHESIA

Total intravenous anaesthesia (TIVA) techniques for induction and maintenance of anaesthesia are widely used. The pharmacokinetic and pharmacodynamic profile of agents such as propofol, alfentanil and remifentanil permit rapid titration of drug dose to the required effect in individual patients. Most general anaesthesia is still maintained using inhalational techniques, partly for historical reasons, but mainly because the non-invasive measurement of end-expired partial pressure of the agent gives a useful estimate of the partial pressure of the agent at the effector site in the central nervous system. However, drug delivery systems have been developed which give improved control of intravenous anaesthesia.

Target controlled infusion (TCI) devices (e.g. Diprifusor) enable the theoretical drug concentration in the plasma of propofol to be controlled continuously and administered without the need for complex calculation by the anaesthetist. The pharmacokinetic data for propofol have been obtained from measurement in patient populations of different age, sex and weight, to create a pharmacokinetic model. The computer program in the TCI device continuously calculates the distribution and elimination of propofol and automatically adjusts the infusion rate to maintain a predicted plasma drug concentration.

Advantages of TIVA include the avoidance of some of the complications of inhalational anaesthesia such as distension of gas-filled spaces, diffusion hypoxia and production of fluoride ions. It may be used safely in patients susceptible to malignant hyperthermia. There is also a reduced incidence of postoperative nausea and vomiting. The main disadvantage is that the actual plasma concentration of the intravenous agent is subject to biological variability; gross variation in the patient's physiological state reduces the model's predictive value. Therefore, the predicted plasma concentration must be adjusted to control the depth of anaesthesia assessed clinically, in the same way as the end-expired partial pressure would be adjusted when using an inhalational technique.

Opioid infusions

Remifentanil, an ultra-short acting opioid may be used as an adjunct to inhalational anaesthesia or in total intravenous anaesthesia, as part of a balanced technique, therefore reducing the amount of anaesthetic agent required and/or avoiding the need for nitrous oxide. Remifentanil is an ester and undergoes rapid hydrolysis by esterases in the plasma. Its short half-life is a useful property in specialities such as neurosurgery where analgesic requirements are high intraoperatively but where rapid recovery is needed postoperatively. Recommended infusion rates for remifentanil are published as part of its data sheet. An initial bolus dose (1 μg kg⁻¹) may be used followed by an infusion which is titrated to patient response. Where postoperative pain is likely to be significant, another type of analgesia must be given before discontinuation of remifentanil as its offset of action is rapid.

HYPOTENSIVE ANAESTHESIA

This may be defined as the deliberate reduction of systemic arterial pressure in order to reduce bleeding and facilitate surgery. Induced hypotension is seldom an absolute requirement but may confer some advantages in some types of surgery (Table 16.8). It should, however, be only part of a strategy which includes maintaining a normal haemostatic response and reducing venous pressure. This may be achieved by wound elevation, e.g. head-up position, avoidance of venous obstruction and maintaining low intrathoracic pressure. It should be remembered that blood flow to the brain is maintained by autoregulatory vasodilatation. In the coronary and cerebral circulations, maximum vasodilatation is reached when the mean arterial pressure decreases to 50–60 mmHg, and further reductions in pressure result in parallel decreases in organ blood flow. Induced hypotension should be avoided in patients with ischaemic heart disease or fixed cardiac output, e.g. in aortic stenosis, and in patients with carotid artery stenosis or a previous cerebrovascular accident.

Induced hypotension may be achieved by a reduction in either systemic vascular resistance or cardiac output (CO). A decrease in systemic vascular resistance may occur as a result of the anaesthetic agent used, e.g. propofol. Drugs may be used that interfere with the sympathetic reflex arc, e.g. adrenergic antagonists such as phentolamine, or which act on the vessel wall, e.g. sodium nitroprusside. A reduction in CO is less desirable as oxygen delivery may be reduced,

Table 16.8   Indications for controlled hypotensive anaesthesia

Expected major blood loss	Pelvic surgery for malignancy
	Head and neck surgery requiring reconstruction
	Large vessel vascular surgery
	Revision of hip prosthesis
	Reconstructive spinal surgery, e.g. scoliosis correction
Complex neurosurgery	Excision of intracranial or spinal meningiomas
	Arteriovenous malformations
	Pituitary surgery
	Craniofacial reconstruction
Microsurgery	Middle ear surgery
	Endoscopic sinus surgery
	Nerve and microvascular surgery
	Plastic free flap grafting
Intraocular surgery	Vitrectomy
	Choroidal surery

but may be achieved using a beta blocker, e.g. esmolol or labetalol.

CONDUCT OF EXTUBATION

This may take place with the patient supine if the anaesthetist is satisfied that airway patency can be maintained by the patient in this position and there is no risk of regurgitation. In patients at risk of regurgitation and potential aspiration, the lateral position is preferred. However, it is safer to use the lateral recovery position after extubation (Fig. 16.7). Return of respiratory reflexes is signified by coughing and resistance to the presence of the tracheal tube.

Tracheobronchial suction via the tracheal tube is carried out using a soft sterile suction catheter with an external diameter less than half the internal diameter of the tube. Preoxygenation precedes suctioning, as the oxygen stores may be depleted by tracheal suction. The catheter is occluded during insertion and suction applied during withdrawal.

Pharyngeal suction is performed best under direct vision, avoiding trauma to the pharyngeal mucosa, uvula or epiglottis. This should take place before antagonism of residual neuromuscular block.

Oxygen 100% replaces the anaesthetic gas mixture before extubation to avoid the potential effects of diffusion hypoxia (p. 30) and to provide a pulmonary reservoir of oxygen in case breath-holding or coughing occurs.

Extubation is performed preferably during inspiration when the larynx dilates; the cuff is deflated and the tube is withdrawn along its curved axis, as careless withdrawal in a straight line may damage laryngeal

structures. Some anaesthetists generate a positive pressure in the trachea during this manoeuvre by 'squeezing the bag' in order to propel secretions into the pharynx.

After extubation, the patient's ability to maintain the airway is ensured, the ability to cough and clear secretions is assessed and an oropharyngeal airway is inserted if required. Administration of oxygen is continued by face mask. Preparations are made for recovery.

COMPLICATIONS OF TRACHEAL EXTUBATION

Laryngeal spasm

This may follow stimulation during extubation. Extubation during deep anaesthesia and subsequent maintenance with a mask may be used. Local anaesthetic spray to the larynx may block the reflex, and pharyngeal suction before extubation removes secretions which may cause stimulation.

Regurgitation/inhalation

Aspiration via the nasogastric tube (if present) should be performed before tracheal extubation to remove gastric liquid. In emergency patients, extubation should be performed with the patient awake so that airway control is continuous. Partial incompetence of laryngeal reflexes may occur in the immediate post-extubation period, especially if local anaesthetic spray has been used. In this event, recovery should take place with the patient in the lateral head-down position, with facilities at hand for suction, oxygenation and reintubation.

Current practice is usually to extubate the trachea as the patient regains response to command as this minimises the risks of both laryngospasm and inhalation of gastric material.

EMERGENCE AND RECOVERY

After completion of surgery, anaesthetic agents are withdrawn and oxygen 100% is delivered. Following removal of the tracheal tube or LMA, the patient's airway is supported until respiratory reflexes are intact. The patient's muscle power and coordination are assessed by testing hand grip, tongue protrusion or a sustained head lift from the pillow in response to command. Adequacy of neuromuscular transmission may also be assessed before the patient is conscious (see

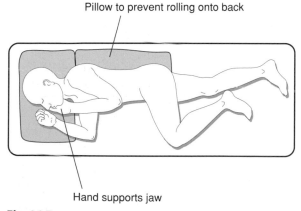

Pillow to prevent rolling onto back

Hand supports jaw

Fig. 16.7
Recovery position.

Ch. 6). Return of adequate muscle power must be ensured before the patient leaves theatre. Full monitoring of the patient should not be discontinued before recovery of consciousness.

The patient is then ready for transfer from the operating table to a bed or trolley. Oxygen is delivered by face mask during transport, and further recovery takes place in a recovery area of theatre or in the recovery ward (see Ch. 24).

The lateral recovery position (see Fig. 16.7) is adopted unless the anaesthetist is satisfied that this is unnecessary. The patient is turned on one side, upper leg flexed and lower extended; the head is on one side and the tongue falls forward under gravity, thus avoiding airway obstruction.

FURTHER READING

Association of Anaesthetists of Great Britain and Ireland 1992 HIV and other blood borne viruses. AAGBI, London

Association of Anaesthetists of Great Britain and Ireland 2003 Suspected anaphylactic reactions associated with anaesthesia. AAGBI, London

Association of Anaesthetists of Great Britain and Ireland 2004 Checking anaesthetic equipment. AAGBI, London

Brimacombe J R, Brain A I J, Berry A M 1996 The laryngeal mask airway instruction manual, 3rd edn. Intavent, Pangbourne

Department of Health 2004 Protecting the breathing circuit in anaesthesia – Report of an expert group on blocked anaesthetic tubing. www.dh.gov.uk

Henderson J J, Popat M T, Latto I P, Pearce A C 2004 Difficult Airway Society guidelines for management of the unanticipated difficult intubation. Anaesthesia 59: 675–694

Latto I P, Vaughan S 1997 Difficulties in tracheal intubation, 2nd edn. WB Saunders, London

Martin J T, Warner M A 1997 Positioning in anesthesia and surgery, 3rd edn. WB Saunders, Philadelphia

Local anaesthetic techniques 17

Local anaesthetic techniques are becoming more popular both for operative anaesthesia and for providing postoperative analgesia. This is a result of advances in drugs, equipment and the anatomical approaches to nerve blocks supported by better techniques of localization, including nerve stimulation and ultrasonic location. In addition, there is a greater appreciation of the need to improve postoperative pain control using techniques that not only reduce pain but have the ability to abolish it and potentially improve outcome. This chapter outlines the basic principles of patient management and the methods used in the performance of a variety of blocks which are commonly undertaken by the trainee anaesthetist.

Regional techniques for obstetrics and dental surgery are described in other chapters.

FEATURES OF LOCAL ANAESTHESIA

Regional anaesthetic techniques may be used alone or in combination with sedation or general anaesthesia depending on individual circumstances. Where there is significant coexisting morbidity, regional anaesthesia may have distinct advantages over general anaesthesia, e.g. in the use of axillary block for hand surgery in a respiratory cripple.

Preservation of consciousness is often considered to be a significant advantage of regional anaesthesia. For example, the patient undergoing caesarean section is able to protect her own airway and experience the birth of the child. The severely arthritic rheumatoid patient can protect the neck and may be positioned safely and comfortably. The head injured, the diabetic or the patient having carotid endarterectomy may have their neurological status continually assessed, whilst in the elderly, acute cognitive impairment may be limited by reducing or avoiding psychoactive drugs and maintaining contact with surroundings. However, some patients may be unhappy at the prospect of

being awake, and in this situation the combination of a regional block with target-controlled intravenous sedation or general anaesthesia may be valuable. Similarly, this combination works well for prolonged surgery and when uncomfortable positioning exists or operation at several sites is necessary.

Of major benefit to all patients is the quality of early postoperative analgesia, which may be prolonged by using catheter techniques either centrally or peripherally, although this may carry some disadvantages, such as delaying the diagnosis of a compartment syndrome or evaluating neurological function. Some patients may be distressed by the accompanying numbness and motor block, but correct preoperative explanation should minimize this concern; in addition, it is important that nursing staff and patient are aware of the risk of trauma to the blocked segments. Simple techniques such as supporting the arm in a sling after brachial plexus block may help prevent injury and encourage earlier mobilization.

Other features of regional anaesthesia include simplicity of administration, sympathetic blockade, attenuation of the stress response, minimal respiratory impairment, less nausea and vomiting, earlier feeding and more rapid mobilization and discharge. There are now several studies suggesting that the net effect of these features may be a reduction in the incidence of major postoperative complications, particularly respiratory, but claims of other pathophysiological benefits are more controversial.

COMPLICATIONS OF LOCAL ANAESTHESIA

The incidence of complications may be minimized by ensuring adequate supervision and training in local anaesthetic techniques, and by exercising care in the performance of each block. Many anaesthetists recommend performing all blocks, in the awake or lightly sedated patient, except in children. This encourages careful practice, provides the trainee with valuable information on block onset and efficacy, and also alerts the anaesthetist to early complications such as inadvertent intravenous injection or intraneural injection. Sufficient expertise and equipment must always be available to deal with potential complications. Complications common to many techniques are discussed in this section; more specific problems are considered later.

LOCAL ANAESTHETIC TOXICITY

This usually results from accidental intravascular injection, an excessive dose of local anaesthetic or faulty technique, particularly during performance of Bier's block.

Features and treatment

These are described in Chapter 4.

Prevention

Correct technique, careful and repeated aspiration and the use of a test dose are important, but the main safety measure is *slow injection* of the local anaesthetic. This prevents rapid production of very high plasma concentrations even if the injection is intravascular. By this means, toxicity may be diagnosed early, the injection discontinued and a major reaction avoided. Fast injection of local anaesthetic is not necessary for the performance of any block.

Test dose

This may be used before administration of the main dose of local anaesthetic drug. It is indicated particularly for epidural block, where it should be capable of demonstrating inadvertent intravenous (i.v.) or subarachnoid injection. A test dose of 4 mL of 2% plain lidocaine is sufficient to cause mild symptoms in most patients after accidental i.v. injection, and any features of local anaesthetic blockade 2 min after injection are good evidence of accidental subarachnoid block. No test dose is infallible; slow administration of the main dose is the most important factor in avoiding local anaesthetic toxicity.

HYPOTENSION

There are several possible mechanisms by which a local anaesthetic technique may cause hypotension. The anaesthetist must always remember that surgical factors may be responsible.

Sympathetic blockade

A limited sympathetic block may be produced by peripheral nerve anaesthesia, but only central blocks are likely to produce hypotension by this mechanism.

Total spinal blockade

This is discussed on page 331. It occurs occasionally during subarachnoid block if excessive spread of local anaesthetic solution occurs, and is a recognized complication of epidural block if the dura has been penetrated. Apnoea may occur if local anaesthetic solution reaches the cerebrospinal fluid (CSF) during interscalene brachial plexus block, or the ventricular system during retrobulbar nerve block.

Vasovagal attack

This is likely to occur particularly in an anxious patient with a rapidly ascending spinal block. Pallor, nausea and bradycardia are associated with the hypotension. The supine position is no guarantee against this complication. Rapid resolution results from placing the patient head-down and administration of i.v. ephedrine 5–6 mg or atropine 0.3–0.6 mg. Cautious i.v. sedation (e.g. midazolam 1–2 mg) may be helpful.

Anaphylactoid reaction

This is very rare with amide local anaesthetics.

Local anaesthetic toxicity

This is considered above and in Chapter 4.

MOTOR BLOCKADE

To avoid unnecessary distress, patients must be warned of the possibility of limb weakness or paralysis which may persist for some time after operation.

PNEUMOTHORAX

This is a potential hazard of supraclavicular brachial plexus, intercostal and paravertebral blocks. The possibility of its occurrence is an absolute contraindication to the use of these techniques in outpatients and also to the performance of these blocks bilaterally.

URINARY RETENTION

This may follow the use of central blocks. It is important to avoid overhydration, as bladder distension may require catheterization. The use of large volumes of crystalloid in the treatment of hypotension often has a very transient effect and predisposes patients to urinary retention, or worse, pulmonary oedema, when the block regresses.

NEUROLOGICAL COMPLICATIONS

Carefully performed blocks rarely result in neurological complications.

Neuritis with persisting sensory changes and/or weakness may result from trauma to the nerve, intraneural injection or bacterial, chemical or particulate contamination of the injected solution. Injection of the incorrect solution has caused some of the most severe neurological complications. To avoid this serious error, all drugs must be checked personally by the anaesthetist immediately before injection.

Anterior spinal artery syndrome may follow an episode of prolonged, severe hypotension and results in painless permanent paraplegia. *Adhesive arachnoiditis* has been described after subarachnoid and epidural blockade and may lead to permanent pain, weakness and bladder or bowel dysfunction. It is suspected that this complication results from injection of the incorrect solution. *Haematoma* or *abscess* formation in the spinal canal after subarachnoid or epidural anaesthesia results in weakness and sensory loss below the level of spinal cord compression. It is associated with intense back pain and is a neurosurgical emergency which demands immediate decompression to avoid permanent disability.

EQUIPMENT PROBLEMS

Needles are most likely to break at the junction with the hub and therefore should never be inserted fully. Catheters may also break, but exploratory surgery to find small pieces of catheter is inappropriate, as complications are very unlikely.

GENERAL MANAGEMENT

PATIENT ASSESSMENT AND SELECTION

Careful preoperative evaluation is as important before a local anaesthetic as it is before general anaesthesia, and the same principles of preoperative management apply. Therapy to improve the patient's condition before surgery should be commenced if appropriate. It is inappropriate to proceed with surgery under local anaesthesia for the sake of convenience in the poorly prepared patient. A decision should be made on the need for immediate surgical intervention before the anaesthetic technique is chosen.

The preoperative visit should be used to establish rapport with the patient. A clear description of the proposed anaesthetic should be given in simple terms, but there is rarely a need for excessive detail. Patients require an explanation of the reasons for selecting a regional technique before accepting it, but there should be no attempt at coercion.

Potential problems related to the intended block should be sought. Anatomical deformities may render some blocks impractical. A history of allergy to amide local anaesthetics is rare, but is an absolute contraindication, as is infection at the site of needle insertion. For most blocks, anticoagulant therapy and bleeding diatheses are also absolute contraindications, and the use of major blocks in patients with distant infection or receiving low-dose subcutaneous (s.c.) heparin, especially low molecular weight heparin, requires careful consideration. Sympathetic blockade with consequent vasodilatation may lead to profound hypotension in patients with significant aortic or mitral stenosis because of the relatively fixed cardiac output. Hypovolaemia must be corrected before contemplating subarachnoid or epidural anaesthesia.

There is no evidence that neuromuscular disorders or multiple sclerosis are adversely affected by local anaesthetic techniques, but most anaesthetists use regional anaesthesia in such patients only if there are obvious benefits to be gained; any perioperative deterioration in the neurological condition is often associated by the patient with the local anaesthetic procedure. Raised intracranial pressure is a contraindication to central blockade but peripheral techniques may be considered.

SELECTION OF TECHNIQUE

Local anaesthetic drugs may be administered by:

- single dose
- intermittent bolus:
  - repeated injections
  - indwelling catheter for repeat administration
- continuous infusion (with optional bolus doses) via a catheter.

If regional anaesthesia has been selected primarily to provide analgesia during and after surgery under general anaesthesia, a distal technique is appropriate and is usually associated with the fewest complications.

Because a local anaesthetic technique renders only part of the body insensible, it is essential that the method employed is tailored to, and sufficient for, the planned surgery. Account must be taken of the duration of surgery, its site (which may be multiple, e.g. the need to obtain bone grafting material from the iliac crest), and the likelihood of a change of procedure in mid-operation. The problem of multiple sites of surgery may be met by one block which covers both sites, or by more than one regional procedure. The duration of anaesthesia may be tailored to the anticipated duration of surgery by selection of an appropriate local anaesthetic agent, or may require the use of a technique which allows further administration of drug.

PREMEDICATION

Manipulation of fractures and other short emergency procedures are often carried out using a local anaesthetic technique in the unpremedicated patient, as rapid recovery is desirable. However, premedication is helpful before inpatient elective or emergency surgery. An oral benzodiazepine allays anxiety, but an opioid (e.g. morphine) alleviates the discomfort of prolonged immobility which may be required during a long procedure. Preoperative analgesia may be required before definitive fixation. A nerve block may be useful in these circumstances, e.g. femoral block to alleviate the pain from a fractured femur, but often the administration of opioids, preferably i.v. in a controlled manner, is more appropriate at this time.

Patients should be fasted for all but the most minor peripheral nerve blocks.

TIMING

It is essential that sufficient time is allowed to perform the block without undue haste on the part of the anaesthetist. This is largely a matter of organization, and the experienced practitioner seldom causes delay to an operating list. Any preoperative delay is compensated for by the ability to return the patient to bed immediately after completion of surgery.

RESUSCITATION EQUIPMENT

A full range of resuscitation equipment must be in working order and immediately available. This includes:

- an anaesthetic breathing system through which oxygen may be administered under pressure via a face mask or tracheal tube
- a laryngoscope with two sizes of blade, a range of tracheal tubes and an introducer
- a table which may be rapidly tilted head-down
- suction apparatus

- intravenous cannulae and fluids
- thiopental to control convulsions
- drugs to treat hypotension, especially atropine, ephedrine and either metaraminol or phenylephrine.

A cannula must be inserted intravenously before any local anaesthetic block is performed in case emergency therapy is required.

REGIONAL BLOCK EQUIPMENT

Regional anaesthesia may be used with basic equipment, but some special items increase the success rate and reduce the risk of complications.

Needles

The use of very fine spinal needles (26G) has significantly reduced the incidence of post-spinal headache as has the use of pencil-point 25G Whitacre and 24G Sprotte needles (Fig. 17.1A). The 27G Whitacre needles appear to be associated with the lowest incidence of post-spinal headache but confident and successful use of these needles requires greater expertise than is needed for the use of larger needles. For peripheral blocks, short-bevelled needles allow greater tactile appreciation of fascial planes and appear to reduce the likelihood of nerve damage. A variety of insulated needles are available for plexus and peripheral nerve blockade using a nerve stimulator (Fig. 17.1B).

Immobile needle technique

For plexus and major nerve blocks, local anaesthetic drug is drawn into labelled syringes and connected to the block needle by a short length of tubing (Fig. 17.2). This allows the anaesthetist to hold the needle steady while aspiration tests are performed and syringes changed. The system must be primed to avoid air embolism.

Catheters

Continuous administration of local anaesthetic drugs has been made possible by the development of high-quality catheters, which are introduced through a needle (occasionally over needle: Fig 17.1A) and may be left in position for hours or even days. Careful fixation is essential to maintain the position of the catheter in the postoperative period. Catheters, in particular spinal catheters, should be labelled clearly to prevent accidental overdosage.

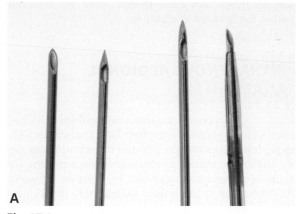

Fig. 17.1
A. Left to right: Quincke, Whitacre, Sprotte and Spinocath needles.

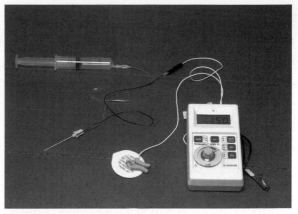

Fig. 17.2
Nerve stimulator and insulated stimulating needle attached to syringe.

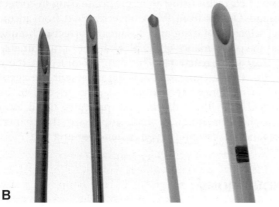

Fig. 17.1
B. Left to right: standard-bevelled, short-bevelled, insulated short-bevelled and insulated Tuohy needles.

Nerve stimulators

Many anaesthetists still prefer to elicit paraesthesiae when performing a major nerve block, but most now tend to use the nerve stimulator (Fig. 17.2) which is especially useful for teaching and improving efficacy. It is important to explain to the patient the sensation elicited by stimulation. It causes little discomfort unless the contracting muscle crosses a fracture site, when duration of stimulation should be kept to the absolute minimum necessary to confirm needle position. The incidence of paraesthesia with short-bevelled insulated needles is very low because of their ability to stimulate without direct neural contact. They also tend to displace nerves rather than penetrate them.

Stimulators that deliver a constant current and give a digital display of the current used are readily available. One lead is attached to an electrocardiogram (ECG) electrode on the patient's skin, and the other to the needle.

After skin puncture, the stimulator is set to a frequency of 1 Hz and an initial current of 2 mA. Most stimulators have a visual display to confirm a complete circuit when needle touches patient. If this fails, connections should be checked or the ECG electrode changed if dry. Failure to confirm a complete circuit could result in unwanted paraesthesiae or potential nerve injury.

As the nerve is approached, motor fibre stimulation causes muscle contraction in the appropriate distribution. The current is reduced until maximal contraction is still present at a current of, optimally, around 0.5 mA. At this point, a gentle aspiration test is performed and 2 mL of local anaesthetic solution injected. Movement should cease immediately. If it does not, and an insulated needle is being used, the tip may be beyond the nerve or intravascular; gentle aspiration should be repeated, the needle withdrawn slightly and the procedure repeated. Severe pain on injection suggests intraneural injection, in which case the needle should be repositioned. When the correct position has been found, the remainder of the anaesthetic solution should be injected slowly with repeated aspiration tests. Performance of the block in the awake patient allows better assessment of early intravascular toxicity and intraneural injection in addition to encouraging gentle and careful technique.

ASEPSIS

A 'no-touch' technique is essential. Drapes should be used for all major blocks and gloves and gown should be worn by the beginner. Gown, gloves, hat and mask are recommended for all central blocks even with a 'no-touch' technique, especially when a catheter is inserted. Taking precautions seriously fosters good practice.

MONITORING

It is essential that the anaesthetist remains with the patient. Monitoring equipment should be appropriate to the anaesthetic technique and surgical procedure.

SUPPLEMENTARY TECHNIQUES

A local anaesthetic may be the only drug administered to the patient, or it may form part of a balanced anaesthetic technique. During surgery, patients may be awake, or sedated by i.v. or inhalational means. Propofol, midazolam or low concentrations of nitrous oxide are commonly used. General anaesthesia may be used as a planned part of the procedure. A combination of regional and general anaesthesia may be useful to obtain advantages from both, particularly for prolonged procedures or where positioning is difficult because of additional trauma or significant arthritis.

When a surgical tourniquet is used, the chosen block must extend to the tourniquet site unless the procedure is brief. Discomfort from prolonged immobility on a hard table is relieved by the administration of an opioid either as a premedicant or i.v. during surgery; this type of discomfort is not relieved by sedative drugs, which often result in the patient becoming agitated, confused and uncooperative. Remifentanil infusion is being used increasingly for this purpose although this technique is not for the beginner and requires careful respiratory monitoring, preferably continuously by nasal capnography.

AFTER-CARE

Clear instructions should be given to the nurses caring for the patient.

After day-case surgery, the patient must be in a safe condition at the time of discharge. Plexus blockade with a long-acting agent is inappropriate because of the risk of the patient injuring the anaesthetized limb, but is suitable for postoperative pain relief in supervised inpatients following major surgery, particularly when the limb is immobilized or conversely when continuous passive mobilization is required. Patients who have received central blockade should have routine nursing observations at least until the block has worn off.

Continuous infusion techniques are suitable for use only by experienced anaesthetists. When used correctly, administration by infusion is safer than repeated bolus injection of drug, but regular observations are essential and the nursing staff must have an adequate level of knowledge to appreciate possible complications. An anaesthetist must be available within the hospital at all times.

INTRAVENOUS REGIONAL ANAESTHESIA

Ideally, intravenous regional anaesthesia (IVRA) (Bier's block) should be the first local anaesthetic technique learnt by a trainee, because its technical simplicity allows the trainee to concentrate on acquiring the skills of patient management. In practice, however, this technique is being used increasingly by accident and emergency staff and less frequently by anaesthetists, who often prefer to block the brachial plexus. Bier's block is simple, safe and effective when performed correctly using an appropriate drug in correct dosage. Deaths from IVRA have resulted from incorrect selection of drug and dosage, incorrect technique and the performance of the block by personnel unable to treat toxic reactions. The drug involved in these deaths, bupivacaine, was not the most suitable agent and is no longer recommended. The lessons to be learned from these deaths are applicable to all local anaesthetic techniques, and emphasize that expert guidance is essential even when learning the most basic blocks.

INDICATIONS

Intravenous regional anaesthesia is suitable for short procedures when postoperative pain is not marked, e.g. manipulation of Colles' fracture or carpal tunnel decompression. Recovery is rapid, and the technique is appropriate for outpatient surgery. Premedication may delay patient discharge and a reassuring visit preoperatively from the anaesthetist is usually sufficient in these circumstances.

METHOD

Intravenous regional anaesthesia involves isolating an exsanguinated limb from the general circulation by means of an arterial tourniquet and then injecting local anaesthetic solution intravenously. Analgesia and weakness occur rapidly and result predominantly from local anaesthetic action on peripheral nerve endings.

An orthopaedic tourniquet of the correct size is applied over padding on the upper arm. All connections must lock, and the pressure gauge should be calibrated regularly. A cannula is inserted intravenously in the contralateral arm in case administration of emergency drugs is required. An indwelling cannula is inserted into a vein of the limb to be anaesthetized. A vein on the dorsum of the hand is preferred; injection into proximal veins reduces the quality of the block and increases the risk of toxicity. Exsanguination by means of an Esmarch bandage improves the quality of the block and increases the safety of the technique by reducing the venous pressure developed during injection. In patients with a painful lesion (e.g. Colles' fracture), elevation combined with brachial artery compression is adequate. The tourniquet should be inflated to a pressure 100 mmHg above systolic arterial pressure.

In an adult, 40 mL of prilocaine 0.5% is injected over 2 min with careful observation that the tourniquet remains inflated. Analgesia is complete within 10 min, but it is important to inform the patient that the feeling of touch is often retained at this time. The anaesthetist must be ready to deal with toxicity or tourniquet pain throughout the surgical procedure. The tourniquet should not be released until at least 20 min after injection, even if surgery is completed. This delay allows for diffusion of drug into the tissues so that plasma concentrations do not reach toxic levels after release of the tourniquet. The technique of repeated reinflation and deflation of the cuff during release has little effect on plasma concentrations and is not necessary.

Reinstitution of the block within 30 min of tourniquet release is possible using 50% of the initial dose, because some drug is retained within the limb. Bilateral blocks may be performed without exceeding the maximum recommended doses, but it is preferable to do this consecutively rather than concurrently.

Tourniquet pain

This may be troublesome if the cuff remains inflated for longer than 30–40 min. It is sometimes alleviated by inflating a separate tourniquet below the first on an area already rendered analgesic by the block; the first cuff is then deflated. Failing this, general anaesthesia is preferable to administration of large and often ineffective doses of opioids and sedatives.

CHOICE OF DRUG

The agent of choice for this procedure is prilocaine 0.5% plain. It has an impressive safety record with no major reactions reported after its use, although minor side-effects such as transient light-headedness after release of the tourniquet are not uncommon. The drug has distinct pharmacokinetic advantages in IVRA (see Ch. 4). Methaemoglobinaemia does not result from the doses used for IVRA.

LOWER LIMB

Intravenous regional anaesthesia of the foot may be produced using the same dose of prilocaine and a calf tourniquet positioned carefully at least 10 cm below the tibial tuberosity to avoid compression of the common peroneal nerve on the fibular neck.

CENTRAL NERVE BLOCKS

Spinal anaesthesia is a term that may be used to denote all forms of central blockade, although it usually refers to intrathecal administration of local anaesthetic. The term subarachnoid block (SAB) avoids ambiguity. The technique of SAB is basically that of lumbar puncture, but knowledge of factors which affect the extent and duration of anaesthesia, and experience in patient management are essential. Epidural nerve block may be performed in the sacral (caudal block), lumbar, thoracic or cervical regions, although lumbar block is used most commonly. Local anaesthetic solution is injected through a needle after the tip has been introduced into the epidural space, or may be injected through a catheter placed in the space.

PHYSIOLOGICAL EFFECTS OF SUBARACHNOID BLOCK

Differential nerve blockade

Local anaesthetic solution injected into the CSF spreads away from the site of injection and the concentration of the solution decreases as mixing occurs. A differential blockade of fibres occurs because small fibres are blocked by weaker concentrations of local anaesthetic solution. Sympathetic fibres are blocked to a level approximately two segments higher than the upper segmental level of sensory blockade. Motor blockade may be several segments caudal to the upper level of sensory block. A sensory level to T3 with SAB may be associated with total blockade of the T1–L2 sympathetic outflow.

Respiratory system

Low SAB has no effect on the respiratory system and the technique is an important part of the anaesthetist's armamentarium for patients with severe respiratory disease.

Motor blockade extending to the roots of the phrenic nerves (C3–5) causes apnoea.

Blocks which reach the thoracic level cause loss of intercostal muscle activity. This has little effect on tidal volume (because of diaphragmatic compensation), but there is a marked decrease in vital capacity resulting from a significant decrease in expiratory reserve volume. The patient may experience dyspnoea, and difficulty in taking a maximal inspiration or in coughing effectively. A thoracic block may lead to a reduction in cardiac output and pulmonary artery pressure and increased ventilation/perfusion imbalance, resulting in a decrease in arterial oxygen tension ($P_a o_2$). Awake patients with a high spinal block should always be given oxygen-enriched air to breathe.

Cardiovascular system

The cardiovascular effects are proportional to the height of the block and result from denervation of the sympathetic outflow tracts (T1–L2). This produces dilatation of resistance and capacitance vessels and results in hypotension. In awake patients, vasoconstriction above the height of the block may compensate almost completely for these changes, thereby maintaining arterial pressure, but general anaesthetic agents may reduce this compensatory response, with consequent profound hypotension.

Hypotension is augmented by:

- the use of head-up posture
- any degree of hypovolaemia – pre-existing or induced by surgery
- administration of sedatives, opioids or especially induction agents which should be given in greatly reduced dosage.

Prevention of hypotension

Both the incidence and the degree of hypotension are reduced by limiting the height of the block and, in particular, by keeping it below the sympathetic supply to the heart (T1–5).

It is common practice to attempt to minimize hypotension during SAB or epidural anaesthesia by preloading the patient with 500–1000 mL of crystalloid solution i.v. before or during the performance of the block. These volumes are usually ineffective even in the short term, may risk causing pulmonary oedema in susceptible individuals either during the procedure or when the block wears off, and may lead to postoperative urinary retention. Appropriate fluid should be given to replace blood and fluid losses and prevent dehydration.

Bradycardia may occur because of:

- neurogenic factors, particularly in awake patients, i.e. vasovagal syndrome
- block of the cardiac sympathetic fibres (T1–4).

Careful patient positioning, maintenance of a normal circulating volume and the use of pharmacological agents (see later), if required, should minimize the incidence of hypotension.

SAB has no direct effect on the liver or kidneys, but reductions in hepatic and renal blood flow occur in the presence of hypotension associated with high spinal blocks.

Gastrointestinal system

The vagus nerve supplies parasympathetic fibres to the whole of the gut as far as the transverse colon. Spinal blockade causes sympathetic denervation (proportional to height of block), and unopposed parasympathetic action leads to a constricted gut with increased peristaltic activity. This is regarded by some as advantageous for surgery.

Nausea, retching or vomiting may occur in the awake patient and are often the first symptoms of impending or established hypotension. If nausea or retching occurs, the anaesthetist must measure arterial pressure and heart rate immediately and take appropriate measures.

PHYSIOLOGICAL EFFECTS OF EPIDURAL BLOCK

The physiological effects of epidural blockade are similar to those following SAB, but may develop more slowly. Additional effects may occur from the much larger volumes of anaesthetic solutions used, as there may be appreciable systemic absorption of local anaesthetic and adrenaline if an adrenaline-containing solution is used.

INDICATIONS FOR SUBARACHNOID BLOCK

Blockade is produced more consistently and with a lower dose of drug by the subarachnoid route than by epidural injection. Duration of analgesia is usually limited to 2–4 h depending on surgical site and may be prolonged by catheter techniques, which appear to be increasing again in popularity. Catheter techniques may also be used to establish block height more carefully in more compromised patients. SAB is most suited to surgery below the umbilicus and in this situation the patient may remain awake. Surgery above the umbilicus using SAB is less appropriate and would necessitate a general anaesthetic in addition, in order to abolish unpleasant sensations from visceral manipulation resulting from afferent impulses transmitted by the vagus nerves.

Types of surgery

Urology

Subarachnoid block is very appropriate for urological procedures such as transurethral prostatectomy, but it should be remembered that a block to T10 is required for surgery involving bladder distension. Perineal and penile operations may also be carried out using peripheral blockade or caudal anaesthesia.

Gynaecology

Minor procedures such as dilatation and curettage may be performed reliably with a block to T10. Pelvic floor surgery and vaginal hysterectomy may also be carried out readily with an SAB extending to T6, but for procedures requiring laparoscopic assistance, general anaesthesia is usually necessary.

Obstetrics

The introduction of the pencil point spinal needle with a reduction in the incidence of post-lumbar-puncture headache has led to an increased use of SAB in obstetric practice to the extent that this is considered the technique of choice for the majority of elective caesarean sections and a large proportion of emergency ones. SAB may also be used for evacuation of retained products, avoiding the risks of general anaesthesia. Further details of obstetric practice are discussed in Chapter 35.

Any surgical procedure on the lower limbs or perineum

For patients with medical problems, low SAB may be the anaesthetic technique of choice:

Metabolic disease. Diabetes mellitus.

Respiratory disease. Low SAB has no effect on ventilation and obviates the requirement for anaesthetic drugs with depressant properties. There is some evidence that SAB may reduce the incidence of chest infection and atelectasis.

Cardiovascular disease. Low SAB may be valuable in patients with ischaemic heart disease or congestive cardiac failure, in whom a small reduction in preload and afterload may be beneficial. SAB is effective in preventing cardiovascular responses to surgery (e.g. hypertension, tachycardia) which are undesirable, particularly in patients with ischaemic heart disease.

INDICATIONS FOR EPIDURAL BLOCKADE

The indications for epidural anaesthesia are widespread, because it is an extremely versatile technique which may be tailored to suit a variety of situations. The duration of analgesia may be prolonged as necessary by means of an indwelling catheter and the use of intermittent top-ups or a continuous infusion. Bupivacaine, levobupivacaine or ropivacaine are the drugs of choice when one of these continuous techniques is used. Their pharmacokinetic properties are such that, with the doses necessary to maintain adequate blockade, systemic accumulation of drug is slow and the risk of toxicity is small. Ropivacaine and levobupivacaine are considered to be safer alternatives to racemic bupivacaine, particularly with regard to cardiotoxicity following inadvertent intravenous administration. Either local anaesthetic drugs or opioids, or frequently a combination of both, may be used epidurally. Opioids are most suited to provision of postoperative analgesia and are inadequate for surgery in most circumstances. Almost all opioids have been tried by the epidural route with success but diamorphine or fentanyl are perhaps the most common additives in the UK. Clonidine combined with local anaesthetic has also been used successfully.

CONTRAINDICATIONS TO SUBARACHNOID BLOCK AND EPIDURAL ANAESTHESIA

Most contraindications are relative, but are best regarded by the trainee as absolute:

- bleeding diathesis
- hypovolaemia
- sepsis – local or systemic
- severe stenotic valvular heart disease – the patient may be unable to compensate for vasodilatation because of a fixed cardiac output
- pre-eclamptic toxaemia – epidural block has been used with great benefit in this condition but a platelet count of less than 100×10^9 L^{-1} usually precludes epidural or subarachnoid anaesthesia
- acute neurological diseases/raised intracranial pressure
- lack of patient consent.

PERFORMANCE OF SUBARACHNOID BLOCK

Intravenous access

Intravenous access must be secured before lumbar puncture is performed.

Positioning the patient

Lumbar puncture for SAB may be performed with the patient sitting or in the lateral decubitus position (Table 17.1) (Fig. 17.3). If it is anticipated that lumbar

Table 17.1 Techniques of subarachnoid block

Type of block	Upper level of analgesia	Position during lumbar puncture	Volume of solution
Saddle block	S1	Sitting 5 min	1 mL hyperbaric solution
Low thoracic	T10–12	Sitting/lateral decubitus	3–4 mL*
Mid thoracic	T4–6	Lateral decubitus/ sitting (immediately supine)	2–3 mL hyperbaric solution
Unilateral	A unilateral block, or at least a differential block between limbs, may be achieved by the slow injection of small volumes (1–1.5 mL) of hyperbaric solution in the lateral position. This position then has to be maintained for at least 15 min to minimize spread. On return to the supine position there may still be some contralateral spread and the necessity for smaller volumes and dosage may increase block failure rate.		

*Plain bupivacaine is slightly hypobaric at body temperature and although it usually results in a low thoracic block, it may occasionally be unpredictable.

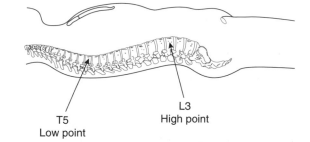

A

T5
Low point

L3
High point

Female

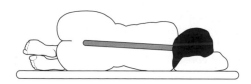

Male

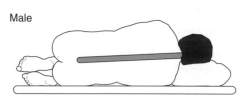

B

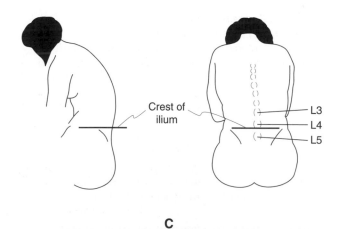

Crest of ilium

L3
L4
L5

C

Fig. 17.3
Spinal curvature. **(A)** Supine position. **(B)** Lateral position. **(C)** Sitting position.

puncture may be difficult, the midline is usually more discernible with the patient in the sitting position, but the risk of hypotension in the sedated patient or following development of the block is increased. The technique of lumbar puncture for the patient in the lateral position is described in the next section.

Technique of lumbar puncture

For the right-handed anaesthetist, the patient is positioned on the operating table in the left lateral position. The patient's back should lie along the edge of the table and must be vertical. A curled position opens the spaces between the lumbar spinous processes. An assistant stands in front of the patient to assist with positioning and to reassure the patient. The anaesthetist must inform the patient before performing each part of the procedure.

A line between the iliac crests lies on the fourth lumbar spinous process; lumbar puncture should be performed at the L3/4 or L4/5 space. A full sterile

technique (with gown, gloves and surgical drapes) is adopted. All drugs should be drawn into syringes directly from sterile ampoules using a filter needle to prevent the injection of glass particles into the subarachnoid space. A selection of spinal needles (22–27 gauge) should be available.

The skin and subcutaneous tissues are infiltrated with local anaesthetic using a small needle. The spinal needle is inserted in the midline, midway between two spinous processes. In the well-positioned patient, the needle is directed at right angles to the skin. Passage through the interspinous ligament and ligamentum flavum into the spinal canal is appreciated easily with a 22-gauge needle (Fig. 17.4A). With some practice, these structures are usually discernible with a 26-gauge needle or 25G pencil-point needle, which all anaesthetists should aspire to use. The use of an introducer (19-gauge needle) is advisable to brace the smaller needles, which are very flexible. When the needle tip has entered the spinal canal, the stilette is withdrawn from the needle and the hub is observed

A

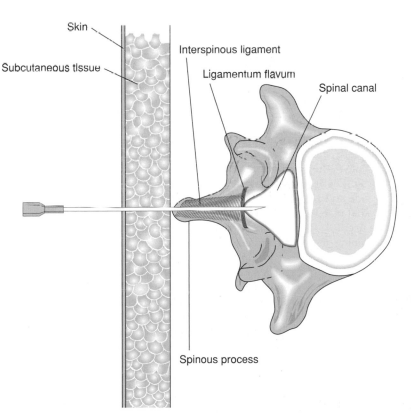

Skin

Subcutaneous tissue

Interspinous ligament

Ligamentum flavum

Spinal canal

Spinous process

Fig. 17.4
Midline approach for subarachnoid block. **(A)** Correctly angled.

Continued

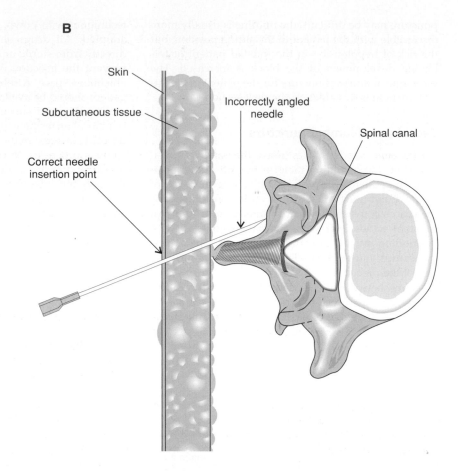

B

Skin

Subcutaneous tissue

Incorrectly angled
needle

Spinal canal

Correct needle
insertion point

Fig. 17.4—Contd
(B) Incorrectly angled.

for flow of CSF; a needle with a transparent hub makes this easier. A gentle aspiration test should be performed if a free flow of CSF is not observed.

The three most common reasons for difficulty are poor patient position, failure to insert the needle in the midline and directing the needle laterally (Fig. 17.4B). This last fault is seen most easily from one side and is usually apparent to onlookers, but not to the anaesthetist, who looks only along the line of the needle.

When CSF is obtained, the syringe containing the local anaesthetic solution should be attached firmly to the needle. Gentle aspiration confirms the needle position and the solution is injected at a rate of 1 mL every 5–10 s. Aspiration after injection confirms that the needle tip has remained in the correct place. Needle and introducer are withdrawn and the patient placed supine.

Factors affecting spread

The most important factor which affects the height of block in SAB (Table 17.2) is the baricity of the solution, which may be made hyperbaric (i.e. denser than CSF)

by the addition of glucose. The specific gravity (SG) of CSF is 1.004. The addition of glucose 5% or 6% to a local anaesthetic produces a solution with SG of 1.024 or greater. A patient who assumes the sitting position for 5 min after injection of 1 mL of hyperbaric solution develops a saddle block which affects the perineum only. Conversely, a patient placed supine immediately after injection of 2-3 mL develops a block to the mid-thoracic region. Slightly larger volumes are advisable to ensure spread above the lumbar curvature (see Fig. 17.3).

Within the range normally used for SAB (2–4 mL), the volume of solution has only a minor effect on spread. Obesity, pregnancy and a high site of injection are minor factors which increase the height of the block; lower volumes may be desirable in these situations. Barbotage and rapid injection may produce high blocks, but increase the unpredictability of spread.

Factors affecting duration

The duration of anaesthesia depends on the drug used and the dose of drug injected. Vasoconstrictors added

Table 17.2   Factors influencing spread of hyperbaric spinal solutions

Factor	Effect
Position of patient	Sitting position produces perineal block only, provided that small volumes are used
Spinal curvature	With standard volumes (2–3 mL) the block often spreads to T4. With small volumes (1 mL) the block may affect only the perineum even when the patient is placed supine immediately
Dose of drug	Within the range of volumes usually employed (2–4 mL), increasing the dose of drug increases the duration of anaesthesia rather than the height of the block
Interspace	Minor factor affecting height of block
Obesity	Minor factor affecting height of block. Obese patients tend to develop higher blocks
Speed of injection	Rapid injection makes the height of block more variable
Barbotage	No longer used. Makes the height of block more variable

to the local anaesthetic solution significantly increase the duration of action of tetracaine, which is widely used in the USA, but this is not so for other agents.

Agents

Only three agents are readily available for SAB in the UK: plain bupivacaine, heavy bupivacaine and plain levobupivacaine. Ropivacaine is currently undergoing evaluation and seems to have a shorter duration of action compared with both racemic bupivacaine and levobupivacaine. Plain bupivacaine 0.5% is slightly hypobaric at body temperature and spread tends to be more unpredictable, although it does tend to produce a lower maximal block height when used in the lateral position, making it a popular choice for lower limb orthopaedic and vascular surgery. It is used in volumes of 3–4 mL and lasts 2–3 h. Hyperbaric bupivacaine 0.5% is more predictable for abdominal procedures and consistently produces a block to the umbilicus (and usually to T5) in supine patients. As with all hyperbaric solutions, hypotension is encountered more frequently because of higher levels of sympathetic blockade. Volumes of 2–3 mL are used and a duration of 2–3 h is usually assured.

Complications

Acute

Hypotension. Significant hypotension should be anticipated with SAB. Changes in position, e.g. turning the patient from the supine to the prone position, may result in a sudden increase in the height of block, with consequent extension of sympathetic blockade. This may occur even after 15–20 min. Treatment (Table 17.3) may not be necessary; moderate hypotension may help to reduce operative blood loss and is tolerated well by most patients. Severe or unwanted hypotension may be treated by i.v. fluids or drugs. The use of large volumes of crystalloid or colloid in this situation is not recommended, as urinary retention may occur postoperatively or circulatory overload may result when the block wears off. However, it is essential that operative blood losses are replaced promptly, and when blood losses are expected (e.g. caesarean section) it is wise to administer fluid in advance of the loss. Hypotension is associated commonly with bradycardia, and ephedrine 5–6 mg i.v. is the most appropriate treatment. Atropine may be useful, but sympathomimetic drugs are usually more effective than vagolytics.

Oversedation. This may occur when sedative drugs have been administered before performance of SAB. When the block is established, the previously satisfactory level of sedation may become excessive, with the

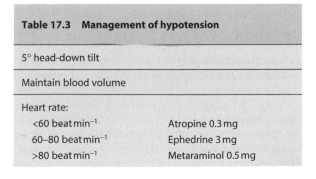

Table 17.3   Management of hypotension

5° head-down tilt	
Maintain blood volume	
Heart rate:	
<60 beat min⁻¹	Atropine 0.3 mg
60–80 beat min⁻¹	Ephedrine 3 mg
>80 beat min⁻¹	Metaraminol 0.5 mg

attendant risks of respiratory obstruction or aspiration. Some reports of cardiac arrest associated with SAB may be related to hypoxaemia produced in this manner.

Postoperative

Headache. This is more common in young adults and particularly in obstetric patients. It may present up to 2–7 days after lumbar puncture, and may persist for up to 6 weeks. Characteristically, it is worse on sitting, occipital in distribution and very disabling. The incidence is reduced by using small-gauge or pencil-point needles and may be reduced by aligning the bevel of the needle to penetrate the dura in a sagittal plane. Simple analgesics may be the only treatment required, but occasionally an epidural blood patch is necessary. The incidence of post-spinal headache is not reduced by keeping the patient supine for 24 h; the patient should remain supine only until the anaesthetic has worn off and the risk of postural hypotension is minimal. If headache is severe and persistent, an epidural blood patch may be performed by removing 20 mL of the patient's own blood under aseptic conditions and injecting it epidurally at the same interspace as SAB was performed. Injection should be stopped if discomfort is experienced. This is 70–80% effective for lumbar puncture headache and appears to be remarkably free from adverse effects.

Other complications. These include:

- Urinary retention – this may be associated with the surgical procedure. Large volumes of i.v. fluids may increase the frequency of this complication.
- Labyrinthine disturbances.
- Cranial nerve palsy – sixth nerve palsy may occur and is usually temporary. This complication is more common with larger needles.
- Meningitis and meningism.
- Spinal cord trauma caused by inserting the needle at too high an interspace – fortunately these conditions, giving rise to permanent neurological damage or paraplegia, are rare.

CONTINUOUS SPINAL ANAESTHESIA

Subarachnoid blockade can be produced incrementally or prolonged by using an indwelling spinal catheter. It may be performed using either a small catheter passed through a 19-gauge Tuohy needle or using a purpose-made catheter-over-wire kit such as the Spinocath (see Fig 17.1A). With the latter, the epidural space is located using a loss of resistance technique with a Crawford-type epidural needle and the 22-gauge Spinocath with

guide wire, inserted through it to puncture the dura. The guide wire is then withdrawn, leaving the catheter in the subarachnoid space. There is, therefore, minimal CSF leak around the catheter, reducing the risk of post-dural-puncture headache.

Spinal catheter techniques fell out of favour in the early 1990s following reports of cauda equina syndrome occurring in association with the use of 28-gauge and 32-gauge microcatheters and large doses of hyperbaric lidocaine 5%. It is postulated that the problem arose through pooling of high concentrations of lidocaine around the sacral nerve roots because of a slow injection rate, leading to permanent neurological damage. Hyperbaric lidocaine 5% and catheters finer than 24-gauge should be avoided and, because of the additional technical difficulty and potential for infection, the technique should be limited to more experienced practitioners in specific circumstances.

PERFORMANCE OF EPIDURAL BLOCK

By virtue of its great versatility, epidural analgesia is probably the most widely used regional technique in the UK. It may be used for procedures from the neck downwards and the duration of analgesia can be tailored to meet the needs of surgery and postoperative pain relief by using a catheter system.

The major differences between SAB and epidural block are summarized in Table 17.4. Further expansion of the technique has taken place with the advent of epidural administration of opioids and other agents such as clonidine or ketamine may have a place in providing postoperative epidural analgesia.

Equipment

Epidural anaesthesia is usually performed using a Tuohy needle (Fig. 17.5). The needle is marked at 1 cm intervals and has a Huber point which allows a catheter to be directed along the long axis of the epidural space. Disposable catheters are available with a single end-hole or with a sealed tip and three side-holes distally.

Technique

Epidural block may be performed at any level of the vertebral column to provide segmental analgesia over an area that can be predetermined with reasonable success. Initial experience should be gained in the lumbar region before progressing to sites above the termination of the spinal cord.

The pressure in the epidural space was originally considered to be subatmospheric, particularly in the

Table 17.4 Differences between subarachnoid and epidural block

	Subarachnoid	*Epidural*
Dose of drug used	Small: minimal risk of systemic toxicity	Large: possibility of systemic toxicity after intravascular injection or total spinal blockade after subarachnoid injection
Rate of onset	Fast: 2–5 min for initial effect, 20 min for maximum effect	Slow: 5–15 min for initial effect, 30–45 min for maximum effect
Intensity of block	Usually complete anaesthesia	Often not complete anaesthesia for all segments
Pattern of block	May be dermatomal for first few minutes, but rapidly develops appearance of cord transection	Dermatomal
Addition of vasoconstrictor	Reliably prolongs block with tetracaine, but not with other drugs	Reliably prolongs block with lidocaine. May prolong block with bupivacaine, but not in all patients

thoracic region. In fact, it is slightly positive, but negative pressures are induced by tenting of the epidural space from the Tuohy needle and account for the rapid inward entry of saline using the hanging-drop method. Some older methods of identifying the epidural space (e.g. Odom's indicator, Macintosh's balloon) relied on detection of this *subatmospheric* pressure in the epidural space. However, methods which depend on loss of resistance to injection of air or saline as the tip of the needle penetrates the ligamentum flavum and enters the epidural space have become more popular. A midline lumbar approach is described here, using loss of resistance to saline to detect the epidural space.

The patient is positioned as for SAB and the vertebral level is identified from the iliac crests. The skin and subcutaneous tissues of the third lumbar interspace are infiltrated with local anaesthetic solution in the midline. A sharp needle is used to puncture the skin and the Tuohy, round-ended epidural needle is introduced through the skin puncture, subcutaneous tissue and supraspinous ligament. The common reasons for difficulty are the same as those for SAB. When inserted into the interspinous ligament, the unsupported needle remains steady. The stilette is withdrawn and a 10 mL plastic syringe filled with saline is attached and advanced using firm but gentle pressure on the plunger. The needle must be gripped tightly at all times (Fig. 17.6) to prevent sudden forward movement. When the needle penetrates the ligamentum flavum, there is a sudden loss of resistance to pressure on the plunger, but the needle must not be allowed to advance further. The needle must not be rotated after its tip has entered the epidural space, as this increases the risk of penetration of the dura.

Single-dose technique

The syringe containing local anaesthetic is connected to the epidural needle, and after aspiration a test dose is administered to detect intravascular or subarachnoid placement. After an appropriate pause, the remainder of the solution is injected at a rate not exceeding $10\,\mathrm{mL\,min^{-1}}$ while verbal contact is maintained with the patient.

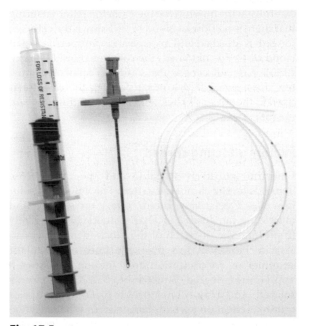

Fig. 17.5
16-Gauge Tuohy extradural needle with loss of resistance syringe and catheter.

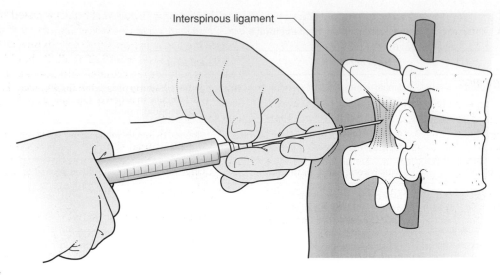

Interspinous ligament

Fig. 17.6
Loss of resistance technique to identify the epidural space. See text for details.

Catheter insertion

An epidural catheter should pass freely through the needle into the epidural space. If the catheter does not thread easily, the needle should be repositioned, as forcing the catheter into the epidural space makes intravascular placement more likely. When a sufficient length of catheter (3–4 cm) is in the space, the needle is carefully withdrawn over the catheter. After ensuring that there is no flow of blood or CSF down the catheter, the hub is attached and an aspiration test performed; if blood or CSF is obtained, the catheter should be reinserted in an adjacent space. A filter is connected and a test dose given. If this is satisfactory, the catheter is fixed to the patient's back with adhesive strapping and the main dose is administered.

Factors affecting spread

Epidural spread is variable and the initial dose depends on the clinical situation. The volume of solution has a relatively minor effect on spread, and increasing the dose of local anaesthetic is more likely to prolong the duration of the block than to increase spread. However, this principle does not hold for extremes of concentration and volume, nor does it apply to the degree of motor block as this is closely related to drug concentration. Posture has a minimal effect on spread, but patients who are pregnant or aged over 60 years may have an increased likelihood of a high block with a given dose of local anaesthetic.

Factors affecting onset

Onset time is reduced by increasing the concentration of the local anaesthetic and by the addition of adrenaline 1:200 000.

Factors affecting duration

The choice of local anaesthetic agent has a major effect on the duration of anaesthesia. The concentration of the drug also has an effect; the higher concentrations of bupivacaine produce a more prolonged block. To some extent this is a reflection of increased dose, which is known to increase the duration of anaesthesia. The addition of adrenaline 1:200 000 to lidocaine increases duration.

Agents

Lidocaine

This drug is used in concentrations of 1.5–2% with or without adrenaline 1:200 000. Without adrenaline, the duration of action is approximately 1 h; a duration of approximately 2–2.5 h may be expected when solutions containing adrenaline are used.

Bupivacaine

This agent is available in concentrations of 0.25% and 0.5%. Increasing the concentration to 0.75% results in a faster onset, a denser block, more profound motor block (and therefore muscle relaxation) and increased duration of anaesthesia, but this concentration is not now freely available for use in the UK.

Levobupivacaine

This agent is the pure S-isomer of bupivacaine and is less cardiotoxic than the racemic mixture, but otherwise appears equipotent in terms of sensory and motor blockade. Levobupivacaine is available as a 0.25%, 0.5% and 0.75% solution. The advantages of a 0.75% solution as described above may be broadly applicable to the use of levobupivacaine although clinical and research experience is limited. A block lasting more than 4 h may be achieved with a 0.75% solution.

Ropivacaine

This long-acting agent is less cardiotoxic than bupivacaine and may produce less motor block for a similar degree of sensory blockade. It is less potent than bupivacaine and slightly higher concentrations/doses are used.

Complications

Intraoperative

Dural tap. The incidence should be less than 0.5% in experienced hands. It usually occurs with the needle rather than the catheter and is immediately obvious because of the free flow of CSF. If this occurs, epidural block should be instituted at an adjacent space and managed cautiously, although experienced anaesthetists, particularly in the obstetric environment, may choose to pass the 'epidural' catheter into the subarachnoid space and manage as a continuous SAB (see Ch. 35). Puncture of the dura with a large epidural needle leads to a high incidence of headache, of up to 70%. Simple analgesics and adequate hydration may suffice if headache occurs; if not, an epidural blood patch should be performed. Accidental total spinal anaesthesia (see below) is rare because the dural tap is usually obvious.

Total spinal anaesthesia

This may occur if the large volume of solution used for epidural anaesthesia is injected into the subarachnoid space. The consequences may be:

- profound hypotension
- apnoea, unconsciousness and dilated pupils secondary to local anaesthetic action on the brainstem.

Paralysis of the legs should alert the physician to the possibility of subarachnoid injection. When using a test dose, motor function should be tested by asking the patient to raise the whole leg and not merely to wiggle the toes; movement of the toes may not be abolished for 20 min after SAB, if at all. It should be noted that relatively large volumes of local anaesthetic solution, e.g. 10 mL of bupivacaine 0.25%, may be injected into the subarachnoid space without total spinal anaesthesia occurring.

Provided that skilled resuscitation is undertaken rapidly, a total spinal should be followed by complete recovery. Appropriate personnel and equipment should be present before epidural analgesia is undertaken and whenever top-up injections are administered.

Massive epidural block and subdural block

A very high block may occur in the absence of subarachnoid injection. This may be associated with Horner's syndrome.

Other complications. These include:

- intravenous toxicity (see Ch. 4)
- hypotension
- urinary retention
- shivering
- nausea/vomiting – this may result from hypotension or visceral manipulation in the awake patient.

Postoperative

- *Headache* following dural tap.
- *Epidural haematoma.* The spinal canal acts as a rigid box, and an expanding haematoma within the canal compresses the spinal cord, resulting in loss of neurological function unless the compression is relieved surgically at a very early stage. Decompression within 6 h is completely effective in virtually all patients, but after 12 h it is almost totally ineffective.
- *Epidural abscess.*
- *Other neurological complications,* e.g. damage to a single nerve root or paraplegia following accidental administration of potassium chloride.

ANTICOAGULANTS AND SUBARACHNOID BLOCK OR EPIDURAL ANAESTHESIA

Oral anticoagulants

Anticoagulation should be stopped at an appropriate time before surgery if SAB or epidural anaesthesia is planned. The degree of anticoagulation most appropriate for the patient depends on a balance between the risk of withholding anticoagulation and the nature of the surgery, in particular the associated risk of bleeding.

Platelets

The platelet count should ideally be in excess of $150 \times 10^9 \text{ L}^{-1}$.

Antiplatelet agents

Concern has been expressed about the antiplatelet effect of aspirin, NSAIDs and dipyridamole with respect to increased risk of vertebral canal haematoma. There is little evidence to support this concern but clopidogrel should be stopped at least 7 days before surgery unless there are overwhelming clinical circumstances, as reports of both serious surgical bleeding and vertebral canal haematoma have been associated with its use.

Heparin

The half-life of heparin given i.v. is 50–160 min, depending on dose. When given s.c., blood concentrations vary widely; in some patients plasma concentrations are in the anticoagulant range. At present, it is regarded as imprudent to use SAB or epidural analgesia when subcutaneous heparin has already been given, especially the low molecular weight variety. Removal of an epidural catheter should be timed to precede, rather than follow, administration of a further dose of subcutaneous heparin.

Guidelines for the use of low molecular weight heparin and epidural anaesthesia are given in Table 17.5.

Intraoperative heparinization

Epidural analgesia and SAB offer advantages for major vascular surgery, but the routine use of heparin introduces the theoretical risk of haemorrhage if an epidural catheter is in place. The precise risk is unknown, as prospective trials would require in excess of 10 000 cases. Some large series (3000 patients) have been conducted under epidural analgesia without haematoma formation.

CAUDAL ANAESTHESIA

Caudal block involves injection of local anaesthetic into the epidural space through the sacral hiatus to obtain anaesthesia of sacral and coccygeal nerve roots. Injection of very large volumes to obtain anaesthesia of lumbar and thoracic roots, although described, is seldom practised because of a high incidence of side-effects and failure to achieve a sufficiently high block. With appropriate volumes, caudal blockade affects the lower limbs infrequently, does not cause sympathetic

---

Table 17.5 Guidelines for the insertion and removal of epidural catheters in association with low molecular weight heparins (LMWH)

1	Patients who need DVT prophylaxis before theatre should receive LMWH the day before at approximately 18.00h.
2	LMWH should not be given on the day of surgery – this allows 12 h before catheter placement; although the LMWH is providing DVT prophylaxis at this time, plasma concentrations are below peak activity and therefore less likely to create a problem.
3	LMWH may be given 2h after placement of an epidural catheter.
4	The epidural catheter should be removed 12h after the last dose of LWMH and the next dose should not be given until 2h have elapsed.
5	Antiplatelet drugs and anticoagulant drugs should not be used concurrently with LMWH.
6	The smallest effective dose of LMWH should be used.
7	Patients should have regular (every 4h) neurological examination after removal of the epidural catheter. This should include sensation, power and reflexes.
8	In cases of traumatic or repeated epidural puncture, administration of LMWH should be delayed for more than 24h; an alternative method of DVT prophylaxis should be used.
9	Epidural mixtures should contain a low concentration of bupivacaine so that motor function may be assessed.
10	If the patient develops a neurological abnormality either during epidural infusion or within 48h of epidural catheter removal, an urgent MRI scan is required and a neurosurgical opinion should be obtained.

blockade and has a low risk of dural puncture. The anatomy is variable and difficulty is experienced in approximately 5% of subjects.

Indications

Caudal anaesthesia is suitable for perineal operations, e.g. haemorrhoidectomy, although in practice a subarachnoid saddle block is usually preferred. It is frequently used in paediatric practice for postoperative analgesia following circumcision, orchidopexy, and inguinal hernia and hypospadias repairs.

Method

Caudal blockade may be performed with the patient in the prone position, but the left lateral position is usually more acceptable to the patient and easier in the anaesthetized paediatric patient. Palpation down the sacral spine leads to the depression of the sacral hiatus at S5, flanked by the sacral cornua, through which the needle is inserted. A 21-gauge hypodermic needle or 22-gauge cannula is introduced through skin and sacrococcygeal ligament in a cephalad direction at 45° to the skin (Fig. 17.7). When the membrane is penetrated, injection may be performed or the needle hub may be depressed toward the natal cleft, and inserted a further 2–3 mm along the sacral canal; it must be remembered that the dura may extend to S3. Lidocaine 2%, with or without adrenaline, and bupivacaine 0.5% are suitable agents. In an adult, 10 mL of solution blocks anal sensation consistently.

In conjunction with general anaesthesia, caudal anaesthesia provides smooth operating conditions and good postoperative analgesia. With this combined technique, the advantages of performing caudal block before induction of general anaesthesia are as follows:

- The patient does not need to be repositioned while anaesthetized.
- Subperiosteal injection is reported by the patient.

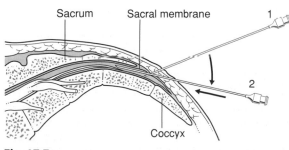

Fig. 17.7
Needle position for caudal anaesthesia.

- Accidental i.v. injection may be detected before the full dose is given.

For patients undergoing haemorrhoidectomy, many surgeons rely on the tone in the anal sphincter to identify it accurately and avoid damage. In these patients, general anaesthesia may be supplemented by a short-acting opioid such as alfentanil for the intraoperative period, and caudal anaesthesia given following the procedure. Extremely effective postoperative analgesia lasting several hours is provided.

Complications

Misplaced needle. Injection into subcutaneous tissue causes a swelling with fluid, or surgical emphysema with 2–3 mL of air. Intraosseous or subperiosteal injection results in marked resistance to injection. Penetration of rectum and fetal head (in obstetric practice) have been reported but should not occur if the technique is performed carefully.

Dural tap. This is rare, but the procedure should be abandoned if CSF is aspirated.

PERIPHERAL BLOCKS

HEAD AND NECK BLOCKS

These are mostly specialized blocks which are used in ophthalmic and plastic surgery. Only the technique of local anaesthesia for awake intubation is described here. Blocks used in ophthalmic surgery are discussed in Chapter 32.

Awake intubation

This may be the safest option in a patient with known or anticipated difficulty with intubation from a variety of causes, anatomical or otherwise. Pretreatment with an antisialagogue such as glycopyrrolate 0.2 mg may be useful to decrease secretions and improve anaesthesia obtained with topical application. Sedation with midazolam or a combination with fentanyl is desirable if this is not likely to exacerbate airway obstruction. A blind, fibreoptic or retrograde technique may be used, and experience and training in these techniques are now more widespread.

The nose is prepared with topical lidocaine 2% with or without a vasoconstrictor such as phenylephrine. The patient may then either suck a benzocaine lozenge, or the posterior tongue and pharynx are sprayed with lidocaine 4%. Cricothyroid injection is performed through either a 23-gauge needle or 22-gauge cannula inserted through the cricothyroid membrane (Fig. 17.8A,B) and air is aspirated to confirm the position. Two millilitres of lidocaine 4% are injected and the needle is withdrawn immediately. A vigorous cough results and spreads the solution. Although absorption of lidocaine from mucous membranes is rapid, in practice, significant amounts tend to be lost or swallowed and rarely cause systemic toxicity.

UPPER LIMB BLOCKS

The upper limb is well suited to local anaesthetic techniques and these remain among the most useful and commonly practised peripheral regional techniques. Percutaneous approaches to the brachial plexus were first described in 1911. In recent times, approaches

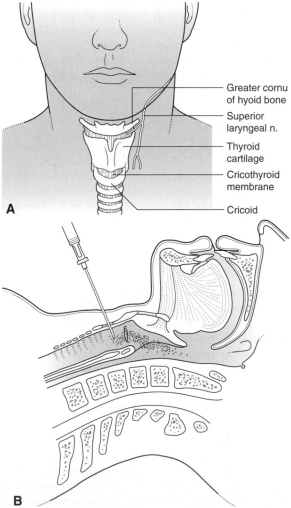

A

B

Fig. 17.8
(A) Cricothyroid anatomy. **(B)** Cricothyroid injection.

Greater cornu of hyoid bone
Superior laryngeal n.
Thyroid cartilage
Cricothyroid membrane
Cricoid

based on the concept of a continuous sheath surrounding the brachial plexus from roots to the distal axilla became more popular, before further advances in imaging and location techniques illustrated the limitations of this approach, despite its undoubted simplistic appeal. It is possible to block almost the whole arm with a single injection, but increasingly, multiple injection techniques are used with either nerve stimulation or ultrasound to achieve rapid and complete blockade with the lowest possible failure rates and minimal complications. With appropriate training, these techniques may now be expected to provide successful surgical anaesthesia in more than 90% of patients using a variety of anatomical approaches.

Anatomy of the brachial plexus

The nerve supply of the upper limb is derived mainly from the brachial plexus, which is formed from the anterior primary rami of the fifth to eighth cervical and first thoracic nerve roots. The roots of the plexus divide repeatedly and recombine to form trunks, divisions, cords and terminal nerves (Fig. 17.9). The roots emerge from the intervertebral foramina and combine into three trunks above the first rib. Each trunk separates above the clavicle into anterior and posterior divisions; anterior divisions supply the flexor structures of the arm and posterior divisions the extensor structures. The divisions recombine into three cords, which surround the second part of the axillary artery behind the pectoralis minor and then form the terminal nerves.

The roots lie between the anterior and middle scalene muscles and are invested in a sheath, derived from the prevertebral fascia, which splits to enclose the scalene muscles. The cutaneous and deep nerve supplies of the upper limb are depicted in Figure 17.11.

Part of the cutaneous nerve supply of the upper limb is not derived from the brachial plexus; the upper medial part of the arm is supplied by the intercostobrachial nerve (T2). The reader is referred to standard texts for a more detailed anatomical description.

Axillary block

This technique represents perhaps the safest approach to the brachial plexus for the trainee to learn. It is useful for elbow, forearm and hand surgery, but traditional single-injection approaches are limited by high failure rates of both musculocutaneous and radial nerves. The orientation of nerves around the axillary artery is shown in Figure 17.10A, as are the needle positions necessary for successful complete blockade. Dense blockade with greater efficacy may often be achieved within 10 min compared with the 20–30 min often

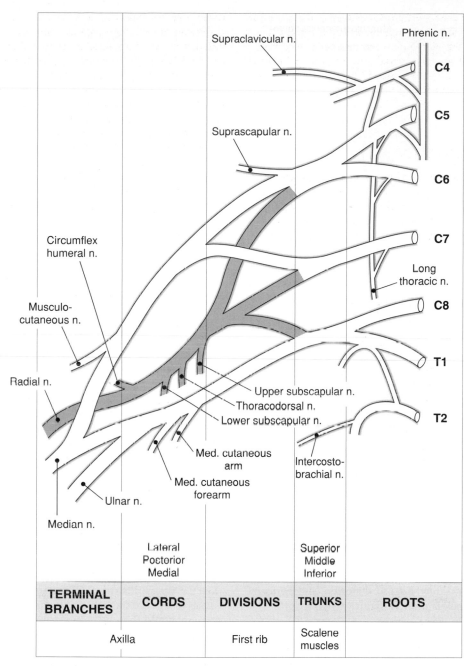

Fig. 17.9
Formation of the brachial plexus.

required for single-injection approaches. Whilst the triple injection appears optimal for success, the trainee may initially choose to locate the musculocutaneous nerve (biceps contraction) with one of the anterior nerves, either median or ulnar nerve (finger flexion), until more experience is gained.

Positioning

The patient lies supine with the arm to be blocked abducted to no more than 90° and the elbow bent to 90° (see Fig. 17.10B). Further abduction with the hand placed behind the head is convenient, but the axillary

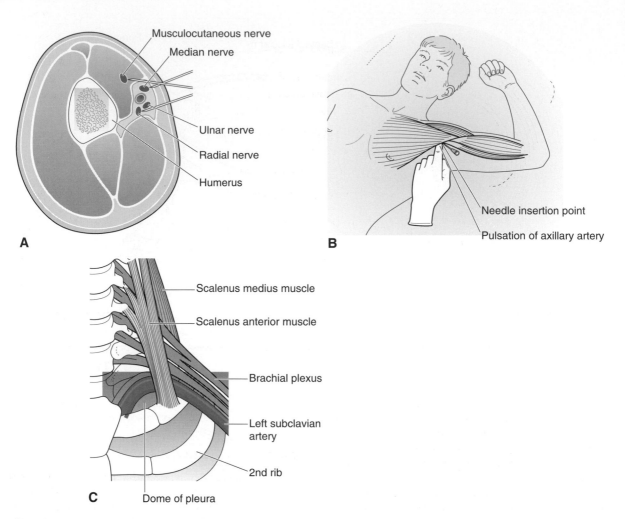

Fig. 17.10
(A) Cross-sectional relationship of the brachial plexus nerves to the axillary artery. **(B)** Correct position and approach for axillary block. The axillary artery is palpated by the finger. **(C)** Relationships of the brachial plexus in the neck.

vessels become stretched and distorted, and performance of the block is more difficult.

Method

The axillary artery is palpated and traced to a point 1–2 cm distal to the lateral border of pectoralis major (see Fig. 17.10B). A 2 mL subcutaneous wheal of local anaesthetic is raised over and inferior to the artery at this point, which also blocks the intercostobrachial nerve. A 22-gauge insulated short-bevelled needle is introduced through this wheal after puncturing the skin with a standard needle. The nerve stimulator is set to deliver a current of 2 mA and the needle directed immediately above the artery (almost parallel to the floor). Stimulation of the musculocutaneous nerve causes biceps contraction and flexion of the elbow. The current should then be reduced until optimal contraction is obtained at a current of around 0.5 mA; 5 mL of the local anaesthetic is injected following gentle aspiration. The needle is then withdrawn and redirected through the same puncture, in a more inferior direction with the current again set to deliver 2 mA. Flexion of wrist and fingers occurs following a distinct fascial click as the needle enters the sheath and stimulates the median nerve. Current is again reduced to optimize muscle contraction at 0.5 mA and 15 mL of local anaesthetic solution injected in 5 mL increments, each preceded by careful aspiration. Finally, the needle is withdrawn and redirected below the artery

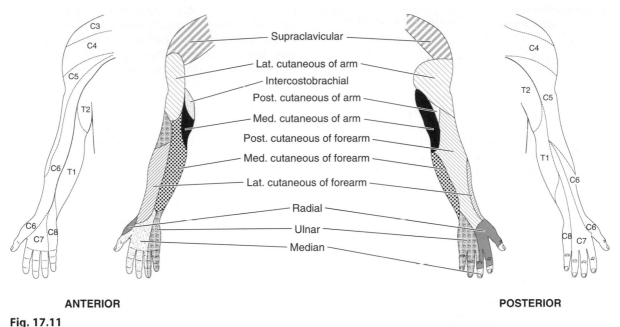

ANTERIOR   **POSTERIOR**

Fig. 17.11
Innervation of the upper limb: outer, dermatomal innervation of the skin; inner, cutaneous nerve supply to the upper limb.

until extension of the fingers is obtained and again current reduced from 2 mA to 0.5 mA. Ten millilitres of solution is then injected in two, 5 mL increments. A total of 30 mL of local anaesthetic solution is therefore used. For most routine upper limb surgery, lidocaine 1.5% with adrenaline 1:200 000 is used, but for major painful procedures, ropivacaine or levobupivacaine 0.5% with adrenaline 1:300 000 may be substituted. Addition of adrenaline allows more obvious detection of intravascular injection, which may occur despite a negative aspiration test and can be prepared by adding 1 mL of fresh 1:10 000 adrenaline to 30 mL of local anaesthetic solution. After completion of injection, the arm should be returned to the patient's side.

Disadvantages and complications

Access is occasionally problematic if arm abduction and external rotation are limited by either additional shoulder trauma or severe arthritis. This approach rarely blocks the axillary nerve unless large volumes of solution are used. If blockade of this nerve is required, a more proximal approach to the plexus should be considered. Puncture of the axillary artery is rarely a problem, but may lead to haematoma formation or inadvertent intravascular injection. Nerve damage occurs rarely and usually results from malpo-

sition of the anaesthetized limb or failure to recognize a compartment syndrome postoperatively.

Infraclavicular block

This is an increasingly popular approach which blocks the three cords of the plexus as they surround the second part of the axillary artery deep to pectoralis minor. There are a variety of approaches, but most locate the plexus below the midpoint of the clavicle or medial and caudad to the coracoid process, using either nerve stimulation or, increasingly, ultrasound.

Advantages

Using ultrasonic location, excellent efficacy and complete block within 10 min can be achieved. For highest possible success rates, a multiple injection technique locating all three cords is recommended, as described by Sandhu & Capan (2002). This approach does not, therefore, depend on surface landmarks which may be variable and difficult to appreciate in the overweight patient. A 5–12 MHz probe not only shows the important vascular structures with which the nerves are intimately related, but with experience also demonstrates the three neural cords. The approach is useful if complete blockade of the arm including the axillary nerve is required or if a catheter is sited for postoperative use, because of greater ease of secure fixation below the clavicle.

Disadvantages

Pneumothorax has been reported although the risk appears to be low. Vascular puncture is fairly common using nerve stimulator techniques because of the close proximity of nerves to both axillary artery and vein in this location. Ultrasonic location reduces this to a minimum. Success rates decrease if a single injection is used, but administering 40 mL rather than 30 mL of local anaesthetic solution may improve success rates with a single-injection approach.

Supraclavicular block

Supraclavicular approaches to the brachial plexus are favoured by many anaesthetists and the description by Winnie (1984) of the subclavian perivascular approach has increased the safety of this technique by reducing the incidence of pneumothorax. The key to successful block is accurate palpation of the interscalene groove (see Fig. 17.10C) above the clavicle, which helps delineate the position of the first rib and lateral border of pleura as well as locating the plexus.

Advantages

This approach provides the best overall efficacy of complete block from a single injection although success may not be as high as the multiple-injection approaches mentioned above. Onset time may be as short as 10–15 min, analgesia of the whole arm is more likely and 25–30 mL of solution is sufficient in an adult.

Disadvantages

The risk of pneumothorax is always present, but is very small (< 0.5%) in experienced hands. The safety and success depend on the accurate localization of the interscalene groove which may not always be straightforward, particularly in the obese. Phrenic nerve paralysis may occur in around one-third of patients, but is usually asymptomatic. However, axillary block is the method of choice if there is diminished respiratory reserve or if bilateral blocks are required. Recurrent laryngeal nerve block may result in hoarseness. Sympathetic block is relatively common and results in Horner's syndrome.

Interscalene block

This is the most proximal approach to the brachial plexus and the only approach which reliably blocks the plexus above C5. With adequate volume (25–30 mL) interscalene injection usually extends to block the cervical plexus roots C2, 3 and 4. Block of the C8 and T1 roots may, however, prove difficult, and this approach is therefore most suitable for shoulder and upper arm surgery and rather less suitable for hand surgery. Complications are similar to those for supraclavicular block but phrenic nerve block occurs almost universally. Pneumothorax, vertebral artery puncture and direct intraspinal injection are also possibilities. Seizures may occur from direct vertebral artery injection with as little as 1–2 mL of local anaesthetic solution.

Agents

Lidocaine 1.5%, with adrenaline 1:200 000, and bupivacaine, ropivacaine or levobupivacaine 0.375–0.5% are suitable. The more dilute solutions are necessary when larger volumes or additional nerve blocks are required, or may be used when the block is combined with general anaesthesia, particularly if a postoperative infusion is planned.

BLOCKS IN THE TRUNK

Intercostal and paravertebral blocks are useful in providing analgesia following abdominal, breast and thoracic surgery and also provide good analgesia for rib fractures. The analgesic area may be extended using multiple injections or by spread of a larger single bolus, usually via an indwelling catheter, which may then be employed for repeat administrations. There is a significant risk of pneumothorax when these blocks are performed by unskilled personnel. Paravertebral block is a relatively difficult procedure, only suitable for the more experienced anaesthetist. It is gaining popularity for analgesia following breast and inguinal hernia surgery but is not considered further here.

Intercostal nerve block

Anatomy

Intercostal nerves are formed from the ventral rami of segmental thoracic nerves after communicating with the associated sympathetic ganglia through white and grey rami communicantes (Fig. 17.12). An intercostal nerve has three main branches: the lateral cutaneous branch divides into anterior and posterior branches; the anterior terminal branch supplies the anterior thorax, rectus muscle and overlying skin; and a collateral branch arises from most nerves in the posterior intercostal space. This may rejoin the main nerve or form a separate anterior cutaneous nerve. Fibres from T1 join

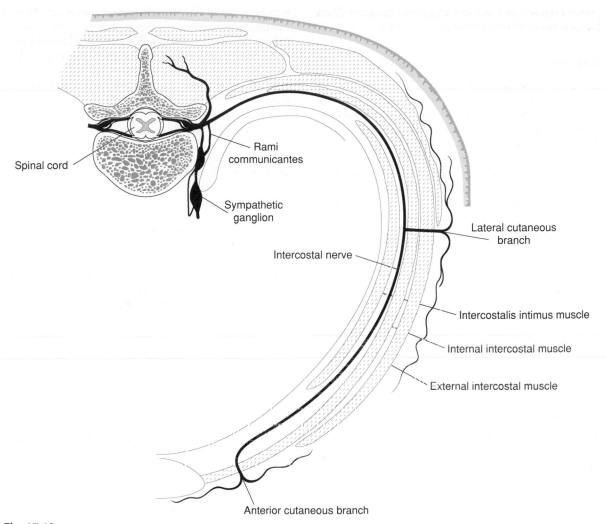

Fig. 17.12
Anatomy of the intercostal nerve.

the brachial plexus, T2 and T3 supply fibres to form the intercostobrachial nerve, and T12, together with L1, contribute to the iliohypogastric, ilioinguinal and genitofemoral nerves.

Method

The optimal place to block the intercostal nerve is proximal to the formation of the lateral cutaneous branch, posterior to the mid-axillary line. With the patient in the lateral position, nerve blocks may be conveniently performed immediately following surgery for unilateral procedures such as open biliary and gallbladder surgery. In awake patients, for example following unilateral rib fractures, a sitting position with the patient leaning forward to abduct the scapulae is often con-

venient. A 23-gauge needle is inserted perpendicular to the skin to make contact with an appropriate rib. The needle is then 'walked' caudally until it can be inserted under the lower border of the rib. After passing through the external intercostal muscle, up to 5 mL of local anaesthetic solution should be injected freely, following a negative aspiration test. Rapid absorption of local anaesthetic solution may produce high systemic concentrations after multiple intercostal nerve blocks and the dose and concentration of drug need to be chosen carefully; 0.25–0.5% levobupivacaine or ropivacaine with or without 1:200 000 adrenaline is recommended, depending on the number of intercostal nerves being blocked. A single injection of 20 mL using a catheter technique may block up to five adjacent segments (approximately two above and three below).

Pneumothorax and haemorrhage are the most likely complications after intercostal nerve block.

Field block for inguinal hernia repair

The main nerves which supply the groin are the subcostal (T12), iliohypogastric (L1) and ilioinguinal (L1). Their blockade produces good postoperative analgesia, but supplementary infiltration, especially around the internal ring and hernial sac, is usually necessary during surgery if this is the only anaesthetic employed.

A needle is inserted 1.5 cm medial and inferior to the anterior superior iliac spine. Using a regional block needle, the external oblique aponeurosis is readily appreciated as the needle is advanced. Fifteen millilitres of local anaesthetic are injected deep to the aponeurosis, down to the inner surface of the ilium between the abdominal muscle layers. Another 5 mL of solution are deposited superficial to the external oblique aponeurosis medially from this point. Bupivacaine 0.5% is a suitable agent for postoperative analgesia.

Local infiltration is used routinely as the sole anaesthetic in some centres and may be the method of choice in the unfit patient or in the day-case unit, but only when surgeons are experienced with this technique.

Penile block

The dorsal nerves to the penis are derived from the pudendal nerves and are blocked with 5–10 mL of local anaesthetic solution injected inferior to the symphysis pubis in the midline at a depth of 3–4 cm. Care must be taken to avoid intravascular injection in this area and vasoconstrictors *must not* be used. Plain bupivacaine 0.5% is suitable. The base of the penis is innervated by the genital branch of the genitofemoral nerve, which may be blocked if necessary by s.c. infiltration around the penis.

Penile block is quick and simple, produces a limited effect and is the block of choice for circumcision or other minor penile surgery such as meatotomy. It is commonly used in combination with light general anaesthesia and provides good postoperative pain relief. However, a simpler technique is to smear lidocaine jelly over the wound on a regular 4- to 6-hourly basis in the postoperative period.

LOWER LIMB BLOCKS

Lower limb blocks are practised less frequently than upper limb blocks for three reasons:

- It is not possible to block the whole of the lower limb with one injection.

- Subarachnoid or epidural anaesthesia may prove simpler.
- There is an impression among some anaesthetists that lower limb blocks are difficult and unreliable.

However, new approaches to the peripheral nerves of the lower limb have simplified the subject and the blocks considered below are appropriate for the trainee anaesthetist.

Sciatic nerve block

Anatomy

The sciatic nerve (L4, L5, S1–3) arises from the sacral plexus, passes through the great sciatic foramen and descends in the posterior thigh to the popliteal fossa, where it divides into the tibial and common peroneal nerves. In the thigh, it supplies muscles and the hip joint. The posterior cutaneous nerve of the thigh (S1–3) may run with the sciatic nerve or separate from it proximally; this nerve supplies the skin of the posterior thigh and upper calf. The tibial and common peroneal nerves, together with the saphenous nerve, supply all structures below the knee.

Method

There are several approaches to the sciatic nerve; the posterior approach described by Labat is the most straightforward but requires the patient to be turned to a lateral semi-prone position; the limb to be blocked is uppermost and flexed at the knee. A line is drawn from the posterior superior iliac spine to the tip of the greater trochanter of femur. At the midpoint, a second perpendicular line is drawn caudally for 4–5 cm to mark the point of needle insertion (Fig. 17.13). Following aseptic preparation, the skin is infiltrated with 2 mL of local anaesthetic and a 100 mm, 21G insulated block needle inserted perpendicular to skin with the stimulator set to deliver 2 mA. After some initial twitches in the gluteal area, further advancement usually results in hamstring contraction. The current is then best reduced to 0.5–1 mA before further subtle advancement produces either dorsiflexion or plantar flexion in the foot at 0.5 mA. Fifteen to 20 mL of local anaesthetic is then injected in 5 mL aliquots after negative aspiration.

This block has a high success rate with few complications, although intravascular placement may be difficult to detect because of the length of the needle. The posterior cutaneous nerve of thigh is usually blocked with this approach. Sciatic block may often be used alone for several procedures in the foot, e.g. hallux valgus operations, using a below-knee tourniquet. This must be

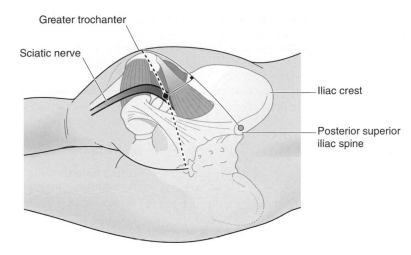

Greater trochanter

Sciatic nerve

Iliac crest

Posterior superior iliac spine

Fig. 17.13
Posterior approach to sciatic nerve block. The greater trochanter and posterior superior iliac spine are marked.

positioned at least 10 cm below the tibial tuberosity to avoid compression of the common peroneal nerve as it courses around the fibular neck. The block is particularly useful for the medically compromised, arteriopathic patient requiring peripheral or forefoot amputation. This may require additional saphenous block at the ankle to complete cutaneous analgesia on the medial aspect. Sciatic block may also be combined with either lumbar plexus or femoral block to allow use of a thigh tourniquet or to complete analgesia of the lower limb.

Lidocaine 1.5–2% with adrenaline 1:200 000, or ropivacaine, levobupivacaine or bupivacaine 0.375–0.5% are suitable agents. Fifteen to 20 mL of solution is necessary. The more dilute solutions are required when other blocks are performed concurrently.

Femoral nerve block

Anatomy

The femoral nerve (L2–4) arises from the lumbar plexus and runs between psoas and iliacus to enter the thigh beneath the inguinal ligament, 1–2 cm lateral to the femoral artery and at a slightly greater depth. Branches of the anterior division include the intermediate and medial cutaneous nerves of the thigh and the supply to the sartorius. The posterior division supplies the quadriceps and the hip and knee joints and terminates as the saphenous nerve, which supplies the skin of the medial side of the calf as far as the medial malleolus and sometimes the medial side of the dorsum of the foot.

Method

The patient lies supine and the inguinal ligament and femoral artery are identified. The skin is anaesthetized lateral to the femoral artery, 1 cm below the inguinal ligament. A 22-guage, short-bevelled insulated needle is inserted parallel to the artery in a cephalad direction of approximately 45° with respect to skin (Fig. 17.14). With the nerve stimulator set to deliver 2mA, two distinct fascial pops are generally appreciated before muscle contractions occur. Patellar ascension or 'tapping' is observed when the femoral nerve is accurately located with the current reduced to around 0.5mA. Observation of this patellar movement should prevent confusion with the contractions obtained by direct stimulation of the sartorius. Fifteen to 20 mL of solution are required for satisfactory blockade.

Femoral nerve block is usually combined with sciatic block for operative procedures. Analgesia following femoral fracture or knee surgery may be satisfactory with femoral nerve block alone, although complete analgesia following knee replacement is best achieved initially with additional sciatic block.

The inguinal perivascular technique of lumbar plexus anaesthesia (the so-called 3-in-1 block) was reported to provide anaesthesia in the distribution of the femoral, lateral cutaneous and obturator nerves from the single injection of 20–30 mL of solution with distal digital pressure. In practice, however, careful assessment has shown that the obturator nerve is not blocked routinely by this approach.

Suitable local anaesthetic agents for femoral or '3-in-1' block are the same as for sciatic nerve block.

Lumbar plexus block

A paravertebral approach to the lumbar plexus provides, in many ways, a more logical approach to blockade of the three main terminal branches – femoral,

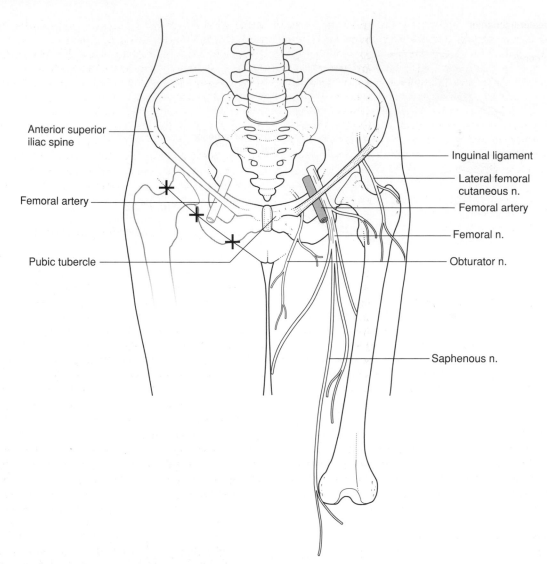

Anterior superior
iliac spine

Inguinal ligament

Lateral femoral
cutaneous n.

Femoral artery

Femoral artery

Femoral n.

Obturator n.

Pubic tubercle

Saphenous n.

Fig. 17.14
Position and approach for femoral nerve block. The anterior superior iliac spine and femoral artery are marked.

obturator and lateral cutaneous nerve of thigh – than the inguinal 3-in-1 approach mentioned above. It may be used in combination with sciatic block to complete analgesia of the lower limb and has been used as the sole technique for femoral neck surgery in addition to providing postoperative analgesia after major hip or revision surgery carried out under general anaesthesia or central neuronal blockade.

Anatomy

The lumbar plexus is formed from the ventral rami of the first three and large part of the fourth lumbar nerves. The nerves run from the vertebral column in an inferolateral direction within psoas major muscle. The femoral and lateral cutaneous nerves then emerge from the lateral aspect and the obturator from the medial aspect of this muscle and may be blocked within psoas or in a fascial plane between it and quadratus lumborum at the L3/4 level or L4/5 level. Local anaesthetic injected within this plane, or close to the nerves within psoas muscle, should block all three nerves.

Method

The patient is positioned either sitting or more commonly in the lateral decubitus position with operative side uppermost. The spine of the fourth lumbar vertebra is identified by palpating the iliac crests. A point 3 cm caudad and 5 cm lateral to this is then identified and infiltrated with local anaesthetic. This should be medial to the posterior superior iliac spine. A 21-guage insulated short-bevelled needle is then introduced perpendicular to skin until contact with the lumbar transverse process is made. The needle is then withdrawn and redirected in a cephalad direction (or occasionally in a caudad direction) until the needle glides over the transverse process. The depth from skin is variable but contact with the plexus, resulting in quadriceps contraction, is usually found at a depth of 1.5–2 cm from the transverse process. Following careful aspiration, 25–30 mL of local anaesthetic, usually levobupivacaine 0.375–0.5% or ropivacaine 0.4–0.5%, is injected in 5 mL increments.

Disadvantages

Care must be taken in selecting an appropriate concentration of local anaesthetic, particularly when combined with sciatic block, to ensure maximum dosage is not exceeded, resulting in systemic toxicity. Epidural spread has been reported, particularly in paediatric practice.

Ankle block

Anatomy

Five nerves supply the forefoot. The medial and lateral plantar nerves are the terminal branches of the posterior tibial nerve, which enters the foot posterior to the medial malleolus; they supply deep structures within the foot and all of the sole. The common peroneal nerve divides into deep and superficial branches; the deep peroneal nerve supplies the web space between first and second toes and the superficial branch supplies the dorsum of the foot. The saphenous nerve may supply a variable area of skin on the medial side of the dorsum of the foot. The sural nerve is a branch of the tibial nerve; it runs posterior to the lateral malleolus and supplies skin over the lateral side of the foot and fifth toe.

Method

To block the posterior tibial nerve, the posterior tibial artery is palpated behind the medial malleolus as far distally as possible. Injection of 3 mL of local anaesthetic to each side of it, below deep fascia, blocks medial and lateral plantar nerves. Alternatively, the posterior tibial nerve may be blocked with 5 mL of local anaesthetic injected at a point distal and posterior to the sustentaculum tali, particularly when there is no vascular landmark. Injection of 2 mL of local anaes-

thetic to each side of the dorsalis pedis artery, below deep fascia, blocks the deep peroneal nerve. The saphenous and superficial peroneal nerves are blocked by s.c. infiltration at the level of the ankle joint in a line extending from a point anterior to the medial malleolus to the lateral malleolus. The sural nerve is blocked with a subcutaneous infiltration behind the lateral malleolus. A complete block of the foot requires 15 mL of solution; ropivacaine, levobupivacaine or racemic bupivacaine are most suitable for postoperative analgesia. It is probably advisable to avoid all five blocks when the circulation to the foot is impaired although selective blockade is useful for vascular amputations.

CONTINUOUS PERIPHERAL NERVE BLOCK

These techniques are growing in popularity for both upper and lower limb blocks, as a method of prolonging postoperative analgesia and facilitating rehabilitation without the side-effects associated with opioids and with fewer unwanted cardiorespiratory complications compared with epidural analgesia. Postoperative care is simplified and may usually be carried out in a general ward environment. The anaesthetist should be proficient in single-shot peripheral blocks – brachial plexus, femoral, lumbar plexus and sciatic – before advancing to catheter techniques. Equipment has improved greatly in recent years and insulated Tuohy needles (see Fig. 17.1) and facet-tipped needles are available to assist catheter placement. Local anaesthetic agents, usually levobupivacaine or ropivacaine, because of their reduced systemic toxicity, are most commonly used in concentrations of 0.1–0.25% and may be continuously infused, or administered by intermittent bolus either by medical staff or as part of a patient-controlled system with or without a background infusion.

SPECIAL SITUATIONS

PAEDIATRIC TECHNIQUES

Most blocks used in adult practice are suitable for use in children, but because of the nature of most paediatric surgery and the understandable difficulties that may be experienced with patient cooperation, only a limited, but increasing number, of techniques are commonly used. Many of these are used for postoperative analgesia and are performed after induction of general anaesthesia; they should only be performed by experienced anaesthetists.

The disposition of local anaesthetic agents in children differs from that in adults. Recent work suggests that, in children of less than 1 year of age, and particularly in the neonate, very high plasma concentrations of local anaesthetic may ensue after standard doses based on weight. In children exceeding 1 year of age, plasma concentrations are consistently lower than would be expected from adult data.

Agents and doses for paediatric blocks are shown in Table 17.6. Caudal block for subumbilical surgery may be prolonged usefully in the postoperative period by the addition of preservative-free S (+)-ketamine 0.5 mg kg^{-1}.

TOPICAL ANAESTHESIA

This may be achieved with either EMLA (eutectic mixture of local anaesthetics) or Ametop (tetracaine) cream, held in place with an occlusive dressing. Both provide anaesthesia of intact skin which is particularly useful before venepuncture in children. EMLA cream must remain in contact with the skin for at least 1 h to be effective and may be left in place for up to 5 h. Ametop is generally effective within 30–45 min, after which time the cream and occlusive dressing should be removed and the site marked.

Table 17.6   Agents and doses of local anaesthetics used in paediatric practice

Caudal anaesthesia	
0.25% bupivacaine	
0.5 mL kg^{-1}	Sacral block
1.0 mL kg^{-1}	Low thoracic block
0.19% bupivacaine (three parts bupivacaine 0.25%:one part saline)	
1.25 mL kg^{-1}	Mid-thoracic block

Penile block	
0.5% bupivacaine *plain*	
Body weight	*Dose*
2.5 kg	0.5 mL
10 kg	1.0 mL
20 kg	2.0 mL
40 kg	4.0 mL

Axillary block	
0.25% bupivacaine	
Body weight	*Dose*
10 kg	6 mL
20 kg	12 mL
30 kg	18 mL
40 kg	24 mL

FURTHER READING

Brown D C 2006 Atlas of regional anesthesia, 3rd edn. WB Saunders, London

Checketts M R, Wildsmith J A W 2004 Regional block and DVT prophylaxis. Continuing Education in Anaesthesia, Critical Care and Pain, 4(2): 48–51

Chelly J E, Casati A, Fanelli G 2001 Continuous peripheral nerve block techniques; an illustrated guide. Mosby, London

Cousins M J, Bridenbaugh P O 1998 Neural blockade in clinical anesthesia and management of pain, 3rd edn. Lippincott, Philadelphia

Coventry D M, Barker K, Thomson M 2001 Comparison of two neurostimulation techniques for axillary brachial plexus blockade. British Journal of Anaesthesia. 86: 80–83

Ellis H, Feldman S, Harrop Griffiths W 2004 Anatomy for anaesthetists, 8th edn. Blackwell Publishing, Oxford

Fischer H B J, Pinnock CA 2004 Fundamentals of regional anaesthesia. Cambridge University Press, Cambridge

Hahn M B, McQuillan P M, Sheplock G J 1996 Regional anesthesia; an atlas of anatomy and technique. Mosby, London

Neal J M, Hebl J R, Gerancher J C, Hogan Q H 2002 Brachial plexus anesthesia: essentials of our current understanding. Regional Anesthesia and Pain Medicine 27: 402–408

Peutrell J M, Mather S J 1997 Regional anaesthesia for babies and children. Oxford University Press, Oxford

Pinnock C A, Fischer H B J, Jones R P 1996 Peripheral nerve blockade. Churchill Livingstone, Edinburgh

Rigg J R A, Jamrozik K, Myles P S, Silbert B S, Peyton P J, Parsons R W, Collins K S. MASTER Anaesthesia Trial Study Group 2002 Epidural anaesthesia and analgesia and outcome of major surgery: a randomised trial. Lancet 359: 1276–1282

Sandhu N S, Capan L M 2002 Ultrasonic-guided infraclavicular brachial plexus block. British Journal of Anaesthesia 89: 254–259

Turnbull D K, Shepherd D B 2003 Post-dural puncture headache: pathogenesis, prevention and treatment. British Journal of Anaesthesia 91: 718–729

Wildsmith J A W, Armitage E N, McClure J H 2003 Principles and practice of regional anaesthesia, 3rd edn. Churchill Livingstone, Edinburgh

Winnie A P 1984 Plexus anesthesia, vol I. Perivascular techniques of brachial plexus block. Churchill Livingstone, New York

The ability to monitor the physiology of patients during anaesthesia has increased rapidly in recent years. While the increase in the numbers of monitors has increased the amount and quality of information available, the risks of misinformation and risks of patient harm have increased correspondingly. It is essential that those who use monitors understand their limitations and are able to justify their risks

GENERAL PRINCIPLES

Although monitors provide information on patient physiology and anaesthetic machine function, it is important to realize that most monitors do not directly measure the displayed variable. For example, an electrocardiograph (ECG) does not measure cardiac function and therefore a normal ECG trace does not guarantee that the heart is pumping effectively. An understanding of how a monitor works usually allows an operator to recognize when a monitor is not producing reliable readings.

In principle, each monitor consists of four components (Table 18.1): (1) a device that connects to the patient – this may either be a direct attachment or via a tube or lead; (2) a measuring device, often a transducer that converts the properties of the patient into an electrical signal; (3) a computer that may amplify the signal, filter it and integrate the signal with other variables to produce a variety of derived variables; (4) a display that may show the results as a wave, a number or a combination.

Currently, monitors are becoming increasingly more compact and integrated. This implies that information from different measuring modules may be shared and the reliability of readouts improved. To avoid misinterpretation of results, the following questions should be asked.

- *What is being measured?* In the case of arterial pressure, there is an obvious answer. However, in

some cases, for example 'depth of anaesthesia', it may not be clear what the monitor is measuring. In addition, many monitors use data from a variety of sources. For example, heart rate is usually derived from the ECG. However, if the ECG fails to provide the data required, the monitor often switches automatically to a rate from either a pulse oximeter or an arterial pressure waveform. Thus, the displayed value may change rapidly despite the patient remaining stable.

- *How is it measured?* Arterial pressure is often measured by either a transducer attached to an arterial cannula or an automated oscillometer. Although a transducer is often regarded as the most accurate, the readings must be compared with the preoperative values recorded on the ward, usually with an oscillometer. Therefore, where accurate control of arterial pressure is essential, it is advisable to start invasive pressure monitoring before anaesthesia to avoid any confusion with non-invasive measures.

- *Is the environment appropriate?* Many monitors have been designed for use in operating theatres and do not function correctly if exposed to the cold and vibration in an ambulance or helicopter. Another example is the strong magnetic field produced by magnetic resonance imaging (MRI) scanners. The electrical currents induced may damage not only noncompatible monitors but even produce burns to a patient's skin.

- *Is the patient appropriate?* Monitors designed for adult use often fail to produce reliable readings when used on small children. Particularly obese adults may require a large blood pressure cuff, and poor-quality readings may be obtained from ECGs.

- *Has the monitor been applied to the correct part of the patient?* For example, in aortic coarctation, arterial pressure may be markedly different in each arm. Pulse oximeters also fail to work reliably if placed on a limb distal to a blood pressure cuff.

- *Is the variable within the range of the monitor?* Most monitors are validated on healthy patients in

Table 18.1	Four components of a monitor
Connection to patient	
Measuring device	
Electronic filter/amplifier	
Display	

Table 18.2	Premonitoring checks
What is being measured?	
What method is being used?	
Has the monitor been serviced and calibrated?	
Is the environment appropriate?	
Is the patient appropriate?	
Is it attached to the appropriate part of the patient?	
Is the range appropriate?	
Can the display be read?	
Are the alarms on and have the limits been set?	

laboratories. Whether such monitors continue to provide accurate results during the extreme physiological changes of, for example, anaphylaxis is uncertain. This does imply that the usefulness of monitors declines with the health of the patient: that is, they are least reliable when needed most. In most cases of acute perioperative patient deterioration, additional monitoring is needed.

● *Has the monitor been checked, serviced and calibrated at the correct intervals?* To reduce costs, departments often re-use single-use equipment and fail to ensure service checks are carried out. All equipment should be tagged with a service sticker. This should identify the date serviced, when the next service is due and who to contact in case of malfunction. Equipment that has not been serviced or is past its service date should not be used.

Table 18.2 shows the checks which the anaesthetist should follow before using a patient monitor

DISPLAYS

The purpose of a monitor is not only to measure an aspect of the physiology of the patient but also to transmit that information to the anaesthetist (Fig. 18.1). The change from an assortment of boxes made by different manufacturers to a single, integrated monitoring system with a single display panel has made this less of a problem. In addition, current systems that use multiple measuring modules inserted into a larger display unit have also enabled additional functions to be added quickly and defective monitors changed.

Most of the current monitoring systems follow good ergonomic principles, with different variables separated consistently by position on the screen and by colour. This allows the most important information to be placed centrally in large symbols or fonts and in bold colours, with less important data either relegated to small print, or placed in submenus. However, the flexibility of most monitors implies that it is still possible for individuals to change colours and priorities, often making the monitor much less effective. Whenever possible,

departments should ensure that all monitors have identical default settings to reduce confusion (these are usually password protected). Unfortunately, the lack of international standards means that confusion may still occur where monitors from multiple sources are used in the same unit.

Despite many attempts to simplify patient data into geometric shapes or bar graphs, data continue to be displayed most often as simple numbers, supported by waveforms where desired. In many cases, trends over time may be displayed to make gradual change more obvious. Trends are particularly useful where

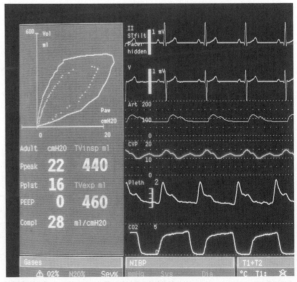

Fig. 18.1
Standard anaesthetic monitoring screen.

clinical problems may produce gradual change. For example, in neurosurgery a gradual decrease in end-tidal carbon dioxide concentration is often associated with multiple air emboli.

ALARMS

All monitors now include alarms which sound (and illuminate) when a variable moves outside the range set. These limits are usually set by the manufacturer as part of the monitoring system's basic functions and may be changed by the user (although the default values are often protected by a password).

This is a desirable function, as it may alert the anaesthetist to a developing physiological change and allow it to be corrected. However, alarms may not respond to a serious problem. For example, marked hypotension in an elderly hypertensive patient may still fall within the range of a 'normal' arterial pressure as set for the monitor.

More commonly, alarms are triggered by artefacts: for example, the electrical interference produced by diathermy often triggers an alarm for arrhythmia from the ECG. Also common is the production of alarms by spurious problems such as an apparently low end-tidal carbon dioxide concentration during induction of anaesthesia, produced by the gas leak around a face mask. The frequency of such false alarms implies that many alarms are ignored, or may lead the anaesthetist to concentrate on the monitoring equipment, and ignore the patient.

Further, because of the lack of standardization of alarm signals and the uniformity of alarms, in a genuine crisis, the cacophony of multiple alarms and series of flashing lights may cause staff to concentrate on a relatively unimportant complication, such as bradycardia, with the cause, such as a disconnection in the breathing system, going unnoticed.

ASSESSMENT OF THE CARDIOVASCULAR SYSTEM

CLINICAL

The principal aim of an anaesthetist is to ensure the delivery of oxygen to the patient's tissues. In physiological terms, oxygen delivery is the product of the cardiac output, the concentration of haemoglobin and its oxygen saturation. Clinically, if the patient is pink, with a normal volume pulse and has warm extremities, then these aims are being met. When combined with a urine output of greater than 0.5 mL h^{-1} it is unlikely that the patient has any cardiovascular problems. A further confirmatory test, especially useful in children, is the capillary refill time. When an extremity is compressed for 5 s, if capillary refill occurs in less than 1.5 s, cardiac output is adequate. If the refill time is greater than 5 s, then shock is likely to be present.

The need for direct patient observation cannot be overestimated. Literally having a 'finger on the pulse' and being able to see the patient are the most important safety factors. While factors such as drapes and dimmed theatre lights may make direct observation difficult, there should not be complete reliance on electronic monitoring.

ELECTROCARDIOGRAPHY

The ECG is a recording of the voltage difference produced between two electrodes placed on the body surface. In the three-lead system commonly in use, the third lead is used as a reference electrode. The voltage changes are very small and require amplification before being displayed as the familiar waveform. Also, different lead positions detect electrical activity from different parts of the myocardium. The commonest position of the electrodes used in the operating theatre is the CM5 arrangement, as this is the best position to detect ischaemia of the left ventricle (Fig. 18.2).

The ECG is a standard monitor used on all patients. The visible waveform allows the cardiac rhythm to be identified and may often be printed for further analysis. Alarms may be set to identify arrhythmias and brady/tachycardias. Many monitors are able to display a numerical value of the heart rate in addition to a measure of any ST segment depression/elevation

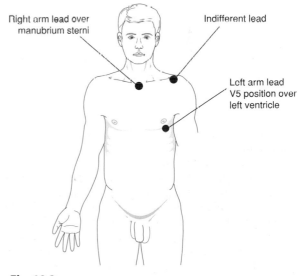

Fig. 18.2
CM5 configuration for electrocardiograph monitoring.

produced by cardiac ischaemia/infarction. This may be displayed as a trend over time and the success of treatment observed.

Unfortunately, the relatively small voltages measured are easily swamped by skeletal muscle activity or surgical diathermy, often leading to false alarms. The signal may also be severely degraded if the gel of the electrodes has been allowed to dry out or if the weight of the leads is allowed to pull on the electrodes. In addition, the monitor only identifies ischaemia in a single area; multiple lead systems are required to monitor the whole myocardium. While the ECG has become a standard monitor, it adds little to the information provided by palpating the pulse. It must be remembered that electrical activity does not always produce a cardiac output. Complications are rare, although the electrode adhesive may produce skin damage in susceptible patients.

ARTERIAL PRESSURE

Clinical methods

An adequate arterial pressure is essential for tissue perfusion; even when perfusion is adequate, hypotension may lead to renal failure. Arterial pressure may be most rapidly estimated by palpating a pulse, although this method is too unreliable as a single technique. While pressure may be estimated reliably by using a pressure gauge and inflatable cuff and either palpating the artery (systolic only) or listening to the Korotkov sounds, these methods are too time consuming during anaesthesia and often impossible because of poor patient access.

Automated oscillometer

The original automatic oscillometers used two cuffs. The upper cuff was inflated to occlude the arterial flow and then gradually deflated. As the blood flow began to pass under the upper cuff, the small changes in volume were detected by the lower cuff. Modern machines use a single cuff with two tubes for inflation/measurement. To avoid high cuff pressures and long deflation times, monitors inflate the cuff to just above a normal systolic pressure and then decrease the pressure until a pulse is detected. If a pulse is not detected, the cuff is then inflated to a higher pressure. This process may be repeated several times before a measurement is made (Fig. 18.3).

These monitors are now used for all except the shortest cases as they measure arterial pressure automatically, reading up to once every minute. In addition, the cuff may be applied under drapes to either an arm or leg.

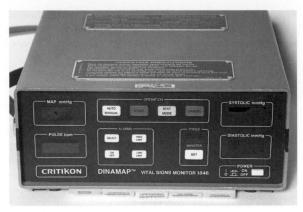

Fig. 18.3
An automated oscillometer.

The disadvantages of automated oscillometry are shown in Table 18.3.

Several other techniques have been used to measure arterial pressure, but have failed to find widespread usage. These include the Penaz technique, which measures the effect of external pressure on the blood flow through a finger, and other devices relying on pressure measurements over an artery, Doppler probes or detection of Korotkov sounds with a microphone.

Invasive arterial pressure

To measure arterial pressure, a cannula (usually 20–22G parallel-sided Teflon) must first be inserted into the artery. This is connected to a transducer by a continuous column of saline contained within a tube.

Table 18.3   Disadvantages of automated oscillometry
Delayed measurement with arrhythmias or patient movement
Inaccuracy with systolic pressure <60 mmHg
Inaccurate if the wrong size cuff used
May be inaccurate in obese patients
Discomfort in awake patients
Skin and nerve damage in prolonged use
Delay in injected drugs reaching the circulation
Backflow of blood into i.v. cannulae
Pulse oximeter malfunction as cuff is inflated

The radial artery is most often chosen as occlusion of the artery is usually compensated for by flow through the ulnar artery. As fluids are incompressible, the pressure in the artery should be transmitted directly to the transducer, which converts pressure into an electrical signal that is displayed by the monitor. To prevent the cannula blocking, the system includes a pressurized bag of heparinized saline that produces a flow of 1–3 mL h^{-1} through a restrictor. Systems also include the facility to allow a higher flow rate to flush the system, for example after a sample has been taken. The transducer should be at the level of the left ventricle and the transducer opened to the atmosphere to provide a zero reading before use. Monitors usually display systolic and diastolic pressures. The waveform can also provide a rapidly appreciated estimate of pressure. The variability or 'swing' in pressure produced during positive pressure ventilation is commonly used to detect relative hypovolaemia.

The advantage of such systems is that they provide a real-time measure of arterial pressure, which is essential when administering drugs such as vasopressors to sick patients (Table 18.4). They also provide a means for obtaining samples for arterial blood gas analysis and other blood tests. The use of arterial cannulae has therefore become standard practice for severely ill patients, both in the operating theatre and in the intensive care unit.

However, errors are common as a result of malpositioning of the transducers and failure to zero the transducer before use. For example, if the operating table is moved upwards while the transducer remains static, the difference in height artificially increases the pressure reading. Further, while modern disposable sets are usually reliable and accurate, they may occasionally malfunction. Unusual readings should therefore be checked against a reading from a non invasive monitor.

Although modern pressure monitoring sets are carefully designed to avoid the problems of resonance, damping may still be produced by air bubbles, clots and damaged cannulae. In particular, failure to ensure that the cannula is continuously flushed results in clot formation. Damage to the arterial intima can result in partial blockage and failure to read accurately within days of cannula insertion.

Complications relating to arterial cannulae are shown in Table 18.5.

CENTRAL VENOUS PRESSURE

Central venous pressure is often considered a measure of the amount of blood within the venous system; a pressure less than normal (2–3 mmHg) indicates hypovolaemia and a higher pressure indicates volume overload. While such a view is reliable for healthy patients with acute blood loss, it is not so simple in other circumstances. For example, patients with damage to the right side of the heart may have raised central venous pressure even when the filling pressure of the left side of the heart is low. Single measurements rarely provide an accurate reflection of the fluid status of the patient. However, repeated measurements taken while a fluid challenge is given are often very informative.

There are four common routes for central venous catheterization.

Long catheters inserted via the antecubital fossa are relatively easy and safe to insert but are of small diameter. Catheters inserted via the basilic vein often cannot be advanced past the shoulder and even catheters inserted into the cephalic vein may encounter resistance. It is also difficult to determine if the tip of the catheter is within a central vein without X-ray imaging.

Table 18.4 Advantages of direct arterial pressure measurement
Accuracy of pressure measurement
Beat-by-beat observation of changes when blood pressure is variable or when vasoactive drugs are used
Accuracy at low pressures
Ability to obtain frequent blood samples

Table 18.5 Complications relating to arterial cannulae
Requires skill to insert
Bleeding
Pain on insertion
Arterial damage and thrombosis
Embolization of thrombus or air
Ischaemia to tissues distal to puncture site
Sepsis
Inadvertent injection of drugs
Late development of fistula or aneurysm

Thrombosis of the veins is common if the catheter is left in situ for more than 24 h.

Femoral venous catheters are inserted just below the inguinal ligament. They are also relatively easy to insert and may be of large gauge to allow rapid transfusion of fluids. This route is often chosen in children. However, the site of insertion is often within a skin fold, making skin sepsis more likely.

Internal jugular catheters are used most commonly as the vein is superficial, of larger diameter, and easily managed. This is the route that is often most appropriate for use in an emergency. However, the insertion point is adjacent to several vital structures, including the carotid artery, lung, brachial plexus and cervical spine, with the result that direct needle trauma to these structures is common. Recent guidelines have made the use of an ultrasonic probe advisable for insertion of a catheter via the internal jugular route.

Subclavian catheters suffer the same problems as those in the internal jugular vein, although the point of insertion under the clavicle may make it easier to anchor the catheter to the skin. However, if accidental arterial puncture occurs, the overlying clavicle obscures bleeding and makes direct compression of the artery impossible. The proximity of the pleura is associated with a risk of accidental lung puncture. The subclavian route should therefore be used only when the internal jugular approach is contraindicated.

As the central venous pressure is relatively low, it may be measured using a simple manometer (Fig. 18.4). A vertical tube is filled with saline from an intravenous fluid bag via a three-way tap. The three-way tap is then rotated so that the column of saline is attached to the central venous cannula and the level of saline allowed to fall until it equilibrates with the venous pressure. If the base of the column has been previously aligned with the mid axillary line, then the height of the column can be read directly to give the central venous pressure. Unfortunately, as central venous pressure is normally only a few centimetres of water, great care is required to ensure that the pressure is read relative to the correct zero point (the right atrium) on the patient (Fig. 18.5). Unless a spirit level and great care are employed, large errors may occur. This method is also time consuming and requires easy access to the patient, so is suitable only for ward use.

When used perioperatively, a central venous catheter is usually connected to the same type of transducer and flush system described for arterial cannulae. This provides a continuous readout of pressure, allowing the effect of infusions of fluids to be assessed in real time. Although a single reading of central venous pressure is of little diagnostic use, changes in

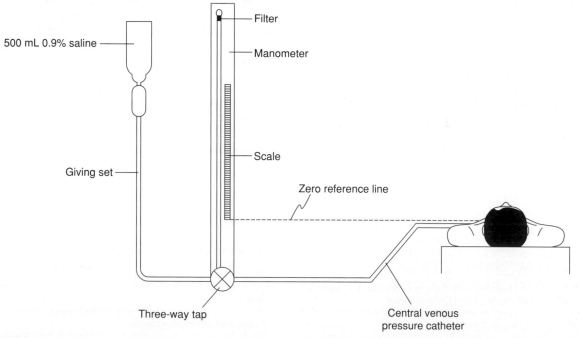

Fig 18.4
Measurement of central venous pressure using a manometer.

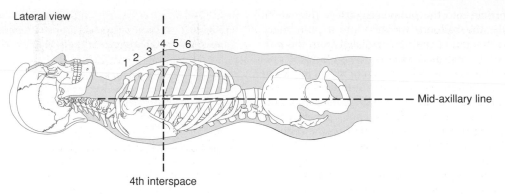

Fig. 18.5
Surface markings used to identify the position of the right atrium.

response to fluid challenge is much more informative. In general, if a fluid challenge has little effect on the central venous pressure, the patient is likely to be hypovolaemic. In contrast, a marked increase in pressure indicates fluid overload.

Complications are infrequent but potentially serious, and are shown in Table 18.6.

PULMONARY ARTERY PRESSURE

Although a central venous cannula may be used to estimate venous volume, it measures the filling of the right side of the heart. However, cardiac output and systemic arterial pressure are determined primarily by the filling pressure of the left side of the heart.

When introduced, the pulmonary artery flotation catheter (PAFC), with its ability to measure cardiac output and left atrial pressure, appeared to be a major advance. Recently, however, frequent complications and a lack of evidence of improved survival have led to a decline in its use. The PAFC is also known as a Swan-Ganz or balloon tip catheter (Fig. 18.6).

A PAFC is a long catheter with three or four lumens, and a thermistor near the tip. It is inserted into a neck vein through a large cannula. A flexible plastic sheath allows the catheter to be inserted, withdrawn and rotated after insertion without desterilizing it. After insertion into the superior vena cava, saline is injected to inflate a balloon at the tip. The pressure at the tip is measured via a transducer and displayed on a monitor. The catheter is then advanced slowly so that the blood flow directs the catheter toward the pulmonary artery. As the catheter is advanced, a series of changes in pressure is observed, marking the progression through the right atrium and

Table 18.6 Complications of central venous catheterization
Acute
Arrhythmias
Bleeding
Air embolus
Pneumothorax
Damage to thoracic duct, oesophagus, carotid artery, stellate ganglion
Cardiac puncture
Catheter embolization
Delayed
Sepsis
Thrombosis
Cardiac rupture

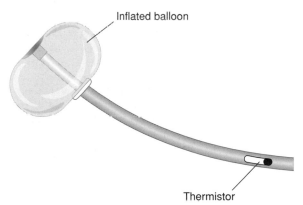

Fig. 18.6
Distal end of a pulmonary artery catheter showing inflated balloon and thermistor.

right ventricle into the pulmonary artery (Fig. 18.7). Eventually, the balloon 'wedges' into a pulmonary artery. At this point, the tip is isolated from the pulmonary artery and measures the pressure in the pulmonary capillaries, which is taken to reflect left atrial pressure. Although the ability to estimate left atrial pressure is useful, the interpretation of measurements is as problematic as for central venous pressure (see above). For the same reasons, measuring the changes after a fluid challenge is more useful than a single reading.

The ability to measure the filling pressure of the left ventricle as well as as the cardiac output was a major advance, and has led to many advances in our understanding of cardiac physiology and the mechanisms and treatments of diseases such as sepsis.

However, the process of insertion described above is not always straightforward and prolonged manipulation may be needed to direct the catheter into the pulmonary artery.

Arrhythmias are extremely common with catheter insertion and the technique carries all the risks of central venous catheterization noted above in addition to the risks shown in Table 18.7.

CARDIAC OUTPUT

Cardiac output is closely linked to oxygen delivery; in addition, studies have shown that low cardiac output is linked to increased mortality. However, it must be remembered that cardiac output is intermittent and not continuous and that factors such as the pressure changes caused by respiration (especially positive pressure ventilation), changes in heart rate and arrhythmias produce complex changes. Therefore, monitors do not produce consistent results even when used carefully.

Dilution techniques have been regarded as the 'gold standard' against which other methods are compared. In simple terms, a marker is injected into

Table 18.7   Risks of pulmonary artery catheterization (in addition to those shown in Table 18.6)
Arrhythmias with catheter manipulation
Damage to tricuspid and pulmonary valves
Knotting of catheter
Pulmonary infarction if balloon left inflated
Pulmonary artery rupture with balloon inflation
Cardiac rupture

a central vein and its concentration measured distally. If the cardiac output is large, the marker is diluted by a large volume of blood and the concentration is low. If the cardiac output is low, the marker is diluted less and the concentration is greater. In practice, a computer is used to convert the measured concentrations into a blood flow. The original studies used a dye, indocyanine green, which was injected into a central vein, with its concentration measured via an arterial catheter. The main problem with this technique is that when the dye has been measured at the artery it passes back to the heart and then back to the arteries (known as recirculation), making the calculations more complex. As the dye is cleared from the circulation only slowly, repeated measurements are impossible. Recently, monitors that use an injection of lithium as a marker have been introduced. These measure the blood lithium concentration with a modified arterial catheter.

Thermodilution method

This requires a PAFC to be inserted into the pulmonary artery. In the 'intermittent' technique, a bolus

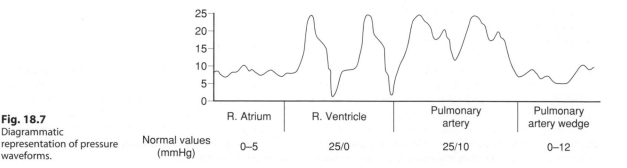

Fig. 18.7
Diagrammatic representation of pressure waveforms.

	R. Atrium	R. Ventricle	Pulmonary artery	Pulmonary artery wedge
Normal values (mmHg)	0–5	25/0	25/10	0–12

of cold saline is injected into the proximal lumen (entering the circulation at the right atrium) which then mixes with the blood flow and passes into the pulmonary artery where the small decrease in temperature is measured by a thermistor. The smaller the temperature drop, the larger is the cardiac output. The advantage of this technique is that recirculation of the marker is not a problem. More recently, monitors have been developed which do not require a pulmonary arterial catheter. These use a bolus of iced saline injected into a modified central venous catheter and a peripheral arterial catheter with a built-in thermistor.

In practice, the method is time-consuming as three separate readings are required to produce a reliable mean result. The procedure also needs to be repeated after each change of therapy.

More recently, 'continuous' cardiac output monitors have been introduced. These use a similar principle, but instead of using a bolus of cold saline, the catheter has an electrical coil which is heated at intervals, creating a bolus of warm blood that passes into the pulmonary artery. This eliminates much of the operator error and produces frequently updated measurements of cardiac output, allowing the effect of interventions to be observed. Most of the current monitors allow the data to be integrated with other measurements such as arterial pressure to provide calculated values of, for example, systemic vascular resistance and stroke volume. This aids the choice and administration of drugs such as vasoconstrictors.

Unfortunately, many factors make the readings prone to error. First, cardiac output is not a continuous flow, and measurements should be synchronized to the heartbeat and respiratory cycle to be accurate. Further, it appears that the mortality associated with the use of a PAFC may outweigh any improvements in care. They should be used only by experienced staff when there is a clear indication for their use.

Transthoracic/oesophageal Doppler probes

These use the principle that when ultrasound waves bounce off a moving object their frequency is changed and the amount of change is proportional to the speed of the object. In practice, a beam of ultrasonic waves is focused on the descending aorta and reflections from red cells are measured by a transducer in the same probe. Probes may be transthoracic (usually placed in the sternal notch) or placed in the oesophagus. The speed of the red cells and some assumptions about the diameter and shape of the aorta are then used to derive a value for the cardiac output. Note that flow in the descending aorta is not the whole cardiac output, as major arteries have already branched to the upper body.

The advantages of these systems is that they produce an almost real-time reading of cardiac output so that changes in output in response to drugs or fluids are seen almost immediately.

These systems are reliant on the ultrasound beam being directed at the centre of the aorta and the aorta being a smooth tube. In practice, even small movements of the sensor may lead to marked changes in readings as the speed of red cells near the aortic wall is measured. Abnormalities of the aorta such as atheroma may also affect readings. Oesophageal probes are more accurate, but are not always tolerated well by conscious patients. Most machines now provide a visual (and audible) measure of signal strength to allow the user to identify when the probe has moved.

These probes are especially useful in high-risk patients who require relatively minor surgery as they may be used to monitor cardiac output during anaesthesia without the risks associated with the insertion of multiple intravascular catheters. However, although they may be used to determine whether a change in therapy has had a positive or negative effect, they are unable to provide reliable estimates of cardiac output in absolute terms. Complications are rare.

Transoesophageal echocardiography

Transoesophageal echocardiography uses a miniaturized ultrasonic probe inserted into the oesophagus under anaesthesia. It provides a real-time picture of all four cardiac chambers and valves. Its advantage is that it can identify any malfunctioning valves in addition to any wall-motion abnormalities related to myocardinal ischaemia. It can also identify if therapy has successfully treated the ischaemia.

However, these probes are expensive to purchase and require an operator who is trained both to use the equipment and to interpret the results. They are especially useful as patients come off bypass after cardiac surgery to ensure that both the myocardium and valves are functioning correctly. Although they cannot provide a numeric value for cardiac output, they are useful in estimating cardiac preload. They are rarely used in non-cardiac surgery.

Pulse contour

These monitors use the principle that the shape of the arterial pulse (the pulse contour) is a product of the rate of ejection of blood into the aorta and the elasticity of the arterial tree. Therefore, if some assumptions are made about the arterial tree, the volume ejected at each heartbeat may be calculated from the shape of the arterial pulse contour.

This system has the advantage of being able to calculate the cardiac output in near real time using an arterial cannula alone.

However, the technique relies on assumptions on arterial tree elasticity that may not always be correct in every patient. Therefore, these systems often require calibration by another method such as thermodilution every 8–12 h to ensure accuracy. The costs of the computer and consumables are also considerable.

Currently, there is no entirely satisfactory method for the measurement of cardiac output, as those methods with high accuracy and reliability are cumbersome and have high complication rates.

PULSE OXIMETRY

Pulse oximeters measure the pulse rate and haemoglobin oxygen saturation by measuring changes in light absorbed by an extremity. The method relies on the principle that the amount of light absorbed by a solution is proportional to the concentration. Therefore, if the absorption can be measured, the concentration may be calculated. Each organic molecule absorbs light of different wavelengths to varying degrees. When plotted as a graph of absorption against wavelength, this is known as an absorption spectrum (see Fig. 12.12).

This implies that if the absorption spectra of a mixture of molecules in solution are known and the absorption of light of different wavelengths is measured, then it is possible to calculate the proportion of each molecule present. In practice, some tissues such as an ear, toe or finger are treated as a chamber containing a solution of haemoglobin and the probe is place around it. One side of the probe contains an array of light-emitting diodes (LEDs) and the other contains a light sensor.

The monitor then progresses through the following steps.

1. The sensor first measures the ambient light and subtracts this value from all other measurements. This implies that sudden changes in ambient light levels, e.g. after drapes are moved, may cause transient errors.
2. An LED is turned on and off rapidly. The absorption of transmitted light is then measured and the variations with time are recorded. The result is a waveform with a trough as blood flows into the finger (more absorption) during systole and a peak as blood flows into the veins in diastole. The monitor requires around eight heartbeats to make a calculation and then assumes the frequency of this waveform is the heart rate. Frequent ectopic

beats or atrial fibrillation may lead to a delay in calculation or unreliable results.
3. The monitor then analyses the measurements and splits the absorption into two components. The fixed or unchanging absorption is assumed to result from tissues such as skin, muscle and bone (Fig. 12.13). The varying absorption is then assumed to be caused by arterial blood moving into the tissue. In situations such as hypotension, hypovolaemia or hypothermia, pulsation may be reduced to the point where the monitor is not able to make any calculations and it fails to read. When a patient is on cardiac bypass the tissues are perfused, but if the flow is non-pulsatile pulse oximeters cannot provide a reading.
4. Steps 1–3 are repeated sequentially using light of at least two different wavelengths at around 120 cycles s^{-1}. When the absorptions of each different wavelength are known, the proportion of oxygenated and deoxygenated haemoglobin may be calculated. The measurements are processed and a new value displayed around every 8 s. However, these calculations are based on the assumption that the blood only contains normal haemoglobin and that no abnormal light-absorbing substances (dyes) are present. For example, if the patient has breathed carbon monoxide, the monoxycarboxyhaemoglobin (as it has a similar absorption spectrum) is measured as oxyhaemoglobin. The result is that patients suffering from carbon monoxide poisoning usually give a reading close to 100% saturation, even though they have severe hypoxaemia. The use of intravascular dyes as markers, or even nail varnish, may produce unpredictable results. Lastly, if the probe slips partially off the patient, some light passes directly from the LEDs to the light sensor and also through the sensor. This also causes unreliable readings.

Pulse oximeters provide rapid, non-invasive measurement of pulse rate and estimate of oxygen saturation. The pulse oximeter has become one of the most widely used monitors and is particularly useful in situations in which it is difficult to identify cyanosis: for example if light levels are low, in pigmented patients and in areas where access is difficult such as CT/MRI scanners. Pulse oximeters are also used to measure the oxygen saturation in patients with intermittent respiratory problems: for example, postoperative patients and those with sleep apnoea. Advances in technology have resulted in several small battery-powered devices becoming available for out-of-hospital use. The accuracy of pulse oximeters is around ± 2% above an oxygen saturation of 70%.

Accuracy below 70% is not known precisely, because it is not ethical to conduct trials at these levels. It is important to note that, especially when oxygen therapy is used, normal oxygen saturation does not equate to normal ventilation. For example, in opioid overdose, hypoventilation may lead to potentially fatal hypercapnia without any decrease in oxygen saturation if the patient is breathing a high concentration of oxygen. Complications are rare. The major drawbacks of pulse oximetry are listed in Table 18.8.

ASSESSMENT OF RESPIRATORY FUNCTION

CLINICAL

Continuous visual monitoring of the colour and the pattern of ventilation of the patient are essential for safe anaesthesia. When the patient is breathing spontaneously, observation should detect signs of airway obstruction, e.g. tracheal tug, paradoxical movement and failure of the anaesthetic reservoir bag to move.

Maintenance of the airway in an anaesthetized patient is a skilled task. Although the introduction of the laryngeal mask has led to a reduction in the frequency of need for airway skills, airway maintenance still remains one of the most basic tasks for the anaesthetist. Auscultation of the chest with a stethoscope may confirm the presence of normal breath sounds and also detect additional sounds caused by secretions, oedema or bronchospasm. Although useful, clinical signs cannot reliably disprove oesophageal placement of a tracheal tube.

Oesophageal stethoscope

This consists of a balloon-tipped catheter that may also carry a temperature probe. It is connected to either an earpiece or stethoscope and inserted into the patient's oesophagus. The catheter is advanced until the heart sounds are maximal and then taped at the nose. It provides a constant monitor of both heart rate and ventilation and is said to be able to identify the characteristic 'millwheel murmur' of an air embolus. It is most often

used in children. In addition to being inexpensive, it carries little morbidity and has the great advantage of forcing the anaesthetist to remain beside the patient.

Respiratory rate

The rate may be timed clinically or more often derived from the capnograph. Many ECG monitors use the leads to pass a very small high-frequency alternating current across the chest; the increase in electrical impedance (resistance to an alternating current) produced by the inhalation of gas into the lungs is measured and the respiratory rate calculated.

Airway pressure

The lungs are damaged easily and although anaesthetic machines incorporate pressure relief valves, these are designed to protect the machine rather than the patient. Although electronic ventilators usually allow a maximum airway pressure to be set to protect the patient, excessive pressure may still be exerted by manual compression of the bag. The self-inflating bags used for resuscitation are often capable of exerting extremely high pressures. As even transient peaks of pressure may lead to lung trauma or pneumothorax, a pressure monitor should be used whenever positive-pressure ventilation is used.

As all ventilators now incorporate pressure monitors, separate airway pressure monitors are rarely used. Most ventilators include a pressure transducer in the form of a piezoelectric crystal that converts pressure to an electrical potential, which is then measured by the monitor and displayed.

Although such monitors are both accurate and reliable, it must be remembered that they measure the pressure within the monitor and not the airway pressure. Therefore, the measured pressure may not be reliable if narrow tracheal tubes, long circuits or high-frequency ventilation are used. High lung pressures may be a particular problem in obese patients, those positioned head down and those with bronchospasm.

In devices without electronic components, such as ventilators used for transport, pressure is measured by devices in which the air pressure deforms a bellows or a metal tube. The deformation is linked to a needle with the pressure read from a scale. These are simple devices and are usually reliable, but are susceptible to damage by excess pressure.

Tidal volume

This principally involves the measurement of gas flow, which is then integrated with time to produce a calculated volume. Most monitors process a variety of measurements

Table 18.8	Disadvantages of pulse oximetry
Damage to skin caused by pressure from probe	
Failure to detect hypoxaemia in carbon monoxide poisoning	
Failure to detect hypoventilation	

to produce calculated variables such as compliance, minute volume and pressure/volume loops. There are three methods of measuring gas flow in common use and these rely on Poiseuille's law, rotating vanes or hot wire.

A hot wire anemometer consists of a wire stretched across a tube. A constant electrical current is passed across the wire causing it to heat, increasing its electrical resistance. As gas flows down the tube it cools the wire and decreases its resistance. The rate of flow of the gas may then be calculated from the resistance of the wire. This method is inexpensive, robust, reliable and works over a wide range of flows. However, it is not able to determine the direction of gas flow.

Devices relying on Poiseuille's law consist of one or more tubes with a pressure monitor at each end. Poiseuille's law states that for laminar flow of gas through a tube, the flow rate is directly proportional to the pressure difference across the tube, so, when calibrated, the flow may easily be calculated from the pressure difference. The Fleisch pneumotachograph consists of a series of narrow tubes associated with heating elements (to reduce condensation) and pressure sensors at each end. The Datex D-lite sensor consists of a plastic connector that is fitted into a breathing system. The connector incorporates a slight narrowing, with tubes at each end connected to pressure sensors in the main module. These devices are robust and accurate, but are susceptible to partial blockage of the tubing, especially by water condensation. They also have a limited response range.

Rotating vane flow meters use a system of vanes to deflect the airflow to a rotor. The rotor spins faster as the airflow increases, and this is detected electronically. The device most often used is the Wright respirometer, which usually incorporates a gauge to measure tidal and minute volumes. It is a simple and reliable device, but has a tendency to underread low flows and overread high flows. It is also susceptible to rough handling and accumulation of moisture.

DISCONNECTION ALARMS

Although these alarms were previously mandatory when positive-pressure ventilation was used, they are now rarely used as separate devices because ventilators incorporate monitoring and alarm systems based on failure to detect tidal volume or a change in carbon dioxide tension. Disconnection alarms usually measured cyclical changes in pressure; failure of the airway pressure to change cyclically then triggered an alarm.

TISSUE OXYGENATION

Transcutaneous oxygen sensors are applied to the skin, which is heated to around 42°C. An oxygen sensor is allowed to equilibrate with the tissue. These probes may be used in neonates, but not in adults, because the skin is too thick. They have a very slow response time and are rarely used in anaesthetic practice. It is also possible to estimate arterial carbon dioxide tension using the same principles.

GAS MONITORING

Measurement of the concentration of gases and vapours in anaesthetic breathing systems is vital to prevent hypoxaemia and ensure the delivery of anaesthetic agents.

Oxygen concentration

Oxygen concentration in a breathing system is measured using either a fuel cell or a paramagnetic analyser.

The fuel cell is the more common device. It contains a lead anode within a small container of electrode gel. When exposed to oxygen, the lead is converted to lead oxide, producing a small voltage that may be measured and amplified. Fuel cells are small, robust and reliable, although they require calibration at regular intervals. After a period of around 6 months, they require replacement as the lead becomes oxidized. Accuracy is better than ± 1% with a response time of <10 s.

The principle of the paramagnetic analyser is that oxygen molecules are attracted weakly to a magnetic field (paramagnetic). Most other anaesthetic gases are repelled by a magnetic field (diamagnetic). In the analyser, a powerful magnetic field is passed across a chamber that contains two nitrogen-containing spheres suspended on a wire. When oxygen is introduced into the chamber, it tends to displace the spheres, causing them to rotate. The degree of rotation is measured to estimate the oxygen concentration. These monitors are accurate, reliable and do not need frequent maintenance. However, they are more bulky and less robust than a fuel cell.

In both cases, the monitors measure the partial pressure of oxygen, but display oxygen as a percentage. If the pressure within the circuit is increased, for example when a gas-driven ventilator is employed, they overestimate the oxygen concentration.

Carbon dioxide and anaesthetic gases

Carbon dioxide, nitrous oxide and anaesthetic vapours are usually measured using infrared absorption. This uses the principle that each gas absorbs light at different wavelengths. Therefore, a cell is arranged with light sources on one side of a chamber and photoelectric cells on the other. The test gas is then passed through the chamber and the amount of light absorbed is measured. According to Beer–Lambert laws, the amount of light absorbed is proportional to the concentration of the gas. In practice, the chambers have mirrors on each side so the light passes across the chamber many times to amplify the absorption. The chamber is also heated to avoid condensation. Accuracy is around 0.5% with a response time of <0.5 s. Unfortunately, interactions between different molecules can cause interference; for example, the presence of nitrous oxide results in overestimation of the concentration of carbon dioxide. This was a problem with early monitors that used a single light source. Modern monitors use multiple light sources at different wavelengths so that the gases present may be identified accurately. However, the presence of large amounts of unexpected vapours, such as ethanol from an intoxicated patient, may still introduce errors.

Most analysers pump a small flow of gas out of a circuit to be analysed in the main monitoring box, a 'main stream' system. This involves some delay while the gas is pumped to the monitor. The movement of gas may also reduce accuracy if mixing of inspiratory and expiratory gas occurs. In most cases, the sampled gas is passed into the scavenging system, but when low flows are required it may be returned to the circuit. This arrangement allows the sensing chamber to be housed within a monitor, making it more robust.

The alternative 'side stream' system places the sensing chamber in a connector within the patient breathing system and so reduces any delay in measurement. However, it also makes the sensor more prone to accidental damage.

The carbon dioxide concentration in respired gases is displayed most often as a graph of concentration against time (capnogram). This provides visual confirmation that the airway is patent and that ventilation is occurring. It also provides the only reliable guarantee after intubation that the tube is not in the oesophagus.

At the start of expiration the carbon dioxide concentration is zero (dead space gas). The concentration then increases to a plateau level (alveolar gas). The end-tidal value of carbon dioxide concentration is used usually as a measure of the adequacy of ventilation because it approximates to alveolar and therefore arterial carbon dioxide partial pressure. However, when the respiratory rate is high, if tidal volume is low, if the sampling point is distant from the airway or if the gases tend to mix in the circuit, the 'end-tidal' value tends to be low. This may give the impression that the lungs are being hyperventilated. For these reasons, it is difficult to measure end-tidal carbon dioxide meaningfully in small children. This is also true in patients, often smokers, who have marked ventilation/perfusion mismatch; there is often a prolonged upstroke on the capnograph trace and the relationship between end-tidal and arterial carbon dioxide tensions becomes less reliable. If the capnograph trace does not appear to resemble a square wave, problems should be suspected and the arterial carbon dioxide partial pressure should be checked by blood gas analysis (Fig. 18.8).

If lung perfusion is compromised, either by a low cardiac output or by pulmonary emboli or an air embolus, the end-tidal carbon dioxide tension decreases as carbon dioxide delivery to the lungs decreases. Paradoxically, arterial carbon dioxide partial pressure increases. Therefore, in situations where air emboli are likely, for example in neurosurgery, any alteration in end-tidal carbon dioxide should be investigated by blood gas analysis.

Other gas monitors

Although infrared analysers are used usually for measuring the concentration of anaesthetic agents, other methods are used occasionally either for calibration or for complex analyses.

When a sample is introduced into a mass spectrometer, it passes into a vacuum where it is bombarded with high-energy electrons. These break up larger molecules and strip off their outer electrons. The resulting positively charged ions are accelerated in an electric field into a magnetic field. The magnetic field causes the

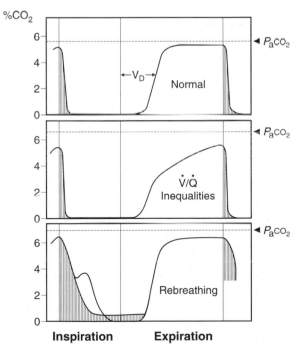

Fig. 18.8
Carbon dioxide traces recorded from the connector of the tracheal tube. $\dot{V}/\dot{Q}$, ventilation/perfusion.

moving particles to curve depending on how heavy they are. A row of sensors then measures the number of molecules and their sizes. Mass spectrometers are expensive to purchase and maintain, but are extremely accurate and can identify a wide range of compounds. They may be sited centrally within large theatre complexes as part of a calibration and quality control system.

A gas chromatograph consists of a column packed with inert beads covered in a thin film of oil, through which a constant stream of inert gas passes. When a sample of gas is introduced at one end, the mixture passes into the column and past the oil. Insoluble gases tend to stay in the carrier gas and move through the column quickly, while soluble gases tend to dissolve in the oil, slowing their progress. At the other end of the column is a flame through which the gas passes. As the test gases pass through the column and into the flame, they cause an increase in luminescence that may be measured. Thus, any gas may be identified by the time it takes to pass through the column and its quantity measured by the amount of luminescence. Their chief advantage is the ability to identify the components in a mixture of unknown compounds.

Lastly, a high-powered laser can be passed through a sample of gas. In a process known as the 'Raman effect', the light interacts with the molecules, causing a scattering of light of different wavelengths. The change in wavelength is characteristic of the molecule under study. Thus, sensors placed at the side of the chamber may detect this radiation and identify the gases present. The size and complexity of this technique have restricted its use.

THE NERVOUS SYSTEM

The best monitor of cerebral function is the patient, who is able to report symptoms such as numbness, loss of function or pain. During general anaesthesia, this monitoring function is lost and it is possible for patients to develop major neurological deficits during anaesthesia that become evident only during the recovery phase. For example, patients who have suffered head trauma may develop undiagnosed cerebral oedema under anaesthesia if appropriate monitoring, such as intracranial pressure measurement, is not used. During procedures that carry a high risk of ischaemia or seizure activity, such as carotid endarterectomy, this problem may be avoided by performing the procedure under local anaesthesia; however, this may not always be acceptable to patients or possible because of unrelated medical problems. In general, therefore, patients at risk of cerebral malfunction should be anaesthetized only if there is no alternative.

Where general anaesthesia is used, estimating the 'depth of anaesthesia' has always been a function of the anaesthetist using clinical signs such as heart rate, blood pressure, sweating and pupillary dilatation. Unfortunately, especially in the presence of autonomic neuropathy, such clinical signs are not reliable enough to avoid the risk of awareness during surgery.

It should be noted that there is no widely accepted definition of what 'anaesthesia' represents. Although it may be characterized in terms of lack of perception, lack of responsiveness and inability to recall, these are all poorly defined concepts. Therefore, any monitor cannot measure 'depth of anaesthesia' in the same way as arterial pressure. Further, what is required is not a monitor that can detect awareness, but a monitor that can predict the onset of awareness and allow the anaesthetist to act before awareness occurs. Another reason to measure depth of anaesthesia is the ability to ensure that each patient receives only the minimum amount of anaesthetic required to maintain unconsciousness. This may have the potential to greatly reduce the side-effects of anaesthesia and improve recovery times.

THE ISOLATED FOREARM TECHNIQUE

In this method, a patient is anaesthetized, and then a tourniquet is applied to the upper arm and inflated to above systolic arterial pressure. A muscle relaxant is then administered (if required as part of the appropriate anaesthetic technique). As the tourniquet prevents the muscle relaxant passing to the arm, the forearm muscles still function and are supplied by nerves passing under the tourniquet. If awareness occurs, the patient is able to signal by moving the forearm. Unfortunately, the technique signals only that the patient is already awake and its duration is limited by the ischaemia caused by the tourniquet.

THE ELECTROENCEPHALOGRAM AND EVOKED POTENTIALS

The electroencephalogram (EEG) is a complex signal that is recorded usually from at least four electrodes fixed to specially prepared sites around the head. The complexity of the raw EEG signals makes its use in the operating theatre impractical.

Two methods are used currently to make the signal easier to interpret. Spectral analysis uses the principle that any complex wave may be broken down into a series of sine waves. Fast Fourier analysis produces an analysis in terms of the proportion of each frequency that contributes to the total signal. Bispectral analysis uses relationships between the phase and power of different frequencies within the original signal.

Initial attempts using spectral analysis showed that general anaesthesia produces a reduction in the mean frequency and spectral edge (frequency below which 95% of activity occurs). Ultimately, increasing doses of anaesthesia produce a suppressed or isoelectric EEG. Unfortunately, these changes have not proved to be reliable as a measure of depth of anaesthesia.

The bispectral index (BIS monitor) is a number from 100 (awake) to 0 (deeply anaesthetised) produced by a commercially available monitor. Although the exact methods used have not been published, it identifies patterns within 30-s periods of EEG, by first excluding episodes likely to be produced by diathermy or muscle activity and periods of burst suppression. The remaining activity is subjected to bispectral analysis with the final result adjusted to take account of the proportion of suppressed EEG. It appears to provide reliable measurements in clinical use. However, it is not clear how factors such as different anaesthetic agents, hypoxaemia or epileptic activity affect the results.

AUDITORY EVOKED POTENTIALS

Auditory evoked potential monitors measure the slowing of auditory information processing produced by anaesthetic agents. The patient wears headphones that repeatedly play soft 'clicks'. Each click produces neuronal activity in the auditory cortex. While the signal from a single click is masked by other brain activity, the signal from repeated clicks may be averaged to isolate the auditory signal. The activity in the auditory cortex may therefore be displayed as the auditory evoked potential, which has a characteristic waveform (Fig. 18.9). The time delay for some waves can then be measured and the result converted into a value typically from zero to 100, reflecting depth of anaesthesia. The equipment cannot be used in patients who have impaired hearing and may require several seconds to generate enough data to process. Monitors using this principle are commercially available, but have yet to be used widely. Equipment using either visual or somatosensory stimulation have also been developed.

Respiratory sinus arrhythmia is the normal variation in heart rate related to the respiratory cycle. This variability is reduced by anaesthesia and has formed the basis of a commercially available monitor. However, it has not achieved widespread use.

Monitors based on physiological measures such as frontalis muscle myography and lower oesophageal contractility have not proved reliable enough for clinical use.

BRAIN OXYGENATION

The crucial need to ensure brain oxygenation and the inability to monitor consciousness during anaesthesia imply that an electronic monitor would be especially valuable, especially during neurosurgery and in head-injured patients. Unfortunately, none of the currently available techniques has proved suitable for general use.

Near infrared spectroscopy (NIRS) uses a pulse oximeter probe attached to the patient's head to detect light reflected from the patient's brain. While the technique may be used in small children, whose skull is thin, doubts remain in adults as to whether this technique reflects brain oxygenation or merely scalp blood flow.

Transcranial Doppler involves a trained operator using a Doppler probe to measure the speed of red cells in cerebral arteries. It may detect vasospasm after subarachnoid haemorrhage, but has little use in routine anaesthesia apart from during carotid endarterectomy when it may be used to demonstrate adequacy of blood flow in the circle of Willis during contralateral carotid artery clamping.

Jugular venous saturation involves passing a catheter retrogradely up the internal jugular vein into the jugular venous sinus. A saturation of less than 55% indicates increased oxygen extraction and therefore relative ischaemia. It is a useful technique in the intensive care unit but only measures global perfusion and fails to detect small areas of ischaemia.

TEMPERATURE

The body is considered to have an inner core temperature and an outer peripheral temperature. In reality, the temperature decreases with distance down limbs and proximity to the skin. The difference between core and peripheral temperatures is related strongly to the cardiac output and degree of vasoconstriction. In practice, a core–periphery difference of > 2°C indicates a low cardiac output state and has been used as a marker of hypovolaemia.

Temperature probes consist of a semiconductor, the electrical resistance of which varies with temperature.

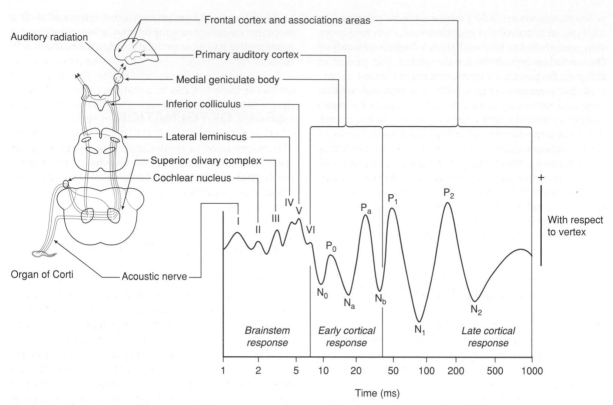

Fig. 18.9
The auditory evoked response consists of a series of waves generated from specific anatomical sites in the auditory pathway as indicated. Activity passes from the cochlea through the brainstem to the cortex.

They are covered with a smooth coating to reduce the trauma of insertion and prevent damage to the probe. The probes may be re-used after sterilization, but are now more commonly single-use.

Probes used to measure core temperature are inserted into the nasopharynx, oesophagus or rectum. Peripheral temperature is measured by attaching a probe to either a finger or toe. Although complications are rare, it is possible to cause mucosal trauma, bleeding and even penetration of the pharynx or rectum. When used for prolonged periods, mucosal damage is possible as a result of pressure-related ischaemia. Many monitors accept two probes and automatically display the temperature difference. Care must be taken to avoid the peripheral probe being exposed to warmth from heating blankets.

Alternatively, temperature may be measured by an ear probe. These are inserted into the external ear with the tip protected by a disposable sheath. They measure the infrared radiation produced from the eardrum and produce a digital readout in less than 3 s. Unfortunately, because of factors such as earwax and variations in the angle of insertion, results are less reliable than fixed probes and they cannot produce continuous readings. They are therefore used principally in recovery and ward areas.

Traditional mercury-in-glass thermometers are no longer used because of the risk of breakage and mercury contamination.

ELECTROLYTE AND BLOOD GAS ANALYSIS

During long operations, or when there is a need for infusion of large volumes of fluid, it may be necessary to measure physiological variables such as pH, haemoglobin and electrolyte concentrations and carboxyhaemoglobin. These have traditionally been performed on samples sent to laboratories and analysed by trained staff. The machines used are often complex and subject to regular servicing and quality control. More recently, it has become possible to use a variety of devices for 'bedside' analysis.

These devices usually comprise a small disposable cartridge that contains a combination of reagents and often some electronic circuitry. A sample is placed in the cartridge, which is then inserted into a larger analyser. Serum glucose concentration may be measured by a reagent strip which is compared with a colour chart or by insertion into a reader. These machines provide rapid results at the bedside and avoid the delays of transporting samples to the laboratory. However, the accuracy of the results produced by such devices are usually dependent on the skill of the operator and they may be affected by poor storage of the reagent or monitor. They also usually lack the organized quality control checks used in laboratories. Results are therefore less reliable and should be confirmed by laboratory analysis where possible.

BLOOD LOSS AND TRANSFUSION

During surgery, blood loss is common; it may be difficult to estimate as blood may soak into surgical drapes and swabs or find its way into suction bottles, or fall onto the floor. Although it is usually impossible to measure the blood loss accurately, an attempt should be made in all cases. This is particularly important in paediatric cases, where, for example, in a 2 kg child, a major haemorrhage equates to a blood loss of more than 20 mL.

RED CELL LOSS

This may be estimated by weighing the swabs after use, but is notoriously inaccurate. Measuring the haemoglobin concentration of a known volume of solution after all the swabs have been washed in it provides a more accurate result, but usually too late to be of immediate clinical use. Regular estimation of blood haemoglobin concentration is the only reliable method of determining the effect of blood loss.

BLOOD CLOTTING

Clotting efficacy is assessed by measuring the platelet count, prothrombin time (intrinsic system), activated partial thromboplastin time (extrinsic system) and fibrinogen concentration. Although these are traditional laboratory-based tests, there are increasing numbers of methods of analysing blood clotting in the operating theatre. These require the user to add a sample of blood to a reagent in a chamber, which is then inserted into a measuring device. The Sonoclot™ device uses a probe that is moved up and down in the sample. As the clot

forms, the increasing resistance is measured and plotted as a graph against time. In thromboelastography, a pin is lowered into the sample and rotated intermittently. As a clot forms, there is increasing resistance to rotation.

Laboratory-based tests of clotting should be used whenever there is a risk of a clotting defect and after a significant blood transfusion. The main advantage of these tests is that they may be interpreted by haematologists who provide advice on suitable treatments. Bedside monitors are used increasingly to measure clotting in procedures such as coronary artery surgery, where anticoagulants are usually used and significant blood loss is common.

MONITORING STANDARDS

The presence of an appropriately trained and experienced anaesthetist is the most essential patient monitor. However, human error is inevitable and there is substantial evidence that many incidents are attributable, at least in part, to error by anaesthetists.

Appropriate monitoring will not prevent all adverse incidents in the perioperative period. However, there is substantial evidence that it reduces the amount of harm to patients, not only by detecting problems as they occur but also by alerting the anaesthetist that an error has occurred. In one study, the introduction of modern standards of monitoring halved the number of cardiac arrests, principally because of the reduction in arrests caused by preventable respiratory causes. In the Australian Incident Monitoring Study, 52% of incidents were detected first by a monitor and in more than half of these cases, it was the pulse oximeter or capnograph that detected the problem.

There has never been a study comparing outcomes from anaesthesia with and without monitoring, and now that there are mandatory standards of monitoring in most countries, it will be impossible to prove that monitors make a difference.

The current recommendations from the Association of Anaesthetists of Great Britain and Ireland are shown in Table 18.9. However, it is not sufficient that the monitors are available. Departmental heads are responsible for ensuring not only that equipment is available but also that it works correctly, is maintained to appropriate standards, staff are trained and that it is used appropriately.

All anaesthetists must ensure that they are familiar with the equipment used in their hospital and that all equipment has been checked before use. The need for training and practice cannot be overemphasized because the increasing complexity of modern monitoring devices

Table 18.9   Summary of recommendations for standards of monitoring during anaesthesia and recovery

1. The anaesthetist must be present throughout the conduct of an anaesthetic

2. Monitoring devices must be attached before induction of anaesthesia and their use continued until the patient has recovered from the effects of anaesthesia

3. The same standards of monitoring apply when the anaesthetist is responsible for a local anaesthetic or sedative technique for an operative procedure

4. All information provided by monitoring devices should be recorded in the patient's notes. Trend display and printing devices are recommended so they allow the anaesthetist to concentrate on managing the patient in emergency situations

5. The anaesthetist must check all equipment before use. All alarm limits must be set appropriately. Infusion devices and their alarm settings must be checked before use. Audible alarms must be enabled when anaesthesia commences

6. The anaesthetist should make observations of the patient's mucosa, pupil size, response to surgical stimuli and movements of the chest wall and reservoir bag. The pulse should be palpated and the lungs auscultated and, where appropriate, urine output and blood loss should be measured. A stethoscope must always be available

7. Monitoring devices supplement clinical observation. The following monitoring devices are essential in every case:
   – an oxygen analyser with an audible alarm
   – measurement of airway pressure, with upper and lower alarm limits, when IPPV is used
   – a vapour analyser during maintenance of anaesthesia whenever a volitle anaesthetic agent is in use
   – pulse oximetry
   – non-invasive blood pressure measurement
   – electrocardiography
   – capnography

8. The following devices must also be available in every case:
   – a nerve stimulator whenever a muscle relaxant is used
   – a means of measuring the patient's temperature

9. Additional (mainly invasive) monitoring devices may be required for some patients or for some types of operation, e.g. invasive monitoring of vascular or intracranial pressures, cardiac output or biochemical variable

10. When handing over to recovery staff, anaesthetists should issue clear instructions concerning monitoring during postoperative care. Monitoring of arterial oxygen saturation and non-invasive monitoring of blood pressure are essential. An electrocardiograph, nerve stimulator, capnograph and a means of measuring temperature must be immediately available

11. Standards of care and monitoring during transfer of sedated, anaesthetized or unconscious patients should be as high as during administration of anaesthesia. Oxygen saturation, the electrocardiogram and arterial pressure should be monitored in all patients. Additional monitors may be required in some circumstances. Airway pressure, tidal volume and expired carbon dioxide concentration should be monitored continuously if the lungs are ventilated artificially.

Reproduced with permission from the Association of Anaesthetists of Great Britain and Ireland 2000.

implies that they can behave in unexpected ways at inopportune moments.

ALARMS

All the electronic monitors described below have alarms (set to default values on start-up) that usually incorporate both audible and visual components. Failure to reset the alarm limits to appropriate values before starting anaesthesia is a common cause of false alarm signals. This often results in the anaesthetist cancelling a series of false alarms, with the risk that an alarm for a real problem is also cancelled without any action being taken.

Alarms must therefore be set to appropriate levels before induction so that they are triggered only by real abnormalities. This is particularly true during procedures involving children, when values for respiratory rate, for example, are not within the 'normal' adult range.

Oxygen supply

The use of an oxygen analyser with an audible alarm is mandatory for all patients breathing anaesthetic gases. The sampling port must be placed so that the gas mixture delivered to the patient is monitored continuously. The analyser should provide a clearly visible readout of the concentration of oxygen in the inspired gas and sound an audible alarm if a hypoxic mixture is delivered.

Breathing systems

The principal problems are of disconnection, leak or excessive pressure. During spontaneous ventilation, the movement of a reservoir bag usually provides evidence of continuing ventilation. However, a capnograph is required to ensure that ventilation is adequate. When positive-pressure ventilation is used, a measure of airway pressure and appropriate alarms are also required.

Monitors do not always detect every abnormality. For example, if a capnograph is attached to an airway filter in a spontaneously breathing patient, the breathing system may become disconnected from the filter, leading to a risk of awareness. However, because the patient continues to breathe room air through the filter, the capnograph trace is unchanged and no alarm is triggered.

Vapour analyzer

A vapour analyser is essential whenever anaesthetic vapours are used, both to prevent accidental overdose and also to prevent awareness. A particular problem with current vaporizers is that they are not able to detect when the vaporizer is empty. During a long procedure, it is possible for a vaporizer to become empty without warning unless an agent monitor is in place.

Cardiovascular

Non-invasive arterial pressure and ECG are always required as monitors of the cardiovascular system. Although these provide useful information, clinical measures such as capillary refill and urine output are more reliable monitors.

Infusion devices

Increasingly, anaesthetic drugs are being delivered by infusion devices. As with most equipment, individual devices are becoming more complex. For example, rather than using simple infusion pumps, anaesthesia may be delivered using devices containing computers, allowing the infusion to maintain a constant plasma concentration, e.g. the Diprifusor™ infusion pump.

These devices contain sophisticated alarm systems and usually need to be programmed with a variety of patient data to function effectively. Anaesthetists also need to be trained and must understand how these devices work before attaching them to a patient. In particular, it must be emphasized that although many infusion devices display information about the amount of drug administered and/or plasma concentration, these are dependent on absence of leaks and on assumptions about the patient. A common problem is disconnection of the infusion line under surgical drapes, leading to underdosage. A further problem is that, in sick patients, factors such as the size of fluid compartments or rate of drug transport may differ greatly from those assumed by the pump, leading to over- or underdosage.

GENERAL GUIDELINES FOR MONITORING DURING ANAESTHESIA

INDUCTION OF ANAESTHESIA

- oxygen analyser
- pulse oximeter
- non-invasive arterial pressure monitor
- ECG
- capnograph.

The following must also be available:

- nerve stimulator if muscle relaxants are used
- means of measuring the patient's temperature.

Monitors should be applied to the awake patient and readings taken to ensure that they are functioning correctly before induction of anaesthesia. If uncooperative patients make application of monitoring impossible before induction, the monitors should be applied as soon as possible after induction and the reason recorded on the anaesthetic chart.

For short procedures such as electroconvulsive therapy (ECT) or orthopaedic manipulations, the above standards are appropriate. However, if the procedure is prolonged then the standards for maintenance of anaesthesia should be applied.

MAINTENANCE OF ANAESTHESIA

The following must be applied to the patient:

- oxygen analyser
- pulse oximeter
- non-invasive arterial pressure monitor
- ECG
- capnograph
- vapour analyser (if anaesthetic vapours are used).

The following must also be available:

- nerve stimulator if muscle relaxants are used
- means of measuring the patient's temperature.

RECOVERY FROM ANAESTHESIA

A high standard of monitoring should be applied continuously until the patient has recovered fully from anaesthesia. Direct clinical observation should be supplemented by:

- pulse oximeter
- non-invasive arterial pressure monitor.

The following must also be available:

- ECG
- capnograph
- nerve stimulator
- means of measuring the patient's temperature.

If the recovery room is not immediately adjacent to the operating theatre, or if the patient's condition is poor, equipment should be available so that the above standards are applied during transfer of the patient.

ADDITIONAL MONITORING

The above standards are the minimum acceptable levels and apply to healthy patients undergoing minor surgery. If the patient is unwell before surgery or major surgery is planned, additional monitoring should be applied. It is difficult to give strict guidelines on what conditions or surgery should prompt the use of each monitor. Suggestions are given in Table 18.10.

MONITORING DURING TRANSFER

It is essential that the standard of care and monitoring during transfer is as high as that applied in the operating theatre and that staff with appropriate training and experience accompany the patient.

During transfer, vibrations may make devices that rely on pressure change, such as non-invasive arterial pressure monitors, inaccurate or non-functional. Vibration may also cause connections to work loose and equipment may suffer physical damage. Movement may make an ECG trace useless for diagnosis of arrhythmias. Noise and poor lighting make the displays of many monitors difficult to read and make audible alarms inaudible. Adequate supplies must be taken for the entire journey, together with additional supplies to anticipate any unforeseen delays. This includes oxygen

Table 18.10 Variables that it may be appropriate to monitor during anaesthesia in some patients in addition to the essential monitoring for all anaesthetized patients

Indications	Monitors
Operative duration > 3 h	Direct arterial pressure measurement
Blood loss > 10% blood volume	Central venous pressure
Operations on: Chest Central nervous system Cardiovascular system	Pulmonary capillary wedge pressure Cardiac output Transoesophageal echocardiography Blood loss measurement
Clinically significant coexisting disease	Urine output Temperature: Patient Blood warmer, mattress Inspired gas Blood gas analysis Serum electrolyte concentrations Haemoglobin concentration Coagulation status

cylinders, batteries (the internal batteries of a monitor may have short lives) and anaesthetic drugs.

Before transfer the patient should be in a stable physiological state. The patient should be moved onto the transport trolley and all the transport monitors applied to the patient and their functions checked. All equipment should then be fastened securely and all catheters and leads taped into position. It should be checked that from a single position, the anaesthetist is able to attend to the airway, see all the monitors and be able to administer drugs and fluids. The process is made much easier and safer with a dedicated transport trolley, so that all the equipment is fixed permanently in place.

ANAESTHETIC RECORD-KEEPING

It is the professional responsibility of every doctor to maintain accurate records of the treatment which patients receive, and their response to it. The anaesthetic record forms a part of a patient's medical record. The principal purpose of the anaesthetic chart is to provide details of the anaesthetic technique used, of the physiological changes which were associated with the technique and with surgery, and of complications or problems which were encountered during the procedure. This information may assist other doctors if complications ensue, or if anaesthesia is required in the future. In addition, the anaesthetic record may be a valuable source of information if a subsequent complication results in litigation; the absence of a full record makes it difficult for an anaesthetist to demonstrate, for example, that postoperative renal failure was not attributable to untreated intraoperative hypotension.

The design of anaesthetic records varies widely, and is probably unimportant provided that it facilitates recording and display of all the relevant data. Suggestions for the reasonable content of an anaesthetic record data set are shown on Table 18.11.

In addition to the data described above, the record should include details of the techniques discussed with the patient, together with any risks or benefits outlined and the management plan agreed. If the patient has any specific requests or concerns, such as a desire to avoid blood transfusion, it is also best to record them in writing.

Table 18.11   Suggested data for inclusion on anaesthetic records

PREOPERATIVE INFORMATION	**Place and time**
Patient identity	Place
Name/ID number/gender	Date, start and end times
Date of birth	**Personnel**
Assessment and risk factors	All anaesthetists named
Date of assessment	Operating surgeon
Assessor, where assessed	Qualified assistant present
Weight (kg) [height (m) optional]	Duty consultant informed
Base vital signs (BP, HR)	
Medication, incl. contraceptive drugs	**Operation planned/performed**
Allergies	**Apparatus**
Addiction (alcohol, tobacco, drugs)	Check performed, anaesthetic room, theatre
Previous GAs, family history	
Potential airway problems	**Vital signs recording/charting**
Prostheses, teeth, crowns	Monitors used and vital signs, recorded not less frequently than every 5 min
Investigations	
Cardiorespiratory fitness	**Drugs and fluids**
Other problems	Dose, concentration, volume
ASA grade ± comment	Cannulation
	Injection site(s), time & route
Urgency	Warmer used
Scheduled – listed on a routine list	Blood loss, urine output
Urgent – resuscitated, not on a routine list	
Emergency – not fully resuscitated	**Airway and breathing system**
	Route, system used
PERIOPERATIVE INFORMATION	Ventilation: type & mode
Checks	Airway type, size, cuff, shape
Nil by mouth	Special procedures, humidifier, filter
Consent	Throat pack
Premedication, type and effect	Difficulty

Continued

Table 18.11   Suggested data for inclusion on anaesthetic records — Contd

Regional anaesthesia	Special airway instructions, incl. oxygen
Consent	Monitoring
Block performed	
Entry site	***Untoward events***
Needle used, aid to location	Abnormalities
Catheter: y/n	Critical incidents
	Preoperative, perioperative, postoperative
Patient position and attachments	Context, cause, effect
Thrombosis prophylaxis	***Hazard flags***
Temperature control	Warnings for future care
Limb position	
Postoperative instructions	
Drugs, fluids and doses	
Analgesic techniques	

Based on recommendations of the Royal College of Anaesthetists and Association of Anaesthetists of Great Britain and Ireland.

AUTOMATED RECORDS

It has been estimated that up to 20% of the anaesthetist's time is taken up with documentation. While the anaesthetic record is usually completed as the anaesthetic proceeds, there are times, such as during induction or a crisis, when it is not possible to complete the chart contemporaneously. This delay lead to inaccuracies. In addition, studies have shown that anaesthetists tend to record 'normalized' data: that is, the record tends to minimize any physiological changes that occur.

To counteract these problems, most anaesthetic monitors and anaesthetic machines may be connected to automatic data recording systems. These log all the monitoring data and have the facility for the anaesthetist to add data such as drugs used and comments on events such as the start of surgery. The data may be stored electronically for later study and printed out in a variety of formats. They have the potential to interact with other sources of information so that patient details, laboratory results, scans and outpatient letters can all be accessed. These systems have the potential to make audits and quality control much easier to perform.

However, these systems are expensive and it must be recognized that all monitors have numerous sources of error; while most anaesthetists tend to ignore erroneous readings, they are recorded and printed by an automated system. Printouts should therefore be checked and errors marked before being included in the patient's medical record.

FURTHER READING

Association of Anaesthetists of Great Britain and Ireland 2004 Checklist for anaesthetic apparatus. AAGBI, London

Association of Anaesthetists of Great Britain and Ireland 1998 Risk management 1998. AAGBI, London

Association of Anaesthetists of Great Britain and Ireland 2006 Recommendations for standards of monitoring during anaesthesia and recovery 4. AAGBI, London

Sykes M K, Vickers M D, Hull C J 1991 Principles of measurement and monitoring in anaesthesia and intensive care. Blackwell Scientific, Oxford

Complications during anaesthesia

19

Complications are unexpected and unwanted events. They occur in approximately 10% of anaesthetics. Only the minority of these complications cause lasting harm to the patient. Death complicates five anaesthetics per million given in the UK (0.0005%). Every complication has the *potential* to cause lasting harm to the patient. Therefore, deviations from the norm must be recognized and managed promptly and appropriately.

The most frequent complications during anaesthesia are arrhythmia, hypotension, adverse drug effects and inadequate ventilation of the lungs. Inadequate ventilation may be caused by poorly managed or difficult tracheal intubation, pulmonary aspiration of gastric contents, breathing system disconnections or gas supply failure. These complications are also the major causes of anaesthetic mortality, preventable intraoperative cardiac arrest and permanent neurological damage. In particular, hypotension and hypoxaemia are implicated consistently in studies of adverse outcome from anaesthesia.

CAUSES OF COMPLICATIONS

HUMAN ERROR

A common contributor to, and cause of, anaesthetic complications is human error, often in association with poor monitoring, equipment malfunction and organizational failure. Human error is commonly associated with poor training, fatigue, inadequate experience and poor preparation of the patient, the environment and the equipment. These conditions are entirely avoidable, and good organization should prevent such circumstances. When complications do occur, effective monitoring and vigilance allow a greater period for action before the complication grows in severity. During this 'window', when the complication is apparent, but has not yet damaged the patient, the anaesthetist must act with precision. Such precision of

action may be obtained through the use of prerehearsed 'action plans' or 'drills'.

Communication failure

Failure of communication is frequently implicated in the generation of complications during anaesthesia. Poor working relationships, varying levels of training amongst staff and poor working conditions make such failure more likely. Team training and simulation-based training are effective in reducing this type of error.

Equipment failure

Equipment failure may result in significant risk to the patient. In particular, failures of breathing systems, airway devices and gas supplies have resulted in several deaths in recent years. In addition, malfunction of mechanical infusion pumps and infusion pressurizing devices have caused injury and death in several cases. Meticulous checking of equipment before use is mandatory. The anaesthetist must not only ensure the correct functioning of items of equipment that may be life-saving or of critical importance but must also ensure that alternative devices are available should the primary device fail.

Coexisting disease

Some complications stem from the deterioration of the patient's medical condition, which may have existed before the anaesthetist's involvement. While such deterioration may be coincidental, it must be recognized that anaesthesia and surgery frequently introduce altered conditions into a patient's finely balanced combination of pathology and compensatory physiology. This may be sufficient to generate instability in the patient's condition, and result in sudden worsening of an apparently stable pathology. Typical examples include diabetes, angina, hypertension and asthma.

Inevitable complications

There exists a subgroup of complications that may be classed as 'inevitable'. Despite excellent surgical and anaesthetic practice, the patient may still experience a complication that brings morbidity or even death. While we must, at all times, make stringent efforts to save our patients from harm, it is also important to recognize that it is not always necessary to place the blame for a complication on a healthcare provider.

AVOIDANCE OF COMPLICATIONS

The most effective steps in preventing harm from complications are implemented before the complication occurs. Thorough preparation should prevent the majority of complications. This preparation includes:

- preoperative assessment, investigation and counselling of the patient
- preoperative checking of equipment and the provision of backup equipment
- ensuring the availability of an appropriately trained assistant
- preoperative consultation with more experienced personnel, where necessary, regarding the most appropriate anaesthetic technique
- the use of appropriate monitoring techniques.

Experience

Complications occur more commonly in inexperienced hands. Clearly, finite resources exist, and appropriately experienced personnel are not always allocated to appropriate patients and procedures. It is the individual anaesthetist's responsibility to ensure that he or she has adequate training for the task presented. If the anaesthetist does not have the necessary experience, then senior assistance must be sought.

Record-keeping

The maintenance of accurate records of a patient's treatment and vital signs is of paramount importance in preventing complications. It allows the observation of trends in vital signs, often providing valuable clues to a gradual deviation from a stable physiological state, and allowing early intervention before a harmful condition arises. Accurate record-keeping also allows safer sharing of care between anaesthetists, facilitating hand-over of care during long cases and allowing better teamwork in complex cases where two anaesthetists are required.

Redundant systems

The use of redundant systems helps prevent complications. The availability of at least two working laryngoscopes illustrates this. Should one system fail, another may be put in its place. The insertion of two or more intravenous cannulae if significant blood loss is expected, and monitoring of expired volatile agent concentration in addition to bispectral index to minimize the risk of awareness, also illustrate the use of redundant systems.

Monitoring

Monitoring systems have been designed to detect and prevent complications during anaesthesia. Aspects of the patient should be monitored that are *likely* to deviate from the norm, or that are *dangerous* if they deviate from the norm. The Association of Anaesthetists of Great Britain and Ireland (AAGBI) has produced guidelines stipulating the acceptable minimum level of intraoperative monitoring (see Ch. 18).

Modern monitoring systems have automatically activated alarms, and the anaesthetist chooses the values at which these alarms sound. The default values are not always the optimal choices. Thought should be applied to the values at which the anaesthetist gains useful insight into the patient's deviation from the healthy *status quo*, without generating unnecessary noise pollution, which may detract from the anaesthetist's concentration and reduce the effectiveness of the monitor. In general, alarms should sound before the value in question reaches a potentially damaging level, but should not sound at values that would be considered within the patient's expected range. Clearly, this is different for each patient, whose coexisting disease, age, anaesthesia and surgical procedure vary greatly. The repeated sounding of an alarm should not trigger reflex silencing of the alarm, but should cause the anaesthetist to consider if treatment of the patient is required or if the alarm limit should be altered.

MANAGEMENT OF COMPLICATIONS

Generic management of complications

The majority of complications that result in serious harm to the patient compromise the delivery of oxygen to tissues. Organs which are damaged most rapidly by a deficiency in oxygen supply include the brain and heart. Less fragile, but potentially at risk from even short interruptions of oxygen supply, are the liver and kidneys. Cessation of perfusion results in more rapid damage to organs than low levels of oxygenation with maintained perfusion. Treatment must be provided rapidly when organ perfusion is threatened or when arterial oxygenation is impaired. The management of virtually any significant complication should include the provision of a high inspired oxygen fraction and the assurance of an adequate cardiac output.

In general, complications should be dealt with through a sequence of:

1. Continual vigilance and monitoring.
2. Recognition of the occurrence of a problem.
3. Creation of a list of differential diagnoses.
4. Choice of a *working diagnosis*, which is either the most *likely* or the most *dangerous* possibility.
5. Treatment of the *working diagnosis*.
6. Assessment of the response of the problem to the administered treatment.
7. Refinement of the list of differential diagnoses, especially if the response has not been as expected.
8. Confirmation or refutation of the choice of *working diagnosis*; if the response to treatment has been unexpected then replacement with a more *likely* working diagnosis is indicated.
9. Go to step 5 and repeat until the problem is resolved.

The evolving problem

The early recognition of an evolving problem allows the anaesthetist time to manage a complication before it damages the patient. Careful selection of monitoring alarm limits and the anaesthetist's vigilance should allow a larger window in which pre-emptive treatment may be provided to reduce the impact of the complication.

The first response to an emerging complication should be to minimize the potential harm to the patient. Such harm may be produced by the anaesthetist's treatment or by a pathological source. It is important to ensure that an abnormal reading from a monitor is not an artefact; inaccurate information may be displayed if, for example, a pulse oximeter probe slips or if an ECG electrode becomes displaced, and the anaesthetist should ensure, through rapid clinical assessment of the patient, that the values shown on the monitor screen are consistent with the patient's clinical appearance and the context. For example, a sudden reading of arterial oxygen saturations of 80% when the values have been greater than 96% throughout the procedure should prompt a rapid examination of the patient; if the patient is not cyanosed, the position of the pulse oximeter probe

should be checked, particularly if the plethysmograph trace is poor.

In most situations where complications present, the diagnosis is simple, and treatment may progress in a linear fashion. Such linear treatment of complications is detailed later in this chapter. However, the causes of some complications, such as hypoxaemia, are not always immediately clear, and several potential aetiologies may exist. Where the differential diagnoses relating to a problem appear equally likely, the anaesthetist should treat the problem that threatens the most harm to the patient. During the management of problems during anaesthesia, the anaesthetist must constantly be reconsidering the list of differential diagnoses, re-arranging them mentally in order of likelihood, and treating the most likely and most dangerous possibilities first.

Record-keeping

Record-keeping, while useful in preventing complications, is also important *during* complications. Trends in a patient's physiological data may become apparent only when charted, and new differential diagnoses may be generated through examination of the recorded data. Review of critical incidents and complications is vitally important in preventing future repetitions of the incident and in providing continuing education to individual practitioners and to Departments of Anaesthesia. Thorough record-keeping is vital in allowing informed review of these cases. Finally, some complications result in harm to the patient, and it is very important for the practitioner and the patient that detailed records are available for later review. In a minority of such cases, legal action may result and detailed, legible records are vital in defending one's actions and in providing an adequate explanation to the patient (and possibly to the court) of what happened in the operating theatre.

MEDICOLEGAL ASPECTS OF COMPLICATIONS

A minority of complications result in a formal complaint, but litigation by patients who feel that they have been wronged by the healthcare system is becoming increasingly common. Defensive practice is consequently becoming widespread. Such practice aims to reduce the potential culpability of the anaesthetist should complications arise. In some situations this may lead to overinvestigation of patients and even to the provision of care that is not necessarily optimal for the patient. The culture of blame in which we now practise dictates that anaesthetists must protect themselves as well as their patients. Meticulous record-keeping, pre-operative information and consent, and frank discussion of risks with the patient are vital.

Management of the medicolegal aspects of complications

Complications must be recognized promptly and treated efficiently, with the patient's best outcome the aim of treatment. Record-keeping must continue to be meticulous, even during the occurrence of problems during an anaesthetic. Help should be sought early if there is any doubt about the anaesthetist's ability or experience.

Complaints by patients should be dealt with promptly and professionally. The complaint and the anaesthetist's response must be recorded clearly in the patient's records. The anaesthetist should express regret that the complication has occurred, and explain why. A frank discussion of the difficulties that occurred during an anaesthetic may provide the patient with sufficient information. If human error has occurred, then the anaesthetist should apologize, and assure the patient that further information will be provided when it becomes available. If the anaesthetist is a trainee, then it is prudent to enlist the assistance of a consultant to attend discussions with the patient. The clinical director should be informed of all discussions with the patient. It may be prudent that the clinical director accompanies the anaesthetist during their dealings with the patient.

Any complaint that goes further than an informal conversation should be referred to the hospital's complaints department and the anaesthetist's defence organization should be informed. The defence organization should provide advice on subsequent action. It must be emphasized that throughout this distressing process, meticulous and professional record-keeping may make the difference between exoneration and condemnation, irrespective of the true origin of blame.

COMPLICATIONS

The presentation, causes and management of the most common and most dangerous complications that occur during anaesthesia are described below. Complications are classified, where possible, according to the body system involved. Some complications (such as hypothermia) do not fit easily into this classification and are described separately. This list of complications is not exhaustive, and the reader is encouraged to consult the texts listed at the end of the chapter.

RESPIRATORY SYSTEM

Respiratory obstruction

Table 19.1 details the common causes of respiratory obstruction during anaesthesia. Obstruction may occur at any point from the gas delivery system through the patient's airway and bronchi to the expiratory parts of the breathing system and the scavenging tubing. It is common and potentially very dangerous. The commonest sites for obstruction are the larynx (e.g. laryngospasm), the tracheal tube (e.g. biting or secretions) and the bronchi (e.g. bronchospasm). Respiratory obstruction causes inadequate ventilation and impaired gas exchange. This causes hypercapnia, hypoxaemia and reduced uptake of volatile anaes-

Table 19.1 Causes of respiratory obstruction during anaesthesia

Equipment	
Breathing system	Valve malfunction, kinking
Tracheal tube	External compression (surgical gag/manipulation, kinking, biting)
	Occlusion of lumen (secretions, blood)
	Cuff (overinflation, herniation)
	Oesophageal or bronchial intubation
Patient	
Oropharynx	Soft tissue (oedema from trauma/infection, reduced muscle tone)
	Secretions (blood, surgical packs)
	Tumour
Larynx	Laryngospasm
	Recurrent laryngeal nerve palsy
	Oedema (drug hypersensitivity, pre-eclampsia, infection)
	Tumour
Trachea	Laryngotracheobronchitis
	External compression (surgical, haematoma, thyroid tumour)
	Stricture (radiotherapy, scarring from previous tracheostomy)
Bronchi	Secretions
	Pneumothorax
	Bronchospasm
	Tumour
	Surgical manipulation

thetic agent. Respiratory obstruction prevents the mass inflow of ambient gas that occurs during apnoea and thus produces hypoxaemia more rapidly than does apnoea with an open airway.

Partial obstruction is indicated by noisy breathing or stridor, while complete obstruction is silent. In spontaneously breathing patients, tracheal tug, paradoxical chest and abdominal movement ('see-saw' ventilation) and reduced movement of the reservoir bag are other signs. The generation of a large negative intrathoracic pressure during powerful attempts to inspire may cause pulmonary oedema in some patients, particularly young adults. In patients whose lungs are mechanically ventilated, respiratory obstruction may be associated with increased inflation pressure, a prolonged expiratory phase, hypercapnia and alteration of the end-tidal carbon dioxide waveform.

Management

Any significant airway obstruction should be treated by gentle, manual ventilation of the patient's lungs with oxygen. Location of the site of obstruction should be sought urgently. In the absence of a laryngeal mask airway (LMA) or tracheal tube, apposition of the tongue and pharyngeal soft tissue is a common cause of upper airway obstruction. This may be overcome by jaw lift or neck extension. It may require the use of an oral or nasopharyngeal airway, although these devices may themselves provoke laryngospasm or pharyngeal abrasion. Absolute obstruction suggests an equipment problem. Easy passage of a suction catheter through the tracheal tube confirms its patency. If obstruction persists and no obvious cause is identified, then the tracheal tube or laryngeal mask may be the site of obstruction and should be replaced.

Suction removes accumulated secretions in the pharynx, but may cause laryngospasm during light anaesthesia. The presence of symmetrical chest movements and breath sounds should be confirmed. Other causes of obstruction such as laryngospasm, bronchospasm, aspiration and pneumothorax should be excluded.

The most common airway complication is partial respiratory obstruction during spontaneous ventilation or during assisted manual ventilation in the absence of a formal airway. A gentle jaw thrust, head tilt and chin lift usually clears a partially obstructed airway, and insertion of an oropharyngeal or nasopharyngeal airway resolves almost all of the remainder. In the rare situation of complete inability to ventilate the patient's lungs manually, and after equipment failure has been excluded, the insertion of a laryngeal mask airway or tracheal tube may be necessary.

Allowing the patient to awaken is prudent if there is no urgency to proceed with the operation. If it is necessary to continue the operation or if the patient cannot be wakened, and insertion of a laryngeal mask airway and tracheal tube have proved impossible, then it becomes necessary to establish a *surgical airway*. This may take the form of a cricothyroid cannula, a surgical cricothyrotomy or an emergency tracheostomy. These procedures must be learned and practised *before* the occurrence of the incident. They are technically demanding and are themselves potentially life-threatening to the patient.

Laryngospasm

Laryngospasm is a reflex, prolonged closure of the vocal cords. It occurs usually in response to a trigger, and this is often airway stimulation by airway devices, secretions or gastric contents during light anaesthesia. Laryngospasm is most common during induction and emergence. It may also be produced by surgical and visceral stimuli such as incision, peritoneal traction and anal or cervical dilatation. Children are particularly prone to laryngospasm. The use of intravenous barbiturates inhibits laryngeal reflexes to a lesser extent than propofol and increases the risk of laryngospasm. Poor management of laryngospasm may lead to inadequate ventilation with hypoxaemia, hypercapnia and reduced depth of anaesthesia. Crowing inspiratory noises with signs of respiratory obstruction suggest laryngospasm. Complete obstruction caused by severe laryngospasm is silent.

Management

Where possible, airway and surgical stimulation should be avoided during light anaesthesia and the lateral position should be used for control of secretions during extubation and transfer. Surgical stimuli should be anticipated, and anaesthetic depth should be adjusted accordingly. The anaesthetist should remove the stimulus to laryngospasm, administer 100% oxygen and provide a clear airway. Gentle pharyngeal suction should be applied. Where appropriate, anaesthetic depth may be increased by administration of an intravenous anaesthetic agent and the lungs ventilated manually, applying continuous positive airway pressure (CPAP). Most episodes of laryngospasm respond to this treatment. If laryngospasm persists and hypoxaemia ensues, a small dose of succinylcholine (e.g. 25 mg in adults) relaxes the vocal cords and allows manual ventilation and oxygenation. A full dose of succinylcholine may be given if tracheal intubation is indicated, but this is usually unnecessary.

Doxapram, an analeptic and respiratory stimulant, has also been used successfully in the treatment of laryngospasm.

Bronchospasm

General anaesthesia may alter airway resistance by influencing bronchomotor tone, lung volumes and bronchial secretions. Patients with increased airway reactivity from recent respiratory infection, asthma, atopy or smoking are more susceptible to bronchospasm during anaesthesia. Bronchospasm may be precipitated by the rapid introduction of a pungent volatile anaesthetic agent (e.g. desflurane), the insertion of an artificial airway during light anaesthesia, stimulation of the carina or bronchi by a tracheal tube or by drugs causing β-blockade or release of histamine. Drug hypersensitivity, pulmonary aspiration and a foreign body in the lower airway may also present as bronchospasm. Bronchospasm causes expiratory wheeze, a prolonged expiratory phase (evident from the upwardly sloping end-tidal carbon dioxide plateau) and increased ventilator inflation pressures. Wheezing may occur in association with other causes of respiratory obstruction, such as pneumothorax, and these should be excluded. If bronchospasm is very severe, ventilation may be quiet and wheeze may not be apparent.

Management

Bronchospasm during anaesthesia results in hypercapnia, hypoxaemia and pulmonary gas trapping, which may cause hypotension. Management is aimed at preventing hypoxaemia, and resolving the bronchospasm. Initially, 100% oxygen should be given, anaesthesia deepened if appropriate and any aggravating factors removed (e.g. the tracheal tube should be repositioned and surgery stopped). If further treatment is necessary, a bronchodilator should be given in increments according to the response. Recommended drugs include intravenous aminophylline (up to 6 mg kg^{-1}) or salbutamol (up to 3 μg kg^{-1}). Volatile anaesthetic agents and ketamine are also effective bronchodilators. Epinephrine is indicated in life-threatening situations, and may be given via the tracheal tube. Steroids and H$_1$-receptor antagonists have no immediate effect but may be indicated in the later management of severe cases of bronchospasm.

If hypoxaemia develops in the spontaneously breathing patient, then tracheal intubation and artificial ventilation should be considered. Mechanical ventilation should incorporate a long expiratory phase to prevent the development of high end-expiratory alveolar pressures, which may cause hypotension, alveolar barotrauma and further hypoventilation. Severe gas trapping (intrinsic PEEP) may result in thoracic hyperexpansion, poor ventilation and pulmonary barotrauma. A very long expiratory phase or disconnection from the ventilator for up to 30 s may be necessary to allow thoracic depressurization. Positive end-expiratory pressure (PEEP) and high ventilatory rates should be avoided if bronchospasm is present because these favour the development of gas trapping. Hypercapnia may have to be tolerated in order to avoid gas trapping and barotrauma.

COMPLICATIONS ASSOCIATED WITH TRACHEAL INTUBATION

Difficult intubation

Some difficulty is experienced during tracheal intubation in about one in ten patients (10%). Approximately one in ten of these patients (1%) presents significant difficulty in intubation. Intubation is impossible in about one in ten of these patients (0.1%), and both intubation and ventilation are impossible in about one in ten of these (0.01%). In most instances, the cause of difficulty with the airway is difficulty in attaining an adequate view of the laryngeal inlet at laryngoscopy.

Poor management of difficult intubation is a significant cause of morbidity and mortality during anaesthesia. Sequelae include dental and airway trauma, pulmonary aspiration, hypoxaemia, brain damage and death. Table 19.2 shows the commonest causes of difficulty in intubation. The single most important cause is an inexperienced or inadequately prepared anaesthetist, and the difficulty is often compounded by equipment malfunction. The anatomical features associated with difficult laryngoscopy are listed in Table 19.3. Of these, the atlanto-occipital distance is the best predictor of difficulty but requires a lateral, cervical X-ray. Many of these factors are normal anatomical variations, but extreme abnormalities do occur. A cluster of normal variations in an apparently healthy patient may be sufficient to cause major difficulties in laryngoscopy.

Management

Preoperative examination of the airway (Table 19.4) is essential. Identification of patients with a potentially difficult airway (see Tables 19.2 and 19.3) before anaesthesia allows time to plan an appropriate anaesthetic technique. The Mallampati test is a widely used and simple classification of the pharyngeal view obtained during maximal mouth opening and tongue

Table 19.2 Causes of difficult intubation

Anaesthetist

Inadequate preoperative assessment

Inadequate equipment preparation

Inexperience

Poor technique

Equipment

Malfunction

Unavailability

No trained assistance

Patient

Congenital	Syndromes (Down, Pierre Robin, Treacher Collins, Marfan)
	Achondroplasia
	Cystic hygroma
	Encephalocele
Acquired	Reduced jaw movement:
	Trismus (abscess, infection, fracture, tetanus)
	Fibrosis (post-infection, post-radiotherapy, trauma)
	Rheumatoid arthritis
	Ankylosing spondylitis
	Tumours
	Jaw wiring
	Reduced neck movement:
	Arthritis
	Ankylosing spondylitis
	Cervical fracture, instability, fusion
	Airway:
	Oedema (infection, trauma, angio-oedema, burns)
	Compression (goitre, haematoma)
	Scarring (radiotherapy, infection, burns)
	Tumours, polyps
	Foreign body
	Nerve palsy
	Others:
	Morbid obesity
	Pregnancy
	Acromegaly

Table 19.3 Anatomical factors associated with difficult laryngoscopy

Short, wide, muscular neck

Protruding incisors

High, arched palate

Receding lower jaw

Poor mobility of the mandible

Increased anterior depth of mandible

Increased posterior depth of mandible (reduces jaw opening, requires X-ray)

Decreased atlanto-occipital distance (reduces neck extension, requires X-ray)

Table 19.4 Preoperative assessment of the airway

General appearance of the neck, face, maxilla and mandible

Jaw movement

Head extension and neck movement

Teeth and oropharynx

Soft tissues of the neck

Recent chest and cervical spine X-rays

Previous anaesthetic records

Mallampati classification

Thyromental distance

protrusion (see p. 308). In practice, this test suggests a higher likelihood of difficult laryngoscopy if the posterior pharyngeal wall is not seen. The predictive value of this test may be strengthened if the thyromental distance (the distance between the thyroid cartilage prominence and the bony point of the chin during full head extension) is less than 6.5 cm.

Premedication with an antisialagogue reduces airway secretions. This is advantageous before inhalational induction and essential for awake fibreoptic laryngoscopy to maximize the effectiveness of topical local anaesthesia. An anxiolytic may also be given (but is contraindicated in patients with airway obstruction, e.g.

caused by burns, trauma, tumour or infection affecting the larynx or pharynx). The presence of a trained assistant is essential and the availability of an experienced anaesthetist and a 'difficult intubation' trolley with a range of equipment such as bougies, a variety of laryngoscopes and tracheal tubes, and cricothyrotomy needles is desirable.

A variety of options exists for the patient in whom a difficult laryngoscopy is anticipated. If the procedure can be carried out under local or regional anaesthesia (see Ch. 17) then this technique should be used as the first choice. However, the patient, anaesthetist and equipment must be prepared for general anaesthesia in case a complication arises.

If general anaesthesia is necessary for the procedure, or if the patient refuses local or regional anaesthesia despite a frank discussion of the risks, then steps must be taken to secure the airway safely. Unless tracheal intubation is essential for airway protection or to enable muscle relaxation and ventilation, the use of an artificial airway such as the laryngeal mask with spontaneous ventilation is usually a safe technique. If intubation is essential, the appropriate anaesthetic technique depends on the anticipated degree of difficulty, the presence or absence of airway obstruction and the risk of regurgitation of gastric fluid.

There is no place for the use of a long-acting muscle relaxant to facilitate tracheal intubation if difficulty is anticipated. Correct positioning of the head and neck is essential and the lungs should be denitrogenated after establishing intravenous access and appropriate monitoring.

The safest anaesthetic technique may usually be chosen from the following clinical examples.

Patients with an increased risk of regurgitation and aspiration (e.g. full stomach, intra-abdominal pathology, pregnancy). An inhalational induction is inappropriate in these patients. Regional anaesthesia is preferable in the parturient (see Ch. 35). Denitrogenation (preoxygenation) and a rapid-sequence induction including administration of succinylcholine may be used if the anticipated difficulty is slight. If intubation is unsuccessful, no further doses of muscle relaxant should be used; the patient should be allowed to awaken and senior assistance should be sought. If significant difficulty is anticipated, an awake technique is recommended.

Patients with little anticipated difficulty and no airway obstruction (e.g. mild reduction of jaw or neck movement). After either intravenous or inhalational induction and confirmation of the ability to ventilate the lungs manually by mask, succinylcholine may be given to provide the best conditions for tracheal intubation. If difficulty is encountered, the patient is allowed to awaken and the procedure is re-planned. Where appropriate, anaes-

thesia may be deepened by spontaneous ventilation using a volatile anaesthetic agent and alternative techniques used to facilitate tracheal intubation.

Patients with severe anticipated difficulty and no airway obstruction (e.g. severe reduction of jaw or neck movement). Appropriate techniques include inhalational induction with halothane or sevoflurane, or the use of fibreoptic laryngoscopy either awake or after inhalational induction. A muscle relaxant must not be used until the ability to ventilate the lungs manually and view the vocal cords is confirmed.

Patients with airway obstruction (e.g. burns, infection, trauma). An inhalational induction may be used, but an awake technique should be considered. A muscle relaxant should not be given until tracheal intubation is confirmed.

Extreme clinical situations. Tracheostomy performed under local anaesthesia may be the safest technique.

Prophylactic insertion of a cricothyroid cannula before induction of anaesthesia in the patient with an expected difficult airway ensures the delivery of oxygen during prolonged airway management. Insertion of a cricothyroid cannula *during* the management of a difficult airway may be very stressful, and markedly more difficult than elective insertion.

Inhalational induction

Premedication with an antisialagogue is desirable. Depth of anaesthesia is increased carefully by spontaneous ventilation of increasing concentrations of a volatile anaesthetic agent in 100% oxygen until laryngoscopy may be performed safely. Sevoflurane currently provides the best conditions for this purpose. If the larynx is viewed easily, intubation may be performed with or without muscle relaxant. If the view is limited, a suitable bougie may be inserted to assist passage of the tracheal tube through the larynx. Correct insertion of the bougie in the trachea may be confirmed by detecting the palpable bumps of the tracheal rings or resistance when the carina is encountered. The tracheal tube is then passed over the bougie into the trachea. This manoeuvre is facilitated by rotating the tracheal tube 90° anticlockwise (to align the bevel) as it passes through the glottis. If intubation during direct laryngoscopy is unsuccessful, anaesthesia may be maintained and the use of fibreoptic laryngoscopy, blind nasal intubation or a retrograde technique considered.

Awake intubation

Fibreoptic laryngoscopy and intubation require special equipment, skill and time. The procedure may be performed by the nasal or oral route after topical anaesthesia has been achieved by spraying the nasal and oropharyngeal mucosa or gargling viscous preparations of local anaesthetic. The injection of 3–5 mL of 2% lidocaine through the cricothyroid membrane induces coughing and anaesthetizes the tracheal and laryngeal mucosa. The technique is described in detail on pages 333 and 546.

Conventional laryngoscopy can also be performed in conscious patients under local anaesthesia. After cricothyroid injection of lidocaine, laryngoscopy is performed in stages. The oropharynx is progressively anaesthetized with lidocaine spray until the patient tolerates deep insertion of the laryngoscope, enabling the larynx to be viewed.

Failed intubation

The total incidence of failed tracheal intubation is approximately 1 in 1000 (0.1%), but about 1 in 300 (0.3%) in obstetric patients. However, failed intubation in obstetric patients is now a rare event because of the high percentage of obstetric surgical patients operated on under regional anaesthesia.

Most failed intubations result from the anaesthetist failing to insert the tube, but occasionally the tube may be misplaced, most commonly in the oesophagus. This complication has resulted in many deaths since the advent of tracheal intubation. It should be suspected whenever difficulty has been experienced in inserting a tracheal tube, particularly when direct visual confirmation of the passage of the tube into the larynx has not been possible. Auscultation of the chest is recommended, although inflation of the stomach may occasionally mimic breath sounds. Auscultation over the stomach usually detects a bubbling sound if the oesophagus has been intubated.

Observation of a normal capnogram usually provides assurance of tracheal placement of the tube, but cases have been described of patients who have 'expired' carbon dioxide briefly despite oesophageal intubation, having ingested carbonated drinks or bicarbonate antacids shortly before anaesthesia. A normal and *persistent* expiratory capnogram should be sought as confirmation of tracheal tube placement.

Fibreoptic bronchoscopy provides an excellent method of assuring the location of the tube, but is not usually available in every operating theatre. The 'Wee' oesophageal intubation detector tests for the free aspiration of air via the tracheal tube into a rubber bulb. The device is cheap, easy to use and accurate, but total reliance should not be placed on this device. The capnogram is the 'gold standard' for confirming correct tracheal intubation.

Poor management of failed intubation is a significant cause of serious morbidity and mortality. The aims of management are to maintain oxygenation and prevent aspiration of gastric contents. The 'failed intubation drill' is now established as an important skill for safe anaesthetic practice. An early decision to use a failed intubation protocol and to call for assistance is essential, because continued attempts at tracheal intubation may result in trauma to the airway, pulmonary aspiration or hypoxaemia. Figure 19.1 shows a drill for managing failed intubation. The obstetric patient is a special case and is considered in Chapter 35.

If the airway is obstructed and ventilation is inadequate during management of a failed intubation, then insertion of an LMA should be considered (see Fig 19.1). It has been used successfully to provide an airway and allow ventilation when attempts to intubate the trachea and ventilate the lungs by other means have failed. Alternatively, it may be possible to pass a small-diameter tracheal tube or a bougie through the LMA into the trachea; a variant of the LMA, the intubating LMA (ILMA) is designed specifically to facilitate tracheal intubation. The LMA should not be regarded as providing protection against pulmonary aspiration, although it is claimed that the ProSeal™ LMA, which has a rearward port for the downward passage of a gastric tube or the upward passage of gastric contents, is better in this regard. The oesophageal obturator airway and similar devices are alternatives in an emergency, but there are doubts about their efficacy and there have been reports of misplacement and oesophageal rupture associated with their use. A recent innovation is an ILMA which incorporates a video camera and LCD screen, allowing direct visualisation of the introduction of a tracheal tube through the larynx.

When consciousness cannot be restored rapidly for pharmacological reasons, then transtracheal ventilation can be life-saving. A cannula or small-diameter tracheal tube may be passed via the cricothyroid membrane. Ventilation through a cannula requires high-pressure, 'jet' ventilation from a Sanders injector or the high-pressure oxygen outlet of the anaesthetic machine. More conventional ventilation is possible through a small-diameter tube placed via the cricothyroid membrane, but the procedure, which requires a transcutaneous scalpel incision, requires some practice and may result in haemorrhage. Both techniques allow adequate oxygenation for many minutes, and should provide time to allow the patient to awaken. Exhalation through a cricothyroid cannula may be inadequate, and if the laryngeal inlet is not patent then inadequate ventilation and barotrauma may result. In this situation, an additional cannula should be inserted to allow gas to escape.

If it is essential that surgery proceeds without the patient awakening then oxygenation and carbon diox-

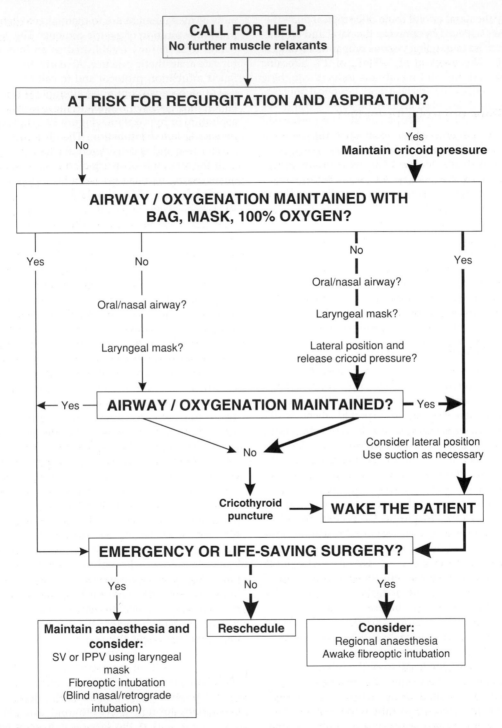

Fig. 19.1
Failed intubation drill. Make an early decision to enter the drill. Basic monitoring, optimal head positioning and the use of a bougie/stilette are assumed. This drill is not applicable to obstetric patients.

ide elimination must be maintained while ensuring an adequate depth of anaesthesia. Any of the rescue techniques described above may be used, but usually the laryngeal mask or the fibreoptic bronchoscope prove most useful.

Unintentional bronchial intubation

Bronchial intubation results in the ventilation of one lung and denial of ventilation to the other. This causes hypoxaemia through the inevitably large pulmonary shunt caused by atelectasis and collapse of the unventilated lung. Intubation of the right main bronchus is more common because of its smaller angle with the trachea. This complication is avoided by cutting the tracheal tube to an appropriate length before intubation, observation of the passage of the tube through the vocal cords and adjusting the length of the tube at the patient's incisors, and by confirmation of its position by auscultation after intubation and after changes in position of the patient on the operating table.

Aspiration of gastric contents

Regurgitation of gastric contents is common during anaesthesia. Frequently, regurgitation proceeds only as far as the mid-oesophagus, but occasionally gastric contents enter the oropharynx. This is particularly likely in patients with a hiatus hernia or a full stomach. The latter may result from recent eating or drinking or may be the result of gastric outlet or bowel obstruction, pain, stress or drugs, such as morphine or alcohol, which delay gastric emptying. Once gastric contents enter the oropharynx, there exists the potential for aspiration into the lungs. This is uncommon, but remains an important cause of morbidity and mortality associated with anaesthesia. Aspiration of oropharyngeal contents is more likely if those contents are allowed to remain in the oropharynx for a significant time, and if laryngeal reflexes are depressed. Aspiration may occur also in the sedated patient, whose laryngeal reflexes are diminished. Aspiration is more common during difficult intubation, emergency cases and in obese or pregnant patients.

Mortality is high after aspiration of large quantities of gastric contents, and the aspiration of solids, in particular, is associated with a poor prognosis. The acidity of gastric contents is also important in determining the degree of severity of the pulmonary reaction to aspiration, with highly acid material being particularly inflammatory. Bronchospasm may be the first sign of pulmonary aspiration. If a large quantity of gastric material is aspirated, respiratory obstruction, ventilation–perfusion mismatch and intrapulmonary shunt-ing may produce severe hypoxaemia, with later development of chemical pneumonitis and/or infection.

Management

At-risk patients should be managed actively to prevent the aspiration of gastric contents. The volume and acidity of the gastric contents should be reduced as far as possible. Preoperative fasting, histamine H_2-receptor blockers and a gastric prokinetic drug (e.g. metoclopramide) are recommended. If general anaesthesia is essential, then the trachea must be intubated. Most commonly, this is achieved using a rapid-sequence induction with cricoid pressure (see Ch. 28), but awake intubation is advisable if difficulty in intubation is predicted. During emergence, the tracheal tube should not be removed until protective airway reflexes are regained when the patient is awake.

If aspiration occurs during anaesthesia, further regurgitation should be prevented by immediate application of cricoid pressure, and the patient should be placed in a head-down position. The left lateral position should also be considered to encourage the drainage of gastric contents out of the mouth. In all but the mildest cases, the trachea should be intubated to facilitate removal of the aspirated material by suction before the use of positive-pressure ventilation. However, ventilation should not be delayed if significant hypoxaemia is present. Bronchodilator therapy may be required and the inspired oxygen concentration should be increased. Positive end-expiratory pressure may be used if hypoxaemia is refractory to increasing inspired oxygen fraction. Surgery should be abandoned if significant morbidity develops. Flexible bronchoscopy permits the removal of liquids, although rigid bronchoscopy may be necessary for the removal of solid matter. Intravenous steroids and pulmonary lavage with saline via a flexible bronchoscope may reduce the post-aspiration inflammatory response. A chest X-ray and arterial blood gas measurement help in the assessment of the severity of injury. The patient should be transferred to a critical care unit for further monitoring and respiratory care.

Hiccups

Regular and repeated spasmodic diaphragmatic movements may occur after i.v. induction of anaesthesia and in association with vagal stimulation during light anaesthesia. Anticholinergic premedication reduces the incidence of hiccups. Although difficult to treat, hiccups are of little consequence unless surgery, or rarely oxygenation, is compromised. Persistent hiccups may be abolished by deepening anaesthesia, stimulating the nasopharynx with a suction catheter or administering metoclopramide. Profound muscle relaxation may be justified to stop all diaphragmatic movement if hiccups are causing surgical difficulty.

Hypoxaemia

Hypoxaemia is an inadequate partial pressure of oxygen in arterial blood. Hypoxia is oxygen deficiency at the tissue level. A practical classification of the causes of hypoxaemia is shown in Table 19.5. Hypoxaemia threatens tissues globally, and if allowed to persist, risks permanent damage to those organs most delicately dependent upon continued oxygen supply. The first organs to be damaged, most commonly, are the brain and heart, and any pathological impairment of their blood supply increases the risk of early and permanent damage. There is no categorically *safe* or *unsafe* level of arterial oxygen tension (P_aO_2). The risk presented by a level of hypoxaemia is dependent upon the patient's haemoglobin concentration, cardiac output, state of hydration, concurrent disease processes (especially vasculopathic diseases) and the duration of exposure to the lowered P_aO_2. In general, few patients are harmed by arterial oxyhaemoglobin saturations of greater than 80%, but clearly, this low level provides very little margin for safety should any other complication occur. Most anaesthetists choose to set the arterial oxygen saturation alarm limits at 92–94%.

Severe hypoxaemia produces tachycardia, sweating, hypertension and arrhythmias, although bradycardia is the commoner response in children. Tachypnoea occurs in spontaneously breathing patients. There may also be clinical signs associated with the cause. As arterial desaturation progresses, bradycardia and hypotension (caused by myocardial depression) develop. Eventually, cardiac arrest occurs, usually in asystole. By this stage, the heart, brain, kidneys and liver may have incurred irreversible, ischaemic damage.

Hypoventilation is very common during anaesthesia, but in the presence of an adequate inspired oxygen concentration (i.e. over 30%) must be very severe to cause hypoxaemia. Reduction of the ventilatory

---

Table 19.5   Causes of hypoxaemia during anaesthesia

Hypoxic inspired gas mixture		
Equipment	Oxygen supply (cylinder or pipeline failure, misconnection)	
	Flowmeters (inaccurate settings, leak)	
	Breathing system (obstruction, leak)	
Hypoventilation		
Equipment	Ventilator failure, inadequate ventilatory minute volume	
	Breathing system (obstruction, leak, disconnection)	
	Tracheal tube (obstruction, oesophageal intubation)	
Patient	Respiratory depression (spontaneously breathing)	
	Obstruction	
V̇/Q̇ mismatch		
Patient	Inadequate ventilation	Bronchial intubation
		Secretions
		Atelectasis
		Pneumothorax
		Bronchospasm
		Pulmonary aspiration
		Pulmonary oedema
	Inadequate perfusion	Embolus (gas, thrombus, amniotic fluid)
		Low cardiac output
Other	Methaemoglobinaemia	
	Malignant hyperthermia	

minute volume from a normal value of 5 L min^{-1} to 2 L min^{-1} in the presence of an inspired oxygen concentration of 30% causes arterial oxygen saturation to decrease to only around 90% in an otherwise healthy patient. This represents severe hypoventilation, and produces an arterial carbon dioxide tension of approximately 13 kPa. The pulmonary shunting and atelectasis that occur during anaesthesia are much more likely to cause hypoxaemia than is hypoventilation.

Management

Hypoxaemia occurring during anaesthesia is almost invariably treatable, and its complications are preventable. Cyanosis should seldom be witnessed by the vigilant anaesthetist because the routine use of pulse oximetry allows early detection and treatment of hypoxaemia. If hypoxaemia is detected, the following drill should be instituted:

1. A-B-C. Ensure an adequate airway, ensure adequate ventilation and check for an adequate cardiac output by feeling the carotid pulse.
2. Exclude delivery of a hypoxic gas mixture using an oxygen analyser. Increase the inspired oxygen concentration to 100%.
3. Test the integrity of the breathing system by manual ventilation of the lungs and confirm bilateral chest movement and breath sounds. Blow down the tracheal tube if necessary.
4. Confirm the position and patency of the tracheal tube by assessing the capnogram, passing a suction catheter through the tracheal tube and auscultating the chest.
5. Search for clinical evidence of the causes of $\dot{V}/\dot{Q}$ mismatch with early exclusion of pneumothorax. If atelectasis or reduced functional residual capacity (FRC) is contributory, gentle hyperinflation of the lungs should improve oxygenation. Lung volume may be maintained by applying PEEP.
6. If the diagnosis is difficult, measure core temperature and consider arterial blood gas analysis and chest X-ray examination.

Apnoea

Apnoea occurs during most anaesthetics. It is eminently treatable, and usually results in no harm to the patient. The occurrence of hypoxaemia, hypercapnia and acidaemia are predictable consequences of prolonged apnoea. The development of hypoxaemia after induction of anaesthesia is often delayed by preoxy-genation of the patient's lungs. However, when hypoxaemia becomes evident, it progresses swiftly and inexorably unless oxygenation of the lungs is restored. Rapid progression of hypoxaemia occurs in the presence of airway obstruction, high oxygen consumption and small FRC. Such factors may appear in combination in small children, pregnancy and obesity. Carbon dioxide is retained during apnoea, and P_aCO_2 increases by 0.4–0.8 kPa min^{-1}, while arterial pH decreases by approximately 1.5 h^{-1} or 0.025 min^{-1}. Atelectasis develops quickly during apnoea under anaesthesia, particularly in obese patients.

As a consequence of its water solubility, very little carbon dioxide enters the lungs during apnoea and the net flow of ambient gas through an open airway and into the alveoli is very nearly equal to the rate of oxygen consumption (i.e. 250 mL min^{-1}). Consequently, adequate oxygenation may be assured for many minutes by the provision of 100% oxygen to the open airway during apnoea. If the airway is obstructed then this mass flow cannot occur and hypoxaemia develops much more quickly. In addition, the intrathoracic pressure may become significantly hypobaric if the airway is obstructed, and this further reduces the alveolar and arterial oxygen tensions.

Management

Unless required for surgery (e.g. during cardiopulmonary bypass or delicate lung surgery), apnoea should not be allowed to persist untreated. Significant atelectasis, hypercapnia and acidaemia may develop silently. If atelectasis develops, then recruitment manoeuvres may be successful in reversing it (see p. 381).

The development of hypoxaemia during apnoea is greatly slowed by the provision of 100% oxygen to an open airway. Therefore, it is mandatory that periods of apnoea (e.g. during rapid-sequence induction) are accompanied by an airway open to a breathing system supplying 100% oxygen. This is of particular importance during periods of high oxygen consumption (e.g. during fasciculations associated with administration of succinylcholine). Following the rescue of an obstructed airway there is a rapid influx of ambient gas into the previously hypobaric thorax. Provision of 100% oxygen at this point may significantly restore depleted oxygen reserves and arterial oxygen saturation.

Hypercapnia

Hypercapnia is an abnormally high partial pressure of carbon dioxide in arterial blood (P_aCO_2). Typically, this is indicated by a P_aCO_2 greater than 6 kPa. Hypercapnia is caused by either inadequate carbon dioxide removal (e.g. caused by hypoventilation or increased pulmonary dead space) or excessive carbon dioxide production. During anaesthesia, hypercapnia may also result from an inadequate fresh gas flow rate into an anaesthetic breathing system, or by exhausted carbon dioxide absorbent in a circle system, resulting in rebreathing of carbon dioxide.

Carbon dioxide production increases during pyrexia, malignant hyperthermia and shivering. Inadvertent or excessive carbon dioxide delivery from the anaesthetic machine and absorption of carbon dioxide during laparoscopic procedures are other causes of hypercapnia.

Hypercapnia stimulates activity of the sympathetic nervous system and causes tachycardia, sweating and arrhythmias (usually ectopics or tachyarrhythmias), increased cerebral blood flow, increased intracranial pressure, tachypnoea and alterations in arterial pressure. As anaesthetic drugs suppress autonomic responses, these signs may not occur during anaesthesia until P_aCO_2 is markedly increased. Acute respiratory acidosis produces an increase in serum potassium concentration.

Management

Mild degrees of hypercapnia are usually tolerated well by spontaneously breathing patients unless there is a contraindication such as head injury. If signs of significant hypercapnia occur, the anaesthetist should control ventilation and provide an appropriate ventilatory minute volume to normalize P_aCO_2.

Hypocapnia

Hypocapnia is an abnormally low P_aCO_2 (less than 4.5 kPa). The most common cause is mechanical hyperventilation. Decreased carbon dioxide production may occasionally be responsible if the patient is cold or deeply anaesthetized. Hypocapnia produces respiratory alkalosis with a decrease in serum potassium concentration. There is generalized vasoconstriction, and reductions in cerebral blood flow, cardiac output and tissue oxygen delivery. Patients with critical cerebrovascular stenosis may risk cerebral ischaemia, but otherwise hypocapnia tends not to produce significant morbidity. There may be a delay in onset of spontaneous ventilation at the conclusion of anaesthesia, while P_aCO_2 increases to levels that stimulate ventilation.

Management

Decreasing the ventilatory minute volume or increasing the breathing system dead space reduces removal of carbon dioxide from the blood. It is important to note that the most accessible representation of P_aCO_2 currently available to anaesthetists is the end-tidal carbon dioxide tension ($P_{E'}CO_2$). This is usually approximately 0.5–1.0 kPa less than P_aCO_2, but this gap varies significantly with the site of sampling of expired gas and with variations in the alveolar dead space fraction. The latter is affected by alterations in arterial pressure, cardiac output, posture and tidal volume. The anaesthetist should not assume, therefore, that a low value of end-tidal carbon dioxide tension necessarily reflects a low P_aCO_2. Such an assumption could result in significant hypoventilation if the minute volume is reduced inappropriately.

Pneumothorax

The causes of pneumothorax include trauma, central venous cannulation especially via the subclavian route, brachial plexus blockade, cervical and thoracic surgery and barotrauma. Occasionally, pneumothorax may develop spontaneously in patients with asthma, chronic obstructive pulmonary disease, congenital cystic pulmonary disease or Marfan's syndrome. During anaesthesia, very high, mechanically generated, peak inspiratory airway pressures greatly increase the risk of pulmonary barotrauma and pneumothorax. Patients with recent chest trauma, asthma or chronic lung disease (particularly with bullae) are most at risk. Pneumothorax significantly reduces ventilation of the affected lung with resultant carbon dioxide retention. Simultaneously, pulmonary shunting often occurs, with resultant hypoxaemia.

Nitrous oxide diffuses into air-filled spaces more rapidly than nitrogen diffuses out, and causes pneumothoraces to expand. Mechanical ventilation forces gas into the pleural space if the lung has been punctured, with a rapid increase in the size of the pneumothorax. Increasing $\dot{V}/\dot{Q}$ mismatch and hypoxaemia follow. If the pneumothorax is under tension, hypoxaemia, mediastinal shift, reduced venous return and impairment of cardiac output may be life-threatening. A pneumothorax should be excluded during anaesthesia if unexplained tachycardia, hypotension, hypoxaemia, hypoventilation (in the spontaneously breathing patient) or high inflation pressures (in the ventilated patient) occur intraoperatively. Examination may reveal unequal air entry, asymmetrical chest movement, wheeze, surgical emphysema, elevated jugular or central venous pressure, or mediastinal shift. Chest X-ray examination provides a definitive diagnosis, but treatment should not be delayed for this investigation if severe hypoxaemia or hypotension exist and a pneumothorax is suspected.

Management

If pneumothorax is suspected prior to anaesthesia, then it should be excluded by chest X-ray. A chest X-ray should be performed preoperatively in all patients who have suffered recent chest trauma and in those in whom a central venous catheter has recently been inserted. Occasionally, a chest X-ray fails to show a small pneumothorax which may expand rapidly with the use of nitrous oxide and positive-pressure ventilation. In patients with recent chest trauma, including rib fractures, regional analgesia or an anaesthetic technique using spontaneous ventilation is advisable where possible. If tracheal intubation and mechanical ventilation are required in a patient with a pneumothorax, a chest drain should be inserted before induction of anaesthesia. If there is a chest drain in situ, its patency and position should be checked before induction of anaesthesia.

If a pneumothorax is suspected intraoperatively, *treatment should not be delayed to confirm the diagnosis by chest X-ray examination*. Administration of nitrous oxide should be discontinued and the lungs ventilated with 100% oxygen, using low inflation pressures. The presence of air in the pleural space may be confirmed by careful aspiration through an intravenous cannula inserted through the chest wall on the suspected side via the second intercostal space in the mid-clavicular line or in the fifth space in the mid-axillary line. If the pneumothorax is under tension, there may be a hiss as air is released. Temporary decompression using one or more large intravenous cannulae may be life-saving. If a pneumothorax is confirmed, the intravenous cannula should be left in place while a formal chest drain is inserted.

The presence of a bronchopleural fistula with substantial air leak may make ventilation ineffective. In this situation, hypoventilation ensues, resulting in carbon dioxide retention. A tension pneumothorax may result. The affected lung may be isolated by insertion of a bronchial tube (either single- or double-lumen) or gas exchange improved by the use of high-frequency ventilation. A chest drain allows decompression of the pneumothorax.

Atelectasis

The reduction in functional residual capacity and the tendency to hypoventilation that occur during general anaesthesia make alveolar collapse, or atelectasis, common. Atelectasis causes impairment of gas exchange and increases the risk of postoperative chest infection. Risk factors for its development include pre-existing lung disease, lengthy anaesthesia, spontaneous ventilation, high abdominal pressures, high inspired oxygen fractions and the head-down position. Extended exposure of the open airway to atmospheric pressure adds significantly to the risk of alveolar collapse. In particular, prolonged apnoea during anaesthesia (e.g. while awaiting the onset of spontaneous ventilation) causes atelectasis.

Management

Atelectasis may be reduced through the use of mechanical ventilation during lengthy operations, the incorporation of nitrogen into the inspired gas mixture, the use of a head-up position where possible and the use of PEEP during mechanical ventilation or continuous positive airways pressure (CPAP) during spontaneous ventilation. If atelectasis is suspected (usually through observation of a gradual downward drift in arterial oxygen saturation or a gradual increase in peak inspiratory pressure during mechanical ventilation), several gentle, manual hyperinflations of the lungs usually re-inflate the collapsed alveoli (alveolar recruitment) and result in an increase in arterial oxygen saturation. Inflation for up to 20 s at 40 cmH_2O is often required for a successful recruitment manoeuvre. Such a recruitment manoeuvre is probably best performed using a mechanical ventilator.

If atelectasis becomes established during general anaesthesia then the patient is at increased risk of pulmonary dysfunction postoperatively. In this situation, the provision of good analgesia (to encourage coughing and mobilization), use of the sitting position and physiotherapy reduce postoperative morbidity.

CARDIOVASCULAR COMPLICATIONS

Hypertension

Intraoperative hypertension may be defined as an arterial pressure (systolic, mean or diastolic) 25% greater than the patient's preoperative value. Systolic hypertension increases myocardial work by increasing afterload and left ventricular wall tension. It is often associated with tachycardia, which places additional metabolic demands upon the myocardium. Patients with ischaemic heart disease or left ventricular hypertrophy may be placed at risk of myocardial ischaemia or infarction. Chronic hypertension is associated with impaired organ perfusion through atherosclerosis. Intraoperative, acute hypertension increases the risks of ischaemia, infarction and haemorrhage in other organs, and in particular, the brain.

Table 19.6 shows the commonest causes of hypertension during anaesthesia. In the absence of pre-existing hypertension, the majority of instances of intraoperative

Table 19.6   Causes of hypertension during anaesthesia

Pre-existing

Undiagnosed or poorly controlled hypertension

Pregnancy-induced hypertension

Withdrawal of antihypertensive medication

Increased sympathetic tone

Inadequate analgesia

Inadequate anaesthesia

Hypoxaemia

Airway manipulation (laryngoscopy, extubation)

Hypercapnia

Drug overdose

Vasoconstrictors (norepinephrine, phenylephrine)

Inotropes (dobutamine)

Mixed inotropes/vasoconstrictors (epinephrine, ephedrine)

Ketamine

Ergometrine

Other

Hypervolaemia

Aortic cross-clamping

Phaeochromocytoma

Malignant hyperthermia

hypertension are related to increased activity of the sympathetic nervous system. This may be associated with tachycardia and arrhythmias. The commonest causes of hypertension are inadequate analgesia, light anaesthesia, surgical stimulation and airway manipulation. However, all instances of intraoperative hypertension must prompt exclusion of awareness and malignant hyperthermia as the cause.

Management

Preoperative preparation reduces the incidence of unexpected intraoperative hypertension. Adequate pharmacological treatment of chronic hypertension is essential. Poorly controlled chronic hypertension may result in exaggerated vascular responses during anaesthesia and these patients may suffer greater intraoperative and postoperative morbidity and mortality from arrhythmias and myocardial ischaemia. A calm, relaxed patient is less likely to experience intraoperative hypertension, so consideration should be given to anxiolytic premedication. Where possible, surgery

should be postponed until adequate control is achieved (e.g. arterial pressure less than 180/100 mmHg) and organ function (e.g. heart and kidneys) assessed. Perioperative β-blockade has been demonstrated to reduce mortality in patients at risk of perioperative myocardial infarction.

Stimulating events during anaesthesia and surgery cause surges in sympathetic tone, which may result in significant increases in arterial pressure. These events may usually be anticipated and a short-acting opioid (e.g. alfentanil 10 μg kg^{-1}), β-blocker (e.g. esmolol 0.5 mg kg^{-1}), lidocaine (1 mg kg^{-1}) or temporary deepening of the anaesthetic may be used to obtund potentially damaging hypertension. Such events include laryngoscopy, surgical incision, extubation and aortic cross-clamping. Hypertension which occurs despite normoxaemia, adequately deep anaesthesia and adequate analgesia should prompt the exclusion of the causes listed in Table 19.6. If no pathological cause is found, the use of an antihypertensive agent such as labetalol or hydralazine may be indicated for persistent hypertension. The effect of negatively inotropic and vasodilating drugs is potentiated by anaesthetic agents, so careful titration is required.

Hypotension

During anaesthesia, hypotension is usefully defined as a mean arterial pressure 25% less than the patient's usual, resting value. Hypotension may impair perfusion and, consequently, oxygenation, of vital organs. During anaesthesia, myocardial and cerebral metabolic rates are reduced significantly, and intraoperative hypotension is less likely to cause permanent damage to these organs than would be the case in the conscious state. However, pathological processes (e.g. atherosclerosis) commonly compromise the arterial supply to organs, and hypotension during anaesthesia occasionally results in critical loss of flow to vital organs. Left ventricular coronary artery flow occurs predominantly in diastole, and diastolic arterial pressure is particularly important in determining myocardial viability in patients with ischaemic heart disease.

Hypotension is caused by decreases in cardiac output or systemic vascular resistance. Table 19.7 shows the common causes of intraoperative hypotension. Most anaesthetic agents cause vasodilation and have a negative inotropic effect, and moderate hypotension is very common during anaesthesia, particularly before the start of surgery when there is no physical stimulation to counteract the effects of anaesthetic drugs. Concurrent hypovolaemia caused by preoperative fluid restriction, in combination with haemorrhage or

Table 19.7   Causes of hypotension during anaesthesia

Decreased cardiac output		
Decreased preload	Hypovolaemia	Inadequate preoperative resuscitation
		Gastrointestinal fluid loss
		Haemorrhage
	Obstruction	Pulmonary embolus
		Aorto-caval compression (surgery, pregnancy, tumour)
		Pericardial effusion/tamponade
	Raised intrathoracic pressure	Mechanical ventilation, PEEP
		Pneumothorax
	Head-up position	
Myocardial	Reduced contractility	Drugs (most anaesthetic agents, β-blockers, calcium antagonists)
		Acidosis
		Ischaemia/infarction
		Arrhythmias
		Pericardial tamponade
Decreased afterload		
Drugs	Relative or absolute overdose (most anaesthetic agents, antihypertensives)	
	Hypersensitivity (drugs, colloids, blood)	
	Direct histamine release (morphine, atracurium)	
	Central regional blockade (local anaesthetics)	
Septicaemia		

concurrent antihypertensive drugs may result in decreases in mean arterial pressure during anaesthesia and surgery. A mean arterial pressure of 50 mmHg or less is potentially damaging, even in healthy individuals, and should not be allowed to persist. The patients most at risk from the effects of hypotension are, unfortunately, often the patients most likely to develop it because of concurrent medications, poor myocardial reserve and atherosclerosis. Elderly or hypertensive patients should, therefore, be observed carefully for the development of hypotension, and it should be treated promptly.

Management

Preoperative correction of hypovolaemia helps to avoid excessive reduction in arterial pressure following induction of anaesthesia. The cardiovascular effects of anaesthetic agents are predictable, and judicious doses of drugs should be used.

Artefactual measurements are not uncommon when using oscillometric devices to measure arterial pressure. If intraoperative hypotension occurs and the measurement is validated, then a working diagnosis should be established, and treatment should be commenced, aimed at correcting the cause of the hypotension. Most commonly, this involves administering intravenous fluids or decreasing the concentration or infusion rate of anaesthetic agents, although care must be taken to ensure delivery of sufficient anaesthetic agent to avoid awareness. This treatment is effective in most patients. Persistent hypotension, where significant pathological causes (e.g. arrhythmia, anaphylaxis, concealed haemorrhage or pneumothorax) have been excluded, may be treated with a cautious dose of a vasopressor agent (e.g. ephedrine 5 mg or metaraminol 1 mg). Treatment of hypotension should follow the sequence of assess → treat → re-assess. Unexpected responses to treatment should prompt a re-evaluation of the diagnosis and suspected aetiology.

Hypovolaemia

Hypovolaemia is a common intraoperative cause of hypotension. Its common aetiologies are listed in Table 19.8. The additive effects of anaesthesia, positive-pressure ventilation and hypovolaemia may cause sudden and severe hypotension, which may be life-threatening. All patients who are undergoing surgery, and in particular patients who require emergency surgery, should be assessed preoperatively with regard to intravascular fluid volume and fluid balance. Signs of hypovolaemia include thirst, dryness of mucous membranes, cool peripheries, oliguria (urine output < 0.5 ml kg^{-1} h^{-1}), reduced tissue turgor, tachycardia and postural hypotension. Patients treated with a β-blocking drug may not develop a compensatory tachy-

cardia despite being hypovolaemic. Fluid deficit and replacement are easily underestimated, especially in patients with intestinal obstruction or concealed haemorrhage. Surgery, unless immediately life-saving, should be delayed to allow adequate fluid resuscitation and restoration of intravascular volume. The response of central venous pressure (CVP) to fluid challenges is a useful guide when assessing and treating patients with significant hypovolaemia. Hypokalaemia and other electrolyte abnormalities are often associated with fluid deficits, particularly when there have been gastrointestinal losses.

In the presence of hypovolaemia, hypotension after induction of anaesthesia is often exaggerated in the elderly and in patients with decreased cardiac reserve or pre-existing hypertension. It is made less likely by fluid preloading and by titration of the induction agent to effect. Etomidate and ketamine produce less cardiovascular depression than do other induction agents.

Blood loss during surgery may be concealed. The anaesthetist must note carefully the total loss in suction jars, swabs and spillage. Body water is lost during anaesthesia and surgery in urine, sweat and exhaled breath. Adequate intraoperative fluid replacement must account for all of these losses. During abdominal surgery, up to 5 mL kg^{-1} h^{-1} may be required to replace evaporative and third-space losses in addition to maintenance requirements and replacement of blood loss.

Haemorrhage

Haemorrhage is the loss of blood and is inevitable during most forms of surgery. Loss of a significant proportion of the total intravascular volume threatens the patient's well-being. Hypovolaemia causes reduced tissue perfusion, while loss of red cell mass causes reduced oxygen carriage in arterial blood. There is no *safe* degree of haemorrhage, in that patients differ in their ability to tolerate blood loss. Anaemic or hypovolaemic patients are less able to compensate for haemorrhage than healthy patients. Patients with pre-existing compromise of vital organ perfusion (e.g. patients with diabetes mellitus or hypertension) suffer deleterious consequences of haemorrhage sooner than healthy patients. In general, adults who have lost 15% of circulating blood volume may require red blood cell transfusion to maintain oxygen-carrying capacity.

Blood loss can be estimated by weighing swabs, measuring the volume of blood in suction bottles and assessing the clinical response to fluid therapy. Estimation is often difficult if large volumes of irrigation fluid have been used, e.g. during transurethral resection of the prostate. Intraoperative measurement

Table 19.8   Causes of hypovolaemia and fluid loss
Preoperative
Haemorrhage
Trauma
Obstetric
Gastrointestinal
Major vessel rupture (aortic aneurysm)
Gastrointestinal
Vomiting
Obstruction
Fistulae
Diarrhoea
Other
Fasting
Diuretics
Fever
Burns
Intraoperative
Haemorrhage
Insensible loss
Sweating
Expired water vapour
Third-space loss
Prolonged procedures
Extensive surgery
Prolonged retraction
Drainage of stomach, bowel, or ascites

of haemoglobin concentration aids estimation of blood loss and guides therapy. With severe or ongoing haemorrhage, maintenance of intravascular volume is essential. When the cardiac output is preserved, very severe anaemia is often well tolerated for short periods, but low tissue blood flow in the presence of anaemia may produce rapid and irreversible organ damage.

Massive blood loss may require the administration of stored blood, fresh frozen plasma, clotting factors and electrolytes. The problems of massive transfusion are discussed in Chapter 22.

Disturbances of heart rate

Bradycardia

Bradycardia is commonly defined as a heart rate less than 60 beat min^{-1}. Heart rate very commonly decreases during anaesthesia because much afferent input is lost and because many anaesthetic agents and opioids have parasympathomimetic actions. Surgical manipulations such as traction on the eye, cervical or anal dilatation and peritoneal traction may increase vagal tone, producing bradycardia and occasionally sinus arrest. Several drugs may cause bradycardia. Succinylcholine may produce a profound decrease in heart rate, especially following repeat doses. Bradycardia occurs in some patients after intravenous injection of rapidly acting opioid analgesics such as remifentanil, alfentanil and fentanyl. There have been several reports of profound bradycardia in association with the use of propofol. Finally, neostigmine and β-blockers may cause profound bradycardia. Anaesthesia-induced bradycardia often leads to an *escape* rhythm, with a wandering suprajunctional pacemaker. Hypothermia and hypothyroidism also cause bradycardia.

Bradycardia reduces cardiac output, although the longer diastolic filling time and lower afterload may result in a larger ejection fraction. Diastolic pressure usually decreases and, consequently, myocardial perfusion is reduced. The concurrent reduction in myocardial oxygen demand protects against myocardial ischaemia, and myocardial damage caused by bradycardia is very rare. However, other organs may suffer; in particular, the brain, kidneys and liver may become ischaemic if a very low heart rate is allowed to persist.

Management Healthy patients usually tolerate a heart rate of 30 beat min^{-1} without organ damage. Patients with impaired organ perfusion or impaired oxygen carriage may not tolerate such low heart rates well. The risk of sinus arrest or asystole is heightened at this low rate, and most anaesthetists treat bradycar-

dia if the heart rate decreases to 40 beat min^{-1} or less. Bradycardia becomes particularly significant if associated with significant hypotension. Bradycardia may be treated by administration of an anticholinergic, antimuscarinic agent such as glycopyrronium or atropine. If bradycardia is refractory to antimuscarinic agents, intravenous isoprenaline or cardiac pacing may be indicated. Atropine or glycopyrronium may be given prophylactically where surgical stimulation increases the risk of bradycardia (e.g. ophthalmic surgery) or before a second dose of succinylcholine.

Tachycardia

During anaesthesia, tachycardia may be defined as a heart rate greater than 100 beat min^{-1}. Tachycardia is a normal sign of increased sympathetic nervous system activity. It is observed in most patients at some time during the perioperative period. Sympathetic nervous system activity is increased by hypoxaemia, hypercapnia, inadequate anaesthesia, inadequate analgesia, hypovolaemia, hypotension and noxious stimulation such as airway manipulations or surgical incision. Other signs of sympathetic nervous activity may be present, including hypertension. Tachycardia is associated also with an increase in metabolic rate (e.g. fever, sepsis, burns, hyperthyroidism, malignant hyperthermia), or the administration of vagolytic drugs (e.g. atropine, pancuronium) or sympathomimetic drugs (e.g. ephedrine, epinephrine). Isoflurane and desflurane may also increase heart rate, particularly if introduced rapidly in a high concentration. Tachycardia reduces diastolic coronary perfusion and simultaneously increases myocardial work. This may precipitate myocardial ischaemia in patients with coronary artery or hypertensive heart disease.

Management. The cause of the tachycardia should be determined and treated, e.g. by providing additional analgesia, deepening anaesthesia or giving intravenous fluids for hypovolaemia. Sinus tachycardia may be associated with myocardial ischaemia despite exclusion or treatment of other causes. In this situation, the tachycardia may be controlled by careful intravenous titration of a β-blocker such as esmolol.

Arrhythmia

Arrhythmias are not infrequent during anaesthesia, and common causes are listed in Table 19.9. Extracellular potassium concentration has a profound effect on myocardial electrical activity. Hypokalaemia increases ventricular irritability and the risks of ventricular ectopics, tachycardia and fibrillation. This effect is potentiated in patients with ischaemic heart disease and

Table 19.9   Causes of arrhythmia during anaesthesia

Cardiorespiratory

Hypoxaemia

Hypotension

Hypocapnia

Hypercapnia

Myocardial ischaemia

Metabolic

Catecholamines:

   Inadequate analgesia

   Inadequate anaesthesia

   Airway manipulation

Sympathomimetics

Hyperthyroidism

Electrolyte disturbance:

   Hypokalaemia/hyperkalaemia

   Hypercalcaemia/hypocalcaemia

Malignant hyperthermia

Surgical

Increased vagal tone (traction on eye, anus, peritoneum)

Direct cardiac stimulation (chest surgery, CVP cannulae)

Dental surgery

Drugs

Vagolytics (atropine, pancuronium)

Sympathomimetics (epinephrine, ephedrine)

Volatile anaesthetic agents (halothane, enflurane)

Digoxin

its use is recommended for routine ECG monitoring. As the ECG gives no indication of cardiac output or tissue perfusion, the detection of an abnormal cardiac rhythm should be followed by rapid assessment of the circulation. An absent pulse, severe hypotension or ventricular tachycardia or fibrillation should be treated as a cardiac arrest. The anaesthetist must exclude hypoxaemia, hypotension, inadequate analgesia and light anaesthesia as possible causes of arrhythmia. Correction of the precipitating factor is often the only treatment required. If the arrhythmia persists and causes a significant decrease in cardiac output, if it is associated with myocardial ischaemia or if it predisposes to ventricular tachycardia or fibrillation, intervention with a specific antiarrhythmic agent or electrical cardioversion is indicated. Serum potassium concentration should be measured if ventricular arrhythmias occur, especially if the patient is receiving digoxin.

Atrial arrhythmias

These may reduce the atrial contribution to left ventricular filling, resulting in a decrease in cardiac output. Premature atrial contractions and wandering atrial pacemakers are common and of little consequence.

Junctional rhythm is associated usually with the use of halothane. Reduction in concentration or change of volatile agent is indicated. Administration of an anticholinergic drug may be required to restore sinus rhythm.

Accelerated nodal rhythm may be precipitated by an increase in sympathetic tone in the presence of a sensitizing volatile anaesthetic agent. Adjusting the depth of anaesthesia or changing the anaesthetic agent is appropriate treatment.

Supraventricular tachycardia (SVT) may occur at any time during the perioperative period in susceptible patients, such as those with Wolff–Parkinson–White or other 'pre-excitation' syndromes. If attempts to increase vagal tone and terminate the SVT by carotid sinus or eyeball massage are unsuccessful, the treatment of choice is adenosine by rapid intravenous injection. This is safe and effective during haemodynamic instability because its duration of action is less than 60 s. It blocks atrioventricular conduction without compromising ventricular function. Adenosine should not be given to patients with asthma or atrioventricular conduction block. If adenosine is unavailable and the patient is normotensive, intravenous verapamil or esmolol may be given in increments. Verapamil may cause prolonged hypotension and depression of ventricular function, especially in the presence of anaesthetic agents which cause myocardial depression;

in those receiving digoxin. Hyperventilation alters acid–base balance, with acute transmembrane redistribution of potassium. Serum potassium concentration decreases by approximately 1 mmol L^{-1} for every 2.5 kPa reduction in P_aCO_2. Life-threatening hyperkalaemia with atrioventricular conduction block or ventricular fibrillation may occur if succinylcholine is used in patients with burns or denervating injuries. Electrolyte disorders are discussed further in Chapter 21.

Management.   Preoperative correction of fluid, electrolyte and acid–base imbalance is essential. Optimization of coronary artery disease and hypertension is also helpful in avoiding intraoperative arrhythmias (Ch. 23).

Continuous intraoperative ECG monitoring is mandatory during anaesthesia because arrhythmias are so common. Lead II best demonstrates atrial activity and β-blockers should not be used in conjunction with verapamil because of their unpredictable synergy, which may result in profound bradycardia. DC cardioversion is indicated if the SVT is associated with hypotension and adenosine is unavailable.

Atrial flutter or fibrillation may be observed during anaesthesia de novo or as a paroxysmal increase in ventricular rate in patients with pre-existing atrial flutter or fibrillation. After correcting any precipitating factors, digoxin by slow intravenous injection is the treatment of choice if the patient was not taking digoxin preoperatively. Alternative therapy with amiodarone or a β-blocker may be necessary to control the ventricular rate in patients already taking digoxin. Immediate cardioversion should be considered if the ventricular rate is fast with a significant reduction in cardiac output.

Ventricular arrhythmias

Premature ventricular contractions (PVCs) are common in healthy patients and may be present preoperatively. If associated with a slow atrial rate (escape beats), increasing the sinus rate by administration of an anticholinergic drug should abolish them. In other situations, an underlying cause should be sought before antiarrhythmic agents are considered, as PVCs rarely progress to more serious arrhythmias unless they are multifocal and frequent or if there is underlying myocardial ischaemia or hypoxaemia. Halothane lowers the threshold for catecholamine-induced ventricular arrhythmias, and this effect is exacerbated by hypercapnia. Halothane should be used with care in patients receiving sympathomimetic drugs (including local anaesthetics containing epinephrine) and in patients taking aminophylline or drugs that block norepinephrine re-uptake, such as tricyclic or other antidepressants. The maximum recommended dose of epinephrine for infiltration in the presence of halothane is 100 μg (10 mL of 1 in 100 000) during any 10-min period, although the rate of absorption depends on the site of injection. The use of enflurane or isoflurane carries a much lower risk of development of arrhythmias, and sevoflurane has an even lower potential to cause myocardial sensitization to catecholamines.

Heart block. Impulses from the atria may be variably conducted to the ventricles. Degrees of impairment range from a small time delay in onward transmission to complete failure of onward propagation of impulses. Heart block may result in bradycardia and reduced cardiac output. Treatment is seldom necessary during anaesthesia, but minor degrees of atrioventricular block may progress to complete heart block, in which atrial impulses do not reach the ventricles. In this situation, bradycardia is usually severe and the atria no longer assist in filling the ventricle before ventricular systole. Cardiac output may fall to life-threateningly low levels, and immediate treatment is necessary. This includes intravenous isoprenaline and transcutaneous or transvenous cardiac pacing.

Ventricular tachycardia is uncommon during anaesthesia. If it is not causing significant hypotension, administration of intravenous lidocaine (1.5 mg kg^{-1}) may be effective, but direct current cardioversion is often necessary. Cardiac massage may be required if the cardiac output is inadequate.

Ventricular fibrillation is very uncommon in association with anaesthesia. It requires immediate DC cardioversion.

Any arrhythmia that causes the loss of a palpable pulse should be treated as for cardiac arrest, with immediate external (or internal, if appropriate) cardiac massage, ventilation of the lungs with 100% oxygen and drug treatment as specified in the appropriate Advanced Life Support protocol.

Myocardial ischaemia

The heart has the highest oxygen consumption per tissue mass of all the organs (second only to the carotid body). Resting coronary blood flow is 250 mL min^{-1} and represents 5% of the cardiac output. The oxygen extraction ratio of the myocardium is 70–80%, compared with an average of 25% for other tissues. Increased oxygen consumption must be matched by an increase in coronary blood flow. Ischaemia results when the oxygen demand outstrips supply. Even very brief reductions in supply result in ischaemia, which may lead rapidly to infarction and permanent loss of muscle function in the affected area.

Myocardial oxygen delivery is the product of arterial oxygen content and coronary artery blood flow. The diastolic pressure time index (DPTI) reflects coronary blood supply. It is the product of the coronary perfusion pressure (predominantly diastolic arterial pressure) and diastolic time. Oxygen demand is represented by the tension time index (TTI), the product of systolic pressure and systolic time.

The ratio of DPTI/TTI is the endocardial viability ratio (EVR) and represents the myocardial oxygen supply–demand balance. The EVR is usually greater than one. A value of less than 0.7 is associated with subendocardial ischaemia. Such a value may be reached in a patient with the data shown in Table 19.10.

It is clear from the above that tachycardia is particularly dangerous in generating myocardial ischaemia,

Table 19.10 Patient data generating a dangerously low endocardial viability ratio

Arterial pressure: 180/90 mmHg	
Heart rate (HR): 130 beat min^{-1}	
LVEDP	10 mmHg
DPTI	= (90 − 10) mmHg × (60 s/130 − 0.2 s)
	= 21 s mmHg
TTI	= 180 mmHg × 0.2 s
	= 36 s mmHg
EVR	= 0.58

Systolic time is typically fixed at 0.2 s, and diastole occupies the remaining time.

while systolic hypertension and diastolic hypotension may also contribute. Patients with coronary artery disease are most at risk. Intraoperative myocardial ischaemia may manifest clinically as arrhythmia, hypotension or pulmonary oedema. It is diagnosed by ECG ST-segment changes (usually depression), although these are not always detected reliably without computer-assisted analysis. The use of the V5 electrode is recommended for ECG monitoring in susceptible patients (e.g. the CM5 configuration; see Ch. 18) because it is the most sensitive ECG lead for the detection of left ventricular ischaemia. When used alone, it may detect up to 85% of the ST abnormalities on a standard 12-lead ECG.

Transoesophageal echocardiography may detect abnormal myocardial wall motion, which is a sensitive indicator of ischaemia and is associated with increased perioperative morbidity. Regional wall dysfunction often persists into the postoperative period without clinical signs. Increased myocardial work during this period, e.g. from pain, may precipitate further ischaemia or infarction in susceptible patients. While the risk of infarction in the general surgical population is low, the overall mortality rate following perioperative myocardial infarction approaches 50%.

Management

Preoperative preparation of the at-risk patient includes optimization of antianginal and antihypertensive medication, suppression of anxiety and assurance of normal intravascular volume. During anaesthesia, the risks associated with ischaemia are minimized by the use of an appropriate anaesthetic technique and early detection by the use of appropriate monitoring in susceptible patients.

If ischaemia is detected, arterial oxygen content should be increased by optimizing P_aO_2 and haemoglobin concentration. Tachycardia should be controlled by ensuring that analgesia, anaesthesia and intravascular volume are satisfactory. If systolic hypertension, diastolic hypotension or tachycardia exist, then these may be controlled pharmacologically; most commonly, increments of a vasodilator or β-blocker are administered to treat hypertension or tachycardia. If signs of myocardial ischaemia persist, the use of a venodilator such as glyceryl trinitrate by intravenous infusion should be considered.

EMBOLUS

An embolus is the passage of a non-blood mass through the vascular system. Venous emboli usually become lodged in the lung, where they impair gas exchange and cause a local inflammatory reaction. Arterial emboli cause obstruction, which may result in distal ischaemia.

Thromboembolus

Embolization of thrombus occurs usually from the deep veins of the legs or pelvis. It is uncommon during anaesthesia. It is often preceded by a period of immobilization, so that patients whose hospital stay is extended or who have suffered major trauma are at highest risk. Other risk factors include malignancy, smoking, pelvic and limb surgery, the oral contraceptive or hormone replacement therapy, and a past history of venous thromboembolism. Venous stasis caused by venous compression, hypovolaemia, hypotension, hypothermia or the use of tourniquets also increases the risk of deep venous thrombosis. Veins may sustain trauma during positioning and surgery, and increased blood coagulability, with a consequent increase in the risk of venous thrombosis, is a consequence of the stress response to surgery.

During anaesthesia, pulmonary thromboembolism may present with tachycardia, hypoxaemia, arrhythmia, hypotension, bronchospasm, an acute decrease in the end-tidal carbon dioxide concentration, or cardiovascular collapse.

Management

Patients with risks factors should be managed actively to prevent deep venous thrombosis. The oral contraceptive pill or hormone replacement therapy should be stopped at least 6 weeks before elective surgery in patients at risk. Prophylactic heparin, graduated compression stockings and intraoperative, intermittent calf compression reduce the likelihood of new thrombosis. The use of subarachnoid or epidural anaesthesia reduces the risk of postoperative venous thromboembolism in some surgical groups.

If intraoperative pulmonary embolism is suspected, the lungs should be ventilated with 100% oxygen and bronchodilator therapy, fluid loading and inotropic support of the circulation should be considered. In extreme presentations, cardiac arrest protocols should be used. After management of the initial haemodynamic disturbance, thrombolytic therapy (if not contraindicated), anticoagulation and, rarely, surgical removal of the embolus may be indicated.

Gas embolus

Gas usually enters the circulation through a surgical wound. A subatmospheric venous pressure greatly encourages the entrainment of air into the venous system. Therefore, positions that place the operative site above the right atrium carry an increased risk of this complication. Such positions include sitting, park bench, knee-chest and head-up. Vascular catheters are another potential route for air entry, particularly during their insertion. Gas embolism (usually carbon dioxide) may also occur during laparoscopy and thoracoscopy.

Clinical presentation varies with the volume and rate of gas entry into the circulation. An entry rate of 0.5 mL kg^{-1} min^{-1} has been reported to produce clinical signs. If a significant volume of gas enters the right side of the heart, an airlock may develop, preventing ejection of blood and effectively halting cardiac output. A 'millwheel murmur' may be heard via a precordial or oesophageal stethoscope, although this is reported to be a late sign and only occurs with very large emboli. The sudden decrease in right ventricular output results in a rapid decrease in end-tidal carbon dioxide concentration. Hypoxaemia, tachycardia, ECG changes (especially arrhythmia) and an increase in pulmonary artery pressure follow.

Transoesophageal echocardiography and precordial Doppler ultrasound are the most sensitive monitors for gas embolus. Clinical and ECG signs have a low sensitivity for detection of gas embolism. As the foramen ovale is potentially patent in more than 25% of the population, an increase in right heart pressure may open the foramen in these patients. Paradoxical gas embolism via this route or across the pulmonary capillary bed to the coronary or cerebral circulations may cause myocardial or cerebral ischaemia and infarction.

Management

Prevention of intraoperative air embolus requires adjustment of the patient's position and the site of the operative field with respect to the right atrium. If air embolism is detected, further air entry is prevented by flooding the operative site with saline. During head and neck procedures, the venous pressure at the surgical site may be increased by compressing the jugular veins. If possible, the operative site should be lowered relative to the right atrium. The application of PEEP increases venous pressure and reduces further ingress of air.

During insufflation procedures, the surgeon should be instructed to depressurize the insufflated body cavity. If the gas embolus is symptomatic, administration of nitrous oxide should be discontinued to avoid expansion of gas bubbles and the lungs should be ventilated with 100% oxygen. Occasionally, gas may be aspirated from the right ventricle or atrium via a venous catheter. However, insertion of a catheter is usually impractical and time-consuming, and this is only worth attempting if a catheter is already in place. Expansion of the intravascular fluid volume, inotropic support of the circulation and internal or external cardiac massage may be necessary. Placing the patient in a head-down left lateral position may help by allowing gas from the right ventricle to escape into the atrium and vena cava.

Other emboli

Fat dislodged from long bone fractures may embolize to the lungs. Patients typically develop sudden mental disturbance, shortness of breath, hypoxaemia and axillary and subconjunctival petechiae. Onset is usually 2–48 h after the injury. Fat globules may be seen in the urine and sputum, or in the retinal vessels during fundoscopy. There should be a high index of suspicion if unexpected haemodynamic events or hypoxaemia occur in patients undergoing surgery for pelvic or lower limb fractures. Treatment is with intravenous fluids, steroids and ventilatory support as necessary. The use of intravenous albumin to bind free fat is controversial.

Other material that may embolize includes tumour fragments, amniotic fluid and orthopaedic cement. Air or clot may embolize via arterial cannulae and produce distal ischaemia.

NEUROLOGICAL COMPLICATIONS
Awareness

Recall of intraoperative events occurs in 0.03–0.3% of anaesthetics. Such recall may be spontaneous, or may be provoked by postoperative events or questioning. Awareness during anaesthesia may be a very distressing event for a patient, particularly if it is accompanied by awareness of the painful nature of an operation. However, the majority of recalled events are not painful, and 80–90% of patients recalling intraoperative events have not experienced pain. Awareness may have psychological sequelae including insomnia, depression and post-traumatic stress disorder (PTSD) with distressing flashbacks.

The risk of awareness correlates with depth of anaesthesia. Light anaesthesia, particularly when the patient is paralysed by muscle relaxants, is associated with the highest risk of awareness. Awareness is associated frequently with poor anaesthetic technique. Errors include the omission or late commencement of volatile agent, inadequate dosing or failure to recognize the signs of awareness. Underdosing of anaesthetic agent may occur during hypotensive episodes, when anaesthetic is withheld in an attempt to maintain arterial pressure. Breathing system malfunctions and disconnections have been associated with awareness.

The signs of awareness in a paralysed patient arise from activation of the sympathetic nervous system (sweating, tachycardia, hypertension, tear formation), and dilatation and reactivity to light of the pupils. Unparalysed patients experiencing noxious stimulation may move or grimace. Depth of anaesthesia may be assessed through clinical examination, monitoring of the patient's expired volatile agent concentration or using specialized monitoring equipment. Such equipment includes processed electroencephalography such as the bispectral index and auditory evoked potential monitoring systems. If the end-tidal concentrations of inhaled anaesthetic agents equate to a total of greater than about 0.8 MAC, it is exceptionally unlikely that a patient experiences intraoperative awareness.

Awareness is more likely to occur during emergency and obstetric surgery, during neuromuscular paralysis, during periods of hypotension and in patients treated with a β-blocker. The use of intravenous drugs for maintenance of anaesthesia (e.g. propofol target-controlled infusion) may be associated with an increased risk of awareness compared with the use of inhaled anaesthetic agents. It is not possible currently to monitor, in real time, the concentration of intravenous agents in blood, while it is possible to monitor exhaled volatile agents. Additionally, the scatter about the mean of the minimum inhibitory concentration (MIC) for intravenous agents is greater than the equivalent for inhaled agents (MAC).

Management

If the anaesthetist suspects intraoperatively that a patient may be experiencing awareness, anaesthesia should be deepened immediately. If the arterial pressure is low despite an inadequate dose of anaesthetic agent, then the arterial pressure should be supported through the use of intravenous fluids, modification of ventilatory pattern or intravenous administration of a vasopressor, and anaesthesia deepened appropriately. Consideration should be given to the use of an intravenous benzodiazepine (e.g. midazolam 5 mg). Some retrograde amnesia may be gained and further recall is made less likely through the anterograde amnesic effect.

If a patient complains in the postoperative period of intraoperative awareness, the anaesthetist should be informed and should visit the patient. The anaesthetist should establish the timing of the episode and try to distinguish between dreaming and awareness. If there is genuine awareness and a clear anaesthetic error, then a prompt apology and explanation should be provided. All details should be recorded in the case notes. The situation may be exacerbated if staff refuse to believe the patient. It is essential to offer follow-up counselling for the patient and to inform the patient's general practitioner. See *Medicolegal aspect of complications* section above for further detail of dealing with any subsequent formal complaints.

Awareness occasionally occurs despite apparently excellent practice and in the absence of equipment malfunction. Successful defence against litigation requires that the anaesthetist has made thorough records. It is advisable that the anaesthetist always records the timing (absolute and relative to surgery) and dose of anaesthetic agents (inhaled or intravenous).

NEUROLOGICAL INJURY

Ischaemia of the central nervous system

Transient disruptions of central nervous system (CNS) perfusion and oxygenation are common during anaesthesia. However, prolonged reduction in oxygenation of the CNS may result in ischaemia or infarction. Ischaemic injury varies from minimal, focal dysfunction to stroke or death. The mechanism is related usually to hypoxaemia and/or hypotension. The risk of ischaemic brain damage related to hypotension is increased in patients with atherosclerosis, and, in particular, cerebrovascular disease. A history of previous transient ischaemic attacks or stroke makes CNS injury much more likely during anaesthesia.

Rarely, intracerebral haemorrhage may occur during anaesthesia, with consequent local compression and downstream ischaemic injury. Although the risk is increased if arterial pressure has been very high, there have been reports of intracerebral haemorrhage during anaesthesia without episodes of hypertension. It is likely that previously undetected vascular abnormalities were present in these cases.

The cervical spinal cord may be damaged during tracheal intubation and positioning in patients with cervical spine instability from fractures, rheumatoid arthritis or congenital conditions such as Down syndrome. Extreme rotation, flexion or extension of the neck may cause cerebral ischaemia because of vertebrobasilar insufficiency in susceptible patients. Ischaemic spinal cord injury may also occur during major vascular and spinal surgery, when the local arterial supply may be compromised.

Management

Hypoxaemia and hypotension should not be allowed to persist, particularly in patients at risk of CNS ischaemic injury. Severe hypocapnia should be avoided, because of its potential for global cerebral vasoconstriction. Deep anaesthesia results in a greatly lowered cerebral metabolic rate, and this confers some protection against cerebral ischaemia.

Peripheral nerve injury

Peripheral nerves may be injured through hypotension and hypoxaemia, but they are far more resistant than is the CNS. Peripheral injuries occur more commonly because of poor positioning or direct injury during nerve blockade or vascular catheter placement. This topic is dealt with in more detail later in this chapter.

TEMPERATURE

Hypothermia

Body temperature very commonly decreases during anaesthesia. A decrease to a core temperature below 36°C represents hypothermia. Hypothermia causes physiological derangement and increases perioperative morbidity (see also Ch. 20).

Heat production is decreased during anaesthesia. Anaesthetic agents alter hypothalamic function, reduce metabolic rate, abolish behavioural responses to heat loss and abolish shivering. Heat loss increases during anaesthesia and surgery because of heat redistribution to the peripheries by vasodilatation and increased radiation by the exposure of large, moist surfaces. Evaporative heat loss is increased by ventilation of the lungs with cold, dry gas, the use of wet packs and operations on open body cavities. Heat loss is exacerbated by low ambient temperature, and high air flow in the operating theatre promotes convective and evaporative loss. Irrigation and intravenous infusion of cold fluids are also associated with increased heat loss. The risks of hypothermia are greatest in neonates and infants, patients with a low metabolic rate (such as the elderly) and patients with burns.

The effects of hypothermia are dependent upon the change in core temperature. Metabolic rate reduces by approximately 10% for each 1°C reduction in core temperature. Cardiac output decreases and the affinity of haemoglobin for oxygen is increased, causing a reduction in tissue oxygenation. Significant hypothermia is associated with metabolic (lactic) acidosis, oliguria, altered platelet and clotting function, and reduced hepatic blood flow with slower drug metabolism. The MAC of volatile agents is reduced (also by approximately 10% for each 1°C decrease) and muscle relaxants have a longer and more variable duration of effect. Postoperative shivering increases oxygen consumption and myocardial work. Peripheral vasoconstriction increases afterload, further increasing the risk of myocardial ischaemia. Hypothermia also increases the risk of postoperative infections because of suppression of function of the immune system.

Management

Ambient temperature and humidity should be maintained as high as is comfortable for staff working in the operating theatre. The patient should be protected from the cool, ambient environment during all phases of anaesthesia and during transfers. A convective warming blanket (e.g. Bair Hugger™), which surrounds the patient with a microenvironment of warm air, is particularly effective. The head and any exposed, moist viscera lose heat particularly quickly, and wrapping these is effective in preventing radiation and evaporative heat loss. Cold intravenous fluids should be warmed where possible, although this should not compromise the administration of adequate volumes. Inspired gases should be warmed and humidified. A heat and moisture exchanging device is very effective in this regard, and is often combined with a microbial filter.

In all but very short operations, the above measures should be commenced as soon as possible after induction of anaesthesia, and core temperature should be monitored both to detect hypothermia and to adjust the warming devices to prevent hyperthermia developing. If core temperature remains significantly below 35°C at the end of surgery then consideration should be given to keeping the patient anaesthetized until temperature is normalized. This applies particularly to patients with cardiovascular or cerebrovascular disease, or metabolic abnormalities.

Induced, deep hypothermia (as low as 16°C) may be used for neurosurgical, aortic or cardiac procedures where circulatory arrest is required to provide the necessary operating conditions. Large reductions in the metabolic rate reduce tissue oxygen consumption and allow a short period of circulatory arrest. Hypothermia reduces cerebral oxygen consumption and is occasionally used in the management of severe head injury.

Hyperthermia

Hyperthermia during anaesthesia may be defined as a core body temperature greater than 37.5°C, and is usually caused by an increase in heat production. Common causes include sepsis and infection, drug reactions (anaphylaxis, incompatible blood transfusion), excessive catecholamine activity (phaeochromocytoma, thyroid storm) and malignant hyperthermia. Elevated metabolic rate may lead to acidosis. Without treatment, sweating and vasodilatation produce hypovolaemia and tissue hypoxia. Seizures and CNS damage may ensue.

Management

General measures include exposure of the body surface, application of ice packs, use of fans and administration of cold intravenous fluids. Specific measures depend on the cause. Paracetamol and non-steroidal anti-inflammatory agents may reduce core temperature if the cause is sepsis-related. The occurrence of any unexplained increase in temperature, especially if temperature is increasing rapidly, must prompt the urgent exclusion of malignant hyperthermia.

Malignant hyperthermia

Malignant hyperthermia (MH) is an inherited disorder of muscle. The incidence varies geographically from 0.02% to 0.002% (1 in 5000 to 1 in 50 000). MH had a mortality rate of 75% at the time it was identified in 1960. Treatment consisted of cooling the patient and treating complications as they arose. The cause was then unknown, and could not be treated. Currently, mortality is approximately 5%. Increased awareness amongst anaesthetists has resulted in earlier diagnosis and treatment. Since 1979, dantrolene has been available for the treatment of MH and has resulted in the dramatic decline in death and disability from the condition.

Malignant hyperthermia is an inherited disorder. Mutations in the human ryanodine receptor in skeletal muscle (a calcium-release channel with a role in excitation–contraction coupling) are apparent in some families. Predisposition to MH has been identified in only three rare clinical myopathies. Abnormal calcium release and re-uptake by the sarcoplasmic reticulum leads to myofibrillar contraction, depletion of high-energy muscle phosphate stores, accelerated metabolic rate, increased carbon dioxide and heat production, increased oxygen consumption and metabolic acidosis. The usual triggering agents are succinylcholine or any volatile anaesthetic agent.

The MH syndrome may present at any time during the perioperative period. The clinical features and their severity vary considerably. The most consistent and early signs are unexplained tachycardia and an increase in the end-tidal $P\text{CO}_2$. Spontaneously breathing patients may present with tachypnoea. MH should be considered in any anaesthetized patient if core temperature increases during anaesthesia. Core temperature increases typically by $2°C\,h^{-1}$ and may exceed 40°C. Muscle rigidity is common and usually involves the limbs and jaw. Without treatment, the full MH syndrome may develop, with sweating, cyanosis, mottled skin, hypoxaemia, ventricular arrhythmias and severe metabolic and respiratory acidosis. Muscle injury causes significant potassium release, with ECG signs of hyperkalaemia. Coagulopathy, hypocalcaemia, oliguria, myoglobinuria and acute renal failure are other sequelae.

Masseter muscle rigidity (MMR) occasionally complicates anaesthesia, particularly following administration of succinylcholine. This progresses to MH in approximately 10% of cases.

Management

Administration of a volatile anaesthetic agent should be discontinued immediately and the lungs hyperventilated with 100% oxygen. The anaesthetic breathing system should be replaced with an unused (and therefore uncontaminated) system. Anaesthesia should be maintained with an intravenous agent. The trachea should be intubated at the earliest opportunity if a tracheal tube is not already in place. Experienced help should be obtained in both the operating theatre and the laboratory, and the operation must be abandoned as soon as possible. Intravenous dantrolene should be given in doses of $1–2\,mg\,kg^{-1}$ every 5 min until the increase in $P_{E'}\text{CO}_2$ is controlled; typically, a total dose of $2.5\,mg\,kg^{-1}$ is required, although doses up to $10\,mg\,kg^{-1}$ may be needed. Dantrolene is packaged as a powder which takes several minutes to reconstitute. It is a skeletal muscle relaxant and causes muscle weakness in large doses. The massive increase in metabolic rate commonly produces severe acidosis, and large amounts of intravenous fluids and sodium bicarbonate may be required. Ice packs should be placed around the neck, axillae and groin and chilled saline should be infused intravenously. If necessary, gastric, rectal and peritoneal lavage with iced saline may be life-saving if hyperthermia is severe. Cardiopulmonary bypass has been used in severe cases.

Core temperature, CVP, direct arterial pressure and urine output should be monitored. Acid–base status, arterial gas tensions, coagulation status and serum electrolyte concentrations should be measured frequently. Hyperkalaemia is common, and should be treated with intravenous glucose and insulin. Arrhythmias usually resolve after treatment of hyperkalaemia and acidosis, but specific antiarrhythmic drugs may be required. Renal hypoperfusion and medullary hypoxia may result rapidly in acute tubular necrosis. Urine output should be maintained by ensuring an adequate circulating blood volume and using intravenous mannitol. Haemofiltration may be required to correct severe biochemical abnormalities or renal dysfunction. The syndrome often persists beyond the initial acute episode, and hyperthermia may return up to 48 hours later. The patient should be managed in a high-dependency area and oral dantrolene should be continued during this time.

Following an episode of MH, the patient should be referred to a specialist centre for further assessment. The tests used to identify individuals with MH susceptibility vary among centres. The most common test is halothane and caffeine-induced contracture of a muscle specimen. Less-invasive genetic tests are being developed. First-degree family members should also be screened for MH.

Anaesthesia for the MH-susceptible patient

A 'clean' anaesthetic machine is used, and this may be prepared by flushing the machine for 12 hours with 100% oxygen and by using a new breathing system. Contact with volatile agents and succinylcholine is absolutely contraindicated. Regional anaesthesia should be used if possible. If general anaesthesia is unavoidable, then total intravenous anaesthesia with propofol is recommended. Dantrolene is not usually used as a premedicant, but should be immediately available throughout the perioperative period. Monitoring of end-tidal carbon dioxide concentration, ECG, arterial pressure, oxygen saturation and core temperature is mandatory.

EQUIPMENT MALFUNCTION

About a third of all critical incidents are related to equipment failure and most are preventable. Most equipment problems have implications for the patient and some have been described above (e.g. leaks and disconnections involving the anaesthetic machine and gas delivery system). Meticulous preparation of equipment prevents most malfunctions, while a systematic approach to identifying problems as they arise should prevent most potentially serious complications.

Monitoring equipment may provide inaccurate and misleading data. Non-invasive arterial pressure devices and pulse oximeters often produce inaccurate readings. Movement, diathermy and poor contact with the patient may contribute to artefact in monitored values. Incorrect data may lead to incorrect treatment of the patient, and artefact must always be borne in mind as a cause for a sudden change to a value outside the acceptable range. Data supplied by monitors must always be used in conjunction with clinical examination of the patient and should be considered in context (e.g. type of surgery, patient's pre-existing illnesses).

DRUG REACTIONS

Hypersensitivity

Susceptible patients may display an enhanced immunological reaction to a trigger, which may be a drug or an environmental agent. These *hypersensitivity* reactions may be anaphylactic or anaphylactoid. Some drugs produce histamine release directly, without an immunological basis.

The incidence of anaphylaxis varies according to the antigen involved. Of the intravenous drugs, reactions are most commonly to muscle relaxants (1 in 5000 to 1 in 10 000). Succinylcholine is the most immunogenic, although reactions to all non-depolarizing relaxants have also been reported. The majority of reactions are IgE-mediated. There is significant cross-reactivity between muscle relaxants and other drugs which contain a quaternary ammonium group. Pancuronium appears to be the least likely muscle relaxant to cause anaphylaxis.

Reactions to intravenous induction agents are far less common (1 in 15 000 to 1 in 50 000). Hypersensitivity to benzodiazepines and etomidate is rare and these drugs do not cause direct histamine release.

Hypersensitivity to local anaesthetics is very rare. Reactions are more likely to be the result of dose-related toxicity, sensitivity to the effects of added vasoconstrictor or a reaction to preservatives such as paraben and benzoates. Amide local anaesthetic agents are less allergenic than esters.

Antibiotics are frequently implicated in allergic reactions. Penicillins are most often to blame, and there is cross-reactivity with cephalosporin antibiotics in 10% of penicillin-allergic patients.

Latex is emerging as one of the more important causes of anaphylaxis during anaesthesia and surgery. Reactions usually begin 30–60 min following exposure, and may be very severe. Previous frequent exposure to latex (e.g. spina bifida) is a strong risk factor for latex allergy. There is often a history of intolerance to some foods, including banana and avocado. Many medical devices contain latex (e.g. arterial pressure cuffs, surgical gloves), and it is important that all such products are eliminated from the care of latex-susceptible patients.

Anaphylaxis also occurs in response to radiocontrast media, blood products, colloid solutions, protamine, streptokinase, aprotinin, atropine, bone cement and opioids. Allergic reactions to volatile agents are exceptionally uncommon.

Anaphylaxis (type 1 hypersensitivity) is an IgE-mediated reaction to an antigen. Antibodies bind to mast cells, which degranulate, releasing the chemical mediators of anaphylaxis. These include histamine, prostaglandins, platelet-activating factor (PAF) and leukotrienes. The signs produced by the actions of these mediators of anaphylaxis include urticaria, cutaneous flushing, bronchospasm, hypotension, arrhythmia and cardiac arrest. *Only one of these signs may be present*, and it is important to have a high index of suspicion. Anaphylaxis has been reported in patients without apparent previous exposure to the specific antigen, probably because of immunological cross-reactivity. This is true particularly of reactions to muscle relaxants; cosmetics and some foods contain structurally similar compounds.

Anaphylactoid reactions are not IgE-mediated, although the clinical presentation is identical to anaphylaxis. The precise immunological mechanism is not always evident, although many reactions involve complement, kinin and coagulation pathway activation.

Non-immunological histamine release is caused by the direct action of a drug on mast cells. The clinical response depends on both the drug dose and the rate of delivery but is usually benign and confined to the skin. Anaesthetic drugs which release histamine directly include d-tubocurarine, atracurium, doxacurium, mivacurium (all of similar chemical derivation), morphine and pethidine. Clinical evidence of histamine release, usually cutaneous, occurs in up to 30% of patients during anaesthesia. However, some very serious reactions have been reported in association with administration of atracurium and mivacurium.

Hypersensitivity reaction should be considered in the differential diagnosis of any major cardiorespiratory problem during anaesthesia. Reactions are more common in women, and in patients with a history of allergy, atopy or previous exposure to anaesthetic agents. Over 90% of reactions occur immediately after induction of anaesthesia. There is a clinical spectrum of severity from the mildest urticaria to immediate cardiac arrest. Coughing, skin erythema, difficulty with ventilation and loss of a palpable pulse are common early signs. Reactions often involve a single, major physiological system (e.g. bradycardia and profound hypotension without bronchospasm). This may make diagnosis confusing, but every instance of bronchospasm, unexpected hypotension, arrhythmia or urticaria should be considered to be due to anaphylaxis until proved otherwise. Erythema of the skin may be short-lived or absent because cyanosis from poor tissue perfusion and hypoxaemia may be occur rapidly and be profound. The conscious patient may experience a sense of impending doom, dyspnoea, dizziness, palpitations and nausea. The differential diagnosis includes anaesthetic drug overdose and other causes of bronchospasm, hypotension or hypoxaemia.

Management

Death may result from tissue hypoxia secondary to inadequate perfusion and/or hypoxaemia. Early recognition and treatment are essential. The aims of management are to obtund the effect of the anaphylaxis mediators and to prevent their further release. A management 'drill' should be used (Table 19.11). The early use of epinephrine is life-saving during anaphylactic reactions because it treats the symptoms (through peripheral vasoconstriction, increased cardiac output and bronchodilation) and the cause (through mast cell re-stabilization). Corticosteroids and histamine H_1-receptor antagonists have a delayed onset of action, but have a role in later management.

Anaphylaxis may persist, despite a promising initial response to management. Therefore, subsequent management should be in a critical care area (e.g. an intensive care unit). An infusion of epinephrine may be required to treat persistent hypotension or bronchospasm, and in the interests of preventing further mast cell degranulation. Progressive oedema involving the airway may develop rapidly and tracheal intubation and mechanical ventilation of the lungs are recommended until the patient is clinically stable and

Table 19.11 Drill for the management of major anaphylaxis
Initial therapy
Stop administration of drug(s) likely to have caused the anaphylaxis
Maintain airway. Give 100% oxygen
Lay patient supine with feet elevated
Give epinephrine. This may be given intramuscularly in a dose of 0.5–1 mg (0.5–1.0 mL of 1:1000) and may be repeated every 10 min according to the arterial pressure and pulse until improvement occurs. Alternatively, epinephrine may be administered intravenously. The dose given depends upon the severity of the reaction. Minor symptoms may be treated with 50 μg boluses, while cardiovascular collapse requires a bolus dose of 1000 μg. Further doses are likely to be required
Start intravascular volume expansion with crystalloid or colloid
Secondary therapy
Antihistamines (chlorpheniramine 20 mg i.v.)
Corticosteroids (hydrocortisone 100 mg i.v.)
Catecholamine infusions (starting doses: epinephrine 0.05–0.1 μg kg^{-1} min^{-1}, norepinephrine 0.05–0.1 μg kg^{-1} min^{-1})
Consider bicarbonate (0.5 mmol kg^{-1} i.v.) for acidosis, repeated as necessary
Airway evaluation (before extubation)
Bronchodilators (salbutamol 2.5 mg kg^{-1}) may be required for persistent bronchospasm

airway patency guaranteed after a period of observation. Blood coagulation status, serum electrolyte concentrations and arterial gas tensions should also be measured regularly.

Venous blood samples should be obtained as early in the reaction as possible, and subsequently should be taken every 4 h for the first 24-h period. The most important sample is 1 h after the beginning of the reaction. The sample should be separated and stored at −20°C for subsequent measurement of serum tryptase concentration. Serum tryptase is a specific marker of mast cell degranulation, and has replaced the measurement of serum IgE as the test of choice for confirming a diagnosis of anaphylaxis. However, a negative test does not exclude a hypersensitivity reaction.

The patient should be reviewed at a later date by an appropriate clinician (e.g. a clinical immunologist) and further investigations performed. Skin prick tests are recommended to identify the culpable agent and any associated cross-reactivity. Such cross-reactivity is commonly found when the reaction has been to muscle relaxants, and the patient is frequently allergic to several related compounds. If allergy is confirmed, then a MedicAlert® bracelet should be worn by the patient. The details of the reaction must be recorded in the medical records and reported to the patient's general practitioner and the appropriate adverse drug reactions body.

Anaesthesia in the susceptible patient

Unless the patient is allergic to local anaesthetics, regional anaesthesia should be used if possible. If the patient requires general anaesthesia, the preoperative use of corticosteroids and histamine H$_1$- and H$_2$-receptor antagonists should be considered as prophylaxis. The anaesthetic technique chosen should avoid re-exposure to implicated agents. Drugs should be chosen that have a low potential for hypersensitivity and direct histamine release. Typically safe drugs include volatile agents, etomidate, fentanyl, pancuronium and benzodiazepines. All drugs should be given slowly in diluted form, and resuscitation facilities must be immediately available.

Other drug reactions

An idiosyncratic drug reaction is a qualitatively abnormal and harmful drug effect which occurs in a small number of individuals and is precipitated usually by small drug doses. There is often an associated genetic defect and the reaction may be severe or even fatal.

Succinylcholine sensitivity (see page 83), malignant hyperthermia (see above) and acute intermittent porphyria are important examples of drug idiosyncrasy in anaesthetic practice.

Acute intermittent porphyria

Acute intermittent porphyria (AIP) is a rare but serious metabolic disorder caused by an inherited deficiency of an enzyme required for haem synthesis. Porphyrin precursors accumulate and cause acute neuropathy, abdominal pain (mimicking an acute abdomen), delirium and death. These precursors are produced in the liver by δ-amino laevulinic acid synthetase, and this enzyme may be induced by barbiturates, amongst other drugs. If an at-risk patient is identified, porphyrinogenic drugs (including barbiturates) must be avoided. Drugs considered safe include propofol, midazolam, succinylcholine, vecuronium, nitrous oxide, morphine, fentanyl, neostigmine and atropine.

REGIONAL ANAESTHESIA

Central techniques

Epidural and subarachnoid anaesthesia are often chosen to reduce the patient's perioperative risk. However, these techniques may pose independent risks.

Hypotension

Arterial and venous dilatation caused by sympathetic pharmacological denervation reduce cardiac afterload and preload. Systemic hypotension results, and may be severe enough to compromise organ perfusion. Signs include tachycardia, low arterial pressure, confusion, nausea and dizziness. Fluid preloading may reduce the incidence of hypotension, and the left lateral position is helpful in pregnant patients. Intravenous titration of a vasopressor agent (e.g. bolus doses of ephedrine 5 mg or metaraminol 1 mg) usually restores arterial pressure rapidly. Directly acting arterial constrictors are more appropriate than indirectly acting sympathomimetics if tachycardia is present and in patients with severe ischaemic heart disease.

Nerve injury

Nerve injury may result from direct trauma caused by the needle, or through chemical toxicity. It is widely held that epidural and subarachnoid block should be undertaken in the conscious patient to allow early identification of impingement upon a nerve or the spinal cord.

Infection and haematoma

Spinal abscess presents as sudden, painless loss of motor function, and is a devastating complication of central nervous blockade. Meticulous aseptic technique helps reduce the incidence of this complication, but some cases arise spontaneously, probably as a result of bacteraemia caused by surgery and inoculation of a small epidural haematoma. Urgent magnetic resonance imaging and referral to a neurosurgeon are indicated if spinal abscess is suspected.

Epidural haematoma is a common complication of epidural catheter placement. The large majority of haematomata are asymptomatic and resolve spontaneously. They may be apparent only upon spinal imaging. Large haematomata may cause permanent nerve injury. As with spinal abscesses, urgent imaging and referral to a neurosurgeon are indicated. Epidural catheters should not be inserted in patients who are receiving warfarin or intravenous heparin, or who

have abnormal coagulation for some other reason. Caution should be exercised if a patient is receiving low-dose heparin for thrombosis prophylaxis. At least 12 h should be allowed to elapse between receipt of low molecular weight heparin prophylaxis and epidural block. If blood is obtained via the needle or catheter during insertion and the patient is expected to be fully heparinized (e.g. during cardiac or major vascular surgery), then the procedure should be postponed for 24 h.

Peripheral nerve blocks

There is a risk of direct damage to nerves in association with any peripheral nerve block. Paraesthesia or pain in the distribution of a nerve are signs of the proximity of a nerve and should prompt needle withdrawal. Pain during injection of local anaesthetic, or the failure to abolish the muscular twitch from a nerve stimulator, may indicate intraneural positioning of the needle and should prompt immediate cessation of injection and withdrawal of the needle.

Local anaesthetic toxicity

Local anaesthetic drugs may cause toxic side-effects when excessive serum concentrations are achieved. This is most commonly caused by accidental intravenous injection, excessively rapid absorption or absolute overdosage. Some sites of injection display a much more rapid uptake into the systemic circulation, usually because of local vascularity. Intercostal nerve blocks result in higher serum concentrations than subcutaneous infiltration, which produces higher serum concentrations than plexus blocks.

Cerebral symptoms occur first. Dizziness, drowsiness, confusion, tinnitus, circumoral tingling and a metallic taste are common signs of toxicity. Patients should be asked about the presence of these symptoms. In severe toxicity, tonic-clonic convulsions occur. Cardiovascular symptoms include bradycardia with hypotension, although solutions which contain epinephrine may produce tachycardia and hypertension. Cardiovascular collapse occurs usually at 4–6 times the serum concentration at which convulsions occur. Local anaesthetics directly depress the myocardium and cause systemic vasodilatation. Cardiovascular collapse occurs earlier with bupivacaine than with lidocaine because of myocardial binding. Severe and intractable arrhythmias may occur with accidental intravenous injection. The toxicity of local anaesthetics is increased by a rapid rate of increase of serum concentration. Thus, a rapid intravenous injection of a small dose has the potential to cause toxicity.

Management

Intravenous access should be secured and adequate resuscitation equipment and drugs should be immediately available before a local anaesthetic block is undertaken. The patient should be adequately monitored. The lowest dose of the least toxic drug available should be used to achieve the effect required (Table 19.12). The total dose should be reduced in frail patients and in patients otherwise at risk of toxicity (e.g. patients with epilepsy or heart block). Local anaesthetics should always be injected slowly, with repeated aspiration for blood, and with constant verbal contact with, and observation of, the patient. Any change in the patient's apparent mental state should prompt immediate cessation of injection. Injection of a test dose of a local anaesthetic which contains epinephrine usually results in sudden tachycardia if intravascular injection has occurred.

The addition of epinephrine reduces the speed of absorption, allowing larger maximum doses, reducing the potential for toxicity and prolonging the action of the local anaesthetic. Epinephrine (1:200 000) typically reduces the maximum serum concentration by approximately 50%. However, the addition of epinephrine does not reduce local anaesthetic toxicity following intravenous injection.

If toxicity occurs, the injection must be stopped, assistance summoned and the patient assessed. The airway should be checked and oxygen should be administered; this prevents hypoxaemia, which makes fitting more likely and makes arrhythmias more difficult to control. If hypoventilation or apnoea ensue, the lungs should be ventilated using a self-inflating bag or anaesthetic breathing system. Tracheal intubation is required if the patient is unconscious or unable to maintain an airway. Intravenous fluids and vasopressors (e.g. ephedrine 10 mg) may be required to treat hypotension. Arrhythmias may occur and should be treated appropriately (see above). Severe heart block may require an infusion of isoprenaline or pacing. Chest compressions are required if there is no palpable pulse. Convulsions are very common in significant toxicity and administration of an anticonvulsant (e.g. diazepam 10 mg, thiopental 50 mg) is often necessary.

Survival from local anaesthetic toxicity should approach 100%. Good preparation, early recognition and prompt treatment are vital in preventing progression to a situation of poor tissue oxygenation and organ damage.

INJURY

Direct, physical injury of the patient is a fairly common event in the perioperative period. Most of these injuries are preventable. Tracheal intubation and poor patient positioning are commonly to blame. Nerve, dental and ophthalmic injuries are common causes of litigation against anaesthetists. Thermal and electrical injuries are less common but potentially disastrous. Neurological deficits presenting during the postoperative period have usually been sustained intraoperatively.

Cutaneous and muscular injury

Skin is damaged easily by poor or prolonged positioning, the use of highly adhesive tape and incautious movement of the patient. In particular, elderly patients and patients who have been treated with steroids for a prolonged period may have very fragile skin, and this must be protected. These patients also tend to heal very slowly, and an apparently minor skin injury may produce many months of suffering postoperatively. Muscle injury is produced most commonly by poor positioning, but tourniquets may also cause direct muscle damage.

Peripheral nerve injury

Peripheral nerves may be injured directly, through peripheral nerve blockade, vascular catheter insertion or surgery, or indirectly, by poor positioning during anaesthesia, or through ischaemia during severe hypoxaemia or hypotension. Peripheral nerve injury occurs during 0.1% of anaesthetics. The position of the patient during general anaesthesia is the commonest cause of injury. The brachial plexus and superficial nerves of the limbs (ulnar, radial and common

Table 19.12 Maximum safe doses of local anaesthetics in common use

Drug	Maximum dose
Lidocaine	4 (7) mg kg^{-1}
Bupivacaine	2 (2) mg kg^{-1}
Levobupivacaine	2.5 (2.5) mg kg^{-1}
Prilocaine	6 (8) mg kg^{-1}

Maximum doses in the presence of 1:200 000 epinephrine are given in parentheses.

peroneal) are the most frequently affected nerves. The usual mechanism of injury to superficial nerves is ischaemia from compression of the vasa vasorum by surgical retractors, leg stirrups or contact with other equipment. Nerve injury may occur as part of a compartment syndrome after ischaemia from poor positioning, particularly when the legs are placed in Lloyd-Davies supports and the patient is positioned head down. Ischaemic injury is more likely to occur during periods of poor peripheral perfusion associated with hypotension or hypothermia. Nerves may also be injured by traction (e.g. the brachial plexus during excessive shoulder abduction).

Meticulous care is necessary when positioning the patient. Padding should be used beneath tourniquets and to protect pressure points. Extreme joint positions should be avoided. Close surveillance of tourniquet ischaemia times is essential. Although many injuries recover within several months, all patients with a peripheral nerve injury must be referred to a neurologist for assessment and continuing care. Many ulnar nerve palsies occur in patients with an anatomical predisposition, and this may be deduced from a history of numbness after sleep or as a result of posture at work. In these patients, the elbows should not be placed in flexion during surgery.

Injury during airway management

Dental damage is the most frequently reported anaesthetic injury and is usually sustained during laryngoscopy. Damage to teeth is much more likely if laryngoscopy is difficult. Most dental injuries result from a rotational force applied to the laryngoscope during attempts to lever the tip of the laryngoscope blade upwards using the upper incisors as a fulcrum. The correct, and much safer, practice is to apply a force upwards and away from the anaesthetist without any leverage on the incisors. Injuries vary from chipped teeth to complete avulsion. The upper incisors are most commonly involved. Preoperative assessment and documentation of dentition are essential. Patients with poor dentition, or in whom a difficult laryngoscopy is anticipated, should be warned of the possibility of dental injury. If a tooth is accidentally avulsed, it should be reimplanted in its socket with minimal interference and a dental surgeon consulted at the earliest opportunity.

Mucosal damage is common during airway management, and mucosal abrasion may be very painful postoperatively. Overinflation of the cuff of a tube in the larynx or trachea may produce local ischaemia, with consequent scarring and stenosis. Cuff pressures should be checked regularly, particularly during prolonged surgery and when nitrous oxide is used. Other reported injuries include dislocated arytenoid cartilages (intubation), recurrent laryngeal nerve damage (laryngoscopy), uvular ischaemia (Guedel airway), epistaxis and nasal turbinate fracture (nasal intubation).

Ophthalmic injury

Retinal ischaemic injury may follow prolonged pressure on the orbit from equipment or the use of the prone position. Permanent blindness may result. Corneal abrasions are associated with inadequate eye protection, especially during transfer or use of the prone position. The use of adhesive tape to close the eyelids is also a risk factor. Lubricated dressings such as sterile paraffin gauze may be a preferable method of securing the eyelids.

Thermal and electrical injury

The high-density electrical current of surgical diathermy is a potential source of injury. If the return current path is interrupted by incorrect application of the diathermy pad, then the ECG electrodes or other points of contact between skin and metal may provide an alternative electrical path, producing serious burns. Failure of thermostatic control on warming devices is a potential source of thermal injury. Warming devices should always be used in accordance with the manufacturer's guidelines. In particular, hot air hoses used to inflate convective warming blankets must never be used alone to blow hot air under the patient's blankets, as serious thermal injury may result. Ignition of alcohol-based surgical preparation solutions is possible, especially if they are not allowed to evaporate fully and if diathermy is used. Airway fires have occurred during laser surgery to the larynx; it is advisable to use a low inspired oxygen fraction and omit nitrous oxide in this situation.

Fires should be extinguished immediately and the area should be soaked in cool saline or covered with saline-soaked swabs. If the burned area is significant, the opinion of a burns surgeon should be sought.

Vascular injury and tourniquets

Arterial catheters may produce significant arterial injury, resulting in ischaemia and, potentially, loss of the distal limb. Arterial tourniquets reduce surgical bleeding, but also rob the distal tissue of its perfusion. An absolute maximum duration of 2 h should be observed, and inflation pressures should be just high enough to occlude arterial flow. Typically, a pressure of 200–250 mmHg is adequate for the upper limb, and 250–300 mmHg for the lower limb. Vascular occlusion (e.g. during tourniquet use, aortic cross-clamping) risks distal ischaemia and infarction. Assurance of an adequate arterial pressure and oxygen saturation is important in facilitating distal oxygenation via collateral flow. Parts distal to an arterial occlusion should never be warmed, because this raises local metabolic rate and causes the onset of ischaemia to be more rapid.

FURTHER READING

Atlee JL (ed) 2006 Complications in anesthesia, 2nd edn. Saunders, NewYork

Benumof JL, Saidman LJ (eds) 1999 Anesthesia and perioperative complications, 2nd edn. Year Book Medical Publications, NewYork

Contractor S, Hardman JG 2006 Injury during anaesthesia. CEACCP 6: 67

Finucane BT (ed) 1999 Complications of regional anesthesia. Elsevier, NewYork

Gravenstein N (ed) 2006 Complications in Anesthesia. Lippincott Williams & Wilkins, Philadelphia

Hardman JG, Aitkenhead AR 2005 Awareness during anaesthesia. CEACCP 5: 183

20 Metabolism, the stress response to surgery and perioperative thermoregulation

METABOLISM

Metabolism may be defined as the chemical processes which enable cells to function. Basal metabolic rate (BMR) is the minimum amount of energy required to maintain basic autonomic function and normal homeostasis. For example, energy is required by the myocardium to maintain heart rate and stroke volume and by nerve and muscle membranes to maintain membrane potentials. In a healthy resting adult, BMR is in the region of 2000 kcal day^{-1} (equivalent to 40 kcal m^{-2} h^{-1}). One calorie is the energy required in joules to raise the temperature of 1 g of water from 15°C to 16°C. Because this is a very small unit, a more practical measure in human physiology is the kcal or Calorie (C).

Adenosine triphosphate (ATP) is the 'energy currency' of the body. It contains two high-energy phosphate bonds and is present in all cells. Most physiological processes acquire energy from it. Oxidation of nutrients in cells releases energy, which is used to regenerate ATP. Conversion of one mole of ATP to adenosine diphosphate (ADP) releases 8 kcal of energy. Additional hydrolysis of the phosphate bond from ADP to AMP also releases 8 kcal (Fig. 20.1). Other high-energy compounds include creatine phosphate and acetyl CoA. The generation of energy through the oxidation of carbohydrate, protein and fat is termed catabolism, whereas the generation of stored energy as energy-rich phosphate bonds, carbohydrates, proteins or fats is termed anabolism (Fig. 20.2). The amount of energy released by carbohydrate, protein and fat metabolism is: carbohydrate 4.1 kcal g^{-1}, protein 4.1 kcal g^{-1} and fat 9.3 kcal g^{-1}.

CARBOHYDRATE METABOLISM

The final product of carbohydrate digestion is glucose, which is used to form ATP in cells. Because the cellular membrane is impermeable to glucose, it is transported by a carrier protein (GLUT 4) across the membrane in a process termed *facilitated diffusion*. Activation of insulin receptors speeds translocation of GLUT 4-containing endosomes into the cell membrane which then mediate glucose transport into the cell. Facilitated diffusion of glucose into cells is increased 10-fold in the presence of insulin, without which the rate of uptake would be inadequate. This is a passive process (i.e. it does not require energy expenditure by the cell). In contrast, glucose absorption in the gastrointestinal tract and reabsorption in the renal tubule are both active processes (i.e. are energy-consuming processes). They involve co-transport with sodium ions via sodium-dependent glucose transporters (SGLT).

After absorption into cells, glucose may be used immediately or stored in the form of glycogen, particularly in liver and muscle. The process of releasing glucose molecules from the glycogen molecule in times of high metabolic demand is termed *glycogenolysis*. This process is initiated by an enzyme *phosphorylase*, which is activated in the presence of epinephrine (adrenaline) and glucagon. Epinephrine is released by the sympathetic nervous system, while glucagon is released from the α cells of the pancreas in response to hypoglycaemia.

The mechanism of glucose catabolism involves an extensive series of enzyme-controlled steps, rather than a single reaction. This is because the oxidation of one mol of glucose (180 g) releases almost 686 kcal of energy, whereas only 8 kcal is required to form one molecule of ATP. Therefore, an elaborate series of reactions, termed the *glycolytic pathway*, releases small quantities of energy at a time, resulting in the synthesis of 38 mol of ATP from each mol of glucose (Fig 20.3). As each molecule of ATP releases 8 kcal, a total of 304 kcal of energy in the form of ATP is synthesized. Hence, the efficiency of the glycolytic pathway is 44%, the remainder of the energy being released as heat.

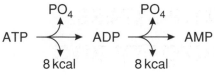

Fig. 20.1
Hydrolysis of adenosine triphosphate (ATP). ADP-adenosine diphosphate; AMP-adenosine monophosphate.

The glycolytic pathway may be summarized as:

1. *Glycolysis,* i.e. splitting the glucose (6 carbon atoms) molecule into two molecules of pyruvic acid (3 carbon atoms each). This results in the net formation of two molecules of ATP anaerobically but also generates two pairs of H^+ for entry into the respiratory chain (see below) (Fig. 20.4).
2. *Oxidation* of each of the pyruvic acid (3 carbon atom) molecules in the Krebs citric acid cycle results in the generation of 5 pairs of H^+ per 3 carbon moiety, i.e. 10 pairs of H^+ per 6 carbon glucose molecule (Fig. 20.5).
3. *Oxidative phosphorylation,* i.e. the formation of ATP by the oxidation of hydrogen to water. This process is also known as the respiratory chain. For each molecule of glucose, a total of 12 pairs of H^+ are fed into the respiratory chain, each pair generating three molecules of ATP. Thus, oxidative phosphorylation results in 36 molecules of ATP per molecule of glucose. A further two molecules of ATP are produced anaerobically. Therefore, one molecule of glucose generates 38 molecules of ATP.

ANAEROBIC GLYCOLYSIS

This is the process of ATP formation in the absence of oxygen and is possible because the first two steps of glycolysis do not require oxygen. In the absence of oxy-gen, pyruvic acid molecules and hydrogen ions accumulate, which would normally stop the reaction. However, pyruvic acid and hydrogen ions combine in the presence of the enzyme *lactic dehydrogenase* to form lactic acid, which diffuses easily out of cells, allowing anaerobic glycolysis to continue. Lactic acidosis is a feature of shock caused by, for example, severe sepsis. This is a highly inefficient use of the energy within glucose. When oxygen is again available to the cells, lactic acid is reconverted to glucose or used directly for energy.

The glycolytic pathway metabolizes 70% of glucose. A second mechanism, the phosphogluconate pathway (also known as the hexose monophosphate shunt) is responsible for metabolism of the remaining 30%. The importance of this pathway is that ATP is formed independently of the enzymes needed in the glycolytic pathway, and hence an enzymatic abnormality in the glycolytic pathway does not completely inhibit energy metabolism. It also provides for the production of pentoses, which are needed for nucleic acid production.

GLUCONEOGENESIS

This is the formation of glucose from amino acids, which are usually used for protein formation. It occurs when stores of glycogen are depleted. Prolonged hypoglycaemia is the main trigger for this process, but ACTH, glucocorticoids and glucagon also have a role.

PROTEIN METABOLISM

Proteins are composed of amino acids, of which there are more than 20 different types in humans. All amino acids have a weak acid group (-COOH) and an amine

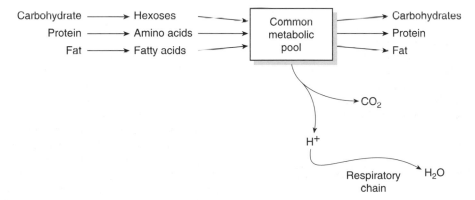

Fig. 20.2
Overview of metabolism.

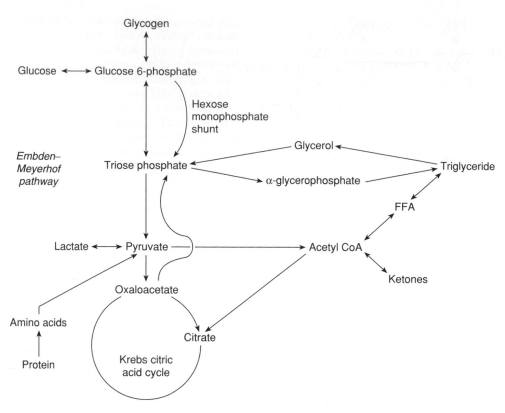

Fig. 20.3
Summary of the glycolytic pathway. Krebs citric acid cycle; FFA=free fatty acid. Note that two molecules of pyruvic acid are produced for each molecule of glucose metabolized. Each pyruvic acid molecule enters the Krebs citric acid cycle.

group (-NH₂). They are joined by peptide linkages to form *peptide chains (primary structure)*, a reaction which releases a molecule of water in the process. The blood concentration of amino acids is approximately 1–2 mmol L⁻¹. Entry into cells requires facilitated or active transport using carrier mechanisms. They are then conjugated into proteins by the formation of peptide linkages. Formation of the peptide link requires 0.5–4.0 kcal derived from ATP. Large proteins may be composed of several peptide chains wrapped around each other (secondary structure) and bound by weaker links, e.g. hydrogen bonds, electrostatic forces and sulphydryl bonds (tertiary structure).

Some amino acids present in the body are not present in proteins to any appreciable extent including, for example, ornithine, 5-hydroxytryptophan, L-Dopa and thyroxine. Catecholamines, histamine and serotonin are formed from specific amino acids. Sulphur-containing amino acids are the source of urinary sulphate and provide sulphur for incorporation into various proteins, e.g. Coenzyme A.

There is equilibrium between the amino acids in plasma, plasma proteins and tissue proteins. Proteins may be synthesized from amino acids in all cells of the body, the type of protein depending on the genetic material in the DNA, which determines the sequence of amino acids formed and hence controls the nature of the synthesized proteins. Essential amino acids must be ingested as they cannot be synthesized in the body. Table 20.1 lists the eight essential amino acids. If there is dietary deficiency of any of these, the subject develops negative nitrogen balance. Others are *non-essential* (i.e. may be synthesized in the cells). Synthesis is by the process of *transamination*, whereby an amine radical (-NH₂) is transferred to the corresponding α-keto acid. Breakdown of excess amino acids into glucose (gluconeogenesis) generates energy or storage as fat, both of which occur in the liver. The breakdown of amino acids occurs by the process of *deamination*, which takes place in the liver. It involves the removal of the amine group with the formation of the corresponding ketoacid.. The amine radical may be recycled to other molecules or released as ammonia. In the liver, two molecules of ammonia are combined to form urea (Fig. 20.6). Amino acids may also take up ammonia to form the corresponding amide.

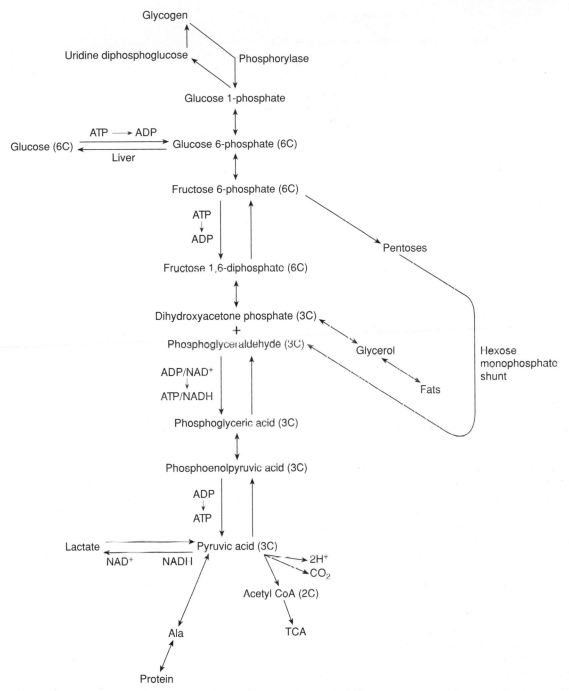

Fig. 20.4
The metabolism of glucose.

During starvation or when no protein is ingested (e.g. after major surgery), 20–30 g day^{-1} of protein is catabolized for energy purposes. This occurs despite the continuing availability of some stored carbohydrates and fats. When carbohydrate and fat stores are exhausted, the rate of protein catabolism is increased to > 100 g day^{-1}, resulting in a rapid decline in tissue function. During the systemic inflammatory response syndrome (SIRS) or after major surgery, there is functional catabolism also. Several hormones influence

403

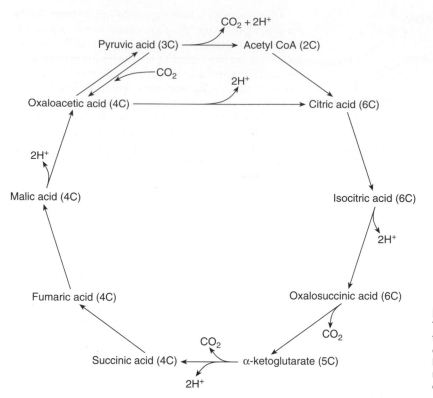

Fig. 20.5
The Krebs citric acid cycle. Note that five pairs of H⁺ are generated by the oxidation of each pyruvate molecule. Each pair of H⁺ generates three molecules of ATP in the respiratory chain in the mitochondria.

protein metabolism. Growth hormone, insulin and testosterone are anabolic, i.e. they increase the rate of cellular protein synthesis. Other hormones, e.g. glucocorticoids, are catabolic, i.e. they decrease the amount of protein in most tissues, except the liver. Glucagon promotes gluconeogenesis and protein breakdown. Thyroxine indirectly affects protein metabolism by affecting metabolic rate. If insufficient energy sources are available to cells, thyroxine may contribute to excess protein breakdown. Conversely, if adequate amino acid and energy sources are available, thyroxine may increase the rate of protein synthesis.

LIPID METABOLISM

Lipids are a diverse group of compounds characterized by their insolubility in water and solubility in non-polar solvents such as ether or benzene. They include fats, oils, steroids, waxes, etc. They serve as an immediate energy source but also provide storage energy. They include cholesterol, which is a precursor of steroids. They provide electrical insulation for nerve conduction and when combined with protein they are known as lipoproteins, an important component of cell membranes. Lipoproteins are also the predominant means for the transport of bloodstream lipids.

Lipids include triglycerides (TGs), phospholipids (PLs) and cholesterol. The basic structure of TGs and PLs is the *fatty acid*. Fatty acids are long-chain hydrocarbon organic acids. TGs are composed of three long-chain fatty acids bound with one molecule of glycerol (Fig. 20.7). Phospholipids have two long-chain fatty

Table 20.1   Essential amino acids

Leucine
Isoleucine
Lysine
Methionine
Phenylalanine
Threonine
Tryptophan
Valine

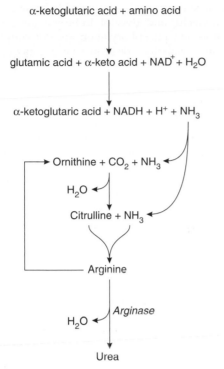

Fig. 20.6
Deamination is the process of metabolizing amino acids. Ammonia is the end product. Two molecules of ammonia combine as shown to form urea. This occurs in the liver.

After absorption in the gastrointestinal tract, lipids are aggregated into droplets (diameter 90–1000 nm), termed chylomicrons, composed mainly of TGs. These molecules are too large to pass the endothelial cells of the portal system and so enter the circulation via the thoracic duct. Chylomicrons are metabolized by lipoprotein lipase adherent to the endothelium of many tissues throughout the body, including adipose tissue but not adult liver. Chylomicrons carry cholesterol to the liver. The fatty acids and lipoproteins released from the liver into the circulation are derived from secondary products of chylomicron metabolism.

Transport of lipids from the liver or adipose cells to other tissues that need it as an energy source occurs by means of binding to plasma albumin. The fatty acids are then referred to as *free fatty acids* (FFAs), to distinguish them from other fatty acids in the plasma. After 12 h of fasting, all chylomicrons have been removed from the blood, and circulating lipids then occur in the form of *lipoproteins*. Lipoproteins are smaller particles than chylomicrons but are also composed of TGs, PLs and cholesterol. They may be classified as:

- very low-density lipoproteins (VLDLs), consisting mainly of TGs
- low-density lipoproteins (LDLs), consisting mainly of cholesterol
- high-density lipoproteins (HDLs), consisting mainly of protein.

CHOLESTEROL

Cholesterol is a lipid with a sterol nucleus and is formed from acetyl CoA. It may be absorbed from food (animal sources only) but is also synthesized in the liver and to a lesser extent other tissue. Its function is predominantly the formation of bile salts in the liver, which promote the digestion and absorption of lipids. The remainder is used in the formation of adrenocortical and sex hormones and it is deposited also in the skin, where it resists the absorption of water-soluble chemicals.

Serum cholesterol is correlated with the incidence of atherosclerosis and coronary artery disease. Prolonged elevations of VLDL, LDL and chylomicron remnants are associated with atherosclerosis. Conversely, HDL is protective. Factors affecting blood cholesterol concentrations are outlined in Figure 20.8.

There is a feedback mechanism whereby increased cholesterol absorption from the diet results in inhibition of the enzyme *HMG-CoA reductase*, which regulates synthesis of cholesterol. There are many hormonal influences in cholesterol metabolism also, including increased plasma concentrations in response

acids bound to glycerol with the third fatty acid replaced by attached compounds such as inositol, choline or ethanolamine. Although cholesterol does not contain fatty acid, its sterol nucleus is formed from fatty acid molecules.

Some polyunsaturated fatty acids are considered essential because they cannot be synthesized in humans and because they are precursors for eicosanoids. They must be acquired from plant sources. These essential fatty acids are linolenic acid and linoleic acid which together with their derivative arachidonic acid form prostaglandins, lipoxins and leukotrienes (collectively termed eicosanoids).

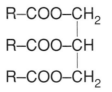

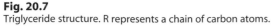

Fig. 20.7
Triglyceride structure. R represents a chain of carbon atoms.

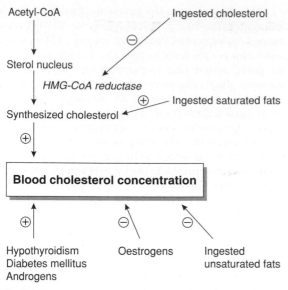

Fig. 20.8
Factors affecting blood cholesterol concentration.

to abnormally low concentrations of thyroid hormone, insulin and androgens. Oestrogen reduces cholesterol concentration by an unknown mechanism. The family of cholesterol-lowering drugs termed statins are inhibitors of the enzyme HMG-CoA reductase.

Lipids are ingested in similar proportions to carbohydrates and may be used as an energy source immediately or stored in the liver or adipose cells for later use as an energy source. The stages in the use of TGs as an energy source are as follows. TG is hydrolysed to its constituent glycerol and three fatty acids; glycerol is then conjugated to glycerol 3-phosphate and enters the glycolytic pathway, which generates ATP as described above. Fatty acids need *carnitine* as a carrier agent to enter mitochondria where they undergo beta oxidation. The precise number of ATP molecules formed from a molecule of TG depends on the length of the fatty acid chain, longer chains providing more acetyl CoA and hence more molecules of ATP. Newborns have a special fat termed brown fat, which on expo-

sure to a cold stressor is stimulated to break down into free fatty acids and glycerol. In brown adipose tissue, oxidation and phosphorylation are not coupled and therefore metabolism of brown fat is especially thermogenic.

KETONES

Initial degradation of fatty acids occurs in the liver, but the acetyl-CoA may not be used either immediately or completely. Ketones, or keto acids, are either *acetoacetic acid*, formed from two molecules of acetyl CoA, *β-hydroxybutyric acid*, formed from the reduction of acetoacetic acid, or acetone, formed when a smaller quantity of acetoacetic acid is decarboxylated (Fig. 20.9). These three substances are collectively termed ketones. They are organic acids formed in the liver, from where they diffuse into the circulation and are transported to the peripheral tissues where they may be used for energy. Their importance is that they accumulate in diabetes and starvation, such as may occur in the perioperative period. In both circumstances, no carbohydrates are being metabolized. In diabetes, decreased insulin results in a reduction in intracellular glucose, and in starvation, carbohydrates are lacking simply because they are not being ingested. The ensuing breakdown of fat as described above results in large quantities of ketones being released from the liver to the peripheral tissues. There is a limit to the rate at which ketones are used by the tissues, because depletion of essential carbohydrate intermediate metabolites slows the rate at which acetyl CoA can enter the Krebs cycle (see Fig. 20.5). Hence, blood ketone concentration may increase rapidly, causing metabolic acidosis and ketonuria. Acetone may be discharged on the breath to give a characteristic sweet odour.

MEASURING METABOLIC RATE

Basal metabolic rate (BMR) is determined at complete mental and physical rest 12–14 h after food ingestion, if body temperature is within the normal range. Metabolic rate increases by approximately 14% for every 1°C rise

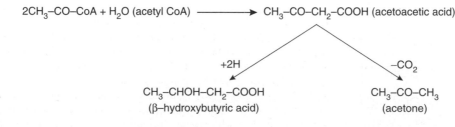

Fig. 20.9
Ketone formation.

of body temperature. BMR may be measured by indirect calorimetry, which involves the measurement of water, CO_2 or protein breakdown products produced to enable the metabolic rate to be quantified. Alternatively, the O_2 consumption can be measured. A total of 4.82 kcal of energy is produced per litre of O_2 consumed although accurate assessment depends on information about the type of food being consumed. Factors influencing BMR are listed in Table 20.2.

THE STRESS RESPONSE TO SURGERY

Surgery or trauma consistently elicits a characteristic neuroendocrine and cytokine response in proportion to the extent of injury or metabolic insult. Therefore, minor surgery on a limb has a negligible stress response, in contrast to major surgery such as a laparotomy or thoracotomy. The characteristics of the stress response to surgery are summarized in Table 20.3. There are two principal components to the stress response to surgery: the *neuroendocrine* response and the *cytokine* response. The neuroendocrine response is stimulated by painful afferent neural stimuli reaching the CNS. It may be diminished and sometimes eliminated altogether by dense neural blockade from a regional anaesthetic technique.

The cytokine component of the stress response is stimulated by *local tissue damage* at the site of the sur-gery itself and is not inhibited by regional anaesthesia. It is diminished by minimally invasive surgery, especially laparoscopic techniques. Triggers are listed in Table 20.4.

There is growing evidence that the stress response is detrimental and is associated with postoperative morbidity. It has adverse effects on several key physiological systems, including the cardiovascular, respiratory and gastroenterological systems.

CONSEQUENCES OF THE NEUROENDOCRINE ELEMENT OF THE STRESS RESPONSE

Protein catabolism

Major surgery results in a net excretion of nitrogen-containing compounds, referred to as negative nitrogen balance, reflecting catabolism of protein into amino acids for gluconeogenesis. This is partly because of perioperative starvation, but mainly because of the stress response, which causes decreased total protein synthesis, in addition to protein breakdown. Peripheral skeletal muscle is predominantly affected, but visceral protein may also be catabolized. Catecholamines, cortisol, glucagon and interleukins (IL-1 and IL-6) are involved in proteolysis and gluconeogenesis. Protein catabolism contributes to weight loss and impaired wound healing, and may delay overall postoperative recovery. Up to 0.5 kg day^{-1} of lean muscle mass may be lost postoperatively because of this aspect of the stress response.

Carbohydrate mobilization

Hyperglycaemia and insulin intolerance are major features of the stress response and may persist for several days postoperatively. They result from increased blood concentrations of catecholamines, cortisol and glucagon and also from sympathetic nervous system stimulation (by further increasing catecholamine release from the adrenal medulla). These hormones also inhibit insulin and therefore glucose uptake into muscle, fat and liver. Moreover, there is decreased sensitivity of muscle and liver to circulating insulin during the stress response. Blood glucose concentrations may increase by about 10 mmol L^{-1}, leading to glycosuria and osmotic diuresis.

Fat metabolism

The net effect of the hormonal alterations listed in Table 20.3 is lipolysis, stimulated by catecholamines acting at α_1-adrenoreceptors, with resultant increased concentrations of FFAs in the circulation. FFAs may be

Table 20.2 Factors influencing metabolic rate
Malnutrition (20%)
Sleep (15%)
Exercise (up to 2000 × BMR)
Protein ingestion
Age: < 5 years has × 2 BMR of > 70
Thyroid hormone imbalance (increase or decrease by 50%)
Sympathetic stimulation
Testosterone (by 15%)
Temperature
Anaesthesia (20% reduction) (regional anaesthesia – no effect)

Table 20.3 Components of the stress response to surgery

Neuroendocrine response	Consequence	Result
Hypothalamic–pituitary–adrenal	ACTH, GH, ADH, β-endorphin, prolactin all increased	Activation of adrenocortical hormones
		Mobilization of glucose reserves
		Water retention
		Protein catabolism and gluconeogenesis
Sympathetic nervous system stimulation	Catecholamines increased	Heart rate and cardiac output increased
		SVR and arterial pressure increased
	Hypothalamic–pituitary–adrenal	Activation of adrenocortical hormones; mobilization of glucose reserves; water retention; protein catabolism and gluconeogenesis
	Renin–angiotensin–aldosterone	Increased SVR, retention Na^+ and H_2O, secretion K^+
	Increased glucagon	Increased plasma glucose, lipolysis and insulin resistance
	Decreased insulin, testosterone	Hyperglycaemia, catabolic state
	Increased acute-phase proteins (liver)	Decreased liver synthesis of albumin
Cytokine response		
Cytokine and inflammatory mediator release	IL-1, IL-6, TNF-α	Platelet adhesion
	Prostaglandins increased	Increased coagulation
		Increased hypothalamic–pituitary–adrenal activity
	Neutrophils increased	Local inflammation, pain
	Lymphocytes decreased	
Pyrexia (due to increased IL-1)	Increased metabolic rate	Increased demand on cardiovascular system

ACTH, adrenocorticotrophic hormone; GH, growth hormone; ADH, antidiuretic hormone; SVR, systemic vascular resistance; TNF-α, tumour necrosis factor alpha.

oxidized in the liver to form ketones (e.g. acetoacetate), which may be used as a source of energy by peripheral tissues.

Cardiovascular effects

The stress response to surgery and postoperative pain activates the sympathetic nervous system (SNS), which may increase myocardial oxygen demand by increasing heart rate and arterial pressure. Activation of the SNS may also cause coronary artery vasoconstriction, reducing the supply of oxygen to the myocardium, which in turn would predispose to myocardial ischaemia. This effect may be aggravated by the fact that there is a hypercoagulable state postoperatively and the stress response is an important factor in causing this. Antidiuretic hormone (ADH),

increased during the stress response, is known to contribute to increased platelet adhesiveness (Fig. 20.10).

Respiratory effects

Postoperative pulmonary dysfunction may also result from pain and the stress response to major surgery. The most important alteration in respiratory function caused by the stress response is reduction in functional residual capacity (FRC). This is the amount of air remaining in the lungs at the end of a normal expiration. The cause of reduction in FRC is postoperative pain, which reduces the depth and rate of breathing. When FRC is reduced, it may become less than the closing capacity, the volume of air in the lungs required to prevent alveolar collapse. When FRC is less than closing capacity, airway closure occurs, with resultant

Table 20.4 Triggers of the neuroendocrine and cytokine response in patients after surgery

Noxious afferent stimuli (especially pain)
Local inflammatory tissue factors, especially cytokines
Pain and anxiety
Starvation
Hypothermia and shivering
Haemorrhage
Acidosis
Hypoxaemia
Infection

ventilation–perfusion mismatch, shunting of blood and hypoxaemia.

Gastrointestinal effects

The stress response to surgery stimulates both afferent nociceptive input and efferent SNS output, resulting in ileus and excessive SNS stimulation relative to parasympathetic nervous system (PNS) stimulation. Postoperative ileus is a temporary impairment of gastrointestinal motility after major surgery. It delays resumption of an enteral diet, and this starvation itself prolongs the stress response to surgery.

Immunological system effects

Many mediators of the stress response (cortisol, interleukins, prostaglandins, etc.) are cellular and humoral immunosuppressants. It is not known if stress response-mediated immunosuppression, which occurs for several days after surgery, influences patient outcome.

Afferent neural stimuli

Afferent noxious stimuli (such as pain, pressure, burning, distension) are transmitted by Aα and C nerve fibres. They enter the spinal cord via the dorsal root and synapse in the dorsal horn.

Local factors and the immunological (cytokine) response

Afferent neural stimuli are not the sole means of eliciting the stress response to surgery. Severe injury in a denervated limb also elicits the response, suggesting

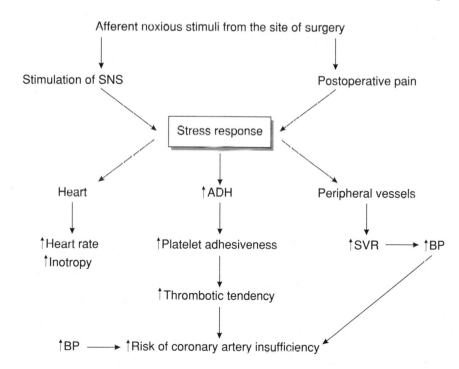

Fig. 20.10
Potential effect of the surgical stress response on coronary arterial blood flow. ADH, antidiuretic hormone; SVR, systemic vascular resistance; SNS, sympathetic nervous system.

a non-neural stimulus. Cytokines and mediators of inflammation are released in response to local tissue destruction or trauma, increasing peripheral nociceptive activity. The magnitude of this response is proportional to the extent of tissue damage.

EFFECT OF GENERAL ANAESTHESIA ON THE STRESS RESPONSE

Intravenous and inhalational anaesthetic agents have no appreciable effect on either the neuroendocrine or the cytokine elements of the stress response, irrespective of dose. However, high-dose opioid analgesia (e.g. morphine $4\,mg\,kg^{-1}$ or fentanyl $50-100\,\mu g\,kg^{-1}$) may completely inhibit the neuroendocrine element. If the opioid is given *after* the surgical incision, it does not prevent the emergence of the stress response. These high doses of opioids are impractical for most operations.

EFFECT OF REGIONAL (EPIDURAL) ANAESTHESIA ON THE STRESS RESPONSE

Neuroendocrine element

While only very high-dose, opioid-based general anaesthesia completely inhibits the stress response to upper abdominal surgery, epidural anaesthesia, commenced before the surgical incision and continued postoperatively, significantly reduces it. Epidural anaesthesia and analgesia for lower limb or pelvic surgery completely suppresses the response. Administration of local anaesthetic drugs into the epidural space is more effective than administration of opioids alone.

Cytokine element

The systemic release of cytokines in response to local tissue damage is not influenced by any anaesthetic technique, including epidural anaesthesia and analgesia. However, the cytokine element of the stress response is reduced by limiting the extent of the surgical incision, in particular, by use of laparoscopic techniques.

THERMOREGULATION AND ANAESTHESIA

PHYSIOLOGY

It is useful to consider thermoregulatory physiology in terms of a two-compartment model. A central core compartment, comprising the major trunk organs and the brain, accounts for two-thirds of body heat content. It is maintained within a narrow temperature

range (36.5–37.5°C), which facilitates cellular enzyme function. The peripheral compartment consists of skin and subcutaneous tissues over the body surface, and the limbs. It amounts to about one-third of total body heat content. In contrast with the core, peripheral tissues have wide variability of temperature, ranging from 2–3°C below to more than 20°C below core temperature in extreme conditions. Under normal conditions, this temperature gradient between core and peripheral compartments is maintained by tonic vasoconstriction. On induction of anaesthesia, normal vasoconstrictor tone is lost, and vasodilatation occurs, allowing heat to flow down its concentration gradient from the core to the periphery, causing an inadvertent, mild core hypothermia (core temperature about 35.5–36.0°C). Note that this core hypothermia occurs because of *redistribution* of body heat on induction of anaesthesia, not because of any significant net loss of heat from the body.

HEAT BALANCE

Maintaining core temperature within a narrow range requires balancing heat production and loss. It is achieved by a control system consisting of afferent thermal receptors, central integrating systems and efferent control mechanisms (Fig. 20.11). It was formerly believed that the spinal cord and brainstem were passive conductors of afferent signals to the pre-

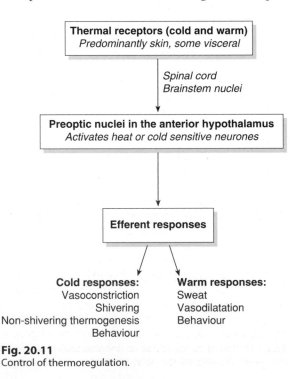

Fig. 20.11
Control of thermoregulation.

optic area of the hypothalamus, but it is now accepted that thermoregulation is a 'multi-level, multiple-input' system with the spinal cord, nucleus raphe magnus and locus subcoeruleus involved both in generating afferent thermal signals and also modulating efferent thermoregulatory responses.

Body heat is produced by metabolism, shivering and exercise. Basal metabolic rate cannot be manipulated by thermoregulatory mechanisms. Vasoconstriction and shivering are the principal autonomic mechanisms of preserving body heat and increasing heat production. Shivering may increase heat production six-fold. *Non-shivering thermogenesis* is an important mechanism in increasing heat production, particularly in neonates. Non-shivering thermogenesis occurs mainly in brown adipose tissue (BAT). This subtype of adipose tissue contains large numbers of mitochondria in its cells and these are supplied by an extensive SNS innervation. When sympathetic stimulation occurs, oxidative metabolism of the mitochondria is stimulated. However, it is *uncoupled* to phosphorylation, so that heat is produced instead of generating ATP. In adults, the amount of BAT is small, and non-shivering thermogenesis increases the rate of heat production by less than 10–15%. In infants, it may double heat production. Exercise may increase heat production by as much as 20-fold for a short time at maximal intensity.

Perioperative heat loss occurs predominantly by radiation (60%), convection (25%) and evaporation of body fluids (10%). Radiation and convective heat loss depend on the difference between peripheral body temperature and ambient temperature. Convection depends also on the velocity of air movement around the body. Vasodilatation and sweating are the major autonomic mechanisms of increasing heat loss. Maximal sweating rates may reach over 1 L h^{-1} for a short time, resulting in heat loss of up to 15 times BMR.

Thermoregulation is achieved by a physiological control system consisting of peripheral and central thermoreceptors, an integrating control centre and efferent response systems (see Fig. 20.11). Afferent thermal input comes from anatomically distinct cold and heat receptors, located predominantly in the skin, but also centrally. The central control mechanism, situated in the hypothalamus, determines mean body temperature by integrating thermal signals from peripheral and core structures and comparing mean body temperature with a predetermined 'set point' temperature.

The afferent thermal input may be central or peripheral. The peripheral input is by thermally sensitive receptors located in the skin and mucous membranes that mediate thermal sensation and contribute to thermoregulatory reflexes. Cold-specific receptors are innervated by Aδ fibres. Heat receptors are innervated by C fibres. Cold receptors in the skin outnumber heat receptors 10-fold and are the major mechanism by which the body protects itself against cold temperatures. Afferent input from these cold receptors in the skin is transmitted ultimately to the posterior hypothalamus.

Afferent thermal signals provide feedback to temperature-regulating centres in the hypothalamus. The preoptic area of the hypothalamus contains temperature-sensitive and temperature-insensitive neurones. The temperature-sensitive neurones, which predominate by 4:1, increase their discharge rate in response to increased local heat and this activates heat loss mechanisms. Conversely, cold-sensitive neurones increase their rate of discharge in response to cooling. Detection of cold differs from detection of heat, in that the principal mechanism of detection of cold is input from cutaneous cold receptors.

The set point or physiological 'thermostat' of the thermoregulatory system is the temperature at which the system requires zero action to maintain that temperature (36.5–37.5°C). The limits of this range represent the thresholds at which cold or heat responses are instigated, and hence it has been termed the 'interthreshold range.' Normally it is no more than 1°C, but is increased to 4°C during general anaesthesia.

EFFECTORS

In normal adults, the first response to a decrease in core temperature below the normal range (36.5–37.5°C) is peripheral vasoconstriction. If core temperature continues to decrease, shivering commences. Vasoconstriction and shivering are characterized by *threshold onset, gain and maximal response intensity. Threshold* is the temperature at which the effector is activated. *Gain* is the rate of response to a given decrease in core temperature. Normally, the threshold temperature for thermoregulatory vasoconstriction is 36.5°C, and shivering would commence at 36.0–36.2°C. General anaesthesia reduces these thresholds by 2–3°C, i.e. shifts them 'to the left', but gain and maximal response intensity are unaffected.

In addition to these autonomic responses to a cold challenge, behaviour is quantitatively more effective in preventing hypothermia. In extreme cold conditions, vasoconstriction and shivering are of limited effect compared to behavioural measures such as taking shelter and wearing protective clothing.

Shivering and non-shivering thermogenesis

Adjacent to the centre in the posterior hypothalamus on which the impulses from cold receptors impinge, there is a motor centre for shivering. It is normally inhibited by impulses from the heat-sensitive area in the anterior hypothalamus, but when cold impulses exceed a certain rate, the motor centre for shivering becomes activated by 'spillover' of signals and it sends impulses bilaterally into the spinal cord. Initially, this increases the tone of skeletal muscles throughout the body, but when this muscle tone increases above a specific level, shivering is observed.

Two patterns of muscular activity, seen in electromyography studies, contribute to the phenomenon of postanaesthetic shivering; first, a tonic pattern (4–8 cycles min^{-1} characteristic of the response to hypothermia in awake patients) is observed, and then a phasic (6–7 Hz) pattern resembling clonus.

MEASUREMENT OF TEMPERATURE

Core temperature may be evaluated reliably by an infrared thermometer at the tympanic membrane and by thermistors positioned in the distal oesophagus, nasopharynx or pulmonary artery. Skin surface temperature varies with ambient temperature and induction of anaesthesia and is usually also measured with a thermistor, or alternatively with a liquid crystal thermometer. Rectal and bladder temperature may lag behind changes in core temperature because these organs are not perfused well enough to reflect rapid changes in body heat content.

EFFECT OF GENERAL ANAESTHESIA ON THERMOREGULATION

General anaesthesia causes thermoregulatory impairment characterized by an increase in heat-response thresholds and a decrease in cold-response thresholds, such that the normal interthreshold range (between which no effector response occurs) is increased from approximately 1°C to 4.0°C. Both heat-response and cold-response thresholds are affected (Fig. 20.12). Thresholds are reduced by 2–3°C. However, gain (the rate of response to a given decrease in core temperature) and maximal response intensity are unaffected. All general anaesthetic agents impair thermoregulatory responses to a similar, but not identical, extent. Mild hypothermia during general anaesthesia follows a distinctive pattern and occurs in three phases (Fig. 20.13): phase 1, an initial rapid decrease in core temperature of approximately 1°C over the first 30 min; phase 2, a slower linear decrease to 34–35°C over the next 2 h; and phase 3, a core temperature plateau (or thermal equilibrium), where heat loss to the periphery equals heat gained from core metabolic heat production.

The initial rapid reduction in core temperature is greater than that which would be explained by a

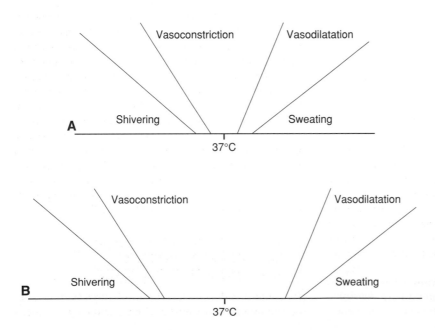

Fig. 20.12
Thresholds for thermoregulatory effectors. **(A)** Under normal conditions, note that the range of core temperature within which no effector is active, i.e. normal temperature, is approximately 0.5°C. **(B)** During general anaesthesia, note that the range of core temperature within which no effector is active is increased to approximately 4.0°C.

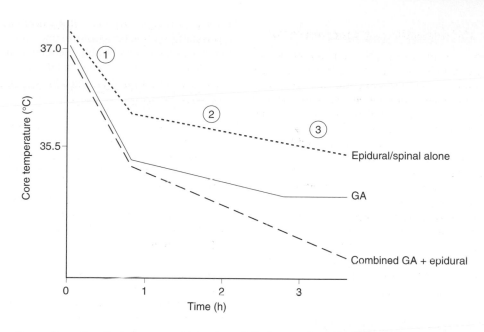

Fig. 20.13
Characteristic patterns of hypothermia during general anaesthesia (GA) alone, epidural or spinal anaesthesia alone and combined general and epidural anaesthesia. Patients in this last category are more likely to develop profound hypothermia than others (see text).

lowering of metabolic rate and heat loss, and is attributable to *core-to-peripheral redistribution* of body heat. Mean body temperature and body heat content remain constant during this 30 min. The subsequent core temperature plateau largely results from thermoregulatory vasoconstriction, triggered by a core temperature of 33–35°C.

EFFECT OF REGIONAL ANAESTHESIA ON THERMOREGULATION

As with general anaesthesia, redistribution of body heat during spinal or epidural anaesthesia is the main cause of hypothermia. Because redistribution during spinal or epidural anaesthesia is confined usually to the lower half of the body, the initial core hypothermia is not as pronounced as in general anaesthesia (approximately 0.5°C). Otherwise the pattern of hypothermia during spinal or epidural anaesthesia follows a similar pattern to that of general anaesthesia for the first two phases. The major difference in spinal or epidural anaesthesia is that the plateau phase does not emerge because vasoconstriction is blocked (see Fig. 20.13). Heat loss continues unabated during epidural anaesthesia despite the activation of effector mechanisms above the level of the block. Therefore, patients undergoing long procedures with combined general and epidural anaesthesia are at risk of a greater degree of hypothermia.

CONSEQUENCES OF PERIOPERATIVE HYPOTHERMIA

In particular circumstances, hypothermia may have a protective effect in terms of reducing basal metabolic rate. The use of moderate hypothermia is routine practice in many centres during cardiopulmonary bypass. It is generally agreed, however, that the deleterious consequences of mild hypothermia outweigh the potential benefits, with evidence emerging that hypothermia per se is responsible for adverse postoperative outcomes. In particular, hypothermic patients are more likely to have postoperative wound infections than normothermic patients. The initial 3–4 h after bacterial contamination are thought to be crucial in determining if clinical infection ensues. In vitro studies suggest that platelet function and coagulation are impaired by hypothermia, and mildly hypothermic patients lose > 25% more blood in the perioperative period than do normothermic patients. In addition, perioperative thermal discomfort is often remembered by patients as the worst aspect of their perioperative experience (Table 20.5).

PHYSICAL, ACTIVE AND PASSIVE STRATEGIES FOR AVOIDING PERIOPERATIVE HYPOTHERMIA

Preventing redistribution-induced hypothermia may be achieved by physical and pharmacological means

Table 20.5 Consequences of perioperative hypothermia

Cardiac	CO↓, HR↓, BP↓ PR duration↑, QRS duration↑, QT prolongation, J waves Viscosity↑ Cardiac work↑ MI risk↑
Respiratory	Increased dead space Respiratory fatigue
Wound infection	Caused by vasoconstricion and hence low subcutaneous tissue oxygen tension (P_tO_2)
Prolonged drug action	
Negative nitrogen balance, metabolism↓, 8% per 1°C below normal temperature	
Prolonged coagulation	
DVT/PE risk↑	
Oxyhaemoglobin dissociation curve shifted to right	
Stress response↑	
Patient discomfort/shivering	

(Table 20.6). Redistribution of heat results when anaesthetic-induced vasodilatation allows heat to flow from the core to the periphery down its concentration gradient. Pre-emptive skin surface warming does not increase core temperature but increases body heat content, particularly in the legs, and removes the gradient for heat loss via the skin. This approach is rarely used in clinical practice, however, because it requires 1 h of prewarming. A similarly impractical approach rarely used but shown to reduce redistribution heat loss by 50% is the preoperative use of nifedipine.

Passive insulation with a single layer of any insulating material reduces cutaneous heat loss by 30%. Because only 10% of metabolic heat production is lost in heating and humidifying inspired gases, this method is relatively ineffective. Heat and moisture exchange filters retain significant amounts of moisture and heat within the respiratory system, but are only 50% as effective as active mechanisms. Ambient temperature determines the rate of heat loss by radiation and convection and maintains normothermia if close to initial, preinduction, core temperature (36°C).

However, this is usually impractical, as operating room staff find this temperature uncomfortable. Water mattresses are demonstrably ineffective at preventing heat loss, possibly because relatively little heat is lost from the back. Moreover, decreased local tissue perfusion associated with local temperatures of 40°C may lead to skin necrosis. Losses may be reduced if intravenous fluids are warmed before or during administration.

Forced air warming systems are undoubtedly the best way to maintain normothermia during long procedures and are particularly effective when used intraoperatively for vasodilated patients, allowing heat applied peripherally to be rapidly transferred to the core. Their use increases core temperature and reduces the incidence of postanaesthetic shivering (Table 20.6).

POSTANAESTHETIC SHIVERING

Postanaesthetic shivering affects 5–65% of patients after general anaesthesia and 33% during epidural regional anaesthesia. It is usually defined as readily detectable tremor of the face, jaw, head, trunk or extremities lasting longer than 15 s. Apart from the obvious discomfort, postanaesthetic shivering, in common with hypothermia, is associated with several potentially deleterious sequelae (see Table 20.5). Postanaesthetic shivering is usually preceded by core hypothermia and vasoconstriction.

While hypothermia is one factor in the aetiology of postanaesthetic shivering, not all patients who shiver are hypothermic. Studies on postoperative patients have indicated that male gender, age (16–60 years) and anticholinergic premedication are risk factors for postanaesthetic shivering, while the intraoperative use of pethidine virtually abolishes it. The use of propofol reduces the incidence of postoperative shivering compared with thiopental.

Postoperative shivering should not be treated in isolation from perioperative hypothermia. Not all

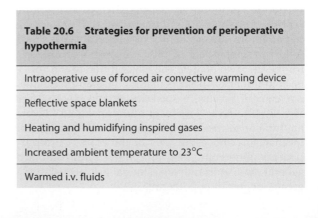

Table 20.6 Strategies for prevention of perioperative hypothermia

Intraoperative use of forced air convective warming device
Reflective space blankets
Heating and humidifying inspired gases
Increased ambient temperature to 23°C
Warmed i.v. fluids

Table 20.7	Treatment of postanaesthetic shivering
Pethidine 0.33 mg kg^{-1} (other opioids to a lesser extent)	
Doxapram 1.5 mg kg^{-1}	
Clonidine 2 µg kg^{-1}	
Methylphenidate 0.1 mg kg^{-1}	
Physostigmine 0.04 mg kg^{-1}	
Ondansetron 0.1 mg kg^{-1}	

patients who shiver are hypothermic, but most are, and successful treatment of shivering in these patients without concomitant management of hypothermia may result in deepening hypothermia. However, the mainstay of symptomatic treatment of postoperative shivering is pharmacological (Table 20.7).

A wide range of drugs is effective and it would be surprising if all worked on a single part of the thermoregulatory mechanism. Pethidine is remarkably effective in treating postoperative shivering, 25 mg being sufficient in the majority of adults. There is evidence that this may be the result of an action at the κ opioid receptor.

One hypothesis for the mechanism of postanaesthetic shivering is that, because the brain recovers later than the spinal cord, uninhibited spinal clonic tremor occurs, resulting in shivering. Consistent with this hypothesis, doxapram (a cerebral stimulant) has also been shown to be an effective treatment, but it is not as effective as pethidine. Various drugs, the mechanism of action of which are unclear, are also effective. Physostigmine prevents the onset of postanaesthetic shivering, implying that cholinergic pathways are involved in the thermoregulatory mechanisms that lead to shivering. Clonidine, an α_2-adrenergic agonist and ondansetron, a serotonergic antagonist, are also effective.

FURTHER READING

Buggy D J, Crossley A W A 2000 Thermoregulation, perioperative hypothermia and post-anaesthetic shivering. British Journal of Anaesthesia 84: 615–628

Buggy D J, Smith G 1999 Epidural anaesthesia and analgesia – better outcome after major surgery? British Medical Journal 316: 530–531

Frank S M, et al 1997 Perioperative maintenance of normothermia reduces the incidence of morbid cardiac events. JAMA 277: 1127–1134

Guyton A C, Hall J E 2005 Metabolism and temperature regulation. In: Guyton A C, Hall J E (eds) Textbook of medical physiology, 11th edn. WB Saunders, Philadelphia

Kehlet H 1998 Modification of responses to surgery by neural blockade. In: Cousins M J, Bridenbaugh P J (eds) Neural blockade in clinical anesthesia and management of pain, 3rd edn. Lippincott-Raven, Philadelphia, pp 128–175

Kurz A, Sessler D I, Lenhardt R 1996 Perioperative normothermia to reduce the incidence of surgical wound infection and shorten hospitalisation. New England Journal of Medicine 334: 1209–1215

Schmied H, Kurz A, Sessler D I, Kosek S, Reiter A 1996 Mild hypothermia increases blood loss and transfusion requirements during total hip arthroplasty. Lancet 347: 289–292

Sessler D I 2000 Temperature monitoring. In: Miller R D (ed) Anesthesia, 5th edn. Churchill Livingstone, Philadelphia, pp 1367–1389

21 Fluid, electrolyte and acid–base balance

The realization that the enzyme systems and metabolic processes responsible for the maintenance of cellular function are dependent on an environment with stable electrolyte and hydrogen ion concentrations led Claude Bernard, over 100 years ago, to describe the 'milieu interieur'. Complex homeostatic mechanisms have evolved to maintain the constancy of this internal environment and thus prevent cellular dysfunction.

BASIC DEFINITIONS

Osmosis refers to the movement of *solvent* molecules across a membrane into a region in which there is a higher concentration of *solute*. This movement may be prevented by applying a pressure to the more concentrated solution – the effective osmotic pressure. This is a colligative property; the magnitude of effective osmotic pressure exerted by a solution depends on the number rather than the type of particles present.

The amounts of osmotically active particles present in solution are expressed in *osmoles*. One osmole of a substance is equal to its molecular weight in grams (1 mol) divided by the number of freely moving particles which each molecule liberates in solution. Thus, 180 g of glucose in 1 L of water represents a solution with a molar concentration of 1 mol L^{-1} and an *osmolarity* of 1 osmol L^{-1}. Sodium chloride ionizes in solution and each ion represents an osmotically active particle. Assuming complete dissociation into Na^+ and Cl^-, 58.5 g of NaCl dissolved in 1 L of water has a molar concentration of 1 mol L^{-1} and an osmolarity of 2 osmol L^{-1}. In body fluids, solute concentrations are much lower (mmol L^{-1}) and dissociation is incomplete. Consequently, a solution of NaCl containing 1 mmol L^{-1} contributes slightly less than 2 mosmol L^{-1}.

The term *osmolality* refers to the number of osmoles per unit of total weight of solvent and, unlike osmolarity, is not affected by the volume of various solutes in solution. Confusion regarding the apparently interchangeable use of the terms osmolarity (measured in osmol L^{-1}) and osmolality (measured in osmol kg^{-1}) is caused by their numerical equivalence in body fluids; plasma osmolarity is 280–310 mosmol L^{-1} and plasma osmolality is 280–310 mosmol kg^{-1}. This equivalence is explained by the almost negligible solute volume contained in biological fluids and the fact that most osmotically active particles are dissolved in water, which has a density of 1 (i.e. osmol L^{-1} = osmol kg^{-1}). As the number of osmoles in plasma is estimated by measurement of the magnitude of freezing point depression, the more accurate term in clinical practice is osmolality.

Cations (principally Na^+) and anions (Cl^- and HCO_3^-) are the major osmotically active particles in plasma. Glucose and urea make a smaller contribution. Plasma osmolality (P_{OSM}) may be estimated from the formula:

$$P_{OSM} = 2\,[Na^+]\,(mmol\ L^{-1}) + blood\ glucose\ (mmol\ L^{-1})$$
$$+ blood\ urea\ (mmol\ L^{-1})$$
$$= 290\ mosmol\ kg^{-1}$$

Osmolality is a chemical term and may be confused with the physiological term, *tonicity*. This term is used to describe the effective osmotic pressure of a solution relative to that of plasma. The critical difference between osmolality and tonicity is that *all* solutes contribute to osmolality, but only solutes that do not cross the cell membrane contribute to tonicity. Thus, tonicity expresses the osmolal activity of solutes restricted to the extracellular compartment, i.e. those which exert an osmotic force affecting the distribution of water between intracellular fluid (ICF) and extracellular fluid (ECF). As urea diffuses freely across cell membranes, it does not alter the distribution of water between these two body fluid compartments and does not contribute to tonicity. Other solutes that contribute to plasma osmolality but not tonicity include ethanol and methanol, both of which distribute rapidly throughout the total body water. In contrast, mannitol and sorbitol are restricted to the ECF and contribute to both osmolality and tonicity. The tonicity of plasma may be estimated from the formula:

$$\text{Plasma tonicity} = 2\,[Na^+]\,(mmol\ L^{-1}) + \text{blood glucose}\ (mmol\ L^{-1})$$
$$= 285\ mosmol\ kg^{-1}$$

COMPARTMENTAL DISTRIBUTION OF TOTAL BODY WATER

The volume of total body water (TBW) may be measured using radioactive dilution techniques involving either deuterium or tritium, both of which cross all membranes freely and equilibrate rapidly with hydrogen atoms in body water. Such measurements show that approximately 60% of lean body mass (LBM) is water in the average 70 kg male adult. As fat contains little water, females have proportionately less TBW (55%) relative to LBM. TBW decreases with age, decreasing to 45–50% in later life.

The distribution of TBW between the main body compartments is illustrated in Figure 21.1. One third of TBW is contained in the extracellular fluid volume (ECFV) and two-thirds in the intracellular fluid volume (ICFV). The ECFV is subdivided further into the interstitial and intravascular compartments. In addition to the absolute volumes of each compartment, Figure 21.1 shows the relative size of each compartment compared with body weight.

SOLUTE COMPOSITION OF BODY FLUID COMPARTMENTS

EXTRACELLULAR FLUID

The capillary endothelium behaves as a freely permeable membrane to water, cations, anions and many soluble substances such as glucose and urea (but not protein). As a result, the solute compositions of interstitial fluid and plasma are similar. Each contains sodium as the principal cation and chloride as the principal anion. Protein behaves as a non-diffusible anion and is present in a higher concentration in plasma. The concentration of Cl^- is slightly higher in interstitial fluid in order to maintain electrical neutrality (Donnan equilibrium).

INTRACELLULAR FLUID

This differs from ECF in that the principal cation is potassium and the principal anion is phosphate. In addition, there is a high protein content. In contrast to the capillary endothelium, the cell membrane is permeable *selectively* to different ions and freely permeable to water. Thus, equalization of osmotic forces occurs continuously and is achieved by the movement of water across the cell membrane. The osmolalities of ICF and ECF at equilibrium must be equal. Water moves rapidly between ICF and ECF to eliminate any induced osmolal gradient. This principle is fundamental to an understanding of fluid and electrolyte physiology.

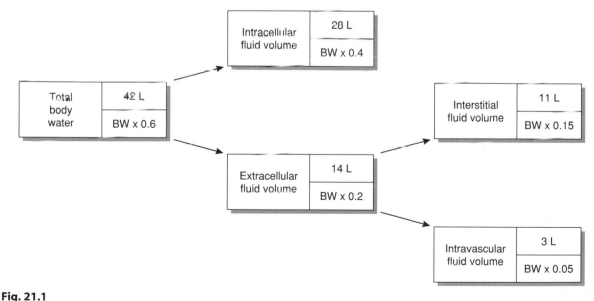

Fig. 21.1
Distribution of total body water in a 70 kg male, and related to body weight (BW).

Figure 21.2 shows the solute composition of the main body fluid compartments. Although the total concentration of intracellular ions exceeds that of extracellular ions, the numbers of osmotically active particles (and thus the osmolalities) are the same on each side of the cell membrane (290 mosmol kg^{-1} of solution).

WATER HOMEOSTASIS

Normal day-to-day fluctuations in TBW are small (< 0.2%) because of a fine balance between input, controlled by the thirst mechanisms, and output, controlled mainly by the renal–ADH (antidiuretic hormone) system.

The principal sources of body water are ingested fluid, water present in solid food and water produced as an end-product of metabolism. Intravenous fluids are another common source in hospital patients. Actual and potential outlets for water are classified conventionally as sensible and insensible losses. Insensible losses emanate from the skin and lungs; sensible losses occur mainly from the kidneys and gastrointestinal tract. Figure 21.3 depicts the daily water balance in a 70 kg adult in whom input and output balance. It should be noted that sources of potential loss are not evident in this diagram. For example, over 5 L of fluid are secreted daily into the gut in the form of saliva, bile, gastric juices and succus entericus, yet only 100 mL of fluid is present in faeces. This illustrates the potential that exists for significant fluid loss in the presence of disease.

PRACTICAL FLUID BALANCE

Calculation of the daily prescription of fluid is an arithmetic exercise to balance the input and output of water and electrolytes.

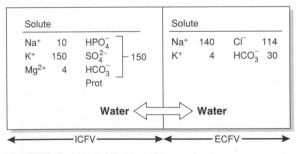

Fig. 21.2
Principal solute composition of body fluid compartments. All concentrations are expressed in mmol L^{-1}.

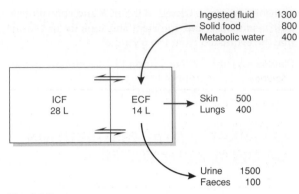

Fig. 21.3
Daily water balance. Input and output in millilitres.

Table 21.1 shows the electrolyte contents of five intravenous solutions used commonly in the United Kingdom. These solutions are adequate for most clinical situations. Two self-evident but important generalizations may be made regarding solutions for intravenous infusion.

Rule 1

All infused Na$^+$ remains in the ECF; Na$^+$ cannot gain access to the ICF because of the sodium pump. Thus, if saline 0.9% is infused, all Na$^+$ remains in the ECF. As this is an isotonic solution, there is no change in ECF osmolality and therefore no water exchange occurs across the cell membrane. Thus, saline 0.9% expands ECFV only. However, if saline 0.45% is given, ECF osmolality decreases; this causes a shift of water from ECF to ICF. If saline 1.8% is administered, all Na$^+$ remains in the ECF, its osmolality increases and water moves from ICF to ECF to maintain osmotic equality.

Rule 2

Water without sodium expands the TBW. After infusion of a solution of glucose 5%, the glucose enters cells and is metabolized. The infused water enters both ICF and ECF in proportion to their initial volumes.

Table 21.2 illustrates the results of infusion of 1 L of saline 0.9%, saline 0.45% or glucose 5% in a 70 kg adult.

Assessment of daily fluid requirements may be allocated usefully into three processes:

- normal maintenance needs
- abnormal losses resulting from the underlying pathology
- correction of pre-existing deficits.

Table 21.1   Electrolyte contents of commonly used intravenous fluids

Solution		Electrolyte content (mmol L^{-1})			Osmolality (mosmol kg^{-1})
Saline 0.9% ('normal saline')	Na$^+$	154	Cl$^-$	154	308
Saline 0.45% ('half-normal saline')	Na$^+$	77	Cl$^-$	77	154
Glucose 4%/saline 0.18% (glucose–saline)	Na$^+$	31	Cl$^-$	31	284
Glucose 5%		Nil			278
Compound sodium lactate (Hartmann's solution)	Na$^+$ K$^+$ Ca^{2+}	131 5 4	Cl$^-$ HCO$_3^-$ (as lactate)	112 29	281

NORMAL MAINTENANCE NEEDS

Water. Regardless of the disease process, water and electrolyte losses occur in urine and as evaporative losses from skin and lungs. It is evident from Figure 21.3 that a normothermic 70 kg patient with a normal metabolic rate may lose 2500 mL of water per day. Allowing for a gain of 400 mL from water of metabolism, this hypothetical patient needs about 2000 mL day^{-1} of water. As a rule of thumb, a volume of 30–35 mL kg^{-1} day^{-1} of water is a useful estimate for daily maintenance needs.

Sodium. The normal requirement is 1 mmol kg^{-1} day^{-1} (50–80 mmol day^{-1}) for adults.

Potassium. The normal requirement is 1 mmol kg^{-1} day^{-1} (50–80 mmol day^{-1}) for adults.

Thus, a 70 kg patient requires daily provision of 2000–2500 mL of water and approximately 70 mmol

Table 21.2   Compartmental expansion resulting from infusion of 1 L of saline 0.9%, saline 0.45% or glucose 5%

Intravenous infusion of 1000 mL	Change in volume (mL)		Remarks
	ECF	ICF	
Saline 0.9%	+1000	0	Na$^+$ remains in ECF
Glucose 5%	+333	+666	66% of TBW is ICF
Saline 0.45%	+666	+333	33% of TBW is ECF

each of Na$^+$ and K$^+$. This could be administered as one of the following:

- 2000 mL of glucose 5% + 500 mL of saline 0.9%
- 2500 mL of glucose 4%/saline 0.18%; plus potassium as KCl, 1 g (13 mmol) added to each 500 mL of fluid.

ABNORMAL LOSSES

These are common in surgical patients. They may be sensible or insensible and either overt or covert.

Losses from the gut are common, e.g. nasogastric suction, diarrhoea and vomiting or sequestration of fluid within the gut lumen (e.g. intestinal obstruction). Although the composition of gastrointestinal secretions is variable, replacement should be with saline 0.9% with 13–26 mmol L^{-1} of potassium as KCl. If losses are considerable (> 1000 mL day^{-1}), a sample of the appropriate fluid should be sent for biochemical analysis so that electrolyte replacement may be rationalized.

Increased insensible losses from the skin and lungs occur in the presence of fever or hyperventilation. The usual insensible loss of 0.5 ml kg^{-1} h^{-1} increases by 12% for each degree Celsius rise in body temperature.

Sequestration of fluid at the site of operative trauma is a form of fluid loss which is common in surgical patients. Plasma-like fluid is sequestered in any area of tissue injury; its volume is proportional to the extent of trauma. This fluid is frequently referred to as 'third-space' loss because it ceases to take part in normal metabolic processes. However, it is not contained in an anatomically separate compartment; it represents an expansion of ECFV. Third-space losses are not measured easily. Sequestered fluid is reabsorbed after 48–72 h.

EXISTING DEFICITS

These occur preoperatively and arise primarily from the gut. The difficulty in correcting these deficits relates to an inability to quantify their magnitude accurately. Fluid and electrolyte deficits occur directly from the ECF. If the fluid lost is isotonic, only ECFV is reduced; however, if water alone or hypotonic fluid is lost, redistribution of the remaining TBW occurs from ICF to ECF to equalize osmotic forces.

Dehydration with accompanying salt loss is a common disorder in the acute surgical patient.

Assessment of dehydration

This is a clinical assessment based upon the following.

History. How long has the patient had abnormal loss of fluid? How much has occurred, e.g. frequency of vomiting?

Examination. Specific features are thirst, dryness of mucous membranes, loss of skin turgor, orthostatic hypotension or tachycardia, reduced jugular venous pressure (JVP) or central venous pressure (CVP) and decreased urine output. In the presence of normal renal function, dehydration is associated usually with a urine output of less than 0.5 mL kg^{-1} h^{-1}. The severity of dehydration may be described clinically as mild, moderate or severe and each category is associated with the following water loss relative to body weight:

- *mild*: loss of 4% body weight (approximately 3 L in a 70 kg patient) – reduced skin turgor, sunken eyes, dry mucous membranes
- *moderate*: loss of 5–8% body weight (approximately 4–6 L in a 70 kg patient) – oliguria, orthostatic hypotension and tachycardia in addition to the above
- *severe*: loss of 8–10% body weight (approximately 7 L in a 70 kg patient) – profound oliguria and compromised cardiovascular function.

Laboratory assessment

The degree of haemoconcentration and increase in albumin concentration may be helpful in the absence of anaemia and hypoproteinaemia. Increased blood urea concentration and urine osmolality (> 650 mosmol kg^{-1}) confirm the clinical diagnosis.

PERIOPERATIVE FLUID THERAPY

In addition to normal maintenance requirements of water and electrolytes, patients may require fluid in the perioperative period to restore TBW after a period of fasting and to replace small blood losses, loss of ECF into the 'third space' and losses of water from the skin, gut and lungs.

Blood losses in excess of 15% of blood volume in the adult are usually replaced by infusion of stored blood. Smaller blood losses may be replaced by a crystalloid electrolyte solution such as compound sodium lactate; however, because these solutions are distributed throughout ECF, blood volume is maintained only if at least three times the volume of blood loss is infused. Alternatively, a colloid solution (human albumin solution or a synthetic substitute) may be infused in a volume equal to that of the estimated loss.

Third-space losses are usually replaced as compound sodium lactate. In abdominal surgery (e.g. cholecystectomy), a volume of 5 mL kg^{-1} h^{-1} during operation, in addition to normal maintenance requirements (approximately 1.5 mL kg^{-1} h^{-1}) and blood loss replacement, is usually sufficient. Larger volumes may be required in more major procedures, but one should be guided by measurement of CVP.

In the postoperative period, normal maintenance fluids should be administered (see above). Additional fluid (given as saline 0.9% or compound sodium lactate) may be required in the following circumstances:

- if blood or serum is lost from drains (colloid solutions should be used if losses exceed 500 mL)
- if gastrointestinal losses continue, e.g. from a nasogastric tube or a fistula
- after major surgery (e.g. total gastrectomy, repair of aortic aneurysm), when additional water and electrolytes may be required for 24–48 h to replace continuing third-space losses
- during rewarming if the patient has become hypothermic during surgery.

Normally, potassium is not administered in the first 24 h after surgery as endogenous release of potassium from tissue trauma and catabolism warrants restriction. The postoperative patient differs from the 'normal' patient in that the stress reaction modifies homeostatic mechanisms; stress-induced release of ADH, aldosterone and cortisol causes retention of Na$^+$ and water and increased renal excretion of potassium. However, restriction of fluid and sodium in the postoperative period is inappropriate because of increased losses by evaporation and into the 'third space'.

This syndrome of inappropriate ADH secretion may persist for several days in elderly patients, who are at risk of symptomatic hyponatraemia if given hypotonic fluids in the postoperative period. Elderly, orthopaedic patients taking long-term thiazide diuretics are especially at risk if given 5% glucose postoperatively. Such patients may develop water intoxication and permanent brain damage as a result of relatively modest reductions in serum sodium concentration.

After major surgery, assessment of fluid and electrolyte requirements is achieved best by measurement of CVP and serum electrolyte concentrations. Fluid and electrolyte requirements in infants and small children differ from those in the adult (see Ch. 36).

Patients with renal failure require fluid replacement for abnormal losses, although the total volume of fluid infused should be reduced to a degree determined by the urine output.

SODIUM AND POTASSIUM

SODIUM BALANCE

Daily ingestion amounts to 50–300 mmol. Losses in sweat and faeces are minimal (approximately 10 mmol day^{-1}) and the kidney makes final adjustments. Urine sodium excretion may be as little as 2 mmol day^{-1} during salt restriction or may exceed 700 mmol day^{-1} after salt loading. Sodium balance is related intimately to ECFV and water balance.

DISORDERS OF SODIUM/WATER BALANCE

Hypernatraemia

Hypernatraemia is defined as a plasma sodium concentration of more than 150 mmol L^{-1} and may result from pure water loss, hypotonic fluid loss or salt gain. In the first two conditions, ECFV is reduced, whereas salt gain is associated with an expanded ECFV. For this reason, the clinical assessment of volaemic status is important in the diagnosis and management of hypernatraemic states. The common causes of hypernatraemia are summarized in Table 21.3. The abnormality common to all hypernatraemic states is intracellular dehydration secondary to ECF hyperosmolality. Primary water loss resulting in hypernatraemia may occur during prolonged fever, hyperventilation or severe exercise in hot, dry climates. However, a more common cause is the renal water loss that occurs when there is a defect in either the production or release of ADH (cranial diabetes insipidus) or an abnormality in response to ADH (nephrogenic diabetes insipidus).

The administration of osmotic diuretics results temporarily in plasma hyperosmolality. An osmotic diuresis may occur also in hyperglycaemia. During an osmotic diuresis, the solute causing the diuresis (e.g. glucose, mannitol) constitutes a significant fraction of urine solute, and the sodium content of the urine

Table 21.3 Causes of hypernatraemia

Pure water depletion	
Extrarenal loss	Failure of water intake (coma, elderly, postoperative)
	Mucocutaneous loss
	Fever, hyperventilation, thyrotoxicosis
Renal loss	Diabetes insipidus (cranial, nephrogenic)
	Chronic renal failure
Hypotonic fluid loss	
Extrarenal loss	Gastrointestinal (vomiting, diarrhoea)
	Skin (excessive sweating)
Renal loss	Osmotic diuresis (glucose, urea, mannitol)
Salt gain	Iatrogenic (NaHCO$_3$, hypertonic saline)
	Salt ingestion
	Steroid excess

becomes hypotonic relative to plasma sodium. Thus, osmotic diuretics cause hypotonic urine losses which may result in hypernatraemic dehydration.

Hypertonic dehydration may occur also in paediatric practice. Diarrhoea, vomiting and anorexia lead to loss of water in excess of solute (hypotonic loss). Concomitant fever, hyperventilation and the use of high-solute feeds may combine to exaggerate the problem. ECFV is maintained by movement of water from ICF to ECF to equalize osmolality, and clinical evidence of dehydration may not be apparent until 10–15% of body weight has been lost. Rehydration must be undertaken gradually to prevent the development of cerebral oedema.

Measurement of urine and plasma osmolalities and assessment of urine output help in the diagnosis of hypernatraemic, volume-depleted states. If urine output is low and urine osmolality exceeds 800 mosmol kg^{-1}, then both ADH secretion and the renal response to ADH are present. The most likely causes are extrarenal water loss (e.g. diarrhoea, vomiting or evaporation) or insufficient intake. High urine output and high urine osmolality suggest an osmotic diuresis. If urine osmolality is less than plasma osmolality, reduced ADH secretion or impairment of the renal response to ADH should be suspected; in both cases, urine output is high.

Usually, hypernatraemia caused by salt gain is iatrogenic in origin. It occurs when excessive amounts of hypertonic sodium bicarbonate are administered during resuscitation or when isotonic fluids are given to patients who have only insensible losses. Treatment comprises induction of a diuresis with a loop diuretic if renal function is normal; urine output is replaced in part with glucose 5%. Dialysis or haemofiltration is necessary in patients with renal dysfunction.

Consequences of hypernatraemia

The major clinical manifestations of hypernatraemia involve the central nervous system. Severity depends on the rapidity with which hyperosmolality develops. Acute hypernatraemia is associated with a prompt osmotic shift of water from the intracellular compartment, causing a reduction in cell volume and water content of the brain. This results in increased permeability and even rupture of the capillaries in the brain and subarachnoid space. The patient may present with pyrexia (a manifestation of impaired thermoregulation), nausea, vomiting, convulsions, coma and virtually any type of focal neurological syndrome. The mortality and long-term morbidity of sustained hypernatraemia ($Na^+ > 160$ mmol L^{-1} for over 48 h) is high, irrespective of the underlying aetiology. In many cases, the development of hypernatraemia can be anticipated and prevented, e.g. cranial diabetes insipidus associated with head injury, but in situations where preventative strategies have failed, treatment should be instituted without hesitation.

Treatment of hypernatraemia

The magnitude of the water deficit can be estimated from the measured plasma sodium concentration and calculated total body water:

Water deficit = (measured [Na^+]/140 x TBW) – TBW

Thus in a 75 kg patient with a serum sodium of 170 mmol L^{-1}:

Water deficit = (170/140 x 0.6 x 75) – (0.6 x 75)

= 54.6 – 45

= 9.6 L

For hypernatraemic patients *without* volume depletion, 5% glucose is sufficient to correct the water deficit. However, the majority of hypernatraemic patients are frankly hypovolaemic and intravenous fluids should be prescribed to repair both the sodium and the water deficits. Regardless of the severity of the condition, isotonic saline is the initial treatment of choice in the volume-depleted, hypernatraemic patient, as even this fluid is *relatively* hypotonic in patients with severe hypernatraemia. When volume depletion has been corrected, further repair of any water deficit may be accomplished with hypotonic fluids. Fluid therapy should be prescribed with the intention of correcting hypernatraemia over a period of 48–72 h to prevent the onset of cerebral oedema.

Hyponatraemia

This is defined as a plasma sodium concentration of less than 135 mmol L^{-1}. Hyponatraemia is a common finding in hospital patients. It may occur as a result of water retention, sodium loss or both; consequently, it may be associated with an expanded, normal or contracted ECFV. As in hypernatraemia, the state of ECFV is important in determining the cause of the electrolyte imbalance.

As plasma osmolality decreases, an osmolal gradient is created across the cell membrane and results in movement of water into the ICF. The resulting expansion of brain cells is responsible for the symptomatology of hyponatraemia or 'water intoxication': nausea, vomiting, lethargy, weakness and obtundation. In severe cases (plasma $Na^+ < 115$ mmol L^{-1}), seizures and coma may result.

A scheme depicting the causes of hyponatraemia is shown in Figure 21.4. True hyponatraemia must be distinguished from pseudohyponatraemia. Sodium ions are present only in plasma water, which constitutes 93% of normal plasma. In the laboratory, the concentration of sodium in plasma is measured in an aliquot of whole plasma and the concentration is expressed in terms of plasma volume (mmol L^{-1} of whole plasma). If the percentage of water present in plasma is decreased, as in hyperlipidaemia or hyperproteinaemia, the amount of Na^+ in each aliquot of plasma is also decreased, even if its concentration in plasma water is normal. A clue to this cause of hyponatraemia is the finding of a normal plasma osmolality. Pseudohyponatraemia is not encountered when plasma sodium concentration is measured by increasingly used ion-specific electrodes, because this method assesses directly the sodium concentration in the aqueous phase of plasma.

True hyponatraemic states may be classified conveniently into *depletional* and *dilutional* types. Depletional hyponatraemia occurs when a deficit in TBW is associated with an even greater deficit of total body sodium. Assessment of volaemic status reveals hypovolaemia. Losses may be *renal* or *extrarenal*. Excessive renal loss of sodium occurs in Addison's disease, diuretic administration, renal tubular acidosis and salt-losing nephropathies; usually, urine sodium concentration

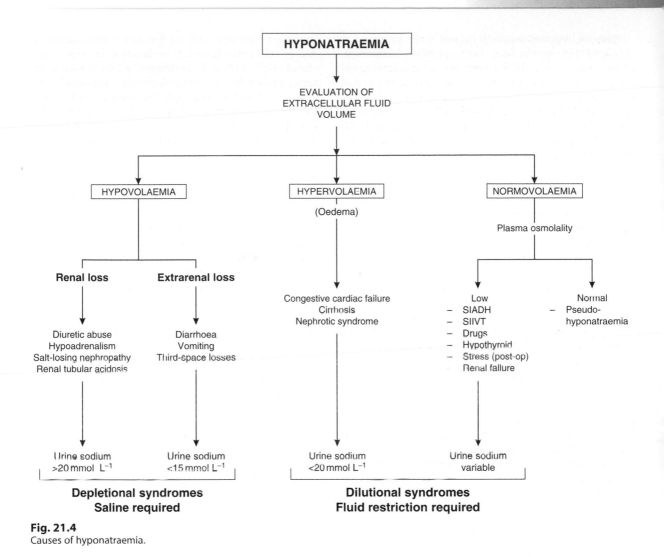

Fig. 21.4
Causes of hyponatraemia.

exceeds 20 mmol L^{-1}. Extrarenal losses occur usually from the gastrointestinal tract (e.g. diarrhoea, vomiting) or from sequestration into the 'third space' (e.g. peritonitis, surgery). Normal kidneys respond by conserving sodium and water to produce a urine that is hyperosmolal and low in sodium. In both situations, treatment should be directed at expanding the ECFV with saline 0.9%.

Dilutional hyponatraemic states may be associated with hypervolaemia and oedema or with normovolaemia. Again, assessment of volaemic status is important. If oedema is present, there is an excess of total body sodium with a proportionately greater excess of TBW. This is seen in congestive heart failure, cirrhosis and the nephrotic syndrome and is caused by secondary hyperaldosteronism. Treatment comprises salt and water restriction and spironolactone.

In normovolaemic hyponatraemia, there is a modest excess of TBW and a modest increase in ECFV associated with normal total body sodium. Pseudo-hyponatraemia is excluded by finding high protein or lipid levels and a normal plasma osmolality. True normovolaemic hyponatraemia is commonly iatrogenic in origin. The syndrome of inappropriate intravenous therapy (SIIVT) is caused usually by administration of intravenous fluids with a low sodium content to patients with isotonic losses.

A more chronic water overload may occur in patients with hypothyroidism and in conditions associated with an inappropriately elevated concentration of ADH. The syndrome of inappropriate ADH secretion (SIADH) is characterized by hyponatraemia, low plasma osmolality and an inappropriate antidiuresis, i.e. a urine osmolality higher than anticipated for the degree of hyponatraemia. It occurs in the presence of malignant tumours (e.g. lung, prostate, pancreas), which produce ADH-like substances, in neurological disorders (e.g. head injury, tumours, infections) and in some severe pneumonias. A number of drugs are associated with increased ADH secretion or potentiate the effects of ADH (Table 21.4). In patients with SIADH, the urine is concentrated in spite of hyponatraemia. Management comprises restriction of fluid intake to encourage a negative fluid balance. In severe or refractory cases, demeclocycline or lithium may result in improvement. Both drugs induce a state of functional diabetes insipidus and have been used effectively in SIADH if the primary disease cannot be treated.

Consequences of hyponatraemia

Symptoms vary with the underlying aetiology, the magnitude of the reduction of plasma sodium and the rapidity with which the plasma sodium concentration decreases. Serious consequences involve the central nervous system and result from intracellular overhydration, cerebral oedema and raised intracranial pressure. Nausea, vomiting, delirium, convulsions and coma result.

Treatment of hyponatraemia

Acute symptomatic hyponatraemia is a medical emergency and requires prompt intervention using hypertonic saline. The rapidity with which hyponatraemia should be corrected is the subject of controversy because of observations that rapid correction may cause central pontine myelinolysis, a disorder characterized by paralysis, coma and death. As a causal relationship between this syndrome and the rate of

increase of plasma sodium has not been established and it is clear that there is a prohibitive mortality associated with inadequately treated water intoxication, rapid correction of the symptomatic hyponatraemic state is warranted. Sufficient sodium should be given to return the plasma concentration to 125 mmol L^{-1} only and this should be administered over a period of no less than 12 h. The amount of sodium needed to cause the desired correction in the plasma sodium can be calculated as follows:

$$Na^+ \text{ required (mmol)} = TBW \times (\text{desired } [Na^+] - \text{measured } [Na^+])$$

Hypertonic saline (3%) contains 514 mmol L^{-1} of Na^+ and administration poses the risk of pulmonary oedema, especially in oedematous patients, in whom renal dialysis is preferable.

POTASSIUM BALANCE

The normal daily intake of potassium is 50–200 mmol. Minimal amounts are lost via the skin and faeces; the kidney is the primary regulator. However, the mechanisms for the retention of potassium are less efficient than those for sodium. In periods of K^+ depletion, daily urinary excretion cannot decrease to less than 5–10 mmol. A considerable deficit of total body potassium occurs if intake is not restored. Hypokalaemia is a more common abnormality than hyperkalaemia.

Hypokalaemia

This is defined as a plasma potassium concentration of less than 3.5 mmol L^{-1}. Non-specific symptoms of hypokalaemia include anorexia and nausea, effects on skeletal and smooth muscle (muscle weakness, paralytic ileus) and abnormal cardiac conduction (delayed repolarization with ST-segment depression, reduced height of the T wave, increased height of the U wave and a widened QRS complex).

The causes of hypokalaemia are summarized in Table 21.5. Management includes diagnosis and treatment of the underlying disorder in addition to repletion of total body potassium stores. As a general rule, a reduction in plasma K^+ concentration by 1 mmol L^{-1} reflects a total body K^+ deficit of approximately 100 mmol. Potassium supplements may be given orally or intravenously. The maximum infusion rate should not exceed 0.5 mmol kg^{-1} h^{-1} to allow equilibration with the intracellular compartment; much slower rates are generally used.

The potassium salt used for replacement therapy is important. In most situations, and especially in the presence of alkalosis, potassium should be replaced as

Table 21.4   Drugs associated with antidiuresis and hyponatraemia
Increased ADH secretion
Hypnotics – barbiturates
Analgesics – opioids
Hypoglycaemics – chlorpropamide, tolbutamide
Anticonvulsants – carbamazepine
Miscellaneous – phenothiazines, tricyclics
Potentiation of ADH at distal tubule
Paracetamol
Indometacin
Chlorpropamide

Table 21.5 Causes of hypokalaemia

Cause	Comments
Reduced intake	Usually only contributory
Tissue redistribution	Insulin therapy, alkalaemia, β_2-adrenergic agonists, familial periodic paralysis, vitamin B_{12} therapy
Increased loss	
Gastrointestinal (urine K^+ < 20 mmol L^{-1})	Diarrhoea, vomiting, fistulae, nasogastric suction, colonic villous adenoma
Renal	Diuretic therapy, primary or secondary hyperaldosteronism, malignant hypertension, renal artery stenosis (high renin), renal tubular acidosis, hypomagnesaemia, renal failure (diuretic phase)

Table 21.6 Causes of hyperkalaemia

Factitious (pseudohyperkalaemia)	*Tissue redistribution*
In vitro haemolysis	Tissue damage (burns, trauma)
Thrombocytosis	Rhabdomyolysis
Leucocytosis	Tumour necrosis
Tourniquet	Hyperkalaemic periodic paralysis
Exercise	
	Massive intravascular haemolysis
Impaired excretion	Succinylcholine
Renal failure	
Acute or chronic hyperaldosteronism	*Excessive intake*
Addison's disease	Blood transfusion
K^+-sparing diuretics	Excessive i.v. administration
Indometacin	

the chloride salt. Supplements are available also as the bicarbonate and phosphate salts.

Hyperkalaemia

This is defined as a plasma potassium concentration exceeding 5 mmol L^{-1}. Vague muscle weakness progressing to flaccid paralysis may occur. However, the major clinical feature of an increasing plasma potassium concentration is the characteristic sequence of ECG abnormalities. The earliest change is the development of tall, peaked T waves and a shortened QT interval, reflecting more rapid repolarization (6–7 mmol L^{-1}). As plasma K^+ increases (8–10 mmol L^{-1}), abnormalities in depolarization become manifest as widened QRS complexes and widening, and eventually loss, of the P wave; the widened QRS complexes merge finally into the T waves (*sine wave pattern*). Plasma concentrations in excess of 10 mmol L^{-1} are associated with ventricular fibrillation. The cardiac toxicity of K^+ is enhanced by hypocalcaemia, hyponatraemia or acidaemia. The causes of hyperkalaemia are summarized in Table 21.6.

Immediate treatment is necessary if the plasma potassium concentration exceeds 7 mmol L^{-1} or if there are any serious ECG abnormalities. Specific treatment may be achieved by four mechanisms:

- chemical antagonism of the membrane effects
- enhanced cellular uptake of K^+
- dilution of ECF
- removal of K^+ from the body.

Methods by which the plasma potassium concentration may be reduced are summarized in Table 21.7.

ACID–BASE BALANCE

The concentration of hydrogen ions (H^+) in body fluids is extremely low and the pH notation was adopted for the sake of practicality. This system expresses H^+ concentration [H^+] on a logarithmic scale:

$$pH = -\log_{10}[H^+]$$

A more logical arithmetic convention which expresses [H^+] in nmol L^{-1} is gaining popularity. Table 21.8 compares values of [H^+] expressed as pH and

Table 21.7 Treatment of hyperkalaemia

Calcium gluconate 10% i.v. (0.5 ml kg^{-1} to maximum of 20 mL) given over 5 min. No change in plasma [K^+]. Effect immediate but transient
Glucose 50 g (0.5–1.0 g kg^{-1}) plus insulin 20 units (0.3 unit kg^{-1}) as single i.v. bolus dose. Then infusion of glucose 20%, plus insulin 6–20 units h^{-1} (depending on blood glucose)
Sodium bicarbonate 1.5–2.0 mmol kg^{-1} i.v. over 5–10 min
Calcium resonium 15 g p.o. or 30 g p.r. 8-hourly
Peritoneal or haemodialysis

nmol L^{-1} and reveals several disadvantages of the pH notation. The most obvious disadvantage is that it moves in the opposite direction to [H$^+$]; a decrease in pH is associated with increased [H$^+$] and vice versa. It is also apparent that the logarithmic scale distorts the quantitative estimate of change in [H$^+$]; for example, twice as many hydrogen ions are required to reduce pH from 7.1 to 7.0 as are needed to reduce it from 7.4 to 7.3. The pH scale gives the false impression that there is relatively little difference in the sensitivity of biological systems to an equivalent increase or decrease in [H$^+$]. However, when [H$^+$] is expressed in nmol L^{-1}, it becomes apparent that tolerance is limited to a reduction in [H$^+$] of only 24 nmol L^{-1} from normal, but to an increase of up to 120 nmol L^{-1}. Nevertheless, the pH notation remains the most widely used system and is used in the remainder of this chapter.

BASIC DEFINITIONS

An *acid* is a substance that dissociates in water to produce H$^+$; a *base* is a substance that can accept H$^+$. Strong acids dissociate completely in aqueous solution, whereas weak acids (e.g. carbonic acid, H$_2$CO$_3$) dissociate only partially. The *conjugate base* of an acid is its dissociated anionic product. For example, bicarbonate ion (HCO$_3^-$) is the conjugate base of carbonic acid:

$$H_2CO_3 \dashrightarrow H^+ + HCO_3^-$$

A *buffer* is a combination of a weak acid and its conjugate base (usually as a salt) which acts to minimize any change in [H$^+$] that would occur if a strong acid or base were added to it. Buffers in body fluids represent an important defence against [H$^+$] change. The carbonic acid/bicarbonate system is an important buffer in blood. The pH of a buffer system may be determined from the Henderson–Hasselbalch equation, which, for the carbonic acid/bicarbonate system, relates pH, [H$_2$CO$_3$] and [HCO$_3^-$]:

$$pH = pK + log_{10}([HCO_3^-]/[H_2CO_3])$$

where K = dissociation constant and pK = $-log_{10}K$.

This equation shows that [H$^+$] in body fluids is a function of the *ratio* of base to acid. For the bicarbonate buffer system, pK is 6.1. As most of the carbonic acid pool exists as dissolved CO$_2$, the equation may be rewritten:

$$pH = 6.1 + log_{10}\{[HCO_3^-]/(0.225 \times P_{CO_2})\}$$

The value 0.225 represents the solubility coefficient of CO$_2$ in blood (mL kPa^{-1}). Normally, [HCO$_3^-$] is 24 mmol L^{-1} and P_aCO$_2$ is 5.3 kPa. Thus:

$$pH = 6.1 + log_{10}[24/(0.225 \times 5.3)] = 7.4$$

Most acid–base disorders may be formulated in terms of the Henderson–Hasselbalch equation. The pH of plasma is kept remarkably constant at 7.36–7.44, i.e. a hydrogen ion concentration of 40 ± 5 nmol L^{-1}. This is achieved by:

- regulation of H$^+$ excretion and bicarbonate regeneration by the kidney
- regulation of CO$_2$ by the alveolar ventilation of the lungs.

Cellular metabolism poses a constant threat to buffer systems by the production of 'volatile acid', i.e. CO$_2$, from cellular respiration and the formation of 'fixed' or 'non-volatile' acids by intermediary metabolism. Thus, the acid–base status of body fluids reflects the metabolism of both H$^+$ and CO$_2$.

ACID–BASE DISORDERS

The normal pH of body fluids is 7.36–7.44. Conventional acid–base nomenclature involves the following definitions:

- *acidosis* – a process that causes acid to accumulate
- *acidaemia* – this is present if pH < 7.36

Table 21.8 Comparison of logarithmic and arithmetic methods of expressing hydrogen ion concentration in the range of blood [H$^+$] compatible with life

pH	[H$^+$] (nmol L^{-1})	
7.8	16	
7.7	20	
7.6	25	Alkalaemia
7.5	32	
7.4	**40**	Normal
7.3	50	
7.2	63	
7.1	80	
7.0	100	Acidaemia
6.9	125	
6.8	160	

- *alkalosis* – a process that causes base to accumulate
- *alkalaemia* – this is present if pH > 7.44.

Simple acid–base disorders are common in clinical practice and their successful management requires logical analysis of pH, $[HCO_3^-]$ and P_aCO_2. The first step involves diagnosis of the primary disorder; this is followed by an assessment of the extent and appropriateness of any compensation.

Primary acid–base disorders are either *respiratory* or *metabolic*. The disorder is respiratory if the primary disturbance involves CO_2, and metabolic if it involves HCO_3^-. Thus, four potential primary disturbances exist (Table 21.9) and each may be identified by analysis of pH, $[HCO_3^-]$ and P_aCO_2. Both pH and P_aCO_2 are measured directly by the blood gas machine. $[HCO_3^-]$ is measured directly on the electrolyte profile but is derived in most blood gas machines. Other derived parameters include *standard bicarbonate* and *base excess*. The standard bicarbonate is not the actual bicarbonate of the sample but an estimate of bicarbonate concentration after elimination of any abnormal respiratory contribution to $[HCO_3^-]$, i.e. an estimate of $[HCO_3^-]$ at a P_aCO_2 of 5.3 kPa. The base excess (in alkalosis) or base deficit (in acidosis) is the amount of acid or base (in mmol) required to return the pH of 1 L of blood to normal at a P_aCO_2 of 5.3 kPa; it is a measure of the magnitude of the metabolic component of the acid–base disorder.

After the primary disorder has been identified, it is necessary to consider if it is acute or chronic and if any compensation has occurred. The body defends itself against changes in pH by compensatory mechanisms, which *tend* to return pH towards normal. Primary respiratory disorders are compensated by a metabolic mechanism and vice versa. For example, a primary respiratory acidosis is compensated for by renal retention of HCO_3^-, whereas a primary metabolic acidosis is compensated for by hyperventilation and a decrease in P_aCO_2. Thus, in each case, the *acidaemia* produced by the primary acidosis is reduced by a compensatory alkalosis. The response to a respiratory alkalosis is increased renal elimination of HCO_3^-, and metabolic alkalosis results in hypoventilation and increased P_aCO_2, pH being restored towards normal by the compensatory respiratory acidosis. In each case, the efficiency of compensatory mechanisms is limited; compensation is usually only partial and rarely complete. Overcompensation does not occur.

Metabolic acidosis

The cardinal features of a metabolic acidosis are a decreased $[HCO_3^-]$, a low pH and an appropriately low P_aCO_2. The extent of the acidaemia depends upon the nature, severity and duration of the initiating pathology in addition to the efficiency of compensatory mechanisms. The magnitude of the compensatory response is proportional to the decrease in $[HCO_3]$. The lower limit of the respiratory response is a P_aCO_2 of 1.3 kPa. In a steady state:

$$\text{predicted } P_aCO_2 = (0.02 \times \text{observed bicarbonate}) + 1.1 \text{ (kPa)}$$

If the observed P_aCO_2 differs from the predicted value, then an independent respiratory disturbance is present.

In most instances, establishing the presence and the cause of a metabolic acidosis is straightforward. In difficult cases, an important clue to the nature of the abnormality is given by the measurement of the *anion gap* in plasma:

$$\text{anion gap} = ([Na^+] + [K^+]) - ([Cl^-] + [HCO_3^-])$$

In reality, the numbers of cations and anions in plasma are the same and an anion gap exists because

---

Table 21.9 Compensatory mechanisms in acid–base disturbances

Primary disorder	pH	HCO_3^-	P_aCO_2	Compensation
Metabolic acidosis	↓	↓↓		Hyperventilation ↓ P_aCO_2
Metabolic alkalosis	↑	↑↑		Hypoventilation ↑ P_aCO_2
Respiratory acidosis	↓		↑↑	Renal retention of HCO_3^-
Respiratory alkalosis	↑		↓↓	Renal elimination of HCO_3^-

↓↓ or ↑↑ denotes the primary abnormality.
The final pH depends on the degree of compensation. Respiratory compensation for metabolic disorders is rapid; renal compensation for respiratory disorders is slow.

negatively charged proteins, together with phosphate, lactate and organic anions (which maintain electrical neutrality), are not measured. The normal anion gap is 12–18 mmol L^{-1}.

Clinically, it is useful to divide the metabolic acidoses into those associated with a normal anion gap and those with an increased anion gap. The former are caused by loss of HCO_3^- from the body and replacement with chloride. In acidoses associated with an increased anion gap, HCO_3^- has been titrated by either endogenous, e.g. lactic, or exogenous acids, thus increasing the number of unmeasured plasma anions without altering the plasma chloride concentration (Table 21.10).

Clinical effects and treatment

Metabolic acidosis results in widespread physiological disturbances, including reduced cardiac output, pulmonary hypertension, arrhythmias, Kussmaul respiration and hyperkalaemia; the severity of the disturbances is related to the extent of the *acidaemia*. Treatment should be directed initially at identifying and reversing the cause. If acidaemia is considered to be life-threatening (pH < 7.2, $[HCO_3^-]$ < 10 mmol L^{-1}), measures may be required to restore blood pH to normal. Overzealous use of sodium bicarbonate may lead to rapid correction of blood pH, with the risks of tetany and convulsions in the short term and volume overload and hypernatraemia in the longer term. The required quantity of bicarbonate should be calculated:

$$\text{bicarbonate requirement (mmol)} = \text{body weight (kg)} \times \text{base deficit (mmol } L^{-1}) \times 0.3$$

Administration of sodium bicarbonate should be followed by repeated measurements of plasma $[HCO_3^-]$ and pH. Sodium bicarbonate is available as isotonic (1.4%; 163 mmol L^{-1}) and hypertonic (8.4%; 1000 mmol L^{-1}) solutions. Slow infusion of the hypertonic solution is advisable to minimize adverse effects.

When considering the use of sodium bicarbonate in the context of metabolic acidaemia, it is important to realize that carbon dioxide is generated during the buffering process. This may result in a superimposed respiratory acidosis, especially in those patients with impaired ventilatory reserve or at the limit of compensation. It is also important to distinguish those acidoses associated with tissue hypoxia (e.g. cardiac arrest, septic shock) from those where tissue hypoxia is not a factor. It appears that therapy with sodium bicarbonate often exacerbates the acidosis if tissue hypoxia is present. For example, in patients with type A lactic acidosis, $NaHCO_3$ increases mixed venous $P_a co_2$, which rapidly crosses cell membranes resulting in an intracellular acidosis, particularly in cardiac and hepatic cells. Theoretically, this could result in decreased myocardial contractility and cardiac output and decreased lactate extraction by the liver, aggravating the lactic acidosis. Current guidelines for the management of cardiopulmonary arrest no longer recommend the routine use of sodium bicarbonate. However, if the acidosis is not associated with tissue hypoxaemia (e.g. uraemic acidosis) then the use of sodium bicarbonate results in a potentially beneficial increase in arterial pH.

Metabolic alkalosis

The cardinal features of a metabolic alkalosis are an increased plasma $[HCO_3^-]$, a high pH and an appropriately raised $P_a co_2$. The compensatory response of hypoventilation is limited and not very effective. For diagnostic and therapeutic reasons, it is usual to subdivide metabolic alkalosis into the chloride-responsive and chloride-resistant varieties (Table 21.11). The differential diagnosis of metabolic alkalosis, and in particular the classification of patients on the basis of the urinary chloride concentration, is important because of the differences in treatment of the two groups. In chloride-responsive alkalosis, the administration of saline causes

Table 21.10 Types and causes of metabolic acidosis	
High anion gap	
Overproduction of acid	Diabetic ketoacidosis
	Lactic acidosis type A (hypoxia, shock) or type B (biguanides)
	Starvation
Exogenous acid	Salicylates
	Methanol
	Ethylene glycol
Reduced excretion	Renal failure
Normal anion gap	
Bicarbonate loss	*Extrarenal*
	Diarrhoea
	Biliary/pancreatic fistula
	Ileostomy
	Ureterosigmoidostomy
	Renal
	Renal tubular acidosis
	Carbonic anhydrase inhibitors
Addition of acid (with chloride)	HCl, NH_4Cl, arginine or lysine hydrochloride

Table 21.11 Types and causes of metabolic alkalosis

Chloride-responsive (urine chloride < 20 mmol L^{-1})

Loss of acid
  Vomiting
  Nasogastric suction
  Gastrocolic fistula
Chloride depletion
  Diarrhoea
  Diuretic abuse
Excessive alkali
  $NaHCO_3$ administration
  Antacid abuse

Chloride-resistant (urine chloride > 20 mmol L^{-1})

Primary or secondary hyperaldosteronism
Cushing's syndrome
Severe hypokalaemia
Carbenoxolone

volume expansion and results in the excretion of excess bicarbonate; if potassium is required, it should be given as the chloride salt. In patients in whom volume administration is contraindicated, the use of acetazolamide results in renal loss of HCO_3^- and an improvement in pH. H_2-receptor antagonists may be helpful if nasogastric suction is contributing to hydrogen ion loss.

Severe alkalaemia with compensatory hypoventilation may result in seizures or CNS depression. In life-threatening metabolic alkalosis, rapid correction is necessary and may be achieved by administration of hydrogen ions in the form of dilute hydrochloric acid. Acid administration requires central vein cannulation, as peripheral infusion causes sclerosis of veins. Acid is given as 0.1 normal HCl in glucose 5% at a rate no greater than 0.2 mmol kg^{-1} h^{-1}.

Respiratory acidosis

The cardinal features of a respiratory acidosis are a primary increase in $P_a co_2$, a low pH and an appropriate increase in plasma bicarbonate concentration. The extent of the acidaemia is proportional to the degree of hypercapnia. Buffering processes are activated rapidly in acute hypercapnia and may remove enough H^+ from the extracellular fluid to result in a secondary increase in plasma $[HCO_3^-]$.

Usually, hypoxaemia and the manifestations of the underlying disease dominate the clinical picture, but hypercapnia per se may result in coma, raised intracranial pressure and a hyperdynamic cardiovas-

cular system (tachycardia, vasodilatation, ventricular arrhythmias) resulting from release of catecholamines.

There are many causes of respiratory acidosis, the most important of which are classified in Table 21.12. Treatment consists of reversing the underlying pathology if possible and mechanical ventilatory support if required.

Respiratory alkalosis

The cardinal features of respiratory alkalosis are a primary decrease in $P_a co_2$ (alveolar ventilation in excess of metabolic needs), an increase in pH and an appropriate decrease in plasma bicarbonate concentration. Usually, hypocapnia indicates a disturbance of ventilatory control (in patients not receiving mechanical ventilation). As in respiratory acidosis, the manifestations of the underlying disease usually dominate the clinical picture. Acute hypocapnia

Table 21.12 Causes of respiratory acidosis

Central nervous system
Drug overdose
Trauma
Tumour
Degeneration or infection
Cerebrovascular accident
Cervical cord trauma

Peripheral nervous system
Polyneuropathy
Myasthenia gravis
Poliomyelitis
Botulism
Tetanus
Organophosphorus poisoning

Primary pulmonary disease
Airway obstruction
  Asthma
  Laryngospasm
  Chronic obstructive airways disease
Parenchymal disease
  ARDS
  Pneumonia
  Severe pulmonary oedema
  Chronic obstructive airways disease
Loss of mechanical integrity
  Flail chest

results in cerebral vasoconstriction and reduced cerebral blood flow and may cause light-headedness, confusion and, in severe cases, seizures. Circumoral paraesthesia, hyperreflexia and tetany are common. Cardiovascular manifestations include tachycardia and ventricular arrhythmias secondary to the alkalaemia.

The causes of respiratory alkalosis are summarized in Table 21.13. Treatment comprises correction of the underlying cause and thus differential diagnosis is important.

RECENT DEVELOPMENTS IN ACID–BASE THEORY

The 'traditional' model of acid–base theory based on the renal and pulmonary regulation of hydrogen ion concentration is relatively easy to understand and to apply in common clinical situations. However, problems have been identified with its interpretation, which is dependent upon normal plasma electrolyte and protein composition. Recently, alternative methods of assessing acid–base derangements have been described based on the work of Stewart. This 'modern' approach to acid–base theory is based on a more complex mathematical model and proposes that three independent variables determine acid–base balance: (1) the strong ion difference (SID) given by the total concentration of fully dissociated cations (Na^+, K^+, Ca^{2+} and Mg^{2+}) minus the concentration of fully dissociated anions (Cl^-, lactate); (2) the Pa_{CO_2}; and (3) the total weak acid concentration (consisting of mostly albumin and phosphate). It is apparent in this modern approach that bicarbonate cannot be considered as an independent variable. Bicarbonate concentration changes not only in response to the pulmonary ($P_a{CO_2}$) and renal (SID) systems but also to the liver and gastrointestinal tract (total weak acid).

Strong ion theory does explain some clinical observations such as the metabolic acidosis that occurs in postoperative patients after large infusions of 0.9% saline (reduced SID and bicarbonate) and the metabolic alkalosis of chronic hypoalbuminaemia (low weak acid concentration) and it is difficult to apply in the clinical arena. It is unclear if this novel approach will find a place in mainstream clinical practice.

Table 21.13 Causes of respiratory alkalosis
Supratentorial
Voluntary/hysterical hyperventilation
Pain, anxiety
Specific conditions
CNS disease
Meningitis/encephalitis
Cerebrovascular accident
Tumour
Trauma
Respiratory disease
Pneumonia
Pulmonary embolism
Early pulmonary oedema or ARDS
High altitude
Shock
Cardiogenic
Hypovolaemic
Septic
Miscellaneous
Cirrhosis
Gram-negative septicaemia
Pregnancy
IPPV
Drugs/hormones
Salicylates
Aminophylline
Progesterone

FURTHER READING

Arieff A I 1991 Indications for the use of bicarbonate in patients with metabolic acidosis. British Journal of Anaesthesia 67: 165–178

Lane N, Allen K 1999 Hyponatraemia after orthopaedic surgery. British Medical Journal 318: 1363–1364

Sirker A A, Rhodes A, Grounds R M, Bennett E D 2002 Acid–base physiology: the 'traditional' and the 'modern' approaches. Anaesthesia 57: 348–356

Swales J D 1991 Management of hyponatraemia. British Journal of Anaesthesia 67: 146–154

Thomson W S T, Adams J F, Cowan R A 1997 Clinical acid–base balance. Oxford University Press, Oxford

Wooten EW 2004 Science review: quantitative acid-base physiology using the Stewart model. Critical Care 8: 448-452

Haematological disorders and blood transfusion 22

In the United Kingdom both medical and surgical specialities make major demands on blood banks and transfusion services. The clinicians most commonly responsible for administering blood transfusions and blood products in the surgical setting are anaesthetists. Therefore, anaesthetists need a thorough working knowledge of common haematological and bleeding disorders together with a sound knowledge of good transfusion practice.

Historically, blood has been a readily available resource, and the level of risk associated with transfusion has been perceived as low. This position is rapidly changing. Transfusion is probably safer nowadays than previously, but there is a much greater awareness of the not inconsiderable hazards of transfusion. Moreover, blood and blood products are rapidly becoming a scarce resource in the United Kingdom and other Western countries. This resource should be used carefully and within appropriate professional frameworks (see Transfusion practice, below).

BONE MARROW AND BLOOD CONSTITUENTS

HAEMOPOIESIS

In the fetus, the main site for haemopoiesis is the yolk sack until 6 weeks of gestation. Thereafter the liver and spleen are the primary sites until about 7 months. Around this stage, bone marrow becomes the major site of blood cell production, although the liver and spleen continue to produce red cells in normal individuals until 2 weeks after birth. In extreme situations the liver may retain haemopoietic potential until much later.

In infants, most bones are involved in haemopoiesis. By adult life, this is confined to the vertebrae, ribs, sternum, sacrum, pelvis, proximal femur and skull. A common pluripotential stem cell is the progenitor of the cells of the circulation. The pluripotential stem cell differentiates into specific progenitor cells for the three main bone marrow cell types: erythropoietic cells, granulocytic cells (including monocytes) and megakaryocytic cells. Progenitor cells can respond to a number of stimuli to produce increased numbers of cells of their cell line.

Red blood cells arise from the pronormoblast. Cell division results in smaller normoblasts with each generation having a higher haemoglobin content. There is progressive loss of RNA from the cytoplasm, and ultimately the cell nucleus is extruded from late normoblasts, resulting in the reticulocyte. Early reticulocytes within the bone marrow have low cytoplasmic levels of RNA but are still capable of synthesizing haemoglobin. By the time the cell enters the circulation as a mature erythrocyte, the ability to synthesize haemoglobin has been lost. The mature red cell is a biconcave disc with no nucleus. It has a diameter of 8 μm and a lifespan of approximately 120 days. The cell is extremely flexible and easily deformable, so it can pass through vessels in the microcirculation whose diameter is less than that of the cell, down to 3.5 μm. The enzyme methaemoglobin reductase is associated with the red cell membrane. This enzyme is important for maintaining the iron in haemoglobin in the ferrous (Fe^{2+}) oxidative state. Oxidation to the ferric form (Fe^{3+}) results in conversion of haemoglobin to methaemoglobin, which is ineffective as an oxygen carrier.

Marrow red cell production is governed predominantly by the hormone erythropoietin. Relative hypoxaemia in the kidney stimulates expression of a nuclear transcription factor. This in turn gives rise to increased expression of the erythropoietin gene. Erythropoietin is released, and this has its effect on the bone marrow. It increases the number of stem cells committed to red cell production. Precursors required for this process include the haematinics, B group vitamins, vitamin C and E, and a number of essential metals (iron, manganese, cobalt) together with the essential amino acids. Shortage of haematinics can result in either microcytic anaemia (typically associated with iron deficiency), or macrocytic anaemia (typically associated with deficiency of vitamin B_{12} or folic acid). Anaemia may also occur with amino acid or androgen deficiency. A number of anaemias of chronic disease may fall into this category.

HAEMOGLOBIN

Haemoglobin is the red cell protein responsible for transport of oxygen and to some extent carbon dioxide. It consists in the adult of four polypeptide chains, two α-chains and two β-chains. Each of these is associated with a haem group. In addition, adult blood contains traces of fetal haemoglobin (haemoglobin F) and haemoglobin A2. These haemoglobins contain normal α-chains but the β-chains are replaced with γ-chains in the case of fetal haemoglobin and δ-chains in case of haemoglobin A2. Each haemoglobin chain has a molecular weight of 68 000.

Haem synthesis occurs predominantly in the mitochondrion. The process begins with condensation of glycine with succinyl CoA, producing the protoporphyrin ring. This combines with iron to form haem. In functional iron deficiency, iron may be replaced by a zinc (Zn^{2+}) ion. The resultant production of zinc protoporphyrin can be used as an index of functional iron deficiency. Each haem molecule associates with a globin chain. Finally a tetramer forms, made up of two α- and two β-chains, each with its haem ring.

WHITE BLOOD CELLS

These are divided into two broad categories: phagocytes and lymphocytes. The phagocyte group includes neutrophil polymorphs, eosinophils, basophils and monocytes. Neutrophils are slightly larger than red blood cells, having a diameter of 12–15 μm. They have a characteristic multilobular nucleus and a cytoplasm filled with fine granules. Primary granules contain myeloperoxidase and acid phosphatase, and secondary granules contain alkaline phosphatase and lysosyme. In times of sepsis and stress, there is an increase in the number of immature neutrophils in the circulation (known as 'band' or 'juvenile' forms).

Lymphocytes are small cells (7–15 μm in diameter). These subdivide into T and B lymphocytes. The lymphocyte population increases following antigenic stimulation.

PLATELETS

Platelets are derived from the pluripotential stem cell, which divides to produce megakaryocytes. Each of these is capable of rapid nuclear replication without cell division. A cell with a slight increase in cytoplasm and cell size is produced, having up to eight nuclei. At this stage the cytoplasm becomes granular and produces microvesicles. The microvesicles coalesce, resulting in platelet demarcation membranes. The megakaryocyte fragments, releasing up to 4000 platelets. Immature platelets spend 24h in the spleen before finally entering the circulation, where they have a lifespan of 2 weeks.

PLASMA

Blood cells are suspended and transported in plasma, which is a solution of electrolytes and proteins, including albumin, globulins, carrier proteins and clotting factors. In addition, lipids and lipoproteins are carried in the plasma. Plasma is an essential vehicle for supporting the circulation, coagulation, immune function and transport of essential nutrients.

GENETIC ABNORMALITIES OF HAEMOGLOBIN

There are very many genetic abnormalities of haemoglobin synthesis. These arise from a great variety of gene mutations. Not all of these are compatible with survival. They can be classified broadly into those genetic defects which result in impaired production of normal globin chains (thalassaemias); and those which result in the synthesis of an abnormal haemoglobin (haemoglobinopathies).

THALASSAEMIAS

The thalassaemias are characterized by a quantitative defect. There is reduced production (or no production if extreme) of the affected globin chain. The production of the other chains is quantitatively and qualitatively normal.

In α-thalassaemia there is failure of production of the α-chain. The homozygous form results in fetal death. In the heterozygous form there is a spectrum of severity, the least severe of which results in a mild hypochromic anaemia. Patients with three of the four α-chains deleted suffer haemoglobin H disease. This is of intermediate severity and may require intermittent transfusion.

In β-thalassaemia, production of the β-chain is reduced. There are three clinical forms. The least severe of these is known as β-thalassaemia trait or thalassaemia minor. This results from heterozygous disease and clinically is relatively insignificant. The condition may present as a mild microcytic anaemia, often detected during pregnancy. Double heterozygotes or homozygotes with less severe mutations may suffer thalassaemia intermedia. This has a more marked anaemia than thalassaemia trait, and may require transfusion. Homozygotes who inherit severe β-chain mutations will have significantly reduced β-chain production, or absence. This results in thalassaemia major, characterized by severe anaemia. This condition requires frequent transfusion, and untreated is usually fatal in childhood. Life expectancy is reduced because of the risk of iron overload.

SICKLE CELL DISEASE

Well over a hundred variants of this condition have been described. The most significant of these clinically is haemoglobin S. In this condition, β-chains are qualitatively different from normal haemoglobin β-chains. The condition is found in African and some Mediterranean countries and also in some parts of the Indian subcontinent. Ten per cent of subjects of African extraction carry the gene for haemoglobin S. Valine is substituted for glutamine at position six of the β-chain. In the heterozygote this may produce mild anaemia of little clinical significance, provided oxygenation and hydration are reasonably well maintained. However, in homozygotes, haemoglobin becomes insoluble at oxygen partial pressures in the venous range (approximately 5.5 kPa). This results in conversion to a crystalline form, which causes deformation and increased rigidity of the red blood cell. This in turn reduces the ability of the red blood cell to transit through capillaries, and leads to occlusion and in severe cases tissue infarction. These episodes are known as crises, and may be precipitated by surgery, anaesthesia, hypoxia, dehydration, intercurrent infection or mild illnesses, and may even arise spontaneously. The condition is accompanied by anaemia, a result of reduced red cell survival. Increased cell turnover may also result in jaundice.

Patients with haemogobinopathies are of particular interest to the anaesthetist, as they carry a substantially increased perioperative risk. Diagnosis is made by haemoglobin electrophoresis, and this should be carried out as a screening test in all patients thought to be at risk. Intraoperative management should be discussed with a haematologist. Consideration should be given to pretransfusion of homozygotes electively, or exchange transfusion. The object of transfusion or exchange transfusion is to increase the percentage of haemoglobin A compared with haemoglobin S to around 40%. Simple transfusion can achieve 35% HbA, whereas exchange transfusion can achieve up to 50%

HbA. The overall incidence of complications in sickle cell disease patients undergoing minor surgery is around 18%. Those undergoing major surgery have a much higher complication rate (up to 35% in one recent study), whereas this can be reduced to very low levels by preoperative exchange transfusion.

THROMBOSIS AND HAEMOSTASIS

Coagulation is a major haemostatic function responsible for the prevention and termination of bleeding following injury. It represents a dynamic interaction between the vessel wall and the clotting factors in the circulation and the platelet. The processes of coagulation are tightly controlled by both positive and negative feedback loops, but predominantly by a process of amplification. The coagulation system is balanced by the fibrinolytic system. This is responsible for breakdown of fibrin and fibrinogen and prevention of excessive thrombi.

Traditional views of the coagulation system divided the process into extrinsic and intrinsic pathways (Fig. 22.1). These pathways remain useful for understanding in vitro tests of clotting, but do not relate usefully to the complex interaction occurring in vivo. This is better summarized by the schema depicted in Figure 22.2. There is a cyclical feedback loop with thrombin generation occurring as a consequence. Extracellular matrix proteins, such as collagen in the vessel wall and subendothelial tissues, are crucial to the initiation of clot formation. Platelet adhesion occurs at the site of vessel injury. Furthermore, endothelial cells have a major influence through synthesis of von Willebrand factor, prostacyclin, antithrombin, protein S, thrombomodulin and tissue plasminogen activator.

PLATELET FUNCTION

Platelets form mechanical plugs during haemostasis. To do this they exhibit a number of functions: adhesion, degranulation (release), aggregation, fusion and platelet procoagulant activity. The rate of adhesion of platelets to exposed subendothelial collagen depends on the presence and function of platelet surface membrane glycoproteins. Exposure to collagen at the point of vascular injury, or exposure to activated thrombin (see Fig. 22.2), induces platelet degranulation. The granules contain adenosine diphosphate (ADP), serotonin, fibrinogen, heparin neutralizing factor and lysozyme. The release process depends on prostaglandin synthesis. This is a function of the platelet membrane under

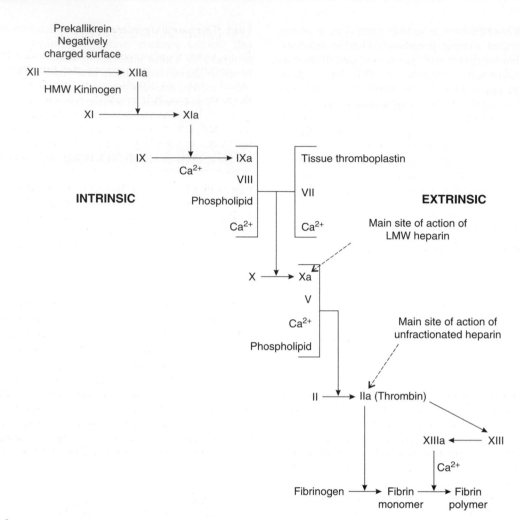

Fig. 22.1
Intrinsic and extrinsic coagulation pathways – useful in understanding in vitro tests of clotting.

conditions of peroxidation. Thromboxane A_2 reduces cyclic adenosine monophosphate (cAMP) and initiates the release reaction. Thromboxane A_4 promotes platelet aggregation and vasoconstriction. These processes are balanced by the effects of vasodilator prostaglandins synthesized by vascular endothelium. Following platelet aggregation, ADP triggers platelet swelling and adhesion of adjacent platelet membranes. This in turn promotes a positive feedback loop with further release of ADP and thromboxane A_2, giving rise to secondary platelet aggregation. This process is sufficient in itself to produce a large enough platelet plug to seal the breach in vascular endothelium.

Platelets have procoagulant activity; during platelet plug formation a membrane phospholipid, platelet factor 3 (PF3), is exposed. PF3 provides a template for

the orientation and interaction of proteins of the coagulation cascade. Inactive glycoprotein IIb/IIIa receptors on the platelet surface membrane are activated and available for binding of fibrinogen and von Willebrand factor. This leads to cross-linking and stabilization of the platelet plug. Finally, fibrin formation reinforces the stability of the platelet plug, which undergoes clot retraction and stabilization.

COAGULATION PATHWAY

This is summarized in Figure 22.2. The initial phase is known as initiation and involves a number of processes broadly similar to the old 'extrinsic pathway'. Initiation occurs following vessel or tissue injury and exposure of tissue factor to blood. This binds acti-

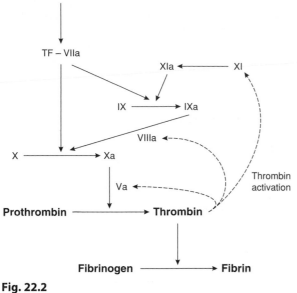

Fig. 22.2
More complex coagulation pathways – more applicable to in vivo situations.

vated factor VII (VIIa), small quantities of which are normally found free in the circulation. This in turn activates factors IX and X, and generates small, 'priming' quantities of thrombin. This is the primer that initiates coagulation and activates platelets. There is then further activation and assembly of coagulation factors on the platelet surface.

Until this stage, however, the quantities of thrombin and coagulation factors activated are very small. The process of amplification follows. This involves numerous feedback mechanisms. Production, of factor VIIa has a positive feedback effect on itself, resulting in further activation of tissue factor bound factor VII. Thrombin activates a number of nonenzymatic cofactors, including factors V and VIII. These increase the rate of production of prothrombin. The final phase of the cascade is propagation, during which large amounts of factor X associate with factor VIIIa on the surface of the activated platelet. This results in activation of factor X. This process requires PF3 (see above) and calcium. In the presence of activated factor V on the surface of an activated platelet, factor Xa converts prothrombin to thrombin, resulting in cleavage of fibrinogen to fibrin. The process is completed by clot stabilization, another thrombin-dependent process in which large quantities of thrombin activate factor XIII. Factor XIIIa in turn leads to cross-linking of soluble fibrin monomers to a stable matrix.

THE FIBRINOLYTIC SYSTEM

If coagulation were to continue uncontrolled, then clot propagation and spontaneous clot formation would rapidly result in a pathological state. The process of fibrinolysis results in breakdown of fibrin and fibrinogen, and limitation of further clot propagation. This is a cascade process summarized in Figure 22.3. The fibrinolytic cascade may be initiated by several routes, including vessel injury, or shear forces, resulting in the release of tissue plasminogen activator; or by the action of the kinin system. These processes in turn have their own inhibitors (for example plasminogen activator inhibitors, PAI1 and PAI2). The activators of fibrinolysis are responsible for cleavage of plasminogen to plasmin. This process normally occurs in association with plasminogen binding to fibrin, which serves as a template for its cleavage. Activated plasmin can break down fibrin or fibrinogen before being released as a free molecule. Unchecked, free plasmin has a systemic fibrinolytic effect. However, its action is rapidly terminated under normal circumstances by a number of circulating inhibitors. These include α_2-antiplasmin, α_2-macroglobulin, α_1-antitrypsin and antithrombin. Several drugs may mimic this effect pharmacologically. These include tranexamic acid and aprotinin (which also has inhibitory effects on the kinin system). The process of fibrinolysis results in fibrin degradation products. These are anticoagulant in themselves, and interfere with fibrin polymerization.

THE BLEEDING PATIENT

Anaesthetists are from time to time presented with patients with a pre-existing coagulopathy or bleeding diathesis. Involvement of a haematologist to establish

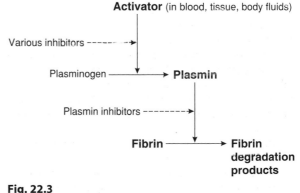

Fig. 22.3
The fibrinolytic system.

the fitness of the patient for surgery is advisable from an early stage.

INHERITED ABNORMALITIES OF COAGULATION

These include haemophilia A (factor VIII deficiency) and Christmas disease (haemophilia B; factor IX deficiency). These two syndromes are clinically indistinguishable. Related to these is von Willebrand's disease. This results from a deficiency of von Willebrand factor which confers stability on factor VIII. Inherited coagulation factor deficiencies have been described for each of the coagulation factors, but these are rare.

The bleeding tendency in patients with haemophilias is directly related to the degree of deficiency and the activity of the relevant factor. In subjects with severe haemophilia, i.e. factor VIII or factor IX levels < 1 unit/dL, spontaneous haemorrhage into joints and muscles is common. Levels of 1–5 units/dL are associated with less spontaneous bleeding, and in patients who are only mildly affected (levels > 5 units/dL) spontaneous bleeding is uncommon. Patients with mild disease may remain undiagnosed until late in life. However, any haemophilia patient, whatever the grade of severity of their disease, is likely to bleed excessively during trauma or surgery. This may lead to incidental clinical diagnosis. Involvement of an experienced haematologist at an early stage is essential for safe surgery. The usual approach is to raise the level of the deficient clotting factor by use of factor concentrate to a haemostatic value. The precise therapeutic regimen will depend on the nature of the deficiency, the severity of the deficiency and on the surgery proposed. In some patients with mild haemophilias and type 1 von Willebrand's disease, treatment with desmopressin (DDAVP) may be effective. This can increase concentrations of factor VIII by 2–6 times and von Willebrand factor by 2–4 times within 30 min of injection. The effect is possibly mediated by a mobilization of existing von Willebrand factor from vascular endothelium. However, the effect is not always clinically reliable or sustained and may be less effective on subsequent dosing. Some patients will require plasma products. Types 2 and 3 von Willebrand's disease are rare but likely to require treatment with factor concentrates or cryoprecipitate; involvement of a haematologist is essential. Type 3 disease is completely resistant to DDAVP.

Some haemophiliacs who have been exposed to clotting factor replacement develop antibodies to these. This may make treatment of their haemophilia extremely difficult. Specialist advice should be sought. Treatment options include high-dose human factor VIII, porcine factor VIII or treatment by use of factors occurring 'further down' the coagulation cascade. Activated factor VII (now available as a recombinant preparation) has been particularly effective in this setting.

In the UK, many haemophiliacs have been infected with HIV and hepatitis C by transfusion with infected products, especially those treated in the 1980s, before routine screening for hepatitis C became available. Patients diagnosed and treated in recent years are at much less risk because of improvements in the screening of blood products, heat treatment of products, and the wider availability of 'pure' recombinant products.

THROMBOCYTOPENIA

Most laboratories have a reference range for blood platelet count of approximately $150–400 \times 10^9/L^{-1}$. A count $< 100 \times 10^9/L^{-1}$ is considered thrombocytopenic. The risk of haemostatic failure increases as the platelet count decreases. Counts $< 20–30 \times 10^9/L^{-1}$ may result in spontaneous bleeding. There are numerous causes of thrombocytopenia including drug therapy, immune reactions (including heparin-induced thrombocytopenia), effects of sepsis and chronic disease, and a number of specific disease processes including disseminated intravascular coagulation and thrombotic thrombocytopenic purpura.

Treatment of thrombocytopenic patients with platelet transfusion should be carried out after discussion with the haematologist. It is not generally necessary to treat a numerical deficiency in the platelet count in the absence of active bleeding. Many patients with pathological conditions and thrombocytopenia can undergo surgery without vigorous platelet supplementation. Furthermore, repeated and unnecessary platelet transfusion may result in production of antiplatelet antibodies, so that the platelet count increment arising from a transfusion may become ineffective.

However, there is general agreement that very low platelet counts (for example below $20 \times 10^9/L^{-1}$) should be treated to prevent the risk of haemorrhage, including spontaneous haemorrhage. Otherwise, during surgery, tests of platelet function and dynamic clot formation (for example the thromboelastogram) may provide a useful guide to platelet and clotting factor transfusion. This is because laboratory values do not always give an accurate prediction of dynamic clot function. Neuraxial blockade should be avoided in patients with significant thrombocytopenia.

DISORDERS OF PLATELET FUNCTION

In addition to platelet numbers, primary haemostasis requires intact function. Drug-induced and metabolic disorders of platelet function occur frequently. Aspirin and nonsteroidal antiinflammatory drugs are prime examples. Aspirin causes irreversible inhibition of the enzyme cyclooxygenase with impaired thromboxane synthesis. Because this effect results from covalent binding, its duration is that of the platelet. Its effect on platelet function measured in vitro lasts up to 10 days and is dependent on production of 'new' platelets. Nonsteroidal antiinflammatory drugs have a similar but reversible effect whose duration and degree of platelet dysfunction are dependent on blood levels of the drug.

In addition, a number of newer drugs used in the secondary prevention and treatment of coronary artery disease and peripheral vascular disease act by inhibiting the function of platelet surface glycoproteins. Examples of such drugs include clopidogrel (which is now in common use). The effect of nonsteroidal antiinflammatory drugs on platelet function is relatively minor, and is generally not a bar to surgery. However, clopidogrel may produce intractable bleeding at surgery and is not necessarily reversed by platelet transfusion. Consideration should be given to its discontinuation 7 days before surgery in high-risk patients. Clopidogrel acts by inhibiting the binding of ADP to its receptors in platelets. This prevents up-regulation of the platelet glycoprotein IIb/IIIa receptor and reduces the amount of fibrinogen that can bind to these receptors. It also reduces thrombosis from shear stress and abolishes cyclic flow variations.

Several new drugs directly inhibit the glycoprotein IIb/IIIa receptor. These include the monoclonal antibody abciximab and the drugs eptifibatide and tirofiban. Again, there is little specific therapy which can be used to limit bleeding caused by these drugs apart from administration of platelets.

Abnormalities of platelet function are also seen in patients undergoing extracorporeal circulation (for example renal dialysis or cardiopulmonary bypass) and patients with uraemia and renal failure.

THE ANTICOAGULATED PATIENT

A commonly encountered problem is that of the patient receiving oral anticoagulants, who presents either for elective or emergency surgery. Clinically significant anticoagulation is generally considered a contraindication to central neuraxial blockade because of the increased risk of spinal haematoma. In all patients there is a balance of risks, though this risk increases with the degree of anticoagulation. Few anaesthetists would consider performing neuraxial blockade at all in patients with an INR > 1.7, and many would place the cut-off value below this level. The drug most commonly encountered is warfarin, although the dicoumaride anticoagulants are still occasionally seen. Warfarin and related drugs act by inhibition of the vitamin K-dependent clotting factors (II, VII, IX, X, but also protein C). The action of warfarin is prolonged and may take many days to reverse after discontinuation of therapy.

Many surgeons are reluctant to proceed without at least partial reversal of anticoagulation. Many hospitals have developed protocols for this situation. Ideally, advice should be sought from a haematologist where time permits.

In the elective situation it is usually reasonable to discontinue warfarin 4 or 5 days prior to surgery until the INR has fallen to approximately 2.0. Surgery with careful haemostasis can usually proceed at this level. In some patients, a decision may be made to introduce perioperative heparinization at a low dose where continuous anticoagulation is deemed desirable. In an emergency, this can easily be reversed with protamine.

In the acute situation, there are a number of options. These include correction of anticoagulation by the use of specific factor concentrates. The current recommendation is to use prothrombin complex rather than fresh frozen plasma. Fresh frozen plasma does not always completely reverse the effect of warfarinization, and carries all the risks of exposing the recipient to multiple donors of blood products. Vitamin K may occasionally be used where the INR is very high. Vitamin K should, however, be used cautiously in increments of 2.5 mg, with the INR being rechecked after 30–60 min before a further dose is given. This is because it can lead to rapid over-correction, with the risk of thrombosis. Further treatment with vitamin K may result in warfarin resistance for many days.

DISSEMINATED INTRAVASCULAR COAGULATION

Disseminated intravascular coagulation (DIC) is also known as consumptive coagulopathy. The latter term reflects pathogenesis. The process can be triggered by a number of proinflammatory, septic or ischaemic or similar states, including shock, major haemorrhage and amniotic fluid embolism (Table 22.1). The process is complex. It involves activation of clotting within the microvasculature and results in a failure of microcirculation, with tissue damage. Simultaneously, there is a 'consumptive coagulopathy'. Normal clotting fails to take place because of depletion of circulating factors. The process is accompanied by activated fibrinolysis, with clot instability.

Table 22.1   Clinical associations of disseminated intravascular coagulation

Release of tissue thromboplastin	Eclampsia
	Placental abruption
	Fetal death in utero
	Amniotic fluid embolism
	Disseminated malignancy including acute leukaemia
	Head injury
	Burns
Infection	Malaria
	Bacteria, especially Gram-negative
	Viruses
Miscellaneous	Incompatible blood transfusion
	Extracorporeal circulation
	Antigen–antibody complexes
	Fat embolism
	Pulmonary embolism
	Shock

Treatment of DIC presents a major challenge. The management is focused on treatment of any predisposing condition. Direct treatment of the coagulopathy may be ineffective and indeed counterproductive. Fresh frozen plasma, cryoprecipitate and platelets may be used as directed both by laboratory tests and clinical endpoints (bleeding). Historically, heparin has also been used to prevent intravascular coagulation and protect the microcirculation. However, this practice has now been largely abandoned because there is a risk of major haemorrhage. There is no place for the use of antifibrinolytic drugs.

LIVER DISEASE

Patients with liver disease frequently present for surgery. This group of patients may have an increased bleeding tendency for a variety of reasons. First, patients with cirrhotic liver disease may also have portal hypertension and varices. This includes varices throughout the abdomen and abdominal wall, with an increased risk of surgical bleeding. Second, this patient population may have a reduced platelet count either because of a reduced level of a thrombopoietin or hypersplenism. Third, they are frequently deficient in vitamin K-dependent clotting factors (II, VII, IX, X, protein C), because of a reduction in bile-dependent absorption. Further, they may have reduced synthesis

of other clotting factors, because of hepatocellular dysfunction. Finally, such patients have increased activity of the fibrinolytic system at rest, due to increased circulating levels of activators of fibrinolysis and reduced levels of its inhibitors, including antithrombin. Fresh frozen plasma, cryoprecipitate, platelets and vitamin K may all be of value in treating this group of patients. Consideration should also be given to use of an antifibrinolytic agent, for example tranexamic acid. Use of clotting products is generally guided by thromboelastography in patients with severe liver disease. This has been shown to reduce the overall product requirement while simultaneously optimizing coagulation profile. Expert advice should be sought.

THE THROMBOTIC PATIENT

The balance between coagulation and fibrinolysis is essential for normal haemostasis and integrity of the blood vessel and microcirculation. Derangement of these mechanisms can give rise to arterial or venous thromboembolism. The risk factors are well recognized (Table 22.2). Thrombosis normally results from an interplay between these factors. Hypercoagulability follows major surgery and represents an interplay between fluid shifts and the stress response. In addition, the components of Virchow's triad (blood constituents, vessel wall and circulatory flow characteristics) play a major contribution. The risk of thrombosis must be assessed on an individual basis, taking into account pre-existing patient variables and the nature of the illness, as well as the presence of trauma, including the surgery planned. For low-risk patients, simple measures such as support stockings or early mobilization are generally sufficient. For patients at greater risk, low molecular weight heparin or subcutaneous low-dose unfractionated heparin are frequently used. Low molecular weight heparins have the advantage of increased bioavailability and therefore a more consistent effect following standard dosing. They are equally as effective as unfractionated heparins in preventing deep vein thrombosis and in some settings, e.g. orthopaedic surgery, are more effective. Anticoagulation should begin before surgery and be continued until after full mobilization. Epidural anaesthesia has been shown to be effective at reducing deep vein thrombosis during orthopaedic surgery of the lower limb.

In patients who have been therapeutically heparinized, normalization of clotting is generally possible within a few hours by discontinuing heparin therapy. Where emergency reversal is required, prota-

Table 22.2 Risk factors for venous thrombosis

Hereditary thrombophilias

Factor V Leiden

Prothrombin mutation

Hyperhomocysteinaemia

Protein C deficiency

Protein S deficiency

Antithrombin III deficiency

Dysfibrinogenaemia

Hypercoagulable states due to physiological stimuli

Pregnancy

Oestrogen therapy

Surgery

Immobilization

Advancing age

Obesity

Hypercoagulable states associated with pathological conditions

Antiphospholipid antibodies

Hyperhomocysteinaemia

Previous venous thromboembolism

Congestive cardiac failure

Malignancy

Nephrotic syndrome

Heparin-induced thrombocytopenia

Paroxysmal nocturnal haemoglobinuria

Myeloproliferative disorders

mine can be used in a dose of 1 mg of protamine per 100 units of heparin administered. Care should be exercised when administering protamine as this can result in hypotension, flushing and wheezing. Large doses of protamine may in themselves have an anticoagulant effect. Protamine is less effective in reversing low molecular weight heparins than it is in reversing unfractionated heparin.

HEPARIN-INDUCED THROMBOCYTOPENIA

Heparin-induced thrombocytopenia exists in two forms. The milder form (type 1 heparin-induced platelet deficiency) is transient and self-limiting, and is probably a result of direct heparin-induced platelet agglutination. In type 1 – the more benign form – the effect is dose related and rapidly reversible on discontinuation of heparin. Type 2 deficiency overlaps with heparin-induced thrombosis. Up to 2–3% of patients receiving unfractionated heparin for 5 or more days develop type 2 deficiency, an immune-mediated reaction. It causes a relatively sudden decrease in platelet count. This is caused by production of antibodies to the heparin-platelet factor 4 complex on the surface of platelets. In the more severe form, the condition is idiosyncratic and long lasting. Further, if heparin is reintroduced during the recovery phase there can be a very rapid recurrence of the condition. In severe cases, platelet activation may lead to circulatory occlusion and major vascular thrombosis, including arterial thrombosis. Renal haemorrhage, infarction and skin necrosis at the site of heparin injection have been described. Where anticoagulation is essential, alternative therapies should be considered. These include hirudin, a thrombin-specific inhibitor.

BLOOD TRANSFUSION

Blood has traditionally been used as a therapy for anaemia and major haemorrhage. There are significant risks associated with blood transfusion and the perception of these risks has heightened in recent years. Additionally, blood and blood products are becoming an increasingly scarce and expensive resource, because screening programmes and donor deferral have limited the number of individuals prepared and able to donate blood while at the same time increasing the cost and complexity of the process. Consequently, blood transfusion should be used in an extremely conservative and responsible fashion. Many centres now advocate a restrictive transfusion policy, and indeed, there is good evidence to suggest that patients tolerate anaemia much better than was previously thought. For patients who do not have ischaemic heart disease, transfusion is unnecessary where the haemoglobin content remains above 8g dL^{-1}.

Hospitals in the UK are now required to establish hospital transfusion teams, which are charged with developing and implementing suitable policies and educational programmes to achieve the aims set out in the Chief Medical Officer's circular *Better Blood Transfusion 2*.

BLOOD DONATION

Extensive screening procedures exist before a unit of blood from a prospective donor can enter the supply. These include health questionnaires and screening to exclude high-risk donors together with bacteriological and virological screening of the donated blood. Because of the risk of variant Creutzfeldt–Jakob disease (vCJD) transmission by blood transfusion, potential donors in the UK who have previously themselves been the recipients of blood transfusion have now been removed from the donor panel. This and other safety measures are dramatically reducing the availability of blood for transfusion in the UK. Should a blood test for variant CJD become available, this is likely to reduce the donor panel even further. This is because, although the number of positive individuals is expected to be small, many potential donors would not wish to donate in the knowledge that this would involve compulsory screening for vCJD – a move which might affect eligibility for life insurance and have a significant impact on employment and credit potential.

Blood donations in the UK are currently screened for hepatitis B and C as well as HIV1, HIV2 and syphilis. Since August 2002, blood in the UK has also been screened for human lymphotropic virus (HTLV). These measures have resulted in almost negligible risk of transfusion-transmitted disease. This is likely to be reduced even further as polymerase chain reaction (PCR)-based screening becomes standard; this further shortens the 'window' periods.

Blood is collected into sterile, plastic bags containing CPD-A (citrate, phosphate, dextrose, adenine), which acts both as an anticoagulant and as a preservative. Units are placed in a centrifuge to separate different components, including red cells. Blood components are leucodepleted to eliminate white cell-associated infections, e.g. CMV and transfusion reactions. There may also be a small reduction in the theoretical risk of vCJD transmission as a result of leucodepletion. However, prion disease is also likely be transmitted through plasma components. Because of this, fresh frozen plasma sourced in the UK is used only for adults and children born before the introduction of the specified offal ban. Plasma for children born after this date (December 1996) is currently sourced from countries thought to be free of variant CJD. Other plasma products are obtained from similar sources. Currently in the UK, plasma for children is additionally virally inactivated using methylene blue and ultraviolet light; the methylene blue is subsequently removed from the plasma.

RED CELL PRODUCTS

Only a small proportion of blood is issued as whole blood. Most red cells are issued as cell concentrates. Some red cell concentrates are suspended in plasma and are produced by the removal of 150–200 mL of plasma from the final donated volume. Most units have a much greater percentage of plasma removed

and are resuspended in a preservative solution. The additive used in the UK is SAGM (saline, adenine, glucose, mannitol). Red cell concentrates have a higher viscosity than whole blood and a higher haematocrit. The preparations have a shelf-life of 35 days. Blood issued to hospitals and by blood banks for transfusion may be of any age up to almost 35 days. Paradoxically, when blood stocks are high, older blood tends to be issued; when blood stocks are low, storage times are shorter, so fresher blood is issued. Red cell storage should be at 4°C in blood bank refrigerators with inbuilt alarm systems. There should be a full and comprehensive audit trail and tracking process, so that blood can be tracked all the way from the donor to the recipient. Adequate handling and storage at all stages of this journey are essential to inhibit bacterial replication, slow red cell glycolysis and, as far as possible, preserve 2,3-DPG. It is important to prevent blood freezing as this results in cell lysis. Blood should be transfused cold except in situations where large volume or rapid transfusion is required or in patients with cold haemagglutinin disease. In such situations, a blood warmer is required. For very rapid transfusion, devices with counter-current warming columns, such as the rapid infusion system or the 'Level 1' warmer, are advisable.

All hospitals must have adequate protocols for checking blood prior to transfusion. The commonest complication of blood transfusion remains the wrong blood being given to the wrong patient. Consequently, protocols must be very strictly followed. When a sample is taken for cross-matching the label on the bottle must be hand written, copying details from the patient's wristband (not the notes) to minimize the chance of errors. Adhesive patient identification labels should not be used, as it is easy to place the wrong label on the bottle. When blood is received from the laboratory, whatever local forms and paperwork are in place, it is absolutely mandatory additionally to check the name and details on the unit of blood against the name and details on the patient's wristband. These checking procedures are even more important in the emergency situation, such as the patient in theatre with massive haemorrhage, because this is the situation in which transfusion error is most likely to occur.

BLOOD GROUPS

The ABO blood groups first described in 1901 by Landsteiner and the Rhesus system (Rh) described by Landsteiner and Weiner in 1940 form the important blood group systems for those practising blood transfusion primarily at the bedside. However, there are many other clinically important blood group systems of more immediate concern to the transfusion laboratory. Problems relating to these groups are normally resolved by the laboratory, well before blood products are issued as compatible for use in the patient. Nevertheless, some patients, particularly those who have received previous transfusions, may have formed an extensive range of antibodies and so may be extremely difficult to cross-match. It may therefore be necessary to use blood which fulfils only a partial cross-match; this must be given very carefully under clinical trial. The laboratory will normally advise the clinician in such a situation.

ABO groups

In the UK, 47% of the population is blood group O (in some countries called group zero, '0'). Blood group A is the second most common (42%), and group B constitutes 8% of the population; group AB is rare (3%). The distribution varies elsewhere in the world; there is an increased gene frequency for blood group B in the Mediterranean and Eastern countries. ABO blood group proteins may also be found on leucocytes and platelets, in body fluids and on several other cell lines. A and B antigens are present on red cells early in fetal development, but the corresponding antibodies appear only after birth (3–6 months). These occur naturally; they are a constant feature of the system in all people, and do not depend on previous exposure to the other blood group antigens.

Traditionally, group O blood (universal donor) was used in emergency situations, where there was insufficient time for a patient to be cross-matched. However, this may result in haemolysis and some transfusion reactions. Where there is inadequate time for cross-matching, most laboratories still produce group-specific blood very rapidly and then phone through a cross-match on individual units subsequently. This emergency procedure is greatly preferable to the indiscriminate use of blood group O. Because group AB is so infrequent, many blood banks do not carry stocks of this blood group. Commonly, therefore, group AB recipient patients are cross-matched against donor units from group A or group B donors. Likewise, group O blood is occasionally used for group B recipients.

ABO-incompatible transfusion accidents are the most serious. They result in complement activation and significant morbidity and mortality. Patients present with symptoms of distress, chest or abdominal pain, loin pain and breathlessness. These symptoms are masked during anaesthesia. Transfusion reactions may therefore progress to hypotension, DIC, uncontrollable bleeding and renal failure before being detected. Incompatible transfusion is frequently fatal.

Such reactions almost always arise from incorrect labelling of the sample or request form, or inadequate checks before administration of blood (see above).

Rhesus antigens

Shortly after discovery of the Rhesus antigens it was recognized that some haemolytic transfusion reactions and haemolytic disease of the newborn resulted from incompatibilities in the Rhesus system. In clinical transfusion practice, the Rhesus D antigen is the most important, although others exist (Cc, Ee). Rhesus factors are inherited in a linked form, one from each parent. Each linkage contains one of each pair of alleles for the C, D and E loci. The commonest genes are 'Cde' (gene frequency 0.41) and 'cde' (0.39), followed by 'cDE' (0.14). The other genes are much less common.

Antibodies of clinical significance occur in the Rhesus system. Spontaneous natural occurrence is rare; more usually there is prior exposure to a foreign antigen. The commonest significant antibody is anti-D, usually as a result of a D-negative mother bearing a Rhesus D-positive fetus. The UK programme for prevention of Rhesus immunization in pregnancy has reduced the incidence of this problem. Undetected, the condition may result in delayed haemolytic transfusion reactions, with impaired survival of the transfused cells.

Other blood groups

The known number of blood group antigens is increasing constantly, usually because of the prior discovery of the corresponding antibody. The majority are of little clinical significance, although some may cause immediate or delayed haemolytic reactions. Specificity and the ability to react at 37°C characterize those antibodies in recipient serum which mandate provision of red cells lacking the specific antigen.

BLOOD GROUPING AND CROSS-MATCHING

In most centres, this is now carried out by automated patch testing and with electronic cross-matching. This is possible because of the widespread introduction of gel-based technologies. In principle, ascertaining a patient's blood group by this method takes only a few minutes, but in practice, because of patch processing, there is usually a delay of a few hours. However, this confers considerable economies of scale. Once a patient has been blood grouped, an antibody screen is also performed using similar technology. This can be carried out well in advance of elective surgery. Information is then available both on ABO and Rhesus

D grouping of the patient. It is further possible to detect, characterize and record details at 37°C of common atypical antibodies in the recipient serum which could result in a transfusion reaction or reduced red cell survival. Verification of the recipient results is then cross-checked either manually, or more commonly by reference to a computerized database, with previous serum samples taken from the patient.

This process removes a significant number of errors in the cross-matching process and, interestingly, regularly in most large laboratories reveals discrepancies with the old record. Investigation of these generally shows that there has been an error in sample collection or labelling – the commonest cause of transfusion accidents. Consequently, comparison of a patient's sample with old records provides an additional, although imperfect, safety check.

When these procedures are performed in accredited laboratories, it is usually possible to select a suitable unit of donor blood very rapidly, which is theoretically compatible with the recipient serum. A simple 'immediate spin' of donor cells with recipient serum at room temperature provides the final cross-match to exclude major mistakes and confirm ABO compatibility.

In the emergency situation, it is generally possible to provide group-specific blood within a few minutes, and follow this with a full cross-match. Where time does not permit this, it is still possible to use group O donor blood, although such situations are extremely rare. When uncross-matched blood is being given to women of childbearing potential, it should also be Rhesus D negative to minimize the risk of subsequent haemolytic disease of the newborn.

TRANSFUSION REACTIONS

The majority of transfusion-related accidents and reactions occur as a result of the wrong blood being given to the wrong patient. All transfusion-related critical incidents, adverse events and near misses should be reported nationally under the SHOT scheme (serious hazards of transfusion). The annual SHOT report is produced and is widely circulated through the Transfusion Committee. It is also freely accessible on the Internet.

The commonest type of transfusion reaction is the non-haemolytic febrile reaction, also known as a white cell reaction. This occurs as a result of the interaction between recipient anti-HLA antibodies to donor white cells, and occurs in up to 2% of red cell or platelet transfusions. Fever and rigors can occur within 30–60 min of the transfusion commencing. The majority are benign and self-limiting. Such reactions may prevent an increment in platelet count following a platelet transfusion. In patients who suffer such reactions or who have had multiple transfusions, it is generally desirable to transfuse HLA-compatible platelets. These problems are thought to have become much less common since the introduction in the UK of universal leucodepletion.

Allergic reaction to donor plasma proteins may cause skin rashes, urticaria and itching. Anaphylaxis to donor plasma fractions is rare but may be serious and indeed life-threatening. It results from the interaction between IgA in the donor serum and anti-IgA in the recipient.

TRANSFUSION-ASSOCIATED ACUTE LUNG INJURY

Transfusion-associated acute lung injury (TRALI) has traditionally been underreported. The true incidence may be as high as 1–2% of all transfusions. This reaction occurs as a consequence of the interaction between antibodies in the donor plasma and foreign white blood cells. Consequently, TRALI can be caused by transfusion of fresh frozen plasma and plasma components as well as by transfusion of blood. The risk depends largely on the donor; those blood donors who have been exposed to previous multiple transfusions, or who have been pregnant, are thought to have a greater risk of developing anti-white cell antibodies. When products from such donors are transfused into a susceptible recipient, the anti-white cell antibodies result in an interaction with white cell activation, which can lead to an increase in capillary permeability and leakage, and a syndrome similar to the acute respiratory distress syndrome (ARDS). The diagnosis can be confirmed by sending samples of the causative blood product and from the recipient to a reference laboratory. Once the diagnosis has been established, the donor of the high-risk products is removed from the donor panel. Management of TRALI may require intensive care admission and artificial ventilation and is largely supportive. Other complications of blood transfusion are listed in Table 22.3.

TRANSFUSION PRACTICE

There is currently considerable debate regarding optimal transfusion practice and the appropriate strategy for minimizing unnecessary transfusions. Several recent studies have suggested that the traditional practice of liberal blood transfusion is not advantageous in all patient groups. Indeed, one major study has suggested that critically ill patients without cardiovascular risk factors are more likely to survive when transfused to a haemoglobin between 8 and 10g dL^{-1},

Table 22.3 Complications of blood transfusion

Transmission of disease, e.g. viral hepatitis, syphilis, malaria, HIV
Bacterial contamination
Pyrogenic reactions
Incompatibility reactions
Haemolytic reactions
Allergic reactions
Citrate toxicity
Hypothermia
Hyperkalaemia
Metabolic acidosis
Circulatory overload
Air embolism
Microaggregate embolism

rather than a higher value. Such information has become available at the same time as the cost of transfusion (both financial and social) has started to rise sharply, and the availability of blood and blood products has begun to fall.

All hospitals in the UK should have in place appropriate transfusion policies administered by a hospital transfusion team. Further, there should be an emergency blood management plan developed and overseen by a senior hospital committee. Transfusion should be given according to locally decided guidelines, which should be evidence based. These should take into account the condition and specific requirements of individual patients as well as evidence, where available, from the literature. Specific measures include the use of transfusion triggers and thresholds, techniques such as acute normovolaemic haemodilution (ANH), and the use of cell-saver devices and autotransfusion. These devices take two forms: those which salvage red cells intraoperatively for immediate reinfusion, and those which salvage red cells from wound drains postoperatively for reinfusion. The former are complex devices and are relatively expensive. They involve a suction unit where blood is mixed, usu-

ally with heparinized saline, and stored in a reservoir. From here it is drained into a centrifuge, which is computer-controlled. The centrifuge separates the red cell component from the other components, and the fluid supernatant is progressively removed. The red cells are simultaneously washed and resuspended in saline to a predetermined haematocrit (usually approximately 50%). Finally, the resuspended red cells are pumped into a bag for reinfusion into the patient. There is controversy as to the safety of such devices in patients with active local infection (e.g. peritonitis), or malignancy.

Jehovah's Witnesses

Much has been learnt about transfusion minimization and avoidance from Jehovah's Witnesses. Although the specific views of individual Witnesses vary, a great deal of experience, and indeed insight, has been gained from working with this group. Jehovah's Witnesses will not accept red cell transfusion, either of bank blood or of their own predonated blood, although many will accept the use of a cell-saver, provided that the blood returned to them is reinfused during the same treatment session. Equally, fresh frozen plasma and platelets are viewed as banned blood products. Many Jehovah's Witnesses will accept minor plasma fractions and recombinant preparations, although this is a matter for the conscience of the individual. When treating Jehovah's Witness patients, it is of paramount importance to respect the wishes of the individual and practise within the framework of appropriately informed consent. The Jehovah's Witness hospital liaison committees are skilled and knowledgeable groups of people, who are prepared to advise both Witnesses and doctors on the appropriate standards of care; their help is invaluable.

FURTHER READING

Better blood transfusion 2. Health service circular, Department of Health, 2002, HSC 2002/009, London, UK; http://www.doh.gov.uk/publications/coinh.html
Bombeli T, Spahn D R 2004 Updates in perioperative coagulation: physiology and management of thromboembolism and haemorrhage. British Journal of Anaesthesia 93(2): 275–287
Mallett S V, Cox D J 1992 Thrombelastography. British Journal of Anaesthesia 69(3): 307–313
Mollison P L, Engelfriet C P, Contresus M 2005 Blood transfusion in clinical medicine, 11th edn. Blackwell Sciences, Oxford, UK
National Blood Service hospitals website; http://www.blood.co.uk/hospitals/index.htm

23 Intercurrent disease and anaesthesia

An increasing proportion of patients presenting for anaesthesia and surgery suffer from intercurrent disease. Patients are often receiving a variety of medications. Many are elderly with limited physiological reserve. All these factors influence the conduct of anaesthesia and surgery and must be considered when assessing and managing a patient perioperatively for the following reasons:

- the course of the disease may be modified by anaesthesia and surgery
- the disease may influence the effects of anaesthesia
- concurrent drug therapy may influence the effects of anaesthesia
- the choice of anaesthetic technique is affected
- normal compensatory responses may be affected.

The aims of anaesthetic management in such patients are to:

- assess the extent of the medical problem
- optimize the patient's condition as far as possible before surgery, depending on the time available, (emergency versus elective procedures)
- tailor the anaesthetic technique to the patient, considering both regional and general techniques
- determine an appropriate level of monitoring
- continue the optimal level of care throughout the perioperative period.

The ability to achieve these aims varies widely depending on the urgency of surgery and thus the time available. All patients presenting for surgery should have a full clinical history and examination. Past medical history, including previous anaesthesia, regular medications and allergies (including food) are important. Ideally, previous anaesthetic records should be reviewed. Appropriate specific investigations may then be planned depending on the age and fitness of the patient and the nature and urgency of the surgery (see Ch. 15).

Assessing the patient's risk from surgery and anaesthesia and planning subsequent management appropriately require consideration of three main issues.

- *Comorbidity*: Does the patient's coexisting pathology increase the risk of surgery and may it be improved to reduce this?
- *Physiological reserve*: What is the patient's functional capacity and is there adequate reserve to undergo anaesthesia and surgery at the level planned? The capacity of the cardiorespiratory system to respond to perioperative stress may be assessed in terms of metabolic equivalents (METs). If a patient can achieve over 4 METs of activity without significant symptoms then the perioperative risk of a cardiac event is low (Table 23.1).
- *Extent of surgery*: High-risk operations include aortic and other major vascular procedures, and also procedures anticipated to be prolonged and to involve significant fluid shifts and blood loss. Following discussion with the patient and surgeon, it may be appropriate in some cases to consider alternatives to surgery or a less major operation if the patient is considered at too high a risk.

The above issues are considered in the context of several common medical problems.

CARDIOVASCULAR DISEASE

ISCHAEMIC HEART DISEASE

The presence of coronary, cerebral or peripheral vascular disease defines a group of patients at increased risk from anaesthesia and surgery, manifesting as postoperative cardiovascular events such as myocardial ischaemia and myocardial infarction. It is considered that the stress response to surgery, increased sympathetic activity and activation of the coagulation cascade combine to increase myocardial oxygen requirements and promote coronary thrombosis.

Table 23.1 Metabolic equivalent (MET) levels for readily assessed activity levels

MET score	Approximate level of activity
1	Dress, walk indoors
2	Light housework, slow walk
4	Climb one flight of stairs, run a short distance
6	Moderate sport, e.g. golf, doubles tennis or dancing
10	Strenuous sports or exercise

One MET is approximately equivalent to an oxygen consumption of 3.5 mL kg^{-1} min^{-1}.
Adapted from ACC/AHA Guidelines for the Perioperative Cardiovascular Evaluation for Noncardiac Surgery. *J Am Coll Cardiol* 1996; 27:910–948. Copyright 1996 The American College of Cardiology Foundation and American Heart Association, Inc.

The presence of left ventricular failure and a low ejection fraction are also risk factors. This is a result partly of the close association with coronary vascular disease and also of the resultant limitation of function.

Hypertension alone is now considered to be a relatively low risk factor. However, it is often a marker of significant underlying vascular disease.

Preoperative assessment

The aims of preoperative assessment in this group are to:

- define the fitness of the patient for the proposed anaesthetic and surgery
- delineate the level of risk of the procedure
- decide on the most appropriate anaesthetic technique
- assess the requirement for preoperative therapy to be initiated, for example beta-blockade or blood transfusion
- assess the level of perioperative monitoring required
- decide on the patient's postoperative management, including where this should take place.

The revised Goldman cardiac risk index for patients undergoing non-cardiac surgery identifies high-risk groups as defined below. If a patient fits into three or more of these groups, there is an estimated 10% risk of cardiac morbidity or death perioperatively:

- high-risk surgery
- ischaemic heart disease diagnosed either from the history or investigation
- congestive cardiac failure
- evidence of cerebrovascular disease, e.g. previous stroke
- insulin-dependent diabetes mellitus
- renal impairment (creatinine >177 μmolL^{-1}).

History

Symptoms of cardiovascular disease include chest pain, dyspnoea, palpitations, ankle swelling and intermittent claudication. The severity of symptoms, combined with an estimate of exercise tolerance, is the most useful assessment of cardiovascular disease and associated perioperative risk.

Past medical history and medical records usually reveal the nature and severity of disease, as many patients with cardiovascular symptoms have undergone relevant investigations before.

Examination

Preoperative cardiovascular examination should include measurement of heart rate, arterial pressure and assessment of peripheral pulses and perfusion. Signs of heart failure should be sought, including a third heart sound, elevated jugular venous pressure and fine basal crepitations on auscultation of the lung fields. The heart should be auscultated for murmurs indicative of valvular disease.

Testing the patient's exercise capacity in the ward or on a flight of stairs is a simple, but very useful, assessment of functional reserve.

Risk stratification

Assessment of the patient's risk of a perioperative cardiac event provides prognostic information (Table 23.2). These issues may be discussed with the patient and appropriate written information provided. Adequate provision of information and the opportunity to ask questions has been shown to allay preoperative anxiety. Assessment also guides perioperative investigation and management.

For patients stratified into the major-risk group, only emergency or very urgent procedures should be considered. Elective procedures should be postponed until such time as the procedure may be undertaken more safely.

For example, patients who have sustained a myocardial infarction (MI) within the 6 weeks before proposed surgery are a high-risk group. As a result of

Table 23.2 Stratification of risk factors for patients undergoing non-cardiac surgery

Major

Unstable coronary syndromes

MI within last 6 weeks

PCI within last 6 weeks

Decompensated heart failure

Significant/compromising arrhythmias

Severe valvular disease

Moderate

MI > 6 weeks < 3 months

Angina

Compensated heart failure

Diabetes mellitus

Renal insufficiency

Low

Elderly

Hypertension

Poor functional reserve (< 4–6 MET)

Arrhythmia

Previous CVA

After American College of Cardiology/American Task Force on Practice Guidelines – guideline update for perioperative cardiovascular evaluation for non cardiac surgery, 2002.

increased sympathetic stimulation and the coagulation activation secondary to surgery, such patients have a greater than 5% incidence of perioperative MI, which carries a very high (30%) mortality. A history of MI more than 6 weeks before surgery is no longer considered an absolute contraindication to elective surgery. Provided that the patient is symptom-free and has a good exercise capacity, this is considered moderate risk (see Table 23.2).

If there is no urgency, it is best to wait until 3 months post-infarct after which time, if patients are asymptomatic with a good exercise capacity, they join the low-risk group.

Asymptomatic patients who have undergone successful coronary artery bypass grafting more than 6 weeks before surgery constitute a low-risk group. Indeed, the mortality in this group is less than in a matched group with well-controlled angina on medical therapy. However, the risk of coronary artery surgery itself negates this benefit. It is therefore recognized that major cardiac interventions such as

bypass grafting are indicated prior to non-cardiac surgery only if the patient's underlying cardiac condition merits intervention for its own sake. This is the case for patients with severe triple vessel disease or significant left main stem stenosis.

Many patients now undergo percutaneous coronary interventions (PCI). There is again no proven benefit for carrying out this procedure before non-cardiac surgery unless clinically indicated. In this case, the subsequent risk of noncardiac surgery is also high within the first 6 weeks following the procedure and should preferably be deferred for at least 3 months. Activation of coagulation secondary to major surgery may be more likely to lead to occlusive thrombus in the presence of atheromatous plaque disruption secondary to angioplasty and stenting.

There is also the requirement for ongoing antiplatelet therapy. If this is stopped, the risk of stent thrombosis (which carries a 7% mortality), is high but patients are at risk of major bleeding if antiplatelet therapy is maintained during major surgery.

Diabetes mellitus and compensated heart failure represent independent risk factors as they are associated frequently with myocardial ischaemia which may be silent; these groups may merit further investigation (see below).

Investigations

Routine investigations including haematology, biochemistry, an ECG and chest X-ray are necessary in all patients with proven or suspected cardiovascular disease. A coagulation screen may be indicated.

Subsequent investigations depend on the assessed risk for the patient and the clinical findings.

All patients found to have a murmur should have preoperative echocardiography. Significant aortic stenosis, for example, is associated with an increased risk of perioperative cardiovascular events and may be difficult to confirm on clinical grounds alone. Echocardiography may also provide useful information on left ventricular function.

Additional cardiovascular investigations are indicated only if they influence patient management. The incidence of coronary artery disease in asymptomatic members of the population is considered to be 4%. Screening tests are unlikely to be helpful in this group. Patients in high-risk groups where specific management of their cardiovascular disease is indicated independent of the need for noncardiac surgery should undergo coronary angiography and further treatment as indicated.

Between these two extremes lies a group of patients at increased risk of perioperative cardiovascular events where further assessment is indicated as perioperative care is influenced by the results. Moreover, accurate determination of risk to the patient may help decision-making with regard to the need for surgery and/or the type of operation and anaesthetic.

Patients who should be considered for further preoperative testing include:

- those in the intermediate-risk group for whom major surgery is planned
- patients with poor functional capacity
- patients undergoing high-risk surgery, e.g. major vascular surgery
- patients with diabetes mellitus
- patients with poor left ventricular function.

The choice of preoperative test is dictated by local and patient factors, but it includes exercise stress testing, dobutamine stress echocardiography and dipyridamole thallium scanning. Cardiological advice should be sought for both the test required and interpretation of the results with regard to predicting the perioperative risk of a serious cardiovascular event.

Preoperative therapy

There are two main areas to be addressed. Pre-existing cardiovascular disease should be treated and management optimized where necessary. In addition, there may be interventions which, appropriately initiated in patients at risk, may improve outcome.

Pre-existing cardiovascular disease

Ischaemic heart disease. Medical therapy should be reviewed and optimized if symptoms are poorly controlled.

Hypertension. Raised arterial pressure is a major cause of morbidity and mortality in the general population because of the detrimental effects on the myocardial and cerebrovascular circulations and on renal perfusion. It is now recognized that both hypertension and isolated systolic hypertension should be treated because effective control of arterial pressure reduces the incidence of complications from target organ damage. The British Hypertension Society guidelines recommend starting antihypertensive therapy for sustained pressures above 140/90 mmHg. However, in the perioperative setting, there is little evidence that patients with isolated hypertension of less than 180/100 mmHg have a significantly increased risk of cardiovascular complications and isolated hypertension below this level is classified as a low-risk factor. If hypertension is identified preoperatively, then evidence of target organ damage should be

sought. If target organ damage is found, then the risks of anaesthesia and surgery are dependent on this. Subsequent investigation and management should be based on target organ function rather than on the hypertension per se. Postoperative follow-up and treatment are indicated.

For non-urgent surgery, patients with severe hypertension, i.e. > 180/100 mmHg, should be treated to lower the arterial pressure in a controlled manner before embarking on surgery. In the case of urgent surgery, more rapid control may be achieved. In light of their beneficial effects in high-risk cardiovascular patients, beta-blockers are the agents of choice. Care must be taken, however, because rapid decreases in arterial pressure may be detrimental.

Antihypertensive therapy should be continued as far as possible throughout the perioperative period.

Many patients seen at preadmission clinic or admitted to hospital have hypertension which subsequently settles or which is not in keeping with the recordings made by their general practitioner. There is no evidence that so called 'white coat hypertension' carries an increased perioperative risk. Often, these patients benefit from a benzodiazepine premedication.

Cardiac failure. Cardiac failure and low left ventricular ejection fraction are intermediate risk factors. Treatment should be optimized as far as possible preoperatively and investigation of underlying coronary artery disease undertaken as appropriate, as outlined above.

Treatment and additional interventions

Beta-blockers. Established beta-blocker therapy should be maintained throughout the perioperative period either orally or intravenously if necessary. Sudden preoperative cessation may be associated with rebound effects such as angina, myocardial infarction, arrhythmias and hypertension. The dose of beta-blocker may be reduced if there is undue bradycardia preoperatively (< 50 beat min^{-1}). Intraoperative bradycardia usually responds to intravenous atropine or glycopyrrolate. Several studies have shown a significant reduction in perioperative cardiovascular sequelae and longer-term beneficial effects on survival if beta-blocker therapy is initiated preoperatively in patients with definite evidence of ischaemic heart disease undergoing high-risk surgery.

For example, in Poldermans et al's (1999) study of major vascular surgery, patients with a positive stress echocardiogram preoperatively had a 10-fold reduction in fatal and non-fatal myocardial infarction if they received perioperative beta-blockade. These advantages are not seen in patients receiving chronic therapy and do not appear to be restricted to any particular beta-blocker. The optimal time to begin therapy and duration of beta blockade are uncertain, as is the benefit conferred in lower-risk situations. In a non-urgent situation, it may be preferable to introduce beta blockade cautiously over several weeks, particularly if there is evidence of left ventricular dysfunction.

Angiotensin-converting enzyme inhibitors and angiotensin II receptor blockers. These agents have beneficial effects in patients with vascular disease, cardiac failure and diabetes, with a reduction in cardiac morbidity and mortality. They may predispose to renal failure and hyperkalaemia and may be associated with intractable intraoperative hypotension. There is currently no consensus as to whether or not these agents should be continued intraoperatively.

Antiplatelet agents. Aspirin and clopidogrel are used increasingly in combination to maintain vessel patency following PCI and to reduce thrombosis in patients with unstable angina or recent MI. Both agents have irreversible effects on platelet action and their effect therefore continues for the life of the platelet. Aspirin inhibits cyclo-oxygenase-mediated production of thromboxane. Clopidogrel is a noncompetitive antagonist of platelet ADP receptors. They have a synergistic effect in inhibiting platelet aggregation. Both agents need to be stopped for at least 7 days to see these effects reversed by new platelet production. Whether or not these agents are continued preoperatively depends on the perceived risk of bleeding versus increased cardiovascular events. If these agents are continued then both the surgeon and anaesthetist must be aware of the increased risk of haemorrhage and take appropriate anticipatory measures. Platelet transfusion is the only effective therapy for uncontrolled haemorrhage secondary to these agents.

In general, if a patient is anticoagulated (see below) or receiving clopidogrel, then neuraxial blockade is contraindicated because of the increased risk of haematoma and neurological damage. Aspirin alone is not considered a significant risk factor.

Anticoagulants. Where long-term therapy is indicated, perioperative control must be monitored closely. Warfarin should be stopped at least 48 hours preoperatively and the prothrombin time monitored daily. The prothrombin time should be less than 1.5 times control at the time of surgery. If prolonged, the use of vitamin K may be considered; however, this takes 6–12 h to act and may compromise subsequent anticoagulation, so its use depends on the reasons for anticoagulation in the first place. In an emergency or where excessive haemorrhage occurs, fresh frozen plasma should be given to supply coagulation factors. For patients at high risk from thrombosis, e.g.

with a prosthetic heart valve, an intravenous heparin infusion should be started when the prothrombin time decreases and continued until 2 h preoperatively. After minor surgery with low risk of haemorrhage, warfarin may be restarted postoperatively. After major surgery, an infusion of unfractionated heparin should be used to maintain anticoagulation until warfarin therapy is reinstituted safely. The heparin infusion may be titrated to thrombin time to maintain good control and if necessary may be reversed rapidly with intravenous protamine. Protamine should be given slowly to avoid hypotension and if given in excessive dose is itself an anticoagulant.

Statins. Statin therapy provides a beneficial reduction in morbidity and mortality in high-risk vascular patients even in the presence of a normal cholesterol level. This is thought to result from stabilization of atheromatous plaques. There is increasing evidence in patients undergoing high-risk vascular surgery that initiating statin therapy may reduce cardiovascular complications. The introduction of a statin preoperatively should therefore be considered in this group. Again, the optimal timing of this intervention is unknown but it has been suggested that therapy should be commenced 1 month preoperatively.

α_2-Agonists. Drugs such as clonidine reduce sympathetic activity, reduce arterial pressure and heart rate and have analgesic properties. There is provisional evidence to suggest they may be of benefit in patients at high risk of perioperative cardiovascular events, but this is insufficient to recommend their routine use.

Continued administration mandates a greater degree of cardiovascular monitoring, particularly with regard to maintenance of intravascular volume. Vasoactive agents may be required to maintain an adequate arterial pressure.

Preoptimization. Measures to improve cardiac output and oxygen delivery have been shown to improve outcome in some high-risk patients with limited physiological reserve undergoing major surgery. These measures include monitored fluid therapy, vasoactive support, blood transfusion and ventilation, and are aimed at improving tissue oxygen delivery and hence oxygen delivery/consumption balance. The level of monitoring required, patient selection and the risk/benefit balance of increasing myocardial oxygen demand in the face of ischaemic heart disease versus improving cardiac output and hence oxygen delivery need to be considered on an individual basis.

This management strategy may be undertaken in a critical care area or in the anaesthetic room and requires close cooperation between relevant medical staff.

It is not known yet if combining preoptimization with preoperative therapy with agents such as beta-blockers is helpful. However, the two approaches are not necessarily mutually exclusive.

Premedication

Anxiety is a cause of sympathetic activation which may be detrimental in patients with cardiovascular disease. While not all patients require anxiolytic premedication, there should be a low threshold for use in this group of patients. A benzodiazepine such as temazepam is usually satisfactory. In patients with low or fixed cardiac output states, e.g. mitral or aortic stenosis, constrictive pericarditis or congestive cardiac failure, and other poor-risk patients, it is important to avoid hypotension or excessive sedation, respiratory depression and hypoxaemia which could result from premedication. It may therefore be preferable to omit sedative premedication.

The patient's usual cardiac medications and any additional therapy commenced preoperatively should be continued and included in the premedication.

High-risk patients benefit from oxygen therapy before transfer to the anaesthetic room.

Anaesthesia: general principles

- Anaesthesia should comprise a balanced technique aimed at maintaining cardiovascular stability. A variety of options may be suitable, including both general and regional anaesthetics or a combination.

- Tachycardia should be avoided and an adequate arterial pressure maintained (there should not be a sustained reduction in arterial pressure of more than 20% of the patient's normal pressure). Coronary perfusion and myocardial oxygen delivery are thus maintained without increasing myocardial work and oxygen requirements.

- For patients identified as high risk, consideration should be given to stress reduction. Measures to achieve this are dictated by patient and operative factors. These include:
  - Use of neuraxial blockade. This has been associated with reduced perioperative myocardial ischaemia and infarction. However, this must be balanced against the sympathetic block and associated hypotension. This may be pronounced, particularly with a high spinal block. Early judicious use of vasopressors coupled with maintenance of intravascular volume should limit this problem. However, neuraxial blockade, particularly spinal block, is relatively contraindicated where there is severely limited cardiovascular reserve and where maintenance of adequate arterial pressure is critical: for example, severe aortic stenosis (see below).
  - Perioperative beta blockade.
  - High-dose opioids, e.g. remifentanil.

- The level of intraoperative monitoring should be dictated by risk assessment. The following should be considered in addition to standard monitoring:
  - Five-lead ECG. The usual ECG configuration for anaesthetic monitoring is standard limb lead II. Whilst this is useful for differentiating arrhythmias, myocardial ischaemia occurs most commonly in the left ventricle and is detected more sensitively with a CM5 configuration (see Fig. 18.2).
  - Direct arterial pressure recording.
  - CVP monitoring with or without central venous oxygen saturations.
  - Oesophageal Doppler, providing a measurement of cardiac output and intravascular filling.
  - Pulmonary artery flotation catheter with continuous cardiac output and mixed venous oxygen saturation monitoring.
  - A variety of less-invasive cardiac output monitors are now available and may prove useful as intraoperative monitors in the future.

- Patients should be well oxygenated and normocapnic.

- Close attention to fluid balance is mandatory. This begins preoperatively when fluid depletion secondary to factors such as excessive fasting times and bowel preparation should be corrected. As far as possible, patients should be maintained normovolaemic. While intravascular volume depletion is known to compromise organ perfusion and oxygen delivery, there is increasing evidence that postoperative recovery is also compromised by excessive volume and sodium loading in the immediate perioperative period.

- Patients at high risk from cardiovascular disease do not tolerate anaemia. The optimal level of haemoglobin is the subject of much discussion but is probably around 10g dL^{-1} for this group.

- Patients should be actively warmed to avoid hypothermia, which activates the stress response, predisposes to arrhythmias and increases oxygen consumption postoperatively as a result of shivering.

- Effective perioperative analgesia is essential. Pain is a potent stimulator of the stress response and uncontrolled sympathetic activation increases myocardial work and oxygen demand, predisposing to myocardial ischaemia or infarction.

- Before embarking on anaesthesia and surgery, consideration needs to be given to the patient's management and destination postoperatively, e.g. would benefit be derived from a period of artificial ventilation or continued close monitoring in an intensive care area postoperatively?
- Good communication between all of the relevant carers, including cardiology, critical care and the surgical team is important.

Anaesthetic agents

Most intravenous induction agents are cardiovascular depressants causing both vasodilatation and myocardial depression. This is exaggerated in patients with low fixed cardiac output states and by concurrent hypovolaemia. Of the agents in regular use, etomidate is the least cardiac depressant. Care with dosing and rate of administration limits the hypotension caused by agents such as propofol or thiopental. Coinduction with more than one agent may be beneficial in reducing the dose requirements of each and limiting hypotension. Concurrent administration of midazolam and a short-acting opioid (alfentanil or fentanyl) is often used. The ultra-short-acting opioid remifentanil may be useful in these patients, in a low-dose infusion of $0.1–0.2\,\mu g\,kg^{-1}\,min^{-1}$. It limits the dose of induction agent required and blunts the cardiovascular response to laryngoscopy and tracheal intubation. However, used in high doses, it may induce respiratory muscle stiffness and make bag and mask ventilation difficult before the onset of neuromuscular blockade.

For patients naive to beta-blockers, esmolol (a short- acting i.v. beta-blocker) may be used to obtund the cardiovascular response to airway manoeuvres.

Of the neuromuscular blocking agents, rocuronium and vecuronium are the most cardiostable.

Brief periods of cardiac ischaemia provide protection against the damaging effects of subsequent more prolonged episodes: this is known as ischaemic preconditioning. Much is now known about the physiology of this in experimental situations, including the fact that volatile anaesthetic agents and opioids help to induce ischaemic preconditioning, while other agents, for example the sulphonylureas, inhibit it.

There is clinical evidence of its relevance, e.g. patients with preinfarct angina generally have a better prognosis than those who are asymptomatic, and this may be a result of preconditioning. The clinical application of these findings is as yet unknown, but may favour the use of volatile agents in this high-risk group.

Arrhythmias

Preoperative arrhythmias should be treated before surgery. The patient should be screened for predispos-

ing factors such as ischaemic or valvular heart disease and electrolyte and endocrine abnormalities. In atrial fibrillation, the ventricular rate should be controlled preoperatively if possible.

Antiarrhythmic therapy should continue throughout the perioperative period.

The indications for antiarrhythmic therapy and pacing are those which are applicable in the absence of surgery and anaesthesia.

Indications for preoperative temporary pacing include:

- bradyarrhythmia unresponsive to atropine if associated with syncope, hypotension or ventricular arrhythmias
- risk of asystole
- complete heart block
- second-degree heart block (Mobitz 2)
- first-degree heart block associated with bifascicular block
- sick sinus syndrome.

Intraoperative arrhythmias

Arrhythmias are common in the perioperative period and are often self-limiting and require no specific treatment. However, precipitants of these arrhythmias should be sought and corrected if possible as they are more likely to occur and cause cardiovascular compromise in patients with underlying heart disease.

Factors predisposing to intraoperative arrhythmias include:
Patient factors:

- hypoxaemia
- hypo- and hypercapnia
- acidosis
- hypo- and hyperthermia
- electrolyte abnormalities, particularly of potassium and magnesium
- hypovolaemia.

Autonomic effects:

- surgical stimulation and pain
- vagal stimulation, e.g. anal and cervical dilatation, traction on mesentery, traction on extraocular muscles
- laryngoscopy
- insertion of laparoscopy ports with peritoneal stretching.

Direct stimulation:

- CVP catheters and guide wires
- PA catheters.

Drugs:

- epinephrine
- local anaesthetic toxicity (bupivacaine)
- halothane.

Management

This depends on the nature of the arrhythmia, likely causes and the degree of haemodynamic compromise.

- The precipitant should be removed if possible. Reflex arrhythmias tend to occur more commonly during light anaesthesia and may often be prevented by deepening anaesthesia.
- Physiological abnormalities should be corrected, as specific antiarrhythmic therapy may be ineffective in the presence of uncorrected hypoxaemia, hypovolaemia and electrolyte abnormalities. Treatment of these should be concurrent with specific management of the arrhythmia.

Intraoperative bradyarrhythmias

Bradyarrhythmias may often be prevented and may be treated using intravenous anticholinergics, e.g. atropine or glycopyrrolate.

External pacing defibrillators are now widely available and can be used for temporary cardiac pacing for patients unresponsive to anticholinergics pending placement of a transvenous pacemaker.

Intraoperative tachyarrhythmias

These are either supraventricular or ventricular in origin. Generally, but not exclusively, supraventricular arrhythmias are narrow-complex in distinction to broad-complex ventricular arrhythmias.

Supraventricular tachycardia. If there is haemodynamic compromise, the treatment of choice is synchronized DC cardioversion (100 J, 200 J, 360 J, or biphasic equivalents), particularly as the patient is already anaesthetized. This applies to all supraventricular tachyarrhythmias.

If the patient is not severely compromised, management depends on the individual arrhythmia:

- Atrial fibrillation: this is the commonest supraventricular arrhythmia seen intraoperatively. Often a return to sinus rhythm cannot be achieved until the underlying precipitants are resolved. However, the ventricular rate should be controlled effectively using either digoxin or amiodarone. When surgery is complete, anticoagulation should

be considered to avoid the embolic complications of atrial fibrillation.
- Atrial flutter: this should be managed in the same way as for atrial fibrillation if it occurs intraoperatively.
- AV node/AV re-entry tachycardia and atrial tachycardia. Vagal manoeuvres, e.g. carotid sinus massage, may be tried and also intravenous adenosine. Adenosine transiently slows AV conduction and may convert SVT to sinus rhythm. Alternatively, it may aid diagnosis by revealing flutter or fibrillation waves. A rapid i.v. bolus of 6 mg is given, followed by 12 mg a maximum of three times at 2-min intervals. Adenosine is contraindicated in asthmatics, patients with second- and third-degree heart block, patients receiving carbamazepine or dipyridamole and patients with denervated hearts, e.g. following cardiac transplant. Care must be taken with its use if the patient has Wolff–Parkinson–White syndrome.

Verapamil, beta-blockers and amiodarone may control the ventricular rate. Intravenous verapamil should never be given to a beta-blocked patient.

Ventricular tachycardia. Synchronized DC cardioversion is the treatment of choice (100 J, 200 J, 360 J, or biphasic equivalents).

Lidocaine or amiodarone may be used if the arrhythmia is well tolerated.

Permanent pacemakers

Many patients with these devices have underlying heart disease which should be managed accordingly

Permanent pacemakers are placed in an increasing number of patients and are becoming increasingly complex. Pacemakers are classified by a series of 5 letters relating to the functions they possess (Table 23.3).

Specific issues in anaesthetic management

- Preoperative assessment: the indication for pacemaker insertion should be known, any evidence of malfunction sought and mode of action of the pacemaker noted. Routine investigations should include ECG, chest X-ray and electrolytes
- The pacemaker should be checked preoperatively if there is any doubt about its function
- Because of the complexity of programming available, it is no longer acceptable practice to use a magnet to return the pacemaker to a fixed rate mode. Magnets should not be used, as they have an unpredictable effect on programming

Table 23.3   Pacemaker classification

Letter position	Function	Chamber/function
1st	Chamber paced	Atrium/ventricle/both
2nd	Chamber sensed	Atrium/ventricle/both
3rd	Response to sensing	None/triggered/inhibited/both
4th	Programmable? Rate modulation?	Simple/multiple/communicating Yes/no
5th	Antitachyarrhythmia functions	None/pacing/shock/both

For example: a VVI pacemaker both paces and senses with a ventricular wire and is inhibited by a patient's own heart beat.

- Some pacemakers have a rate modulation facility. This implies that they can vary the rate of pacing with the patient's activity detected usually by muscle activity or respiratory activity so that heart rate may be increased with exercise. Ideally, rate modulation should be switched off before anaesthesia and surgery, as shivering and muscle fasciculation may be misinterpreted and lead to inappropriate increases in heart rate
- Central venous or pulmonary artery catheters may dislodge pacing leads, particularly if the pacemaker has only recently been inserted. Consideration should be given to use of the femoral vein for central venous access and to alternative monitors of cardiac output
- Alternative pacing should be available in the event of pacemaker failure; external pacing is a rapid and effective back-up
- Pacemakers should be routinely checked postoperatively either before discharge or via an early appointment at the pacemaker clinic

Electromagnetic interference may unpredictably reprogram the pacemaker or cause damage to it.

- Diathermy: bipolar diathermy should be used if possible. If unipolar diathermy is used, the diathermy and ground plate should be as far from the pacemaker as possible and the current pathway should be placed at right angles to the pacing wire(s)

- Lithotripsy: the lithotriptor should be at least 12 cm away from the pacemaker and rate modulation should be deactivated
- Peripheral nerve stimulators and transcutaneous electrical nerve stimulators (TENS) should be kept at least 12 cm from the pacemaker
- Defibrillator paddles should be 12 cm away from the pacemaker
- MRI is contraindicated

Implantable cardioverter defibrillators (ICDs)

Increasingly, these devices are used for the management of patients with recurrent life-threatening episodes of VF and VT. ICDs may also have a pacemaker function. As with permanent pacemakers, they may be subject to electromagnetic interference and the same precautions apply.

The antitachycardia and defibrillator actions should be switched off before surgery involving diathermy. Diathermy could be interpreted as VF and a shock delivered unnecessarily. An external defibrillator must be available and the patient should be in a high-dependency area postoperatively until the ICD is checked and reactivated.

VALVULAR HEART DISEASE

In both aortic and mitral stenosis there is a low fixed cardiac output which leaves no reserve to compensate for changes in heart rate or vascular resistance.

Regurgitant lesions are usually better tolerated.

As with ischaemic heart disease, specific intervention such as valve replacement or valvuloplasty is indicated before non-cardiac surgery only if the valvular lesion merits intervention anyway. Clearly, in an emergency situation, this is not an option.

General principles:

- The patient's functional reserve is a good indicator of the severity of a valve lesion
- All patients with valvular heart disease should receive appropriate antibiotic prophylaxis
- Patients with valvular heart disease may be receiving anticoagulants; perioperative heparinization is necessary in this group
- No specific anaesthetic technique is preferred for valvular heart disease. The aim is to maintain cardiovascular stability. In severe disease, this is often best achieved using a general anaesthetic technique with opioids and controlled ventilation
- Invasive monitoring is often required in these patients

Aortic stenosis

Isolated aortic stenosis is associated most commonly with calcification, often on a congenital bicuspid valve. In rheumatic heart disease, aortic stenosis occurs rarely in the absence of mitral disease and is combined usually with regurgitation. The diagnosis is suggested by the findings of an ejection systolic murmur, low pulse pressure, and clinical and ECG evidence of left ventricular hypertrophy. It is important to distinguish between aortic stenosis and the murmur of aortic sclerosis found in some elderly patients. Clinical signs provide a guide; a slow-rising, low-volume pulse with reduced pulse pressure, reduced intensity of the second heart sound and the presence of a click are suggestive of stenosis, as is evidence of left ventricular hypertrophy on ECG. However, echocardiography with Doppler flow monitoring is essential for confirmation. The heart size on chest X-ray is normal until late in the disease, while symptoms of angina, effort syncope and left ventricular failure indicate advanced disease.

Perioperative mortality is increased in patients with aortic stenosis.

Left ventricular systolic function is usually good but the hypertrophied ventricle is less compliant. Tachycardia and arrhythmias which compromise ventricular filling are poorly tolerated and should be avoided. Normally, 30% of ventricular filling results from atrial systole; therefore, maintenance of sinus rhythm is important. Tachycardia also reduces the duration of coronary perfusion, compromising blood supply to the hypertrophied ventricle, particularly if there is concomitant coronary artery disease. The resulting myocardial ischaemia causes further cardiovascular deterioration, which may be catastrophic. Excessive bradycardia also compromises cardiac output. Adequate venous return must be maintained to ensure ventricular filling and hypotension, which compromises coronary flow, must be avoided.

Mitral stenosis

This is usually a manifestation of rheumatic heart disease. Characteristic features include atrial fibrillation, arterial embolism, pulmonary oedema, pulmonary hypertension and right heart failure. Acute pulmonary oedema may follow the onset of atrial fibrillation.

Patients with mitral stenosis who present for surgery are frequently receiving digoxin, diuretics and anticoagulants. Preoperative control of atrial fibrillation, treatment of pulmonary oedema and management of anticoagulant therapy (see Ch. 22) are necessary. During anaesthesia, control of heart rate is important. Tachycardia reduces diastolic ventricular filling and thus cardiac output, while bradycardia also results in decreased cardiac output because stroke output is limited. As with aortic stenosis, drugs which produce vasodilatation may cause severe hypotension.

As a result of pre-existing pulmonary hypertension, patients are particularly vulnerable to hypoxaemia. Both hypoxaemia and acidosis are potent pulmonary vasoconstrictors and may produce acute right ventricular failure. Thus, opioid analgesics should be prescribed cautiously, and airway obstruction avoided.

Aortic regurgitation

Acute aortic regurgitation, e.g. resulting from infective endocarditis, causes rapid left ventricular failure and may require emergency valve replacement, even in the presence of unresolved infection.

Chronic aortic regurgitation is asymptomatic for many years. Left ventricular dilatation occurs, with eventual left ventricular failure.

Patients with mild or moderate aortic regurgitation without left ventricular failure or massive ventricular dilatation tolerate anaesthesia well. A slightly increased heart rate of approximately 100 beat min^{-1} is desirable because this reduces left ventricular dilatation. Bradycardia causes ventricular distension and should be avoided. Vasodilator therapy increases net forward flow by decreasing afterload and is useful in severe aortic regurgitation; isoflurane anaesthesia may be beneficial. Vasopressors should be avoided. Careful monitoring is required, and in severe cases a pulmonary artery catheter may be useful to aid management.

Mitral regurgitation

Acute mitral regurgitation commonly results from infective endocarditis, or myocardial infarction with papillary muscle dysfunction or ruptured chordae tendineae. Acute pulmonary oedema results, and urgent valve replacement is required. Left ventricular failure with ventricular dilatation may cause functional mitral regurgitation.

Chronic mitral regurgitation is commonly associated with mitral stenosis. In pure mitral regurgitation, left atrial dilatation occurs with a minimal increase in pressure. The degree of regurgitation may be limited by reducing the size of the left ventricle and the impedance to left ventricular ejection. Thus, inotropic agents and vasodilators may be useful, while vasopressors should be avoided. A slight increase in heart rate is desirable unless there is concomitant stenosis.

Infective endocarditis

This is caused predominantly by the viridans group of streptococci, occasionally by Gram-negative organisms or enterococci and also by staphylococci, especially after cardiac surgery or in intravenous drug abusers. *Coxiella burnetii* also accounts for some cases. Patients with rheumatic or congenital heart disease, including asymptomatic lesions, e.g. bicuspid aortic valve, are at risk. Infection is caused by transient bacteraemia, most frequently after dental extraction or genitourinary investigation or surgery.

Antibiotic cover should be given for all surgical procedures in at-risk patients (see *British National Formulary*). Flucloxacillin or an alternative antistaphylococcal agent should be included in regimens for cardiac surgery.

Hypertrophic cardiomyopathy

Hypertrophic cardiomyopathy (HOCM) is a genetic cardiac disorder affecting 1 in 500 adults. There is a variable degree of ventricular muscle hypertrophy affecting mainly the interventricular septum. Patients may remain asymptomatic, or they may suffer dyspnoea, angina and syncope as a result of muscle hypertrophy and subsequent left ventricular outflow obstruction. HOCM is also a cause of sudden cardiac death caused by arrhythmias.

Diagnosis is confirmed by echocardiography.
Anaesthetic issues include:

- Antibiotic cover is required as prophylaxis against endocarditis
- Acute changes in volume status cause severe haemodynamic consequences and hypovolaemia should be avoided
- Outflow obstruction is exacerbated by catecholamines so that inotropic agents should be avoided
- Patients are usually receiving a beta-blocker and these should be continued perioperatively
- Patients with previous malignant ventricular arrhythmias are likely to have an ICD in situ.

RESPIRATORY DISEASE

Successful anaesthetic management of the patient with respiratory disease is dependent on accurate assessment of the nature and extent of functional impairment and an appreciation of the effects of surgery and anaesthesia on pulmonary function.

ASSESSMENT

History

Of the six cardinal symptoms of respiratory disease (cough, sputum, haemoptysis, dyspnoea, wheeze and chest pain), dyspnoea provides the best indication of functional impairment. Specific questioning is required to elicit the extent to which activity is limited by dyspnoea. Dyspnoea at rest or on minor exertion clearly indicates severe disease. A cough productive of purulent sputum indicates active infection. Chronic copious sputum production may indicate bronchiectasis. A history of heavy smoking or occupational exposure to dust may suggest pulmonary pathology.

A detailed drug history is important. Long-term steroid therapy within 3 months of the date of surgery necessitates augmented cover for the perioperative period and may cause hypokalaemia and hyperglycaemia. Bronchodilators should be continued during the perioperative period. Patients with cor pulmonale may be receiving digoxin and diuretics.

Examination

A full physical examination is required, with emphasis on detecting signs of airway obstruction, increased work of breathing, active infection which may be treated preoperatively, and evidence of right heart failure. The presence of obesity, cyanosis or dyspnoea is noted. In addition, a simple forced expiratory manoeuvre may reveal prolonged expiration, and a simple test of exercise tolerance may be useful, e.g. a supervised walk up stairs.

Measurement of oxygen saturation provides a quick useful indication of oxygenation; an $S_pO_2 > 95\%$ on air excludes significant hypoxaemia and, by inference, hypercapnia.

Investigations

Chest X-ray

The preoperative chest X-ray is a poor indicator of functional impairment but may be indicated in certain situations:

- when history and/or examination suggest acute disease, e.g. infection, effusion, neoplasm
- in patients with chronic lung disease
- in patients from tuberculosis-endemic countries.

ECG

This may indicate right atrial enlargement or ventricular hypertrophy (P pulmonale in II; dominant R wave in III, V_{1-3}). Associated ischaemic heart disease is common, and ECG abnormalities may confirm this.

Haematology

Polycythaemia occurs secondary to chronic hypoxaemia, while anaemia aggravates tissue hypoxia. Leucocytosis may indicate active infection.

Sputum culture

Sputum culture is essential in patients with chronic lung disease or suspected acute infection.

Pulmonary function tests

Peak expiratory flow rate, forced expiratory volume in 1 s (FEV_1) and forced vital capacity (FVC) may be measured easily at the bedside. The FEV_1:FVC ratio is decreased in obstructive lung disease and normal in restrictive disease. In the presence of obstructive disease the test should be repeated 5–10 min after administration of a bronchodilator aerosol to provide an indication of reversibility. An FVC < 1–1.5 L is indicative of limited ability to take large sigh breaths, expand lung bases and clear secretions by coughing.

Fuller investigation involves measurement of functional residual capacity (FRC), residual volume and total lung capacity, but these are rarely of value in determining clinical management.

Blood gas measurement

Arterial blood gas measurement is indicated in patients with chronic respiratory disease undergoing significant surgery and also if there is suspected acute hypoxaemia. It is also advisable when pulmonary function tests are markedly abnormal, e.g. in obstructive disease where the FEV_1 is less than 1.5 L. A raised P_aCO_2 with normal pH indicates chronic hypercapnia with renal compensation; a combined raised P_aCO_2 and acidosis indicates an acute event. Hypercapnia, particularly if acute, associated with acidosis, is likely to be associated with postoperative pulmonary complications. With a P_aCO_2 of 6.7 kPa (50 mmHg) or greater, elective controlled ventilation may be required after major surgery. The combination of a low preoperative arterial oxygen tension (P_aO_2) and dyspnoea at rest is also associated with a high likelihood of the need for planned ventilation after abdominal surgery.

Effects of anaesthesia and surgery

The effects of anaesthesia alone on respiratory function are generally minor and short-lived, but may tip the balance towards respiratory failure in patients with severe disease. These effects include:

- mucosal irritation by anaesthetic agents
- ciliary paralysis
- introduction of infection by aspiration or tracheal intubation
- respiratory depression by relaxants, opioid analgesics or volatile anaesthetic agents.

In addition, anaesthesia is associated with a decrease in FRC, especially in the elderly and in obese patients, which leads to basal airways closure and shunting of blood through underventilated areas of lung, an effect which is magnified by inhibition of the hypoxic pulmonary vasoconstrictor reflex. Following recovery from anaesthesia, residual concentrations of anaesthetic agents inhibit the hyperventilatory responses to both hypercapnia and hypoxaemia, so that without close monitoring, e.g. with pulse oximetry, serious hypoxaemia and hypercapnia may occur. Following thoracic and upper abdominal surgery, the decrease in FRC is more profound and persists for 5–10 days after surgery, with a parallel increase in alveolar–arterial oxygen tension difference ($P_{A-a}O_2$). Complications including atelectasis and pneumonia occur in approximately 20% of these patients.

Regional anaesthesia

The use of appropriate regional anaesthetic techniques, where possible, confers several advantages in patients with respiratory disease both intra- and postoperatively, including:

- possible avoidance of tracheal intubation and controlled ventilation
- reduced or absent requirement for respiratory depressant agents such as volatile agents and opioids
- epidural analgesia may reduce postoperative hypoxaemia by diminishing the decrease in FRC associated with anaesthesia and abdominal surgery
- effective analgesia, allowing the patient to undergo chest physiotherapy, early mobilization and avoid prolonged bedrest.

The effects of surgery are dependent on its type and magnitude. Clearly, patients with pre-existing respiratory disease are at much greater risk following upper abdominal and thoracic surgery than after limb, head and neck or lower abdominal surgery.

Laparoscopic surgery

The use of laparoscopic techniques for cholecystectomy, fundoplication and other abdominal procedures has markedly reduced postoperative pulmonary morbidity, with the result that patients with severe pulmonary disease can usually undergo these procedures without the need for postoperative ventilatory support. The reasons for reduced morbidity include the relative lack of postoperative pain and the preservation of lung volumes postoperatively. These techniques should be encouraged in patients with chronic pulmonary disease. Nevertheless, cardiopulmonary function may be considerably compromised intraoperatively by raised intra-abdominal pressure, and judicious use of invasive haemodynamic monitoring has been recommended in patients with severe cardiorespiratory disease.

OBSTRUCTIVE PULMONARY DISEASE

This includes both chronic obstructive pulmonary disease and bronchial asthma. Patients with bronchiectasis and cystic fibrosis may also demonstrate marked airways obstruction, and justify a similar approach to management.

CHRONIC OBSTRUCTIVE PULMONARY DISEASE

Chronic obstructive pulmonary disease (COPD) is characterized by the presence of productive cough for at least 3 months in two successive years. Airways obstruction is caused by bronchoconstriction, bronchial oedema and hypersecretion of mucus. In the postoperative period, pulmonary atelectasis and pneumonia result if sputum is not cleared. COPD may be classified into two groups – the bronchitis group (blue bloaters) and the emphysematous group (pink puffers) – although in practice most patients have mixed pathologies. The former group is characterized by hypoxaemia, hypercapnia and right ventricular failure, while patients in the latter group are usually markedly dyspnoeic.

ASTHMA

Asthma may affect all age groups; it is characterized by recurrent generalized reversible airways obstruction, caused by bronchial smooth-muscle spasm, mucus plugs and bronchial oedema. Asthma may be classified into two types: *extrinsic*, where an external allergen is demonstrable, and *intrinsic*. Intrinsic asthma tends to occur in adults, is more chronic and continuous and often requires long-term steroid therapy. There is an overlap between intrinsic asthma and COPD.

Preoperative management

The current state of the patient's disease is assessed by:

- History – frequency and severity of attacks, factors provoking attacks, recent episodes of infection, drug history.
- Examination – presence or absence of wheeze, prolonged expiratory phase, overdistension, evidence of infection (temperature, WBC, cough, sputum).
- Pulmonary function tests – peak expiratory flow rate or FEV_1/FVC before and after inhalation of bronchodilator.
- Blood gas analysis.
- The patient's ventilatory response to carbon dioxide by serial blood gas measurements with different concentrations of inspired oxygen.

Treatment of airways obstruction

Elective surgery should not be undertaken unless or until airways obstruction is well controlled. Existing bronchodilator therapy should be continued perioperatively. Asthmatic patients are more likely to respond to inhaled β_2-adrenoceptor agonists, e.g. salbutamol, either by metered dose inhaler or nebulizer. Chronic asthmatics and patients with COPD may benefit from an inhaled anticholinergic agent (ipratropium bromide). The role of the phosphodiesterase inhibitor aminophylline is still controversial; it remains useful in the treatment of acute bronchospasm. If patients are receiving long-term theophyllines, the plasma concentration should be checked. Magnesium i.v. may be beneficial in acute asthma.

Corticosteroids are also important in the prevention and treatment of bronchospasm in asthmatics. Patients prescribed long-term inhaled or systemic steroid therapy who are suboptimally controlled may require a course of augmented steroid therapy, e.g. prednisolone 40–60 mg daily or hydrocortisone 100 mg four times daily, to cover the anaesthetic and postoperative periods. Equivalent doses of steroid preparations are shown in Table 23.4. The steroid dose should be gradually reduced postoperatively, titrated against the severity of the asthma.

Treatment of active infection

Amoxicillin, co-amoxiclav or ceftriaxone are appropriate, the common infecting organisms being *Streptococcus pneumoniae* and *Haemophilus influenzae*. Sputum for culture and sensitivities should be obtained to allow an

Table 23.4 Equivalent doses of glucocorticoids

Glucocorticoid	Dose (mg)
Betamethasone	3
Cortisone acetate	100
Dexamethasone	3
Hydrocortisone	80
Methylprednisolone	16
Prednisolone	20
Triamcinolone	16

appropriate choice of antibiotic. Chest physiotherapy and humidification of inspired gases aid expectoration.

Treatment of cardiac failure

Biventricular failure resulting from concurrent ischaemic heart disease and cor pulmonale frequently complicates COPD. Diuretics are indicated, while nitrates or digoxin may have a role.

Weight reduction

This should be encouraged before elective surgery in obese patients with respiratory disease.

Smoking

Ideally, smoking should be stopped for at least 6 weeks before elective surgery.

Premedication

A benzodiazepine to allay anxiety is appropriate for asthmatic patients, plus a dose of bronchodilator 30 min before induction of anaesthesia.

Anaesthesia

The anaesthetic technique in obstructive airways disease should be guided by the nature of the surgery, and also the severity of the disease.

A minimal intervention approach

Spontaneous ventilation with the option of local or regional anaesthesia is indicated for minor body sur-

face operations. The use of a laryngeal mask airway (LMA) avoids tracheal intubation with its attendant risk of provoking bronchoconstriction, and if undue respiratory depression occurs, manifested by an increased P_aCO_2, ventilation may be easily assisted via the LMA. Volatile anaesthetic agents, being bronchodilators, are well tolerated in asthmatics. Plexus blocks and low subarachnoid or epidural anaesthesia enable limb, lower abdominal or pelvic surgery in patients with severe respiratory impairment. Sedation should be administered carefully.

Elective mechanical ventilation

A decision may be made to undertake intermittent positive-pressure ventilation (IPPV) during anaesthesia and for a variable period after operation, at least until elimination of muscle relaxants and anaesthetic agents has occurred. This also permits optimal provision of analgesia without fear of opioid-induced depression of ventilation. This technique is usually preferred if the preoperative P_aCO_2 is greater than 6.7 kPa (50 mmHg) or if major thoracic or abdominal surgery is planned. Care should be taken with ventilatory settings. A sufficiently long expiratory phase should be allowed to enable lung deflation, while the inspiratory time should be adequate to avoid unduly high inflation pressures, with the attendant risk of pneumothorax.

Regional anaesthesia

A combined general/epidural anaesthetic technique is often useful for major abdominal or thoracic surgery, as there is good evidence of a reduction in postoperative pulmonary complications with effective epidural analgesia. This approach may avoid a need for postoperative IPPV in some patients.

Anaesthetic agents

Drugs which are associated with histamine release, e.g. atracurium, and morphine are best avoided, whilst vecuronium and fentanyl are preferred. Beta-blocking drugs should also be avoided. If bronchospasm occurs during anaesthesia, it may result from easily remedied causes such as light anaesthesia or tracheal tube irritation and these should be corrected. If bronchospasm persists, nebulized salbutamol 2.5–5 mg should be administered into the anaesthetic breathing system and if this is not immediately beneficial, salbutamol 125–250 μg or aminophylline 250 mg should be administered by slow i.v. injection under ECG monitoring. The aminophylline dose should be modified if the patient is receiving oral theophylline. Thereafter, an infusion of aminophylline, up to 0.5–0.8 mg kg^{-1} h^{-1}, or salbutamol, possibly in combination with nebulized salbutamol by positive-pressure ventilation (solution of 50–100 μg mL^{-1} of water), should be maintained until improvement occurs. Hydrocortisone 200 mg i.v. should be given simultaneously, although it has no immediate effect. Inhaled volatile anaesthetic agents, e.g. sevoflurane, and intravenous ketamine have also been used with success when other agents have failed to relieve acute bronchospasm.

Postoperative care

Postoperative care of the patient with severe COPD or asthma should be conducted in an HDU or an ICU, to allow close respiratory monitoring and ventilatory support if required.

Elective postoperative controlled ventilation allows adequate oxygenation, analgesia without respiratory depression, clearance of secretions by physiotherapy, tracheal suction and, if necessary, fibreoptic bronchoscopy. Cardiac output and peripheral perfusion should be optimized before restoration of spontaneous ventilation. Unless there is pre-existing pulmonary infection, a period of 24 h of elective controlled ventilation is usually adequate and many patients may be weaned to spontaneous breathing much sooner. Analgesia produced by regional, e.g. epidural, blockade often allows earlier return to spontaneous ventilation, and permits pain-free coughing and clearing of secretions.

Oxygen and respiratory care

Asthmatic patients rarely lose carbon dioxide responsiveness, and therefore high inspired oxygen concentrations are tolerated well. In COPD patients with spontaneous ventilation, controlled oxygen is generally required using a 24% or 28% Ventimask with frequent checks on arterial blood gas tensions to ensure an adequate P_aO_2 (> 8 kPa) without excessive carbon dioxide retention (P_aCO_2 < 7.5–8 kPa). Using a pulse oximeter, the F_IO_2 may be titrated to achieve an S_pO_2 of around 90%. Hypoxaemia may seriously aggravate existing pulmonary hypertension and precipitate right ventricular failure.

Percutaneous cricothyroid puncture and insertion of a small-diameter tube into the trachea (minitracheotomy) permits aspiration of secretions while preserving the ability of the patient to cough and speak. This may be indicated postoperatively if sputum retention is a major problem.

The use of non-invasive respiratory support via a face-mask may be beneficial in the postoperative period. Non-invasive ventilation with a bilevel ventilator may aid carbon dioxide clearance and avoid postoperative invasive ventilation, or bridge the gap from invasive ventilation to spontaneous breathing. Face mask CPAP increases lung volumes and may prevent or treat lung atelectasis, with consequent improvement in oxygenation, but without any significant effect on CO_2 clearance.

Intermittent positive-pressure breathing (IPPB), generally supervised by a physiotherapist, also expands the lungs and aids clearance of secretions.

Analgesia

Simple, non-opioid analgesics and/or local and regional techniques should be used if possible. Non-steroidal anti-inflammatory drugs (NSAIDs) such as diclofenac or ibuprofen are useful in reducing the opioid requirements following major surgery and may be adequate on their own after minor surgery. However, NSAIDs may aggravate bronchospasm in some asthmatics as a result of increased leukotriene production. These agents should not be given to patients with a history of aspirin hypersensitivity or to asthmatics who have never taken NSAIDs previously. Opioid analgesics are best administered, where necessary, in small i.v. doses, e.g. morphine 2 mg, under direct supervision, or using patient-controlled analgesia. Physiotherapy, bronchodilators and antibiotics should be continued postoperatively.

BRONCHIECTASIS

The patient should receive intensive physiotherapy with postural drainage for several days before surgery. Appropriate antibiotics, based on sputum culture, should be prescribed. Severe disease localized in one lung should be isolated using a double-lumen tube.

RESTRICTIVE LUNG DISEASE

This category includes a wide range of conditions which affect the lung and chest wall. Lung diseases include sarcoidosis and fibrosing alveolitis, while lesions of chest wall include kyphoscoliosis and ankylosing spondylitis. Pulmonary function tests reveal a decrease in both FEV_1 and FVC, with a normal FEV_1/FVC ratio and decreased FRC and total lung capacity (TLC). Small airways closure occurs during tidal ventilation, with resultant shunting and hypoxaemia. Lung or chest wall compliance is decreased; thus, the work of breathing is increased and the ability to cough and clear secretions is impaired. There is an increased risk of postoperative pulmonary infection.

Anaesthesia causes little additional decrease in lung volumes and is tolerated well, provided that hypoxaemia is avoided. Postoperatively, however, inadequate basal ventilation and retention of secretions may occur, partly as a result of pain, opioid analgesics and the residual effects of anaesthetic agents. High concentrations of oxygen may be used without risk of respiratory depression. A short period of mechanical ventilation may be necessary in patients with severe disease to allow adequate analgesia and clearing of secretions. Minitracheostomy may aid sputum clearance in the postoperative period, while non-invasive ventilation may avert the need for prolonged intubation and IPPV. Effective epidural analgesia helps to reduce postoperative respiratory complications.

BRONCHIAL CARCINOMA

Patients with bronchial carcinoma frequently suffer from coexisting COPD. In addition, there may be infection and collapse of the lung distal to the tumour. Patients with bronchial carcinoma may have myasthenic syndrome (see p. 475), while oat-cell tumours may secrete a variety of hormones, among the commonest being adrenocorticotrophic hormone (ACTH), producing Cushing's syndrome, and antidiuretic hormone (ADH), producing dilutional hyponatraemia (syndrome of inappropriate ADH secretion).

TUBERCULOSIS

Tuberculosis should be considered in patients with persistent pulmonary infection, especially if associated with haemoptysis or weight loss. If active disease is present, all anaesthetic equipment should be changed after use to avoid cross-infection.

GASTROINTESTINAL DISEASE

Gastrointestinal disease presents several problems for the anaesthetist:

- malnutrition
- anaemia
- fluid and electrolyte depletion
- gastro-oesophageal reflux.

Malnutrition cannot usually be corrected fully before surgery, but fluid and electrolyte depletion may be remedied, and appropriate measures may be taken to minimize the risk of regurgitation and aspiration.

MALNUTRITION

This may be caused by decreased nutritional intake, malabsorption or gut losses. Patients are at increased risk of perioperative morbidity and mortality, with infections, poor wound healing and thromboembolic complications being prominent. If patients are undergoing major surgery, consideration should be given to commencing preoperative nutritional support with enteral or total parenteral nutrition (TPN) before surgery. Vitamin supplementation is essential. Anaemia should be corrected.

FLUID AND ELECTROLYTE DEPLETION

This may result from decreased fluid intake caused by dysphagia or vomiting, or diarrhoea, for example. Significant fluid depletion may be caused by preoperative bowel preparation with hypertonic solutions and fluid may be given i.v. preoperatively to maintain hydration before surgery.

Clinical assessment of volume depletion (poor perfusion, decreased tissue turgor, postural hypotension) should be supplemented by serum urea and electrolyte measurement, and fluid and electrolyte deficits replaced. Patients with intestinal obstruction may have extreme fluid and electrolyte depletion with consequent risk of cardiovascular collapse, if vigorous fluid resuscitation is not provided before induction of anaesthesia. These patients require invasive cardiovascular monitoring throughout the perioperative period.

GASTROINTESTINAL REFLUX

Patients at risk include those with symptoms such as heartburn and regurgitation, and those with proven hiatus hernia. Patients with intestinal obstruction, ileus secondary to peritonitis from any cause, and those presenting with vomiting may have a full stomach and be prone to regurgitation.

Other factors associated with reflux include raised intra-abdominal pressure, with obesity, pregnancy and the lithotomy position being particular risk factors.

The risk of aspiration of gastric acid and subsequent pneumonitis is reduced by administration of a histamine H_2-receptor antagonist, e.g. ranitidine, on the night before and morning of surgery, or a proton pump inhibitor, e.g. omeprazole. Sodium citrate 30 mL 5 min before induction neutralizes residual gastric acid. Metoclopramide is sometimes given to promote gastric emptying.

In patients with intestinal obstruction, emptying the stomach before induction of anaesthesia, using a large nasogastric tube, may be attempted. However, this may precipitate vomiting and, even if apparently effective, an empty stomach cannot be assumed.

Prevention of regurgitation and aspiration of gastric contents is based on early securing of the airway; preoxygenation, followed by rapid-sequence induction of anaesthesia with cricoid pressure to prevent regurgitation, is mandatory.

LIVER DISEASE

By far the commonest cause of liver disease in patients presenting for anaesthesia and surgery is alcoholic cirrhosis. This ranges in severity from asymptomatic to hepatic failure. Anaesthesia and surgery may affect liver function adversely, e.g. by decreasing liver blood flow, while pre-existing liver dysfunction may affect the conduct of anaesthesia because of impaired drug metabolism.

PREOPERATIVE ASSESSMENT

Preoperative assessment should be directed both to the degree of liver dysfunction and to the complications of liver disease.

Clinical features of liver disease include jaundice, ascites, oedema and impaired conscious level (encephalopathy).

Preoperative investigations should include full blood count, a coagulation screen, serum urea and electrolytes, bilirubin, alkaline phosphatase and transaminases, protein, albumin and blood sugar concentrations. The patient should also be screened for viral hepatitis. Universal precautions should be taken to protect staff and patients from transmission of viral hepatitis.

As far back as 1963, Child identified an increased mortality in patients with liver disease and classified surgical risk in patients with liver disease on the basis of:

- bilirubin and albumin concentrations
- nutritional state
- presence of ascites
- neurological disturbance
- surgical risk.

Particular problems relevant to the anaesthetist include the following:

Cardiovascular function. Patients with liver disease tend to be vasodilated and hypotensive. This may be aggravated by loss of fluid from the circulation as a result of hypoalbuminaemia and hence low oncotic pressure. Hypotension may also be aggravated by alcoholic cardiomyopathy.

Respiratory function. There may be respiratory compromise caused by diaphragmatic splinting by ascites, and by pleural effusions. In severe disease, intrapulmonary shunting may cause disproportionate hypoxaemia.

Acid–base and fluid balance. Many patients are overloaded with salt and water. Hypoalbuminaemia results in oedema and ascites and predisposes to pulmonary oedema. Secondary hyperaldosteronism produces sodium retention (even though plasma sodium concentration may be low) and also hypokalaemia. Diuretic therapy, often including spironolactone, may also affect serum potassium concentration. In hepatic failure, a combined respiratory and metabolic alkalosis may occur, which shifts the oxygen dissociation curve to the left, potentially impairing tissue oxygenation.

Hepatorenal syndrome. This is defined as acute renal failure developing in patients with pre-existing chronic liver failure. Jaundiced patients are at risk of developing postoperative renal failure. This may be precipitated by hypovolaemia. Prevention involves adequate preoperative hydration, with i.v. fluids for at least 12 h before surgery and close monitoring of urine output, intra- and postoperatively. Intravenous 20% mannitol 100 mL is recommended immediately preoperatively and is indicated postoperatively if the hourly urine output decreases below 50 mL. Close cardiovascular monitoring is essential and may include measurement of cardiac output.

Bleeding problems. Production of clotting factors II, VII, IX and X is reduced as a result of decreased vitamin K absorption. Production of factor V and fibrinogen is also reduced. Thrombocytopenia occurs if portal hypertension is present. Gastrointestinal haemorrhage from gastro-oesophageal varices may cause major management problems. Vitamin K should be administered preoperatively and fresh frozen plasma given to provide clotting factors during surgery, with regular checks made on coagulation. Infusion of platelet concentrate is indicated to cover surgery in cases of severe thrombocytopenia (platelet count $< 50 \times 10^9$ L^{-1}) or if there is overt bleeding in a thrombocytopenic patient. Close liaison with the haematology service is essential and local protocols should be in place for the management of major haemorrhage.

Infection. Impairment of the filtering function of the liver's Kupffer cells leads to a higher incidence of endotoxaemia and infection. Bacterial peritonitis is a potential problem in ascitic patients.

Drug metabolism. Impairment of liver function slows elimination of drugs, including anaesthetic induction agents, opioid analgesics, benzodiazepines, succinylcholine, local anaesthetic agents and many others. Because the duration of action of many of these drugs is determined initially by redistribution, prolongation of action may not become apparent until a subsequent dose has been given.

In addition, many drugs have toxic effects on the liver. Halothane was previously well recognized as a cause of postoperative hepatitis, or even fulminant hepatic failure. Modern volatile anaesthetic agents, e.g. isoflurane, sevoflurane, are minimally metabolized and this complication is now rare.

Hepatic failure. The management of hepatic failure is beyond the scope of this chapter. The main issues are recognition, assessment and initial resuscitation and transfer to a specialist centre.

INITIAL MANAGEMENT ISSUES

- The airway and breathing may be compromised by impaired conscious level, diaphragmatic splinting by ascites or both. Intubation of the trachea and IPPV may be required, especially for transport.
- direct monitoring of arterial and central venous pressures is required. Hypotension requires correction, generally with a vasopressor, e.g. noradrenaline (norepinephrine). Intravascular hypovolaemia and poor cardiac output need to be considered as possible additional factors.
- conscious level: airway protection and IPPV may be required. Blood glucose concentration must be checked, and hypoglycaemia corrected with intravenous glucose infusion. The presence of blood in the gastrointestinal tract following variceal or other haemorrhage is commonly a precipitating factor for encephalopathy; it is treated with lactulose by nasogastric tube.
- electrolyte problems such as hypokalaemia should be corrected.
- active bleeding should, if possible, be controlled before transfer to a specialist centre, e.g. by banding of oesophageal varices, or insertion of a Sengstaken-Blakemore tube.

CONDUCT OF ANAESTHESIA

Anaesthesia with tracheal intubation and IPPV is commonly required to enable procedures to control gastrointestinal bleeding, e.g. upper GI endoscopy with injection or banding of oesophageal varices, to be undertaken safely.

The liver is particularly vulnerable to hypoxia, hypovolaemia and hypotension. During anaesthesia, cardiovascular stability should be maintained as far as possible. Blood loss should be replaced promptly, and overall fluid balance maintained. Close arterial and central venous pressure monitoring is required. Drugs which depress cardiac output or arterial pressure,

including volatile anaesthetic agents and beta-blockers, should be used with caution to avoid reduction in hepatic blood flow.

The muscle relaxants of choice are those with cardiovascular stability and a short duration of action; atracurium may be preferable because its elimination is independent of liver and renal function. Opioid analgesic drugs should be administered with caution unless ventilatory support is planned postoperatively. Short-acting agents such as remifentanil should be infused intraoperatively and fentanyl PCA may be suitable for postoperative analgesia. NSAIDs should be avoided.

Controlled ventilation to a normal $P_a\text{CO}_2$ is important, as hypocapnia is associated with decreased hepatic blood flow. Hypoxaemia should be avoided throughout the perioperative period. In the adequately volume-expanded patient, hypotension may be reversed by infusion of noradrenaline (norepinephrine). However, in the unstable patient, expert help should be sought and monitoring should include measurement of cardiac output and pulmonary artery occlusion pressure (PAOP) with a pulmonary artery catheter.

RENAL DISEASE

Renal dysfunction has several important implications for anaesthesia, and therefore full assessment is required before even minor surgical procedures are contemplated.

Measurement of blood urea and electrolyte concentrations should be undertaken before all major surgery and in all elderly or potentially unhealthy patients; a raised blood urea concentration demonstrated preoperatively may be the first indication of renal disease. Severity of renal dysfunction may be assessed further by measurement of serum creatinine concentration and creatinine clearance, urinary:plasma osmolality ratio and urinary urea and electrolyte excretion (Table 23.5).

PREANAESTHETIC ASSESSMENT

Preanaesthetic assessment of the patient should be directed to several specific problems which require correction before embarking on anaesthesia.

Fluid balance

In acute renal failure, fluid overload may develop suddenly and is uncompensated. In chronic renal failure, overload may be controlled with diuretic therapy or dialysis. Pulmonary oedema and hypertension may result from fluid overload and must be treated before induction of anaesthesia. This may require fluid removal using dialysis or haemofiltration.

In patients with nephrotic syndrome, hypoalbuminaemia results in oedema and ascites. Circulating blood volume in these patients is often decreased, and care should be taken at induction of anaesthesia to avoid hypotension.

Electrolyte disturbances

Sodium

Sodium retention occurs in renal failure, and through increased secretion of ADH is associated with water retention, oedema and hypertension.

Hyponatraemia is also common in renal disease. It is the result either of sodium losses through the kidney or gastrointestinal tract, or of water overload causing dilutional hyponatraemia. The renal tubules may have a reduced ability to conserve sodium, e.g. in pyelonephritis, analgesic nephropathy or recovering acute renal failure, or sodium may be lost through diuretic therapy, vomiting or diarrhoea. Dilutional hyponatraemia is caused by either inappropriate fluid administration (glucose 5%), inappropriate ADH secretion, or both. Following transurethral prostatectomy, hyponatraemia may result from absorption of glycine irrigation fluid. Diagnosis of the cause of hyponatraemia involves measurement of urinary and plasma osmolality and urinary sodium concentration.

Potassium

Hyperkalaemia occurs typically in renal failure, frequently in association with metabolic acidosis. It causes delayed myocardial conduction and, if untreated, leads to cardiac arrest in asystole or ventricular fibrillation.

Hyperkalaemia should be treated promptly when the serum potassium concentration exceeds 6 mmol L^{-1} or when ECG changes are evident:

- calcium chloride 10% titrated up to 20 mL i.v. to antagonize the cardiac effects of hyperkalaemia, under ECG guidance
- glucose 50%, 50 mL with 5 units of soluble insulin followed by an infusion of 20% glucose with insulin as required, depending on BM-test blood sugar estimation
- nebulized salbutamol 5 mg and repeated regularly
- sodium bicarbonate 1.26% to improve the metabolic acidosis
- an ion exchange resin, e.g. calcium polystyrene sulphonate, orally provides longer-term control in chronic renal failure
- haemodialysis or haemofiltration. The former is more effective in lowering serum potassium concentration rapidly, but haemofiltration may be more easily set up as an emergency in a general ICU.

Hypokalaemia occurs commonly in patients receiving diuretic therapy. These patients require preoperative measurement of serum potassium concentration and replacement if necessary. Hypokalaemia is associated with ventricular irritability, notably in patients taking digoxin.

Calcium

Retention of phosphate and vitamin D depletion (1,25-dihydroxycholecalciferol) in chronic renal failure lead to hyperparathyroidism. The development of a parathyroid adenoma leads to hypercalcaemia (tertiary hyperparathyroidism).

Cardiovascular effects

Hypertension may occur for several reasons:

- a raised plasma renin concentration secondary to decreased perfusion of the juxtaglomerular apparatus results in hypertension through increased secretion of angiotensin and aldosterone.
- fluid retention also causes hypertension by increasing the circulating blood volume.

Conversely, hypertension from other causes results in renal impairment. The precise cause of hypertension in these patients should be sought and the hypertension treated. Management of hypertensive patients is discussed on page 447.

Table 23.5 Urinary measurements in prerenal and renal failure

Variable	Prerenal	Renal
Specific gravity	High > 1.020	1.010–1.012
Sodium (mmol L^{-1})	Low < 20	High > 40
U:P urea ratio	High > 20	Low < 10
U:P creatinine ratio	High > 40	Low < 10
U:P osmolality ratio	High > 2.1	Low < 1.2
U, urine; P, plasma.		

Both pulmonary and peripheral oedema may occur from a combination of fluid overload, hypertensive cardiac disease and hypoproteinaemia. Cardiac failure should be treated preoperatively. Uraemia may cause pericarditis and a haemorrhagic pericardial effusion, which may embarrass cardiac output and require aspiration. Good control of blood urea with haemodialysis or haemofiltration usually prevents this complication and is essential for its resolution.

Neurological effects

Uraemia causes drowsiness and eventually coma. Electrolyte disturbances and rapid fluid shifts, e.g. during dialysis, may also affect conscious level by causing cerebral oedema. Sedative drugs, including morphine, should be used with care in these patients, as renally excreted metabolites, in particular morphine-6-glucuronide, accumulate. In addition, a combined motor and sensory peripheral neuropathy may occur in uraemic patients.

Haematology

Patients with chronic renal failure suffer from normochromic anaemia, which results from marrow depression, partly as a result of erythropoietin deficiency. They also have an increased incidence of gastrointestinal bleeding, and so iron deficiency may also be present. These patients are usually well compensated, with an increased cardiac output, so that excessive preoperative blood transfusion should be avoided. Increasingly, such patients are treated with long-term erythropoietin. There is often a bleeding tendency, in part caused by platelet dysfunction. Platelet count and coagulation should be checked. Platelet dysfunction may be improved with cryoprecipitate.

Other factors

Patients with chronic renal failure are frequently undernourished. They tend to be vulnerable to infection. Patients who have received a renal transplant and are immunosuppressed are particularly vulnerable to opportunistic pathogens, e.g. *Pneumocystis carinii*.

Drug treatment

This is important for several reasons:

- patients are frequently receiving concurrent medication for attendant problems, e.g. antihypertensive therapy

- many drugs are excreted renally; dosages require modification, and plasma concentrations may require monitoring, e.g. aminoglycosides, digoxin
- some drugs have active metabolites which are excreted renally, e.g. morphine, midazolam. Dosage requires careful titration, or use of alternative agents should be considered, e.g. fentanyl, oxycodone
- some drugs adversely affect renal function, even in normal dosage. NSAIDs, and the newer specific cyclo-oxygenase 2 inhibitors, inhibit vasodilator prostaglandin production in the kidney and thus reduce glomerular blood flow and sodium excretion. This may be critical in septic or shocked patients, or those undergoing surgery associated with major blood loss. Their use should be avoided in such high-risk patients.

ACE inhibitors dilate the postglomerular arterioles in the kidney and thus reduce glomerular filtration pressure. They may therefore precipitate renal failure in hypotensive patients. Patients receiving these agents should be monitored carefully and fluid should be replaced adequately to avoid hypotension. It may be prudent to omit the immediate preanaesthetic dose in the high-risk patient. ACE inhibitors may also cause hyperkalaemia, particularly in patients with renal dysfunction.

ANAESTHESIA

Minor procedures, e.g. to establish vascular access for dialysis, are carried out most satisfactorily under regional anaesthesia: brachial plexus block for upper limb and combined femoral and sciatic block for lower limb.

Patients who suffer from acute renal failure, and those receiving long-term dialysis for chronic renal failure, may require dialysis before surgery to correct fluid overload, acid–base disturbances and hyperkalaemia. Ideally, there should be some delay before surgery to allow correction of anticoagulation.

The i.v. cannula for induction and fluid infusion should be sited in the contralateral limb from the arteriovenous shunt or fistula in patients undergoing dialysis and care should be taken to protect the fistula during the operation. Careful monitoring of arterial pressure and ECG is required and CVP measurement may be indicated in patients who are clinically fluid overloaded. Intravenous fluid administration should be cautious and in some instances titrated against CVP measurements. Excessive sodium administration and potassium-containing solutions should be avoided in renal failure. If the patient is anaemic preoperatively, intraoperative blood loss should be replaced promptly.

Succinylcholine should be avoided in hyperkalaemic patients in view of its effect of releasing potassium from muscle cells. An increase of up to 0.6 mmol L^{-1} may be expected in normal dosage.

Drugs excreted primarily via the kidneys should be used with caution in renal failure. In anaesthetic practice, the principal drugs involved are the muscle relaxants. Atracurium, elimination of which is independent of kidney and liver function, and which has minimal cardiovascular effects, is the relaxant of choice. All other relaxants depend to some extent on renal elimination and should be avoided, particularly in repeated doses. In addition, many drugs, including morphine, are conjugated in the liver before excretion in the urine. Depending on the activity of the conjugated metabolite, these drugs may have adverse effects following repeated doses. Morphine-6-glucuronide, an active metabolite of morphine, accumulates in renal failure and may result in prolongation of clinical effects after administration of morphine.

Modern volatile anaesthetic agents avoid metabolism to the fluoride ion, and are free of any deleterious effects on renal function.

POSTOPERATIVE RENAL FAILURE

In the absence of severe sepsis or pre-existing renal dysfunction, this is now relatively uncommon. In high-risk patients, such as those undergoing major surgery which involves large blood loss, surgery following trauma, and septic patients, avoidance of renal failure involves close monitoring of the cardiovascular state, including CVP and urinary output, avoidance of hypoxaemia and hypotension, and adequate fluid and blood replacement. In many instances, e.g. in patients with pre-existing renal dysfunction, shock, sepsis or liver disease, a pulmonary artery catheter may be required to optimize cardiac output and oxygen delivery, and to guide vasoactive drug therapy. Low-dose (2–5 µg kg^{-1} min^{-1}) dopamine was formerly recommended to prevent renal failure in such situations, but it has been demonstrated by randomized controlled trial to be ineffective in this role. The only proven therapy in the prevention and early treatment of acute renal failure is adequate fluid resuscitation titrated against CVP or PAOP and maintenance of an adequate cardiac output and mean arterial pressure (> 80 mmHg). This may involve use of a vasoactive agent such as dobutamine, norepinephrine or even dopamine.

Other measures, such as use of an osmotic diuretic (mannitol 100 mL of 20% solution over 15 min) or loop diuretic (furosemide by bolus or infusion), are of doubtful value. Mannitol continues to be recommended in jaundiced patients at risk of developing the hepatorenal syndrome and in patients with rhabdomyolysis. In some cases of oliguric acute renal failure, where adequate resuscitation has failed to achieve diuresis, furosemide i.v. does appear to 'kick-start' a urine output which is then maintained.

Postoperative oliguria may also be the result of postrenal causes. Patients with prostatic enlargement are particularly liable to develop acute urinary retention. Examination to exclude a full bladder and catheterization should always be carried out in the anuric postoperative patient. Abdominal ultrasound may be useful in more complicated cases.

DIABETES MELLITUS

Diabetes mellitus is common. Around 10% of patients admitted to hospital have diabetes either as a cause of admission or coincidentally. Fifty per cent of all diabetic patients present for surgery during their lifetime, most commonly for ophthalmic or vascular disease or for drainage of an abscess. Perioperative morbidity and mortality are greater in diabetic than in nondiabetic patients. This results from several factors:

- hyperglycaemia leading to increased risk of infectious complications and impaired healing (including anastomotic failure)
- hypoglycaemia, the clinical signs of which may be masked completely by anaesthesia
- complications of diabetes:
  - ischaemic heart disease
  - autonomic neuropathy
  - infection
  - renal impairment.

There are two main types of diabetes: type 1, pancreatic β-cell destruction (insulin dependent); type 2, defective insulin secretion and insulin resistance (non-insulin-dependent diabetes mellitus). Both groups suffer from hyperglycaemia. However, the complete lack of insulin in the former group allows unrestrained glycogenolysis, gluconeogenesis, and protein and fat catabolism with subsequent production of keto acids if insulin treatment is interrupted. These effects are limited by residual insulin production in type 2 diabetics. However, additional significant stress such as major surgery or sepsis may be sufficient to precipitate ketoacidosis in this group too.

The specific problems of managing diabetics who undergo surgery are a result of the attendant period of starvation and the stress response to surgery with catabolic hormone release. The aim is to minimize the metabolic disturbance by ensuring an adequate intake of glucose and insulin, thus controlling hyperglycaemia and reducing proteolysis, lipolysis and production of lactate and ketones. Adequate control of blood glucose concentration must be established preoperatively and maintained until oral feeding is resumed after operation.

The availability of accurate near-patient monitoring of blood glucose (e.g. Dextrostix, Ames: BM-Test-Glycemie, Boehringer-Mannheim, preferably used in conjunction with a reflectance colorimeter) have allowed close glycaemic control to be achieved perioperatively and there is now strong evidence that good glycaemic control improves outcome following major surgery.

Precise diabetic management depends upon:

- the nature of the diabetes and its treatment (insulin-dependent or noninsulin-dependent)
- the magnitude of the surgery contemplated, in particular duration of fasting
- the time available for improving control of the diabetes preoperatively if necessary.

PREOPERATIVE ASSESSMENT

Preoperative assessment is aimed at evaluating blood glucose control, the treatment regimen used and the presence of complications.

Control of blood glucose

This is assessed by inspection of the patient's urine-testing or BM-testing records, by random blood glucose measurements and by measurement of glycosylated haemoglobin (HbA$_{1c}$). Whenever possible, blood glucose concentration should be maintained between 6 and 10 mmol L^{-1}. HbA1c should be 7–8% in a well-controlled diabetic patient. In an elective situation, a patient with poor preoperative glycaemic control should benefit from review and optimization of treatment before embarking on surgery.

Treatment regimens

Oral hypoglycaemic agents

- the sulphonylureas, e.g. glipizide, gliclazide, stimulate release of insulin from the pancreatic islets. Hypoglycaemia may be induced by these agents.
- biguanides (metformin), which increase peripheral uptake of glucose and decrease gluconeogenesis, are used in obese maturity-onset diabetics either

alone or in combination with sulphonylureas. These agents may cause lactic acidosis, usually, but not exclusively, in patients with a degree of renal or hepatic impairment. Guidelines for the administration of i.v. contrast media include the instructions to withhold metformin for 24 h before and 48 h after the investigation. Lactic acidosis carries a very high mortality; consequently, metformin, the only biguanide now available, should be discontinued at least 24 h before surgery

- acarbose inhibits intestinal glucosidases, delaying carbohydrate digestion and reducing postprandial glucose surges.

Insulins.

Insulin therapy is required by all type 1 diabetics and some type 2 patients. Most insulins in clinical use are now human insulins produced via recombinant DNA technology. Duration of action of insulin preparations varies:

- Short-acting insulins. Soluble insulins, e.g. Velosulin, Actrapid, have an onset time of 30 min, peak effect 2–4 h, duration 8 h given subcutaneously. Given intravenously, their effect is much shorter, with a half-life of around 2.5 min and a duration of action of 30 min. Insulin aspart (NovoRapid) and insulin lispro (Humalog) are human insulin analogues and have an even faster onset and shorter duration of action.
- Intermediate, e.g. isophane insulin, insulin zinc suspension and long-acting, e.g. insulin glargine, crystalline insulin zinc suspension. These have a duration of action of 18–35 h.
- Biphasic fixed mixtures, e.g. Mixtard (soluble and isophane insulin), Humalog (insulin lispro and insulin lispro protamine), NovoMix (insulin aspart and insulin aspart protamine). These are a combination of soluble and longer-acting insulin available in a variety of different proportions.

Insulin is given by subcutaneous injection and the patient's specific regimen is tailored to provide optimal glycaemic control. Often this is a twice-daily biphasic insulin injection. However, with the increasing requirement to achieve near normoglycaemia, more complex regimens are increasingly seen, e.g. a single 'background' injection of long-acting insulin with soluble insulin given before meals.

In well-controlled diabetics it is not usually necessary to change the insulin regimen on the day before surgery. Often, a change of regimen results in poorer control.

COMPLICATIONS OF DIABETES MELLITUS

- *Cardiovascular disorders* (coronary artery, cerebrovascular and peripheral vascular) are common in diabetic patients and there is an increased risk of perioperative myocardial infarction. There may be significant ischaemic heart disease in the absence of warning symptoms and, as discussed earlier, this is a group which may merit further cardiovascular investigation before major surgery
- *Renal disease*. Microvascular damage produces glomerulosclerosis with proteinuria, oedema and eventually chronic renal failure. Anaesthetic implications of renal disease are discussed on page 461.
- *Ocular problems*. Cataracts, exudative or proliferative retinopathy, vitreous haemorrhage and retinal detachment may occur. In the long term, good blood glucose control has been shown to reduce the frequency of such complications
- *Infection*. Diabetic patients are prone to infection and an increased risk of septicaemia, abscess formation and wound infection. Infection is associated with increased insulin requirements, which return to normal on its eradication, e.g. after surgical drainage of an abscess
- *Neuropathy*. Chronic sensory peripheral neuropathies are common; mononeuropathies and acute motor neuropathies (amyotrophy) are associated with poor control of blood glucose. Loss of sensation together with peripheral vascular disease may lead to ulceration after trivial trauma. Consequently, care in positioning patients in the operating theatre is important. Local anaesthetic nerve or plexus blocks should be avoided in patients with an acute neuropathy, as neurological deficits may be attributed to the local anaesthetic solution
- *Autonomic neuropathy* may cause postoperative urinary retention or vasomotor instability, e.g. postural hypotension or hypotension during anaesthesia. IPPV or subarachnoid or epidural block may be associated with significant hypotension; preoperative intravascular volume status should be assessed and fluids given to achieve normovolaemia before performing a block. Precise cardiovascular monitoring, use of vasopressors and careful anaesthetic management are essential.

CONCURRENT DRUG THERAPY

Thiazide diuretics, adrenergic agents, e.g. salbutamol, and corticosteroids tend to increase the blood glucose concentration. Beta-adrenergic blockers tend to potentiate hypoglycaemia and may mask its clinical signs. Blood glucose concentration should be monitored if any of these drugs is administered, and insulin dosage altered accordingly.

Some drugs, including phenylbutazone, displace sulphonylureas from protein-binding sites and potentiate their hypoglycaemic effect.

PERIOPERATIVE DIABETIC MANAGEMENT

Advice regarding perioperative management of diabetes should always be sought from the metabolic team and local guidelines should be available.

Type 2 noninsulin-dependent diabetics undergoing minor surgery, and who are able to recommence oral intake immediately postoperatively, do not require perioperative insulin therapy. These patients should be scheduled early on the operating list. They should omit the usual morning hypoglycaemic agents. Blood glucose monitoring should continue throughout the fasting period. If hyperglycaemia occurs (blood glucose > 16 mmol L^{-1}) or there is any delay in recommencing normal diet and therapy, insulin treatment should be started.

In type I diabetes, a combination of glucose and insulin is the most satisfactory method of overcoming the deleterious metabolic consequences of starvation and surgical stress in the diabetic patient.

Although satisfactory control of blood glucose may be achieved using a no glucose/no insulin regimen, the raised blood urea concentration which often occurs in the postoperative period is indicative of the increased protein breakdown, accompanying lipolysis and ketosis that occur as a result of lack of insulin. Minor procedures, e.g. cystoscopy, examination under anaesthesia, may be carried out at the start of an operating list by delaying the morning dose of insulin until a late breakfast is taken after recovery from anaesthesia. Attention must be paid to avoiding postoperative nausea and vomiting with adequate hydration, avoiding opioids if possible and with prophylactic antiemetic use. This may be facilitated by the use of regional anaesthesia with or without sedation, which allows the patient to resume normal oral intake earlier than is usually possible following general anaesthesia.

Tables 23.6 and 23.7 describe schemes for the precise management of patients receiving oral hypoglycaemic agents or insulin therapy who require insulin therapy perioperatively. Patients normally receiving oral hypoglycaemics may be very sensitive to insulin therapy.

Table 23.6 Perioperative management of the mature-onset diabetic	
Preoperative	
Check random glucose, urea and electrolyte concentrations	
Poor control	Start insulin (soluble, before meals) and delay surgery
	Urgent surgery: glucose insulin infusion (Table 23.7)
Good control	Chlorpropamide – change to a shorter-acting agent
Day of surgery	
Check fasting blood glucose	
No oral hypoglycaemic agent	
Minor surgery	If blood glucose < 10 mmol L^{-1}, no specific therapy
Major surgery	Treat as insulin-dependent diabetic (Table 23.7)
Postoperative	
Check blood glucose	
Minor surgery	Restart oral hypoglycaemic agent with first meal
Major surgery	Treat as insulin-dependent diabetic (Table 23.7)
	When oral diet is resumed, soluble insulin 8–12 units before each meal; restart oral therapy when daily requirement is less than 20 units

Table 23.7 Perioperative management of the insulin-dependent diabetic	
Preoperative	
Blood glucose profile; Hb A$_{1c}$ urea and electrolytes; urine ketones	
Poor control	Change to soluble insulin before meals and delay surgery
Urgent surgery	glucose/insulin infusion (see below)
Day of surgery	
Check fasting blood glucose; repeat 1–2 hourly	
No subcutaneous insulin	
Start infusion of 10% glucose (500 mL) with soluble insulin 10 units and KCl 10 mmol at 0800 h to run 4–6 hourly. Insulin dose may need to be adjusted dependent on the patient's usual requirements	
Adjust insulin in 500 mL glucose 10% as follows depending on blood glucose:	
< 4 mmol L^{-1}	No insulin
4–6 mmol L^{-1}	Insulin 5 units
6–10 mmol L^{-1}	Insulin 10 units
10–20 mmol L^{-1}	Insulin 15 units
> 20 mmol L^{-1}	Insulin 20 units
Adjust potassium dosage depending on plasma K$^+$concentration:	
< 3 mmol L^{-1}	Add KCl 20 mmol L^{-1}
> 5 mmol L^{-1}	Omit KCl
Postoperative	
Check blood glucose 1–4 hourly; check urea and electrolytes daily	
Continue infusion until oral diet re-established	
When oral diet resumed, soluble insulin s.c. before meals; daily dosage as preoperative	
When requirements stable, restart normal regimen	

There are two methods of delivering insulin and dextrose:

- GKI regimen (Table 23.7):
  - simple regimen with glucose, insulin and potassium in one bag
  - less responsive to requirement for frequent dose changes
  - less suitable for controlling markedly hyperglycaemic patients
  - avoids continued insulin dosing and subsequent hypoglycaemia if the dextrose infusion fails.
- Sliding scale regimen (Table 23.8):
  - ideal for patients who are markedly hyperglycaemic or who require frequent changes in insulin dose
  - there is a risk of hypoglycaemia if the dextrose arm of the infusion fails for any reason and insulin continues to be infused.

In practice the choice of regimen is dictated by local practice.

Glucose 10% is used to provide adequate carbohydrate and energy without excessive volume. Given at 100 mL h^{-1}, this provides 240 g of glucose (1000 kcal) in 24 h. It is essential to use an infusion pump to regulate the rate of infusion This infusion is not designed for volume replacement and should be given separately. Saline infusion will be required to avoid hyponatraemia.

Blood transfusion may increase insulin requirements as the elevated citrate concentration stimulates gluconeogenesis.

Table 23.8 Sliding scale for infusion of insulin

Glucose concentration (mmol L^{-1})	Infusion rate of insulin (unit h^{-1})
< 4.0	0
4–4.9	0.5
5.0–6.9	1.0
7–9.9	2
10–12.9	3
13–15.9	4
> 16	6 (test for ketones)

Insulin administered from syringe pump. Infusion comprises 50 units of human soluble insulin in 50 mL isotonic saline

Commence 10% dextrose with 10 mmol KCl at 100 mL h^{-1}

Blood glucose concentration is measured at 1-hourly intervals (initially) and rate of insulin infusion adjusted according to sliding scale

BMs should remain between 6 and 12 mmol L^{-1}

When stability has been achieved, blood glucose concentration may be measured at 4-hourly intervals

EMERGENCY SURGERY AND DIABETIC KETOACIDOSIS

Diabetic ketoacidosis results from inadequate insulin dosage or increased insulin requirements, often precipitated by infection, trauma or surgical stress. Diabetic patients who require emergency surgery often have a grossly elevated blood glucose concentration and occasionally overt ketoacidosis. Such patients require rehydration, correction of sodium depletion, correction of potassium depletion and i.v. soluble insulin by infusion at an initial rate of 4–8 unit h^{-1}.

Initial fluid replacement should consist of isotonic (0.9%) saline: 1 L in the first 30 min, 1 L in the next hour and an additional 1 L over the next 2 h, guided by clinical reassessment and cardiovascular monitoring.

Progress is monitored by regular measurements of blood glucose, sodium and potassium concentrations, and arterial pH and blood gas tensions. Correction of acidosis with bicarbonate is very rarely, if ever, required. Cellular potassium depletion is present from the outset, but hyperkalaemia or normokalaemia may

be found initially because potassium shifts out of the cells in the presence of acidosis. Potassium replacement is required as the plasma concentration begins to decrease with the correction of the acidosis. Magnesium is also required. An infusion of glucose 5% should be given, in conjunction with continued insulin therapy, when the blood glucose concentration decreases to approximately 15 mmol L^{-1}. When volume resuscitation is under way, and some reversal of acidosis and hyperglycaemia has been achieved, surgery may be carried out while management of the diabetes is continued intra- and postoperatively.

OTHER ENDOCRINE DISORDERS

PITUITARY DISEASE

The clinical features of pituitary disease depend on the local effects of the lesion and its effects on the secretion of pituitary hormones. Local effects include headache and visual field disturbances. The effects on hormone secretion depend on the cells involved in the pathological process.

Acromegaly

Acromegaly is caused by increased secretion of growth hormone from eosinophil cell tumours of the anterior pituitary gland. If this occurs before fusion of the epiphyses, gigantism results. Problems for the anaesthetist include the following:

- upper airway obstruction may result from an enlarged mandible, tongue and epiglottis, thickened pharyngeal mucosa and laryngeal narrowing. Maintenance of a clear airway and tracheal intubation may be difficult, and postoperative care of the airway must be meticulous. Consideration may be given to awake fibreoptic tracheal intubation.
- cardiac enlargement, hypertension and congestive cardiac failure occur commonly and require preoperative treatment.
- growth hormone increases blood sugar concentration. Hyperglycaemia should be controlled perioperatively.
- thyroid and adrenal function may be impaired because of decreased release of thyroid-stimulating hormone (TSH) and ACTH. Thyroxine and steroid replacement may be required.

Treatment involves hypophysectomy, which requires steroid cover preoperatively, and steroid, thyroxine and possibly ADH replacement thereafter.

Cushing's disease

Cushing's disease results from basophil adenomas, which secrete ACTH (see below).

Hypopituitarism (Simmonds' disease)

Causes include chromophobe adenoma, tumours of surrounding tissues, e.g. craniopharyngioma, skull fractures, infarction following postpartum haemorrhage and infection. Clinical features include loss of axillary and pubic hair, amenorrhoea, features of hypothyroidism and adrenal insufficiency, including hypotension, but with a striking pallor, in contrast to the pigmentation of Addison's disease (see p. 470).

The fluid and electrolyte disturbances are not as marked as in primary adrenal failure as a result of intact aldosterone production, but may be unmasked by surgery, trauma or infection. Anaesthesia in these patients requires steroid cover (p. 471), cautious administration of induction agent and volatile anaesthetic agents, and careful cardiovascular monitoring.

Diabetes insipidus

This is caused by disease or damage affecting the hypothalamic posterior pituitary axis. Common causes are pituitary tumour, craniopharyngioma, basal skull fracture and infection, or it may occur as a sequel to pituitary surgery. In 10% of cases, diabetes insipidus is renal in origin.

Dehydration with hypernatraemia follows excretion of large volumes of dilute urine. Patients require fluid replacement and treatment with parenteral vasopressin or desmopressin which can be given orally or intranasally in addition to parenteral routes.

Thyroid disease

Goitre

Thyroid swelling may result from iodine deficiency (simple goitre), autoimmune (Hashimoto's) thyroiditis, adenoma, carcinoma or thyrotoxicosis. Nodules of the thyroid gland may be 'hot' (secreting thyroxine) or 'cold'.

The goitre may occasionally cause respiratory obstruction. Retrosternal goitre may in addition cause superior vena caval obstruction. The presence of a goitre should alert the anaesthetist to the possibility of tracheal compression or displacement. A preoperative X-ray of neck and thoracic inlet may be useful, and a selection of small-diameter, armoured tracheal tubes should be available. Preoperative assessment of thyroid function is essential.

Thyrotoxicosis

This is characterized by excitability, tremor, tachycardia and arrhythmias, (commonly atrial fibrillation), weight loss, heat intolerance and exophthalmos. Diagnosis is confirmed by measurement of total serum thyroxine, tri-iodothyronine (T_3) and TSH concentrations.

Elective surgery should not be carried out in hyperthyroid patients; they should first be rendered euthyroid with carbimazole or radioactive iodine. However, urgent surgery and elective subtotal thyroidectomy may be carried out safely in hyperthyroid patients using β-adrenergic blockade alone or in combination with potassium iodide to control thyrotoxic symptoms and signs. Emergency surgery carries a significant risk of thyrotoxic crisis. Control is best achieved in these circumstances by i.v. potassium iodide and a nonselective β-blocker (e.g. propranolol). If patients are unable to absorb oral medication, i.v. infusion is indicated (for propranolol, the daily i.v. dose is approximately one-tenth of the oral dose).

The doses of sedative drugs for premedication, and of anaesthetic agents, should be increased to compensate for faster distribution and elimination. Larger doses of sedative drugs than normal are required to avoid anxiety when procedures are carried out under regional anaesthesia.

Preparation for thyroidectomy

Previous conventional management involved at least 6–8 weeks administration of carbimazole to render the patient euthyroid, followed by potassium iodide 60 mg 8 hourly for 10 days to decrease the vascularity of the gland.

Many anaesthetists now use a beta-blocker to prepare the hyperthyroid patient for thyroidectomy. Propranolol 160–480 mg daily for 2 weeks preoperatively and a further 7–10 days postoperatively provides adequate control in most patients. However, control with beta-blockers depends on maintaining an adequate plasma concentration of the drug. Because beta-blockers, in common with other drugs, are cleared more rapidly than normal in thyrotoxic patients, propranolol should be prescribed more frequently than usual, e.g. four times daily. Alternatively, a long-acting beta-blocker, e.g. atenolol once daily, continued on the morning of surgery, provides satisfactory control and avoids the problem of impaired drug absorption immediately after operation. A combination of beta-blocker and potassium iodide 60 mg 8 hourly provides reliable control in even the most severely thyrotoxic patient. Postoperatively, laryngoscopy should be carried out to check vocal cord function, and exclude recurrent laryngeal nerve injury.

Hypothyroidism

This may result from primary thyroid failure, Hashimoto's thyroiditis, as a consequence of thyroid surgery, or secondary to pituitary failure. The diagnosis is suggested by tiredness, cold intolerance, loss of appetite, dry skin and hair loss. It may be confirmed by the finding of a low serum thyroxine concentration, associated, in primary thyroid failure, with a raised serum TSH concentration.

Basal metabolic rate is decreased. Cardiac output is decreased, with little myocardial reserve, and hypothermia may be present. Treatment is with thyroxine, which should be started in a small dose of 25–50 µg daily. Rapid correction of hypothyroidism may be achieved using i.v. T_3, but this is inadvisable in elderly patients and those with ischaemic heart disease, which is common in hypothyroidism, as the sudden increase in myocardial oxygen demand may provoke ischaemia or infarction. ECG monitoring is advisable during treatment. Elective surgery should be avoided in myxoedematous patients, but if emergency surgery is necessary, close cardiovascular, ECG and blood gas monitoring is essential. Drug distribution and metabolism are slowed, and thus all anaesthetic agents must be administered in reduced doses.

DISEASE OF THE ADRENAL CORTEX

Clinical symptoms are associated with increased or decreased secretion of cortisol or aldosterone.

Hypersecretion of cortisol (Cushing's syndrome)

Most instances are caused by pituitary adenomas which secrete ACTH and thus cause bilateral adrenocortical hyperplasia (Cushing's disease). In 20–30% of patients, an adrenocortical adenoma or carcinoma is present. Rarely, an oat-cell carcinoma of bronchus, secreting ACTH, is the cause. ACTH and corticosteroid therapy present similar pictures. Clinical features include obesity, hypertension, proximal myopathy and diabetes mellitus. Biochemically, there is a metabolic alkalosis with hypokalaemia. Depending on the cause, treatment may involve hypophysectomy or adrenalectomy.

Anaesthetic management of these patients involves preoperative treatment of hypertension and congestive cardiac failure, and correction of hypokalaemia. Intraoperative management is directed towards careful monitoring of arterial pressure and maintenance of cardiovascular stability, with careful choice and administration of anaesthetic agents and muscle relaxants. Etomidate and atracurium or vecuronium would be an appropriate choice of induction agent and relaxant, respectively. Postoperative steroid therapy is required for hypophysectomy and adrenalectomy (see below). Fludrocortisone 0.1–0.3 mg daily is required after bilateral adrenalectomy.

Primary hypersecretion of aldosterone (Conn's syndrome)

Conn's syndrome is caused by an adenoma of the zona glomerulosa of the adrenal cortex and presents with hypertension, hypernatraemia, hypokalaemia and oliguria. Anaesthetic management involves preoperative treatment of hypertension, administration of spironolactone and potassium replacement; meticulous intra- and postoperative monitoring of arterial pressure is essential.

Adrenocortical hypofunction

Primary adrenocortical insufficiency (*Addison's disease*) may be caused by an autoimmune process, tuberculosis, amyloid, metastatic carcinoma, or bilateral adrenalectomy. Haemorrhage into the glands during meningococcal septicaemia may cause acute adrenal failure in association with septic shock. Secondary failure results from hypopituitarism or prolonged corticosteroid therapy. In secondary failure resulting from pituitary insufficiency, aldosterone secretion is maintained, and fluid and electrolyte disturbances are less marked.

Clinical features include weakness, weight loss, hyperpigmentation, hypotension, vomiting, diarrhoea and volume depletion. Hypoglycaemia, hyponatraemia, hyperkalaemia and metabolic acidosis are characteristic but late biochemical findings. The stress of infection, trauma or surgery provokes profound hypotension. Diagnosis is made by measurement of plasma cortisol concentration and the response to ACTH stimulation.

All surgical procedures in these patients must be covered by increased steroid administration (see below). Patients with acute adrenal insufficiency require urgent fluid and sodium replacement with arterial pressure and CVP monitoring, glucose infusion to combat hypoglycaemia and hydrocortisone 100 mg 6-hourly i.v. They should be cared for in a high dependency or critical care area. Antibiotics are advisable to cover the possibility that infection has provoked the crisis. In cases of primary adrenal failure, mineralocorticoid replacement with fludrocortisone is required.

If emergency surgery is required in acute adrenal failure, all precautions necessary for anaesthetizing the shocked patient should be taken (see Ch. 28).

Congenital adrenal hyperplasia (adrenogenital syndrome)

This is associated with overproduction of androgens as a result of deficiency of the hydroxylase enzyme required for production of cortisol. Hydrocortisone treatment overcomes adrenal insufficiency and, by suppressing ACTH production, decreases androgen accumulation. Augmented steroid cover is required for surgery in these patients.

Steroid therapy

Replacement therapy in cases of primary adrenocortical failure and hypopituitarism is given as oral hydrocortisone 20 mg in the morning and 10 mg in the evening. Fludrocortisone 0.05–0.1 mg daily is given additionally to replace aldosterone in primary adrenocortical failure. Equivalent doses of other steroid preparations are shown in Table 23.4. Prednisolone and prednisone have less mineralocorticoid effect, while betamethasone and dexamethasone have none. Requirements increase following infection, trauma or surgery.

Corticosteroids are also prescribed for a wide range of medical conditions, including asthma and collagen diseases. Prolonged therapy suppresses adrenocortical function.

STEROID COVER FOR ANAESTHESIA AND SURGERY

Indications for augmented perioperative steroid cover and the dosage required are the subject of ongoing debate. Suggested indications:

- patients with pituitary adrenal insufficiency, receiving steroid replacement therapy
- patients undergoing pituitary or adrenal surgery
- patients receiving systemic steroid therapy for more than 2 weeks before surgery
- patients no longer receiving systemic steroid therapy, but who received steroids within the 3 months before surgery.

Topical fluorinated steroid preparations applied widely to the skin and high-dose inhaled steroids may be absorbed sufficiently to produce adrenal suppression. An ACTH stimulation (short synacthen) test can be carried out to assess adrenal function. Preoperative assessment should identify fluid and electrolyte abnormalities, which should be corrected. Evidence of infection should be sought in patients receiving long-term steroid therapy.

Corticosteroid cover for operation should be given as follows:

- minor diagnostic procedures – hydrocortisone 25 mg at induction
- intermediate operations, e.g. inguinal herniorrhaphy – hydrocortisone 50 mg at induction, then 25 mg 6-hourly for 24 h
- major surgery – hydrocortisone 50 mg at induction, then 6-hourly for 48–72 h.

The requirements may need to be increased if infection is present, or be continued beyond 3 days if infection or the effects of major trauma persist. Oral steroid preparations may be preferred for premedication and then resumed after 24 h.

If steroids are prescribed for asthma or other medical conditions, the perioperative dosage may require modification according to the activity of the disease.

DISEASE OF THE ADRENAL MEDULLA

Phaeochromocytoma

This is discussed in Chapter 37.

NEUROLOGICAL DISEASE

GENERAL CONSIDERATIONS

Neurological disease embraces a wide range of differing conditions, the effects of which may influence the conduct of perioperative care in a number of ways:

- a depressed level of consciousness may prejudice airway protection and result in depressed respiratory drive.
- peripheral neuromuscular disease may lead to impaired ventilatory function and reduced ability to clear secretions.
- autonomic dysfunction may result in blood pressure instability, cardiac arrhythmias and dysfunction of gastrointestinal motility.
- there may also be significant adverse effects from specific drug treatment, and there are several important drug interactions which need to be recognized.

ASSESSMENT

In addition to standard history and examination, a detailed drug history should be obtained. Many patients with neurological disease should have their medication continued up to the time of surgery and reinstated as soon as possible thereafter, e.g. epilepsy, Parkinsonism, myasthenia gravis. Respiratory function should be assessed by the use of pulmonary function tests including vital capacity and measurement of arterial blood gas tensions. Erect and supine arterial pressure should be performed where appropriate and a 12-lead ECG performed to assess QT interval and possible heart block.

Respiratory impairment

Inadequate ventilatory function may result from:

- reduced central drive, e.g. because of an impaired conscious level
- motor neuropathy, e.g. Guillain–Barré syndrome, motor neurone disease
- neuromuscular dysfunction, e.g. myasthenia gravis
- muscle weakness, e.g. muscular dystrophies
- rigidity, e.g. Parkinson's disease.

These patients are sensitive to anaesthetic agents, opioids and muscle relaxants. If intraoperative positive-pressure ventilation is undertaken, a period of elective postoperative ventilation may be necessary until full recovery from the effects of anaesthesia has occurred. If appropriate, procedures may be carried out under a regional anaesthetic technique.

Bulbar muscle involvement may lead to inadequate protection of the airway such that regurgitation and aspiration can occur. Chest infection should be effectively treated preoperatively, and in the elective situation this may necessitate postponing surgery.

Altered innervation of muscle and hyperkalaemia

An altered ratio of intracellular to extracellular potassium tends to produce sensitivity to nondepolarizing, and resistance to depolarizing, relaxants. Consideration should be given to the use of short acting agents such as propofol, sevoflurane and remifentanil. If there is widespread denervation of muscle with lower motor neurone damage, e.g. in Guillain–Barré syndrome, disorganization of the motor end-plate occurs, resulting in hypersensitivity to acetylcholine and succinylcholine, with increased permeability of muscle cells to potassium. A similar potassium efflux occurs in the presence of direct muscle damage, widespread burns involving muscle, upper motor neurone lesions, spinal cord lesions with paraplegia and tetanus. In upper motor neurone and spinal cord lesions, the reason for this shift is less clear. Patients undergoing mechanical

ventilation in the ICU who are suffering from sepsis and multiple organ failure may develop a critical illness polyneuropathy, with a similar hyperkalaemic response to succinylcholine.

The resulting increase in serum potassium concentration after succinylcholine may be 3 mmol L^{-1} (in comparison with 0.5 mmol L^{-1} in the normal patient) and may occur from 24 h after acute muscle denervation or damage. In such patients, succinylcholine is clearly contraindicated.

Autonomic disturbances

These may occur as part of a polyneuropathy, e.g. diabetes mellitus, Guillain–Barré syndrome and porphyria, or from central nervous system involvement, e.g. in Parkinsonism. Sympathetic stimulation, e.g. during light anaesthesia, tracheal intubation or following administration of pancuronium or catecholamines, may produce severe hypertension and arrhythmias. More commonly, blood loss, head-up posture, IPPV or neuraxial regional blocks may be associated with severe hypotension. Cardiac arrhythmias may also occur.

Conscious level

Patients with pre-existing marked reduction in conscious level for whatever reason require tracheal intubation and artificial ventilation of the lungs for airway protection and control of CO_2 and O_2 levels.

Increased intracranial pressure

Elective surgery should be postponed if raised intracranial pressure is suspected, until investigation by CT scan and treatment have been undertaken. Anaesthetic agents which cause an increase in cerebral blood flow must be avoided. Hypercapnia must also be avoided, and controlled ventilation to a P_aCO_2 of approximately 4 kPa (30 mmHg) is indicated. This is discussed fully in Chapter 38.

Medicolegal

Perioperative alteration in neurological deficit may be attributed to anaesthesia. This may render subarachnoid or epidural anaesthesia inadvisable in some patients.

EPILEPSY

Epilepsy may be associated with birth injury, hypoglycaemia, hypocalcaemia, drug overdose or withdrawal, fever, head injury, cerebrovascular disease and cerebral tumour, the most likely cause depending on the age of onset. In most patients with epilepsy, no identi-fiable cause is found. Epilepsy developing after the age of 20 years usually indicates organic brain disease.

Anaesthesia

Patients should receive maintenance anticonvulsant therapy throughout the perioperative period. Some anaesthetic agents, e.g. enflurane, have cerebral excita-tory effects and should be avoided. Sevoflurane and isoflurane do not cause cerebral excitation. Convulsions and abnormalities of muscle posture have been reported after operation in patients who have received propofol and it is currently recom-mended that this drug should not be used in known epileptics, although it is an effective anticonvulsant agent. Thiopental is a potent anticonvulsant and is the i.v. induction agent of choice, while isoflurane is cur-rently the volatile agent of choice. Local anaesthetic agents may cause convulsions at lower than normal concentrations and the safe maximum dose should be reduced. The anticonvulsants phenobarbital and phenytoin induce hepatic enzymes and accelerate elimination of drugs metabolized by the liver.

In cases of late-onset epilepsy, where increased intracranial pressure may be present as a result of tumour, controlled ventilation is advisable to avoid any further increase in intracranial pressure.

Status epilepticus

Management is aimed at cessation of the fits while maintaining tissue oxygenation. Initial treatment should be Diazemuls, titrated intravenously in a dose of up to 10–20 mg or until fitting ceases. An alternative is lorazepam 2–4 mg i.v. slowly. A loading dose of phenytoin 10–15 mg kg^{-1} should be administered i.v. under ECG monitoring over 30–60 min. High-concen-tration oxygen should be administered, and a clear air-way maintained throughout. If the convulsions persist or conscious level diminishes to the extent of compro-mising the airway and ventilation, the patient should be anaesthetized, the trachea intubated and mechani-cal ventilation commenced. While propofol has been associated with convulsive episodes when used for standard general anaesthesia, it is also highly effective in the treatment of status epilepticus and indeed may be the anaesthetic agent of choice in this condition. Propofol may be used in seizures refractory to benzo-diazepines and phenytoin both as the anaesthetic induction agent and as maintenance by infusion.

The conventional anaesthetic induction agent used is thiopental. Thereafter, an infusion of propofol may be used to control the fits. This has the advantage over thiopental of being short acting, allowing the patient's conscious level to be assessed readily.

With status epilepticus, patients undergoing mechanical ventilation should not be paralysed, but if they are, a cerebral function monitor/electroen-cephalogram monitor must be used so that continued fitting is noted and treated.

PARKINSON'S DISEASE

The clinical signs of resting tremor, muscle rigidity and bradykinesia characterize Parkinson's disease. This illness affects around 3% of individuals over 66 years of age. It is caused by cell death in areas of the basal ganglia with loss of dopaminergic neurones. Similar symptoms and signs occur with loss of dopaminergic function secondary to drugs such as antipsychotic agents and following encephalitis in some patients.

Patients commonly present for urological, oph-thalmic or orthopaedic surgery. There are various con-siderations for the anaesthetist.

Respiratory. The airway may be difficult because of fixed flexion of the neck. Upper airway muscle dys-function may lead to aspiration. Excessive salivation may necessitate administration of a preoperative dry-ing agent. An obstructive ventilatory pattern is present in around 35% of patients and muscle rigidity and tremor may also impair ventilation.

Cardiovascular. Postural hypotension may be pres-ent and there is an increased risk of cardiac arrhyth-mias. Autonomic failure may cause or exacerbate these problems.

Gastrointestinal. There is an increased risk of reflux.

Medications. These may have cardiovascular side-effects and there are several potential interactions with anaesthetic agents, analgesics and neuromuscular blocking drugs. These are detailed in Table 23.9.

Anaesthetic management

Preoperatively. Medication should be continued up to the time of surgery and reinstated as soon as possi-ble thereafter. Regional techniques offer several advantages such as the avoidance of opioid drugs and less effect on respiratory function. Diphenhydramine may be used for sedation in the awake patient where tremor makes surgery difficult, e.g. ophthalmology.

General anaesthesia. A technique which avoids pul-monary aspiration should be used when appropriate. Isoflurane and sevoflurane are the inhalational agents of choice although hypotension may be a problem, particularly in the presence of autonomic neuropathy and when bromocriptine or selegiline have been

Table 23.9 Potential drug interactions in patients with Parkinson's disease

Drug	Comments
Induction agents	
Propofol	Avoid for stereotactic procedures (dyskinetic, may abolish tremor)
Etomidate	Probably safe
Thiopental	Probably safe
Analgesics	
Fentanyl	Possible muscle rigidity
Morphine	Possible muscle rigidity
Volatile agents	
Isoflurane	Probably safe
Sevoflurane	Probably safe
Neuromuscular blocking agents	
Succinylcholine	Possible hyperkalaemia
Nondepolarizing agents	Probably safe
Antiemetics	
Metoclopramide	Precipitates or exacerbates Parkinsonism

administered. In the patient requiring general anaesthesia, nasogastric L-dopa can be administered in prolonged operations. Where the enteral route is not possible, parenteral apomorphine can be used. This should be preceded by administration of domperidone for 72 h. Parkinsonian patients have an increased risk of postoperative confusion and hallucinations and following general anaesthesia may exhibit abnormal neurological signs such as decerebrate posturing, upgoing plantars and hyperreflexia.

Drugs. Phenothiazines, haloperidol and metoclopramide are contraindicated. Opioids must be used with caution but paracetamol and NSAIDs can be used as normal.

MULTIPLE SCLEROSIS

Deterioration of symptoms tends to occur after surgery, but no specific anaesthetic technique has been implicated. It may be advisable to avoid epidural and subarachnoid anaesthesia, but only for medicolegal reasons, as there is no evidence that these techniques affect the disease adversely. They may be used if indicated strongly, provided that a full explanation has been given to the patient, e.g. in obstetrics.

If a large motor deficit of recent onset is present, there may be increased potassium release from muscle following administration of succinylcholine, which should be avoided.

PERIPHERAL NEUROPATHIES

These may exhibit axonal 'dying back' degeneration or segmental demyelination. They are classified by anatomical distribution, the commonest being a symmetrical peripheral polyneuropathy.

Motor, sensory and autonomic fibres are involved. Causes include:

- metabolic disorders (diabetes, porphyria)
- nutritional deficiency
- toxicity (heavy metals, drugs)
- collagen disease
- carcinoma
- infection
- inflammation
- critical illness polyneuropathy.

Problems for the anaesthetist include the effects of autonomic neuropathy, respiratory and bulbar involvement.

ACUTE DEMYELINATING POLYNEUROPATHY (GUILLAIN–BARRÉ SYNDROME)

This autoimmune polyneuropathy appears some days after a respiratory or gastrointestinal infection. Progression is variable, ranging from nearly total paralysis in 24 h to progression over several weeks. Respiratory and bulbar muscles may be affected and, if so, tracheal intubation and IPPV are necessary. Several techniques may be used for induction of anaesthesia and intubation. We recommend either the combination of an i.v. induction agent with rocuronium or the combination of propofol and alfentanil. The patient's general state, particularly the presence of cardiovascular instability, dictates which agents should be used. Autonomic neuropathy may result in hypotension after commencing IPPV. This may be minimized by adequate fluid preloading and gradual increases in minute volume. Succinylcholine should be avoided. There is evidence that either high-dose immunoglobulin therapy or plasmapheresis beneficially modifies the course of the disease, although mortality is not affected. Severe pain in a girdle distribution and peripheral neuropathic pain are particular problems in many patients and require a multimodal approach to analgesia.

MOTOR NEURONE DISEASE (PROGRESSIVE MUSCULAR ATROPHY, AMYOTROPHIC LATERAL SCLEROSIS, PROGRESSIVE BULBAR PALSY)

Motor neurone disease is characterized by slow-onset and progressive deterioration in motor function. Several patterns of motor loss occur with both upper and lower motor neurone loss. Problems for the anaesthetist include sensitivity to all anaesthetic agents and muscle relaxants, respiratory inadequacy and laryngeal incompetence. Regional techniques may be useful. Long-term IPPV should generally be avoided, but non-invasive ventilation has a definite role in palliation of dyspnoea.

HEREDITARY ATAXIAS

Friedreich's ataxia is the most common. Spinocerebellar, corticospinal and posterior columns are involved, and the course of the disease is slowly progressive. Problems for the anaesthetist include scoliosis, respiratory failure and cardiomyopathy with cardiac failure and arrhythmias.

SPINAL CORD LESIONS WITH PARAPLEGIA

Release of potassium from muscle cells by succinylcholine precludes its use within 6–12 months of cord injury. Assessment of ventilatory function is important, as impaired cough and poor inspiration may indicate a need for postoperative controlled ventilation.

In cervical spine lesions, patients are dependent on the diaphragm for breathing. In the acute situation, the loss of intercostal muscle function, to which patients may take some time to adjust, coupled with general anaesthesia, may lead to postoperative respiratory failure necessitating controlled ventilation.

Regional anaesthetic techniques may be useful in these patients, reducing the autonomic reflexes stimulated by surgery and avoiding compromise of ventilatory function.

HUNTINGTON'S CHOREA

It has been reported that thiopental may cause prolonged apnoea, and decreased serum cholinesterase activity may prolong the action of succinylcholine.

MYASTHENIA GRAVIS

This disease usually presents in young adults and is characterized by episodes of increased muscle fatigability, caused by decreased numbers of acetylcholine receptors at the neuromuscular junction. Treatment comprises an anticholinesterase (pyridostigmine 60 mg 6-hourly or neostigmine 15 mg 6-hourly) with a vagolytic agent (atropine or propantheline) to block the muscarinic side-effects. Steroid therapy is useful in some cases and thymectomy may benefit many patients considerably, especially young women with myasthenia of recent onset.

The principal problems concern adequacy of ventilation, ability to cough and clear secretions, and the increased secretions resulting from anticholinesterase therapy. If there is evidence of respiratory infection, surgery should be postponed. Serum potassium concentration should be normal, as hypokalaemia potentiates myasthenia. Local and regional anaesthesia, including subarachnoid or epidural block, may be suitable alternatives to general anaesthesia, although the maximum dose of local anaesthetic agents should be reduced because of their neuromuscular blocking action. The minimum possible dose of induction agent should be used and relaxants should be avoided if possible. For major procedures requiring relaxation, the anticholinesterase may be omitted for 4 h preoperatively, and a small dose of relaxant may be given if necessary. Atracurium is the relaxant of choice because of its short duration of action, and should be administered in a reduced dose. Succinylcholine has a variable effect in myasthenia and is best avoided.

Postoperatively, the patient's lungs should be ventilated electively after major surgery, usually for a few hours, but in some cases for up to 48 h. Frequent chest physiotherapy and tracheal suction are required. Steroid cover is given if appropriate. If extreme muscle weakness occurs, i.v. neostigmine 1–2 mg and atropine 0.6–1.2 mg may be given. Care must be taken to titrate the doses of anticholinesterase carefully, or a cholinergic crisis may occur, characterized by a depolarizing neuromuscular block, with sweating, salivation and pupillary constriction. An infusion of neostigmine is required if resumption of oral intake is delayed after surgery; 0.5 mg i.v. equivalent to 15 mg neostigmine or 60 mg pyridostigmine orally, which should be combined with an anticholinergic agent. Edrophonium may be used to test the end-plate response to acetylcholine.

A myasthenic state may also be associated with carcinoma, thyrotoxicosis, Cushing's syndrome, hypokalaemia and hypocalcaemia. In these patients, non-depolarizing relaxants should be avoided or used in reduced dosage.

FAMILIAL PERIODIC PARALYSIS

This is also associated with prolonged paralysis after administration of non-depolarizing muscle relaxants.

PROGRESSIVE MUSCULAR DYSTROPHY

Several types of muscular dystrophy exist, of varying patterns of heredity, and described according to their anatomical distribution. Muscle weakness occurs and must be distinguished from myasthenia and lower motor neurone disease. The anaesthetic complications comprise sensitivity to relaxants, opioids and other sedative and anaesthetic drugs, and liability to respiratory infection. Myocardial involvement may occur. These patients may be treated long-term with nocturnal non-invasive ventilation.

DYSTROPHIA MYOTONICA

This is a disease of autosomal dominant inheritance characterized by muscle weakness and muscle contraction persisting after the termination of voluntary effort. Other features may include frontal baldness, cataract, sternomastoid wasting, gonadal atrophy and thyroid adenoma. Problems which affect anaesthetic management include the following:

- *Respiratory muscle weakness*. Respiratory function should be assessed fully before operation. Respiratory depressant drugs, e.g. thiopental or opioids, should be used with care; there is sensitivity also to non-depolarizing relaxants. Planned IPPV may be required after surgery. Postoperative care of the airway must be meticulous. Chest infections are common.
- *Cardiovascular effects*. There may be a cardiomyopathy and conduction defects, including complete heart block. Patients may have a cardiac pacemaker in situ. Arrhythmias are common, particularly during anaesthesia, and may result in cardiac failure. Careful monitoring is essential.
- *Muscle spasm*. This may be provoked by administration of depolarizing muscle relaxants or anticholinesterases; succinylcholine and neostigmine should thus be avoided. The spasm is not abolished by non-depolarizing relaxants.
- *Gastrointestinal*. Oesophageal dysmotility may predispose to regurgitation and aspiration.

PSYCHIATRIC DISEASE

There are several considerations in the anaesthetic management of patients with psychiatric disease:

- Psychiatric patients are frequently depressed, with little understanding of, or interest in anaesthesia.
- Patients are receiving a variety of medications with potential for serious drug interactions with anaesthetic agents.
- Patients may have associated pathology as a result of drug and/or alcohol abuse.
- Repeated anaesthetics are required for electroconvulsive therapy.

ELECTROCONVULSIVE THERAPY

Electroconvulsive therapy (ECT) involves application of an electrical stimulus to the patient's head with the intention of inducing seizure activity. It is a successful treatment for severe depression and some other psychiatric conditions. Anaesthesia is given to render the procedure safe and acceptable. However, it is important that seizure induction and duration are not compromised by the anaesthetic agents such that ECT is ineffective.

Seizure activity dramatically increases cerebral oxygen consumption, associated with an increase in intracranial pressure. Autonomic activation with an initial parasympathetic followed by sympathetic stimulation occurs. This results in an initial bradycardia followed by tachycardia and hypertension. Myocardial ischaemia may result, in susceptible individuals.

Anaesthesia

Preoperative assessment

- Cardiorespiratory function must be assessed in the light of the autonomic effects described.
- Previous anaesthetic records – common in this group.
- Antidepressants with anticholinergic effects slow gastric emptying so that an adequate fasting time (8 h) is important in this group. However, patient reports of fasting time may be unreliable.

Anaesthetic management

- Premedication is not usually given as it may influence seizure activity and prolong recovery time unnecessarily.
- Anaesthesia is induced, usually with either etomidate or propofol. The use of propofol is uncertain because, although it provides suitable anaesthesia, it may impair seizure activity.

- A short-acting muscle relaxant is used to prevent trauma caused by seizure activity, and succinylcholine is the most frequently used agent.
- Hyperventilation by bag and mask before seizure induction lowers the seizure threshold and prolongs duration, whilst ventilation continued in the postictal phase avoids desaturation.

ECT is frequently undertaken in isolated units. However, the availability of monitoring, anaesthetic assistance and recovery facilities should be of an equivalent standard to those required for surgical patients.

Drug interactions

In general, it is usually more likely that a patient may be harmed by discontinuing long-term medications than by continuing them with the risk of drug-related complications. This is provided that potential complications are recognized and the anaesthetic technique is tailored to avoid detrimental interactions. Traditionally, it is recommended that monoamine oxidase inhibitors (MAOIs) are discontinued 2 weeks before surgery. However, it is recognized that since this group of drugs is reserved for patients who have failed on other therapy or have particularly severe symptoms it may be preferable to continue treatment. Stopping MAOIs early is not an option in the emergency situation. There is also a risk of precipitating unpleasant withdrawal symptoms if any antidepressants are discontinued acutely.

Tricyclic antidepressants

Tricyclic antidepressants inhibit reuptake of norepinephrine into the presynaptic nerve terminals, e.g. amitriptyline, dothiepin. These drugs have the following side-effects:

- anticholinergic – dry mouth, constipation, delayed gastric emptying, urinary retention
- arrhythmias and heart block, postural hypotension, which may occur during anaesthesia
- sedation
- the hypertensive response to direct acting sympathomimetics is increased
- increased risk of CNS toxicity with tramadol

Monoamine oxidase inhibitors

- MAOIs inhibit intraneuronal metabolism of sympathomimetic amines, e.g. phenelzine, tranylcypromine.
- Tyramine (norepinephrine precursor) precipitates hypertensive crises ('cheese reaction').

- They inhibit metabolism of indirect-acting sympathomimetic amines, resulting in severe hypertension if these drugs are given concurrently.
- CNS excitation occurs with pethidine: agitation, hypertension, convulsions and hyperthermia. Other opioids appear to be safe although excessive sedation has been described.

Selective serotonin reuptake inhibitors

They selectively inhibit serotonin reuptake, e.g. fluoxetine, sertraline. They have less cardiac and anticholinergic effects than tricyclic antidepressants and may cause CNS toxicity in conjunction with tramadol.

Phenothiazines

This is a broad group of drugs and their therapeutic and side-effects vary considerably, e.g. chlorpromazine, thioridazine, prochlorperazine:

- antipsychotic, antiemetic
- sedation, extrapyramidal effects, antimuscarinic effects, antihistamine, α-adrenoceptor blockade, inhibition of normal temperature regulation
- drug interactions are generally related to enhanced effects such as excess sedation, hypotension and anticholinergic actions.

Lithium

Lithium inhibits release and increases reuptake of norepinephrine:

- lithium is used to treat manic states
- lithium acts as a sodium ion, and may potentiate muscle relaxants
- it is renally excreted, and toxicity is enhanced by hyponatraemia where lithium is conserved along with sodium
- its toxic effects include tremor, ataxia, nystagmus, renal impairment and convulsions
- it is recommended that lithium is discontinued 24 h before major surgery.

CONNECTIVE TISSUE DISORDERS

RHEUMATOID ARTHRITIS

Rheumatoid arthritis is by far the most common connective tissue disorder; it is a multisystem disease, with several implications for anaesthesia which must be considered at the time of preoperative assessment.

Airway problems

The arthritic process may involve the temporomandibular joints, rendering laryngoscopy and intubation difficult. The cervical spine may be fixed or subluxed, and thus unstable, especially when the patient is anaesthetized and paralysed. Cricoarytenoid involvement should be suspected if hoarseness or stridor is present.

Respiratory function

Costochondral involvement causes a restrictive defect with reduced vital capacity. Pulmonary involvement with interstitial fibrosis produces ventilation/perfusion ($\dot{V}/\dot{Q}$) abnormalities, a diffusion defect and thus hypoxaemia.

Cardiovascular system

Endocardial and myocardial involvement may occur. Coronary arteritis, conduction defects and peripheral arteritis are other uncommon features. Immobility caused by arthritis may make assessment of cardiorespiratory function difficult.

Anaemia

A chronic anaemia, hypo- or normochromic, but refractory to iron, occurs. Preoperative transfusion to a haemoglobin concentration of approximately 10g dL^{-1} is advisable before major surgery. Treatment with salicylates or other NSAIDs may cause gastrointestinal blood loss.

Renal function

Renal impairment, or nephrotic syndrome, may occur as a result of amyloidosis or drug treatment. NSAIDs should be used with caution in the perioperative period.

Steroid therapy

Many patients are receiving long-term steroid therapy and require augmented steroid cover for the perioperative period (see p. 471). They are more vulnerable to postoperative infection.

Routine preoperative investigation

This should include full blood count, serum urea and electrolyte concentrations, chest X-ray, cervical spine X-ray and ECG. Other investigations, e.g. pulmonary function tests, may be required in some instances.

Conduct of anaesthesia

Particular care should be taken with venepuncture and placing of i.v. infusions because of atrophy of skin and subcutaneous tissues and fragility of veins. Careful positioning of the patient on the operating table is required because these patients may have multiple joint involvement. Padding may be required to prevent pressure sores.

The anaesthetist should be prepared for a difficult intubation; spinal, epidural or regional techniques are useful for many limb or lower abdominal operations because they obviate the need for tracheal intubation. Where intubation is essential, an awake fibreoptic-assisted intubation is often the technique of choice.

OTHER CONNECTIVE TISSUE DISEASES

Implications for the anaesthetist are similar to those associated with rheumatoid arthritis. Some particular features may, however, be more prominent, e.g. vasculitis, including cerebral vasculitis, glomerulonephritis, pulmonary fibrosis, or peri- or myocarditis. Steroid and immunosuppressive therapy are other potential problems.

Scleroderma

Scleroderma (systemic sclerosis) is particularly associated with restricted mouth opening, lower oesophageal involvement with increased risk of regurgitation, pulmonary involvement, renal failure, steroid therapy and peripheral vascular disease.

Systemic lupus erythematosus

Anaemia, renal and respiratory involvement may be severe. Cardiac involvement may include mitral valve disease. Cerebral vasculitis may occur. Steroid therapy is usual.

Ankylosing spondylitis

The rigid spine makes intubation difficult, and spinal and epidural anaesthesia may be technically impossible. Awake fibreoptic-assisted intubation is often required for airway control and may be difficult. Costovertebral joint involvement restricts chest expansion. Postoperative ventilatory support may be required.

Marfan's syndrome

This is a disorder of connective tissue of autosomal dominant inheritance, which is characterized by long, thin extremities, high arched palate, lens subluxation and aortic and mitral regurgitation. Regurgitation may be severe, and the valve lesions may be complicated by infective endocarditis. Antibiotic cover is necessary for dental and other surgical procedures.

NUTRITIONAL PROBLEMS

OBESITY

Obesity poses several problems to the anaesthetist and surgeon.

Cardiovascular function

Obesity is associated with increased blood volume, increased cardiac work, hypertension and cardiomegaly. Atherosclerosis and coronary artery disease are common. Diabetes mellitus may coexist.

Respiratory function

Vital capacity and FRC are decreased. Closing volume is increased. As a result, increased shunting occurs through underventilated, dependent lung regions, with consequent hypoxaemia. These changes, brought about by abdominal splinting of the diaphragm, are accentuated in the supine, Trendelenburg and lithotomy positions. Total thoracic compliance is decreased, the work of breathing increased, and increased oxygen consumption and carbon dioxide production cause hyperventilation.

Other factors

There may be difficulty in cannulating a vein, and arterial pressure measurement may be inaccurate unless the appropriate size of cuff is used. Direct arterial measurement is often preferable. Assessment of volume state is generally more difficult. Surgery is technically more difficult, with heavy blood loss and increased incidences of wound infection and wound dehiscence. Hiatus hernia with risk of regurgitation is more common, and maintenance of the airway and tracheal intubation may be more difficult.

Obese patients require careful preoperative respiratory and cardiovascular assessment (see Ch. 15). The inspired oxygen fraction should be increased and positive end-expiratory pressure (PEEP) applied. to maintain a satisfactory S_pO_2. Fluid balance should be monitored carefully. Elective postoperative artificial ventilation should be considered, especially after abdominal surgery. Pulmonary, thromboembolic and wound complications are more common, and appropriate prophylactic measures and/or early recognition and treatment are important.

PICKWICKIAN SYNDROME

Pickwickian syndrome is characterized by a combination of obesity, episodic somnolence and hypoventilation with cyanosis, polycythaemia, pulmonary hypertension and right ventricular failure. Avoidance of hypoxaemia is important, and elective postoperative ventilation may be necessary, especially after abdominal surgery.

MALNUTRITION

As a result of persistent anorexia, dysphagia or vomiting, malnourished patients may have severe depletion of fluid and electrolytes. Anaemia and hypoproteinaemia are common. The anaemia may result from iron, vitamin B_{12} or folate deficiency, and if megaloblastic in nature, it may be associated with thrombocytopenia.

Preoperative correction of fluid and electrolyte deficits is required, with CVP monitoring in severe cases. Infusion of albumin may be advisable in some instances to raise the colloid osmotic pressure. A multivitamin preparation should be administered in view of probable thiamine deficiency. Induction agents should be administered carefully to avoid hypotension, while smaller doses of relaxants are required.

ANAESTHETIC CONSIDERATIONS IN THE ELDERLY

With a steady increase in life expectancy, there is an associated increase in the need for surgery and anaesthesia in increasing numbers of elderly people.

The normal ageing process is associated with progressive loss of functional reserve in several vital organ systems, so that an elderly patient may be unable to increase functional capacity adequately to cope with the stress of major surgery. Several other factors increase the risk for elderly patients undergoing anaesthesia and surgery:

- associated comorbidity
- concomitant drug therapy
- increased sensitivity to many drugs

- impaired drug metabolism
- nutritional impairment.

ORGAN SYSTEM CHANGES

Central nervous system

- autonomic dysfunction, leading to attenuated baroreceptor reflexes and susceptibility to hypotension, impaired temperature regulation and impaired gut motility
- cognitive impairment, resulting in a reduced capacity to cope with new situations and increased likelihood of confusional states. This effect may be compounded by sensory deprivation associated with impaired hearing and vision

Cardiovascular

- there is a loss of atrial pacemaker cells, resulting in an increasing tendency to develop atrial fibrillation
- maximum heart rate decreases and the elderly are increasingly dependent on increased stroke volume to increase cardiac output. This renders them more sensitive to hypovolaemia and reduced preload
- peripheral vascular resistance is increased as a result of loss of blood vessel compliance, and compensatory left ventricular hypertrophy is common
- catecholamine receptors are downregulated, resulting in a less predictable response to adrenergic agents used therapeutically

Respiratory system

- closing volume increases and encroaches on tidal volume such that when supine, significant shunting, hypoxaemia and later atelectasis may occur
- obstructive sleep apnoea is more common with associated episodes of desaturation. These episodes may be potentiated by opioid analgesia
- silent regurgitation and aspiration of gastric contents occurs more commonly

Renal

- there is a progressive loss of functioning glomeruli and a resultant reduction in the ability to excrete or conserve sodium and water

ANAESTHETIC CONSIDERATIONS

There is no preferred anaesthetic technique for elderly patients and their management must be tailored to the individual patient in the context of the surgery required.

Conditions limiting mobility such as arthritis and Parkinson's disease make assessment of cardiorespiratory function more difficult. In high-risk situations, dobutamine stress testing may be appropriate for cardiovascular assessment.

Cognitive impairment is associated with reduced cholinergic function and, generally, centrally active anticholinergics should be avoided in the elderly. This includes antiemetics such as cyclizine. The elderly are generally more sensitive to sedative agents, which should be given slowly and titrated to effect. Opioid sensitivity increases with age, so that bolus doses of these agents should be reduced in the elderly and titrated to effect.

The elderly are at increased risk from drug side-effects, e.g. renal compromise and gastrointestinal bleeding with NSAIDs. The elderly are at increased risk of adverse drug interactions because of multiple concurrent therapies. Particular care is required when prescribing. Drug doses must be adjusted where appropriate.

The elderly are less resilient in the face of profound changes in volume status and may require a greater degree of monitoring to effectively guide fluid replacement.

The elderly are also at increased risk of complications such as chest infections and thromboembolic events secondary to prolonged immobilization. Anaesthetic techniques should be used which allow prompt mobilization after surgery, e.g. effective epidural analgesia.

HUMAN IMMUNODEFICIENCY VIRUS

With a steady increase in the prevalence of human immunodeficiency virus (HIV) carriage, there is a commensurate increase in patients who are HIV positive requiring anaesthesia and surgery. This raises issues both for patients and for their carers.

Initial infection with HIV is associated with a high viral load which stimulates an immune reaction that is initially effective in reducing the viral load. HIV replicates in T-helper (CD4) cells. Ten per cent of patients who seroconvert develop aquired immunodeficiency syndrome (AIDS) in the first 2–3 years. The remainder develop it over a median duration of 10 years. Development of AIDS is associated with a reduction of CD4 cells and an increase in viral load.

Transmission of HIV requires a large infecting dose. HIV is present in body fluids and may be transmitted by contamination with body fluids. Of particular relevance to anaesthesia is the risk of transmission via needle stick injury. Wearing gloves reduces the size of the inoculum of virus, and double gloving improves on this further. It is imperative that universal precautions are used in the theatre environment to reduce the risk of blood-borne infection transmission including HIV. Sharps safety is particularly important.

Patient-to-patient transmission via contaminated equipment is also possible and appropriate precautions must be taken to avoid exposure of patients to this risk. Increasingly, a move to single-use-only equipment is being introduced where direct patient contact occurs to avoid the possibility of transmission of infection, including HIV.

In the event of significant exposure to infected body fluids, postexposure prophylaxis should be given. The local occupational health department and/or the local infectious diseases unit should be contacted for advice urgently, because treatment should commence within 1–2 h.

With regard to anaesthesia, there is little specific information available:

- general anaesthesia versus regional anaesthesia? General anaesthesia is known to be immunosuppressant so that theoretically a regional technique, e.g. epidural, might be preferable. However, this must be balanced against the risk of pre-existing immunosuppression leading to epidural abscess and the potential to exacerbate pre-existing neuropathy. At present, individual decisions should be made at the discretion of the anaesthetist and the patient involved.
- pain is a common symptom of late HIV infection and AIDS, and pain should be assessed and treated as part of the patient's perioperative management.
- drug interactions may occur with antiretroviral agents; for example, the protease inhibitors inhibit cytochrome P450, resulting in reduced metabolism of many drugs including fentanyl and benzodiazepines. Conversely, non-nucleoside reverse transcriptase inhibitors induce cytochrome P450. Patients with HIV infection are usually receiving a combination of three agents so that interactions may be complex.

MYELOMA

This neoplastic condition affects plasma cells and has several features of significance to the anaesthetist:

- widespread skeletal destruction occurs and careful handling of the patient on the operating table is essential. Pathological fractures are common
- bone pain may be severe and often requires large doses of analgesics
- hypercalcaemia occurs as a result of bony destruction and may precipitate renal failure.
- chronic renal failure may also result from direct nephrotoxicity
- anaemia is almost invariable, and preoperative blood transfusion is often necessary
- during cytotoxic therapy, thrombocytopenia is common
- patients are liable to infection, including chest infection, especially during chemotherapy
- increased plasma immunoglobulin concentrations may increase blood viscosity, predisposing to arterial and venous thrombosis. Drug binding may be affected
- neurological manifestations include spinal cord and nerve root compression.

PORPHYRIA

The porphyrias are an inherited group of disorders of porphyrin metabolism characterized by increased activity of D-aminolaevulinic acid synthetase with excessive production of porphyrins or their precursors. In the UK, acute intermittent porphyria is the most common type. It is characterized by acute attacks which may arise spontaneously or be precipitated by infection, starvation, pregnancy or administration of some drugs. Inheritance is Mendelian dominant and thus patients with a family history of porphyria require further investigation. Clinical features include the following:

- gastrointestinal – abdominal pain and tenderness, vomiting, constipation and occasionally diarrhoea
- neurological – a motor and sensory peripheral neuropathy is common. It may involve bulbar and respiratory muscles. Epileptic fits and psychological disturbance may occur
- cardiovascular – hypertension and tachycardia often occur during the attacks. Hypotension has also been reported
- fever and leucocytosis occur in 25–30% of patients.

Drugs which provoke the attack include alcohol, barbiturates, chlordiazepoxide, steroid hormones, chlorpropamide, pentazocine, phenytoin and sulphonamides.

Anaesthesia in such patients is directed to avoiding drugs which may provoke attacks. Induction with propofol, followed by muscle relaxation with succinylcholine or vecuronium, ventilation with nitrous oxide, and oxygen and analgesic supplementation with morphine or fentanyl is satisfactory (Table 23.10). If fits occur, diazepam is a suitable anticonvulsant, while chlorpromazine, promethazine or promazine are suitable sedatives.

FURTHER READING

Avidan M S, Jones N, Pozniak A L 2000 The implications of HIV for the anaesthetist and the intensivist. Anaesthesia 55: 344–354

Benumof J L (ed) 1998 Anesthesia and uncommon diseases, 4th edn. WB Saunders, Philadelphia

British Journal of Anaesthesia 2004 Postgraduate educational issue, cardiovascular disease in anaesthesia and critical care. Oxford University Press, Oxford

Table 23.10 Safety of drugs commonly used in clinical anaesthesia for patients with acute porphyrias

Drug group							
Intravenous induction agents	Propofol	PS	Ketamine	C	Barbiturates	U
	Midazolam	PS			Etomidate	PU
Inhalation agents	Nitrous oxide	S	Isoflurane	ND	Enflurane	PU
Muscle relaxants	Succinylcholine	S	Atracurium	ND		
	Vecuronium	PS	Pancuronium	C		
Neuromuscular blockade reversal	Atropine	S	Glycopyrronium	ND		
	Neostigmine	S				
Local anaesthetics			Lidocaine	C		
			Prilocaine	C		
			Bupivacaine	C		
Analgesics	Morphine	S	Alfentanil	ND		
	Fentanyl	S				
	Buprenorphine	S				
	Naloxone	PS				
	Paracetamol	S				
Anxiolytics	Temazepam	S	Diazepam	C	All other benzodiazepines	U
	Lorazepam	PS				
	Phenothiazines	S				
Antiarrhythmics	Beta-blockers	S			Verapamil	U
					Nifedipine	U
					Diltiazem	U
Other cardiovascular drugs	Epinephrine	S	Beta-agonists	ND		
	Phentolamine	S	Alpha-agonists	ND		
Bronchodilators	Corticosteroids	PS			Aminophylline	U
	Salbutamol	S				
Gastric– for caesarean section	Metoclopramide	PS	Ranitidine	C	Cimetidine	PU
	Domperidone	S				

PS, possibly safe; S, safe; C, contentious; ND, no data; U, unsafe; PU, probably unsafe.

British National Formulary 51st edn, 2006 British Medical Association and Royal Pharmaceutical Society of Great Britain, London.

Chassot P G, Delabays A, Spahn D R 2002 Preoperative evaluation of patients with, or at risk of, coronary artery disease undergoing non-cardiac surgery. British Journal of Anaesthesia 89: 747–759

Eagle K A, Berger P B, Calkins H et al 2002 ACC/AHA guidelines for perioperative cardiovascular evaluation for noncardiac surgery – executive summary: a report of the American College of Cardiology/American Heart Association Task Force on Practice Guidelines. Journal of the American College of Cardiology 39: 542–553

McAnulty G R, Robertshaw H J, Hall G M 2000 Anaesthetic management of patients with diabetes mellitus. British Journal of Anaesthesia 85: 80–90

Miller R D 2005 Miller's Anesthesia, 6th edn. Elsevier, London

Nicholson G, Pereira A C, Hall G M 2002 Parkinson's disease and anaesthesia. British Journal of Anaesthesia 89: 904–916

Poldermans D, Boersma E, Bax J J et al 1999 The effect of bisoprolol on perioperative mortality and myocardial infarction in high-risk patients undergoing vascular surgery. New England Journal of Medicine 341:1789–1794

Priebe H J 2000 The aged cardiovascular risk patient. British Journal of Anaesthesia 85: 763–778

Stoelting R K, Dierdorf S R 1993 Anaesthesia and co-existing disease, 3rd edn. Churchill Livingstone, London

24 Postoperative care

In modern anaesthetic practice, the patient is monitored and supervised closely and continuously during induction and throughout the operative procedure. However, many problems associated with anaesthesia and surgery may occur in the immediate postoperative period, and it is essential that supervision by adequately trained and experienced personnel is continued during the recovery period. In addition, some major and minor complications of anaesthesia and surgery may occur at any time in the first few days after operation.

THE EARLY RECOVERY PERIOD

Most hospitals have a recovery ward in close proximity to the operating theatre suite (see Ch. 14). The Association of Anaesthetists of Great Britain and Ireland (AAGBI) recommends that fully staffed recovery facilities must be available at all times in hospitals with an emergency surgical service. Some anaesthetizing locations (e.g. the X-ray department) may not have a recovery ward. This section describes common problems which occur in the immediate postoperative period and refers specifically to their management in a recovery ward; however, the same principles are applicable to recovery in other locations.

The recovery period starts as soon as the patient leaves the operating table and the direct supervision of the anaesthetist. All the complications described below may occur at any time, including the period of transfer from operating theatre to recovery ward; in some operating theatre suites, the transfer to the recovery ward may last for several minutes, and it is essential that the standard of observation does not diminish during the journey. The patient must be supervised and monitored closely *at all times*.

SYSTEMS AFFECTED

Central nervous system

Consciousness may not return for several minutes after the end of general anaesthesia and may be impaired for a longer period of time. During this period, a patent airway must be maintained. There is a risk of aspiration into the lungs of any material, e.g. gastric content or blood, which is present in the pharynx. Consciousness may also be depressed in patients who have received sedation to facilitate endoscopy or regional anaesthesia.

Excitement and confusion may occur during recovery and may result in injury. Pain may be severe if long-acting analgesics have not been given during surgery.

Cardiovascular system

Peripheral resistance and cardiac output may be reduced because of residual effects of anaesthetic drugs in the absence of surgical stimulation. Hypovolaemia may be present because of inadequate fluid replacement during surgery, continued bleeding postoperatively or expansion of capacitance of the vascular system as a result of rewarming. Cardiac output may also be reduced as a result of arrhythmias or pre-existing disease. Hypertension may occur as a result of increased sympathoadrenal activity after restoration of consciousness, especially if analgesia is inadequate.

Respiratory system

Hypoventilation occurs commonly, usually as a result of residual effects of anaesthetic drugs or incomplete antagonism of neuromuscular blocking drugs. Hypoxaemia may result from hypoventilation, ventilation/perfusion imbalance or increased oxygen consumption produced by restlessness or shivering.

Gastrointestinal

Nausea and vomiting are common in the immediate postoperative period.

STAFF, EQUIPMENT AND MONITORING

The recovery ward should be staffed by trained and experienced nurses. One nurse must remain with each patient at all times until consciousness and airway reflexes return. The responsibility for the patient's welfare remains with the anaesthetist. Ideally, an anaesthetist should be available immediately to treat complications detected by the nursing staff in the recovery ward.

The patient is nursed in a bed if a prolonged stay is anticipated, but more commonly on a trolley (Fig. 24.1). All beds and trolleys must have the facility to be tipped head-down. Suction apparatus, including catheters, an oxygen supply with appropriate face mask, a self-inflating resuscitation bag and anaesthetic mask, a pulse oximeter and an automated oscillometer must be available for each patient. In addition, there should be a complete range of resuscitation equipment within the recovery area; this includes an anaesthetic machine, a range of laryngoscopes, tracheal tubes, bougies, intravenous (i.v.) cannulae, fluids, emergency drugs, electrocardiogram (ECG) monitor and defibrillator. Facilities for cricothyroid cannulation, e.g. minitracheotomy set, and for formal tracheostomy should also be available.

A wide range of drugs should be stored in the recovery area for the treatment of common complications and also emergency events (Table 24.1).

On arrival in the recovery ward, the anaesthetist should give the nurse full details of pre-existing medical problems, surgical procedure, anaesthetic technique, drugs, regional blocks, fluids, blood loss/replacement, any untoward events and any anticipated problems during recovery. All patients should be monitored by measurement of pulse rate, arterial pressure, arterial oxygen saturation and respiratory rate and by assessment of level of consciousness, peripheral circulation and adequacy of ventilation. Depending on the nature of work undertaken in the theatre suite, a proportion of bed stations should have the facility for monitoring ECG, systemic and pulmonary arterial pressures and central venous pressure (CVP) continuously; this may be required in high-risk

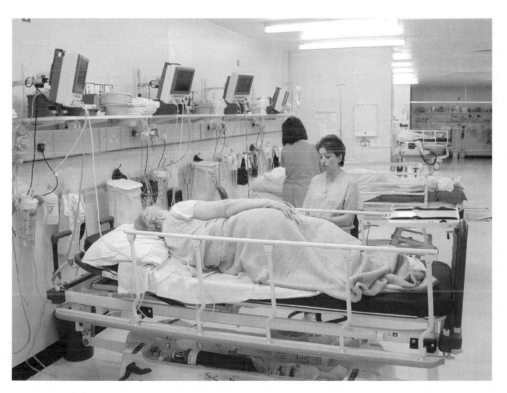

Fig. 24.1
Part of a recovery ward. Many patients are nursed on a trolley, but a bed is used for those who have undergone major surgery and those who need to stay for several hours.

Table 24.1 Drugs which should be available in the recovery room

Adenosine	Digoxin	Isoprenaline (isoproterenol)	Pethidine
Alfentanil	Dobutamine	Ketamine	Phentolamine
Aminophylline	Dopamine	Ketorolac	Phenytoin
Antibiotics	Doxapram	Labetalol	Phytomenadione
Aprotinin	Edrophonium	Lidocaine	Potassium chloride
Aspirin	Ephedrine	Metaraminol	Procainamide
Atracurium	Epinephrine	Methoxamine	Prochlorperazine
Atropine	Fentanyl	Methylprednisolone	Propranolol
Bupivacaine	Flumazenil	Metoclopramide	Protamine
Calcium chloride	Furosemide	Midazolam	Ranitidine
Calcium gluconate	Glucose	Morphine	Salbutamol
Calcium heparin	Glyceryl trinitrate	Naloxone	Sodium citrate
Chlorphenamine (chlorpheniramine)	Glycopyrronium	Neostigmine	Sodium nitroprusside
Co-proxamol	Hyaluronidase	Nifedipine	Succinylcholine
Cyclizine	Hydralazine	Norepinephrine	Tranexamic acid
Dexamethasone	Hydrocortisone	Ondansetron	Verapamil
Diazepam	Hyoscine	Papaverine	
Diclofenac	Insulin	Paracetamol	

patients or those who have undergone major surgery. Capnography should be available for use in patients who require tracheal intubation. At least one mechanical ventilator should be available, although more may be required depending on the workload. Urine output should be measured routinely in patients who have undergone major surgery. Wounds and surgical drains should be inspected regularly for signs of bleeding.

A record should be made of pulse rate, arterial pressure and arterial oxygen saturation, respiratory rate, level of consciousness, pain score, sensory level (if regional anaesthesia has been used), and any other relevant information (such as complications, and drug and fluid administration) obtained while the patient is in the recovery area. In most units, recordings of physiological measurements are made every 5 min, at least until consciousness has returned.

The patient should not be discharged to the surgical ward until the following criteria have been met:

- Consciousness has returned fully, a patent airway can be maintained and protective reflexes are present.
- Ventilation and oxygenation are satisfactory.
- The cardiovascular system is stable with no unexplained cardiac irregularity or persistent bleeding. Consecutive measurements of pulse rate and arterial pressure should approximate to the patient's normal preoperative values or be at an acceptable level commensurate with the planned postoperative care. Peripheral perfusion should be adequate.
- Pain and nausea are controlled.
- Temperature is within acceptable limits.

High-risk patients or those who have undergone major surgery should stay in the recovery ward for up to 24 h. If this is not feasible, or if instability persists for longer than 24 h, the patient should be transferred to a high-dependency or intensive care unit. The level of monitoring and care during transfer should be the same as that in the recovery room.

Although the recovery room nurse undertakes the direct care of the patient, the responsibility for the patient remains with the anaesthetist. Patients must only be discharged to the ward with the anaesthetist's consent.

The remainder of this chapter is devoted to the diagnosis and management of common problems which occur in the postoperative period. Some of these occur most frequently in the immediate recovery period, while others may occur at any time during the patient's convalescence from surgery. Some surgical procedures are associated with specific complications.

CENTRAL NERVOUS SYSTEM

CONSCIOUS LEVEL

Many patients are unconscious on arrival in the recovery ward because of residual effects of anaesthetic drugs. The duration of impaired consciousness depends on:

- *The drugs used.* Recovery of consciousness may be delayed if the following agents have been used:
  - volatile anaesthetics with a high blood/gas solubility coefficient
  - barbiturates, particularly if large total doses have been given
  - benzodiazepines
  - opioids with a long duration of action, including large doses of fentanyl.
- *The timing of drug use.* Delayed recovery may occur if a long-acting i.v. anaesthetic or analgesic drug has been given towards the end of the procedure, or if the more soluble volatile agents have been continued until the end of surgery.
- *Pain.* The presence of pain speeds recovery of consciousness. Recovery may be delayed after minor procedures or if potent analgesia has been provided by administration of opioids or by regional anaesthesia.

Undue prolongation of unconsciousness should not be attributed to these factors alone. Other causes should be considered, as their early recognition may prevent serious sequelae. These are:

- hypoxaemia – in the presence of an adequate circulation, coma occurs only if profound hypoxaemia is present
- hypercapnia – unconsciousness may occur if arterial carbon dioxide tension ($P_a\text{CO}_2$) exceeds 9–10 kPa
- hypotension
- hypothermia.

Hypoglycaemia

This occurs most commonly in diabetic patients treated with oral hypoglycaemic agents or insulin and an inadequate intake of glucose. The perioperative management of the diabetic patient is discussed in Chapter 23.

Hyperglycaemia

Hyperglycaemia in known diabetics may occur as a result of inadequate provision of insulin or injudicious infusion of glucose. However, coma is unusual in acute hyperglycaemia. Undiagnosed diabetics with hyperglycaemia and ketosis may present for surgery because of abdominal pain, and prolonged postoperative coma may occur unless the metabolic defect is diagnosed and treated.

Cerebral pathology

Consciousness may be impaired by functional or structural cerebral damage. Possible causes include:

- episodes of cerebral ischaemia (e.g. carotid artery surgery, profound hypotension) or hypoxia during anaesthesia
- intracranial haemorrhage, thrombosis or infarction – these may occur fortuitously or may have been associated with intraoperative hypertension, hypotension or arrhythmias
- pre-existing cerebral lesions, e.g. tumour, trauma – anaesthetic techniques which increase intracranial pressure are likely to impair cerebral function
- epilepsy – convulsions may have been masked by anaesthesia or neuromuscular blocking drugs
- air embolism
- intracranial spread of local anaesthetic solution after subarachnoid injection – introduction into the subarachnoid space may be accidental, e.g. during epidural block or, rarely, interscalene brachial plexus block; unconsciousness is almost always accompanied by apnoea.

Other causes

- *Hypo-osmolar or TURP syndrome.* This results most commonly from absorption of water from the bladder during transurethral resection of the prostate (TURP). The investigation and management of this condition are described on page 422.
- *Hypothyroidism.*
- *Hepatic or renal failure.*

CONFUSION AND AGITATION

These occur occasionally during emergence from an otherwise uncomplicated anaesthetic. They are more common in elderly patients, particularly if hyoscine has been given as a premedicant. Atropine also crosses the blood–brain barrier and may result in the central anticholinergic syndrome, characterized by restlessness and confusion, together with obvious antimuscarinic effects. Glycopyrronium does not cross the blood–brain barrier and is preferable to atropine for antagonism of the muscarinic effects of neostigmine in elderly patients; in addition to its lack of central effects, it produces less tachycardia and antagonizes the effects of neostigmine for a longer period.

All the factors listed above as causes of prolonged coma may also result in confusion and agitation. Pain may also contribute, although it is seldom responsible alone. Emergence delirium is associated particularly with the use of ketamine and may occur after the administration of etomidate. Septicaemia may result in confusion, as may distension of the stomach or bladder.

A lightly sedated, conscious patient with inadequate antagonism of neuromuscular blocking drugs may appear to the inexperienced observer to be agitated and confused. Movements are uncoordinated. The condition is distressing to the patient and is an indication of a poor anaesthetic technique. It should never be allowed to develop.

PAIN

This subject is discussed fully in Chapter 25. The effects of pain should be differentiated from those of hypercapnia and hypovolaemia (Table 24.2).

RESPIRATORY SYSTEM

HYPOVENTILATION

Common causes of hypoventilation in the immediate postoperative period are listed in Table 24.3. Hypoventilation results in an increase in $P_a\text{CO}_2$ (Fig. 24.2) and a decrease in alveolar oxygen tension ($P_A\text{O}_2$), and thus hypoxaemia, which may be corrected by increasing the inspired concentration of oxygen. The risk factors for developing hypoventilation include:

- old age
- obesity

Table 24.2   Common problems in the recovery room: symptoms and signs

	Pain	Hypercapnia	Hypovolaemia
Conscious level	May be restless May be quiescent if severe pain	Comatose	Restless or quiescent depending on extent of analgesia and residual anaesthesia
Periphery	Vasoconstriction, pallor ± sweating	Warm, flushed with bounding pulse (if normovolaemic)	Vasoconstriction, pallor ± sweating
Heart rate	Tachycardia	Tachycardia	Tachycardia
Arterial pressure	Systolic ↑ Diastolic ↑ Pulse pressure normal	Systolic ↑ Diastolic ↑↓ Pulse pressure ↑	Systolic and diastolic may be normal until marked reduction in stroke volume, then ↓ Pulse pressure ↓

Table 24.3   Causes of postoperative hypoventilation

Factors affecting airway	Factors affecting ventilatory drive	Peripheral factors
Upper airway obstruction	Respiratory depressant drugs	Muscle weakness
Tongue	Preoperative CNS pathology	Residual neuromuscular block
Laryngospasm	Intra- or postoperative cerebrovascular accident	Preoperative neuromuscular disease
Oedema	Hypothermia	Electrolyte abnormalities
Foreign body	Recent hyperventilation ($P_a\text{CO}_2$ low)	Pain
Tumour		Abdominal distension
Bronchospasm		Obesity
		Tight dressings
		Pneumo-/haemothorax

CNS, central nervous system; $P_a\text{CO}_2$, arterial carbon dioxide tension.

- prolonged surgical operations
- opioids
- upper abdominal or thoracic surgery.

Airway obstruction

Airway obstruction caused by the tongue, by indrawing of the pharyngeal muscles or by blood or secre-

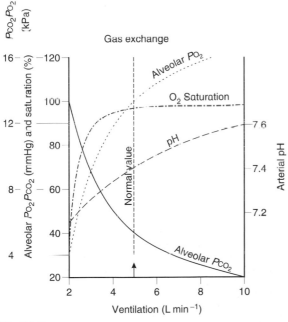

Fig. 24.2
Gas exchange during hypoventilation. Note the relatively rapid increase in alveolar partial pressure of carbon dioxide ($P\text{CO}_2$) compared with the slow decrease in arterial oxygen saturation. $P\text{O}_2$, partial pressure of oxygen.

tions in the pharynx is ameliorated by placing the patient in the lateral or recovery position (see Fig. 16.7). This position should be used for all unconscious patients who have undergone oral or ear, nose and throat surgery, and for patients at risk of gastric aspiration.

Partial obstruction of the airway is characterized by noisy ventilation. As the obstruction increases, tracheal tug and indrawing of the supraclavicular area occur during inspiration. Total obstruction is signalled by absent sounds of breathing and paradoxical movement of the chest wall and abdomen.

In many patients, a clear airway is maintained only by displacing the mandible anteriorly and extending the head. In some, it is necessary also to insert an oropharyngeal airway, although this may stimulate coughing, gagging and laryngospasm during recovery of consciousness. A nasopharyngeal airway is often tolerated better, but there is a risk of causing haemorrhage from the nasopharyngeal mucosa. Occasionally, insertion of a laryngeal mask airway is necessary to maintain the airway until consciousness has returned fully; very occasionally, tracheal intubation is required.

Blood, oral secretions or regurgitated gastric fluid which have accumulated in the pharynx should be aspirated and the patient placed in the recovery position to allow any further fluid to drain anteriorly.

Foreign bodies, such as dentures (particularly partial dentures) or throat packs, may cause airway obstruction. It may be difficult to maintain a patent airway in an unconscious patient with an oral, pharyngeal or laryngeal tumour.

Obstruction of the upper airway occurs intermittently after recovery from anaesthesia. Obstructive sleep apnoea is common in the postoperative period and may result in decreases of arterial oxyhaemoglobin saturation (S_aO_2) to less than 75%. Episodes occur with the greatest frequency in the first 4 h after anaesthesia and are more common and severe in patients who receive opioids for postoperative analgesia than in those in whom analgesia is provided by a regional technique.

Airway obstruction may result from haemorrhage after surgery to the neck, including thyroid surgery; the wound should be opened urgently, and the haematoma drained. Occasionally, tracheal collapse occurs after thyroidectomy in patients who have developed chondromalacia of the cartilaginous rings of the trachea caused by pressure from a large goitre. Inspiratory stridor may be present or there may be total obstruction during inspiration; the trachea must be reintubated immediately.

Laryngeal spasm

This complication is relatively common after general anaesthesia. In particular, children undergoing oropharyngeal surgery are more at risk. It may be partial or complete and is caused usually by direct stimulation of the cords by secretions or blood, or of the epiglottis by an oropharyngeal airway or laryngeal mask. It may follow extubation of the trachea in the semiconscious patient. It may be difficult to differentiate this condition from airway obstruction caused by the pharyngeal wall; if airway obstruction persists despite implementation of the measures described above, laryngoscopy should be undertaken.

Any obvious foreign material causing laryngospasm should be removed by aspiration, and oxygen 100% administered. If obstruction is complete, positive-pressure ventilation by mask may force some oxygen through the cords to maintain arterial oxygenation until the spasm has subsided; there is a significant risk of inflating the stomach with oxygen during this procedure. If attempts to oxygenate the lungs fail, succinylcholine should be administered, and the lungs ventilated with oxygen when the spasm is relieved. When satisfactory oxygenation has been achieved, it may be advisable to intubate the trachea to reduce the risk of regurgitation of gastric contents, as the stomach may have been inflated with oxygen, and to administer 60–65% nitrous oxide in oxygen to minimize the risk of awareness if the patient regains consciousness before muscle power returns. When the effects of succinylcholine have terminated, oxygen 100% is administered and the trachea is extubated when the patient regains consciousness.

Rarely, laryngeal obstruction occurs after thyroid surgery if both recurrent laryngeal nerves have been traumatized.

Laryngeal oedema

This occurs occasionally after tracheal intubation and may result in severe obstruction, particularly in a child. Treatment depends on the severity of the obstruction; immediate reintubation may be required if obstruction is complete, but partial obstruction may subside if the patient is treated with heated humidified gases. Dexamethasone may hasten resolution of the oedema.

Bronchospasm

This may result from stimulation of the airway by inhaled material. It is commoner in asthmatic or bronchitic patients and in smokers. It may result directly from intrinsic asthma or may be part of an anaphylactic reaction. Several drugs used in anaesthetic practice may precipitate bronchospasm either by a direct effect on bronchial muscle or by releasing histamine; these include barbiturates, morphine, mivacurium and atracurium. Treatment comprises the removal of any predisposing factor and the administration of oxygen and bronchodilators.

Ventilatory drive

There are several possible causes of reduced ventilatory drive during recovery from anaesthesia (see Table 24.3). The presence of intracranial pathology, e.g. tumour, trauma or haemorrhage, may affect ventilatory drive in the postoperative period. Ventilation is reduced in the presence of hypothermia, although it is usually appropriate for the metabolic needs of the body. Hypoventilation occurs in the hypocapnic patient, e.g. after a period of hyperventilation until P_aCO_2 is restored to normal, and in the presence of primary metabolic alkalosis.

The most important cause of reduced ventilatory drive during recovery is the effect of drugs administered by the anaesthetist in the perioperative period. All the volatile and i.v. anaesthetic agents – with the exception of ketamine – depress the respiratory centre; significant concentrations of these drugs remain in the brainstem during the early postoperative period.

All opioid analgesics depress ventilation. With most opioids, the effect is dose-dependent, although the agonist-antagonist agents are claimed to have a ceiling effect. In the majority of patients, opioids do not produce apnoea, but result in decreased ventilatory drive and an increase in P_aCO_2, which plateaus at an elevated value. The elderly are particularly sensitive to drug-induced ventilatory depression. The treatment of postoperative pain begins in the recovery area, often by administration of i.v. opioids by the medical or nursing staff, and ventilation must be monitored carefully after each dose.

Spinal (intrathecal or epidural) opioids, particularly lipid-insoluble agents such as morphine, may produce ventilatory depression some hours after administration. Patients who have received subarachnoid or epidural opioids should remain in the recovery ward or in a high-dependency unit for at least 12 h after administration of the last dose of spinal morphine, or at least 3 h after fentanyl, unless protocols and training programmes for surgical ward nurses have been implemented.

Reduced ventilatory drive is easy to diagnose if the ventilatory rate or tidal volume is clearly reduced. However, lesser degrees of hypoventilation may be difficult to detect, and the signs of moderate hypercapnia, e.g. hypertension and tachycardia, may be masked by the residual effects of anaesthetic agents, or misdiagnosed as pain-induced (see Table 24.2).

Mild hypoventilation is acceptable provided that oxygenation remains adequate; this may easily be achieved by a modest increase in fractional concentration of oxygen (F_IO_2; see below). If ventilatory drive is reduced excessively by opioids, resulting in an increasing P_aCO_2 or delayed recovery of consciousness, naloxone in increments of 1.5–3 µg kg^{-1} should be administered every 2–3 min until improvement occurs. Administration of excessive doses of naloxone reverses the analgesia induced by systemic (but not to the same extent by spinal) opioids; large doses may cause severe hypertension and have been associated with cardiac arrest on rare occasions. The effects of i.v. naloxone last only for 20–30 min; in order to prevent recurrence of reduced ventilation after long-acting opioids, an additional dose (50% of the effective i.v. dose) may be administered intramuscularly or an i.v. infusion commenced.

Peripheral factors

The commonest peripheral factor associated with hypoventilation is residual neuromuscular blockade. This may be exaggerated by disease of the neuromuscular junction, e.g. myasthenia gravis, or by electrolyte disturbances. Inadequate reversal of neuromuscular blockade is usually associated with uncoordinated, jerky movements, although these may occur occasionally during recovery of consciousness in patients with normal neuromuscular function. Measurement of tidal volume is not a reliable guide to adequacy of reversal of neuromuscular blockade; a normal tidal volume may be achieved with only 20% return of diaphragmatic power, but the ability to cough remains severely impaired. If the patient is able to lift the head from the trolley for 5 s or maintain a good hand grip, it is likely that there is sufficient return of neuromuscular function for adequate ventilation and maintenance of the airway. Some more objective means of assessment are listed in Table 24.4, but these require the cooperation of the patient. In the unconscious or uncooperative patient, nerve stimulation (see Ch. 6) provides the best means of assessing neuromuscular function, although there are differences among the non-depolarizing relaxants in the relationship between their actions in the forearm and diaphragm.

If residual non-depolarizing blockade is confirmed, further doses of neostigmine may be administered (with atropine or glycopyrronium) up to a total of 5 mg; in higher doses, neostigmine can worsen neuromuscular function. If the block persists, artificial ventilation must be maintained while the cause is sought.

Factors responsible most commonly for difficulty in antagonism of neuromuscular block include overdosage with muscle relaxant, too short an interval between administration of the drug and the antagonist, hypokalaemia, respiratory or metabolic acidosis, administration of aminoglycoside antibiotics, local anaesthetic agents, diseases affecting neuromuscular transmission and muscle disease.

Delayed elimination of all of the non-depolarizing muscle relaxants (except atracurium and cisatracurium) has been reported, and causes prolonged neuromuscular block. Delayed elimination occurs most frequently in the presence of renal or hepatic insufficiency, or in dehydrated patients with low urine output. Muscle paralysis may recur 30–60 min after administration of neostigmine if elimination of the relaxant is inadequate, even if antagonism appears to be satisfactory initially. A similar phenomenon may occur if acidosis develops, or when patients who have been hypothermic are rewarmed.

Prolonged neuromuscular block after succinylcholine or mivacurium occurs in the presence of atypical plasma cholinesterase or a low concentration of normal

---

Table 24.4 Clinical assessment of the adequacy of antagonism of neuromuscular block

Subjective
Grip strength
Adequate cough

Objective
Ability to sustain head lift for at least 5 s
Ability to produce vital capacity of at least 10 mL kg^{-1}

plasma cholinesterase. Paralysis after succinylcholine may persist for up to 8 h, although in most instances recovery occurs within 20–120 min. Neostigmine should not be administered if prolonged neuromuscular block occurs after administration of succinylcholine.

Artificial ventilation of the lungs must be maintained or resumed in any patient who has inadequate neuromuscular function. Anaesthesia should be provided to prevent awareness; this is achieved most easily with nitrous oxide and a low concentration of a volatile anaesthetic agent.

Hypoventilation may be caused also by restriction of diaphragmatic movement resulting from abdominal distension, obesity, tight dressings or abdominal binders. Pain, particularly from thoracic or upper abdominal wounds, may cause reduced ventilation.

The presence of air or fluid in the pleural cavity may result in hypoventilation. Pneumothorax may occur during intermittent positive-pressure ventilation (IPPV). It is an occasional complication in healthy patients, but is a particular risk in those with chronic obstructive airways disease, especially if bullae are present, and after chest trauma. It may complicate brachial plexus nerve block, central venous cannulation or surgery involving the kidney or neck. Haemothorax may result from chest trauma or central venous cannulation. Hydrothorax may be caused by pleural effusions or inadvertent infusion of fluids through a misplaced central venous catheter. These rapidly remediable causes of hypoventilation are often overlooked.

Treatment

This consists primarily of treatment of the cause. Mild or moderate hypoventilation resulting from residual effects of anaesthetic drugs may respond to a bolus dose or infusion of doxapram. Artificial ventilation should be recommended if severe hypercapnia is present or P_aCO_2 continues to increase, or if the clinical condition of the patient is deteriorating.

HYPOXAEMIA

A functional classification of causes of hypoxaemia in the early recovery period is shown in Table 24.5. An inspired oxygen concentration of less than 21% should never occur, although P_aO_2 is decreased when air is breathed at high altitudes.

Ventilation–perfusion abnormalities

These are the commonest cause of hypoxaemia in the recovery room. Cardiac output and pulmonary arterial pressure may be reduced after general or regional

Table 24.5 Functional classification of the causes of hypoxaemia in the postoperative period

Reduced inspired oxygen concentration
Ventilation–perfusion abnormalities
Shunting
Hypoventilation
Diffusion deficits
Diffusion hypoxia after nitrous oxide anaesthesia

anaesthesia, causing impaired perfusion of some areas of the lungs. Functional residual capacity (FRC) is reduced during and immediately after anaesthesia. Patients who are elderly, obese or those undergoing thoracic or upper abdominal surgery are particularly at risk. The closing capacity may encroach on the tidal breathing range, resulting in reduced ventilation of some lung units, particularly those in dependent alveoli. Thus, the scatter of ventilation/perfusion ($\dot{V}/\dot{Q}$) ratios is increased. Areas of lung with increased ratios constitute physiological dead space. Areas of lung with low $\dot{V}/\dot{Q}$ ratios increase venous admixture which results in hypoxaemia unless the inspired oxygen concentration is increased.

Shunt

Physiological shunt may be increased in the immediate postoperative period if small airways closure has been extreme. Shunting may be present also in patients with pulmonary oedema of any aetiology, or if there is consolidation in the lung. Shunt may be increased in the later postoperative period as a result of retention of secretions and underventilation of the lung bases because of pain; these changes lead to alveolar consolidation and collapse.

Hypoventilation

This has been discussed in detail above. Moderate hypoventilation, with some elevation of P_aCO_2, leads to a modest reduction in P_aO_2 (Fig. 24.2). Obstructive sleep apnoea may produce profound transient but repeated decreases in arterial oxygenation. S_aO_2 may decrease to less than 75%, corresponding to a P_aO_2 of less than 5 kPa (40 mmHg). These repeated episodes of hypoxaemia cause temporary, and possibly permanent, defects in cognitive function in elderly patients

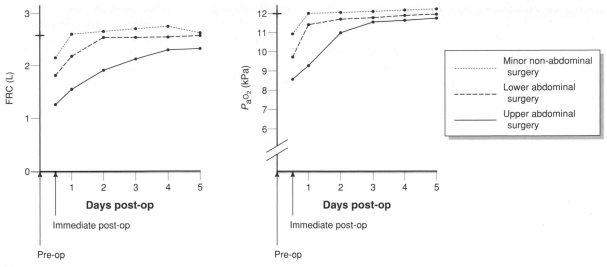

Fig. 24.3
Changes in functional residual capacity (FRC) and arterial oxygen tension (P_aO_2) postoperatively.

and may contribute to perioperative myocardial infarction. Obstructive sleep apnoea is exacerbated by opioid analgesics, and patients who are known to suffer from this condition should be monitored carefully in the postoperative period, preferably in a high-dependency unit. Patients who normally use a continuous positive airways pressure (CPAP) mask to reduce obstructive sleep apnoeic episodes should use the mask at night throughout the postoperative period.

Diffusion defects

Interstitial oedema produced by overtransfusion of fluids or by left ventricular dysfunction may cause hypoxaemia by impairment of oxygen transfer across the alveolar–capillary membrane.

Diffusion hypoxia

Nitrous oxide is 40 times more soluble than nitrogen in blood. When administration of nitrous oxide is discontinued at the end of anaesthesia, nitrous oxide diffuses out of blood into the alveoli in larger volumes than nitrogen diffuses in the opposite direction. Consequently, the alveolar concentrations of other gases are diluted. P_aO_2 is reduced and arterial oxygenation impaired if the patient breathes air; P_aCO_2 decreases as a result of effective alveolar hyperventilation. S_aO_2 is reduced to values as low as 90% for several minutes in normal individuals after breathing 50% nitrous oxide in oxygen. Arterial desaturation is

greater in elderly patients, if higher concentrations of nitrous oxide have been used, or if P_aCO_2 is initially low because of hyperventilation during anaesthesia.

Diffusion hypoxia is avoided by the administration of oxygen for 10 min after discontinuation of nitrous oxide anaesthesia.

Reduced venous oxygen content

Assuming that oxygen consumption remains unchanged, anaemia or reduced cardiac output results in increased oxygen extraction from circulating arterial blood, and consequently in a reduction in mixed venous oxygen content. In the presence of increased $\dot{V}/\dot{Q}$ scatter or intrapulmonary shunt, this causes a variable degree of arterial hypoxaemia. Similarly, if cardiac output remains constant, increased oxygen utilization by the tissues (as may occur during shivering, restlessness or malignant hyperthermia) causes a reduction in mixed venous oxygen content and a worsening of arterial hypoxaemia if any shunt is present.

Tissue hypoxia

Oxygenation of the tissues is a function of arterial oxygenation, oxygen carriage in blood, delivery of blood to the tissues and transfer of oxygen from the blood. It may be impaired by respiratory or cardiovascular dysfunction, by severe anaemia or by a leftward shift of the oxyhaemoglobin dissociation curve (reduced P_{50}).

PULMONARY CHANGES AFTER ABDOMINAL SURGERY

Patients with previously normal lungs suffer impairment of oxygenation for at least 48 h after abdominal surgery. The extent of this impairment is related to the site of operation. It is less marked after lower abdominal surgery, more severe if there has been a large incision in the upper abdomen and worst after thoracoabdominal procedures. In these circumstances, the differences between pre- and postoperative P_aO_2 may be as much as 4 kPa.

Impairment of oxygenation in the postoperative period is related to a reduction in FRC. After induction of anaesthesia, there is an abrupt decrease in FRC. The magnitude of the decrease is similar for anaesthetic techniques in which the patient breathes spontaneously and those in which IPPV is employed. Postoperatively, this decrease is maintained by wound pain, which causes spasm of the expiratory muscles, and abdominal distension, which leads to diaphragmatic splinting. This is also influenced by the site of surgical incision; the greatest reduction follows thoracic or upper abdominal surgery. The supine position also reduces FRC.

The reduction in FRC may lead to closing capacity impinging upon the tidal breathing range. This results in small airways closure during normal tidal ventilation. Gas trapping occurs in the affected airways and subsequent absorption of air may lead to the development of small, discrete areas of atelectasis which are not visible on chest X-ray. This occurs mainly in the dependent parts of the lung and may be demonstrated by CT scan very soon after induction of anaesthesia. The result is an increase in the number of areas of low $\dot{V}/\dot{Q}$ ratio within the lungs. The relationship between changes in FRC and P_aO_2 postoperatively is shown in Figure 24.3.

In most patients, these abnormalities return towards normal by the fifth or sixth postoperative day. However, if the changes have been marked, the areas of low $\dot{V}/\dot{Q}$ ratio may become a focus for infection, particularly in the presence of retained secretions. The following factors contribute to retention of secretions after surgery:

- *Inability to cough*. This results mostly from wound pain. However, excessive sedation may also contribute. Postoperative electrolyte imbalance, especially hypokalaemia or hypophosphataemia, may compound the situation by interfering with muscle function.
- *Suppression of bronchial mucosal ciliary activity*. This results from the use of unhumidified anaesthetic gases.

- *Antisialagogue drugs*. When antisialagogue premedicants have been used, the secretions become more viscid. The dry mucosa itself is more prone to inflammatory reaction. If this occurs, the exudate produced increases the problem still further.
- *Infection*. If pulmonary infection supervenes, impairment of oxygenation may contribute to a lack of cooperation in clearing secretions.

A combination of these factors may result in retention of secretions, leading to areas of visible pulmonary collapse on chest X-ray and an increase in the work of breathing. Ultimately, oxygenation of the blood may become inadequate despite oxygen therapy, or carbon dioxide retention may occur. The sequence of events that culminate in ventilatory failure is shown in Figure 24.4.

Predisposing factors

- *Site of surgery*. Pulmonary complications occur more commonly after upper abdominal or thoracic surgery than after lower abdominal operations.
- *Pre-existing respiratory disease* increases the complication rate. This is particularly so in the presence of concurrent infection or excessive secretions.
- *Smokers* have an increased incidence of pulmonary complications compared with non-smokers.
- *Obesity* is associated with a high incidence of pulmonary complications. Obese patients have a low FRC and increased work of breathing postoperatively.

The anaesthetic technique has little effect on the incidence of postoperative pulmonary complications.

Clinical findings

Collapse of lung units

In patients who develop clinical symptoms, the first signs of atelectasis are usually seen within 24 h of operation. The triad of pyrexia, tachycardia and tachypnoea is often present. Temperature is usually in the range of 38–39°C. There is often a productive cough. If atelectasis is extensive, the patient is cyanosed. On physical examination, localizing signs are uncommon unless the area of involvement is large. Chest X-ray reveals patchy areas of atelectasis.

Pneumonia

Lobar pneumonia is rarely seen postoperatively. Bronchopneumonia is more common, especially in the elderly. The onset of symptoms is not as rapid as in

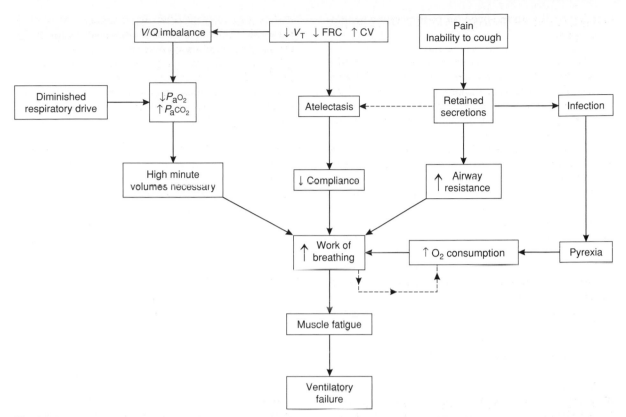

Fig. 24.4

Diagrammatic representation of events that result in postoperative ventilatory failure. V_T, tidal volume; FRC, functional residual capacity; CV, closing volume; V/Q, ventilation/perfusion; P_aO_2, arterial oxygen tension; P_aCO_2, arterial carbon dioxide tension.

atelectasis. There is usually fever and associated tachycardia, with an increase in the ventilatory rate. Physical examination usually reveals areas of consolidation, predominantly at the lung bases, which are evident on chest X-ray.

Treatment

If a pulmonary complication is suspected, a sputum sample should be sent to the laboratory for bacteriological analysis. Appropriate antibiotic therapy may then be started. Intensive physiotherapy should be prescribed in an attempt to remove secretions and re-expand atelectatic areas of the lung.

Patients with pulmonary collapse are usually hypoxaemic, but P_aCO_2 remains normal or may be low as a result of tachypnoea, at least in the early stages. Usually, oxygen in moderate concentrations (30–40%) is sufficient to correct hypoxaemia, but this should be confirmed by blood gas analysis; CPAP given via a tightly fitting face mask is effective in re-expanding the collapsed alveoli and improving the mechanics of

breathing. If the patient fails to respond to these measures, signs of respiratory distress develop. The patient becomes drowsy and ventilation is laboured, with rapid shallow breathing involving the accessory muscles. P_aCO_2 increases and arterial oxygenation deteriorates despite oxygen therapy. The presence of continued deterioration in blood gases is an indication for ventilatory support.

REDUCING PULMONARY COMPLICATIONS

Preoperative

Measures to reduce pulmonary complications should begin preoperatively. Upper and lower respiratory tract infections should be treated before surgery. Dental sepsis and sinus infections should be eradicated. Pre-existing chronic respiratory disorders should be treated so that the patient is in optimal condition before surgery. Spirometry is useful to monitor such treatment, but arterial blood gas analysis is the only assessment which has been demonstrated to correlate well with the need for postoperative ventilatory support. Smoking should be discouraged and weight loss encouraged where indicated. In patients with increased risk factors, heavy premedication should be avoided to ensure minimal ventilatory depression at the end of the procedure.

Intraoperative

At induction, care should be taken not to introduce infection by contaminated equipment. During prolonged procedures, the anaesthetic gases should be humidified. If neuromuscular blocking agents are used, particular care should be taken to ensure that antagonism is adequate.

Postoperative

Analgesia should be optimal to ensure adequate coughing and cooperation during physiotherapy, which should be started as soon as possible after operation.

OXYGEN THERAPY

Hypoxaemia may occur to some degree in any patient during the early recovery period as a result of one or more of the mechanisms described above. Consequently, *all* patients should receive additional oxygen for the first 10 min after general anaesthesia has been discontinued. Oxygen therapy should be continued for a longer period in the presence of any of the conditions listed in Table 24.6.

Oxygen therapy is particularly beneficial in treating hypoxaemia caused by hypoventilation; P_aO_2 is substantially increased by a modest increase in F_1O_2. In contrast, higher concentrations are required in the presence of a shunt fraction in excess of 0.1–0.15 (Fig. 24.5). Known concentrations of oxygen may be administered by a tightly fitting mask supplied with metered flows of air and oxygen via either an anaesthetic breathing system or a CPAP system. In small children, an oxygen tent or headbox may be used. However, oxygen is usually administered by less cumbersome disposable equipment.

Oxygen therapy devices

The characteristics of oxygen face masks depend predominantly on their volume, the flow rate of gas supplied and the presence of holes in the side of the mask. If no gas is supplied, face masks act as increased dead space and result in hypercapnia unless minute volume is increased; the increase in dead space is proportional

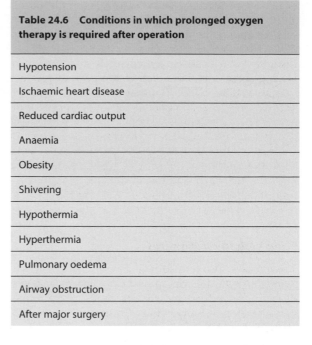

Table 24.6   Conditions in which prolonged oxygen therapy is required after operation
Hypotension
Ischaemic heart disease
Reduced cardiac output
Anaemia
Obesity
Shivering
Hypothermia
Hyperthermia
Pulmonary oedema
Airway obstruction
After major surgery

to the volume of the mask. If the mask contains holes, air is entrained readily during inspiration.

When oxygen is supplied, the inspired oxygen concentration increases, but to an extent which depends upon the relationship between the oxygen flow rate and the ventilatory pattern. If there is a pause between

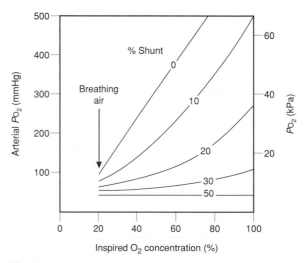

Fig. 24.5
Response of arterial partial pressure of oxygen (Po_2) to increased inspired oxygen concentrations in the presence of various degrees of shunt. Note that, in the presence of shunt, arterial Po_2 remains well below the normal value when 100% oxygen is breathed. Nevertheless, useful increases in arterial oxygenation occur with a shunt of up to 30%.

expiration and inspiration, the mask fills with oxygen and a high concentration is available at the start of inspiration; during inspiration, the inspired oxygen is diluted by air drawn in through the holes when the inspiratory flow rate exceeds the flow rate of oxygen. During normal tidal ventilation, the peak inspiratory flow rate (PIFR) is 20–30 L min^{-1}, but is considerably higher during deep inspiration or in the hyperventilating patient. If there is no expiratory pause, alveolar gas may be rebreathed from the mask at the start of inspiration; this occurs especially when the oxygen flow rate is low or when no holes are present in the mask. A predictable and constant inspired oxygen concentration may be achieved only if the total gas flow to the mask exceeds the patient's PIFR.

Fixed-performance devices

These masks, also termed high air flow oxygen enrichment (HAFOE) devices, provide a constant and predictable inspired oxygen concentration irrespective of the patient's ventilatory pattern. This is achieved by supplying the mask with oxygen and air at a high total flow rate. Oxygen is passed through a jet which entrains air (Fig. 24.6). The mask is designed in such a way that the total flow rate of gas to the mask exceeds the expected PIFR of most patients who require oxygen therapy. For example, if a jet designed to supply 28% oxygen is supplied with an oxygen flow rate of 4 L min^{-1}, approximately 41 L min^{-1} of air is entrained and a total flow of 45 L min^{-1} passes to the patient's face.

Various types of HAFOE device are available; an example is shown in Figure 24.7. Ventimasks are the most accurate, but a different mask is required for each of the range of oxygen concentrations available. Some manufacturers produce masks in which the jet device can be changed by the user, so that the oxygen concentration may be adjusted as appropriate.

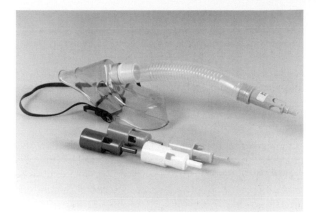

Fig. 24.7
A high air flow oxygen enrichment (HAFOE) face mask.

The air-entraining jets of HAFOE devices provide a relatively constant oxygen concentration irrespective of the flow rate of oxygen. The recommended oxygen flow rates are larger when jets providing a high concentration are used (e.g. 8 L min^{-1} for 40%, 15 L min^{-1} for 60%) so that the total flow rate supplied to the mask remains adequate despite the smaller proportion of air entrained. The total flow rates through masks which deliver more than 28% oxygen are between 20 and 30 L min^{-1} when the recommended oxygen flow rates are provided; higher flow rates of oxygen may be used in patients who are thought to have an increased PIFR.

Because of the high fresh gas flow rate, expired gas is rapidly flushed from the mask. Thus, rebreathing does not occur, i.e. fixed-performance devices do not act as an additional dead space.

Variable-performance devices

All other disposable oxygen masks and nasal cannulae provide an oxygen concentration which varies with the oxygen flow rate and the patient's ventilatory pattern. Although there is no increase in dead space when nasal cannulae are used, all variable-performance disposable face masks add dead space, the magnitude of which depends on the patient's pattern of ventilation. Table 24.7 gives an indication of the range of oxygen concentrations achieved with a number of commonly used variable-performance devices; an example is shown in Figure 24.8.

Oxygen therapy in the recovery ward

The large majority of patients recovering after anaesthesia require only a modest increase in F_1O_2 to overcome the combined effects of mild hypoventilation,

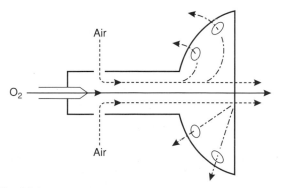

Fig. 24.6
Diagram of high air flow oxygen enrichment (HAFOE) mask (see text for details).

Table 24.7   Oxygen masks, flow rates and approximate oxygen concentration delivered

Type of mask	Oxygen flow (L min⁻¹)	Oxygen concentration (%)
Edinburgh	1	24–29
	2	29–36
	4	33–39
Nasal cannulae	1	25–29
	2	29–35
	4	32–39
Hudson	2	24–38
	4	35–45
	6	51–61
	8	57–67
	10	61–73
MC	2	28–50
	4	41–70
	6	53–74
	8	60–77
	10	67–81

diffusion hypoxia and some degree of increased $\dot{V}/\dot{Q}$ scatter. Usually, an inspired concentration of 30% is adequate and this may be achieved in most instances by supplying an oxygen flow rate of 4 L min⁻¹ to any of the variable-performance devices (see Table 24.7). However, in a small proportion of patients, it is necessary to control the F_IO_2 more strictly.

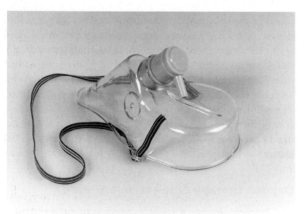

Fig. 24.8
A variable-performance oxygen face mask.

Controlled oxygen therapy

This is required in two categories of patient:

- Some patients with chronic bronchitis develop chronic hypercapnia, and ventilatory drive is produced largely by hypoxaemia. If P_aO_2 increases above the level which stimulates breathing, ventilatory depression may occur. However, these patients may become dangerously hypoxaemic after anaesthesia, and oxygen therapy is required so that adequate oxygenation of the tissues is maintained. The aim of oxygen therapy in these circumstances is to increase arterial oxygen content without an excessive increase in P_aO_2. This is achieved by a modest increase in F_IO_2. In the hypoxaemic patient, the relationship between arterial oxygen tension and saturation (and therefore oxygen content) is represented by the steep portion of the oxyhaemoglobin dissociation curve, and a small increase in oxygen tension results in significant increases in saturation and oxygen content (Fig. 24.9).

  The use of a variable-performance device in these patients is unsatisfactory, as an unacceptably high F_IO_2 may be delivered. A fixed-performance device delivering 24% oxygen should be used initially, and the response assessed. If the patient remains clinically well, and the P_aCO_2 does not increase by more than 1–1.5 kPa, 28% oxygen – and subsequently higher concentrations – may be administered if further increases in P_aO_2 are desirable.

  Most patients with chronic bronchitis do not depend on hypoxaemia for respiratory drive and should not be denied adequate inspired concentrations of oxygen. Patients at risk may usually be detected preoperatively by the presence of central cyanosis; hypoxaemia and hypercapnia are confirmed by blood gas analysis.

- Patients with increased shunt, e.g. those with acute respiratory distress syndrome (ARDS), pulmonary oedema or pulmonary consolidation, may require a high inspired oxygen concentration (see Fig. 24.5), which cannot be guaranteed if a variable-performance device is used. In addition, serial blood gas analysis is normally used to assess improvement or deterioration in their condition. Changes in P_aO_2 and the degree of shunt may be interpreted accurately only if the F_IO_2 is known. Thus, controlled oxygen therapy should be employed, using a fixed-performance device which delivers 40% oxygen or more.

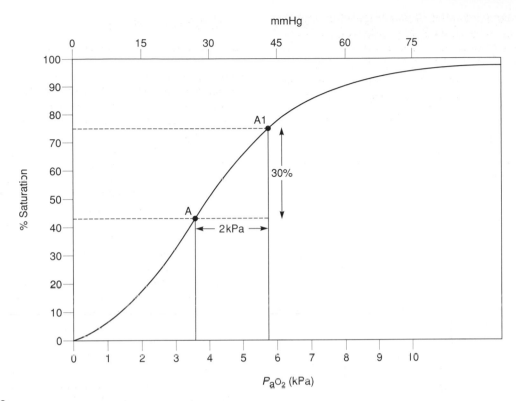

Fig. 24.9
Effect of controlled oxygen therapy on oxygen saturation in a hypoxaemic chronic bronchitic patient. A small increase in inspired oxygen concentration produces a modest increase in arterial oxygen tension (P_aO_2) but a substantial increase in arterial oxygen saturation.

CARDIOVASCULAR SYSTEM

HYPOTENSION

Residual effects of anaesthetic drugs

Hypotension may result from the residual vasodilator effect of i.v. or inhalational anaesthetic drugs, particularly in patients who are experiencing little pain. Subarachnoid or epidural nerve block may also cause hypotension which persists into the postoperative period. Heart rate is seldom elevated, and the peripheries are warm if anaesthetic drugs or regional anaesthesia are the cause of hypotension. Up to 20% decrease in the mean arterial pressure is tolerated well except by the elderly or patients with myocardial disease. No treatment is required in most patients. Elevation of the legs often increases arterial pressure by increasing venous return. Intravenous infusion of 7–10 mL kg^{-1} of colloid solution is usually effective in restoring normotension if there is concern; infusion should be undertaken cautiously in elderly patients and in those with cardiovascular disease.

Other causes of hypotension in the recovery period are more sinister and must be excluded before it may be assumed that residual anaesthesia is responsible.

Hypovolaemia

This may result from inadequate or inappropriate replacement of preoperative or intraoperative fluid and blood losses, or from postoperative haemorrhage. Surgical bleeding may be obvious from inspection of wounds and drains, but may be concealed, particularly in the abdomen, retroperitoneal space or thorax, even when drains are present.

Inadequate surgical haemostasis is the usual cause of postoperative bleeding, but coagulation disorders may be present in the following circumstances:

- after massive blood transfusion, which results in decreased concentrations of clotting factors and reduced platelet numbers
- pre-existing bleeding tendency, e.g. haemophilia

- disseminated intravascular coagulation produced by sepsis, amniotic fluid embolism, etc.
- if anticoagulant drugs have been administered.

A coagulation disorder is frequently associated with prolonged bleeding after venepuncture, oozing from the wound and the development of petechiae or bruises. The investigation and management of coagulation disorders are discussed in Chapter 22.

Hypotension caused by hypovolaemia is accompanied by signs of poor peripheral perfusion, e.g. cold, clammy extremities and pallor. Tachycardia may be present but is masked, not infrequently, by the effects of drugs (e.g. anticholinesterases, β-blockers). CVP may be low or normal. Urine output is reduced (< 30 mL h^{-1}). The effects of hypovolaemia on arterial pressure are more pronounced in the presence of vasodilatation or reduced myocardial contractility resulting from the effects of residual anaesthetic drugs, or antihypertensive, calcium channel or β-blocker therapy. In patients who have undergone prolonged surgery, and particularly if the core temperature is below normal, vasoconstriction may be profound and hypovolaemia may be unmasked at a relatively late stage, as normal vasomotor tone returns with rewarming.

Treatment comprises elevation of the legs and administration of appropriate crystalloid or colloid solutions; in elderly or high-risk patients, or if hypovolaemia is profound, administration of fluids should be monitored by measurement of CVP. Clotting factors or platelets should be administered if appropriate, and surgical bleeding treated by re-operation if necessary.

Arrhythmias

These are discussed below.

Ventricular failure

Left or right ventricular failure may cause hypotension. Right ventricular failure is uncommon in the postoperative period and is secondary usually to acute pulmonary disease, e.g. ARDS.

Left ventricular failure in the postoperative period is associated most commonly with perioperative myocardial infarction or overtransfusion. The peripheral circulation is poor. Usually, tachycardia is present and there is clinical and radiological evidence of pulmonary oedema. Jugular venous pulse and CVP are usually elevated, but they may remain normal despite a substantial increase in left atrial pressure, particularly if right ventricular hypertrophy is present. Thus, left ventricular failure may be misdiag-

nosed as hypovolaemia in some patients, and in some instances the two conditions coexist. If there is doubt about the diagnosis, a small fluid load may be administered (no more than 200 mL) and the response of arterial pressure and CVP monitored; if the diagnosis remains uncertain, echocardiography should be performed or a pulmonary artery catheter should be inserted to measure pulmonary artery and left atrial pressures.

Treatment comprises administration of oxygen, fluid restriction, diuretics and, if necessary, inotropic support or vasodilator therapy. ECG, arterial pressure and CVP should be monitored. The possibility of myocardial infarction should be investigated.

Septic shock

In this condition, hypotension is accompanied by raised cardiac output and peripheral vasodilatation in the early stages, followed by vasoconstriction and reduced cardiac output caused partly by loss of fluid from the circulation. CVP monitoring is essential and a pulmonary artery catheter may be desirable. Treatment includes infusion of appropriate volumes of colloid solutions, inotropic support, antibiotic therapy and, if necessary, surgical treatment of the source.

HYPERTENSION

Arterial hypertension is a common complication in the early postoperative period. The causes include the following:

- pain
- pre-existing hypertension, particularly if controlled inadequately
- hypoxaemia
- hypercapnia
- administration of vasopressor drugs
- after aortic surgery, as a result partly of increased plasma concentration of renin.

A combination of these causes may be present. Hypertension results in increased cardiac work and myocardial oxygen consumption, and may result in myocardial ischaemia or infarction, left ventricular failure or cerebral haemorrhage. The cause should be elicited rapidly and treated if possible. Oxygen should be administered. If no remediable cause is found, vasodilatation with hydralazine (i.v.), nifedipine (sublingual) or glyceryl trinitrate (sublingual or i.v.) should be started. Alternatively, labetalol may be used, particularly if there is a degree of tachycardia. Such treatment may unmask hypovolaemia (see above) and additional i.v. fluids may be required.

ARRHYTHMIAS

These are common during and immediately after anaesthesia (see also Ch. 19). The majority are benign and require no treatment. However, the cause should be sought and its effect on the circulation assessed. Common causes include the following:

- residual anaesthetic agents
- hypercapnia
- hypoxaemia
- electrolyte or acid–base disturbance
- vagal stimulation, e.g. by tracheal tube or suction catheters
- myocardial ischaemia or infarction
- pain.

Sinus tachycardia is common and may be a reflex response to hypovolaemia or hypotension. It also occurs in the presence of hypercapnia, anaemia or hypoxaemia, and if the metabolic rate is elevated by fever, shivering, restlessness or malignant hyperthermia. The commonest cause is pain. Tachycardia increases myocardial oxygen consumption and decreases coronary artery perfusion by reducing diastolic time. The combination of arterial hypertension and tachycardia is dangerous in the presence of ischaemic heart disease and should *not* be allowed to persist, as it may result in myocardial infarction. Sinus tachycardia should be treated specifically only if it persists after therapy for underlying causes has been given; a small i.v. dose of a short-acting β-blocker (esmolol) followed by continuous intravenous infusion should be administered. The ECG must be monitored.

Sinus bradycardia may result from inadequate antagonism by atropine or vagal stimulation by neostigmine, pharyngeal stimulation during suction or the residual effects of volatile anaesthetic agents. Other causes include hypoxaemia (especially in neonates and infants), raised intracranial pressure, myocardial infarction and some cardiac drugs, e.g. β-blockers, digoxin. Oxygen should be administered. Intravenous atropine is usually effective and should be given in a dose of 0.4–0.6 mg in adults if the heart rate is less than 45 beat min^{-1} or if there is associated hypotension. In the presence of severe bradycardia, external cardiac massage is necessary to increase cardiac output.

Bradycardia may also occur as a result of complete heart block; this may require electrical pacing.

Supraventricular arrhythmias, including atrial fibrillation, flutter or supraventricular tachycardia, are treated as in other circumstances. Rapid arrhythmias are best treated by cardioversion, but may require pharmacological therapy to prevent recurrence. Nodal rhythm with a normal heart rate is common in the perioperative period, particularly when volatile anaesthetic agents have been used. Supraventricular arrhythmias may cause moderate hypotension because of the loss of synchronization between atrial and ventricular contractions.

Ventricular arrhythmias. Premature ventricular contractions (PVCs) may require treatment with i.v. lidocaine 1–1.5 mg kg^{-1} if they are frequent (> 5 min^{-1}), multifocal or occur close to the preceding T wave; however, most cardiologists regard PVCs as benign if cardiac output is adequate. Ventricular tachycardia requires immediate treatment with lidocaine or cardioversion.

CONDUCTION DEFECTS

In the perioperative period, these usually occur in patients with pre-existing heart disease. Heart rate and cardiac output in complete heart block may increase in response to isoproterenol, but electrical pacing should be started as soon as possible. Patients who develop second-degree heart block during anaesthesia or in the recovery ward should be transferred to a coronary care or intensive therapy unit for an appropriate period of observation.

MYOCARDIAL ISCHAEMIA

This occurs most commonly in patients with pre-existing coronary artery disease, and most often in the presence of hypoxaemia, hypotension, hypertension or tachycardia. The ECG should be monitored throughout the recovery period in patients known to be at risk, and precipitating factors should be avoided. Angina occurring during the recovery period should be treated by elimination of any predisposing factor and administration of glyceryl trinitrate sublingually or intravenously.

MYOCARDIAL INFARCTION

The average incidence of myocardial infarction (MI) is 1–2% in unselected patients over 40 years of age undergoing major non-cardiac surgery. Pre-existing coronary artery disease and, in particular, evidence of a previous MI result in a higher risk. Mortality in patients who suffer a perioperative MI may be as high as 60%. Perioperative MI occurs most commonly on the third postoperative day, but may happen at any time during or after surgery.

Several factors which may be detected during preoperative assessment are known to increase the likelihood of perioperative MI. The most important of these is the time interval between surgery and a previous MI. One extensive study of risk factors which might predict major cardiac complications (including, but not exclusively, MI) showed that preoperative evidence of cardiac failure, arrhythmias (of any type) or aortic stenosis, and age were also associated with a high risk. In addition, there is evidence that pre-existing uncontrolled hypertension is associated with increased risk. These problems are discussed more fully in Chapter 23.

The incidence of perioperative MI is related also to intraoperative and postoperative factors. The magnitude of surgery is an important determinant; in patients with a history of previous MI, the incidence of perioperative reinfarction associated with major vascular surgery is considerably higher than when surgery is performed outside the thorax and abdomen. In patients with ischaemic heart disease, postoperative MI is more likely if there is evidence of ischaemic changes on ECG during operation. Such changes are associated most commonly with episodes of intraoperative hypotension, hypertension or tachycardia; the last two occur most frequently in response to noxious stimuli, e.g. tracheal intubation, surgical incision. The drugs used and the manner in which they are employed by the anaesthetist influence the incidences of both intraoperative ischaemia and perioperative MI. Regional anaesthesia is not associated with a reduction in risk when major surgery is undertaken.

Reduction of risk

The incidence of perioperative MI may be reduced by the following:

- *Identification of patients at risk.* Elective surgery should be postponed if possible until at least 3 months after a previous MI.
- *Treatment of risk factors.* Cardiac failure, hypertension and arrhythmias should be controlled before surgery. If necessary, the operation should be postponed until control is achieved. Coronary artery bypass grafting or aortic valve replacement may be required in patients with severe coronary artery disease or aortic stenosis, respectively, before other major abdominal or thoracic surgery is undertaken.
- *Avoidance of ischaemia.* The anaesthetic technique and postoperative management should ensure adequate oxygenation of the myocardium and should minimize myocardial oxygen demand (see Ch. 23).
- *Monitoring.* ECG must be monitored throughout anaesthesia, including induction, in all patients at risk; the CM5 electrode configuration (see Fig. 18.2)

is suitable for detection of ischaemic changes. Arterial pressure should be monitored regularly, and continuously in patients undergoing major surgery. Monitoring of right and left atrial pressures by central venous and pulmonary artery catheterization, and prompt treatment of abnormalities which occur during operation and in the early postoperative period reduce the incidence of perioperative MI.

Diagnosis

Perioperative MI may be difficult to diagnose. It occurs most commonly on the third postoperative day. The classic distribution of pain is present in only 25% of patients.

The diagnosis should be considered in any patient at risk who develops an arrhythmia or becomes hypotensive in the postoperative period. Premature ventricular contractions occur in 90% of patients who experience an MI; sinus bradycardia and the development of any degree of atrioventricular conduction defect are also common. There is often a pyrexia of up to 39°C. The diagnosis is confirmed by changes in serial ECG recordings and/or serum troponin concentrations.

OTHER MAJOR POSTOPERATIVE COMPLICATIONS

DEEP VENOUS THROMBOSIS

The main factors postulated by Virchow as contributing to the formation of venous thrombi are:

- changes in the composition of blood
- damage to walls of blood vessels
- decreased blood flow.

However, the exact trigger mechanism which initiates thrombosis remains unknown.

Risk factors

A higher incidence of deep venous thrombosis (DVT) has been reported in patients with:

- extensive trauma
- infection
- heart failure
- blood dyscrasias
- malignancy
- metabolic disorders.

DVT is commoner after hip, pelvic and abdominal surgery than after other types of surgery; regional anaesthetic techniques, with general anaesthesia or in isolation, may reduce the risk There is a well-established association between spontaneous DVT and oestrogen, and DVT may occur in women who take some types of oral contraceptive pill. The number of women who develop this complication is small. However, the incidence increases if surgery is performed while the patient is currently taking the drug. The risk is reduced but not abolished if a low-oestrogen (50 μg or less) preparation is used. Women who take hormone replacement therapy are also at increased risk.

Diagnosis

Approximately 70% of patients with a DVT have neither symptoms nor signs. Fifty per cent of patients with calf pain and tenderness on dorsiflexion of the foot do not have a DVT. Often there is mild pyrexia.

Investigations

Venography

This is an effective method for demonstrating most thrombi of clinical importance.

Radioactive fibrinogen uptake

Iodine-labelled fibrinogen is taken up preferentially by a growing thrombus. The investigation is quick to perform and may detect small thrombi in the calf vessels. Its main disadvantage is that it cannot be used to detect iliac and pelvic vein thrombi, although most thrombi in surgical patients occur in the calf. It does not correlate well with either venography or the development of pulmonary embolism and is associated with a high incidence of false-positive results.

Ultrasonography

This is non-invasive and simple to perform. However, it is insensitive and is useful only for confirming the diagnosis of a major thrombus.

Prophylaxis

Elimination of stasis

The efficacy of early ambulation after operation in reducing the incidence of DVT is not clear. Attempts directed at preventing stasis, including physiotherapy, elastic stockings and elevation of the feet, may reduce the incidence of DVT but have not been shown to influence the incidence of pulmonary embolism.

Two methods are currently used for increasing venous return from the lower limbs during surgery:

- *Electrical stimulation of the calf muscles.* A low-voltage current is applied across the calf to contract the muscles every 2–4 s.
- *Pneumatic compression of the calves.* The legs are encased in an envelope of plastic material, which is inflated and deflated rhythmically, thus squeezing the calves intermittently. This technique may be continued postoperatively.

Although the incidence of DVT is substantially reduced by these techniques, there is no reduction in the incidence of, or mortality from, pulmonary embolism.

Alteration of blood coagulability

Platelet aggregation

Various drugs which interfere with different aspects of platelet function have been investigated. These include dextran 70, dipyridamole, aspirin and chloroquine. There is no evidence to suggest that dipyridamole or aspirin prevents DVT. Infusion of dextran during and after surgery may reduce the incidence of fatal postoperative pulmonary embolism but its role in the prevention of peripheral venous thrombosis is undetermined.

The coagulation mechanism

Oral anticoagulant commenced before operation is the only well-substantiated method of reducing venous thrombosis. However, there is a risk of increased surgical haemorrhage. Low-dose heparin, 5000 units subcutaneously 2 h before operation and subsequently at 8 or 12 h intervals until the patient is mobile, reduces the risk of DVT and carries little risk of major haemorrhage. If DVT does occur, it is more likely to be confined to the calf if heparin has been given. Subcutaneous heparin reduces the incidence of fatal pulmonary embolism. There is evidence that low molecular weight heparins (dalteparin, enoxaparin and tinzaparin) are more effective antithrombotics than standard heparin in orthopaedic surgery, and they are as effective and safe in other types of surgery. They have a longer duration of action and are therefore more convenient.

PULMONARY EMBOLISM

This term covers a range of events from sudden circulatory collapse and death, through minor episodes of pleurisy and haemoptysis, to the long-standing disability of patients with chronic thromboembolic pulmonary hypertension. The acute forms of pulmonary embolism are encountered after anaesthesia and surgery. In the elderly, multiple small pulmonary emboli may be misdiagnosed as bronchopneumonia.

The common sites of origin for thrombi which result in pulmonary embolus are the veins of the pelvis and lower extremities. The most common time for presentation of a postoperative pulmonary embolism is during the second week. In some patients, predisposing factors may have existed preoperatively for some time, and the whole time-scale of events may be shifted; the embolus may occur at the time of, or shortly after, surgery.

Diagnosis

Presenting features

The principal features are circulatory collapse and sudden dyspnoea, often associated with chest pain. If the embolus is large, the pulmonary artery outflow is blocked and sudden death results. If the embolus involves more than 50% of the main pulmonary arteries, it is termed massive.

Physical signs

A low cardiac output state develops. Tachypnoea and central cyanosis are usual. There is arterial hypotension, sinus tachycardia and a constricted peripheral circulation. The jugular venous pressure is elevated. A fourth heart sound is usually present on auscultation.

Investigations

- *ECG* (Fig. 24.10). This reflects acute right ventricular strain, with features that often include right axis deviation, T-wave inversion in leads V_1–V_4 and sometimes right bundle branch block. The classic S1–Q3–T3 pattern is less common.
- *Chest X-ray.* This is often unremarkable but may show areas of oligaemia reflecting pulmonary vascular obstruction.
- *Arterial blood gases.* There is usually hypoxaemia because of ventilation–perfusion imbalance, and hypocapnia resulting from hyperventilation.
- *Perfusion and ventilation lung scans.* The perfusion scan shows uneven circulation, with perfusion defects delineating the emboli. A simultaneous ventilation scan is usually normal.
- *Pulmonary angiography.* This provides a definitive diagnosis of major obstruction in the pulmonary circulation. This investigation is particularly useful if the patient is critically ill and the diagnosis is in doubt, and is essential if pulmonary embolectomy is planned. However, it is invasive and normally requires transfer of the patient to the X-ray department.

Treatment

Deep venous thrombosis

The mainstay of therapy is anticoagulation. Initially, i.v. heparin is infused in a dose of 40 000 units day^{-1}. At the same time, oral anticoagulant therapy is started. Warfarin is used most commonly. Heparin may be discontinued after 48 h. Oral anticoagulants are continued for at least 3 months.

Pulmonary embolism

Immediate treatment consists of administration of oxygen in a high concentration and i.v. heparin. Digoxin is

Pulmonary embolus

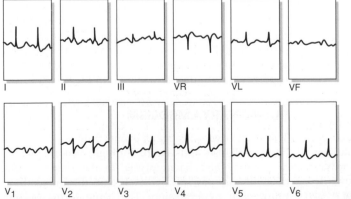

I II III VR VL VF

V_1 V_2 V_3 V_4 V_5 V_6

Fig 24.10
Typical electrocardiogram changes in pulmonary embolism.

often useful. Sometimes it is necessary to use additional inotropic support for the circulation. Heparin is continued for 5–6 days. Oral anticoagulant therapy is started as soon as possible and is continued for at least 6 months.

Massive pulmonary embolus which does not respond to the above measures may warrant the use of thrombolytic agents, e.g. streptokinase. The risk of haemorrhage with these agents is considerably higher than with heparin. If the cardiovascular effects of the embolism are life-threatening, open pulmonary embolectomy under cardiopulmonary bypass may be considered.

POSTOPERATIVE RENAL DYSFUNCTION

The kidney is vulnerable to a wide range of drugs and chemicals. It is particularly susceptible to toxic substances for the following reasons:

- large blood flow per unit mass
- high oxygen consumption
- non-resorbable substances concentrated by tubules
- permeability of tubular cells.

All anaesthetic techniques depress renal blood flow and, secondary to this, interfere with renal function. Provided that prolonged hypotension is avoided, the effects are temporary. However, there is the potential for some anaesthetic agents to produce permanent renal damage.

The administration of the volatile anaesthetic agent methoxyflurane was associated with a relatively high incidence of renal dysfunction. Clinically, the defect was characterized by failure of the concentrating ability of the kidney. In certain instances, this progressed to high-output renal failure. The nephrotoxicity of methoxyflurane was dose-dependent and was caused by inorganic fluoride ions produced during its metabolism. Administration of methoxyflurane in combination with other nephrotoxic drugs, e.g. aminoglycosides, was particularly hazardous.

Large quantities of fluoride ion are also produced during metabolism of enflurane and sevoflurane, although a much smaller proportion of these drugs (2–3%) is metabolized in comparison with methoxyflurane (45%). Concentrations of fluoride ion in blood following administration of sevoflurane may exceed the value associated with renal impairment after anaesthesia with methoxyflurane. However, there has been no evidence to suggest that either enflurane or sevoflurane is associated with renal impairment related to the production of fluoride ions. The reason is probably related to the fact that the very soluble methoxyflurane continues to be metabolized for some days, resulting in prolonged production of fluoride ions, whereas the peak concentrations associated with the use of enflurane and sevoflurane are of short duration because of their relative insolubility in tissues.

POSTOPERATIVE HEPATIC DYSFUNCTION

There are many causes of postoperative hepatic dysfunction (Table 24.8). Most patients show no evidence of hepatic damage after anaesthesia and surgery. If it occurs, it is usually attributable to one of the causes shown in Table 24.8. However, if other causes are excluded, consideration should be given to the possibility of hepatotoxicity from anaesthetic drugs.

Chloroform was the first anaesthetic agent to be suspected of causing hepatic damage. In large doses, chloroform is a direct hepatotoxin, and after anaesthesia a hepatitis-like syndrome, with histological evidence of centrilobular hepatic necrosis, occurred occasionally. Methoxyflurane was also associated with hepatic damage, causing a syndrome clinically similar

Table 24.8 Causes of postoperative hepatic dysfunction

Increased bilirubin load	Hepatocellular damage	Extrahepatic biliary obstruction
Blood transfusion	Pre-existing liver disease	Gallstones
Haemolysis and haemolytic disease	Viral hepatitis	Ascending cholangitis
Abnormalities of bilirubin metabolism	Sepsis	Pancreatitis
	Hypotension/hypoxia	Surgical misadventure
	Drug-induced hepatitis	
	Congestive heart failure	

to viral hepatitis. Two of the volatile agents in current use have been implicated in cases of postoperative hepatic dysfunction.

Halothane

Attention was first focused on halothane-associated hepatitis in the early 1960s. Numerous case reports prompted institution in 1969 of the largest retrospective anaesthetic study ever undertaken (United States National Halothane Study). The incidence and causes of fatal hepatic necrosis occurring within 6 days of anaesthesia were reviewed. The overall incidence was 1 in 10 000; that associated with halothane was 1 in 35 000 and was no greater than the incidence associated with other anaesthetic agents. However, it is believed at present that there is a small number of patients who develop postanaesthetic jaundice in which halothane is the aetiological agent.

The histological picture of halothane-associated hepatitis is similar to that seen in type A viral hepatitis. Clinically, there is hepatocellular jaundice, with elevation of the aminotransferase enzymes. The exact mechanism of liver damage is not known. At present, there are two main hypotheses:

- Metabolites of reductive halothane metabolism bind covalently to hepatocyte macromolecules, causing hepatocellular damage.
- Halothane or its metabolites react with hepatocyte proteins to form antigenic compounds, against which the body mounts an immune response that results in hepatocellular damage.

Antibodies to halothane have been demonstrated in patients who have suffered hepatic damage after administration of the drug. At present, this is the most promising method for evaluating the aetiology of a condition which has been a source of great controversy.

The following groups of patients are believed to be at the greatest risk of developing hepatic dysfunction after halothane anaesthesia:

- patients subjected to repeated halothane anaesthetics, especially within a 3-month period
- patients who have developed unexplained pyrexia or jaundice after a previous halothane anaesthetic
- obese patients, particularly women.

Enflurane

Several causes of unexplained jaundice have been reported after the use of enflurane.

OTHER COMPLICATIONS (Table 24.9)

LOCAL VASCULAR COMPLICATIONS

Haematoma formation is probably the commonest complication of i.v. injection. This usually results from inadequate pressure at the injection site after removal of the needle. Phlebitis, thrombosis or thrombophlebitis may occur after intravenous injections. Most drugs used currently by anaesthetists are associated with low incidences of these complications; intravenous diazepam is a potent cause of phlebitis, although the formulation of diazepam in a fat emulsion (Diazemuls) has overcome this problem.

Table 24.9 Minor morbidity resulting from anaesthesia
Nausea and vomiting
Related to operation site
Females > males
Sore throat
Up to 70% of patients
Hoarseness
Laryngeal granulomata
Headache
Up to 60% of patients
Backache
Discomfort from catheters, drains, nasogastric tubes
Anxiety
Muscle pains
Up to 100% of those who receive succinylcholine
Shivering
Drowsiness
Anorexia
Disorientation
Thrombophlebitis at injection site
Bruised or cut lip
Chipped teeth
Corneal abrasions

Intravenous infusions commonly cause thrombophlebitis. The incidence is related to the duration of infusion, and this is more important than the type of cannula used. Thrombophlebitis is rare if the infusion site is changed every 12 h. If it is changed every 72 h, the incidence of thrombophlebitis is 70%. Cannulae constructed from polytetrafluorethylene (Teflon) appear to be the least thrombogenic of those available.

Arterial cannulation is commonly performed to permit continuous monitoring of systemic arterial pressure during major surgery. Unfortunately, it is not without adverse sequelae. Intimal damage may lead to thrombosis and occasionally aneurysm formation. Recannulation of the vessel generally occurs, even when the vessel has been completely occluded. Nevertheless, gangrene of the extremities is an occasional complication, particularly if the brachial artery is used rather than the radial artery. Ischaemia of the hand or fingers may occur after radial artery cannulation if there is inadequate collateral circulation.

It has been suggested that a modified Allen's test should be performed to assess the adequacy of the collateral circulation through the ulnar artery before radial artery cannulation. The patient is asked to clench the fist, and radial and ulnar arteries are compressed by the examiner. The patient is subsequently instructed to unclench the fist; the examiner releases the ulnar artery and observes the palm of the hand. If there is adequate collateral flow, prompt return of colour to the palm is seen; if there is little or no return of colour within 15 s, the collateral flow is poor. However, there is some doubt about the relationship between the results of Allen's test and the incidence of ischaemic episodes after radial artery cannulation. After an arterial cannula has been inserted, regular checks should be made to ensure that there is no evidence of ischaemia in the area supplied by the artery; if detected at an early stage, permanent damage can be avoided.

The incidence of thrombosis after arterial cannulation is reduced by the use of a cannula made of Teflon and of a diameter that is small relative to the size of the artery. A 20-gauge cannula is appropriate in the adult, and a 22- or 24-gauge cannula in children. Arterial damage is also reduced by avoiding multiple punctures of the artery during cannulation. The incidence of radial artery thrombosis is highest in the presence of sepsis, low cardiac output states and when the duration of cannulation is prolonged beyond 24 h.

NAUSEA AND VOMITING

Although often regarded by medical and nursing staff as only a minor complication of anaesthesia and surgery, nausea and vomiting are frequently the cause of great distress to patients. Many studies have been undertaken to investigate nausea and vomiting after anaesthesia and surgery. The incidence varies from 14% to 82%, the wide range resulting partly from differences in design of studies. Many factors contribute to the aetiology of postoperative nausea and vomiting and these are discussed in detail in Chapter 26.

Prevention and treatment

The incidence of postoperative vomiting may be reduced by careful selection of drugs in the perioperative period, and the prophylactic use of antiemetic agents (see Ch. 26).

HEADACHE

The reported incidence of severe headache after anaesthesia and surgery ranges from 12% to 35%, but up to 60% of patients complain of some headache. Individuals who are susceptible to headaches caused by stress, etc., are more likely to complain of postoperative headache. Most investigations have failed to identify any single agent as being responsible for postoperative headache after general anaesthesia. Severe postural headache may occur after dural puncture (see p. 641).

SORE THROAT

Up to 80% of patients complain of sore throat after anaesthesia and surgery. Some of the common causes include:

- *Trauma during tracheal intubation.* Damage to the pharynx and tonsillar fauces may be caused by the laryngoscope blade.
- *Trauma to the larynx.* This is more likely if a red rubber tracheal tube is used rather than a plastic disposable tube, or if the tube has been forced through the vocal cords. A poorly stabilized tube causes more frictional damage to the larynx than one which is securely stabilized.
- *Trauma to the pharynx.* This may occur during passage of a nasogastric tube or insertion of an oropharyngeal or laryngeal mask airway, and is particularly common when a throat pack has been used. Occasionally, the pharynx or upper oesophagus may be perforated during insertion of a nasogastric tube, or during difficult tracheal intubation, and severe pain in the throat is often the first symptom. Sore throat is likely if a nasogastric tube remains in situ during the postoperative period.
- *Other factors.* The mucous membranes of the mouth, pharynx and upper airway are sensitive to

the effects of unhumidified gases; the drying effect of anaesthetic gases may cause postoperative sore throat. The antisialagogue effect of anticholinergic drugs may also contribute to this symptom.

The use of topical local anaesthetics does not reduce the incidence of sore throat. Lubrication of the tracheal tube is effective in reducing the incidence, although there is no difference in this respect between plain or local anaesthetic jellies. However, there is little difference in the incidence of sore throat between an anaesthetic technique in which tracheal intubation is employed and one in which only an oropharyngeal or laryngeal mask airway is used.

In the absence of a nasogastric tube, postoperative sore throat is usually of short duration; most patients are symptom-free within 48 h.

HOARSENESS

This should not be confused with sore throat. It is almost always associated with tracheal intubation and is caused predominantly by prolonged abduction of, and pressure on, the vocal cords. However, traumatic tracheal intubation can cause direct trauma to the vocal cords, resulting in prolonged hoarseness.

LARYNGEAL GRANULOMATA

These may occur after tracheal intubation, and arise from areas of ulceration, usually on the posterior aspect of the vocal cords. The ulcers are caused by pressure and consequent ischaemia. Granulomata are reported most frequently after thyroidectomy.

If hoarseness persists for longer than 1 week, indirect laryngoscopy should be performed. If ulceration is present, complete voice rest is indicated. Any granulomata present should be excised; untreated granulomata may grow to such a size as to obstruct the airway.

DENTAL TRAUMA

This is the commonest cause of litigation against anaesthetists. Damage usually occurs during laryngoscopy, especially if tracheal intubation is difficult. Loose teeth, crowns, caps and bridges are particularly susceptible to damage. Preoperative enquiry and examination should alert the anaesthetist to the possibility of damage.

OCULAR COMPLICATIONS

Carelessness is the commonest cause of damage to the eyes; corneal abrasion is the most frequent lesion. The eyes are often allowed to remain open during anaes-

thesia. The cornea is thus exposed and vulnerable to the irritant effects of skin preparations, dust and surgical drapes. This type of damage is easily prevented by securing the eyelids in a closed position with adhesive tape.

Retinal infarction has occurred on rare occasions as a result of pressure on the eyeball from a face mask. It can also occur if patients are placed in the prone position in such a way that pressure is exerted on the eye, e.g. by a horseshoe head rest.

MUSCLES

Problems associated with inadequate reversal of neuromuscular blocking drugs are discussed above. The detection and treatment of malignant hyperthermia are described on page 392; it is important to appreciate that this condition may present during recovery.

Shivering

This is a common complication in the recovery room. It may occur in patients who are hypothermic as a result of prolonged surgery, or during injection of local anaesthetic solution into the epidural space. However, in most patients, the onset of shivering is not related to body temperature, and there is evidence from electromyography that the characteristics of postoperative (or postanaesthetic) shivering differ from those of thermoregulatory shivering. The incidence and severity of shivering are increased in patients who have received an anticholinergic premedication, and women are more likely to shiver in the luteal than in the follicular phase of the menstrual cycle.

Shivering increases oxygen consumption and carbon dioxide production and may result in hypoxaemia and hypercapnia if the response of the respiratory centre to carbon dioxide is impaired by drugs. Oxygen should be administered. A small dose of pethidine (20 mg i.v.) is frequently effective in aborting postoperative shivering.

Succinylcholine pains

Muscle pains after succinylcholine are very common, occurring in at least 50% of patients who receive the drug. The muscles involved most frequently are those of the shoulder girdle, neck and thorax. The pain is similar in nature to that caused by viral-related myositis. The incidence is influenced by the following factors:

- *Age*. Succinylcholine pains are unusual in young children and the elderly.
- *Gender*. Women are more susceptible than men. The incidence is reduced during pregnancy.

- *Type of surgery*. There is an increased incidence after minor procedures, when early ambulation is likely.
- *Physical fitness*. The incidence is higher in individuals who are physically fit.
- *Repeated doses*. The incidence is increased if repeated doses of succinylcholine are administered.

The exact cause of muscle pains after succinylcholine is unknown, although it is thought that fasciculations produced by depolarization of the motor nerve end-plate are involved in the pathogenesis. However, the visible extent of fasciculations does not correlate with the severity of subsequent pain. Myoglobinuria occurs after administration of succinylcholine, demonstrating that muscle cell injury does occur.

After minor surgery, the patient may be disturbed by the muscle pains to a greater extent than the discomfort caused by the operative procedure. Analgesics such as paracetamol or NSAIDs may be required for 2–3 days to relieve the pain.

It is possible to reduce, but not to eliminate, the incidence of succinylcholine pains by pretreatment with one of the following agents:

- a small dose of non-depolarizing muscle relaxant (usually 10% of the normal dose) 2–3 min before induction of anaesthesia
- lidocaine 1 mg kg^{-1}

- diazepam 0.15 mg kg^{-1} i.v. before induction of anaesthesia.

SURGICAL CONSIDERATIONS

During the recovery period, several surgical complications may occur. These include haemorrhage, blockage of drains or catheters and soiling of dressings. Prosthetic arterial grafts may block, resulting in ischaemia of the limbs. Recovery ward nurses and anaesthetists must be aware of potential surgical complications, as rapid surgical intervention may be required.

The recovery period may also be used to commence orthopaedic traction before the patient returns to the ward.

FURTHER READING

Association of Anaesthetists of Great Britain and Ireland 2002 Immediate postanaesthetic recovery. AAGBI, London

Mecca R S 2002 Postanesthesia recovery. In: Kirby R R, Gravenstein N, Lobato E B, Gravenstein N (eds) Clinical anesthesia practice. WB Saunders, Philadelphia, pp 83–127

25 Postoperative pain

Pain is an extraordinarily complex sensation which is difficult to define and equally difficult to measure in an accurate, objective manner. It has been defined as the sensory appreciation of afferent nociceptive stimulation which elicits an affective (or autonomic) component; both are subjected to rational interpretation by the patient. It may be represented as a Venn diagram (Fig. 25.1), the shaded area of which represents the quantum of suffering experienced by the patient. The advantage of describing pain by means of the Venn diagram is that it may be seen instantly that the sensation of pain differs among individual patients; the emotional component may vary according to the patient's psychological composition and the rational component varies with the patient's previous experience, insight and motivation.

Postoperative pain differs from other types of pain in that it is usually, but by no means always, transitory, with progressive improvement over a relatively short time-course. Typically, the affective component tends towards an anxiety state associated with diagnosis of the condition and fear of delay in provision of analgesic therapy by attendants. In contrast, chronic pain is persistent, frequently with fluctuating intensity, and the affective component contains a greater depressive element. Thus, acute pain is more easily amenable to therapy than chronic pain. Despite this, a recent survey showed that most adults still expect to have significant postoperative pain after surgery, and that this is their primary concern before surgery. Such concern may be justified, because traditional management of postoperative pain, using intramuscular opioid administration given on demand, often failed to produce good analgesia.

The traditional management of postoperative pain comprised the prescription of a standard dose of an opioid, to be given on demand by a nurse when the patient's pain threshold had been exceeded. This leads to poor control of postoperative pain for the following reasons:

- Responsibility for management of pain is delegated to the nursing staff, who err on the side of caution in the administration of opioids. They tend to give too small a dose of drug too infrequently because of unwarranted fears of producing ventilatory depression or addiction.
- Because the administration of drugs is left entirely to the discretion of the nursing staff, the degree of empathy between nurse and patient affects analgesic administration. This explains the common observation that the mean dosage of morphine given for a standard operation varies among hospitals and even among wards in the same hospital.
- Because the measurement of pain is difficult, it is seldom possible to adjust the dosage of drug to match the extent of pain.
- There are enormous variations in the extent of analgesic requirements depending upon the type of surgery, pharmacokinetic variability, pharmacodynamic variability, etc.

These inadequacies in the traditional management of postoperative pain have been confirmed by a survey of ethical problems nurses face, which showed that they regard pain management to be a significant problem in their clinical practice.

PHYSIOLOGY

The physiology of acute pain is no longer considered to be a simple 'hard-wired' system with a pure 'stimulus–response' relationship. Rather, tissue damage or disease sets up a process involving tissue receptors, the peripheral, central and autonomic nervous systems, and higher centres in the brain that produce the perception of pain.

NOCICEPTORS

Nociceptors are receptors that require a strong (high threshold) stimulus for activation. Most are polymodal,

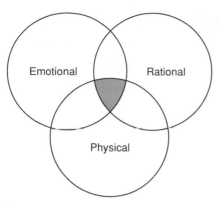

Fig. 25.1
The interrelationship between emotional, rational and physical components of pain. Perceived pain is represented by the area of intersection of all three components.

i.e. respond to a variety of noxious stimuli (heat, mechanical, chemical). The usual stimulus for activation is mechanical distortion of the receptor, followed by local increases in K^+ and H^+ ions. Inflammation leads to a reduction in the threshold for stimulation, and activation of dormant or 'silent' nociceptors. This is termed 'peripheral sensitization'.

PRIMARY AFFERENT FIBRES

Primary afferent fibres conduct impulses from the nociceptor to the spinal cord, and have their cell bodies in the dorsal root ganglion. There are two types of primary afferent fibres from nociceptors, and they are distinguished mainly by their speed of conduction. Aδ fibres have a high speed of conduction, and are responsible for 'immediate', sharp pain and reflex withdrawal. C fibres conduct at a lower speed, and are responsible for persistent pain and central sensitization in the spinal cord (Table 25.1). Most primary afferent fibres terminate by synapsing with dorsal horn neurones (Fig. 25.2).

DORSAL HORN NEURONES

A cross-section of the spinal cord shows 10 anatomically and physiologically distinct layers called Rexed laminae (Fig. 25.3). Laminae 1–6 and lamina 10 are sites at which sensory afferents synapse with *dorsal horn cells*. Laminae 7, 8 and 9 represent the motor horn. Aδ and C fibres terminate in several layers, including the outer (marginal) zone and in particular lamina 2 (substantia gelatinosa).

Some dorsal horn cells respond to painful and non-painful stimuli, and are called 'wide dynamic range' neurones (WDR). They exhibit 'wind up' in which their output *increases* in the presence of a continuous, low-frequency, C fibre (i.e. painful) input. In this case, the C-fibre input has 'sensitized' the dorsal horn cell, and animal models have demonstrated that NMDA (*N*-methyl, D-aspartate) receptor activation is a key feature. This process is termed 'central sensitization'.

ALLODYNIA AND HYPERALGESIA

Allodynia is the term for pain induced by a previously non-painful stimulus. Hyperalgesia is increased pain from a previous painful stimulus. Both occur following peripheral and central sensitization, and they should be regarded as normal physiological processes following tissue injury, designed to encourage the organism to protect the injury.

The receptive field of a dorsal horn neurone refers to the area in the periphery where stimulation triggers action potentials in that dorsal horn neurone. Following tissue injury, the receptive field expands, and minor changes in excitability cause major changes in the size of the receptive field.

ASCENDING TRACTS AND SUPRASPINAL SYSTEMS

Most dorsal horn neurones project to the brain by ascending several segments in the spinal cord before

Table 25.1 Characteristics of primary afferent fibre (Aβ is included for comparison)

	C	Aδ	Aβ
Conductive velocity	IV ($<2m\,s^{-1}$)	III ($10–40m\,s^{-1}$)	II ($>40m\,s^{-1}$)
Myelination	No	Yes	Yes
Receptors	High threshold	High and low threshold	Low threshold

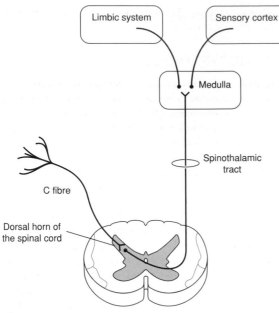

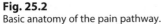

Fig. 25.2
Basic anatomy of the pain pathway.

crossing over to the opposite ventrolateral side, and joining one of three major spinal systems:

- Spinothalamic tract: probably the most important tract for pain transmission, this tract projects to several nuclei in the thalamus. It is the target for treating intractable cancer pain with cordotomy.
- Spinoreticular tract: terminates in the reticular nuclei in the brainstem.
- Spinomesencephalic tract: terminates in the mesencephalic reticular formation and periaqueductal grey.

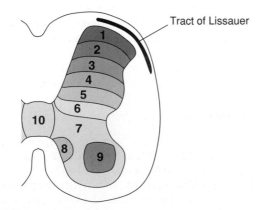

Fig. 25.3
Rexed laminae.

- All the terminal sites of spinal tracts project to the somatosensory cortex, associated with the sensory aspect of pain.
- Limbic system, associated with the affective aspect of pain.

DESCENDING SYSTEMS

Transmission across spinal cord synapses may be modulated by descending inhibitory pathways, originating in particular from the periaqueductal grey in the midbrain, and rostral ventromedial medulla. Both these areas contain high concentrations of endogenous opioids and opioid receptors. Activation of these receptors *increases* activity in descending monoamine (serotonin and norepinephrine) pathways (indirectly, by reducing stimulation of inhibitory interneurones), and reduces transmission across dorsal horn synapses.

VISCERAL PAIN

Afferent C fibres from abdominal viscera travel with autonomic nerves, particularly sympathetic, and synapse with dorsal horn cells. Thus, sympathetic denervation may be useful for intractable visceral pain (e.g. coeliac plexus block for pancreatic cancer). There is no distinct spinothalamic tract for visceral afferents.

REFERRED PAIN

Referred pain is experienced at a site distant from the pain source, and occurs because of *convergence* of different pain afferents onto common dorsal horn neurones. Segmental embryonic innervation remains throughout growth and accounts for the distance between the source of pain and referred site. Referred pain is often described as an ache, and is not accompanied by any other sensory abnormality.

NEUROPATHIC PAIN

This is pain arising from an abnormality in either the peripheral or central nervous systems. It is usually accompanied by other sensory (numbness, paraesthesia), motor (weakness) or autonomic dysfunction, and so may be distinguished from referred pain. Radicular pain is pain arising in the distribution of a spinal nerve, and may be caused by compression of the spinal cord, nerve root, or plexus.

Changes occur within the nervous system following any prolonged, noxious stimulus, as in the postoperative period where the surgical wound sends afferent neuronal information to the central nervous system for some time. Both 'peripheral' and 'central' sensitization occur and alter the body's response to further peripheral sensory input. Moreover, surgery generates a catabolic state by changes in endocrine hormonal control with increased secretion of catabolic hormones and decreased secretion of anabolic hormones. The results include pain; nausea, vomiting and intestinal stasis; alterations in blood flow, coagulation and fibrinolysis; alterations in substrate metabolism; alterations in water and electrolyte handling by the body; and increased demands on the cardiovascular and respiratory systems.

New principles of pain management have been developed to improve analgesia after surgery in the light of our new understanding of the processes involved. These include the recognition of the adverse effects of unrelieved pain, the need for an experienced and flexible approach to the problem by medical and nursing staff, and the necessity of informing the patient about the pain relief process. It is best to make plans for analgesia before surgery takes place, and this is especially important in short-stay surgery where the patient is discharged home soon after the operation. The safety and efficacy of postoperative pain management may be improved by frequent assessment of the patient, good education of the staff and patients about the techniques and drugs used, preparation of protocols and guidelines for staff to follow, and regular evaluation by quality assurance programmes. Whilst acute postoperative pain normally settles over a relatively short time period, it is recognized that there is a significant incidence of chronic, severe pain after surgery including thoracotomy, mastectomy, limb amputation, and the less-invasive operation of vasectomy. The aetiology of ongoing severe pain after surgery must lie in the pathophysiological changes, described above, that occur after tissue damage.

CAUSES OF VARIATION IN ANALGESIC REQUIREMENTS

Using patient-controlled analgesic apparatus (see below), it has been shown that there is marked interindividual variation in analgesic requirements. Thus, after open cholecystectomy, some patients may require no morphine within the first 24 h, whereas others may require as much as 120 mg. Unfortunately, there is no way of predicting in advance the extent of opioid requirements of an individual patient. In clinical practice, requirements are assessed on a trial-and-error basis; anaesthetists are therefore in an ideal position to be involved in prescribing postoperative analgesia, as they obtain a 'feel' for dose requirements during management of anaesthesia.

SITE AND TYPE OF SURGERY

In general, upper abdominal surgery produces greater pain than lower abdominal surgery, which in turn is associated with greater pain than peripheral surgery. This generalization is not entirely accurate; operations on the richly innervated digits may be associated with quite severe pain.

The type of pain may differ with different types of surgery. Operations on joints are associated with sharp pain; in contrast, abdominal surgery is associated with two types of pain: a continuous dull nauseating ache (which responds well to morphine) and sharper pain induced by coughing and movement (which responds poorly to morphine). Pain associated with surgery on the digits may respond relatively poorly to opioids but well to nonsteroidal anti-inflammatory drugs. There is increasing evidence that minimally invasive, laparoscopic surgery produces less-prolonged postoperative pain than do traditional techniques, but the pain may still be severe, especially in the immediate postoperative period.

Table 25.2 provides an approximate guide to the duration and severity of postoperative pain.

AGE, GENDER AND BODY WEIGHT

The analgesic requirements of males and females are identical for similar types of surgery. However, there is a reduction in analgesic requirements with advancing age. Consequently, it is essential that the anaesthetist reduces the dosage of opioid drugs in elderly patients. For example, reasonable starting doses for intramuscular (or subcutaneous) postoperative morphine administration would be 7.5–12.5 mg for patients aged 20–39 years, but the dose should be reduced to only 2.5–5.0 mg for 70–85-year-old patients.

The established anaesthetic practice of prescribing the potent opioid drugs on a milligram or microgram per body weight basis lacks scientific validity. There is no evidence to suggest that variations in body weight in the adult population affect opioid requirements.

PSYCHOLOGICAL FACTORS

The patient's personality affects pain perception and response to analgesic drugs. Thus, patients with a low anxiety and low neuroticism score on a personality scale exhibit less postoperative pain and require smaller doses of opioid than patients who rate highly on these scales. Patients with high scores may exhibit a higher incidence of postoperative chest complications (Table 25.3).

Table 25.2   Duration and severity of postoperative pain

Site of operation	Duration of opioid use (h)	Severity of pain (0–4)
Abdominal		
Upper	48–72	3
Lower	Up to 48	2
Inguinal	Up to 36	1
Thoracotomy	72–96	4
Limbs	24–36	2
Faciomaxillary	Up to 48	2
Body wall	Up to 24	1
Perineal	24–48	2
Hip surgery	Up to 48	2

Table 25.3   Psychological factors which influence postoperative analgesic requirements

Personality – more pain if high neuroticism/extroversion
Social background
Culture
Motivation
Preoperative psychotherapy

The extent of a patient's anxiety also affects pain perception; increased anxiety results in a greater degree of perceived postoperative pain and increased opioid requirements.

These psychological factors help to explain the efficacy of preoperative psychotherapy. Anxiety and postoperative analgesic requirements are reduced if the preoperative assessment by the anaesthetist includes an explanation of forthcoming perioperative events and details regarding the provision of pain relief.

PHARMACOKINETIC VARIABILITY

After the intramuscular injection of an opioid, there is a three- to sevenfold difference between patients in the rate at which peak plasma concentrations of the drug occur and a two- to fivefold difference in the peak plasma concentration achieved. This is illustrated in Figure 25.4, which shows the mean change in plasma concentration after the first and second, and seventh and eighth injections. The variability in the plasma concentration is reflected by the large standard deviation of the mean. In addition, average concentrations increase after each of the first few injections; oscillation around a steady mean concentration does not occur until after approximately the fourth injection.

This pharmacokinetic variability helps to explain the relatively poor response to a single intramuscular injection given in the postoperative period.

PHARMACODYNAMIC VARIABILITY

Although there are widespread pharmacokinetic variations between patients in response to administration of opioids, the major reason for variation in opioid sensitivity is pharmacodynamic, i.e. a difference in the inherent sensitivity of opioid receptors.

Using continuous infusions of opioids to achieve equilibrium between receptor drug concentration and plasma concentration, it is possible to define a steady-state plasma concentration of opioid at which analgesia is produced. This is termed the minimum effective analgesic concentration (MEAC); values of MEAC for the commonly available opioids are shown in Table 25.4. MEAC levels vary four- to fivefold between individual patients and are affected by age and differences in psychological profile.

MEASUREMENT OF PAIN

Although pain measurement is subjective, it is a useful tool to aid assessment of the patient and the effect of treatment. Patient and doctor recall of the effectiveness of previous treatment is an unreliable way of monitoring response to therapy, and it is much better to record some type of repeatable measure. Some simple ways of measuring pain are listed below. It is important to involve the patient in the assessment process, as individual responses to treatment are so variable. Pain should be assessed upon movement, not simply when the patient is lying perfectly still in an attempt to minimize discomfort.

- Verbal rating scales tend to be short, easy to administer and easy to understand (e.g. 'none, mild, moderate or severe').
- The Visual Analogue Scale (VAS) is validated in clinical use, but some patients find it more

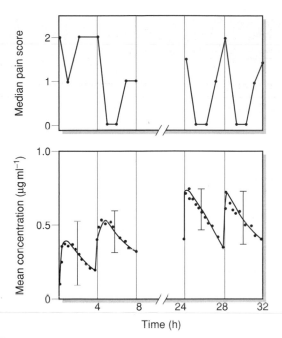

Fig. 25.4
Blood concentrations of pethidine and pain score after surgery; a pain score of 0 indicates no pain. Doses of pethidine 100 mg have been given 4-hourly. Mean blood concentration of pethidine continues to rise for 24 h before a plateau is reached. Little pain relief is provided by the first dose. Even after 24 h, significant pain is present 3 and 4 h after each injection, as blood concentrations decline.

difficult to understand than scales using word descriptors.

- A binary scale is one of the simplest to use. For example, 'Is your pain at least 50% relieved?', to which the patient answers yes or no.

Table 25.4   Minimum effective analgesic concentration (MEAC) in blood for a number of analgesic drugs (Note the wide range of values for each agent)

Drug	MEAC (ng ml⁻¹)
Fentanyl	1–3
Alfentanil	100–300
Pethidine	300–650
Morphine	12–24
Methadone	30–70

METHODS OF TREATING POSTOPERATIVE PAIN

See Table 25.5.

TRADITIONAL ADMINISTRATION OF OPIOIDS

Intramuscular administration of opioids on a pro re nata (p.r.n.; as required) basis was traditionally the method used most commonly for prescribing postoperative analgesia. However, for the reasons noted above, this technique leads frequently to inadequate pain relief. Almost 60% of patients report dissatisfaction with the quality of postoperative analgesia administered in this way.

Intramuscular injection results in variable absorption, particularly in patients with hypothermia, hypovolaemia or hypotension. In addition, there is inevitably a considerable delay between request for analgesia and subsequent administration while controlled drugs are checked and drawn into a syringe. Although it is customary to prescribe opioids on a 4-hourly p.r.n. basis, there are frequently much longer periods between injections and this may lead to considerable 'breakthrough' pain.

The commonest cause of postoperative nausea and vomiting is the administration of opioids either intraoperatively or in the postoperative period. It should therefore be standard practice to prescribe antiemetic drugs regularly for administration with opioids.

Regular administration of intramuscular opioids provides improved analgesia, although care must be taken to avoid overdosage in debilitated patients and those at the extremes of age.

The advantages and disadvantages of repeated p.r.n. administration of opioids are listed in Table 25.6. Drugs used commonly for postoperative pain and antiemesis are listed in Table 25.7; their pharmacological properties are discussed fully in Chapter 5. The use of pethidine for postoperative pain relief is decreasing because of the potential accumulation of the excitatory metabolite, norpethidine with repeated use.

SUBCUTANEOUS ADMINISTRATION OF OPIOIDS

Morphine may be given subcutaneously, and patients prefer this to intramuscular injections. A small-gauge cannula may be inserted subcutaneously and left in place for 2–3 days, avoiding the need for repeated skin punctures. Absorption of morphine from the subcutaneous route is comparable with absorption from the intramuscular route.

Table 25.5 Methods of treating postoperative pain

Traditional administration of opioid
Intramuscular or subcutaneous on-demand bolus

Parenteral administration of opioid
Bolus intravenous administration
Continuous intravenous infusion
Patient-controlled analgesia
    Bolus intravenous
    Bolus + infusion
Subcutaneous

Non-parenteral administration of opioid
Sublingual
Oral
Transmucosal
Rectal
Transdermal
Nasal
Inhalation
Intra-articular opioids

Local anaesthetic techniques
Spinal/extradural opioids
Entonox
Non-steroidal anti-inflammatory drugs (NSAIDs)
COX-2 selective inhibitors
Paracetamol
NMDA antagonists
α_2-Adrenergic agonists
Systemically
Extradurally

Non-pharmacological methods
Cryotherapy
Transcutaneous electrical nerve stimulation (TENS)
Acupuncture
Psychological methods

Table 25.6 Advantages and disadvantages of intramuscular p.r.n. administration of opioids

Advantages	Disadvantages
Familiar practice	Fixed dose not related to pharmacovariability
Gradual onset of side-effects	i.m. administration causes profound pharmacovariability
Nursing assessment before	Painful injections
Inexpensive	Fluctuating plasma concentrations
	Delayed onset of analgesia

Table 25.7 Drugs used systemically for postoperative pain relief and antiemesis

Drug	Dose i.m. or s.c. (healthy adult)
Opioids	
Morphine	10 mg 4-hourly
Pethidine	100 mg 3-hourly
Buprenorphine (sublingual)	0.4 mg 6-hourly
Tramadol	50–100 mg 4–6-hourly
Moderate analgesics	
Ketorolac	10–30 mg 6-hourly
Paracetamol	1 g 6-hourly
Dihydrocodeine	50 mg 4-hourly
Antiemetics	
Prochlorperazine	12.5 mg 6-hourly
Cyclizine	50 mg 6-hourly
Metoclopramide	10 mg 6-hourly
Ondansetron	4 mg i.v. 6-hourly

ALGORITHMS FOR OPIOID ADMINISTRATION

Some acute pain services have constructed algorithms for postoperative intramuscular or subcutaneous opioid administration that other less-experienced members of staff may then follow to provide safe and effective pain relief for their patients. Figure 25.5 is an example. An important aspect of such algorithms is the frequent assessment of the patient to ensure safety and efficacy of the treatment. Clinical assessments include pain (at rest and upon movement) and sedation scores, respiratory rate and arterial blood pressure. The algorithm includes a description of recommended doses

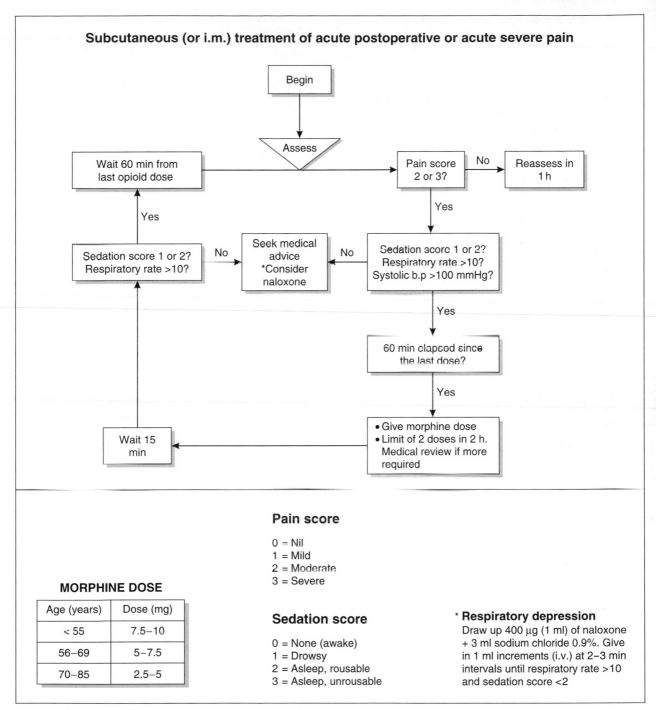

Subcutaneous (or i.m.) treatment of acute postoperative or acute severe pain

Begin

Assess

Wait 60 min from last opioid dose

Pain score 2 or 3? — No → Reassess in 1 h

Yes

Sedation score 1 or 2? Respiratory rate >10? — No → Seek medical advice *Consider naloxone ← No — Sedation score 1 or 2? Respiratory rate >10? Systolic b.p >100 mmHg?

Yes (Sedation score 1 or 2? Respiratory rate >10?)

Yes

60 min elapsed since the last dose?

Yes

- Give morphine dose
- Limit of 2 doses in 2 h. Medical review if more required

Wait 15 min

MORPHINE DOSE

Age (years)	Dose (mg)
< 55	7.5–10
56–69	5–7.5
70–85	2.5–5

Pain score

0 = Nil
1 = Mild
2 = Moderate
3 = Severe

Sedation score

0 = None (awake)
1 = Drowsy
2 = Asleep, rousable
3 = Asleep, unrousable

* Respiratory depression

Draw up 400 µg (1 ml) of naloxone + 3 ml sodium chloride 0.9%. Give in 1 ml increments (i.v.) at 2–3 min intervals until respiratory rate >10 and sedation score <2

Fig. 25.5
Subcutaneous (or intramuscular) treatment of acute postoperative or acute severe pain.

and instructions on how to treat recognized side-effects such as respiratory depression. An important feature of such algorithms is that they permit more frequent opioid administration, e.g. '2-hourly p.r.n.'.

Sites of action and properties of morphine and morphine-like drugs

Opioids act supraspinally (nucleus raphes magnus, periaqueductal and periventricular grey areas), in the spinal cord (around C-fibre terminals in lamina I and the substantia gelatinosa, lamina II), and peripherally (opioid receptors are transported peripherally in axons, and are expressed by immune cells at the site of tissue damage). The actions of morphine are:

- Analgesia – morphine produces analgesia by binding with opioid receptors which are present in high concentrations in the periaqueductal area and limbic system of the brain and in the region of the substantia gelatinosa of the spinal cord
- Ventilatory depression
- Sedation
- Cough suppression
- Vasodilatation
- Release of histamine
- Constipation
- Nausea and vomiting
- Pupillary constriction
- Biliary spasm
- Urine retention
- Tolerance
- Physical dependence (addiction to opioids is rare when they are used for the relief of acute postoperative pain).

The most important side-effects of morphine are ventilatory depression and nausea and vomiting. (As significant hypoxaemia may occur for several days postoperatively, supplemental oxygen is recommended for at least the first 48–72 h following major surgery, and in the elderly or high-risk patient regardless of the analgesic method used.) Morphine should not be administered to patients with biliary or renal colic (occasionally it may precipitate pain in patients with gallbladder disease when administered as premedication) and should be avoided in patients with head injury and perhaps in asthmatics. Tramadol is an interesting synthetic analgesic as it has both opioid and non-opioid mechanisms of action and may produce analgesia with less respiratory depression, sedation, gastrointestinal stasis and abuse potential. Unfortunately, as with morphine, the use of tramadol is associated with nausea and vomiting.

PARENTERAL ROUTES OF OPIOID ADMINISTRATION

Bolus i.v. administration

It is possible to improve the quality of analgesia in the postoperative period by giving small incremental doses of opioid i.v. when required. However, this carries the risk of rapid induction of ventilatory depression and in many hospitals cannot be undertaken by nursing staff in the wards. In general, this technique is employed only by anaesthetists and experienced nursing staff in the immediate recovery period.

Continuous i.v. infusion

Continuous i.v. infusion (Table 25.8) is employed to provide analgesia in patients receiving artificial ventilation in an intensive therapy unit (ITU). An infusion rate designed to exceed MEAC in all patients is clearly safe and ventilatory depression is an advantage in this situation.

Continuous infusions have been used in general surgical wards for the provision of postoperative analgesia in spontaneously breathing patients. The dosage rate is determined by the medical attendant on a trial-and-error basis and a fixed infusion rate prescribed. However, this carries great risks of producing ventilatory depression and cannot be recommended in spontaneously breathing patients outside a high-dependency unit or ITU.

Patient-controlled analgesia

The main problem with continuous i.v. infusion is that there is no way of predicting an individual patient's MEAC. With patient-controlled analgesia (PCA), the patient determines the rate of i.v. administration of the drug, thereby providing feedback control.

Table 25.8 Advantages and disadvantages of continuous i.v. infusions

Advantages	Disadvantages
Rapid onset of analgesia	Fixed dose not related to pharmacodynamic variability
Steady-state plasma concentrations	Errors may be fatal
Painless	Expensive fail-safe equipment required
	May result in less frequent assessment by nursing staff

PCA equipment comprises an accurate source of infusion coupled to an i.v. cannula, and controlled by a patient–machine interface device. Safety features are incorporated to limit the preset dose, the number of doses which may be administered and the 'lockout' period between doses. Advantages and disadvantages of PCA are listed in Table 25.9.

The drug that has been used most commonly with PCA is morphine. The size of the demand dose is usually 1–2 mg with a lockout period of between 5 and 10 min. Fentanyl (10–20 μg), pethidine (10 mg) and hydromorphone (0.2 mg) may also be used for intravenous PCA. Although there may be some theoretical advantage in the use of a continuous low-dose infusion on which the patient may superimpose demand bolus administrations, in practice several clinical investigations have failed to reveal any advantage. Because of the slightly increased risk of overdosage, therefore, it is generally recommended that PCA apparatus be used in the 'bolus alone' mode.

Intravenous PCA is now a standard method of providing postoperative analgesia in many hospitals worldwide. It provides better pain relief than conventional intermittent intramuscular administration. It is essential that monitoring of the patient is not reduced, as respiratory depression may occur with this technique and many patients may require antiemetics for nausea. If the pump is being used to deliver morphine via an intravenous infusion, it is essential that a one-way valve be incorporated between the PCA equipment and the infusion giving set in order to prevent morphine collecting in the giving set if the cannula becomes occluded; if this happens, a large bolus may be delivered at a later time, with possible lethal effects.

The effective and safe use of PCA requires frequent monitoring of the patient by nurses who have had in-service training and accreditation in the use of the drugs and devices. There is evidence that PCA is more effective when it is overseen by an acute pain service involving pain nursing staff and pharmacists. Standard PCA prescription orders and drug dilutions may minimize complications. PCA may also be used to deliver opioids subcutaneously or epidurally.

NON-PARENTERAL OPIOID ADMINISTRATION

Sublingual opioids

Sublingual administration requires cooperation. With buprenorphine, good analgesia may be provided without the need for painful injections, making this route popular with patients and convenient for nursing staff.

This route is confined largely to buprenorphine. Combination with morphine may result in dysphoria and withdrawal phenomena. If this route is chosen, it is preferable to use buprenorphine as the sole opioid in the perioperative period, although, as it is a partial opioid agonist, it has a ceiling effect for analgesia.

Oral route

All the opioids undergo extensive metabolism in the gut wall and liver (first-pass metabolism) and therefore the bioavailability is relatively low (e.g. 20–30% for morphine). Oxycodone (UK; OxyNorm) undergoes less biotransformation, acts rapidly, and is therefore a useful oral opioid for the relief of severe pain (e.g. 5–10 mg, 2–3 hourly). Oxycodone is also available as a sustained-release preparation and an injectable form. In the immediate postoperative period, there is invariably a reduction in the rate of gastric emptying (caused mainly by the intraoperative or preoperative use of opioids). For this reason, care should be taken if opioids are used orally for pain relief in the postoperative period because:

- Absorption may be delayed, with poor analgesia.
- If opioids have been given orally on a regular basis, there is a danger of a large dose being propelled into the upper gastrointestinal tract when gastric motility returns to normal, resulting in overdosage and ventilatory depression.

If normal gastric emptying has resumed, then oral opioids may be used safely and effectively after sur-

Table 25.9 Advantages and disadvantages of patient-controlled analgesia (PCA)	
Advantages	**Disadvantages**
Dose matches patient's requirements and therefore compensates for pharmacodynamic variability	Technical errors may be fatal
	Expensive equipment
	Requires ability to cooperate and understand
Doses given are small and therefore fluctuations in plasma concentration is reduced	
Reduces nurses' workload	
Painless	
Placebo effect from patient autonomy	

gery to provide analgesia without the need for injections.

Transmucosal

Oral transmucosal fentanyl citrate has been prepared as a palatable solid matrix (presented as a lollipop) for use as a pre-anaesthetic medication in children. The time to the onset of pain relief is of the order of 9 min, and both transmucosal (buccal) and gastric routes contribute to the absorption of fentanyl. Side-effects include nausea and vomiting, and hypoxaemia.

The rectal route

The rectal route may be used as a means of delivering morphine but there is marked variability in the plasma concentrations achieved. Venous blood from the lower part of the rectum drains directly into the systemic circulation, but the upper part drains into the portal circulation. Thus, bioavailability varies according to the site of a suppository within the rectum. However, this route avoids the problems of reduced gastrointestinal motility. Probably the best indication for the rectal route is the treatment of chronic intractable pain, particularly where there is dysphagia.

Inhaled/intranasal

Intranasal spray devices for fentanyl are now available in some countries. Inhaled opioid preparations are being developed that have metered inhalers with improved pulmonary drug delivery systems and lockout times, and in the future they may allow noninvasive PCA administration.

Transdermal

Because of the high lipid solubility and high potency of fentanyl, this drug may be absorbed across the skin in sufficient quantities to produce effective plasma concentrations. Transdermal fentanyl patches are available with delivery rates from 25 to 100 μg h^{-1}. Because of the difficulty in matching transdermal patches of differing strengths to the pharmacodynamic variability between different patients, this technique is not suitable for management of acute pain, but is used for the relief of cancer pain. A disposable PCA skin patch for the iontophoretic delivery of fentanyl through the skin has been developed. Preliminary results of clinical trials indicate this is a safe and effective way of administering fentanyl after surgery.

LOCAL ANAESTHETIC TECHNIQUES

Many local anaesthetic techniques, administered for the purpose of operative surgery or during the course of general anaesthesia, may provide excellent analgesia in the early postoperative period. However, it is usually necessary for the anaesthetist to administer an opioid to the patient before the block regresses, to reduce the likelihood of severe pain when the block wears off.

Many local anaesthetic techniques may be used for the primary purpose of providing analgesia in the early postoperative period. However, a major disadvantage is that the duration of blockade with a 'single-shot' technique is relatively short. Bupivacaine (0.25% or 0.5%) has been the drug of choice and may produce peripheral nerve blockade lasting for 8–12 h and occasionally for as long as 18 h. The duration of action for epidural nerve block is 4–6 h. Ropivacaine has similar local anaesthetic characteristics to those of bupivacaine, but with less cardiac toxicity. Ropivacaine is available as 2, 7.5 and 10 mg mL^{-1} preparations; motor blockade is less at low doses than with bupivacaine. Levobupivacaine is the single 'S' isomer derivative of bupivacaine, has similar local anaesthetic properties, but with the theoretical promise of less cardiotoxicity. Levobupivacaine is available as 2, 5 and 7.5 mg mL^{-1} preparations

Epinephrine may be added to a local anaesthetic solution to prolong the block, although this produces relatively little effect on the duration of analgesia produced by bupivacaine or ropivacaine. The most effective means of prolonging the block is by the use of a catheter to permit either repeated bolus doses or a continuous infusion of local anaesthetic to be administered.

Local anaesthetic blocks in common use are described in Chapter 17. The following blocks represent those which are most useful for postoperative analgesia.

Spinal nerve block

Subarachnoid analgesia rarely lasts more than 3–4 h with the drugs currently available and is therefore of limited use for postoperative analgesia, although there is evidence that intrathecal analgesia may modify the physiological changes associated with surgery. Although the insertion of a catheter into the subarachnoid space is used in the USA, this is not a popular manoeuvre in the UK or Australia.

Epidural block

Epidural block is popular for postoperative analgesia because of familiarity with the technique and ease of insertion of a catheter. Epidural analgesic techniques can provide superior postoperative analgesia and modify the physiological changes associated with some forms of surgery. Postoperative epidural analgesia can reduce the incidence of pulmonary morbidity. However, epidural techniques also have uncommon but serious risks attached to catheter insertion and removal (e.g. epidural haematoma) and so the risk–benefit ratio for each patient must be considered. Repeated injections may be made through the catheter or a dilute solution of local anaesthetic infused continuously. Initially, bupivacaine produces analgesia lasting up to 4 h, but by 24–48 h some tolerance develops and single-bolus administrations may last for only 2 h. Ropivacaine, in low doses, may offer the advantage of producing similar sensory block with less motor impairment. Levobupivacaine produces local anaesthetic effects similar to those of bupivacaine.

Bupivacaine 0.25% injected at L2/3 provides good analgesia after lower abdominal or perineal surgery, e.g. hysterectomy or transurethral resection of prostate. Upper abdominal procedures require a higher block; 15 mL of bupivacaine 0.5% produces analgesia up to T7.

For thoracic surgery, an epidural catheter may be inserted in the thoracic region between T6 and T8, and volumes of bupivacaine of 6–12 mL may provide excellent postoperative analgesia.

In general, it is recommended that epidural catheter techniques should be used only when the patient is nursed in a high-dependency unit, because of the risks of hypotension after epidural injections and total spinal block if the catheter migrates into the subarachnoid space. However, in some institutions, continuous infusion epidural techniques are managed on general wards, but only with the benefit of adequate medical and nursing staff experience, and the existence of clear protocols for monitoring and the early detection of side-effects.

Some potential advantages of epidural analgesia

- Superior pain relief.
- Improved postoperative respiratory function.
- Reduction in the stress response to surgery after lower abdominal and lower limb surgery (minimal effect after upper abdominal or thoracic surgery).
- Reduction in the hypercoagulable state after major surgery; there is a decreased incidence of deep venous thrombosis and pulmonary embolism after hip surgery.
- Reduced intraoperative blood loss during surgery on the lower part of the body.
- Improved postoperative gut function, facilitating early enteral nutrition.

Some potential complications of epidural analgesia

- Dural puncture (0.6–1.3%).
- Epidural haematoma – the risk is increased by impaired haemostasis when the catheter is inserted or removed. Guidelines must be followed for concomitant prophylactic low molecular weight heparin and low-dose heparin therapy.
- Epidural abscess, meningitis and direct neurological damage.
- Systemic local anaesthetic toxicity.
- Total spinal anaesthesia.
- Sympathetic blockade (haemodynamic effects), urinary retention and motor block.

Caudal block

Caudal administration of local anaesthetic drugs is useful for child day-case surgery, e.g. circumcision, or in patients undergoing anal or perineal surgery. It is customary to administer only a single dose of local anaesthetic; catheter techniques are unpopular in the UK because of the risk of infection. Suitable doses of local anaesthetic solution for use by the caudal route are shown in Table 25.10.

Other regional blocks used for postoperative analgesia

Intercostal nerve blockade. Blocks from T4 to T8 or 9 provide satisfactory analgesia for pain relief after subcostal incision for cholecystectomy. Intercostal blocks may be repeated at regular intervals; catheters have been used for repeated administration. Bilateral blockade should not be carried out because of the risk of pneumothorax.

Paravertebral block. This may be used to provide analgesia after thoracic or abdominal surgery. Local anaesthetic solution is injected into the region of the paravertebral space to block the dorsal sensory nerve roots as they emerge from the vertebral foramina. This technique may be performed using single or repeated injections or with an indwelling catheter.

Table 25.10 Doses of bupivacaine (0.25% plain) for caudal analgesia	
Adult	**Child**
0.3–0.4 ml kg^{-1}	0.5–0.7 ml kg^{-1} (or 0.1ml year^{-1} for each segment to be blocked)
N.B. Dosage of bupivacaine should *never* exceed 2 mg kg^{-1}.	

Interpleural analgesia may be used to provide unilateral analgesia after thoracotomy, breast surgery, open cholecystectomy and renal surgery. The use of interpleural analgesia can improve postoperative respiratory function, although the presence of intercostal chest drains or haemothorax may diminish the effectiveness of this procedure.

Brachial plexus analgesia, using a catheter placed close to the plexus and a continuous infusion of local anaesthetic, covers almost all of the upper limb and produces a sympathetic block that may be beneficial following plastic surgery.

Femoral nerve block, using a continuous infusion technique, is useful for relief of pain after knee surgery and may facilitate recovery after knee arthroplasty.

Combined ilioinguinal and iliohypogastric nerve block is a safe and effective regional technique for postoperative pain control after inguinal hernia repair.

Wound infiltration after minor or paediatric surgery is an established analgesic technique for pain relief, but the benefit after major surgery is not clear. Portable continuous infusion devices have been developed to allow prolonged administration of local anaesthetics after surgery, e.g. to provide good analgesia after shoulder surgery.

SPINAL AND EPIDURAL OPIOIDS

In recent years, there has been great interest in the use of opioids by the subarachnoid or epidural routes. After injection of opioid into the cerebrospinal fluid (CSF), drug is taken up in the region of the substantia gelatinosa within the dorsal horn. It is thought that opioids act predominantly on the presynaptic enkephalin receptors, although opioid is absorbed from the CSF into the circulation. After epidural administration of opioids, the drug diffuses through the dura into the CSF and produces analgesia by the same mechanism as that associated with subarachnoid injection. However, there is more rapid uptake of opioid into the circulation via the rich network of blood vessels in the epidural space. Consequently, there is a rapid increase in both CSF and blood concentrations of the drug after epidural administration.

Uptake into the dorsal horn and rate of passage through the dura are dependent upon lipid solubility. Thus, the more highly lipid-soluble drugs (e.g. fentanyl) have a more rapid onset and a shorter duration of action. The less lipid-soluble drugs (e.g. morphine) have a slower rate of onset of action; in addition there is a greater dispersion within the CSF because of reduced uptake into spinal cord and the drug may reach the medulla to cause delayed ventilatory depression.

Subarachnoid opioids

This route is less popular than the epidural route of administration for opioids because of the production of spinal headache. However, smaller doses are required than with the epidural route and therefore systemic concentrations are lower. The quality of analgesia is not as good as that achieved with subarachnoid local anaesthetic drugs.

Epidural opioids

The administration of epidural opioids is more popular because spinal headache is avoided and a catheter technique may be used. It is possible to achieve analgesia without the motor or autonomic block produced by local anaesthetic injected into the epidural space. Thus, postural hypotension and changes in heart rate do not occur. Early ventilatory depression may occur as a result of systemic absorption (e.g. within the first 1–2 h), but late ventilatory depression (8–20 h) is a result of rostral spread of opioid within the CSF to the medulla. Prolonged duration of action of analgesia is produced by a single injection (up to 24 h).

Side-effects of epidural opioids

- Early ventilatory depression occurs more commonly with lipid-soluble agents.
- Late ventilatory depression occurs more commonly with agents of lower lipophilicity.
- Coma occurs relatively late, usually in association with late ventilatory depression and can be reversed by naloxone.
- Urinary retention.
- Itching is reversed only partially by naloxone.
- Nausea and vomiting.

Epidural opioids are more effective when used in combination with local anaesthetics to produce a synergistic analgesic action. This reduces the necessary dose and the side-effects that would be associated with the local anaesthetic or the opioid alone. For example, continuous epidural infusion of a combined solution of a low concentration of bupivacaine with fentanyl provides a good postoperative analgesia with minimal side-effects.

INHALATION OF VOLATILE OR GASEOUS ANAESTHETICS

Although volatile anaesthetics were used in the past, the only agent in current use is N_2O. This is administered in the form of Entonox (premixed 50% N_2O, 50% O_2) usually via a demand valve and face mask.

Entonox is used extensively in obstetric analgesia, in the field situation (e.g. by ambulance personnel to provide analgesia at the site of an accident), or occasionally in the wards during change of surgical dressings. The potential spinal cord and haematological adverse effects of nitrous oxide, via interference with vitamin B_{12} metabolism, may prevent repeated use.

NON-STEROIDAL ANTI-INFLAMMATORY DRUGS (NSAIDS) AND SELECTIVE COX-2 INHIBITORS

The use of NSAIDs (cyclo-oxygenase inhibitors) for postoperative pain relief is now routine practice. NSAIDs may be given orally, rectally (e.g. diclofenac 100 mg) or intravenously (e.g. ketorolac 10 mg). NSAIDs produce pain relief without sedation, respiratory depression or nausea and vomiting, but their use is limited by gastric, renal and platelet side-effects. A recent authoritative and extensive review of the published literature concerning NSAIDs drew the following conclusions:

- NSAIDs are not sufficiently effective as the sole analgesic agent after major surgery.
- NSAIDs are often effective after minor or outpatient surgery.
- NSAIDs often decrease opioid requirement. Significant reduction in opioid side-effects has been noted in a few studies only.
- The quality of opioid-based analgesia is often enhanced by NSAIDs.
- NSAIDs increase bleeding time and some studies have shown increased blood loss after surgery.

The major adverse effects of NSAIDs for surgical patients are those involving the gastrointestinal system, renal and platelet function, and aspirin-induced asthma in susceptible patients. The adverse effects of NSAIDs are serious, and contraindications (e.g. peptic ulceration, bleeding diathesis, renal impairment, aspirin-induced asthma) must be respected. The incidence and severity of NSAID-related adverse effects are greater in elderly patients. Aspirin is contraindicated in children less than 12 years old. There have been case reports of sudden renal dysfunction in patients given NSAIDs perioperatively; risk factors for this may include nephrotoxic antibiotics (e.g. gentamicin), raised intra-abdominal pressure during laparoscopy, hypovolaemia, and age greater than 65 years.

New drugs have been developed that selectively inhibit the inducible cyclo-oxygenase enzyme, COX-2, and spare the constitutive, COX-1, enzyme. Most conventional NSAIDs in clinical use are nonselective inhibitors of COX-1 and COX-2, and many of the side-effects of the older drugs may be by COX-1 inhibition and disruption of physiological prostaglandin production. COX-2 is induced by tissue damage and inflammation, and selective inhibitors of this enzyme produce analgesia with fewer side-effects. Studies have confirmed that COX-2 inhibitors produce effective analgesia after surgery, similar to that of the NSAIDs. There is encouraging evidence that COX-2 inhibitors have less gastrointestinal side-effects, but the effect on the kidneys is similar to that of conventional NSAIDs. As platelets produce thromboxane for aggregation via COX-1 only, COX-2 inhibitors do not affect platelet function and have been shown to be associated with lower surgical blood loss. The role of COX-2 inhibitors in producing a tendency to thrombosis, by inhibition of endothelial prostacyclin but no antiplatelet effect, is a significant disadvantage that has led to the withdrawal of rofecoxib and restrictions on the use of other agents. There is encouraging evidence that COX-2 inhibitors are tolerated well by individuals who suffer from aspirin-induced asthma.

PARACETAMOL

Paracetamol is a useful adjunct to opioids in the treatment of postoperative pain, with fewer contraindications than the NSAIDs. It is analgesic and antipyretic, but not anti-inflammatory. The mechanism of action is unclear, but may involve the selective inhibition of prostaglandin synthesis in the central nervous system, perhaps by inhibition of another cyclo-oxygenase subtype, COX-3. In adults with normal hepatic and renal function, the recommended dose is 500–1000 mg orally or rectally every 3–6 h when necessary, with a maximum daily dose of $6 \, g \, day^{-1}$ for acute use and $4 \, g \, day^{-1}$ for chronic use. (Care must be taken to avoid inadvertent paracetamol overdosage and resultant hepatic and renal toxicity.) An intravenous preparation is available and has been shown to be an effective postoperative analgesic.

NMDA ANTAGONISTS

The activation by excitatory amino acids (glutamate) of spinal cord dorsal horn N-methyl-D-aspartate (NMDA) receptors is essential for the development of central sensitization. The anaesthetic agent ketamine is a potent NMDA receptor antagonist. Low-dose subcutaneous or intravenous ketamine infusions (5–$15 \, mg \, h^{-1}$) produce significant pain relief after surgery. Unfortunately, the side-effects of ketamine, including hallucinations, limit the use of this agent. Dextromethorphan is an alternative NMDA receptor antagonist which has been shown to reduce opioid requirements following oral surgery and during abdominal surgery.

NON-PHARMACOLOGICAL METHODS

Cryotherapy

This may be applied to intercostal nerves exposed during a thoracotomy. The nerve is surrounded by an ice-ball produced by intense sub-zero temperatures at the end of a probe. The neuronal disruption produced by this method is temporary and sensation returns after some months, although it may be accompanied by unpleasant paraesthesia and occasionally by persistent neuralgia.

Transcutaneous electrical stimulation

A small alternating current is passed between two surface electrodes at low voltage and at a frequency of 0.2–200 Hz. It is thought that the technique acts by increasing CNS concentrations of endorphins. Acupuncture may work in a similar manner. The technique produces only moderate analgesia.

Acupuncture

Acupuncture has been assessed as a technique for pain relief after surgery. There is evidence that acupuncture reduces pain and analgesic consumption after dental and abdominal surgery, although there is some variability in the method of administration.

PRE-EMPTIVE ANALGESIA

The importance of peripheral and central sensitization in amplifying pain perception has directed research towards preventing these processes. Experimentally, it has been shown that nociceptive stimulation from the periphery causes functional changes in the spinal cord which lead to enhancement and prolongation of the sensation of pain. It has also been shown that prior administration of analgesics may inhibit the development of the hyperexcitability within the spinal cord. Unfortunately, however, in clinical practice, prior administration of analgesics (pre-emptive analgesia) has not been shown to have an important effect on postoperative pain. Further studies are being performed on pre-emptive analgesia, incorporating additional strategies to prevent and modulate the prolonged neuronal input to the spinal cord from the peripheral tissue inflammatory process.

BALANCED (MULTIMODAL) ANALGESIA

The concept of balanced analgesia is analogous to that of balanced anaesthesia. It is possible to block the development of pain by the use of a combination of different drugs acting at different sites: peripherally, on somatic and sympathetic nerves, at spinal cord level and centrally. The benefit of this technique is that not only may superior analgesia be achieved by a combination of drugs but also their individual doses may be reduced, thereby decreasing the incidence of side-effects. For example, after thoracotomy, the addition of an NSAID to a regimen based on intercostal nerve blocks and PCA morphine significantly improves analgesia.

Pain transmission may be blocked clinically at the following sites:

- inhibition of peripheral nociceptor mechanisms using NSAIDs, COX-2 inhibitors, steroids or opioids
- blockade of afferent neuronal transmission using peripheral, epidural or spinal local anaesthetic administration
- interference at both spinal cord level and higher centres using spinal and systemic opioids.

The use of non-opioid analgesics in multimodal analgesia minimizes opioid side-effects including gastrointestinal stasis. After bowel surgery, multimodal analgesia (an epidural infusion of a low-dose local anaesthetic and opioid mixture, and systemic NSAID) produces excellent pain relief, avoids the need for systemic opioids and speeds the recovery of gastrointestinal function. This facilitates early mobilization of the patient and a more rapid return to enteral nutrition.

Typically, for minor surgery, e.g. hernia repair on a day-case basis, the anaesthetist may employ multimodal or balanced analgesia in the form of:

- preoperative administration of a mild oral analgesic, e.g. paracetamol and an NSAID or a COX-2 inhibitor
- administration of fentanyl intraoperatively ± tramadol
- local anaesthetic block using ilioinguinal and iliohypogastric nerve blocks and wound infiltration
- the use of NSAIDs in the form of a diclofenac suppository 100 mg, or a COX-2 inhibitor.

With this technique, patients frequently do not require supplementary opioids postoperatively and may be managed on a day-case basis using simple oral analgesics in the postoperative period, e.g. paracetamol. Oral tramadol may be useful if stronger postoperative analgesia is required.

NEUROPATHIC PAIN IN THE POSTOPERATIVE PERIOD

The possibility of the development of neuropathic pain should be borne in mind after surgery, as it is often missed in patients with acute pain and may require specific therapy (see Ch. 42 for the management of chronic pain). A useful definition of neuropathic pain is 'pain associated with injury, disease or surgical section of the peripheral or central nervous system'. One diagnostic clue after surgery is an unexpected increase in opioid consumption, as neuropathic pain often responds poorly to normal doses of opioids. Features suggestive of neuropathic pain include:

- pain without ongoing tissue damage
- sensory loss
- allodynia (pain in response to non-painful stimuli)
- hyperalgesia (increased pain in response to painful stimuli)
- dysaesthesiae (unpleasant abnormal sensations)
- burning, stabbing or shooting pain
- a delay in onset after injury.

ACUTE PAIN SERVICES

The supervision of postoperative pain relief has been allocated in many hospitals to acute pain services, often staffed by anaesthetists and nurses. The establishment of an acute pain service in a hospital has been shown to improve postoperative pain management. Acute pain services have various roles:

- continuing staff education about pain
- standardization of orders of analgesic prescription and monitoring of patients
- the provision of new or specialized methods of pain relief
- audit and clinical research.

In the future, acute pain services may be better integrated with surgical and other staff to form perioperative care services that can direct all aspects of multimodal analgesia, perioperative nutrition and postoperative mobilization to facilitate the rapid recovery of the patient after surgery.

FURTHER READING

McQuay H, Moore A (eds) 1998 An evidence-based resource for pain relief. Oxford University Press, Oxford

National Health and Medical Research Council of Australia 2005 Acute pain management: scientific evidence, 2nd edn. Commonwealth of Australia, Canberra

Royal College of Anaesthetists 1998 Guidelines for the use of nonsteroidal antiinflammatory drugs in the perioperative period. Royal College of Anaesthetists, London

26 Postoperative nausea and vomiting

Death or serious morbidity resulting directly from anaesthesia is now extremely rare. However, postoperative nausea and vomiting (PONV) is still very common. Surveys have confirmed that PONV is feared considerably by patients undergoing surgery. Indeed, it is often rated above postoperative pain when patients are asked to rank their concerns. Therefore, every anaesthetist must be aware of the physiology of PONV and its consequences, causes, associated factors and management.

VOMITING REFLEX

All reflexes, including the vomiting reflex, consist of afferent inputs, a degree of central processing and motor efferents. The vomiting reflex is summarized in Figure 26.1.

BRAINSTEM

Areas of the brainstem involved in vomiting have been termed the 'vomiting centre'. However, this is not an anatomical entity; it represents several nuclei in the brainstem (e.g. nucleus tractus solitarius, respiratory neural networks) which are responsible for the coordination of the efferent limb of the vomiting reflex. It receives input from the afferent limbs of the reflex and the area postrema.

AREA POSTREMA

The area postrema is located at the caudal end of the floor of the fourth ventricle; this area is also known as the chemoreceptor trigger zone (CTZ). Evidence from ablation studies by Borison and Wang in the 1950s and the fact that the blood-brain barrier is defective in this area suggest that the area postrema is responsible for detecting toxins circulating in the blood and cerebrospinal fluid. However, it may be that a more precise area for this function is the nearby nucleus tractus solitarius where dopamine and opioid receptors are abundant.

AFFERENT LIMBS OF VOMITING REFLEX

Gastrointestinal tract

Information from mechano- and chemoreceptors in the gastrointestinal tract is relayed via the vagus nerve to the nucleus tractus solitarius in the brainstem. Abnormal gastric or intestinal distension, increased smooth muscle contraction and abnormal or toxic gastrointestinal contents can trigger the vomiting reflex. Peripheral $5-HT_3$ receptors are intimately involved in this system. Radiation, chemotherapy and other toxins release 5-HT from chromaffin cells in the gut, which stimulates vagal afferents – a process inhibited by the $5-HT_3$ antagonist antiemetics (see below). Dopamine receptors are also abundant in the upper gastrointestinal tract.

Vestibular system

Input from the vestibular system is responsible for motion sickness, particularly when vestibular and visual signals conflict. Patients with a history of motion sickness and those who are moved excessively in the early postoperative period are more likely to suffer from PONV.

Cardiovascular system

Stimulation of afferents from both cardiac ventricles and blood vessels may lead to vomiting. For example, hypotension and myocardial infarction are often associated with nausea and vomiting.

Higher centres

Input from higher centres often plays a vital role in the genesis of PONV. A calm, well-informed patient who

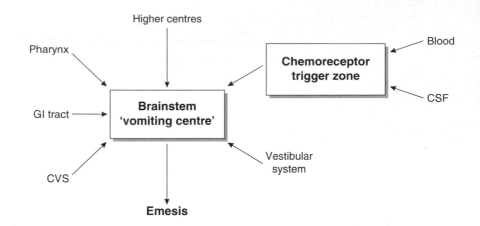

Fig. 26.1
The vomiting reflex.

is denied unpleasant sights, sounds and smells is less likely to experience nausea or vomiting.

Miscellaneous inputs

Nausea and vomiting are frequently induced by stimulation of pharyngeal afferents, e.g. nasopharyngeal tube, endoscopy. Stimulation of the auricular branch of the vagus nerve on examination of the ear with an auroscope may induce sudden vomiting, especially in children. It is advisable to examine the ear from behind.

The role of sympathetic innervation of the gastrointestinal tract in PONV is not clear. However, pain pathways from the viscera reside in the splanchnic nerves and visceral pain is a frequent cause of nausea and vomiting.

EFFERENT LIMB OF THE VOMITING REFLEX

Nausea

Nausea is not an inevitable consequence of vomiting but it is often the most troublesome symptom after surgery and anaesthesia. It is thought to be caused by the same stimuli that are responsible for vomiting, but the nature of the higher centres involved in this sensation are unknown. As a symptom, it is difficult to investigate because it is entirely objective and cannot be measured in animals. However, a consistent finding is that antiemetic therapy is often very effective in reducing the incidence of vomiting or retching, but less so for nausea.

Vomiting

The processes involved in vomiting are summarized in Figure 26.2. In the prodromal or pre-ejection phase, there is a relaxation of the gastric muscles followed by

small intestinal retrograde peristalsis. The latter forces intestinal contents into the relaxed stomach. At the beginning of the ejection phase, the anterior abdominal muscles and the diaphragm contract together, accompanied by retrograde contraction of the striated musculature of the oesophagus. At the same time, the upper oesophageal sphincter becomes widely dilated. During vomiting, the oesophagus is not obstructed by diaphragmatic contraction, as the crural (perioesophageal) muscles of the diaphragm are relaxed. This autonomic and somatic activity is coordinated in the brainstem (see above).

Retching

Retching (i.e. unproductive vomiting) often occurs before vomiting and when the retrograde intestinal peristalsis reaches the stomach. During retching, the

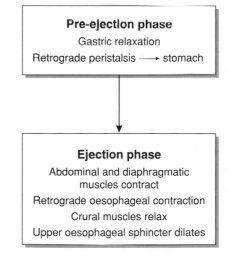

Fig. 26.2
Processes involved in vomiting.

abdominal muscles and diaphragm contract less intensely and there is no retrograde oesophageal contraction or crural relaxation. Clinically, retching is a frequent and distressing symptom, often associated with intense nausea.

ADVERSE EFFECTS

The potential adverse effects of PONV are summarized in Table 26.1. The most important and frequent adverse effect is the profound distress of most patients when they experience nausea and vomiting.

Aspiration of stomach contents is an important cause of anaesthetic mortality and morbidity and can occur in the postoperative period, particularly if the patient is drowsy. Nausea and vomiting make this more likely. PONV may limit significantly the dose of opioid that may be given for pain relief, and prevention with antiemetics often enables effective doses to be administered. Oral administration of drugs (e.g. analgesics, antihypertensives), fluids and nutrients is delayed by PONV and this may cause significant problems if the delay is prolonged. PONV is often more severe on movement and may hinder postoperative mobilization. It is also an important cause of delayed discharge from day-care surgery units, including unscheduled overnight stay.

PONV may be associated with poor surgical outcome; for example, vomiting may disrupt neck, abdominal and eye sutures.

ASSOCIATED FACTORS

Many studies have investigated the relative importance of patient, surgical and anaesthetic factors in the incidence of PONV. Some factors have been associated with an increased risk. However, it is still not possible to predict with any great certainty the likelihood that an individual patient will vomit.

PATIENT FACTORS

Studies have revealed several patient factors which are associated with a relatively high risk of PONV. A previous history of PONV or travel sickness is a strong association. Children and females are at greater risk but there is no difference between the sexes in childhood or old age. The influences of the menstrual cycle and obesity have been investigated but there is no consistent evidence that they are important factors. Smoking seems to protect against PONV.

SURGICAL FACTORS

The surgical factors associated with an increased risk of PONV are summarized in Table 26.2. Major and minor gynaecological procedures have been associated consistently with PONV. Indeed, gynaecological surgery is often used in studies investigating the efficacy of new antiemetics. PONV after ENT surgery

Table 26.1 Adverse affects of PONV

Patient distress

Aspiration of stomach contents

Limitation of analgesia

Poor surgical outcome
   Eyes
   Head and neck
   Oesophageal
   Abdominal wound

Dehydration and/or requirement for intravenous fluids

Delayed oral input
   Drugs
   Nutrition
   Fluids

Delayed mobilization

Delayed discharge from day-care unit

Table 26.2 Surgical factors associated with an increased risk of PONV

Type of surgery
   Gynaecological
   ENT
   Gastrointestinal
   Head and neck
   Squint correction

Duration of surgery

Postoperative antibiotics

may be more frequent because of stimulation of pharyngeal afferents, blood in the gastrointestinal tract and the fact that it is a common procedure in children. In abdominal surgery, almost all the efferent limbs of the vomiting reflex are stimulated. Duration of surgery and anaesthesia may also be important.

ANAESTHETIC FACTORS

Choice of induction agent may influence the incidence of PONV (Table 26.3); etomidate is comparatively more emetogenic. The incidence of PONV associated with induction and/or maintenance of anaesthesia with propofol is lower than that with other intravenous and volatile agents. Indeed, it has been suggested that propofol has antiemetic properties.

Nitrous oxide when used alone, e.g. Entonox, may cause nausea and vomiting, but its effect is uncertain when used as part of a balanced anaesthetic technique. Modern volatile agents, although less emetogenic compared with older agents, contribute to the overall likelihood of PONV.

It is clear that the perioperative use of opioids (oral, i.m., i.v., epidural, spinal) is associated with an increased incidence of PONV and many anaesthetic techniques aim to avoid opioids for this reason. Paradoxically, postoperative pain may cause PONV, which may be alleviated by judicious use of opioids.

Antagonism of neuromuscular blockade with neostigmine has been blamed for PONV but this is controversial. Episodes of hypotension during spinal or epidural anaesthesia are a common cause of nausea and vomiting. Indeed, nausea is often the first sign of this problem. In addition, there is a lower incidence of PONV in patients anaesthetized by experienced anaesthetists compared with those managed by novices. The inexperienced tend to maintain anaesthesia at a deeper plane and are more likely to inflate the stomach with air during manual ventilation.

MANAGEMENT

PREVENTION

Prevention rather than treatment of PONV should be the anaesthetist's aim. Although there is no agreed protocol as to which patients should receive preventative antiemetic therapy, the relative indication for prophylaxis increases as the number of risk factors increase.

There is an important organizational factor in the incidence of PONV. Antiemetics are often prescribed but not given. The overall incidence of PONV in a hospital is reduced if all professionals involved in the care of the patient understand the importance and nature of antiemetic therapy and an agreed management protocol is in place.

TREATMENT

Treat the cause

An important principle in the management of any symptom is to seek and treat the cause before treating the symptom itself. This is relevant when dealing with a patient with PONV. There are many important causes of PONV and these are summarized in Table 26.4.

PONV may indicate postoperative hypotension; simply administering an antiemetic does not help and may mask an important sign. Hypoxaemia should be treated with oxygen and investigated further if necessary. Early fluid intake or mobilization, particularly after day-case surgery is a common cause. Psychological factors, e.g. anxiety, loss of control and illness beliefs, play an important role and may respond to appropriate non-pharmacological management. Occasionally, PONV may herald significant intra-abdominal or other pathology resulting from a surgical complication. This should be borne in mind constantly, particularly before discharge from the day-care unit.

Opioids are a common cause of PONV, particularly if they are administered injudiciously. Changing to a local anaesthetic technique or adopting a more

Table 26.3 Anaesthetic factors associated with an increased risk of PONV
Opioids
Volatile agents

Intravenous induction agents (c.f. propofol)
    Thiopental
    Etomidate
    Methohexital

Experience of anaesthetist
Postoperative pain
Hypotension during epidural/spinal anaesthesia
? N_2O
? Neostigmine

Table 26.4 Important cause of PONV
Hypotension
Hypoxaemia
Drugs
Opioids
Antibiotics
Intra-abdominal pathology
Psychological factors
Mobilization
Fluid intake
Nasogatric tube
Pain

Table 26.5 Types of antiemetic	
Antagonists	
Dopaminergic	
Cholinergic	
Histaminergic	
$5HT_3$	
NK-1	
Agonists	
Dexamethasone	
Cannabinoids	

balanced approach to analgesia may solve the problem. It should be remembered that many other drugs are emetogenic. Antibiotics are a common culprit and their use should be reassessed if PONV is a severe problem.

Antiemetic therapy

In practice, many patients with PONV require parenteral antiemetic therapy. If an antiemetic has been given previously, there are several factors to consider when choosing the appropriate drug. If the previous drug was effective for some time and it is likely that its plasma concentrations are now low, it is probably appropriate to administer the same drug. However, if the drug was administered relatively recently, a different antiemetic is required. In this situation, it makes pharmacological sense to choose a drug which acts at a different receptor (see below).

PHARMACOLOGY OF ANTIEMETICS

TYPES OF ANTIEMETIC

The agonists and antagonists effective as antiemetics are summarized in Table 26.5. Antiemetics may be antagonists at the dopamine (D_2 – e.g. metoclopramide, droperidol, prochlorperazine), 5-HT_3 (e.g. ondansetron, dolasetron, granisetron, tropisetron) and cholinergic (e.g. cyclizine) receptors.

Dexamethasone and cannabinoids (e.g. nabilone, dronabinol) are effective against chemotherapy-induced emesis. The efficacy of cannabinoids for PONV is uncertain but there is increasing evidence that dexamethasone is effective. Antagonists at the NK-1 receptor are antiemetic also and their site of action is probably in the brainstem where there is an abundance of these receptors. They are presently undergoing clinical trials.

Metoclopramide

Metoclopramide acts at the dopamine receptors in the stomach, upper intestine and CTZ. It enhances gastric emptying, intestinal transit and lower oesophageal sphincter pressure. It is still prescribed frequently as an antiemetic, but at the recommended dose (10 mg) it is no better than placebo in many situations.

The bioavailability of metoclopramide after oral administration is unpredictable (Table 26.6) and time to maximum concentration (t_{max}) is 1–2.5 h. Its elimination half-life is approximately 4 h but its redistribution half-life after intravenous administration is short (approximately 5 min).

Side-effects include extrapyramidal reactions, usually dystonia (e.g. facial muscle spasm, trismus, abnormal tongue movements, oculogyric crises, opisthotonus). They occur more commonly in young females (approximately 1 in 5000). Agitation has been reported after metoclopramide premedication. Hypotension, sinus tachycardia, supraventricular tachycardia and sinus bradycardia have been described after intravenous injection. It is recommended that an intravenous dose should be given over a period of 1–2 min.

Phenothiazines

Phenothiazines are antiemetics because of their dopamine receptor antagonist activity. They were synthesized originally by dye chemists in the late

Table 26.6 Approximate pharmacokinetic values of the commonly used antiemetics

	Bioavailability (%)	t_{max} (h)	$t_{1/2}$ (h)
Metoclopramide	80 (range 32–97)	1–2.5	4
Prochlorperazine	14	2.8	6 (range 1–15)
Droperidol			2
Cyclizine			13–20
Ondansetron	60	0.5–2	4
Granisetron	60	2	3–6
Dolasetron		1[a]	7–9[a]

[a] Active metabolite.

nineteenth century, but it was only in the 1930s that the sedative and antiemetic effects of promethazine were discovered. Promethazine is used occasionally as premedication for children but its sedative effect restricts its use as an antiemetic. Perphenazine was used extensively as an antiemetic but was associated with a high incidence of extrapyramidal side-effects and is now used rarely. Prochlorperazine is prescribed frequently for PONV.

Prochlorperazine

Prochlorperazine was synthesized in 1949 and introduced for the prevention of PONV. Although relatively few controlled studies are available, it is likely that prochlorperazine is an effective antiemetic. Elimination half-life is approximately 6 h and oral bioavailability is poor (see Table 26.6).

Extrapyramidal side-effects are similar in nature to those associated with metoclopramide but less frequent. Sedation is not usually a problem in doses used for PONV. Rare side-effects include cholestatic jaundice, skin sensitization and haematological abnormalities.

Butyrophenones

Butyrophenones are used as major tranquillizers and neuroleptics. They are dopamine antagonists. Only droperidol is administered perioperatively but haloperidol is prescribed occasionally as an antiemetic in palliative medicine.

Droperidol

Droperidol is presently unavailable. Chronic administration of droperidol in psychiatric patients was associated with adverse effects on the QT interval of the ECG. Consequently, the only manufacturer withdrew all preparations of droperidol in 2001. There is scant evidence that this is a problem when used as a perioperative antiemetic in relatively low doses.

Droperidol was administered intravenously for PONV. It was developed originally for use in neuroleptic anaesthetic regimens; this technique, which involved the combination of high-dose opioids and droperidol with no volatile agent, has now been abandoned because of concerns regarding awareness. The redistribution half-life of droperidol is approximately 10 min and elimination half-life 2 h (see Table 26.6).

Many studies have confirmed the efficacy of droperidol against placebo, but sedation is often reported. Side-effects are similar to those of the phenothiazines. Extrapyramidal reactions are less frequent compared with metoclopramide. Feelings of apprehension, restlessness and even nightmares are less obvious but occur more frequently. In addition to antagonistic effects at the dopamine receptor, droperidol is also an α-adrenergic antagonist and may cause vasodilatation and hypotension.

Anticholinergics

Hyoscine (scopolamine) and atropine are anticholinergics with antiemetic actions. Cyclizine is anticholinergic but also an antagonist at the histamine type-1 receptor. Cyclizine is administered most frequently for PONV.

Cyclizine

In recent years, cyclizine has become more popular for the prevention and treatment of PONV. Although there are relatively few well-controlled studies, its popularity probably reflects reasonable efficacy combined with a low incidence of side-effects. Its elimination half-life is 13–20 h.

Extrapyramidal side-effects are not associated with cyclizine, but sedation and dry mouth (anticholinergic action) may occur. Other complications include urinary retention, blurred vision, restlessness and hallucinations when given in large doses. In patients with severe cardiac failure, it may increase arterial pressure, heart rate and pulmonary wedge pressure, leading to a reduction in cardiac output.

5-HT₃ receptor antagonists

5-HT$_3$ receptor antagonists were developed as antiemetics when it was realized that the efficacy of high-dose metoclopramide (i.e. 10 mg kg^{-1}) in chemotherapy-induced emesis was the result of some degree of antagonism at the 5-HT$_3$ receptor.

Ondansetron was the first specific potent 5-HT$_3$ receptor antagonist available for PONV. It may be given orally or intravenously. Oral bioavailability is approximately 60% and elimination half-life is 4 h (see Table 22.6). It is available for oral and intravenous administration. Granisetron and tropisetron have similar pharmacological properties to those of ondansetron. Dolasetron relies upon an active metabolite for its activity.

A major advantage of 5-HT$_3$ receptor antagonists is their wide therapeutic index. They are not associated with extrapyramidal side-effects, excessive sedation or significant prolongation of recovery from anaesthesia.

Dexamethasone

The efficacy of dexamethasone for the prevention of chemotherapy-induced nausea and vomiting is well established. Its mode of action is unclear, and the plasma half-life is approximately 3 h. There is now clear evidence that the efficacy of a single intravenous dose (8 mg) of dexamethasone for the prevention of PONV is comparable with that of standard antiemetics. It may be useful particularly when used in combination with 5-HT$_3$ antagonists. Classic steroid side-effects do not occur with a single dose and, to date, no adverse effects have been reported.

COMBINATION THERAPY

The efficacy of antiemetic therapy for the prevention or treatment of PONV may be enhanced by combination therapy. It makes pharmacological sense to administer drugs which act at different receptors. Presently, there is considerable interest in this, and most studies have found combinations to be significantly more efficacious than a single drug.

ACUPUNCTURE

The use of acupuncture was championed in the 1980s by the late Professor Dundee. Acupuncture for nausea is performed at the P6 (Neiguan) point which is situated between the tendons of the flexor carpi radialis and palmaris longus, 2 Chinese inches from the distal skin crease. (A Chinese inch is the width of the interphalangeal joint of the thumb.) Studies using meta-analysis have confirmed that stimulation of the P6 point is indeed effective if applied before or after anaesthesia. It is less effective if applied during anaesthesia. There are no significant side-effects of this therapy and it should be considered as a serious option if personnel are available to administer it.

FURTHER READING

Eberhart L H, Morin A M, Guber D et al 2004 Applicability of risk scores for postoperative nausea and vomiting in adults to paediatric patients. British Journal of Anaesthesia 93: 386–392

Gan T J, Meyer T, Apfel C C et al; Department of Anesthesiology, Duke University Medical Center 2003 Consensus guidelines for managing postoperative nausea and vomiting. Anesthesia and Analgesia 97: 62–71

Gupta A, Wu C L, Elkassabany N et al 2003 Does the routine prophylactic use of antiemetics affect the incidence of postdischarge nausea and vomiting following ambulatory surgery?: A systematic review of randomized controlled trials. Anesthesiology 99: 488–495

Habib A S, Gan T J 2004 Evidence-based management of postoperative nausea and vomiting: a review. Canadian Journal of Anaesthesia 51: 326–341

Strunin L, Rowbotham D J, Miles L (eds) 2003 The effective management of postoperative nausea and vomiting, 2nd edn. Aesculapius Medical Press, London

Day-case anaesthesia 27

A day-case patient is one who is admitted for investigation or operation on a planned non-resident basis. Patients are usually discharged from the hospital or unit later on the day of the procedure. The procedure may require general, regional or local anaesthesia, sedative techniques or a combination of these.

In recent times, there has been rapid expansion in the use of day case surgery. In the last 25 years, the percentage of patients going home the same day has increased from < 10% to approximately 65% in the United States. Procedures that are commonly selected today are those taking < 60 min to complete and which do not cause severe haemorrhage or produce excessive amounts of postoperative pain (Table 27.1). Increasingly complex cases are now performed as day procedures, including laparoscopic cholecystectomy and tonsillectomy. By extending day surgery opening hours and using staggered admission times, patients who would normally require hospital admission may be treated as day cases. The British Association of Day Surgery (BADS) publishes guidelines and protocols for the management of specific issues: for example, day surgery for patients with diabetes. BADS has published a list of 25 procedures that should normally be undertaken as day-cases. The NHS Modernisation Agency audited current day surgery rates for these procedures and set target rates for individual hospitals. The Audit Commission report for the year 2000 (its most recent report on the subject) showed expansion in the number of procedures performed as day cases compared to 1996, but highlighted 120 000 patients treated as inpatients who may have been appropriate as day cases.

To achieve a pain-free ambulant patient requires skilful patient selection and experienced anaesthetists and surgeons working within a day surgery unit. Large-scale reports have indicated that day surgery represents a safe, cost-effective and efficient practice. Advantages include decreased risk of nosocomial infections and deep venous thrombosis, less social disruption to patients and their families and minimal need for inpatient hospital resources. Hence we are now confronted with the challenge of faster recovery, more rapid discharge and better pain relief for outpatients.

PATIENT SELECTION

The selection of patients for day-case surgery is of vital importance if maximum use is to be made of the resources in the day-case unit and also to facilitate smooth running of the unit. The selection of patients must take into account two separate aspects: first, the patient's state of health, and secondly, his or her social circumstances. Patients should normally be ASA I, II, or medically stable ASA III. Recent reviews have shown that patients with body mass index of > 35 kg m^{-2} do not have an increase in unplanned admission rates or postoperative complications. However, Chung et al (1999), in a prospective study of over 17 000 patients, found that obesity was one of five predictors of adverse events in day-case surgery. Obesity, smoking and asthma predicted postoperative respiratory events, while hypertension predicted cardiovascular events and reflux predicted intubation-related events. Elderly patients are more likely to have comorbidities and should be assessed according to physiological rather than chronological age. Careful medical and social preoperative assessment is required in order to help the elderly benefit from shorter hospital stays with less risk of postoperative confusion. The patient should stay a minimum of 1 h drive from the hospital on the following night and should have an adult escort available for the first 24 h after surgery. An example of guidelines used for patient selection for day-case anaesthesia is shown in Table 27.2.

The selection of patients for day-case surgery is made at the time of outpatient consultation and routine measurement of pulse, BP and urine analysis and other relevant investigations (e.g. ECG, full blood count and sickle cell testing) are performed; performance of these

Table 27.1 A selection of surgical procedures commonly undertaken as day cases

Gynaecology

Dilatation & curettage, laparoscopy, vaginal termination of pregnancy, colposcopy, hysteroscopy

Plastic surgery

Dupuytren's contracture release, removal of small skin lesions, nerve decompression

Ophthalmology

Strabismus correction, cataract surgery, lacrimal duct probing, examination under anaesthesia

ENT

Adenoidectomy, tonsillectomy, myringotomy, insertion of grommets, removal of foreign body, polyp removal, submucous resection

Urology

Cystoscopy, circumcision, vasectomy, transurethral bladder resection

Orthopaedics

Arthroscopies, carpal tunnel release, ganglion removal, bunion operation, removal of metal ware

General surgery

Breast lumps, herniae, varicose veins, endoscopy, laparoscopic cholecystectomy, haemorroidectomy, anal fissure dilatation

Paediatrics

Circumcision, orchidopexy, squint, dental extractions

Table 27.2 Guidelines for patient selection for day-case surgery under general anaesthesia

ASA I, II and medically stable ASA III

Age: > 52 weeks post-conceptual age

Weight: body mass index = weight/height^2 (kg m^{-2})

  ≤ 35: acceptable

  > 35: discuss with anaesthetic department

Generally healthy, i.e. can climb two flights of stairs

Patient exclusions

Cardiovascular

  MI/TIA/CVA within 6 months

  Hypertension: persistent diastolic >110 mmHg

  Unstable angina

  Arrhythmias

  Heart failure

  Poor exercise tolerance

  Symptomatic valve disease

Respiratory

  Acute respiratory tract infection

  Asthma requiring regular β_2-agonists or steroids

Metabolic

  Alcoholism /narcotic addiction

  Insulin-dependent diabetes

  Renal failure

  Liver disease

Neurological/musculoskeletal

  Severe arthritis of jaw or neck

  Cervical spondylosis/ ankylosing spondylitis

  Myopathies/ muscular dystrophies/ myasthenia gravis

  Advanced multiple sclerosis

  Epilepsy >3 fits per year

Drugs

  Steroids

  Monoamine oxidase inhibitors

  Anticoagulants

  Antiarrhythmics

  Insulin

routine tests is thought to reduce the number of problems when patients are admitted on the day of surgery. A standardized patient health/anaesthesia questionnaire and preliminary nurse assessment with appropriate referral for anaesthetic consultation minimize problems encountered on the day of surgery. Pre-assessment clinics provide an opportunity to educate patients and have been shown to reduce both patient cancellations and unnecessary preoperative investigations. Children scheduled for day-case procedures should be healthy and usually ASA I or II. Premature babies who have not reached 52 weeks post-conceptual age should not be considered for day-case surgery because of the risk of postoperative apnoea, and special consideration should be given to babies who have been receiving ventilatory support. The parent must be able to cope with the pre-procedure instructions and with the care of the child after treatment. The parent must agree to day treatment and be available to stay

throughout the day, although there may be exceptions for older children who attend regularly. Home facilities and travelling conditions should be taken into account. After a general anaesthetic, the use of public transport is inappropriate.

Following selection of a patient for day-case surgery, the nature of the operation and the routine of management are explained fully to the patient and the consent form may be signed. Many units issue the patient with explanatory leaflets or audio cassettes explaining the procedure. A date for surgery may then be arranged and registration completed as for an in-patient admission. It is wise to book any pathological or radiological investigations that are required well in advance of the day of admission.

The patient should be given written instructions detailing the date and time of attendance at the day unit, with written instructions relating to preoperative starvation and the patient's usual medication, e.g. antihypertensives, should be taken as usual but oral hypoglycaemics must be omitted on the morning of surgery. These instructions should be written clearly in plain English or another appropriate language, and the patient advised not to eat anything from midnight for a morning list.

Recent clinical studies suggest that overnight fasting may not be justified in adults or children. Pulmonary aspiration usually occurs in emergency abdominal and obstetric procedures where there may be complicating factors such as recent food and fluid intake, trauma or administration of opioid analgesics. These factors do not normally apply to healthy elective day-case patients. The universal order of nil by mouth from midnight should only apply to solids. Clear fluids should be allowed until 3 h before the scheduled time of surgery. The effect of giving patients 150 mL clear fluid 2 h before general anaesthesia for termination of pregnancy has been studied; the results showed that clear fluids do not increase the incidence of regurgitation or vomiting during anaesthesia and that preoperative thirst was decreased in the clear fluid group. It is advisable to ask patients who smoke to refrain from smoking for 4–6 weeks before the operation. Patients should be asked to bring with them all tablets and medicines that they take regularly.

ORGANIZATION OF THE DAY-CASE UNIT

TYPES OF UNIT

There are three common types of day-case unit:

- A unit within a hospital complex, but with separate staff, wards and operating theatre; this is functionally the most flexible type as it may be adapted to the varying requirements of day-case patients.
- A unit with a separate ward, but using the hospital's main operating theatre complex.

- Outside the UK, it is common for a separate centre to have its own operating theatres and wards remote from a conventional hospital. This type of unit has now been introduced into the UK.

Ideally, day surgical units should not be freestanding but situated on inpatient hospital sites. The ward area should be close by the theatre, to reduce portering time, particularly when short operations are performed. This arrangement also enables parents to accompany their children to the anaesthetic room if this is desirable.

Preferably, the unit should be near a car park and well signposted to facilitate the prompt arrival of patients and to avoid unnecessary delays.

FACILITIES AVAILABLE

The accommodation should ideally include:

- *An admission area*, which includes reception, treatment and examination rooms, a nurses' station, lavatories, a playroom and a discharge area.
- *An anaesthetic room*, fully equipped and large enough to allow free access around the patient's trolley to permit the use of local or general anaesthesia. There should be good lighting, scavenging, piped gases and suction equipment, anaesthetic machine and monitoring equipment. The hazards and risks of day-surgery general anaesthesia are no less than those for inpatient surgery; indeed, in some respects they may be greater and the facilities provided must be comparable.
- *An operating theatre*, which should be of the same specification as the inpatient equivalent. A good operating light, air-conditioning and piped services are required, in addition to the usual scrub-up and autoclave facilities. There is always the possibility of a minor operation developing unexpectedly into a major operation and this demands that the theatre is well equipped to deal with this eventuality.
- *A fully equipped recovery room*, which must always be equipped and staffed for the safe recovery of patients after general anaesthesia. Piped gas supplies and resuscitation equipment are mandatory and the full range of monitoring and ventilation equipment must be readily available.

Other facilities that should be available include office space, equipment store, staff locker room, a staff room, a pantry to make drinks and lavatories for patients, parents and staff.

ADMISSION

Patients should be admitted to the day ward in adequate time for history-taking and examination. The results of any investigation requested as an outpatient should be available and noted. Patients should receive an identity bracelet and their name should be entered into the nursing record. The surgeon should ensure the indication for surgery is still present, e.g. presence or absence of lumps to be removed, as it may be several months since the clinic appointment; the consent form should be signed if not already done during the outpatient appointment, and the operation site marked. A pregnancy test in women of fertile age may need to be performed if there is any risk of pregnancy. Staggering patient admissions decreases waiting times and improves the efficiency of the unit. Using dedicated paediatric day-case lists ensures appropriate staffing mix for these cases. The use of separate operating lists for local anaesthesia and general anaesthesia may improve throughput, as does the introduction of day-surgery operating trolleys.

ANAESTHESIA

PREMEDICATION

Most anaesthetists do not routinely prescribe premedication for day cases, as it is usually unnecessary. Premedicant drugs that may be used include the following.

Benzodiazepines

It is thought that sedative premedication may prolong the recovery time and delay the patient's discharge from hospital. However, a double-blind study of temazepam premedication for day cases found effective anxiolysis in the groups that received 10 or 20 mg temazepam; there was no delay in recovery times as measured by memory test cards and all patients were discharged from the day unit 3 h after administration of general anaesthesia. Oral midazolam has been used as a premedicant in day surgery, but it was found that it produced delay in immediate and late recovery compared with temazepam.

Antiemetics

If patients are at high risk of postoperative nausea and vomiting (PONV), antiemetics may be administered orally before operation, or via the intravenous or rectal route perioperatively. Apfel et al (1999). developed

a simplified PONV risk score and suggest prophylactic antiemetics for any patient with two or more of the following: female gender; past history of motion sickness or PONV; non-smoker; and use of postoperative opioids. However, risk scores such as this have no better than a 70% chance of predicting PONV.

Antacids

If there is a risk of acid reflux, H_2-antagonists are commonly prescribed as a premedication in day surgery.

Analgesics

Oral non-steroidal anti-inflammatory drugs (NSAIDs) and paracetamol may be given preoperatively if the patient declines rectal administration perioperatively. Oral COX II inhibitors have better gastrointestinal side-effect profiles than NSAIDs and less antiplatelet effects. Patient satisfaction with self-administration of rectal diclofenac preoperatively has been reported. Dermal application of tetracaine (amethocaine) over a vein has a useful role for children and nervous adults or those with a needle phobia as it acts within 20 min and it does not cause local vasoconstriction.

GENERAL AND REGIONAL ANAESTHESIA

General, local or regional anaesthesia may be administered safely to day-case patients. The choice of technique should be determined by surgical requirements, anaesthetic considerations and the patient's physical status and preference.

General anaesthesia

The choice of induction and maintenance agent depends upon the requirements of the patient and the preferences of the anaesthetist. Any induction agent used in day-case anaesthesia should ensure a smooth induction, good immediate recovery with minimal postoperative sequelae and a rapid return to street fitness.

Propofol is now used widely as the primary induction agent in day-case anaesthesia. One of its main advantages is the ease and rapidity with which patients recover. Patients are clear-headed and have a lower incidence of PONV. Inhalational agents used for induction of anaesthesia include halothane and sevoflurane, although halothane is no longer used frequently. Both are non-irritant to the airways, but the latter has the advantage of more rapid induction in both children and adults, minimal cardiovascular side-effects and a rapid recovery profile. However, sevoflurane causes more PONV than propofol.

Which technique should be used for maintenance of anaesthesia? Both sevoflurane and desflurane have been marketed as ideal agents for day-case anaesthesia, with favourable recovery profiles and more rapid awakening than isoflurane. However, both sevoflurane and desflurane have been associated with emergence delirium because of rapid awakening, especially in children. Moreover, desflurane is less suitable for spontaneously breathing subjects as it is more irritant to the airways than both sevoflurane and isoflurane. The use of nitrous oxide for maintenance of anaesthesia has been shown to increase the risk of PONV; however, its use does reduce the requirements for volatile agents and may reduce the risk of intraoperative awareness. Target-controlled infusion (TCI) of propofol with or without the ultra-rapid-acting opioid remifentanil are techniques which have minimal risk of PONV and short recovery times, but these have to be balanced against the cost of the agents.

A clear airway is a fundamental requirement of safe anaesthesia. The laryngeal mask airway (LMA) is used widely and avoids intubation and extubation, which improves turnaround time between cases. Some anaesthetists are using the LMA for cases that traditionally have required tracheal intubation, such as tonsillectomy and laparoscopy. The ProSeal LMA provides a higher pressure seal than a conventional LMA and has an internal lumen that aids aspiration of gastric contents if necessary. However, patients at risk of aspiration still require a rapid-sequence induction technique with tracheal intubation; this is not a contraindication to day surgery.

The choice of muscle relaxant depends on the anticipated duration of surgery. Succinylcholine is associated with muscle pains, especially in ambulant patients, and for all but the shortest procedures is not ideal in the day-case setting. Of the non-depolarizing muscle relaxants (NDMRs) currently available, atracurium and vecuronium have a relatively short duration of action when they are used in appropriate doses and are readily antagonized after 15–30 min. Mivacurium has an even shorter duration of action as it undergoes rapid hydrolysis by plasma cholinesterase, but it must be remembered, as with the use of succinylcholine, that a small number of patients may suffer prolonged muscle paralysis because of plasma cholinesterase deficiency. Rocuronium may have a role as it has a more rapid onset of action than any of the other NDMRs, providing intubating conditions within 60–90 s at a dose of 0.6 mg kg^{-1} and duration of action of 30–45 min. Cisatracurium, the stereoisomer of atracurium, has been introduced with a slightly longer duration of action compared with that of atracurium but without the side-effect of histamine release.

Regional anaesthesia

Spinal anaesthesia has been used for day-case anaesthesia, but the side-effects of post-dural puncture headache (PDPH) and motor weakness may delay discharge. Smaller-gauge pencil-point spinal needles have reduced the incidence of PDPH to < 1% in patients aged > 40 years. Shorter-acting local anaesthetics may increase the use of day-case spinals in the future; however, intrathecal lidocaine has been associated with transient neurological symptoms and is not licensed for intrathecal use in the UK. Prilocaine, mepivacaine and pethidine have also been used for outpatient spinals in other countries, including the United States. The new preservative-free preparation of 2-chloroprocaine may provide acceptable anaesthesia and discharge times with low potential for transient neurological symptoms, but more clinical trials are needed. Low-dose bupivacaine (3 mL 0.17%) has been used successfully for knee arthroscopy with times to discharge of 190 min. The addition of 10 μg fentanyl increases duration of sensory blockade without affecting discharge times.

Local anaesthetic blocks are an excellent choice for day-case patients, because of the low incidence of PONV and the provision of good postoperative analgesia. Inguinal hernia repair is commonly performed under an ilioinguinal nerve block and local infiltration. For operations on the hand or arm, axillary or mid-humeral approach to brachial plexus block is preferable to the supraclavicular approach to minimize the risk of producing a pneumothorax, which may become apparent only after discharge. Intravenous regional anaesthesia (Bier's block) is another alternative for hand operations provided that effective exsanguination of the arm is achieved before performing the block.

Caudal block is used to reduce pain in paediatric patients for circumcision, herniorrhaphy, hypospadias or orchidopexy, using 0.25% plain bupivacaine; this provides excellent postoperative analgesia. Whenever a caudal block is administered for analgesia, care must be taken to ensure that motor strength is not compromised. There does not appear to be any advantage in using more concentrated solutions than 0.25% bupivacaine. Penile blocks and the application of local anaesthetic cream are also effective for circumcision.

Intra-articular local anaesthetics are useful following arthroscopy of the knee or shoulder. Femoral nerve block has been found to give superior analgesia to patients going home after anterior cruciate ligament repair and, combined with sciatic nerve block, reduces admission rates for complex knee surgery. Regional catheter techniques such as continuous interscalene brachial plexus blocks using a portable infusion pump, allow a local anaesthetic infusion to continue at home. Guidance from community outreach teams improves efficacy and patient satisfaction. Overall analgesia is improved and side-effects from opioids minimized. New elastomeric pumps which slowly infuse local anaesthetic solution at a fixed rate and have an air filter incorporated have been used safely on an outpatient basis. These pumps do not need a power source and deliver local anaesthetic directly to the surgical site.

POSTOPERATIVE CARE

Recovery from anaesthesia is an important aspect of day-case anaesthesia. The recovery area should be provided with the same range of monitoring equipment and resuscitation facilities as available in an inpatient facility. Many day-surgery units in the UK now have three separate recovery areas: the first stage is for the immediate postoperative period, when patients require one-to-one nurse-to-patient care and monitoring; the second involves lower nursing dependency care where the patient is not attached to monitoring, but is mobilizing and usually given food and drink; and the third stage is the discharge area. The overall responsibility for assessing when patients are ready to go home is that of the clinicians involved. Often, experienced nursing staff who work regularly in the day unit become very good at detecting potential problems with day-case patients.

Postoperative pain control should be started pre- or intraoperatively by supplementing intravenous or inhalational anaesthesia with a combination of an NSAID, paracetamol (especially in children), shorter-acting opioid analgesics, and local/regional block intraoperatively. The patient's awakening is smoother and discharge home is quicker. The most frequently used drugs to provide intraoperative analgesia are fentanyl and alfentanil; the relatively short duration of action of these drugs makes them suitable for use in day-case anaesthesia. The provision of good postoperative analgesia is primarily the responsibility of the anaesthetist. Anaesthetists may do little to limit the number of patients requiring admission for surgical complications, but play a major role in reducing admissions caused by pain or vomiting. NSAIDs, e.g. diclofenac and ketorolac, are useful for provision of postoperative analgesia in day-case patients. COX II inhibitors are available as intravenous or oral preparations and have better gastrointestinal side-effect profiles than NSAIDs and fewer antiplatelet effects. An intravenous preparation of paracetamol is now available and provides good analgesia without side-effects. Multimodal analgesia reduces the requirement for postoperative opioids.

Factors contributing to postoperative nausea and vomiting include a previous history of PONV, gender (females are more susceptible), the use of longer-acting opioid analgesic drugs such as morphine, the choice of anaesthetic technique or agents, operative procedure, pain, sudden movement or position change, history of motion sickness, hypotension, obesity, day of menstrual cycle and high oestrogen levels. A relationship between pain and the frequency of nausea and vomiting in the postoperative period has been established. There is controversy regarding the use of opioid analgesics in the day-case patient, because they may increase PONV. Several studies have shown that if an opioid-nitrous oxide anaesthetic is given, the occurrence of PONV is greater compared with an inhalational anaesthetic. In contrast, there are studies that have demonstrated that an opioid-supplemented anaesthetic technique results in earlier ambulation and discharge. PONV may be treated with intravenous 5-HT$_3$ antagonists, dexamethasone, or cyclizine and intramuscular prochlorperazine. Adequate hydration and analgesia are also of paramount importance.

In general, discharge of the patient should not take place until the patient is able to sit unaided, walk in a straight line and stand still without swaying. Usually, patients have been able to drink and eat (this also demonstrates the absence of nausea). A responsible person should be present to escort the patient home and both the responsible person and the patient should be given verbal and written discharge instructions and an adequate supply of oral analgesic drugs for at least 3 days. The patient should be advised to refrain from activities such as driving a car, operating machinery and drinking alcohol for 24 h. Communication with the patient's general practitioner is very important to ensure awareness of the operation performed and the requirements for postoperative follow-up. A follow-up telephone call to the patient after discharge should highlight any particular problems. Table 27.3 displays typical discharge criteria for day-case patients.

Patient hotels are a relatively new concept. The patients spend their first postoperative night in a hotel near to the day-surgery unit where there is a resident nurse. These have been used so far for patients who have had, for example, a tonsillectomy. Patient hotels are cheaper than an inpatient overnight stay and are useful for those patients who live too far from the day unit to be considered under normal circumstances for day surgery.

Table 27.3 Discharge criteria for day-case patients
Stable vital signs for at least 1 h
Orientated in time, place and person
Adequate pain control
Minimal nausea, vomiting or dizziness
Adequate oral hydration
Minimal bleeding or wound drainage
Able to pass urine
Responsible escort
Discharge authorized by appropriate staff member
Written and verbal instructions given to patient
Suitable analgesia provided

Each day-care unit should have an established system for audit of outcomes related to anaesthesia and include these outcomes in quality assurance and peer review processes. Reasons for non-attendance, cancellation and unplanned overnight admission should be assessed.

FURTHER READING

Apfel C C, Läärä E, Koivuranta M et al 1999 A simplified risk score for predicting postoperative nausea and vomiting: conclusions from cross-validations between two centers. Anesthesiology 91: 693–700

British Association of Day Surgery *www.bads.co.uk*

Chung F, Mezei G, Tong D 1999 Pre-existing medical conditions as predictors of adverse events in day-case surgery. British Journal of Anaesthesia 83: 262–270

Ilfeld B M, Morey T E, Wright T W 2003 Continuous interscalene brachial plexus block for postoperative pain control at home: a randomized, double-blinded, placebo controlled study. Anesthesia and Analgesia 96: 1089–1095

Millar J M, Rudkin G E, Hitchcock M 1997 Practical anaesthesia and analgesia for day surgery. BIOS Scientific Publishers, Oxford

Modernisation Agency Day Surgery Programme *www.wise.nhs.uk*

Urmey W F 2003 Spinal anaesthesia for outpatient surgery. Best Practice & Research in Clinical Anesthesiology 17: 335–346

White P F, Issioui T, Skrivanek G D 2003 The use of continuous popliteal sciatic nerve block after surgery involving the foot and ankle: does it improve the quality of recovery? Anesthesia and Analgesia 97: 1303–1309

Williams B A, Kentor M L, Vogt M T 2003 Femoral sciatic nerve blocks for complex outpatient knee surgery are associated with less postoperative pain before same day discharge: a review of 1200 consecutive cases from the period 1996–1999. Anesthesiology 98: 1206–1213

28 Emergency anaesthesia

Patients scheduled for elective surgery are usually in optimal physical and mental condition, with a definitive surgical diagnosis and with coexisting medical disease well controlled. In contrast, the patient with a surgical emergency may have an uncertain diagnosis and uncontrolled coexisting medical disease, with associated cardiovascular, respiratory and/or metabolic derangements. Thus, a major principle governing the practice of emergency anaesthesia is to be prepared for all potential complications, including vomiting and regurgitation, hypovolaemia and haemorrhage, and abnormal reactions to drugs in the presence of electrolyte disturbances and renal impairment.

PREOPERATIVE ASSESSMENT

The objective of emergency anaesthesia is to permit correction of the surgical pathology with the minimum of risk to the patient. This requires adequate and accurate preoperative evaluation of the patient's general condition, with particular attention to specific problems that may influence anaesthetic management.

It is essential to ascertain the likely surgical diagnosis, the magnitude of the proposed surgery and how urgently surgery is required, as these dictate both the extent of preoperative preparation and the method of anaesthesia.

A pertinent past medical and drug history is elicited. In particular, enquiry is made into the presence and severity of specific symptoms relevant to cardiopulmonary reserve: angina, productive cough, dyspnoea of effort, orthopnoea or nocturnal coughing bouts. The presence of such symptoms should provoke detailed enquiry into the cardiovascular and respiratory systems (see Ch. 15 on preoperative assessment).

Depending upon the urgency of surgery, physical examination may be selective to identify significant cardiopulmonary dysfunction or any abnormalities that might lead to technical difficulties during anaesthesia. Basal crepitations, triple rhythm and raised jugular venous pulse signify impaired ventricular function and limited cardiac reserve, which increase significantly the risk of anaesthesia. It is also important to exclude arrhythmias and heart sounds indicative of valvular heart disease, as these influence the patient's response to physiological change and thus anaesthetic management. Assessment of respiratory function is particularly difficult, as the patient in pain (with or without peritoneal irritation) may be unable to cooperate with pulmonary function testing.

It is important to cultivate the habit of airway evaluation if a rapid-sequence induction is contemplated, as contingency plans are required for management of the patient in the event of failure to intubate the trachea. Irregular dentition, limitation of mouth opening, poor range of movement at the atlanto-occipital joint and/or reduced distance between the hyoid bone and the mental symphysis are associated with difficult laryngoscopy. A history of difficult intubation is of considerable significance.

Finally, a review of any laboratory investigations is made and urgent requests are made for additional tests which may influence patient management.

ASSESSMENT OF VOLAEMIC STATUS

Assessment of intravascular volume is essential, as underestimated or unrecognized hypovolaemia may lead to circulatory collapse during induction of anaesthesia, which attenuates the sympathetically mediated increases in arteriolar and venous constriction. In any patient in whom fluid is sequestered or lost (e.g. peritonitis, bowel obstruction) or in whom haemorrhage has occurred (e.g. trauma), efforts should be made to quantify the blood volume or extracellular fluid volume and to correct any deficit.

Intravascular volume deficit

Assessment of blood loss may be made from the history and any measured losses, but more commonly the anaesthetist has to rely on clinical evaluation of the patient's circulatory status. Profound circulatory shock with hypotension, poor peripheral perfusion, oliguria and cerebral obtundation is easy to recognize. However, recognition of the early manifestations of haemorrhage, such as tachycardia and cutaneous vasoconstriction, requires a more careful assessment. Useful indices include heart rate, arterial pressure (especially pulse pressure), the state of the peripheral circulation, central venous pressure and urine output. Table 28.1 describes approximate correlations among these clinical indices and the extent of haemorrhage, but it should be stressed that these refer to the 'ideal' patient. In young, healthy adults, arterial pressure may be an unreliable guide to volume status because compensatory mechanisms may preclude a measurable decrease in arterial pressure until more than 30% of the patient's blood volume has been lost. In such patients, attention should be directed to pulse rate, skin circulation and a diminishing pulse pressure. In elderly patients with widespread arterial disease, limited cardiac reserve and a rigid vascular tree (fixed total peripheral resistance), signs of severe hypovolaemia may become evident when blood volume has been reduced by as little as 15%. However, as baroreceptor sensitivity decreases with age, elderly patients may exhibit less tachycardia for any degree of volume depletion.

In general, hypovolaemia does not become apparent clinically until blood volume has been reduced by at least 1000 mL (20% of blood volume). A reduction by more than 30% of blood volume occurs before the classic 'shock syndrome' is produced, with hypotension, tachycardia, oliguria and cold, clammy extremities. Haemorrhage in excess of 40% of blood volume may be associated with loss of the compensatory mechanisms that maintain cerebral and coronary blood flow, and the patient becomes restless and agitated and eventually comatose.

In patients with major trauma, it is valuable to compare the clinical assessment of the extent of haemorrhage with the measured or assumed loss. A marked disparity between these two estimates leads not infrequently to a diagnosis of a further concealed source of haemorrhage.

Extracellular volume deficit

Assessment of extracellular fluid volume deficit is difficult, as considerable losses must occur before clinical signs are apparent. Clinical acumen and a high index of suspicion are necessary to detect the subtle signs of lesser deficits.

Guidance is obtained from the nature of the surgical condition, the duration of impaired fluid intake and the presence and severity of symptoms associated with abnormal losses (e.g. vomiting). At the time of the earliest radiological evidence of intestinal obstruction, there may be 1500 mL of fluid sequestered in the

---

Table 28.1   Clinical indices of extent of blood loss

Class of hypovolaemia	1 Minimal	2 Mild	3 Moderate	4 Severe
Percentage blood volume lost	10	20	30	Over 40
Volume lost (mL)	500	1000	1500	2000+
Heart rate (beat min^{-1})	Normal	100–120	120–140	Over 140
Arterial pressure (mmHg)	Normal	Orthostatic hypotension	Systolic below 100	Systolic below 80
Urinary output (mL h^{-1})	Normal (1 mL kg^{-1} h^{-1})	20–30	10–20	Nil
Sensorium	Normal	Normal	Restless	Impaired consciousness
State of peripheral circulation	Normal	Cool and pale	Cold and pale, slow capillary refill	Cold and clammy Peripheral cyanosis

lumen of the bowel. If the obstruction is well established and vomiting has occurred, the deficit may exceed 3000 mL. At this stage, clinical signs are minimal, but evident to the skilled observer.

For convenience, extracellular fluid volume loss may be graded into four degrees of severity; in each instance, loss is expressed as the percentage of the body weight lost as fluid. It may be seen from Table 28.2 that in minor degrees of extracellular fluid volume loss, diagnosis is dependent on two highly subjective signs: diminished skin elasticity and reduced intraocular pressure. Changes in skin turgor are difficult to assess in elderly patients in whom a natural loss of subcutaneous tissue elasticity may contribute to the impression of reduced turgor. The most reliable sites for interpreting 'tenting' of the skin as a sign of tissue dehydration are the anterior thigh, the forehead, sternum, clavicle or tibia, areas where, under normal circumstances, there is little subcutaneous fat or redundant skin. Soft eyeballs resulting from lower intraocular pressure are assessed by asking the patient to close his or her eyes and look downwards; the examiner presses lightly on the eyeballs (above the tarsal plate) with the index finger of each hand.

It should be noted that the presence of orthostatic hypotension indicates considerable deficit, which, if not corrected, may lead to severe hypotension on induction of anaesthesia. Orthostatic hypotension should be elicited with caution.

Laboratory investigations may help to confirm the extent of extracellular fluid volume deficit. Haemoconcentration results in an increased haemoglobin concentration and an increased packed cell volume. As dehydration becomes more marked, renal blood flow diminishes, reducing renal clearance of urea and consequently increasing the concentration of blood urea. Patients with moderate volume contraction exhibit a prerenal pattern of uraemia characterized by an increase in blood urea out of proportion to any increase in serum creatinine concentration. Under maximal stimulation from ADH and aldosterone, conservation of sodium and water by the kidneys results in excretion of urine of low sodium concentration (0–15 mmol L^{-1}) and high osmolality (800–1400 mosmol kg^{-1}).

After estimation of the extent of blood volume or extracellular fluid volume deficit, correction is accomplished with the appropriate fluid. Hartmann's solution (compound sodium lactate) and 0.9% saline are isotonic, remaining predominantly in the extracellular space, and are suitable for replacement of extracellular fluid losses. Anaemia is treated preferably by blood transfusion, but alternative fluids may be used (see Ch. 21). The optimal time for surgical intervention is when all fluid deficits have been corrected, but if there are urgent indications for surgery (e.g. presence of gangrenous bowel), compromise is necessary. As a general rule, the demonstration of orthostatic hypotension indicates that further fluid replacement is required.

THE FULL STOMACH

Of all the hazards of emergency anaesthesia, vomiting or regurgitation of gastric contents, followed by aspiration into the tracheobronchial tree whilst protective laryngeal reflexes are obtunded, is one of the commonest and most devastating.

Vomiting is an active process that occurs in the lighter planes of anaesthesia. Consequently, it is a potential problem during induction of, or emergence from, anaesthesia, but should not occur during maintenance if anaesthesia is sufficiently deep. In light planes of anaesthesia, the presence of vomited material above the vocal cords stimulates spasm of the

Table 28.2	Indices of extent of loss of extracellular fluid	
Percentage body weight lost as water	mL of fluid lost per 70 kg	Signs and symptoms
Over 4% (mild)	Over 2500	Thirst, reduced skin elasticity, decreased intraocular pressure, dry tongue, reduced sweating
Over 6% (mild)	Over 4200	As above, plus orthostatic hypotension, reduced filling of peripheral veins, oliguria, low CVP, apathy, haemoconcentration
Over 8% (moderate)	Over 5600	As above, plus hypotension, thready pulse with cool peripheries
10–15% (severe)	7000–10 500	Coma, shock followed by death

cords, which prevents material from entering the larynx. Apnoea may persist until severe hypoxaemia occurs, at which point the vocal cords open and ventilation resumes. Thus, the presence of laryngeal reflexes provides a margin of safety provided that the anaesthetist clears the oropharynx of all debris before ventilation resumes.

In contrast, regurgitation is a passive process that may occur at any time, is often 'silent' (i.e. not apparent to the anaesthetist) and, if aspiration occurs, may have clinical consequences ranging from minor pulmonary sequelae to fulminating aspiration pneumonitis and acute respiratory distress syndrome (ARDS). Because regurgitation occurs usually in the presence of deep anaesthesia or at the onset of action of muscle relaxant drugs, laryngeal reflexes are absent and the risk of aspiration is high.

In elective surgery, patients are usually starved of food and drink overnight, or at least for 4–6 h, although the need for such absolute rules concerning clear fluids has been questioned. However, in emergency surgery, it may be necessary to induce anaesthesia urgently before an adequate period of starvation occurs. In addition, the patient's surgical condition is often accompanied by delayed gastric emptying.

The most important factors determining the extent of gastric regurgitation are the function of the lower oesophageal sphincter and the rate of gastric emptying.

THE LOWER OESOPHAGEAL SPHINCTER

The lower oesophageal sphincter (LOS) is an area (2–5 cm in length) of higher resting intraluminal pressure situated in the region of the cardia. The sphincter relaxes during oesophageal peristalsis to allow food into the stomach, but remains contracted at other times. The structure cannot be defined anatomically but may be detected using intraluminal pressure manometry.

The LOS is the main barrier preventing reflux of gastric contents into the oesophagus and many drugs used in anaesthetic practice affect its resting tone. Reflux is related not to the LOS tone per se, but to the difference between gastric and LOS pressures; this is termed the *barrier pressure*. Drugs that increase the barrier pressure decrease the risk of reflux. Prochlorperazine, cyclizine, anticholinesterases, α-adrenergic agonists and succinylcholine increase barrier pressure. For many years it was thought that the increase in intragastric pressure during succinylcholine-induced fasciculations predisposed to reflux. However, there is an even greater increase in LOS pressure with a consequent increase in barrier pressure.

Anticholinergic drugs, ethanol, ganglion-blocking drugs, tricyclic antidepressants, opioids and thiopental reduce LOS pressure and it is reasonable to assume that these drugs increase the tendency to gastro-oesophageal reflux.

GASTRIC EMPTYING

Under normal circumstances, peristaltic waves sweep from cardia to pylorus at a rate of approximately three per minute, although temporary inhibition of gastric motility follows recent ingestion of a meal. The rate of gastric emptying is proportional to the volume of the stomach contents, with approximately 1–3% of total gastric content reaching the duodenum per minute. Thus, emptying occurs at an exponential rate. The presence of some drugs, fat, acid or hypertonic solutions in the duodenum delays significantly the rate of emptying (the inhibitory enterogastric reflex), but both the nervous and humoral elements of this regulating mechanism are still poorly understood. Many pathological conditions are associated with a reduced rate of gastric emptying (Table 28.3). In the absence of any of these factors, it is reasonably safe to assume that the stomach is empty provided that solids have not been ingested within the preceding 6 h, or fluids consumed in the preceding 2 h, and provided normal peristalsis is occurring.

Vomiting and regurgitation during induction of anaesthesia are encountered most frequently in patients with an acute abdomen or trauma. All patients with minor trauma (fractures or dislocations) must be assumed to have a full stomach; gastric emptying virtually ceases at the time of significant trauma as a result of the combined effects of fear, pain, shock and treatment with opioid analgesics. In all trauma patients, the time interval between ingestion of food and the accident is a more reliable index of the degree of gastric emptying than the period of fasting. It is not uncommon to encounter vomiting 24 h or longer after ingestion of food when trauma has occurred very shortly after the meal. Thus, the 4–6 h rule is unreliable.

Injury from aspiration of gastric contents results from three different mechanisms: chemical pneumonitis (from acid material), mechanical obstruction from particulate material and bacterial contamination. Aspiration of liquid with a pH < 2.5 is associated with a chemical burn of the bronchial, bronchiolar and alveolar mucosa, leading to atelectasis, pulmonary oedema and reduced pulmonary compliance. Bronchospasm may also be present. The claim that patients are at risk if they have more than 25 mL of gastric residue with a pH < 2.5 is based on data from animal studies extrapolated to humans and should not be

Table 28.3 Situations in which vomiting or regurgitation may occur
Full stomach
With absent or abnormal peristalsis
Peritonitis of any cause
Postoperative ileus
Metabolic ileus: hypokalaemia, uraemia, diabetic ketoacidosis
Drug-induced ileus: anticholinergics, those with anticholinergic side-effects
With obstructed peristalsis
Small or large bowel obstruction
Gastric carcinoma
Pyloric stenosis
With delayed gastric emptying
Shock of any cause
Fear, pain or anxiety
Late pregnancy
Deep sedation (opioids)
Recent solid or fluid intake
Other causes
Hiatus hernia
Oesophageal strictures – benign or malignant
Pharyngeal pouch

regarded as indisputable fact. Day-case patients often have residual gastric volumes greater than 25 mL.

If aspiration of gastric contents occurs, the first manoeuvre after the airway is secured is to suction the trachea to remove as much foreign material as possible. If particulate matter is obstructing proximal bronchi, bronchoscopy may be necessary. Hypoxaemia is managed with O_2, IPPV and PEEP. Steroids are not recommended and antibiotics should be given if the aspirated material is considered unsterile.

TECHNIQUES OF ANAESTHESIA

It is important to recognize any patient who may have significant gastric residue and who is in danger of aspiration. The anaesthetic management of such a patient may be described in five phases: preparation, induction, maintenance, emergence and postoperative management.

PHASE I – PREPARATION

Whilst postponement of surgery in the emergency patient may be indicated in order to obtain investigations and institute resuscitation with i.v. fluids, there is usually no benefit to be gained in terms of reducing the possibility of aspiration of gastric contents, and the risk of aspiration must be weighed against the risk of delaying an urgent procedure. However, two manoeuvres are available:

- Although not completely effective, insertion of a nasogastric tube to decompress the stomach and to provide a low-pressure vent for regurgitation may be helpful. Aspiration through the tube may be useful if gastric contents are liquid, as in bowel obstruction, but is less effective when contents are solid. Cricoid pressure is still effective at reducing regurgitation even with a nasogastric tube in situ.
- Clear oral antacids (e.g. sodium citrate) may be used to raise the pH of gastric contents immediately before induction. However, this also increases gastric volume. Particulate antacids should not be used, as they may be very damaging to the airway if aspirated. The preoperative administration of H_2-receptor antagonists consistently raises gastric pH and may reduce the chance of chemical pulmonary injury occurring in the event of inhalation. Although this is standard practice in obstetric anaesthesia, few anaesthetists employ these measures for emergency general surgery. The regimens that may be used are described in Chapter 35.

PHASE II – INDUCTION
Rapid-sequence induction

This is the technique used most frequently for the patient with a full stomach, although it contravenes one of the fundamental rules of anaesthesia, namely that muscle relaxants are not given until control of the airway is assured. The decision to employ the rapid-sequence induction technique balances the risk of losing control of the airway against the risk of aspiration. It is therefore imperative to assess carefully whether or not difficulty is likely to be encountered in performing tracheal intubation. The anaesthetist must have prepared a contingency plan for management of the patient should intubation fail. If preoperative evaluation indicates a particularly difficult airway, the anaesthetist should consider alternative methods of proceeding, e.g. local anaesthetic techniques or 'awake intubation' under local anaesthesia.

For rapid-sequence induction to be consistently safe and successful, it should be performed with meticulous attention to detail. The patient *must* be on a tipping trolley or table, preferably with an adjustable headpiece so that the degree of neck extension/flexion may be altered quickly. Ideally, the patient's head should be in the classic 'sniffing position' with the neck flexed on the shoulders and the head extended on the neck. Failure to appreciate this point increases the likelihood of difficult intubation.

The anaesthetist *must* be aided by at least one skilled assistant to perform cricoid pressure, assist in turning the patient, obtain smaller tracheal tubes, supply stilettes for tubes, etc. High-volume suction apparatus *must* be functioning and the suction catheter should be within reach of the anaesthetist's hand.

As with any anaesthetic, the machine should have been checked before starting, the ventilator adjusted to appropriate settings and all drugs drawn up into labelled syringes before induction. The patient should breathe 100% O_2 for 3–5 min while appropriate monitoring devices are attached and an i.v. infusion started (if not already in place). The optimal inclination of the operating table is debatable as some authorities recommend the reverse Trendelenburg (head-up) position (to prevent regurgitation) and others the classic Trendelenburg position (to prevent aspiration of any regurgitated or vomited material). In general, the optimum position is that in which the trainee anaesthetist has gained greatest experience in performing intubation.

Preinduction measurement of heart rate, arterial pressure (and, when appropriate, central venous pressure) and inspection of the ECG are made and a skilled assistant is positioned at the patient's side to perform Sellick's manoeuvre (cricoid pressure). It is important that the assistant can identify the cricoid cartilage, as compression of the thyroid cartilage distorts laryngeal anatomy and may render tracheal intubation very difficult. To perform Sellick's manoeuvre correctly, the thumb and forefinger press the cricoid cartilage firmly in a posterior direction, thus compressing the oesophagus between the cricoid cartilage and the vertebral column. Because the cricoid cartilage forms a complete ring, the tracheal lumen is not distorted (Fig. 28.1).

Opinions differ with regard to the time at which cricoid pressure should be applied. Some prefer to inform the patient and apply it just before administration of the i.v. induction agent; others apply it as soon as consciousness is lost.

With the assistant in position, a predetermined sleep dose of i.v. induction agent is given (usually thiopental 4 mg kg^{-1} or less in the presence of hypovolaemia). Without waiting to assess the effect of the induction agent, a paralysing dose of succinylcholine

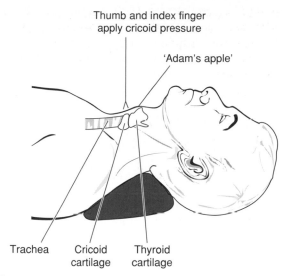

Thumb and index finger apply cricoid pressure

'Adam's apple'

Trachea · Cricoid cartilage · Thyroid cartilage

Fig. 28.1
Sellick's manoeuvre. The cricoid cartilage is palpated immediately below the thyroid cartilage.

(1.5 mg kg^{-1}) is administered immediately. As soon as the jaw begins to relax or after fasciculations have ceased, laryngoscopy is performed and the trachea intubated. Cricoid pressure is maintained until the cuff of the tracheal tube is inflated and correct placement of the tube ascertained by auscultation of both lungs and the presence of end-tidal carbon dioxide. The lungs are gently ventilated manually, as excessive increases in intrathoracic pressure may have harmful effects on circulatory dynamics. One of the main disadvantages of the rapid-sequence induction technique is the haemodynamic instability that may result if the dose of induction agent is excessive (hypotension, circulatory collapse) or inadequate (hypertension, tachycardia, arrhythmia). Unfortunately, selection of the correct dose is difficult and is dependent largely upon the experience of the anaesthetist. For thiopental, a dose of 4 mg kg^{-1} may suffice for healthy, young patients, 2 mg kg^{-1} for the elderly and less for the very frail. An alternative is etomidate 0.1–0.3 mg kg^{-1} (which, in equipotent doses, is less cardiodepressant than thiopental). In very frail patients it may be preferable to avoid i.v. induction agents altogether and consideration should be given to an inhalational induction (see below).

Inhalational induction

If there is reasonable doubt about the ability to perform intubation or to maintain a patent airway in a patient with a full stomach (e.g. the patient with faciomaxillary trauma or the child with epiglottitis or bleeding tonsil), an inhalational induction may be used with oxygen and halothane or sevoflurane. When the patient has reached a deep plane of anaesthesia, laryngoscopy is performed followed by an attempt at tracheal intubation during spontaneous ventilation. Normally, the patient should be placed in the left lateral, head-down position, but if circumstances do not allow the lateral position then the supine posture with cricoid pressure may have to be accepted. Indeed a modification of this technique may be used in any elderly, frail patient who may not tolerate i.v. induction agents. Anaesthesia may be induced by inhalational induction with the maintenance of cricoid pressure and, when the patient is sufficiently anaesthetized, succinylcholine is given and the trachea intubated.

Awake intubation

Although blind nasal intubation is a valuable skill, the introduction of the narrow-gauge fibreoptic intubating laryngoscope has replaced it as the technique of choice in those patients who are likely to develop unrelievable airway obstruction when loss of consciousness occurs (e.g. trismus from dental abscess) or who are a known/probable difficult intubation. Such endoscopic tracheal intubations may be performed via either the nasal route (more commonly used) or the oral route. Before embarking on awake fibreoptic nasal intubation, it is necessary to render the nasopharynx and, to a greater or lesser extent, the upper airway insensitive, so that the introduction of a tracheal tube may be tolerated. The details of the technique differ depending on the preference of the individual anaesthetist and one method that is used commonly is described below:

1. The nasal mucosa is anaesthetized with cocaine solution 4% (maximum 2.5 mL per 70 kg) which is sprayed into the more patent nasal passage. In addition to providing surface anaesthesia, this shrinks the nasal mucosa and reduces the chance of bleeding. A well-lubricated, soft nasopharyngeal airway (size 6 or 7) is then gently inserted into the nasopharynx and left in situ for 3–5 min. Lidocaine is sprayed through the nasopharyngeal airway to anaesthetize the oropharynx and supraglottic area.
2. Anaesthesia of the tracheal mucosa below the vocal cords is accomplished best by transtracheal injection of local anaesthetic. A 21-gauge needle is introduced in the midline through the cricothyroid membrane. Entry into the trachea is confirmed by aspiration of air, and a bolus of 3–5 mL of lidocaine 1% is injected rapidly. Invariably this

results in a bout of coughing, which aids spread of the local anaesthetic over the inferior surface of the vocal cords. This procedure may be omitted if the risk of aspiration is considered high, as anaesthesia of the upper airway increases the risk of pulmonary aspiration if vomiting or regurgitation occurs.

For patients in whom there is a high risk of aspiration, it is possible with experience to perform awake nasal intubation after performing only step 1 above and using a 'spray as you go' technique, injecting aliquots of lidocaine through the suction port of the fibreoptic laryngoscope as it is advanced.

The nasopharyngeal airway is removed and, with the patient's head in the 'sniffing the morning air' position, a well-lubricated, reinforced tracheal tube (size 6 or 7) is inserted gently into the anaesthetized nostril and advanced towards the nasopharynx. The tube should be rotated slowly between thumb and forefinger (pill-rolling movement) and a distinct 'give' is felt on entry into the nasopharynx. Whilst maintaining optimal head position, the fibreoptic laryngoscope is then advanced through the tracheal tube and the pharynx and laryngeal aperture are viewed. As maximal vocal cord abduction occurs during inspiration, the scope is advanced slowly in small steps coordinated with inspiration. Even with good upper airway anaesthesia, entry into the larynx results frequently in a violent cough. After passing through the larynx, the position of the scope is confirmed by visual recognition of tracheal rings and the tracheal tube is railroaded gently over the scope into the trachea. Position is again confirmed by seeing tracheal rings, and the scope is removed.

Although considerable practice is needed in the operation of this instrument to ensure a successful outcome, attention to the details of the technique improves the chance of success.

Regional anaesthesia

Anaesthetic expertise in the use of regional anaesthesia is lacking in many UK hospitals. This is unfortunate, as local blocks are eminently suitable for emergency procedures on the extremities (e.g. to reduce fractures or dislocations).

Brachial plexus block by the axillary, supraclavicular or interscalene approach is satisfactory for orthopaedic manipulations or surgical procedures involving the upper extremity. It satisfies surgical requirements for analgesia, muscle relaxation and immobility. There is minimal effect on the cardiovascular system and there is a prolonged period of analgesia postoperatively. Similarly, i.v. regional anaesthesia is useful for orthopaedic reductions; prilocaine 0.5% plain is the drug of choice, but if not available, then lidocaine 0.5% plain is suitable.

For regional anaesthesia of the lower extremity, techniques available include subarachnoid, epidural and sciatic/femoral blocks. Spinal and epidural blocks are contraindicated if there is doubt about the adequacy of extracellular fluid or vascular volumes, as large decreases in arterial pressure may result from the associated pharmacological sympathectomy.

It is a common surgical misconception that subarachnoid or epidural anaesthetic techniques are safer than general anaesthesia for patients in poor physical condition. It must be emphasized that for the *inexperienced* anaesthetist, these techniques are invariably more dangerous than general anaesthesia for the patient with moderate/major trauma or any intra-abdominal emergency condition.

PHASE III – MAINTENANCE OF ANAESTHESIA

In emergency anaesthesia, there are strong arguments in favour of a balanced technique of anaesthesia combining:

- anaesthesia – loss of awareness
- analgesia to attenuate autonomic reflexes in response to the painful stimulus
- muscle relaxation.

If a rapid-sequence induction has been performed, the patient's lungs are gently ventilated manually whilst heart rate and arterial pressure measurements are repeated to assess the cardiovascular effects of the drugs used and of the insult of tracheal intubation. Nitrous oxide 50–66% (dependent upon the patient's condition) in oxygen contributes to loss of patient awareness but does not ensure it and an appropriate concentration of a volatile anaesthetic agent should be added to the inspired gas mixture.

When there is evidence of return of neuromuscular transmission (by clinical signs or use of a nerve stimulator) as succinylcholine is degraded, a non-depolarizing myoneural blocking agent is administered. The choice is dependent upon the patient's condition and the effect of the induction of anaesthesia on the patient's cardiovascular status. Both rocuronium and atracurium are appropriate drugs for routine use. Pancuronium (dose 50–100 μg kg^{-1}) is useful in patients with hypovolaemia, as it tends to increase arterial pressure and heart rate. (The tachycardia it produces is undesirable in patients with ischaemic heart disease or valvular disease.) Atracurium has virtually no cardiovascular

effects in clinical doses and is useful if renal impairment is present.

When the muscle relaxant has been administered, the tracheal tube is connected to a mechanical ventilator and minute volume adjusted to produce normo- or slight hypocapnia. There are few accurate means of estimating ventilatory requirement, but a minute volume of 75–100 mL kg^{-1} min^{-1} at a tidal volume of 6–10 mL kg^{-1} should be used initially. The inspiratory flow rate should be adjusted to minimize peak airway pressure.

Before the initial surgical incision is made, analgesia may be supplemented by small incremental doses of morphine 1–5 mg or fentanyl 25–100 μg.

The use of supplemental doses of analgesic and muscle relaxant drugs is described in Chapters 5 and 6. The trainee should be aware that during emergency anaesthesia, particularly for intra-abdominal or trauma surgery, much smaller doses of drugs are usually required. As a general rule, it is safe practice to administer half the dose, which might be considered appropriate for an elective patient, and to determine further doses by assessment of the subsequent response. If there are poor or inadequate recovery room facilities, it is also a good general rule to err on the side of caution in the use of i.v. drugs.

Fluid management

During emergency intra-abdominal surgery, there may be large blood and fluid losses, which exceed the patient's maintenance fluid replacement. These include evaporative losses from exposed gut and mesentery, blood loss on to swabs and into suction bottles, and the poorly defined 'third-space' losses caused by sequestration of fluid in inflamed and traumatized tissue. Intraoperatively, maintenance requirements are supplied with Hartmann's solution (compound sodium lactate) at 2 mL kg^{-1} h^{-1}. An appropriate volume of replacement for third-space loss and evaporative gut loss is given in addition. This volume depends on the degree of surgical trauma but is normally in the range 2–7 mL kg^{-1} h^{-1}.

Haemorrhage in excess of 15% blood volume in adults or 10% in children is usually an indication for blood transfusion.

PHASE IV – REVERSAL AND EMERGENCE

After insertion of the last skin suture, the administration of anaesthetic drugs can be discontinued. Direct pharyngoscopy is performed and secretions/debris removed from the pharynx; if a nasogastric tube is in situ, it is aspirated and left unspigoted. Glycopyrrolate and neostigmine are given in one bolus of 20 and 50 µg kg^{-1}, respectively, and ventilation is undertaken manually (with an F_1O_2 of 1.0) so that spontaneous ventilatory activity may be detected. Because the risk of aspiration of gastric contents is as great on recovery as at induction, extubation of the trachea should not be performed until protective airway reflexes are intact. To demonstrate the adequacy of reflexes, both level of consciousness and neuromuscular transmission should be assessed.

Level of consciousness

The patient should be awake and respond appropriately to verbal commands, e.g. eye opening.

Neuromuscular function

The adequacy of reversal of paralysis may be determined by observing the patient's ability to sustain a head lift for 5 s and sustain a firm grip without fade. Preferably, a nerve stimulator is used to define reversal of neuromuscular transmission (see Ch. 6).

Immediately before tracheal extubation, the patient is turned to the lateral position (if possible) and asked to take a deep inspiration while gentle positive pressure is applied to the airway. At the peak of inspiration, the cuff is deflated and the tracheal tube removed as the patient exhales, thus assisting removal of any secretions which may have accumulated above the cuff. Oxygen 100% is administered until a regular ventilatory rhythm is re-established and the patient has demonstrated an ability to cough and maintain a patent airway. Breathing 40% O_2, the patient is transported in the lateral position to the recovery room and remains there until all vital signs are stable, postoperative shivering has ceased, core temperature is normal and there is good perfusion as judged by warm extremities and good urine output.

If there is any doubt about the adequacy of ventilation after reversal of neuromuscular blockade, the patient is taken to the recovery room with the tracheal tube in situ and this is removed from the trachea only when ventilation and gas exchange are adequate.

PHASE V – POSTOPERATIVE MANAGEMENT

Postoperatively, the patient requires analgesics, e.g. morphine 0.2 mg kg^{-1} i.m. or s.c. 4-hourly, or as patient-controlled analgesia, if appropriate. If there is continued concern about the metabolic or volaemic state of the patient, these dosages should be reduced considerably. Fluid balance should take into account maintenance needs plus compensation for abnormal fluid loss

(e.g. gastric aspirate, loss from intestinal fistulae or from surgical drains). This subject is discussed in Chapter 21.

The need for further blood replacement is assessed by regular observation of vital signs and drainage measurements and postoperative Hb or haematocrit measurements.

Prophylactic postoperative IPPV

Continuation of IPPV should be considered electively in several circumstances, some of which are listed in Table 28.4.

EMERGENCY LAPAROTOMY IN THE ELDERLY PATIENT

The NCEPOD (formerly National Confidential Enquiry into Patient Outcome and Death) recommendations suggest that the decision to perform emergency surgery on elderly patients requires the input of a senior clinician from surgery, anaesthesia and critical care. It is unacceptable to subject all infirm, elderly patients to needless, major surgery followed by prolonged intensive care. If it is considered that the burden of surgical treatment and poor prognosis outweigh the likely benefit of surgery, then such intervention is not in the best interests of the patient and should be withheld.

It is emphasized that such decisions must be individualized and must take into account patient/relatives' wishes in addition to surgical, medical and humanitarian considerations.

There are some questions that need to be answered *BEFORE* embarking on emergency, potentially major surgery in frail, elderly and infirm patients with a surgical, acute abdomen:

- Is it likely that the patient will die *with* or *without surgery*? If the answer is yes, then surgery is *not* indicated unless it is likely that it will contribute to

Table 28.4   Indications for continuation of ventilatory assistance postoperatively
Prolonged shock/hypoperfusion state of any cause
Massive sepsis (faecal peritonitis, cholangitis, septicaemia)
Severe ischaemic heart disease
Extreme obesity
Overt gastric acid aspiration
Previously severe pulmonary disease

the physical comfort of the patient during the dying process, i.e. contribute to a 'good death'.

- Is it likely that the patient would survive a laparotomy if the underlying cause were found to be curable/treatable (e.g. perforated duodenal ulcer, appendicitis)? If the answer is yes, then surgery may be indicated and agreement on the appropriate level and duration of postoperative organ support must be reached.
- If, having embarked on surgery, the underlying cause is found to be treatable but not curable (e.g. perforated carcinoma with metastases, gangrenous bowel) would radical surgery be appropriate, given the patients overall physical state? If not, aggressive postoperative intensive care is not indicated. If yes, then what would be an appropriate level and duration of postoperative support? These questions need to be answered by experienced clinicians.

THE ANAESTHETIST AND MAJOR TRAUMA

The management of the patient with major trauma requires a multidisciplinary team effort. Successful treatment is often dependent on the efficacy of the initial resuscitation and rapid formulation of the correct priorities. In many hospitals, the anaesthetic/ICU trainee is an integral member of the 'trauma team', which is called whenever a multiply-injured patient is expected. Increasingly, trauma management is based on advanced trauma life support (ATLS) teaching and it is important that the trainee is familiar with major ATLS protocols.

The suggested scheme for trauma management is as follows:

1. *Rapid primary survey*. Recognition and treatment of any *immediately* life-threatening complications, such as airway obstruction, tension/open pneumothorax, massive haemothorax, haemoperitoneum, flail chest, cardiac tamponade or intracranial injury.
2. *Resuscitation of vital functions*. Control of haemorrhage, intravenous access and volume resuscitation.
3. *Detailed secondary survey*. Recognition of any *potentially* life-threatening injuries, such as ruptured aorta, pulmonary/cardiac contusions, diaphragmatic rupture, haemoretroperitoneum and pelvic disruption.
4. *Definitive care*.

Steps 1 and 2 are performed simultaneously. The anaesthetic trainee may be involved in any or all of the above areas of management.

PRIMARY SURVEY/RESUSCITATION OF VITAL FUNCTIONS

As soon as the patient arrives in the accident and emergency department, rapid primary survey is performed at the same time as resuscitation of vital functions. The approach is similar for all ill patients and the trainee should look for and treat:

- airway obstruction – effective airway management is paramount; hypoxaemia and hypercapnia are extremely undesirable and their avoidance must be guaranteed
- breathing difficulty caused by pneumothorax or flail chest
- circulatory shock and the need for control of obvious bleeding.

Airway/breathing

The first priority for the anaesthetist when confronted with an unconscious trauma victim is to establish the patency of the patient's airway whilst assuring immobilization of the cervical spine. If upper airway obstruction is present, the pharynx is cleared of any debris and the jaw displaced forward (jaw thrust). Neck tilt and chin lift are avoided, as these manoeuvres could displace an unstable cervical spine. Early establishment of a patent airway is paramount to successful resuscitation and although unstable cervical spine injuries are relatively uncommon, *all* patients should be assumed to be at risk until proved otherwise. Exclusion of this injury requires cervical spine radiography and possibly computed tomography (CT). No patient should remain even marginally hypoxaemic for the purposes of clinical assessment, but in the alert patient who is to have semi-urgent tracheal intubation, consideration should be given to clinical exclusion of cervical spine injury, flail chest, abdominal tenderness, etc.

When the airway is clear, attention is directed to the adequacy of ventilation and the need for tracheal intubation. If the patient is apnoeic, ventilation by mask with 100% oxygen is started immediately, as good oxygenation and correction of hypercapnia should be ensured before tracheal intubation is undertaken. The possibility of a cervical spine injury does not contraindicate orotracheal intubation provided it is performed with care *and* in-line immobilization of the cervical spine is maintained throughout the procedure.

In general, airway assessment reveals one of three clinical scenarios:

- *Patient is conscious, alert, talking.* Give high-flow oxygen via face mask. There is no need for immediate airway intervention and a full clinical evaluation can be done. Persisting signs of shock and/or the diagnosis of serious underlying injuries might be an indication for planned endotracheal intubation and mechanical ventilation.
- *Patient has a reduced conscious level but some degree of airway control and gag reflex still present.* If the patient is maintaining the airway and breathing adequately then there is no need for immediate intervention. Endotracheal intubation will be necessary but a clinical evaluation can be done whilst equipment is being readied.
- *Patient has a reduced conscious level, gag reflex absent.* If the patient is unable to maintain the airway or is breathing poorly, tracheal intubation and artificial ventilation should be carried out at once.

All trauma patients should undergo tracheal intubation via the oral route using a rapid-sequence induction with in-line stabilization of the cervical spine. The dose of induction agent is judged bearing in mind the patient's cardiovascular state and the possibility of intracranial injury. If there are clinical signs suggesting a pneumothorax or surgical emphysema and/or a flail segment is apparent, then a chest drain should be inserted simultaneously or before mechanical ventilation is commenced. Persistence of hypoxaemia after institution of mechanical ventilation suggests unrecognized pneumothorax, haemothorax, pulmonary contusion or poor cardiac output caused by hypovolaemia, tamponade, etc.

Patients with severe faciomaxillary trauma who are cooperative and awake despite their injuries may not require immediate tracheal intubation, but do need frequent and regular upper airway evaluation to assess the rate of progress of pharyngeal or laryngeal oedema, which may proceed to complete airway obstruction with alarming rapidity.

When the airway is under control, ventilation is deemed adequate and any obvious external bleeding has been arrested, the next priority is evaluation of the cardiovascular system; this may be classified into assessment of blood volume status and pump function.

Circulation

This has been described earlier in this chapter. Haemorrhage is the most common cause of shock in the injured patient and virtually all patients with multiple injuries have an element of hypovolaemia. Patients with major trauma often require urgent restoration of circulating blood volume. At least two large-gauge (14-gauge) i.v. cannulae are inserted percutaneously into veins in one or two limbs and both cannulae are attached to blood-warming coils. Isotonic electrolyte solutions are used for initial resuscitation and 1–2 L of Hartmann's solution is given as rapidly as possible and the patient's response is assessed. If this does not increase perfusion and arterial pressure significantly and cross-matched blood is not yet available, either plasma or a plasma substitute should be considered. Human albumin solution is very expensive and probably has little advantage in comparison with starch and gelatin solutions. Their half-life in the circulation is approximately 4 h in the normal patient, but is shorter in the presence of shock. As 85% is excreted by the kidneys, gelatin solutions promote an osmotic diuresis and may therefore preserve urine output and renal function. Up to 1500 mL may be given initially; in most circumstances this is adequate to restore circulating blood volume until cross-matched blood is available. Warmed, stored blood is administered subsequently to maintain urine output, arterial pressure and CVP. As soon as possible, a reliable CVP catheter is inserted. The right internal jugular vein is the preferred site for this purpose. Fluid is infused through the peripheral i.v. cannulae to produce a CVP of approximately 5–10 mmHg (zero reference mid-axillary line).

Whilst whole blood is the ideal fluid for restoration of blood volume in haemorrhagic shock, if the patient is exsanguinating (< 40% blood loss), a synthetic colloid (gelatin or hydroxyethylstarch) should be given immediately while cross-matching is undertaken. Type-specific blood may be given, as the chance of a reaction is less than 1% in males (over 2% in parous females), but in this situation the imperative is on the diagnosis and surgical management of the source of haemorrhage. If the breach in the circulation is large, then the prime objective of resuscitation is to maintain cerebral and coronary perfusion whilst control of the source of bleeding is accomplished, *not* to restore a normal blood pressure.

Pump function

The commonest cause of pump failure in major trauma is the presence of a tension pneumothorax, but other possibilities include severe myocardial contusion and traumatic pericardial tamponade.

Tension pneumothorax causes compression of the mediastinum (heart and great vessels) and presents with extreme respiratory distress, shock, unilateral air entry, a shift of the trachea towards the normal side and distension of the veins in the neck, although the last sign may not be seen in hypovolaemic shock. It may be relieved immediately by insertion of a 14-gauge cannula through the second intercostal space in the midclavicular line, but this should be followed by standard chest drainage. If there is any suspicion of tension pneumothorax, IPPV should not be commenced until decompression has been achieved, otherwise mediastinal compression is increased. Patients with blunt chest trauma and fractured ribs may develop a tension pneumothorax rapidly when positive-pressure ventilation is commenced, and consideration should be given to the prophylactic insertion of chest drains in such patients.

DEFINITIVE CARE

Whenever possible, hypovolaemia should be corrected before anaesthesia is induced, but if the rate of haem-

orrhage is likely to exceed the rate of transfusion and continued transfusion results only in further bleeding (e.g. ruptured aorta), it is necessary to induce anaesthesia in a hypovolaemic patient.

On arrival in theatre, the patient is placed on the operating table. One hundred per cent oxygen is given whilst at least two large-gauge cannulae are inserted (each connected to a blood-warming coil), if this has not already been accomplished. In patients with major trauma, anaesthesia should be induced in theatre so that surgery can start as soon as possible. Figure 28.2 illustrates standard monitoring which is necessary for the management of major trauma. In the unconscious patient, the trachea may be intubated after administration of a paralysing dose of succinylcholine. If the patient is conscious, despite being severely hypovolaemic, a controlled rapid-sequence induction using ketamine as the i.v. induction agent is preferred. The dose of ketamine is

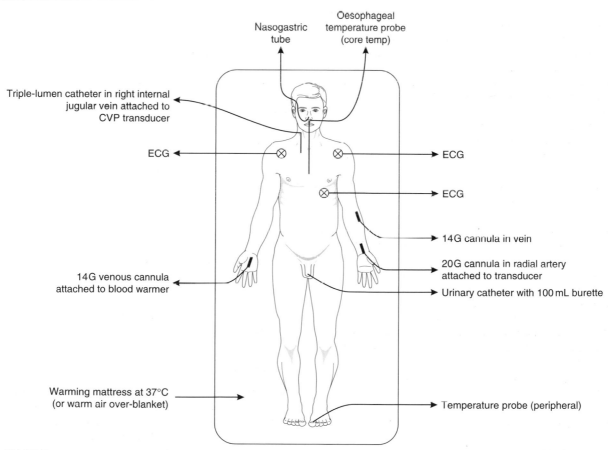

Fig. 28.2
Commonly used monitoring and resuscitation attachments in management of a patient with multiple injuries. Pulse oximetry and capnography are also used during anaesthesia.

critical and often very small doses (0.3–0.7 mg kg^{-1}) suffice. If the dose is misjudged, cardiovascular decompensation similar to that seen with other i.v. induction agents may occur. The depressant effects of i.v. induction agents are exaggerated because the *proportion* of the cardiac output going to the heart and brain is increased. In addition, the rate of redistribution and/or metabolism is decreased as a result of reduced blood flow to muscle, liver and kidneys and thus blood concentrations remain increased for longer periods in comparison with healthy patients. Ketamine should not be used in patients with significant head injury. Etomidate (0.1–0.3 mg kg^{-1}) is an alternative for normovolaemic patients with head injury, but is more likely to attenuate compensatory mechanisms. Even a single bolus dose of etomidate may interfere with adrenal function and recommendations concerning the use of this drug must be guarded.

After tracheal intubation, the lungs are ventilated at the lowest peak airway pressure consistent with an acceptable tidal volume. Pancuronium or rocuronium is given in small incremental doses of 1 or 5 mg, respectively, to maintain relaxation. When the haemodynamic situation has stabilized and systolic arterial pressure exceeds 90 mmHg, consideration may be given to deepening anaesthesia. This should be undertaken cautiously and, in principle, agents which are rapidly reversible or rapidly excreted should be used.

In the shock state, there is very rapid uptake of inhalational agents. Reduced cardiac output and pulmonary blood flow decrease the rate of removal of anaesthetic agent from the alveoli, producing a rapid increase in alveolar concentration. Thus, the MAC value is approached more rapidly than in normovolaemic patients.

Monitoring should be comprehensive in these patients (see Fig. 28.2) and should be commenced before induction of anaesthesia when feasible. Blood may be sampled from the arterial cannula to monitor changes in acid–base state, haemoglobin concentration, coagulation and electrolyte concentrations. Requirements for further colloid replacement may be assessed from CVP measurements and urine output.

When surgical bleeding has been controlled, the patient's cardiovascular status should improve, but if hypotension persists despite apparently adequate fluid administration, other causes of haemorrhage should be sought (Table 28.5). It is important that the anaesthetist assesses the patient regularly during prolonged anaesthesia to exclude these latent complications of major trauma.

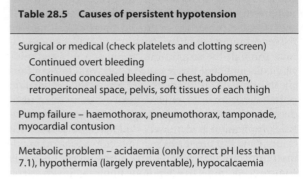

Table 28.5   Causes of persistent hypotension

Surgical or medical (check platelets and clotting screen)
   Continued overt bleeding
   Continued concealed bleeding – chest, abdomen, retroperitoneal space, pelvis, soft tissues of each thigh

Pump failure – haemothorax, pneumothorax, tamponade, myocardial contusion

Metabolic problem – acidaemia (only correct pH less than 7.1), hypothermia (largely preventable), hypocalcaemia

MASSIVE TRANSFUSION

One definition states that if an amount greater than 50% of the patient's blood volume is replaced rapidly, the transfusion is deemed massive, e.g. 5 units of blood in 1 h in a 70 kg adult. This is a life-threatening situation and close communication between a designated member of the anaesthetic team and the blood bank is essential if the goals of restoration of circulating blood volume and effective management of blood component replacement are to be achieved. Disseminated intravascular coagulation (DIC) is a feared complication in the acutely bleeding patient and is associated with significant mortality. Whole blood and plasma-reduced blood contain some residual coagulation activity. However, the UK transfusion service now provides almost all stored blood as red cells in optimal additive solution, containing no plasma, platelets, coagulation factors or leucocytes. Transfusion of red cells in optimal additive solution in quantities approaching the patient's blood volume causes a dilutional thrombocytopenia and some degree of clotting factor deficiency, both of which affect haemostasis adversely and may result in DIC. These abnormalities may be detected by frequent measurement of platelet count, fibrinogen level, prothrombin time (PT) and activated partial thromboplastin time (APTT), reflecting disorders of extrinsic and intrinsic systems as a result of dilutional loss of factors V and VIII. Measurement of fibrinogen degradation products and D-dimers may be useful. Treatment should be directed at correcting the dilutional coagulation change. Coagulation factor deficiency is likely when fibrinogen decreases below the critical level of 1.0 g L^{-1} and is common after 150% blood loss (i.e. 1½ blood volumes). This is followed by decreases in other labile coagulation factors to 200% activity after 20% blood loss. Prolongation of the APTT and PT to more than 1.5 times the normal value is correlated with an increased risk of coagulopathy and requires correction. It has been suggested that 'formula replacement' (fresh frozen plasma (FFP) 1 unit for every 4 units of blood) be used if blood loss is rapid and laboratory turnaround time is excessive. FFP alone corrects fibrinogen and most coagulation factor deficiencies. However, if fibrinogen concentration remains < 1.0 g L^{-1}, cryoprecipitate therapy should be considered. It is necessary to give platelet concentrate for severe thrombocytopenia (platelet count less than 50×10^9 L^{-1}) or milder thrombocytopenia in patients with high-energy trauma or central nervous system injury. A platelet count of 50×10^9 L^{-1} is to be anticipated when approximately two blood volumes have been replaced by plasma-poor red cells. In assessing the requirement for platelets, frequent measurements are needed, as it may be necessary to request platelets at levels above the desired target in order to ensure their availability when needed. Requests for these expensive blood products should be made early as there is often delay in obtaining them and it is better, if possible, to prevent the development of coagulation failure and the resulting bleeding tendency. Although diffuse pathological bleeding may be secondary to dilutional effects, it is also a manifestation of tissue hypoperfusion resulting from shock and inadequate or delayed resuscitation. Clinically, this microvascular bleeding produces oozing from mucosae, raw surfaces and puncture sites and may increase the extent of soft tissue and pulmonary contusions. It is difficult to treat and this underscores the importance of rapid and adequate resuscitation. Frequent estimation of platelet count, fibrinogen, PT and APTT is strongly recommended.

The rapid and effective restoration of an adequate circulating blood volume is crucial in the management of major haemorrhage, as mortality increases with increasing duration and severity of shock. Inadequate volume replacement is the most common complication of haemorrhagic shock. The importance of the prevention of hypothermia during massive transfusion cannot be overstated. Hypothermia causes platelet dysfunction, reduced metabolism of citrate and lactate and an increased tendency to cardiac arrhythmias, which may result in a bleeding diathesis, hypocalcaemia, metabolic acidaemia and cardiac arrest. Core temperature should be measured continuously during massive transfusion and every effort must be made to prevent heat loss. Warm air over-blankets (e.g. Bair Hugger™) are usually effective in maintaining body temperature. Efficient systems for heating stored blood and allowing rapid infusion are available, but all fluids should be warmed to body temperature if possible.

FURTHER READING

American College of Surgeons 1997 Advanced trauma life support program for doctors, 6th edn. American College of Surgeons, Chicago

Stainsby D, MacLennan S, Hamilton P J 1997 Management of massive blood loss: a template guideline. British Journal of Anaesthesia 85(3): 487–496

29 Anaesthesia for gynaecological and genitourinary surgery

Gynaecological and genitourinary surgery have much in common. Both include frequently performed 'minor' procedures. Increasingly, modern narrow-gauge fibreoptic telescopes allow these procedures to be performed at outpatient clinics, with topical anaesthesia administered by the operator. Many other procedures may be undertaken as day cases. Inpatient gynaecological and urological lists comprise an increasing proportion of major oncological surgery. Although patients undergoing gynaecological surgery tend to be young, many presenting in the urology service are elderly and have concurrent medical problems.

POSITIONING THE PATIENT

Many procedures are carried out with the patient in the lithotomy position. Care is needed to avoid damage to the common peroneal nerve because the legs may press against the lithotomy poles. The Lloyd-Davies position provides a variant of the lithotomy position. It is used traditionally for those with osteoarthritis of the hips or the lumbar spine. Before placing patients in these positions, they should be adequately anaesthetized with good airway control, because it is impossible to turn them rapidly onto the side should they regurgitate or vomit stomach contents. During positioning, the patient's head must be supported, and the arms prevented from falling. The anaesthetic breathing tubes should be free to move and monitoring apparatus connected without unnecessary delay. These positions increase the pressure of the abdominal contents on the diaphragm, making spontaneous respiration more difficult and causing closure of basal alveoli. This may lead to a decrease in oxygen saturation, most marked in the obese and when head-down tilt is used. The combination of respiratory obstruction, if allowed to develop, with the expiratory effort of the lower abdominal muscles commonly seen during anaesthesia results in exten-sive movement with respiration, making the view through endoscopic instruments difficult and occasionally too dangerous to allow more extensive surgery.

After surgery, the legs are lowered, resulting in a reduction in venous return and cardiac output. This is exacerbated by some cardiovascular drugs, spinal (subarachnoid block) or epidural anaesthesia and blood loss. The legs should be lowered before recovery from anaesthesia, so that the patient may be turned to the lateral position if necessary.

MINIMALLY INVASIVE SURGERY

The number of operations that may be performed laparoscopically is increasing. Female sterilization, ovarian cystectomy, emergency surgery for ectopic pregnancy, nephrectomy, pyeloplasty, adrenalectomy, vaginal hysterectomy and iliac lymph node dissection may be performed in this way. Most of these procedures require longer operating and anaesthetic times than open versions of the same procedures, but are less painful after surgery, require a shorter duration of stay in hospital and lead to earlier return to normal activities. A pneumoperitoneum is created, most commonly by insufflating the peritoneal cavity with carbon dioxide. As carbon dioxide is soluble in blood, the risk of gas embolus is reduced. It is also inexpensive and non-flammable. Increased pressure and duration of pneumoperitoneum decrease the patient's tolerance of this procedure during surgery.

PHYSIOLOGICAL CHANGES

Respiration

Pneumoperitoneum increases intra-abdominal pressure and reduces both chest wall and lung compliance, and also functional residual capacity. These effects are more marked for patients undergoing surgery in the lithotomy posture. Hypoventilation ensues and intrapulmonary shunt is increased. A decrease in cardiac output increases the ventilation/perfusion ratio and alveolar dead space.

Cardiovascular system

Bradycardia is a common occurrence after peritoneal insufflation, and occasionally asystole occurs. Both decreases and marked increases in arterial pressure may occur during laparoscopic surgery. The increased intra-abdominal pressure decreases venous return, leading to a reduction in cardiac output, but sometimes a compensatory increase in systemic vascular resistance (SVR) maintains systolic arterial pressure. Large increases in arterial pressure are caused by increased concentrations of arginine vasopressin during pneumoperitoneum, causing increases in SVR. A rapid return to normal concentrations occurs after release of the pneumoperitoneum.

COMPLICATIONS OF LAPAROSCOPIC SURGERY

- If the Verres' needle is not inserted fully into the peritoneal cavity, carbon dioxide is forced subcutaneously, leading to surgical emphysema.
- Blood vessels may be punctured by the Verres' needle in the abdominal wall, in the peritoneal cavity or retroperitoneally. Blood loss in the abdominal wall and retroperitoneal space may be considerable before detection.
- Abdominal viscera may be perforated during surgery, causing leakage of intestinal contents, peritonitis and septicaemia.
- If the pressure used to inflate the peritoneum is too high, carbon dioxide may be forced through congenital foramina in the diaphragm, causing pneumomediastinum, pneumothorax or pneumopericardium. Increased ventilation pressures may also lead to pneumothorax by rupturing emphysematous bullae.
- It is possible for insufflating gas to cause gas embolism. The Verres' needle or trocar may be sited in a vessel, or gas may be forced into open venous sinuses by high intra-abdominal pressures. When the carbon dioxide embolus reaches the heart, cardiac output decreases abruptly, less blood is delivered to the lungs and the end-tidal carbon dioxide suddenly decreases.

ANAESTHETIC IMPLICATIONS OF LAPAROSCOPIC SURGERY

A large-gauge cannula should be inserted in case of inadvertent puncture of large blood vessels. The choice of induction and maintenance agent is not important. As there is a risk of severe bradycardia, some anaesthetists give glycopyrrolate 0.2 mg or atropine 0.3 mg at induction. There is a high incidence of postoperative nausea and vomiting (PONV) after laparoscopy, especially following gynaecological procedures. An antiemetic should be given prophylactically.

In several studies of short laparoscopic procedures, there have been no reports of regurgitation and inhalation in patients breathing spontaneously through a laryngeal mask airway (LMA). Spontaneous ventilation through an LMA should be considered only for short procedures (up to about 10 min) in healthy, slim individuals. Pneumoperitoneum increases the work of breathing and obesity exacerbates this. In addition, carbon dioxide absorbed through the peritoneum increases the carbon dioxide load to be excreted. Therefore, intermittent positive-pressure ventilation (IPPV) is necessary for procedures of greater than 10–15 min duration, in patients who have pre-existing respiratory and cardiovascular disease or those who are obese. Ventilation of the lungs may be undertaken via LMA if the patient is slim, with no respiratory or cardiovascular comorbidity. An intra-arterial cannula is useful for carbon dioxide measurement in patients with respiratory disease undergoing prolonged laparoscopic procedures as there is a greater difference between the partial pressure of carbon dioxide in arterial blood and alveoli.

There is more rapid recovery of respiratory function, decreased postoperative pain and consequently smoother recovery after laparoscopic surgery than after open operations. Pain after laparoscopy is caused by the stretching of the peritoneum (which produces an inflammatory response), residual intraperitoneal gas, the effects of the surgery and the 'portholes' or any skin incisions. Pain is treated optimally with local anaesthetic, paracetamol, non-steroidal anti-inflammatory drugs (NSAIDs) and opioids if required. The longer the pneumoperitoneum and the higher the pressure used, the more severe is postoperative pain.

Laparoscopic sterilization

This produces additional pain from tubal ischaemia. Many methods of local anaesthesia have been used: instillation of local anaesthetic through the uterus to the inside of the Fallopian tubes, injection of local anaesthetic into the mesosalpinx, dipping Filshie clips in local anaesthetic jelly, and instillation of local anaesthetic into the pouch of Douglas via an epidural catheter inserted through the abdominal wall. None of these methods is totally effective, and some patients may still require an opioid. One or two doses of intravenous fentanyl may be sufficient. In some centres, patient-controlled analgesia (PCA) with alfentanil is used. Other patients require morphine.

The ischaemic pain diminishes after 2 or 3 h and pain may then be managed with NSAIDs, paracetamol and weak oral opioids, such as dihydrocodeine, codeine or tramadol. Patients who have received opioid drugs and who then travel home are particularly likely to be nauseated. Prophylactic antiemetics are justified.

SURGERY FOR MALIGNANCY

OPEN PELVIC SURGERY

Most urological and gynaecological operations have the same basic anaesthetic requirements. The duration of surgery for Wertheim's hysterectomy, total cystectomy and radical prostatectomy is about 3-6 h. During these operations, there may be extensive blood loss, the patient's temperature decreases and there is considerable postoperative pain. Surgery often offers the best long-term prognosis (debulking tumours increases the efficacy of chemotherapy) and increasingly, more debilitated patients are undergoing extensive surgery. The choice of induction agent is dependent on the patient's condition, whilst the choice of volatile agent is not important. Tracheal intubation and artificial ventilation are necessary. Epidural analgesia or opioid drugs provide intraoperative analgesia. The level of epidural depends on the incision site. As oncological surgery is often tailored to a specific patient's disease, it is wise to ask the surgeon what incision is required. Epidural analgesia provides cardiovascular stability, imparts some protection against deep venous thrombosis, reduces blood loss and decreases some elements of the stress response to surgery. However, there may be precipitate decreases in arterial pressure if bleeding occurs and measurement of central venous pressure (CVP) is useful to prevent hypovolaemia. Monitoring of intra-arterial blood pressure and temperature is also advisable. The patient should be kept warm by maintaining a warm environment, minimizing exposure, especially during insertion of cannulae/catheters, the use of warmed intravenous fluids, warming blankets and warm humidified gases. A high-dependency area is ideal for continuing epidural or other analgesia, supervision of fluid balance and rewarming of the

patient. Younger and more healthy patients may be managed in a general surgical ward, with PCA or other techniques. In patients undergoing cystectomy, the ureters are diverted into a loop of small bowel and the resulting ileus may be prolonged by opioid analgesia. Epidural analgesia is particularly useful in these cases.

RADICAL VULVECTOMY AND TOTAL AMPUTATION OF PENIS

Both these operations are performed with the patient in the Lloyd-Davies or lithotomy position. There is often marked blood loss and heat loss. Tracheal intubation and artificial ventilation are advisable in all but the very healthy and slim. The use of invasive monitoring is dictated by the patient's state of health and the extent and difficulty of the surgery. Temperature should be monitored and the patient kept warm as for open pelvic surgery. Epidural analgesia intra- and postoperatively is ideal for these patients. If this is not possible, spinal anaesthesia using local anaesthetic and intrathecal opioids gives good postoperative analgesia. PCA may be used in the postoperative period.

NEPHRECTOMY

Full assessment of the patient is required with particular reference to renal function and arterial pressure. Anaemia may accompany impaired renal function or chronic infection of the kidney. Computed tomography (CT) of a renal tumour indicates if there is extension along the renal vessels and the inferior and superior venae cavae. The extent of the tumour and its proximity to vessels provide information on the likely duration of surgery and potential blood loss. Patients require tracheal intubation and ventilation of the lungs to allow surgical access, because of the position, and the risk of pneumothorax during surgery. Central venous and direct arterial pressure measurement may be required if extensive blood loss is anticipated or if the patient has significant cardiovascular disease. Temperature should be monitored and the patient kept warm. The patient is placed in the lateral position with the flank raised to open the space between the ribs and the pelvis for surgical access. This is referred to as 'breaking the table' At this point, attention to the patient's head and airway is very important as these may become unsupported as the table moves. The upper arm must not be abducted excessively at the shoulder and all areas of the body in contact with supports should be well padded. After positioning the patient, correct placement of the tracheal tube should be checked in case inadvertent bronchial intubation has occurred. As the legs are dependent, there is a risk of decreased venous return. This may be exacerbated by kinking of the inferior vena cava as a result of the position of the trunk.

There is a risk of pneumothorax from perforation of the pleura by the surgeon. The hole is generally small, so the use of positive-pressure ventilation and manually inflating the lung before closure of the pleura help to prevent postoperative problems. A chest drain may be inserted before the end of surgery. The incision used for these operations is very painful and various methods of local analgesia are used. Thoracic epidural block provides good analgesia. Intercostal blocks may be used but they have a short duration of action and carry a risk of pneumothorax, as does intrapleural analgesia. PCA may be the best available method. If there is renal impairment and morphine is used, a reduced dose, or a longer lockout period, may be necessary, as morphine-6-glucuronide is an active metabolite of morphine excreted by the kidney. The addition of paracetamol and NSAIDs to the analgesic regimen reduces opioid requirement. NSAIDs may be used only if there are no contraindications, the remaining kidney is functioning well and the patient is well hydrated.

TESTICULAR TUMOURS

Orchidectomy may be undertaken through the scrotum or inguinal region. There are no special anaesthetic requirements for this surgery. Assessment of the patient determines if a regional technique, e.g. spinal anaesthetic, or a general anaesthetic is most suitable. In the case of general anaesthesia, the patient's condition determines if intubation and ventilation, laryngeal mask airway or face mask is required. In cases of advanced testicular cancer, dissection of the para-aortic nodes is undertaken; this is a major operation, and the same type of anaesthetic technique as that used for major pelvic surgery is suitable. Epidural analgesia is exceedingly useful for this surgery, which is very extensive.

CERVICAL TUMOURS

Many procedures are undertaken involving diathermy to the cervix. If there is no contraindication, general anaesthesia via a face mask or LMA is satisfactory. Postoperative pain is not usually a problem.

BLADDER TUMOURS

These are often removed repeatedly by diathermy or loop excision. Some destruction by laser may be car-

ried out without a general anaesthetic. Patients may attend regularly for general anaesthesia, as a day case, for several years. It is essential to carry out appropriate preoperative assessment each time, as these are frequently elderly individuals with declining general health. The lithotomy position is used. These procedures may be carried out with spinal anaesthesia. However, they are frequently rapid and unless there is a contraindication, general anaesthesia with a face mask or LMA is suitable. Occasionally, there is rapid blood loss, so a large-gauge cannula should be used. The bladder is irrigated continuously and this makes blood loss difficult to estimate. During diathermy, the obturator nerve is often directly stimulated; this leads to excessive jerking movements of the leg, surgery is made more difficult and there is a risk of perforation of the bladder. Paralysis and ventilation may therefore be required to prevent perforation. If the bladder is perforated, irrigating fluid is absorbed into the perivesical space and may cause TURP syndrome (see below).

There is often postoperative pain which may require opioid analgesia. Blood clots may block the catheter after surgery and cause pain from bladder distension. This may cause hypertension, restlessness and bradycardia.

SURGERY FOR RENAL TRACT STONES

Renal stones are frequently idiopathic but may be caused by hypercalciuria arising from sarcoidosis, malignancy, renal tubular acidosis, hyperparathyroidism, Cushing's syndrome or administration of adrenal corticosteroids. All these diseases may have anaesthetic implications and should be investigated at preoperative assessment. Patients with recurrent urinary tract infection related to bladder malfunction, e.g. neurological diseases or congenital abnormalities, form stones. This type of stone may be large and grow to become a staghorn calculus in the renal pelvis.

Many renal tract stones are removed by extracorporeal shock wave lithotripsy. This uses ultrasound to disintegrate the stone and the procedure may take 1 h or more. Patients are usually awake, experience pain and require analgesia. Occasionally, the procedure is not tolerated and general anaesthesia is required. Administering general anaesthesia in unfamiliar surroundings may be hazardous. The anaesthetist must insist on skilled assistance, adequate lighting and monitoring of arterial pressure, oxygen saturation, ECG and capnography.

PERCUTANEOUS LITHOTRIPSY

This procedure may be undertaken when extracorporeal shock wave lithotripsy has failed. Such patients include those with staghorn calculi and associated infection. The procedure takes place in the X-ray department – a hazardous area for the anaesthetist. It is unfamiliar, dark, often cramped, and it is essential for the anaesthetist to have a trained and experienced assistant. It is usually best to anaesthetize the patient on a trolley as X-ray tables may not tip head-down quickly.

Procedure

First of all, a balloon-tipped ureteric catheter is passed through a cystoscope. The balloon is dilated just below the kidney to enable distension of the renal pelvis. This also prevents stone fragments from passing into the ureter. The patient is then placed in the prone position, a nephrostomy track is created and a nephroscope is passed. The stone may then be removed with forceps or fragmented with an ultrasonic probe. Continuous flushing of the pelvis with normal saline clears fragments of stone, distends the renal pelvis, washes away blood and cools the ultrasonic probe. Normal saline is used to prevent hyponatraemia.

Possible problems

- *Fluid in retroperitoneal space*. This may occur if the renal pelvis is ruptured. Fluid input and collection should be monitored. If a deficit of more than 2 L occurs, the procedure may need to be terminated.
- *Sepsis*. Many patients have chronic urinary infection. Bacteria may be flushed into the venous system of the kidney if the pressure from the irrigation is too great. All patients should receive appropriate i.v. antibiotics, but signs of cardiovascular collapse may suggest Gram-negative septicaemia.
- *Cooling*. Heat loss may be a major problem; in addition to routine methods of maintaining normothermia, the irrigating fluid should be warm, and waterproof drapes applied.
- *Bleeding*. In addition to bleeding at the nephrostomy site, large vessels, spleen and liver may be punctured. A large retroperitoneal haematoma may collect which is difficult to diagnose. All bleeding is harder to detect in the environment of the X-ray department.
- *Pneumothorax*. This may occur whilst performing nephrostomy.
- *Electrical hazards*. Irrigating fluid may cause electrical equipment to 'short circuit'.

Anaesthetic technique

Regional anaesthesia

Epidural blockade should extend to reach the sixth thoracic level. The operation may last up to 3 h and therefore a catheter technique is required. Patients become very uncomfortable lying prone for this duration.

General anaesthesia

As the patient is prone, intubation of the trachea and ventilation of the lungs are necessary. Attention must be paid to positioning of the head, avoidance of pressure on the eyes, and padding of the limbs at vulnerable points. The choice of induction, neuromuscular blocking and maintenance agents is less important than good monitoring, particularly of heat loss.

Open pyelolithotomy and pyeloplasty

Pyelolithotomy is undertaken if all other methods of renal stone removal have failed. Pyeloplasty is a refashioning of the pelvi-ureteric junction to relieve obstruction. These procedures have the same anaesthetic implications as nephrectomy.

PENILE SURGERY

This includes circumcision, procedures for impotence and treatment of Peyronie's disease. Impotence often occurs in diabetic and other arteriopathic patients. It may be treated by insertion of various devices. Peyronie's disease is treated by inflating the penis with saline and reshaping it (Nesbitt's procedure). General anaesthesia and spinal or epidural anaesthesia may be used for all these procedures. A penile block is very useful for analgesia after surgery. A simple ring block with plain bupivacaine is effective.

ENDOSCOPIC SURGERY

TRANSURETHRAL RESECTION OF THE PROSTATE GLAND

Transurethral resection of the prostate gland (TURP) is a common operation, performed in the lithotomy position. Continuous irrigation with glycine is used to allow vision of the operative site. Glycine has reasonable optical properties, does not conduct electricity, but is hypotonic. Chippings are cut from the prostate gland with a wire loop. When enough tissue has been cut away, diathermy is used to stop any further bleeding. A catheter, usually a three-way irrigating type, is inserted after surgery.

Possible problems

Haemorrhage

This is difficult to quantify as blood is mixed with irrigation fluid. If available, estimation of the haematocrit by HemoCue, is very useful. Other suggestions for measuring blood loss include assaying the haemoglobin concentration of the collected irrigating fluid and, from the known volume, calculating the quantity of haemoglobin lost. In practice, methods such as the total weight of prostate chippings or resection time may be used to estimate blood loss More than 40–50 g of prostatic chippings should prompt review of blood requirements. Assiduous monitoring of heart rate and arterial pressure may help to identify bleeding, although this may be a late sign. The decision to transfuse is often made by assessment of the patient's clinical condition.

TURP syndrome

This is a complex syndrome which may encompass hypo-osmolality, hyponatraemia, hyperglycinaemia, hyperammonaemia and intravascular fluid shifts. These changes are caused by absorption of irrigating fluid through open prostatic veins, and later by its absorption from pooled irrigation fluid in the retroperitoneal and perivesical spaces. Hyperammonaemia is caused by metabolism of absorbed glycine, and glycine itself can be toxic.

Massive haemolysis may occur from hypo-osmolality. Haemoglobinaemia from haemolysis, in combination with hypotension, may lead to acute renal failure.

Symptoms of TURP syndrome include hyper- or hypotension and pulmonary oedema. Confusion, bradycardia, convulsions and visual disturbance (all symptoms of cerebral oedema) may occur from as early as 15 min into the resection up to 12 h after operation. The incidence of this syndrome may be decreased by maintaining the height difference between the bladder and the bag of irrigating fluid at 80 cm or less, to decrease intravesical pressure. Continuous irrigating resectoscopes also result in lower intravesical pressure. Restricting the resection time to 1 h decreases the incidence of TURP syndrome. Surgery must be abandoned as soon as possible if TURP syndrome is suspected.

Various methods may be used to estimate fluid absorption. Addition of ethanol to the irrigating fluid followed by measurement of alcohol in expired gas gives an indication of the quantity of fluid absorbed.

Measurements of serum sodium concentration or osmolality are also good guides.

Treatment depends on careful assessment and consists of mannitol, hypertonic saline or loop diuretics. Mannitol does not cause as great a loss of sodium through renal excretion as loop diuretics. Supportive management, including ventilation, is often required until electrolyte abnormalities are corrected.

Sepsis

There is a risk of septicaemia in those patients with urinary tract infection, stones in the bladder or an indwelling catheter. Patients with septicaemia should receive intravenous antibiotics, as should any patient with a joint prosthesis or valvular heart disease.

Anaesthetic technique

Transurethral resection of the prostate gland is frequently performed in very elderly patients. These patients have a high incidence of concomitant disease, especially of the respiratory tract and cardiovascular system.

Spinal anaesthesia is useful particularly for patients with significant respiratory disease, although coughing during the procedure may render surgery difficult. An additional advantage of spinal anaesthesia is postoperative analgesia. Frequently, the worst discomfort has settled by the time spinal anaesthesia has regressed.

One of the main concerns with spinal anaesthesia is hypotension caused by sympathetic blockade, as blood loss may result in precipitate decreases in arterial pressure because of lack of compensatory vasoconstriction. There is often additional hypotension when the legs are lowered at the end of surgery. Reductions in arterial pressure may be treated by fluid or vasoconstrictors. Spinal anaesthesia has traditionally not been used for patients with ischaemic heart disease. However, the incidence of silent myocardial ischaemia is the same whether general anaesthesia or spinal anaesthesia is used and appears to be related to the severity of pre-existing cardiac disease. There is some evidence that the increase in cardiac pre- and afterload when the spinal anaesthetic regresses may induce ischaemia.

A dose of heavy bupivacaine 0.5%, sufficient to produce a block to the eighth thoracic nerve, is needed; this is generally about 2.7–3 mL. Post-dural puncture headache is less common in elderly men than in other groups of patients. The incidence is least with the use of pencil-point needles. The choice between spinal and general anaesthesia depends on the patient's preoperative condition and the preferences of both the patient and the anaesthetist. The usual absolute contraindications to spinal analgesia (anticoagulants, clotting disorders and local sepsis) apply. Any method of general anaesthesia is suitable, depending on the patient's medical condition. A caudal injection of local anaesthetic may be useful for postoperative pain relief.

Careful monitoring of arterial pressure and drainage from the catheter is necessary after surgery and the possibility of TURP syndrome should be borne in mind for 12 h or so, especially if the resection was prolonged.

HOLMIUM LASER DESTRUCTION OF THE PROSTATE

This is a much less invasive operation than TURP. Blood loss is minimal, there is no need for postoperative irrigation, postoperative pain is decreased and the patient requires a urinary catheter for a shorter duration, leading to earlier discharge from hospital. Saline is used intraoperatively for irrigation, as diathermy is not required. Therefore, TURP syndrome is avoided. The disadvantage is a considerably increased theatre time.

TREATMENT OF MENORRHAGIA

Various methods of endometrial ablation may be used, including thermal and microwave techniques. Some of these procedures may be performed with local anaesthesia. If this is not possible, a regional or general anaesthetic technique is suitable. Postoperative pain may be managed with paracetamol, NSAIDs and/or opioid drugs as required. Prophylactic antiemetics are advisable.

INCONTINENCE SURGERY

PROCEDURES FOR THE IRRITABLE BLADDER

Helmstein's procedure

An expandable bag is placed in the bladder at cystoscopy and filled to a pressure just below mean arterial pressure for 6 h with the aim of increasing bladder capacity. The distension is very painful and an epidural infusion of bupivacaine and an opioid is used.

Clam cystoplasty

In this procedure, a segment of small bowel is resected, opened out and used to create a 'patch' in the bladder. The interruption of the bladder by the bowel patch stops transmission of irritable contractions and avoids premature voiding. Muscle relaxation, tracheal

intubation and IPPV are required. The choice of anaesthetic drugs depends on the patient's general health. Postoperative pain may be treated with an epidural or PCA. There is often postoperative ileus, which may be made worse by opioids.

PROCEDURES FOR STRESS INCONTINENCE

Tension-free vaginal tape

This is a technique used increasingly to treat stress incontinence. Two curved needles, joined by a strip of 'tape', are passed through the vaginal vault and out on to the skin of the abdomen, one on each side. The needles are removed and the tape is held at the skin. The tape passes round the bladder neck between the two attachments. It is tightened at the abdominal skin until it is just tight enough to prevent leakage of urine. This procedure may be undertaken with local, epidural/spinal or general anaesthesia. Occasionally, the patient is required to be awake, and able to cough, in order to assess the correct tension. In this case local anaesthesia, administered by the surgeon, is the best choice, supplemented by sedation if necessary. If infiltration is used, a large volume (100 mL) is required, so care must be taken to avoid toxic doses.

Burch colposuspension

This is performed through a Pfannenstiel incision. If there are no contraindications, e.g. obesity, respiratory disease, a spontaneously breathing technique can be used. Spinal or epidural analgesia is equally suitable. Some surgeons perform these operations laparoscopically, as this results in less pain and earlier mobility. If a laparoscopic technique is used, it is sensible to intubate the trachea and ventilate the lungs. If surgery is of the open type, postoperative analgesia with opioid drugs is needed.

Prolapse and pelvic floor repair

These procedures may be undertaken using spinal/epidural or general anaesthesia or a combination of both. In some units, the simpler procedures are performed in healthy patients as day cases.

HYSTERECTOMY

This may be performed abdominally or vaginally. It is essential to check for anaemia. Both of these operations may be performed with spinal or epidural anaesthesia, which decreases blood loss. For abdominal hysterectomy, the spinal or epidural should be combined with a general anaesthetic, as insertion of packs to retract the bowels is very unpleasant. Vaginal hysterectomy is performed in the lithotomy position, and if patients have epidural or spinal anaesthesia, they may be awake, or sedated. A spontaneously breathing general anaesthetic technique is an alternative if the patient does not wish to be awake, and there are no indications for tracheal intubation.

Without regional analgesia, opioid analgesia is required intraoperatively. There is a high incidence of postoperative nausea and vomiting, so prophylactic antiemetics should be given. Postoperative analgesia may be provided by an epidural or opioid drugs via PCA or a subcutaneous cannula, with paracetamol and NSAIDs as supplements. Intrathecal opioid drugs administered with the local anaesthetic during spinal anaesthesia provide some analgesia for 24 hours. The patient should be monitored as if they were using PCA, as there may be late respiratory depression.

SUCTION VAGINAL TERMINATION OF PREGNANCY

This is undertaken between 7 and 15 weeks of gestation. The operation is performed in the lithotomy position. All volatile agents cause relaxation of the uterus, so many anaesthetists use an infusion or intermittent boluses of propofol, supplemented with fentanyl or alfentanil. Other anaesthetists use 0.5 of the minimum alveolar concentration (MAC) of a volatile agent with nitrous oxide. Dilatation of the cervix is very stimulating and if the patient is not anaesthetized adequately, laryngospasm may occur. Alfentanil is useful to prevent this response, as high concentrations of volatile agent are not advisable.

Syntocinon (oxytocin) may be given to encourage contraction of the uterus and this may cause a transient decrease in arterial pressure. There is little postoperative pain. The procedure is usually performed as a day case and paracetamol or an NSAID is suitable for analgesia at home.

GYNAECOLOGICAL AND UROLOGICAL EMERGENCIES

UROLOGICAL

There are not many true urological emergencies: torsion of the testis is the most important. The anaesthetic requirements for this procedure are dictated by the general health of the patient.

GYNAECOLOGICAL

Ectopic pregnancy

If there is not extensive bleeding, a laparoscopic procedure provides a better long-term outcome. The anaesthetic implications of laparoscopy are described earlier in this chapter. A rapid-sequence induction may be required if the patient has a full stomach. If the ectopic pregnancy is bleeding, an open operation is performed. The degree of hypovolaemia should be assessed carefully before surgery. It is essential to resuscitate the patient fully during preparation for surgery. Great care is needed at induction to avoid a precipitate decrease in arterial pressure. If there is excessive bleeding, a clotting screen should be performed and any deficiencies corrected. Postoperative analgesia with PCA and supplementary analgesics is required. Epidural analgesia is not used as the patient is usually hypovolaemic and may develop deranged clotting.

Evacuation of retained products of conception

This is an extremely common emergency procedure, which is usually very brief (5–10 min). However brief and simple the procedure anaesthetically, the patient is often very distressed and the procedure should not be cancelled repeatedly to make way for greater emergencies as this adds to the patient's distress. Surgery is performed in the lithotomy position. Occasionally, there is excessive bleeding, necessitating immediate surgery. Often the operation may be performed at a time when the patient has an empty stomach, thus avoiding tracheal intubation.

Because volatile anaesthetic agents may cause some degree of uterine relaxation, many anaesthetists use an infusion or intermittent boluses of propofol, supplemented with alfentanil or fentanyl. Syntocinon (oxytocin) is often required. The cervix is often already open, so that dilatation is not always necessary. Postoperative pain may be managed with oral analgesics.

FURTHER READING

Alexander J I 1997 Pain after laparoscopy. British Journal of Anaesthesia 79: 369–378

Brichant J F 1995 Anaesthesia for minimally invasive abdominal surgery. In: Adams A P, Cashman J N (eds) Recent advances in anaesthesia and analgesia, 19. Churchill Livingstone, Edinburgh, Ch. 3

Edwards N D, Callaghan L C, White T, Reilly C S 1995 Perioperative myocardial ischaemia in patients undergoing transurethral surgery: a pilot study comparing general with spinal anaesthesia. British Journal of Anaesthesia 74: 368–372

Gravenstein D 1997 Transurethral resection of the prostate (TURP) syndrome: a review of the pathophysiology and management. Anesthesia and Analgesia 84: 438–446

Naef M M, Mitchell A 1994 Anaesthesia for laparoscopy. In: Kaufman L, Ginsburg R (eds) Anaesthesia review, 11. Churchill Livingstone, Edinburgh, Ch. 3

Windsor A, French G W G, Sear JW et al 1996 Silent myocardial ischaemia in patients undergoing transurethral prostatectomy. A study to evaluate risk scoring and anaesthetic technique with outcome. Anaesthesia 51: 728–732

Wong D H, Hagar J M, Mootz J et al 1996 Incidence of perioperative myocardial ischaemia in TURP patients. Journal of Clinical Anesthesia 8: 627–630

Anaesthesia for orthopaedic surgery 30

One in five operations in the United Kingdom is for orthopaedic, spinal or trauma surgery. Anaesthesia for trauma surgery is discussed in Chapter 28. This chapter provides a framework for the conduct of anaesthesia for orthopaedic surgery.

THE PATIENT POPULATION

A large proportion of patients presenting for orthopaedic surgery are young and healthy. Sporting injuries and disease processes without systemic impact are common, and these patients are at low risk of complications relating to anaesthesia or surgery. However, several disease processes are more common in patients presenting for orthopaedic surgery than in the general surgical population, and these are discussed below.

COMORBIDITIES

Rheumatoid arthritis

Rheumatoid arthritis is a chronic inflammatory disease of unknown aetiology, affecting women more often than men. Rheumatoid factor is found in 90% of affected patients, and there exists a genetic predisposition with associated human leucocyte antigen HLA-DR4. It is a multisystem disease that may present the anaesthetist with problems of a difficult airway, cervical spine instability (and cervical cord vulnerability) and widespread vasculitis-induced organ dysfunction. Additionally, drug therapy for rheumatoid disease frequently produces severe and widespread side-effects. These are detailed below (see Concurrent drug therapy). The airway of the rheumatoid patient may present problems because of stiffness of the temporomandibular joint, stiffness or instability of the neck and cricoarytenoid arthritis. Radiological examination shows involvement of the cervical spine in 80% of patients, and 30% have neurological symptoms suggesting instability of the neck. Atlantoaxial subluxation, subaxial subluxation and cervical spine ankylosis are common, and should be investigated through history-taking, clinical examination and cervical X-ray. Flexion-extension views may be necessary to observe instability. Magnetic resonance imaging provides good assessment of the rheumatoid neck. Systemic disease is very common, and includes pericardial effusion, constrictive pericarditis, heart block, aortic and mitral valve disease, pleural effusion, interstitial fibrosis, anaemia, thrombocytopenia and renal and hepatic dysfunction.

A thorough history and examination are important for patients with rheumatoid disease. Careful assessment of the airway and cervical spine should be performed. The range of neck movement should be assessed, and any associated neurological symptoms should be noted. In all patients, a full blood count and serum urea and electrolyte concentrations should be measured, and an ECG and chest X-ray are required. Additionally, all patients should have a lateral cervical X-ray, preferably with flexion-extension views. Systemic disease may require arterial blood gas analysis, lung function tests, echocardiogram or liver function tests to be undertaken. Suspicion of cricoarytenoid involvement should prompt preoperative indirect laryngoscopic examination.

Regional anaesthesia should be used if possible. It has the advantage of avoiding airway and neck manipulation, and may be safer than general anaesthesia in patients with severe systemic disease. However, epidural and spinal anaesthesia may be very difficult because of spinal ankylosis and osteophytes. If general anaesthesia is used, patients with an unstable neck should be managed by an experienced anaesthetist, especially if tracheal intubation is planned. Tracheal intubation is even more difficult if movement of the temporomandibular joint is restricted. The need for tracheal intubation should be considered carefully in patients with severe disease because of the associated risks and difficulty. For many procedures, the use of a laryngeal mask airway is a suitable and potentially less traumatic alternative. If tracheal intubation is required, intubation aids such as the intu-

563

bating laryngeal mask airway or fibreoptic-guided intubation may be safer alternatives to tracheal intubation using direct laryngoscopy.

Osteoarthritis

A reduced range of joint movement may present problems in positioning, airway management, regional blockade and vascular access. Concurrent analgesic therapy may cause increased bleeding and renal dysfunction (non-steroidal anti-inflammatory drugs) or tolerance to opioid analgesia (opioids).

Ankylosing spondylitis

Ankylosing spondylitis causes rigidity of the entire spinal column, and may present problems with tracheal intubation. Unlike rheumatoid arthritis, cervical spine instability does not occur, but the fixed flexion deformity may render direct laryngoscopy utterly impossible. The use of the laryngeal mask airway is a suitable option for many procedures, and fibreoptic laryngoscopy is usually fairly straightforward in these patients. The normal routes of escape of local anaesthetic solution from the epidural space may be obstructed in patients with ankylosing spondylitis, and spinal cord ischaemia with permanent nerve damage has been reported after rapid injection of local anaesthetic into the epidural space in patients suffering from this condition.

CONCURRENT DRUG THERAPY

Many young healthy patients presenting for orthopaedic surgery do not take concurrent medication. However, use of analgesics is very common in the orthopaedic population because of the painful nature of their disease process. Concurrent therapy with antihypertensive, antianginal, antidepressant or cholesterol-lowering medication is common in older patients presenting for orthopaedic surgery. These patients often present for arthroplasty, and this major procedure may place significant demands upon their physiological reserves. Preparation of the patient taking these drugs is discussed in detail in Chapter 15. Patients may also be using orthopaedic disease-modifying drugs such as methotrexate, steroids and gold.

Non-steroidal anti-inflammatory drugs

Thromboxane A_2 and prostaglandin endoperoxide, which are needed for the haemostatic function of platelets, are synthesized from arachidonic acid by the cyclo-oxygenase (COX) enzyme system. Non-steroidal anti-inflammatory drugs (NSAIDs) inhibit this enzyme system, impairing the formation of clots and, consequently, haemostasis. There are two COX isoforms: COX-1 synthesizes prostaglandins, which protect the gastric mucosa; COX-2 is involved with inflammatory responses. Inhibition of these systems ceases rapidly when administration of NSAIDs is stopped. However, the effects of aspirin persist for up to 10 days after treatment because of its covalent bonding with cyclo-oxygenase. Although NSAIDs taken up to the time of surgery may increase surgical blood loss, this does not imply that preoperative administration should be avoided. NSAIDs are valuable in providing analgesia pre- and postoperatively, and increased surgical blood loss is usually modest. Of more concern is gastroduodenal ulceration, of which the first symptom may be life-threatening upper gastrointestinal haemorrhage. The risk of ulceration is dose-related, commoner as age advances and even commoner if corticosteroids are also used to control inflammation. NSAIDs should be avoided in patients who have a history suggestive of gastrointestinal ulceration or bleeding.

Opioid analgesics

Chronic opioid use results in tolerance to the analgesic effects of the drugs and to their undesirable side-effects. When patients have used opioids for more than a few days before surgery, postoperative administration of an opioid is less effective than normal, and a larger dose is required than would be expected in the opioid-naive patient. A useful guide is to provide the regular intake of opioid *in addition* to that prescribed for acute, postoperative pain relief. It is mandatory that frequent observations are made of these patients, and the involvement of an acute pain team is advisable.

Corticosteroids

Regular medication with glucocorticoid drugs (e.g. prednisolone, hydrocortisone, dexamethasone, steroid inhalers) produces suppression of endogenous glucocorticoid production. There is an increase in glucocorticoid concentration as part of the stress response after surgery, and these patients are at risk of an Addisonian crisis because they may not be able to synthesize sufficient endogenous glucocorticoid. Patients who have taken doses of steroids greater than the equivalent of prednisolone 10 mg daily during the past 3 months require replacement corticosteroid therapy. Corticosteroid therapy may cause poor wound healing and gastrointestinal ulceration; consequently, low-dose replacement therapy is currently favoured. Typically, a single, intraoperative, intravenous dose of hydrocortisone 100 mg is given, and further doses of 25 mg are administered four times daily until the patient's usual corticosteroid regimen is re-established.

Immunosuppressant drugs

Drugs such as methotrexate inhibit the immune system, damping the inflammatory response that causes distressing symptoms from some joint diseases. The induced immunosuppression may also render the patient at increased risk of hospital-acquired infection, and strict aseptic techniques should be used during any invasive procedures.

Other drugs

A large variety of potentially toxic drugs are used to reduce the symptoms and retard the disease process in rheumatoid arthritis. Antimalarials, such as chloroquine, may cause retinopathy and cardiomyopathy. Gold and penicillamine cause undesirable side-effects in up to 40% of patients; these include nephrotic syndrome, thrombocytopenia, agranulocytosis, marrow aplasia, hepatitis and pneumonitis. Sulfasalazine may cause haematological toxicity and fibrosing alveolitis. Administration of azathioprine may result in gastrointestinal side-effects, cholestatic hepatitis, leucopenia, thrombocytopenia and anaemia.

It should be apparent that the provision of anaesthesia for any patient with rheumatoid arthritis must be associated with a thorough search for the potentially dangerous side-effects of concurrent drug therapy.

TECHNIQUES OF ANAESTHESIA

GENERAL ANAESTHESIA

This is appropriate for all types of orthopaedic surgery, but regional anaesthesia may be the preferred technique for many procedures, for reasons discussed below. Patients undergoing procedures of long duration (e.g. hip revision) often require general anaesthesia because of the discomfort incurred by remaining in the same position for a prolonged period. In many countries, including the United Kingdom, patients usually expect to receive general anaesthesia, and may not have been aware in advance of their surgery that regional anaesthesia represents a viable option. Thus, the use of general anaesthesia offers the benefit to patients of familiarity. General anaesthesia causes the greatest loss of control for the patient and many patients are pleasantly surprised to find that regional anaesthesia is an option for their operation.

REGIONAL ANAESTHESIA

Central neuraxial block (spinal or epidural anaesthesia) reduces the stress response to surgery and has been shown to reduce some serious complications following many types of surgery. There is a reduction in the incidences of deep vein thrombosis, blood loss, myocardial infarction, respiratory and renal complications and possibly pulmonary embolism. There is a high incidence of thromboembolic events in patients undergoing major lower limb arthroplasty, which makes this type of anaesthesia an attractive option.

Lower limb arthroplasty and minor lower limb procedures are frequently carried out using central neuraxial block. For longer procedures, such as hip arthroplasty, sedation or light general anaesthesia may be added. The combination of general anaesthesia with a central neuraxial block has not been shown to reduce the benefits attributable to this form of regional anaesthesia.

Following central neuraxial block, the patient is usually pain-free in the immediate postoperative period. Careful thought should be given to administration of analgesia after the nerve block has worn off (see below). There is a higher incidence of urinary retention in patients who have undergone joint arthroplasty under central neuraxial block, and this leads to an increased risk of urinary tract infection. Patients may be managed by prophylactic urethral catheterization, or monitoring of bladder volume postoperatively using ultrasound.

Peripheral nerve block is commonly used as a sole technique for many procedures, with the advantages of excellent pain relief, reduction of surgical stress, avoidance of complications of general anaesthesia and earlier discharge in the day-case setting. Peripheral surgery in 'high-risk' patients may also be carried out under peripheral nerve block to avoid the potential complications of general anaesthesia or central neuraxial block. Patients report a high degree of satisfaction following surgery carried out using this form of anaesthesia. Table 30.1 shows the sites at which surgery may be performed in association with specific nerve blocks. This form of anaesthesia requires a high level of expertise and an understanding of the issues of managing a conscious patient during surgery.

Intravenous regional anaesthesia (IVRA) is suitable for manipulation of fractures and brief operations (less than 30 min) on the forearm and lower leg. It is technically easy to perform, but fatalities have occurred as a result of a large dose of local anaesthetic reaching the systemic circulation. Before performing IVRA, it is essential to understand how the risk of complications may be minimized and how they may be treated if

Table 30.1 Peripheral regional anaesthesia and analgesia

Site of surgery	Block
Shoulder	Interscalene brachial plexus
Upper arm	Interscalene or supraclavicular brachial plexus plus intercostobrachial and medial cutaneous nerve of the arm
Forearm and hand	Infraclavicular or axillary brachial plexus, IVRA, elbow or wrist
Fingers	Metacarpal or digital nerve
Hip	Posterior lumbar plexus (psoas compartment), 3-in-1 femoral sheath, proximal sciatic nerve
Knee	Femoral and proximal sciatic nerve
Ankle	Sciatic (popliteal fossa) ± saphenous nerve or IVRA
Foot	Sciatic (popliteal fossa) ± saphenous nerve or ankle or IVRA
Toes	Ankle, metatarsal or digital nerve

IVRA, intravenous regional anaesthesia.

they occur. Details of the technique and safety precautions are described in Chapter 17.

POSTOPERATIVE ANALGESIA

ORAL AND INTRAVENOUS AGENTS

Many patients are already taking regular analgesics for pre-existing bone and joint pain. Paracetamol is very useful in reducing the dose requirements of other analgesics, and may occasionally be sufficient analgesia alone. It is virtually free from side-effects in standard doses, and is contraindicated only in patients with liver dysfunction. If gastric motility is impaired, it may be administered rectally. The addition of NSAIDs, if there are no contraindications, is usually indicated and these reduce the requirement for opioid analgesia.

NSAIDs inhibit the formation of prostaglandins and are widely used as analgesics in the treatment of acute bone-related pain. The newer COX-2 inhibitors widen the number of patients who can benefit from these agents by reducing the potential for gastroduodenal ulceration, although there have been recent concerns about increased incidences of myocardial infarction and stroke in patients taking long-term COX-2 inhibitors, leading to the withdrawal of rofecoxib in September 2004.

Prostaglandins are known to have an important role in bone repair and homeostasis. Animal studies have demonstrated that both non-specific and specific inhibitors of COX impair fracture healing. Some studies have suggested that this impairment results from COX-2 inhibition. This has raised concerns regarding the use of NSAIDs as anti-inflammatory or analgesic drugs in patients undergoing orthopaedic procedures; however, the clinical implications of this are probably minimal and NSAIDs remain extremely important analgesic agents for orthopaedic patients.

NSAIDs also affect platelet function and would therefore be expected to increase perioperative blood loss. The clinical evidence for increased blood loss in major arthroplasty surgery patients receiving NSAIDs is minimal.

Intravenous opioids are frequently used following major joint arthroplasty. Patient-controlled analgesia systems are the most commonly used delivery systems. The doses of opioid required are much reduced by the other analgesic agents prescribed, thus minimizing the risk of side-effects.

CENTRAL NEURAXIAL DRUGS

Single-dose spinal or epidural anaesthesia using local anaesthetic alone usually provides analgesia for only a relatively short period of time after operation. An adjuvant administered into the intrathecal or epidural space with the local anaesthetic improves the quality of the block and extends the duration of analgesia. Table 30.2 describes some of the more commonly administered drugs. Rarely used agents include midazolam and neostigmine.

An epidural (or, rarely, intrathecal) infusion of local anaesthetics may be combined with an opioid to produce excellent analgesia. The combination of local anaesthetic and opioid is synergistic, reducing the side-effects of both and minimizing motor block. However, relatively high incidences of itching, nausea and urinary retention are encountered. It is routine practice in most hospitals to insert a urethral catheter in the anaesthetic room to avoid urinary retention in the postoperative period.

Epidural infusions are commonly used for up to 5 days following surgery. Careful observation for signs of inadequate analgesia (often a result of catheter migration) and infection is required. The involvement

Table 30.2   Central neuraxial block adjuvants

Drug	Action	Duration	Side-effects
Morphine	Opioid receptor agonist	Long	Itching, nausea, urinary retention, respiratory depression
Diamorphine	Opioid receptor agonist	Medium	Itching, nausea, urinary retention, respiratory depression
Fentanyl	Opioid receptor agonist	Short	Itching, nausea, urinary retention, respiratory depression
Clonidine	α_2-adrenoceptor agonist	Extends block duration	Sedation, hypotension, respiratory depression
Ketamine	*N*-methyl D-aspartate receptor antagonist	Long	Dysphoria, sedation, possible intrathecal toxicity
Epinephrine	Adrenoceptor agonist	Extends block duration	Systemic sympathetic activation (tachycardia, hypertension), myocardial ischaemia

of an acute pain team is very useful in this regard. Many units manage these patients in an extended recovery or high-dependency setting to increase the level of nursing care and to facilitate early detection and prompt management of complications.

PERIPHERAL NERVE BLOCKS

Peripheral nerve block, with or without a central neuraxial block or general anaesthesia, often provides excellent pain relief for a number of hours postoperatively, allowing transition to oral or intravenous analgesia when required. The use of continuous 3-in-1 (femoral sheath) nerve block after knee replacement surgery results in better pain relief, faster postoperative rehabilitation and earlier discharge from hospital than opioid analgesia alone. Posterior lumbar plexus block (psoas compartment) or 3-in-1 femoral sheath block combined with proximal sciatic nerve block (e.g. Labat's approach) can be used for hip surgery, although it is difficult to obtain analgesia of the entire surgical area with peripheral blocks alone.

Single-dose peripheral nerve blocks using a long-acting local anaesthetic such as levobupivacaine may last for over 16 h. Additives such as clonidine may be used to prolong the duration of single-dose blocks, although few additives have been shown clearly to be effective in this regard. Alternatively, a catheter may be inserted, allowing an infusion of a low concentration of a local anaesthetic drug (e.g. 0.2% ropivacaine) to allow selective return of motor power.

Nerve injury due to peripheral nerve block is rare (see Ch. 19); it occurs in 1:5000 to 1:10 000 blocks performed. However, the incidence of nerve injury secondary to orthopaedic surgery is more frequent and often occurs in the sensory distribution of the nerve block. This reduces the popularity of peripheral nerve blocks in some institutions lest the block is blamed for nerve damage.

SURGICAL CONSIDERATIONS

POSITIONING

Patients with arthritis frequently have restricted mobility of joints. Positioning at the extremes of the range of movement of diseased joints may cause severe postoperative pain in addition to the pain resulting from the operation. Consequently, a patient's ability to assume the position required for operation must be assessed carefully; it is often useful to ask the patient to adopt that position before induction of anaesthesia if there is concern that mobility of joints may be an issue. Orthopaedic surgery often requires the use of unusual positions, some of which carry risks of nerve damage, soft tissue ischaemia, electrical and thermal injury and joint pain. Care must be taken in protecting areas at risk of injury. These include bony promontories, sites of poor tissue viability and locations where nerves run close to the skin or close to the surface of a bone.

Forceful movement of the patient by the surgeon is often inevitable during orthopaedic surgery. When such movement occurs, it is advisable to re-check the patient's position, ensuring that soft tissues, nerves, eyes and venous access are safe. Although some procedures may be performed under regional anaesthesia alone, long operations may result in discomfort related to posture, and when the block wears off there may be significant discomfort if positioning has been poor during the procedure.

Some positions adopted during orthopaedic surgery are associated with venous air embolism. These postures include the lateral position for hip surgery, the sitting position for shoulder surgery and the prone position for spinal surgery. Monitoring for, and treatment of, air embolism are discussed in detail in Chapter 19.

PROPHYLAXIS AGAINST INFECTION

Prophylactic intravenous antibiotics are used very frequently during orthopaedic surgery. Infection of bone is particularly threatening to the patient and is very difficult to eradicate; consequently, prevention has a high priority. Allergic reactions to antibiotics are not infrequent, and facilities must be available to treat such a reaction when intravenous antibiotics are used.

Laminar flow is used commonly in orthopaedic theatres to provide a constant flow of microscopically filtered air over the surgical field, and to minimize the risk of wound infection by environmental pathogens. This high flow of air over the patient's body surface greatly speeds convective heat loss, and precautions should be taken to avoid hypothermia.

Various in-theatre rituals exist for the prevention of cross-infection. These include the wearing of face masks and hats. Evidence supporting their use is scant.

PROPHYLAXIS AGAINST HYPOTHERMIA

Following induction of general or regional anaesthesia, heat is redistributed from the core to the peripheries. Following induction of general anaesthesia, there is typically a reduction in core temperature of 1°C in the first 30 min of anaesthesia. Core temperature reduces more slowly after this initial redistribution phase, typically by approximately 0.5°C per hour, although the rate of fall is heavily dependent upon ambient temperature, exposure and insulation, and the use of warming devices (see Ch. 20).

Hypothermia is known to be associated with increased blood loss, because of the narrow temperature range in which enzyme-dependent systems work, and perhaps because of platelet sequestration in the spleen. Hypothermia is also associated with poor postoperative wound healing and postoperative hypoxaemia.

The most effective method of reducing heat loss is forced air warming. However, warmed intravenous and surgical irrigation fluids and impermeable surgical drapes to reduce heat loss by evaporation are also useful.

PROPHYLAXIS AGAINST THROMBOEMBOLISM

Deep venous thrombosis (DVT) may complicate any surgery, but is associated particularly with surgery involving the pelvis, hip and knee. Pulmonary embolism (PE) may be fatal and accounts for 50% of all deaths after surgery for hip replacement. Although an infusion of dextran has been shown to reduce the incidence of PE after surgery, there is a relatively high risk of anaphylaxis associated with its administration, and low-dose heparin regimens have become the norm. There is evidence that heparin reduces the incidence of fatal PE in high-risk groups, including patients who undergo surgery on the pelvis, hip or knee. Compared with unfractionated heparins (UFH), low molecular weight heparins (LMWH) inhibit the coagulation enzyme Xa and bind antithrombin-3 to a similar extent, but bind less to thrombin. The use of LMWH might be expected to result in less surgical bleeding than when UFH is used. LMWH probably protects better against DVT after hip replacement, but the evidence for better prophylaxis against PE is less firm. The simplicity of once-daily administration of LMWH is an added advantage compared with UFH.

Dehydration and immobility increase the risk of the development of postoperative DVT. Consequently, adequate hydration and encouragement of early postoperative mobilization are advisable. Good analgesia improves mobilization, and regional anaesthesia may be particularly helpful in this regard.

Epidural anaesthesia reduces fibrinolysis and activation of clotting factors, reduces the risk of DVT and may reduce the risk of PE. These advantages, and the very small risk of epidural haematoma in patients who have received heparin, must be considered in an overall risk–benefit assessment of the use of epidural anaesthesia or analgesia during and after surgery. Current practice is to wait at least 12 h after the administration of LMWH before insertion of an epidural catheter. A similar interval should be used between administration of LMWH and removal of the epidural catheter.

Correctly applied graduated stockings and intermittent calf compression devices reduce the incidence of DVT, but there may be no extra benefit for patients who receive heparin.

ARTERIAL TOURNIQUETS

Effective exsanguination of a limb and application of an arterial tourniquet greatly improve the visibility of the surgical field, as well as minimizing surgical blood loss. Exsanguination may be performed by elevation of the limb or by wrapping it in a rubber bandage. The tourniquet cuff should be 20% wider than the diameter of the limb; this correlates to approximately one-third of the circumference of the limb. To avoid damage by shearing and compression of skin, nerves and other tissues, the tourniquet should be lined with padding and applied over muscle bulk. To avoid injury from chemical burns, entry of spirit cleansing lotions under the cuff must be prevented. This is achieved usually by wrapping adhesive tape round the distal edge of the tourniquet and the adjacent skin.

The pressure in the arterial tourniquet should, in all cases, exceed arterial pressure, but, for reasons explained below, pressures are required that significantly exceed arterial pressure if arterial ooze is to be prevented. For the lower limb, this pressure is typically 300 mmHg (or 150 mmHg above systolic arterial pressure) and for the upper limb, 250 mmHg (or 100 mmHg above systolic arterial pressure). These rather wide margins are used for two reasons:

- First, the pressure on the measuring gauge is not the same as the effective tourniquet pressure; the narrower the cuff, the greater is the difference.
- Second, blood pressure commonly increases about 30 min after the tourniquet is inflated. This is not caused by the autotransfusion during exsanguination or by the increased systemic vascular resistance caused by tourniquet inflation, but results probably from activation of C-fibres by ischaemia (mediating 'slow' pain). This pain may be difficult to relieve, and patients whose operation is conducted under regional anaesthesia may find the pain intolerable, and may require general anaesthesia. Some temporary tolerance may be achieved by administration of a short-acting opioid (e.g. alfentanil 250 µg), inhaled nitrous oxide or intravenous ketamine (e.g. 0.2 mg kg^{-1}). Dense regional anaesthesia, whether spinal, epidural or nerve block, may prevent tourniquet pain. However, despite an apparently adequate block, occasions may arise where the patient becomes intolerant of the tourniquet after some time. The noxious stimulation of tourniquet pain is even apparent during general anaesthesia, when the arterial pressure often increases progressively until the tourniquet is deflated.

Electromyographic and histological changes which follow prolonged application of a tourniquet reverse after deflation. The maximum period of safe ischaemia is not known precisely. Lasting damage is unlikely if a tourniquet time of 90–120 min is not exceeded. Current practice is that 2 h represents the absolute upper limit of tourniquet inflation time. Brief deflation followed by re-inflation of a tourniquet that has been in place for 2 h is not adequate 'rest' for the limb; several hours are required for restoration of metabolic normality within the limb.

When the tourniquet is deflated, the products of anaerobic metabolism in the limb are released. A bolus of cold, acidaemic, hypercapnic and hypoxaemic blood is returned to the circulation. The systemic vascular resistance suddenly decreases, and venous volume increases. This may result in transient cardiovascular changes, including cardiac arrhythmias, myocardial ischaemia and changes in arterial pressure. There may also be an increase in intracranial pressure (which is of importance in patients with reduced intracranial compliance, e.g. as a result of recent head injury). Bleeding may also occur at the operative site. Tourniquets on more than one limb should never be deflated (or inflated) simultaneously.

Tourniquets may cause damage to peripheral tissues, to the tissue underlying the cuff and to the patient as a whole due to the release of altered blood once the tourniquet is deflated. They are contraindicated to differing degrees in patients with poor peripheral circulation, crush injuries, infection and sickle cell disease or trait. The use of a tourniquet in a patient with sickle cell disease may result in within-limb sickling and subsequent ischaemia or thrombosis.

BLOOD CONSERVATION

An arterial tourniquet is used during a large proportion of orthopaedic operations. Consequently, intraoperative blood loss is often slight. However, tourniquets cannot be used for some procedures, such as hip arthroplasty and shoulder surgery, which may result in significant blood loss. Spinal surgery, in particular, is frequently associated with very extensive blood loss; bleeding from epidural veins is often responsible, and the techniques of blood conservation described below have made possible several spinal surgical procedures which were previously too dangerous to contemplate. Transfusion of donated blood carries significant risks, including cross-infection, hypothermia, clotting dysfunction, electrolyte disturbances, mismatched transfusion and allergic reactions. Donor blood is also a very expensive and rapidly dwindling resource. For these reasons, it is considered appropriate to avoid blood transfusion where possible. Various techniques are in popular use.

Avoidance of red cell loss

The use of a tourniquet significantly reduces blood loss associated with limb surgery (see above). Isovolaemic and hypervolaemic haemodilution have been proposed as methods of reducing the requirement for donor blood, but the evidence for these practices is tenuous. Careful positioning may reduce venous bleeding through the assurance of adequate venous drainage at the surgical site. The maintenance of normothermia avoids hypothermia-induced clotting dysfunction. Epidural and spinal anaesthesia are associated with reduced intraoperative blood loss; this association is probably related to reductions in both arterial and venous pressures.

Cell salvage

The collection and retransfusion of blood lost during surgery has become popular in recent years. Few contraindications exist, although some of these are relevant in patients presenting for orthopaedic surgery:

- Salvage and retransfusion of blood from a wound containing malignant cells is contraindicated because of the risk of dissemination of tumour cells. Malignant cells are incompletely removed by washing and filtration.
- Contamination with bowel contents or infection at the site of blood retrieval is a contraindication to salvage and retransfusion. Washing with antibiotic solutions has been shown to be ineffective in neutralizing all bacteria.
- Salvaged blood that contains topical haemostatic agents such as collagen, cellulose, gelatin and thrombin should not be retransfused as it may result in intravascular coagulation.
- Salvaged blood that contains surgical irrigants, liquid methylmethacrylate or antibiotics not licensed for parenteral use (e.g. neomycin) should not be retransfused.

Modified transfusion triggers

Most modern clinical practice guidelines recommend restrictive red blood cell transfusion practices with the goal of minimizing transmission of blood-borne pathogens. The haemoglobin concentration used as a trigger for transfusion has reduced progressively in recent years as awareness has increased that patients are relatively tolerant of anaemia if there are no organs with critical perfusion or oxygenation, and if an adequate cardiac output (and therefore an adequate circulating, intravascular volume) is present. The context of the patient's anaemia is also of importance; if the patient is still losing blood, a haemoglobin concentration of $8\,g\,dL^{-1}$ is less tolerable than if bleeding has ceased. Independent of the patient's coexisting pathology, anaemia is less acceptable half-way through a hip

arthroplasty than it would be at the end of a knee arthroscopy. Thus, the patient's haemoglobin concentration is relevant, but must be considered together with coexisting organ function and oxygenation (e.g. angina, renal dysfunction, transient ischaemic attacks), the nature of the operation and the timing of the measurement in relation to the progress of the procedure.

Healthy patients tolerate a haemoglobin concentration of $7\,g\,dL^{-1}$ well if they have no additional requirements for physiological reserve. It may be safer to use a higher trigger than this for patients with known organ malperfusion. The adoption of lower transfusion triggers for patients undergoing surgery mandates that intravascular volume is maintained meticulously, because anaemia is tolerated poorly in the presence of a reduced cardiac output. It is also necessary to check the patient's haemoglobin concentration frequently during the operation and in the early postoperative period; this is performed easily using a HemoCue® haemoglobinometer.

Hypotensive anaesthesia

Intentional reduction of the systemic arterial pressure is rarely indicated in orthopaedic surgery. The risk of poor perfusion of vital organs makes this a potentially dangerous technique, and other options exist to avoid donor blood transfusion and to maintain a clear surgical field.

SPECIFIC SURGICAL PROCEDURES

PRIMARY HIP ARTHROPLASTY

The operation is performed in either a supine or a modified lateral position. The femoral head is removed, and the new cup and femoral components are fixed to prepared bone with polymethylmethacrylate cement. Application and hardening of the cement, particularly after its insertion into the femoral shaft, are sometimes accompanied by sudden reductions in end-tidal CO_2 concentration and arterial pressure. Although attributable in part to toxic monomers released as the cement polymerizes, the high incidences of these changes reported when the technique was relatively new were probably related to a high frequency of air embolism; air was forced into the circulation as the prosthesis was pushed into the femoral shaft. Techniques such as filling the shaft with cement from the bottom upwards, or venting the shaft with a cannula, have dramatically reduced the incidence of adverse events. However, insertion of cement may still cause embolism of marrow, fat or blood clots. Embolization of air is also possible if the intramedullary pressure increases above venous pressure. Intramedullary pressure reaches its highest values when intact bone is first opened and reamed.

Regional anaesthesia is regarded by many anaesthetists as the preferred technique for hip replacement (see above) and immediate postoperative pain may be controlled by the addition of a spinal opioid. Blood loss is rarely large during primary replacement but vigilance is required, as assessment is made difficult by the large volumes of irrigation fluid used during the operation. Temperature homeostasis should be maintained by the use of active warming devices such as a warm air blanket.

To reduce the risk of dislocation of the new joint, the patient is placed supine in an abduction splint at the end of the procedure. This device makes it difficult to move the patient, and extra assistance is needed if the patient needs to be turned during the immediate recovery phase. After the first few postoperative hours, analgesic requirements are usually fairly low, irrespective of the anaesthetic technique employed.

HIP RESURFACING ARTHROPLASTY

This is a more recently developed surgical technique for primary hip arthroplasty with the advantage that only the joint surfaces are removed during surgery. Most of the normal bone is preserved, including the femoral head and neck. The medullary canal is not opened and no femoral stem prosthesis is necessary. It is an operation designed to postpone definitive joint replacement in younger patients with progressive disease. The operation is intended to interfere minimally with the normal mechanics of the joint and it is also anticipated that the longevity of the prosthesis should be greater than when a rigid stem prosthesis is placed in elastic bone. The anaesthetic management for this procedure is essentially the same as for traditional primary hip arthroplasty. The risk of embolic events is low because of the reduced bone destruction and lack of exposure of the femoral medullary canal.

REVISION OF HIP REPLACEMENT

Hip prostheses have a finite life, and increasing numbers of patients present for removal of the original prosthesis and insertion of a new one. This procedure is of longer duration and usually involves greater blood loss than primary hip replacement. General anaesthesia, often combined with a regional block, is used commonly. In addition to the precautions for primary hip replacement, central venous and invasive arterial pressure monitoring should be considered. A bladder catheter should be inserted to monitor urine output. Greater heat loss is experienced because of the increased length of the procedure and particular attention needs to be paid to maintenance of core temperature to reduce intraoperative coagulation abnormalities and postoperative complications. The use of blood conservation techniques such as intraoperative cell salvage should be considered. Replacement clotting factors may be required to correct abnormalities of coagulation if major blood loss occurs. Patients who have undergone revision of a hip replacement may require a period of high-dependency care postoperatively.

DISLOCATION OF A PROSTHETIC HIP

This needs manipulation and reduction to relieve pain and is more urgent if posterior dislocation threatens the sciatic nerve; this is more likely after trauma. Usually, a brief general anaesthetic without neuromuscular blockade suffices; if reduction is difficult, muscle relaxation may be required. It is often unrealistic to move the patient from the bed before inducing anaesthesia, but precautions against regurgitation and aspiration of gastric fluid, including antacids and rapid-sequence induction, may be indicated if urgent reduction is required or if the patient has been receiving systemic opioid analgesics (which delay gastric emptying). Usually, the patient wakes up with less pain than before manipulation.

KNEE REPLACEMENT

Spinal or general anaesthesia are appropriate techniques for this operation. Knee replacement is performed with the patient in the supine position. Pain after knee replacement is more severe than after most other major joint replacements. Administration of a spinal opioid or performance of sciatic and 3-in-1 (femoral sheath) blocks results in prolonged analgesia. Paracetamol and NSAIDs should be prescribed on a regular basis (if there are no contraindications), together with an opioid.

There is less risk of thromboembolism after knee replacement than after other major joint replacements. Close observation for evidence of hypotension and cardiac arrhythmias, particularly in frail patients, is required following deflation of the tourniquet as the products of cellular metabolism are washed out of the tissues into the circulation. Significant blood loss may occur when the tourniquet is deflated and it may be necessary to reassess fluid and blood transfusion needs in the early recovery period. Specialized drains, which collect postoperative blood loss and allow immediate retransfusion, are often inserted by the surgeon.

Manipulation under anaesthesia is sometimes needed in the postoperative period. Muscle relaxants are not required. Depending on the extent of manipulation, intravenous opioid analgesia may be required to control pain, especially in the first hour after the procedure. Nerve blocks may be given to aid passive mobilization of the joint following the procedure.

SHOULDER REPLACEMENT

Patients undergoing shoulder replacement are often younger than those requiring hip or knee arthroplasty. They usually mobilize more rapidly in the postoperative period and rarely require a prolonged infusion of intravenous fluids or blood transfusion.

During surgery, the patient is placed in a 'deckchair' position. The patient's head is relatively inaccessible during the procedure; tracheal intubation with a reinforced tube provides a secure airway. Surgery often involves vigorous manipulation of the arm, so the head needs to be fixed firmly to the operating table. To avoid sudden hypotension, elevation to the deckchair position should be undertaken with a freely running intravenous infusion, with vasopressors available. Because the shoulder is above the heart during surgery, there is a risk of air embolism. Interscalene brachial plexus block with insertion of a catheter provides effective analgesia after surgery; indeed, it is possible to carry out the whole procedure under this block. Transient neuropraxia may be attributed to these blocks but, as with lower limb surgery, this is more likely to be caused by the surgical procedure. After other operations on the shoulder, when no prosthesis is inserted and the infection risk is lower, intermittent injections of local anaesthetic through a subacromial catheter may be used for pain management.

SPINAL SURGERY

Spinal surgery is a major orthopaedic subspecialty. It provides several challenges for the anaesthetist; these include massive blood loss, difficult airway management, single-lung ventilation and consideration of a variety of pathologies seldom seen outside this surgical population. Spinal surgical procedures include trauma surgery, vertebral fusion, laminectomy and correction of scoliosis. The very young and the very old may present for spinal surgery.

Active warming is required during most procedures to prevent hypothermia caused by extensive surgical exposure through a long wound, blood transfusion and laminar airflow systems.

Airway management may be difficult in patients with cervical spine instability; these patients may have external spinal fixation. Patients with a cervical spinal cord injury may develop autonomic hyperreflexia and cardiovascular instability. Succinylcholine may produce a dangerous increase in serum potassium concentration in patients who have a denervating spinal cord injury which is more than 24 h old. This is caused by a proliferation of nicotinic cholinergic receptors at the neuromuscular junction. Difficult airway management skills are often needed to achieve tracheal intubation in patients with an anatomical abnormality of the spine, e.g. ankylosing spondylitis or scoliosis.

Scoliosis is associated with neuromuscular diseases in many patients. There is some evidence that such diseases (e.g. muscular dystrophies) may be associated with an increased risk of malignant hyperthermia or a malignant hyperthermia-like syndrome of abnormal metabolism in muscles, with a rapid and progressive increase in core temperature. There may also be increased difficulty with spontaneous ventilation in the postoperative period because of muscle weakness.

Patients with scoliosis may have severely limited respiratory function (e.g. a restrictive defect due to scoliosis) and may be at risk of increased intraoperative bleeding. Single-lung ventilation is often required to achieve adequate surgical access during the correction of thoracic scoliosis.

Spinal cord function may be compromised during correction of scoliosis because of ischaemia caused by excessive straightening of the spine. Spinal cord integrity may be tested using an intraoperative wake-up test. This requires preoperative psychological preparation of the patient and a suitable anaesthetic technique. However, the wake-up test has been superseded almost entirely by advances in spinal cord monitoring techniques including somatosensory and motor evoked potential recording, which give an early warning of compromised spinal cord blood supply during surgery to correct scoliosis.

PERIPHERAL SURGERY

Most peripheral orthopaedic surgery may be carried out in the day-case setting. If general anaesthesia is required, a simple inhalational technique usually suffices. Regional techniques provide excellent analgesia postoperatively and reduce the degree of disability which the patient suffers. Regional techniques may obviate the need for general anaesthesia and may lead to earlier discharge and a high level of patient satisfaction. There is increasing interest in the use of regional techniques for both intraoperative and postoperative management; one or more catheters are inserted at the time of operation, and used to infuse a local anaesthetic.

It is easy to underestimate the degree of pain and disability that the patient may experience following peripheral orthopaedic operations. Analgesia should be prescribed on a regular basis postoperatively and additional 'as required' analgesia should be made available. Regular paracetamol, NSAIDs and opioids, if required and not contraindicated, should be prescribed. At the end of many procedures, a plaster cast is applied. If anaesthesia ends before the plaster hardens, the patient may move, break the cast and need to be reanaesthetized.

FURTHER READING

Auroy Y, Narchi P, Messiah A et al 1997 Serious complications related to regional anesthesia: results of a prospective survey in France. Anesthesiology 87: 479–486

Singelyn F J, Deyaert M, Joris D et al 1998 Effects of intravenous patient-controlled analgesia with morphine, continuous epidural analgesia, and continuous three-in-one block on postoperative pain and knee rehabilitation after unilateral total knee arthroplasty. Anesthesia and Analgesia 87: 88–92

31 Anaesthesia for ENT and maxillofacial surgery

ENT SURGERY

Two hundred and seventy thousand ear, nose and throat operations are performed in the UK each year, accounting for approximately 5% of the workload of an anaesthetic department. Patients are usually young and healthy and the average hospital stay is short (less than 2 days). Many operations are performed as day cases, thereby reducing the need for inpatient admission.

Children and young adults are frequently apprehensive and require reassurance. Some may have an atopic history which influences the anaesthetic technique. Older patients may have hypertension or ischaemic heart disease and require careful preoperative assessment.

Smooth anaesthesia and a clear airway are essential, as coughing and straining result in venous congestion which may persist during surgery and cause increased bleeding. Partial obstruction of the airway may lead to hypoxaemia, hypercapnia and unduly light anaesthesia.

The patient's eyes should be protected from corneal abrasions in all ENT procedures by taping the eyelids shut, except for procedures where the periorbital fat may be accessed, e.g. nasal endoscopic surgery

THE SHARED AIRWAY

Special problems are caused when the airway is shared by both anaesthetist and surgeon. If bleeding is anticipated, the airway *must* be protected and the oropharynx packed to avoid contamination of the larynx with blood, pus and other debris. The anaesthetic circuit connections are usually hidden under the drapes and may well be 'knocked' by the surgeon during the procedure. Anaesthetic disconnections are, therefore, a constant threat. It is important to realize that disconnections on the machine side of the capnograph sampling tube, in a patient who is breathing spontaneously, does not lead to a loss of the capno-graph trace and so careful observation of the reservoir bag is mandatory.

At the end of the procedure, the pack must be removed and the pharynx cleared of blood and debris before the trachea is extubated with the patient in a head-down lateral position.

THE LARYNGEAL MASK AIRWAY

The laryngeal mask airway (LMA) has been used for all types of ENT anaesthesia. To justify its use, the anaesthetist must be able to demonstrate that it conveys an advantage over the traditional use of a tracheal tube.

TONSILLECTOMY

Each year 80 000 adenotonsillectomies are performed in the UK, with a rate of 8 per 1000 children under the age of 15. This frequency is 40% of that 15 years ago. In 1968 there were six deaths, a mortality rate of 1 in 28 000, but this has now been reduced to less than 1 in 100 000.

Most children attend for surgery on the day of operation and premedication is often not practical for these children. If premedication is required before tonsillectomy, it is administered most conveniently to the younger child as a syrup (alimemazine (trimeprazine) 1.5 mg kg^{-1} or midazolam (0.5 mg kg^{-1} maximum 15 mg). Some anaesthetists combine this with atropine 20 µg kg^{-1} to a maximum of 600 µg given orally (except in hot weather) to decrease secretions intraoperatively.

Most children are given an i.v. induction of anaesthesia after the application of a patch of local anaesthetic cream; some children, however, may prefer an inhalational induction and this is necessary in the child with poor venous access. Oral intubation is facilitated by succinylcholine or performed under deep inhalational anaesthesia; on occasions it may be difficult to maintain a patent airway because of respiratory obstruction produced by enlarged tonsils.

Analgesia is given during surgery, but good control of postoperative pain is still difficult. Tracheal extubation is performed with the patient slightly head-down in a lateral position after suction has ensured that the pharynx is free from blood. The trachea may be extubated either under deep anaesthesia or when fully awake; with 'deep extubation' the anaesthetist must continue to take responsibility for protecting the airway. Postoperative vomiting is a significant problem (50% of children vomit at least once) and therefore antiemetics should be prescribed.

Blood loss during tonsillectomy is not usually measured but may be deceptively large. Increasing numbers of children under 3 years of age (15 kg) are presenting for tonsillectomy for sleep apnoea syndrome. Particular care is required in this group as blood transfusion is necessary after 100 mL blood loss. Many of these children should have an intravenous infusion until they are ready to take oral fluids.

The reinforced LMA is frequently used for tonsillectomy; however, the Boyle Davis gag is more difficult to place and obstruction to the airway occurs more frequently than when a tracheal tube is used.

In 2001, after discussion with the RCOA, the Department of Health issued guidelines on the use of disposable equipment for adenotonsillectomy. This was in response to the threat to health from bovine spongioform encephalopathy. Despite changes in the advice to surgeons (regarding disposable instruments) this guideline has not been revoked or superseded; it is therefore necessary to dispose of all airway equipment at the end of each case (this includes the LMA). In the case of expensive equipment, e.g. laryngoscopes, the metal blade should be covered by a transparent sheath or a disposable laryngoscope blade used (see AAGBI guidelines on infection, referenced in Ch. 13).

The postoperative bleeding tonsil

These patients fall into two separate groups: those with an acute bleed in the immediate postoperative period (usually in the recovery area) and those who ooze blood slowly from the tonsil bed. This latter group is usually diagnosed on the ward, on the basis of the clinical signs of hypovolaemia – tachycardia, pallor and sweating. Swallowing is not uncommon, followed by vomiting of a large quantity of blood. Anaesthesia for these children is difficult and the assistance of an experienced anaesthetist must be sought. An i.v. infusion is essential and blood transfusion may be required.

The group with an acute bleed present a particularly difficult problem in that there is active bleeding in the airway. Such patients require an inhalational induction of anaesthesia (sevoflurane in oxygen) in the left lateral position with Trendelenburg tilt and frequent pharyngeal suction. Intubation of the trachea is undertaken under deep anaesthesia.

Patients with bleeding on the ward present with the problems of hypovolaemia and a full stomach; after resuscitation, the patient is placed head-down in a lateral position and suction apparatus is positioned within grasp. After preoxygenation, a small dose of thiopental (2–3 mg kg^{-1}) is given followed by succinylcholine 1.5 mg kg^{-1} and cricoid pressure is applied, although this may make laryngoscopy difficult.

When bleeding has been controlled surgically, the stomach is emptied with a nasogastric tube, and the trachea is extubated with the patient in the lateral position.

It should be emphasized that induction of anaesthesia with thiopental or propofol must never be attempted before adequate resuscitation has been undertaken and the intravascular volume restored.

ADENOIDECTOMY

Adenoidectomy is often combined with either tonsillectomy or examination of the ears under anaesthesia. Anaesthesia is induced either by inhalation or via the i.v. route. Oral tracheal intubation is advisable either under deep anaesthesia or facilitated by succinylcholine. A Boyle Davis gag is inserted, the adenoids are curetted and the postnasal space is packed to achieve haemostasis. After 3 min, this pack is removed, the patient is turned into the lateral position and the trachea is extubated.

Increasingly, adenoidectomy in the absence of tonsillectomy is being performed as a day-case procedure. For these patients, rectal paracetamol may be an appropriate analgesic.

MICROLARYNGOSCOPY

The operating microscope has revolutionized the treatment of laryngeal disorders. The Kleinsasser laryngoscope is supported on the chest by rests and the operating microscope allows detailed examination and assessment of the larynx.

The most popular anaesthetic technique uses a Coplan's microlaryngoscopy tube (5 mm ID, 31 cm long, constructed from soft plastic, with a 10 mL cuff volume). Anaesthesia is induced with an i.v. induction agent followed by a non-depolarizing muscle relaxant; the vocal cords are sprayed with 3 mL lidocaine 4% to assist smooth anaesthesia and to minimize the possibility of postextubation laryngospasm. Alternatively, the cords may be 'painted' with 3% cocaine at the end of the procedure, which has the added advantage of reducing bleeding from biopsy sites. The Coplan's tube is passed either orally or nasally. The lungs are ventilated artificially with 66% N_2O in O_2 supplemented with a volatile agent and analgesic drug. The small-diameter tube does not impede the surgeon's view and allows good access to the larynx. The cuff prevents contamination of the trachea with blood or debris.

At the end of the procedure, the pharynx is cleared with suction under direct vision, the muscle relaxant is antagonized and tracheal extubation is performed in a lateral position. Oxygen is administered to minimize the risk of hypoxaemia, particularly if laryngeal stridor occurs.

Other techniques used for microlaryngoscopy include:

- topical analgesia to the larynx with insufflation of N_2O/O_2 and volatile agent via a fine catheter
- Venturi ventilation with O_2 using a catheter and a Sanders injector. Hypnosis is maintained with increments or infusion of a rapidly metabolized induction agent.

In children, microlaryngoscopy is performed using spontaneous ventilation via an oral tracheal tube one size smaller than would be used normally. The larynx should be sprayed with a measured quantity of lidocaine in an attempt to prevent postoperative laryngospasm. Occasionally, the surgeon requests to observe the larynx without a tracheal tube in situ; in these circumstances the tube is removed during deep anaesthesia, allowing examination to take place during emergence or during Venturi ventilation via the operating laryngoscope.

LARYNGECTOMY

The incidence of carcinoma of the larynx is 3–4 per 100 000 population. Many tumours may be treated with radiotherapy and therefore surgery is relatively uncommon for this condition. Airway obstruction by tumour is the major anaesthetic problem; alcohol and smoking are aetiological factors which may influence anaesthesia.

Respiratory function should be assessed preoperatively, although this is difficult to measure accurately if there is airway obstruction. Chest physiotherapy should always be prescribed, as it aids clearance of secretions pre- and postoperatively.

When respiratory obstruction is suspected, opioid or sedative premedication should be avoided. All patients presenting for laryngectomy undergo flexible nasal endoscopy to assess the larynx; the findings of this investigation are of great importance to the administration of the anaesthetic. If there is a risk of mechanical obstruction on induction of anaesthesia, an inhalational technique should be used; if this results in severe respiratory obstruction, awake intubation may be required. A selection of non-cuffed tracheal tubes should be available as the lumen of the trachea may be narrowed at the level of the cords or subglottically. Laryngoscopy and tracheal intubation may be more difficult if preoperative radiotherapy has reduced the mobility of the floor of the mouth.

In the absence of respiratory obstruction, an i.v. induction agent may be used; it should be given slowly in minimal dosage until consciousness is lost. If subsequently the patient's lungs can be inflated using a face mask, succinylcholine may be given to facilitate tracheal intubation; if not, anaesthesia is deepened slowly with nitrous oxide and isoflurane or sevoflurane in oxygen until laryngoscopy is possible. If there is any doubt regarding the ability to maintain a patent airway after loss of consciousness, the anaesthetist must *not* use an i.v. induction agent.

Monitoring of S_pO_2, ECG and arterial pressure is commenced in the anaesthetic room before induction of anaesthesia, which is maintained using controlled ventilation with nitrous oxide in oxygen supplemented by a volatile agent and opioid analgesic. Induced hypotension is often used to facilitate dissection of the neck. When the larynx has been dissected free, it is important to check that a sterile tracheal tube and compatible connections are available before the trachea is divided. The patient's lungs are ventilated with 100% oxygen for 2 min, the tracheal tube is withdrawn into the larynx and disconnected, the trachea is divided and a second tracheal tube is placed rapidly into the open end of the trachea, connected to the anaesthetic circuit and secured firmly. This tube should be positioned carefully within the shortened trachea to prevent inadvertent one-lung anaesthesia.

At the end of surgery, residual neuromuscular block is antagonized and the tracheal tube changed for a tracheostomy tube. Adequate humidification is essential postoperatively. Enteral nutrition is provided via a nasogastric tube.

PHARYNGOLARYNGO-OESOPHAGECTOMY

Pharyngolaryngo-oesophagectomy is performed for tumours of the postcricoid region. The pharynx and larynx are removed and the stomach mobilized and anastomosed in the neck behind the tracheostomy. There are two surgical approaches: in one, after initial laparotomy, the stomach is passed through a mediastinal tract which is formed by blunt dissection; in the other more common procedure, the stomach is mobilized via a thoracoabdominal incision to be anastomosed in the neck. Thus several problems may occur:

- difficulty in tracheal intubation
- temperature loss resulting from a large surgical incision, a prolonged operative procedure and extensive blood loss
- pneumothorax if the pleura is damaged during dissection
- rupture of the trachea causing difficulty in ventilation and mediastinal emphysema.

LASER SURGERY

The laser is used to strip polyps or tumours from the vocal cords accurately and with immediate control of bleeding. There are two major anaesthetic problems:

- *Damage to the tracheal tube.* It has been found that in the presence of oxygen, PVC microlaryngoscopy tubes may be ignited by the intensity of the laser beam. The use of an aluminized PVC tube does not remove this problem completely. The introduction of cuffed flexible stainless steel tubes for nasal or oral use has essentially solved this problem. For added safety, the cuff should be filled with water.
- *Retinal damage.* The DOH recommends that all personnel wear protective spectacles to prevent retinal damage. Anaesthetists are particularly at risk as they are unable to retire behind the operating microscope during the laser procedure.

NASAL OPERATIONS

Preparation of the nose with local anaesthetic

In 1942, Moffatt described a method of topical anaesthesia of the nose using cocaine as an alternative to spraying or packing the nose. There were three advantages of his method: minimal patient discomfort during preparation, a low risk of cocaine toxicity and a bloodless surgical field.

In 1952, Curtiss simplified Moffatt's method as follows. The patient lies supine with the head extended fully over the end of a trolley and supported by an assistant. A round-ended angulated needle is inserted with its tip directed along the floor of the nose. When the angle of the needle is reached, the tip is directed towards the roof of the nose and 2 mL of solution deposited when the tip has made contact. The procedure is repeated in the second nostril. The patient remains in this position for 10 min and is advised not to swallow any solution which may have trickled into the pharynx. The patient then sits upright and spits out any residual solution.

Analgesia is produced by accumulation of cocaine in the region of the sphenopalatine ganglion, thereby blocking most of the sensory supply to the nose, including the anterior ethmoidal nerve. The columella is not affected and requires a separate injection. Arterial blood supply to the nose accompanies the nerve supply and is therefore constricted by the cocaine, producing good haemostasis.

Preparation of the nose in this manner enables any operation to be performed and dispenses with the need to use hypotensive techniques to control surgical bleeding.

In the anaesthetized patient, Moffatt's prescription may be modified further by diluting it into 20 mL of solution: 10 mL is instilled into each nostril with the head extended, after placement of a gauze throat pack. The pack holds the solution in the nose for maximum effect. This method has the advantage of requiring less precise placement of the solution.

Anaesthetic technique for nasal operations

Anaesthesia for nasal surgery has been revolutionized by the introduction of the LMA. Difficulties in maintaining a patent airway in the presence of surgical nasal packing are almost completely eliminated by leaving the LMA in place postoperatively until the patient rejects it in the recovery room.

Anaesthesia for nasal surgery may be maintained using either spontaneous or controlled ventilation, depending on the duration of surgery. The pharynx should be packed with 2-inch ribbon gauze so that blood, pus or debris does not contaminate the larynx or pass into the stomach. The presence of the pack should be marked in writing on the strapping which secures the tube (or LMA) to remind the anaesthetist to remove it at the end of the operation.

The patient is positioned 10° head-up and all breathing system connections are checked before surgery begins. When surgery has been completed, the pack is removed, the pharynx is cleared and the patient is turned into a lateral position.

If a tracheal tube is used, a Guedel airway should be placed in position before the tracheal tube is removed to provide a patent airway in the presence of surgical nasal packing. The advent of cannulated nasal packs has improved the patient's airway, but not all procedures are suitable for these packs.

Epistaxis

Surgical intervention may be necessary to control bleeding from the nose and may involve packing the nose or postnasal space or ligation of the maxillary artery.

The patient is often elderly and may be hypertensive. It is essential that the blood volume is restored before induction of anaesthesia. The problems inherent in haemorrhage from the upper airway and a stomach containing swallowed blood are similar to those of the bleeding tonsil and the anaesthetic technique used is similar.

The sinuses

Bacterial infection of the paranasal sinuses occurs when the self-cleansing mechanism becomes impaired and mucus accumulates and stagnates. Antral washouts and intranasal antrostomies are performed to aid restoration of normal mucosal activity. In a Caldwell Luc operation, radical antrostomy is performed via a buccal incision above the canine tooth. These procedures are becoming less and less common as functional endoscopic sinus surgery replaces them.

In all these procedures, the airway is protected by an LMA and a pharyngeal pack is inserted, provided there is no contraindication.

EARS

Myringotomy

Examination of the ears together with myringotomy and insertion of grommets is carried out commonly in children who have secretory otitis media. This operation is usually performed as a day case. Either inhalational or i.v. induction, following the application of local anaesthetic cream, may be used and anaesthesia is maintained with spontaneous ventilation via a face mask for myringotomy alone; if adenoidectomy is performed also, oral tracheal intubation is required. The use of nitrous oxide increases middle ear pressure significantly, especially when combined with IPPV, and this may alter the appearance of the tympanic membrane.

Middle ear surgery

Relative hypotension is required to minimize haemorrhage in the field of the microscope. Smooth anaesthesia is essential for operations on the middle ear. Coughing, straining or bucking increases venous pressure and produces oozing which may persist for some time. Premedication may be given orally. After induction of anaesthesia with propofol, a muscle relaxant is used to facilitate intubation with a non-kinking oral tracheal tube; the trachea and larynx are sprayed with lidocaine to aid tolerance of the tube. The hypertensive response to intubation may be attenuated with an

opioid such as alfentanil. Often, sufficient reduction in arterial pressure is obtained using nitrous oxide in oxygen with enflurane or isoflurane in combination with a non-depolarizing muscle relaxant, opioid and IPPV. A small dose of a β-blocker to reduce heart rate is an effective adjuvant. A 10° head-up tilt aids venous drainage. When induced hypotension is used, ECG and accurate arterial pressure monitoring are essential. Labetalol, glyceryl trinitrate or sodium nitroprusside may be used as infusions for relative hypotension, but these have now been superseded by an infusion of remifentanil. A 25% reduction in mean arterial blood pressure is usually adequate to produce a good surgical field.

The middle ear is a closed cavity and nitrous oxide diffuses rapidly into it, causing an increase in pressure. The maximum pressure is reached approximately 40 min after induction. There is concern that this may cause grafts to become dislodged. Such complications have led some authors to suggest that O_2/N_2 should be used in place of O_2/N_2O gas mixtures. Surgical techniques have improved and been modified over the years so that an increase in middle ear pressure is no longer a significant surgical problem. It is therefore no longer necessary to turn off the nitrous oxide before the end of the procedure.

Bandaging the ear at the end of surgery involves movement of the head. This should be anticipated and supervised by the anaesthetist to prevent undue movement which may lead to coughing on the tracheal tube. If labyrinthine function is disturbed, an antiemetic may be necessary to control postoperative vertigo and vomiting.

The LMA is used in major ear surgery, but the anaesthetist must be aware that if the airway is lost during the procedure, as a result of movement of the head, the operation may have to be abandoned.

MAXILLOFACIAL SURGERY

Many of the basic principles of anaesthesia for ENT surgery apply to anaesthesia for maxillofacial surgery. The anaesthetist does not have direct access to the patient's airway and may have to share the airway with the surgeon. Great care and attention are required to ensure that all connections are secure and that the tubing is of appropriate length.

Many straightforward cases may be carried out with the patient breathing spontaneously. The anaesthetist must therefore be aware that a disconnection occurring on the machine side of the capnograph attachment results in an adequate capnograph trace and no alarm.

The reservoir bag should therefore be placed in a position where it may be easily observed to ensure a complete anaesthetic circuit is maintained. Maxillofacial surgery includes simple procedures such as dental extractions through to prolonged, complicated head and neck resections with microvascular free flap transfers.

ORAL SURGERY

Many of these procedures may be carried out with the patient breathing spontaneously. After appropriate preoperative assessment, the patient is attached to monitors in the anaesthetic room and receives an intravenous induction. A nasotracheal tube is inserted after the administration of a muscle relaxant. Succinylcholine 1.5 mg kg^{-1} can be used, but many practitioners prefer to use mivacurium 0.2 mg kg^{-1} and provide intermittent positive-pressure ventilation for the first 10 min of the case. When the relaxant has worn off, the patient is allowed to breathe spontaneously and anaesthesia is maintained with oxygen in nitrous oxide supplemented with a volatile agent. Analgesia is provided with incremental doses of opioid and supplemented with infiltration of local anaesthesia by the surgeon.

Bleeding into the pharynx is a common occurrence and ingestion of this blood is prevented by the insertion of a gauze pack to block the pharynx, immediately after intubation. A record should be kept of this manoeuvre both in the anaesthetic notes and also on the theatre 'white-board'. At the end of the procedure, patients are extubated on their side *after the gauze pack has been removed* (this must also be documented). Deep and awake extubation techniques are practised. Some anaesthetists elect to carry out anaesthesia for these procedures using an LMA. This should be done only after consultation with the surgeon to ensure that the oral airway does not compromise the surgery. A gauze pack should still be used when an LMA is used; the pack should be removed before the patient leaves theatre, but the mask is left in situ until it is rejected (in the recovery ward).

FACIAL FRACTURES

Fractures of the mandible and maxilla may affect patients' ability to open the jaw. The cause may be mechanical as a result of oedema or possible disruption of the temporomandibular joint and, in addition, jaw opening may be limited by pain. Careful assessment of mouth opening is essential at the preoperative visit together with assessment of loose or broken teeth. An anaesthetic plan for establishing an airway should be formulated and senior assistance should be requested if appropriate. Tracheal intubation in many

patients may be performed in a conventional manner but some require awake fibreoptic insertion of a nasotracheal tube. If tracheal intubation is carried out under anaesthesia, it is necessary to provide an inhalational induction with either sevoflurane or halothane in oxygen and to laryngoscope the patient under deep anaesthesia to ensure a view of the vocal cords before relaxants are given.

Mandibular fractures

Satisfactory reduction of the fractures may require operative intermaxillary fixation (jaw wiring) and hence it is necessary to insert a nasotracheal tube. Current surgical practice is mainly to plate these fractures and this avoids the need for postoperative intermaxillary fixation and simplifies the anaesthetic management of extubation. Extubation may be achieved after reversal of the neuromuscular blockade with the patient on the side and when the protective reflexes have returned. There are, however, some instances where fixation is required and if this is the case the patient should receive a full explanation of how extubation will be achieved. The patient should be awakened with the tube in situ and it is then removed when the patient is alert and has full return of protective reflexes. Suction of the airway may be achieved using catheters inserted via either the nose or the retromolar space. Prokinetic drugs such as metoclopramide are used intraoperatively and ondansetron may be used as an antiemetic.

Fracture of the zygoma

This surgical procedure does not require intermaxillary fixation and usually a fracture of the zygoma does not interfere with jaw movement. The anaesthetic management therefore focuses on associated injuries, and anaesthesia for an isolated fracture of the zygoma is the same as for any other urgent procedure.

HEAD AND NECK RESECTION AND RECONSTRUCTION

Anaesthesia for these procedures requires detailed preoperative assessment, as the patients are often elderly and suffer multiple comorbidities such as smoking-related diseases, cardiovascular disease and renal impairment. Anaesthesia for these procedures is testing as there are the problems of difficult airway management, tracheostomy, potential large blood loss, long procedures and microvascular anastomosis for free tissue transfer. These patients require at least level 2 care postoperatively. The operation usually proceeds as follows: anaesthetic management of the difficult airway, which on occasions may require awake fibreoptic intubation (it is important to note that fibreoptic intubation is much more difficult in patients who have pathology in the airway which may cause contact bleeding); the next stage is usually to perform surgical tracheostomy, followed by resection of the tumour with the possibility of significant blood loss. Assesssment of the need to transfuse must take into account the need for the relative haemodilution that is beneficial for flow in the free tissue graft. As a result, the patient is usually transfused to maintain a haemoglobin concentration of $10\,g\,dL^{-1}$. The next stage is to raise a free tissue graft followed by microvascular anastomosis of the graft to the operative site, and finally surgical repair of the defect and closure. These procedures may take up to 18 h and require intra-arterial monitoring, possible central venous catheterization (usually from the arm),

measurement of urinary output, temperature monitoring, warming of all i.v. fluids, good airway humidification and external warming of the patient.

FURTHER READING

Cheshire NJ, Knight DJW 2001 Anaesthetic management of facial trauma and fractures. BJACEPD Reviews 2: 100

Hospital Inpatient Inquiry Series MB4, 27. DHSS Office of Population Censuses and Surveys, Welsh Office, ENT Microfiches 24, 25

Puttick N, Van der Walt J H 1987 The effect of premedication on the incidence of postoperative vomiting in children after ENT surgery. Anaesthesia and Intensive Care 15: 158

Van der Spek A L, Spargs P M, Norton M L 1988 The physics of lasers and implications for their use during airway surgery. British Journal of Anaesthesia 60: 709

www.doh.gov.uk/cjd.index.htm

Anaesthesia for ophthalmic surgery 32

Patients who present for eye surgery are frequently at the extreme ends of age. Both neonatal and geriatric anaesthesia present special problems. Some eye surgery may last many hours and repeated anaesthetics at short intervals are often necessary. The anaesthetic technique may influence intraocular pressure (IOP), and skilled administration of either local or general anaesthesia contributes directly to the successful outcome of the surgery. Close cooperation and clear understanding between surgeon and anaesthetist are essential. Risks and benefits must be assessed carefully and the anaesthetic technique selected accordingly.

Ophthalmic surgery can be classified into subspecialties and intraocular or extraocular procedures may be performed (Table 32.1); each has different anaesthetic requirements.

CHOICE OF ANAESTHESIA

Ophthalmic surgery can be carried out under either local or general anaesthesia. The type of surgery, planned duration, age and fitness of the patient influence the choice (Table 32.2). Local anaesthesia is preferred for older and sicker patients, as the stress response to surgery is diminished and complications such as postoperative confusion, nausea, vomiting and urinary retention are mostly eliminated. Younger patients may sometimes be too anxious for local anaesthesia and are usually managed with general anaesthesia.

CONDITIONS FOR INTRAOCULAR SURGERY

For most intraocular operations, the eye must be pain-free and preferably immobile. Except for glaucoma surgery, the pupil should be dilated and intraocular pressure reduced.

INTRAOCULAR PRESSURE

There is a diurnal variation in intraocular pressure. Resting pressure greater than 22 mmHg is considered abnormal.

EXPULSIVE HAEMORRHAGE

In the presence of markedly raised IOP, sudden reduction in pressure on incision of the globe may lead to the expression of the contents. The balance between venous and intraocular pressure is crucial. An increase in venous pressure causes fluid to pool in the choroid and may progress to cause rupture of the ciliary artery with prolapse of the iris. On rare occasions, disastrous expulsive haemorrhage may result in the loss of the entire contents of the eyeball.

CONTROL OF INTRAOCULAR PRESSURE

Factors controlling IOP are very complex but there is a similarity to those that influence intracranial pressure, as both involve manipulation of a volume contained in a semi-rigid container. These factors include external pressure, volume of arterial and venous vasculature (choroidal volume) and the volumes of the aqueous and vitreous humour (Fig. 32.1).

External pressure

Pressure from squeezing the eyes closed or the injection of a volume of local anaesthetic into the orbit is transmitted to the eyeball and increases the IOP.

Venous pressure

Venous congestion increases vascular volume within the eye and reduces aqueous drainage through the

Table 32.1   Categorization of ophthalmic surgery

Ophthalmology subspecialities

Paediatric

Oculoplastic

Retinovitreous

Anterior segment

Glaucoma

Neuro-ophthalmology

Extraocular operations

Globe and orbit

Eyebrow and eyelid

Lacrimal system

Muscles

Conjunctiva

Cornea, surface

Intraocular operations

Iris and anterior chamber

Lens and cataract

Vitreous

Retina

Cornea, full thickness

Table 32.2   Preferred anaesthetic technique for common surgical procedures in ophthalmology

Local anaesthesia

Cataract

Glaucoma techniques

Minor extraocular plastic surgery

Laser dacrocystorhinostomy

Minor anterior segment procedures

Simple vitrectomies

General anaesthesia

Paediatric surgery

Squint surgery

Major oculoplastic surgery

Dacrocystorhinostomy

Penetrating keratoplasty

Orbital trauma repair

Perforating eye injuries

Complex retinovitreous surgery

canal of Schlemm, causing an increase in IOP. During anaesthesia, venous pressure is influenced mainly by posture and transmitted intrathoracic pressure. A 15° head-up tilt causes a significant decrease in IOP.

Raised arterial pressure, anxiety, restlessness, full bladder, coughing, retching and airway obstruction cause an increase in venous pressure which is reflected immediately in the IOP. Intermittent positive-pressure ventilation (IPPV) produces a small increase in venous pressure secondary to the increase in mean intrathoracic pressure, but is compensated for by control of arterial $P\text{CO}_2$.

Arterial blood gas tensions

Arterial $P\text{CO}_2$ is an important determinant of choroidal vascular volume and IOP. A reduction in $P_a\text{CO}_2$ constricts the choroidal vessels and reduces IOP. Elevation of $P_a\text{CO}_2$ results in a proportional and linear increase in IOP. Increases in $P_a\text{CO}_2$ may also increase central venous pressure. Hypoxaemia produces intraocular vasodilatation and an increase in IOP.

Arterial pressure

Stable values of arterial pressure within the physiological range maintain normal IOP. Sudden increases in systolic arterial pressure above the normal autoregulatory range increase choroidal blood volume and consequently IOP. Reduction in arterial pressure below normal physiological levels reduces IOP, but the response is unpredictable in old age when arterial capacitance is reduced.

Aqueous and vitreous volumes

A decrease in either aqueous or vitreous volume reduces IOP. Osmotic diuretics are sometimes used to reduce aqueous and vitreous volume. Acetazolamide reduces the production of aqueous.

Haelan (sodium hyaluronate)

Sodium hyaluronate is used as a soft viscous retractor during surgery. It augments the effect of general anaesthesia by controlling vitreous bulge and compensates for small changes in IOP. Sodium hyaluronate is a large-molecular-weight, clear viscoelastic polysaccharide. The manufactured product is injected by the surgeon at the time of incision and helps to maintain the shape of the anterior chamber and the work space. Haelan with lidocaine admixture has been introduced recently and is used when cataract surgery is conducted under topical anaesthesia.

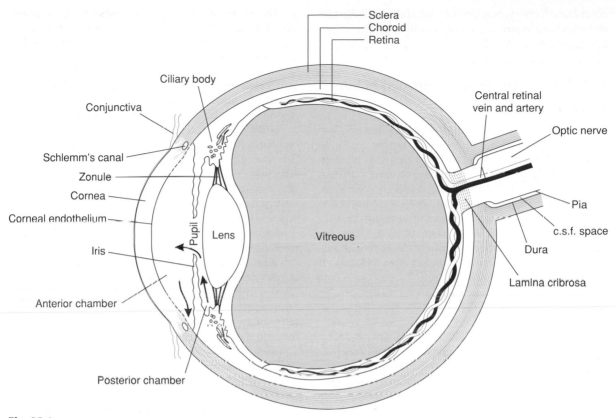

Fig. 32.1
Cross-section through eye and optic nerve. Arrows indicate flow of aqueous.

EFFECT OF ANAESTHETIC DRUGS ON INTRAOCULAR PRESSURE

Premedication

Drugs used for premedication have little effect on intraocular pressure, and the commonly used anxiolytic and antiemetic drugs may be used as preferred.

Induction agents

Most of the intravenous induction agents, with the exception of ketamine, reduce intraocular pressure and may be used as indicated clinically. Ketamine should be avoided if intraocular surgery is planned.

Muscle relaxants

Succinylcholine increases intraocular pressure, with a maximal effect 2 min after i.v. administration, but the pressure returns to baseline values after 5 min. This effect is thought to be caused by the increase in tone of the extraocular muscles and intraocular vasodilatation. Pretreatment with a small dose of a non-depolarizing muscle relaxant does not obtund this response reliably. The problems involved with the use of succinylcholine in the patient with penetrating eye injury are discussed below.

Non-depolarizing muscle relaxants have no significant direct effects on IOP.

Volatile anaesthetic agents

All the volatile anaesthetic agents in use today decrease intraocular pressure. Nitrous oxide has no effect on IOP in the absence of air or a therapeutic inert gas bubble in the globe (for further explanation, see the discussion on retinal surgery below).

Opioids

Opioids cause a moderate reduction in IOP in the absence of significant ventilatory depression. They contribute to postoperative nausea and vomiting and are not often required for postoperative analgesia following eye surgery.

TECHNIQUES OF GENERAL ANAESTHESIA

Premedication

Premedication is not now used routinely for eye surgery, but a short-acting benzodiazepine such as temazepam may be given orally as premedication to anxious patients. These drugs should be used with caution in the elderly as they may result in confusion. Premedication by injection is not necessary. Anticholinergic agents cause a dry mouth and discomfort and do not need to be given with premedication. They are more likely to be needed in strabismus or retinal surgery, but may be given intravenously after induction if necessary.

Induction

The synergistic effects of midazolam with short-acting opioid analgesics such as fentanyl or alfentanil may precede induction. These drugs reduce dose requirements of induction and maintenance agents and modify the cardiovascular response to airway manipulation. This combination should be administered with caution in the elderly, who easily become apnoeic with small doses. Propofol is used widely because of its short duration of action, pleasant induction and reduced postoperative nausea. Etomidate is useful in elderly or unhealthy patients because of its cardiostability, reduction in IOP and rapid recovery. Frequent pain on injection and involuntary movements offset these advantages. Thiopental is still a satisfactory alternative for induction in both adults and children. Inhalational induction with sevoflurane is another alternative and has largely superseded halothane for gaseous induction in children. It may be used in needle-phobic adults or as a cost-effective alternative to propofol induction and maintenance.

Airway management and maintenance of anaesthesia

Most anaesthetists use a balanced anaesthesia technique with IPPV for intraocular surgery. Moderate hyperventilation reduces P_aCO_2 and provides excellent operating conditions. Less anaesthetic is used and the patient should wake up rapidly at the end of surgery. Spontaneous ventilation may need deeper levels of anaesthesia, and CO_2 retention, hypotension and slow recovery may result.

The laryngeal mask has now largely replaced tracheal intubation for intraocular surgery. Insertion is easier and the problems associated with postoperative coughing, straining and laryngospasm are virtually eliminated. The laryngeal mask should be positioned accurately to give unobstructed ventilation. Care should be taken to maintain sufficiently deep anaesthesia so that the laryngeal mask is not rejected.

Early on in the procedure, the surgeon should be encouraged to infiltrate a long-acting local anaesthetic by the sub-Tenon's route. This should successfully eliminate variations in anaesthetic requirements from the surgical stimulus and provide a stable anaesthetic with a reduction in the amounts of general anaesthetic agent required. If topped up towards the end of the procedure, excellent postoperative analgesia should be produced without other analgesic drugs.

The laryngeal mask is unsuitable for patients at risk of aspiration. This group includes the morbidly obese, those with gastro-oesophageal reflux and patients with hiatus hernia. In these patients, preoperative administration of an H_2-receptor antagonist and antacid therapy should be considered and a cuffed tracheal tube is recommended to protect the airway. Preoxygenation with the head elevated and cricoid pressure reduces the risk of aspiration. Muscle relaxants are required for intubation and maintenance, but coughing and straining at extubation are problems for which there is no easy solution. Continuation of the volatile agent until reversal of residual neuromuscular blockade, or the use of i.v. lidocaine, has been recommended to overcome this problem.

PENETRATING EYE INJURY

The anaesthetic management of the patient with a penetrating eye injury and a full stomach creates a dilemma. Rapid-sequence induction with tracheal intubation is advisable, but the use of succinylcholine is contraindicated theoretically as it produces an increase in IOP which could expel the ocular contents. It may be possible to delay surgery for a few hours, but following trauma, gastric emptying is not assured in the usual time-scale. Drugs which facilitate gastric emptying such as metoclopramide may help. In choosing a muscle relaxant for tracheal intubation, the anticipated visual prognosis and the risks of further damage to the eye must be weighed against the life-threatening dangers of pulmonary aspiration. If it is anticipated that tracheal intubation will be uneventful, a large dose of non-depolarizing muscle relaxant (rocuronium may be the most appropriate for this purpose) may be substituted for succinylcholine in the usual rapid-sequence technique. Coughing and straining must be avoided. Care should be taken not to exert pressure on the injured eye with the face mask during preoxygenation. If intubation is difficult and ventilation with a face mask is not efficient, the resulting hypoxaemia and hypercapnia may cause more damage to the eye than a single dose of succinylcholine.

Anaesthetic management during surgery conforms to the pattern used for other intraocular procedures. Extubation should be performed with the patient in the lateral position and almost awake.

RETINAL SURGERY

Retinal surgery may be either extraocular or intraocular or a combination of both. General anaesthesia is used frequently for retinal surgery. Patients are often in younger age groups and the procedures may take longer than anterior segment surgery. Patients are liable to become uncomfortable and restless if required to lie still on a hard operating table for too long. Increasingly, local anaesthesia is used in the medically compromised patient or for vitrectomies and retinal procedures of short duration. Careful monitoring is needed as the oculocardiac reflex is not blocked reliably by local anaesthetic. The surgeon can readily use a sub-Tenon's injection to top up the local anaesthetic if it starts to diminish.

As fundal examination, vitrectomy and laser therapy are carried out in the dark, the anaesthetist must ensure that there is sufficient lighting to conduct anaesthesia safely. Protective goggles of correct filtration specification for the type of laser being used *must* be worn by all theatre staff during laser therapy.

Towards the end of an intraocular vitrectomy retinal detachment procedure, the surgeon may inject a bubble of sulphur hexafluoride (SF_6) or perfluoropropane (C_3F_8) into the eye to tamponade the retina. Some minutes before this is done, the anaesthetist must discontinue administration of nitrous oxide but continue to maintain anaesthesia with air, oxygen and additional volatile agent. The use of a continuous intravenous propofol technique is a suitable alternative. If the nitrous oxide is not eliminated beforehand, it equilibrates with the tamponading gas during the operation, but at the end of the anaesthetic the nitrous oxide diffuses out and reduces the pressure in the gas bubble. The inhaled anaesthetic gas mixture at the time of injection of SF_6 or C_3F_8 should approximate as nearly as possible to room air. As soon as there is sufficient recovery from anaesthesia, the patient is turned to the prone position so that the bubble exerts upward pressure on the area of the retinal detachment.

Silicone oil may be used for a similar effect. These patients have to return at a later date for removal of the oil under anaesthesia. If it stays in the eye too long it may emulsify and obscure vision or block the drainage of the anterior chamber, causing an increase in the IOP. Patients with intraocular tamponading gas bubbles are in danger from the bubble expanding and the globe rupturing if subsequent nitrous oxide anaesthesia is administered for purposes other than surgery on the same eye. This effect may last for several weeks after insertion of the gas bubble and if there is any doubt the ophthalmologist should be consulted beforehand.

LOCAL ANAESTHESIA

Serious reactions to local orbital anaesthesia are rare but have been well documented. The need to monitor patients closely is now well recognized. Better quality of patient care, quicker turnaround times and excellent operating conditions may be achieved by the skilled anaesthetist trained in local orbital anaesthesia techniques. A detailed knowledge of the anatomy of the eye is a prerequisite (Fig. 32.2).

APPLIED ANATOMY OF THE ORBIT

The orbit is a four-sided bony pyramid with its base pointing anteriorly and its apex posteromedially. The medial walls of the right and left orbits are parallel to each other (Figs 32.3, 32.4). The mean distance from the inferior orbital margin to the apex is 55 mm. This has important implications when injections are made into the orbit. The deeper the injection, the narrower is the space, and the greater the chance of causing damage to the structures within. The inferotemporal quadrant is relatively avascular and is probably the safest approach for orbital injections.

Squeezing and closing of the eyelids are controlled by the zygomatic branch of the facial nerve (VII), which supplies the motor innervation to the orbicularis oculi muscle. This nerve emerges from the foramen spinosum at the base of the skull, anterior to the mastoid and behind the earlobe. It passes through the parotid gland before crossing the condyle of the mandible, then passes superficial to the zygoma and malar bone before its terminal fibres ramify to supply the deep surface of the orbicularis oculi. The facial nerve also supplies secretomotor parasympathetic fibres to the lacrimal glands, and glands of the nasal and palatine mucosa.

Movement of the globe is controlled by the six extraocular muscles. The motor nerves which control these muscles emerge from the skull through the superior orbital fissure. The common tendinous ring forms the fibrous origin of the four rectus muscles at the apex of the orbital cone. The trochlear nerve (IV) emerges through the superior orbital fissure *outside* the common tendinous ring and supplies the superior oblique muscle. All the other motor nerves to the extraocular muscles pass *inside* the common tendinous ring and are situated inside the cone. The ophthalmic division of the oculomotor nerve (III) divides into superior and inferior branches before emerging from the superior orbital fissure. The superior branch supplies the superior rectus and the levator palpebrae superioris muscles. The inferior branch divides into three to supply the medial rectus, the inferior rectus and the inferior oblique muscles. The abducent nerve (VI) emerges from the superior orbital fissure beneath the inferior branch of the oculomotor nerve to supply the lateral rectus muscle.

Sensation to the eyeball is supplied through the ophthalmic division of the trigeminal nerve (V). Just before entering the orbit, it divides into three branches: lacrimal, frontal and nasociliary. The nasociliary nerve is sensory to the entire eyeball. It emerges through the superior orbital fissure between the superior and inferior branches of the oculomotor nerve and passes *through* the common tendinous ring. Two long ciliary nerves give branches to the ciliary ganglion and, with the short ciliary nerves, transmit sensation from the cornea, iris and ciliary muscle. Some sensation from the lateral conjunctiva is transmitted through the

lacrimal nerve and from the upper palpebral conjunctiva via the frontal nerve. Both nerves are outside the cone.

The cone is the area between the four rectus muscles and the posterior surface of the globe. The muscles arise from a fibrous ring which bridges over the superior orbital fissure. Through this common tendinous ring pass the optic nerve, the ophthalmic artery, the two divisions of the oculomotor nerve, the nasociliary nerve and the abducent nerve. The superior and inferior ophthalmic veins may also pass through the ring. Tenon's capsule or bulbar fascia is a thin membrane that envelops the eyeball from the optic nerve to the sclerocorneal junction, separating it from the orbital fat and forming a socket in which it moves. The sheaths of the rectus muscles interconnect in the perimysium in a complex and variable manner and form the walls of the cone. Well-defined expansions laterally and medially form the check ligaments, and inferiorly a hammock-like expansion forms the suspensory Lockwood's ligament.

SELECTION OF PATIENTS FOR LOCAL ANAESTHESIA

Local anaesthesia is the usual choice for most people undergoing cataract surgery. This preferred type of anaesthetic should be discussed by the ophthalmologist when he first sees the patient. The young, the mentally unstable and those with physical disabilities that

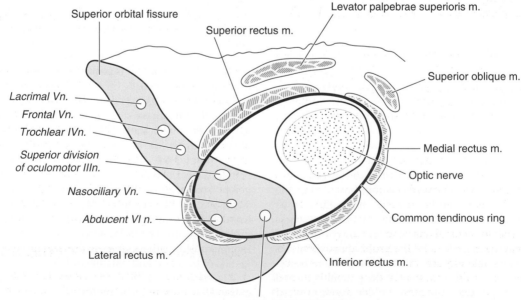

Fig. 32.2
Anatomy of the right orbit: relationship of the four rectus muscles and the apex of the cone to the orbital nerve supply.

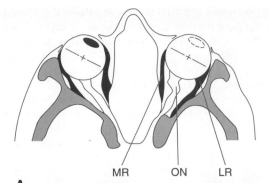

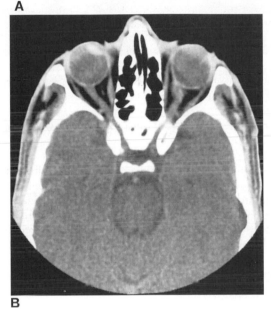

Fig. 32.3
Diagram (**A**) and CT scan (**B**) of orbits taken in coronal view with the subject looking to the right. Note the almost parallel sides of the medial orbital walls; optic nerve movement to left; the optic nerve canal and optic nerve chiasma; the proximity of the midbrain; and that the cataract has been removed from the right eye. MR, medial rectus muscle; LR, lateral rectus muscle; ON, optic nerve.

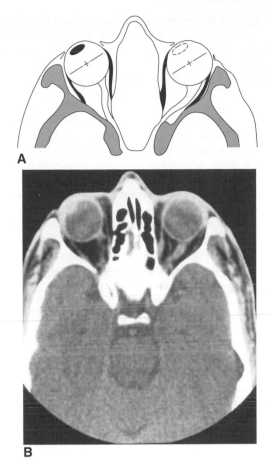

Fig. 32.4
Diagram (**A**) and CAT scan (**B**) of the same patient as in Fig. 32.3, now looking to the left. Note the optic nerve movement to the right.

prevent them from lying still may be unsuitable. Warfarin therapy is not considered an absolute contraindication to local anaesthesia provided that preoperative INR values are in the therapeutic target range. There are some patients whose chronic illness poses too severe a risk for general anaesthesia, but whose quality of life may be improved by the proposed surgery. The chance of having surgery under local anaesthesia need not be denied to this group. Operating conditions may not always be ideal. Surgery of brief duration by an experienced surgeon may be successful.

Premedication is not usually necessary, but if needed may be given intravenously just before the local anaesthetic block is inserted. Caution should be exercised with the dose of benzodiazepine in the elderly. There is a danger that the oversedated patient may fall asleep during surgery, only to wake up suddenly and, in confusion, try to sit up. Very small increments of propofol (10 mg or less) may be given to anxious patients; midazolam in small doses (1 mg or less) or the two in combination may be very effective. If the patient is sufficiently relaxed and not straining at the time of injection of the local anaesthetic, the chances of complications such as orbital haemorrhage may be reduced.

AXIAL LENGTH AND EYE MOVEMENTS

It is good practice at the time of the preoperative visit to check the axial length of the eyeball. All patients scheduled for fitting of an intraocular lens will have an ultrasound scan and this measurement will have been recorded. There is an increased danger of global perforation in the high myope and patients with an axial length in excess of 25 mm should be treated with caution (Figs 32.5, 32.6). Patients scheduled for glaucoma surgery are not usually scanned preoperatively, but rarely have a long axial length. The extraocular movements and facial nerve function should be checked and recorded. It is not unknown for a patient with a pre-existing Bell's palsy to try to implicate a subsequent facial nerve block. Myopathy of one or more of the extraocular muscles following the inadvertent injection of local anaesthetic into the muscle has been recorded. This complication is more likely to occur if the more concentrated long-acting local anaesthetic agents are used. Recent evidence suggests that the addition of hyaluronidase to the local anaesthetic solution will significantly reduce the incidence of this complication.

CONDITIONS FOR PERFORMING LOCAL EYE BLOCKS

The patient's medical history should be obtained and the patient should be in optimal health. The staff

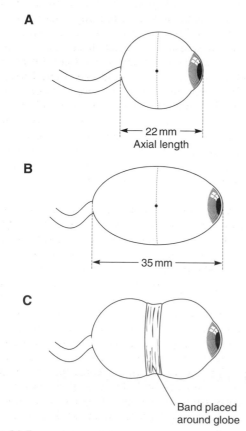

Fig. 32.5
Eyeballs of various shapes. **(A)** Normal eyeball. **(B)** High myope. **(C)** Scleral buckle applied after surgery for retinal detachment.

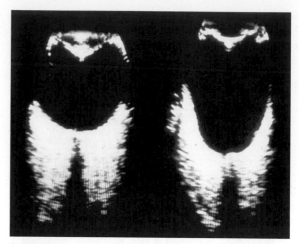

Fig. 32.6
Ultrasound scans of a normal eyeball (left) and a high myope (right).

should establish a friendly rapport with the patient, who should be allowed to keep dentures and hearing aids in place.

A suitable vein should be cannulated if a sharp needle intraorbital technique is planned. It is essential that full cardiopulmonary resuscitation equipment is immediately available and that the medical personnel who undertake these blocks are familiar with resuscitation techniques. Appropriate monitoring should be used.

LOCAL ANAESTHETIC AGENTS AND ADJUNCTS

The ideal local anaesthetic agent should be safe and painless to inject. It should quickly block motor and sensory nerves. The duration should be long enough to perform the operation but not so long as to cause persistent postoperative diplopia.

Lidocaine 2% is safe and produces effective motor and sensory blocks. Bupivacaine has been largely superseded by its isomer levobupivacaine which has less propensity for causing cardiovascular side-effects. It may be used in 0.5% or 0.75% concentrations. Its onset of action is slower than that of lidocaine but it has a longer duration of action. The more concentrated solutions are liable to cause prolonged diplopia until the morning after surgery, or myopathy if injected directly into one of the extraocular muscles.

Prilocaine 2–4% has a rapid onset of action, few side-effects and a duration of action comparable with that of bupivacaine. Ropivacaine 1% has been shown to be effective.

Local anaesthetic mixtures of equal volumes of 2% lidocaine and either 0.5% or 0.75% levobupivacaine are commonly used for longer procedures. This combination has the dual effect of the quick onset of action of lidocaine with the prolonged postoperative analgesic effect of levobupivacaine.

Topical anaesthesia with 1% tetracaine, 0.4% oxybuprocaine eyedrops or other topical local anaesthetic may be used for minor surgery to the conjunctiva if akinesia of the globe is not necessary. Proxymetacaine 0.5% drops sting less on insertion but may not be so efficacious. Topical local anaesthetics may cause dehydration and temporary clouding of the cornea.

The addition of hyaluronidase to the local anaesthetic used for intraconal blocks improves efficacy. With hyaluronidase, an injectate placed more anteriorly (and therefore more safely) in the orbit diffuses to the apex to block the relevant nerves as they emerge. A dose of hyaluronidase of as little as 7.5 units in each 1 mL of local anaesthetic is optimal. The advantage of using hyaluronidase in extraconal anaesthesia has not been clearly shown.

Vasoconstrictors such as epinephrine and felypressin may be added to the injectate. They improve the intensity and duration of the block and may reduce the incidence of haemorrhage. There is a small risk that retinal circulation may be impaired by the vasoconstrictor action on the ophthalmic artery.

pH adjustment of levobupivacaine and lidocaine by the addition of sodium bicarbonate allows more of the local anaesthetic solution to exist in the uncharged form, facilitating faster onset and less discomfort. Warming the anaesthetic solution may lessen the discomfort of injection.

Freshly prepared, preservative-free anaesthetic mixtures are preferable to the preprepared mixtures.

LOCAL ANAESTHESIA TECHNIQUES FOR INTRAOCULAR SURGERY

TOPICAL ANAESTHESIA

Ophthalmic regional anaesthesia should provide conditions appropriate for the surgeon's needs and planned surgery. The rapid advance in surgical techniques in recent years has necessitated rethinking of anaesthesia requirements. These advances have been particularly noticed in the field of cataract surgery. For soft, early cataracts, phacoemulsification of the old lens with an ultrasound probe and the insertion of a small folding plastic artificial lens is now the operation of choice. With this type of surgery, anaesthesia that gives akinesia and a lowered intraocular pressure is no longer an essential requirement. It is less invasive to use topical and intracameral anaesthesia. Topical

viscous local anaesthetic drops containing sodium hyaluronate 0.3% and 2% lidocaine in a phosphate buffered solution last longer and, by hydrating the cornea, prevent clouding which is inherent in other topical formulations. Intracameral analgesia is provided by 1% lidocaine in 1.5% sodium hyaluronate.

EXTRACONAL, INTRACONAL OR SUB-TENON'S ANAESTHESIA

Many different techniques and ingredients may be used to achieve the aims of akinesia, analgesia and a soft eyeball. The anaesthetist must learn a suitable technique under the supervision of an experienced practitioner.

Three different methods are practised: extraconal (peribulbar), intraconal (retrobulbar) and sub Tenon's anaesthesia.

Intraconal anaesthesia places the injectate in the fatty compartment which surrounds the nerve to be blocked, whereas extraconal techniques rely on variable diffusion across connective tissue septa. Periconal techniques were introduced more recently in the expectation that the incidence of complications would be reduced, but this expectation has not been realized. Periconal anaesthesia takes longer to achieve the same degree of akinesia and analgesia than intraconal anaesthesia. In practice the differentiation between retrobulbar and peribulbar is more semantic than actual. If the onset of anaesthesia is rapid with a peribulbar anaesthetic, then the chances are that it has found a direct pathway or been injected directly into the cone. Sub-Tenon's injections involve a minor surgical procedure, and although avoiding some of the complications of the two other techniques, have their own problems.

All orbital blocks should be performed with the patient looking straight ahead in the primary gaze position. This ensures that the optic nerve is slack and out of the direct line of approaching needles (Figs 32.7–32.9) and that the extraocular muscles are relaxed.

The gauge of needle should be the finest that can be used comfortably. In practice, this would be a 25- or 27-gauge needle, as finer needles are difficult to manipulate and larger needles may cause more pain and damage. Sharp needles are used because blunt needles are painful to insert and cause vasovagal syncope. The operator should consistently use the same volume syringe with the same gauge needle, as it is then possible to feel and judge the resistance to injection. A correctly placed injection has minimal resistance.

Following orbital injection, gentle digital pressure and massage around the globe help to disperse the

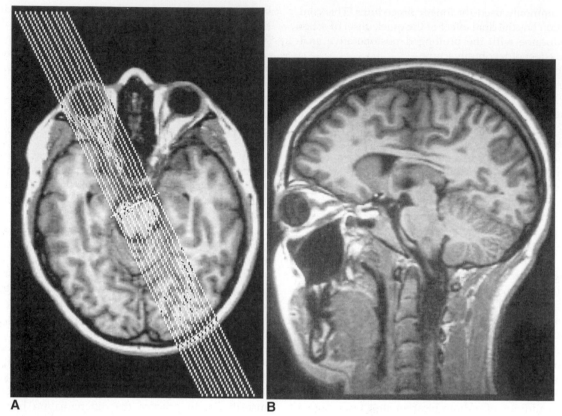

Fig. 32.7
MRI scans of the left orbit. **(A)** Note the oblique angle of scan needed to visualize the optic nerve. **(B)** Note the slackness of the optic nerve with the eyeball in the neutral gaze position.

anaesthetic and reduce IOP. Extraocular volume is reduced further by application of a pressure-reducing device such as Honan's balloon. This may be applied for a period of 20 min or longer, at a pressure of no greater than 35 mmHg. At this pressure, blood supply to the eyeball is assured. The balloon should be removed just before surgery. The low IOP facilitates surgery but the effect lasts for only a short time.

Extraconal (peribulbar) anaesthesia

These techniques rely on the placement of relatively large volumes and high concentrations of local anaesthetic outside the cone. The anaesthetic mixture takes time to diffuse through the connective tissue layers of the cone. Spread of the anaesthetic superficially ensures that the terminal fibres of the facial nerve are blocked as they enter the orbicularis oculi. Most peribulbar methods require two initial injections, each of about 5 mL of local anaesthetic. The volume

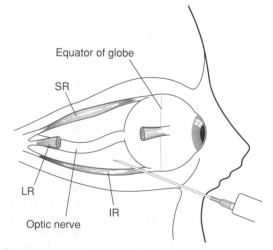

Fig. 32.8
Intraconal injection is placed between the inferior border of the lateral rectus and the inferior rectus. SR, superior rectus; LR, lateral rectus; IR, inferior rectus.

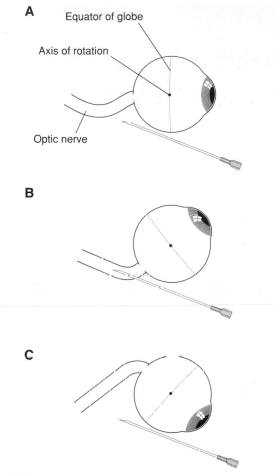

Fig. 32.9
Movements of the optic nerve in relation to eyeball movement when the needle is introduced into the cone from the inferotemporal quadrant. **(A)** Primary gaze. **(B)** Upwards and inwards. **(C)** Downwards and outwards.

injected depends on the shape of the orbit. The inferotemporal injection should be made to a depth of no more than 30 mm from the infraorbital margin using a fine 25-gauge or smaller needle. The safest sites for the injections are in the inferotemporal quadrant and just medial to the medial canthus. The inferotemporal injection may be perconjunctival or percutaneous. Topical local anaesthetic drops should be applied to the conjunctiva before injecting. The superonasal quadrant should be avoided, as injection at this site may damage the trochlear apparatus or cause haemorrhage. After the injections, a pressure-reducing device should be applied to the eye for 10 min before checking again for akinesia. Additional injections may be necessary.

Intraconal (retrobulbar) anaesthesia

Intraconal injection

The intraconal injection may be inserted (see Fig. 32.8) with the patient looking straight ahead. The anaesthetist uses one index finger to palpate the groove between the eyeball and the inferolateral orbital margin and gently displaces the eyeball superiorly. A fine retrobulbar needle on a 5 mL syringe of local anaesthetic is inserted perpendicularly until the point is safely past the equator of the globe. The point is then directed superomedially and floats into the cone with minimal resistance. After aspiration, 2–4 mL of local anaesthetic are injected very slowly. The syringe and needle are then withdrawn in the reverse direction to which they were inserted. The last 1–3 mL of local anaesthetic are injected just under the orbicularis oculi muscle, where it spreads to block the terminal fibres of the facial nerve and enhance the facial nerve block. A single-shot local anaesthetic with intraconal and suborbicularis injection is effective in patients who do not have marked blepharospasm. With marked blepharospasm, a separate facial nerve block may be needed first (see below). Alternatively, if the patient has a very slack lower lid and a wide orbit, the inferotemporal intraconal injection may be made perconjunctivally after prior application of topical anaesthesia.

Facial nerve block

Additional facial nerve blocks are rarely needed but, if required, the facial nerve may be blocked anywhere along its course to the orbit and many different methods have been described. Nadbath described blocking the nerve as it emerges from the stylomastoid foramen, but this technique has many unwanted side-effects. O'Brien blocked the facial nerve as it passed over the condyle of the mandible. Atkinson infiltrated over the zygoma, and Van Lint infiltrated the orbit. The simplest method is to use the most prominent part of the zygoma, midway between the tragus of the ear and the lateral orbital margin, as the landmark. A 25-gauge 30 mm needle on a 5 mL syringe containing the local anaesthetic mixture is inserted perpendicularly down to the zygoma, withdrawn from the periosteum and aspirated. A volume of 3–5 mL is injected lateral to the lateral orbital margin. Gentle massage to the wheal that is raised helps to spread the local anaesthetic and ensures that there is no bleeding.

Sub-Tenon's anaesthesia

This procedure requires some surgical dexterity and a relatively cooperative patient. Its popularity with anaesthetists has increased. Topical anaesthetic drops are applied to the conjunctiva and a speculum inserted. Using forceps and a blunt-pointed pair of scissors, a small incision is made in the inferomedial conjunctiva. A special curved, blunt-pointed cannula is then passed into the sub-Tenon's space and 1–3 mL of anaesthetic are introduced. This method reduces the risk of CNS spread, optic nerve damage and global puncture but may be more likely to cause superficial haemorrhage. Akinesia may take longer to achieve. It cannot be used if the patient has had previous external retinal banding procedures performed; intraconal anaesthesia would be indicated instead.

COMPLICATIONS OF LOCAL ANAESTHESIA

Haemorrhage

Haemorrhage is a serious complication of both intraconal and extraconal anaesthesia, and sub-Tenon's anaesthesia. It occurs with a frequency of between 0.1 and 3%. Despite this, eventual visual outcome after surgery is not significantly worse than in patients who have uncomplicated anaesthesia. The haemorrhage may be either venous or arterial in origin and may be concealed or revealed. Extravasation of blood into the periorbital tissues increases the tissue volume and pressure. This is transmitted to the globe, raising the intraocular tension and creating difficult and dangerous conditions for intraocular surgery (Fig. 32.10).

Venous haemorrhage usually presents as markedly bloodstained chemosis and raised IOP. It may be possible to reduce the IOP by digital massage and cautious application of an IOP-reducing device to such an extent that surgery may proceed safely. Before the decision is made to proceed with surgery or postpone it for a few days, it is advisable to measure and record IOP.

Arterial haemorrhage is a more serious complication and urgent measures must be taken to stop the haemorrhage and reduce the seriously elevated IOP. Firm digital pressure usually stops the bleeding and, when it has been arrested, consideration must be given to reducing the IOP so that the blood supply to the retina is not jeopardized. Lateral canthotomy, intravenous acetazolamide, intravenous mannitol or even paracentesis may need to be considered in consultation with the ophthalmologist.

Prevention of haemorrhage

Unduly anxious patients may strain while the procedure is taking place. The blood vessels behind the eye become engorged and are readily punctured. The anxious,

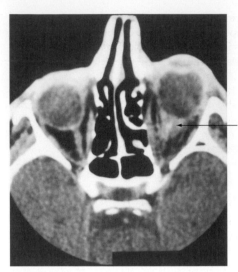

Concealed haemorrhage

Fig. 32.10
CT scan taken in coronal section of a patient following an intraconal haemorrhage. Note the marked proptosis of the right eye and the confined space occupied by the haemorrhage. This was a concealed haemorrhage as, despite elevated intraocular pressure and proptosis, no signs of bleeding or bruising were evident until the next day.

straining patient may need some sedation and should be encouraged to breathe quietly through an open mouth and so prevent the Valsalva manoeuvre. The fewer injections that are made into the orbit, the less is the chance of damaging a blood vessel. Cutting and slicing movements at the needle tip should be avoided. Fine needles are less traumatic than thicker ones. Deep intraorbital injections must be avoided. The inferotemporal quadrant has fewer blood vessels and is less hazardous. It is advisable to apply firm digital pressure to the orbit as soon as the needle is withdrawn after any intraorbital injection, as this reduces any tendency to ooze.

Central spread

Mechanism

The cerebral dura mater provides a tubular sheath for the optic nerve as it passes through the optic foramen. This sheath fuses to the epineurium of the optic nerve and is continuous with the sclera, providing a potential conduit for local anaesthetic to pass subdurally to the brain. Central spread occurs if the needle tip has perforated the optic nerve sheath and injection is made. Even a tiny volume injected under the optic nerve sheath may pass to the central nervous system and/or cross the optic chiasma to the opposite eye and may cause life-threatening sequelae. The time of onset of symptoms is variable, but any major sequelae develop usually in the first 15 min after injection. It is advisable that the patient's face is not covered up on the operating table for at least this interval after the block has been inserted.

Another mechanism for central spread may occur on rare occasions if an orbital artery is cannulated by the needle tip. The local anaesthetic is injected in a retrograde fashion up the artery until it meets a branch, where it can then flow in a cephalad direction. The onset of central nervous system toxicity is almost instantaneous if this mechanism is invoked; in addition, orbital haemorrhage can be expected.

Signs and symptoms of central spread

The symptomatology of central spread is varied and depends upon which part of the central nervous system is affected by the local anaesthetic. As a result of the anatomical proximity of the optic nerve to the midbrain (see Fig. 32.3) it is usual for this area to be involved. A range of different signs and symptoms has been described, involving the cardiovascular and respiratory systems, temperature regulation, vomiting, temporary hemiplegia, aphasia and generalized convulsions. Palsy of the contralateral oculomotor and trochlear nerves with amaurosis (loss of vision) is pathognomonic of central nervous system spread and should be sought in any patient whose response to questions following block are not as crisp as they were beforehand.

Treatment of central spread

The treatment is symptomatic throughout the duration of effect of the local anaesthetic drug. With longer-acting local anaesthetic agents, treatment may be required for 60–90 min. The patient must be monitored intensively. Bradycardia requires treatment with an anticholinergic drug. Asystole has been reported rarely, but if it occurs, intravenous epinephrine and sustained cardiac massage are required. Respiratory depression or apnoea necessitates ventilatory support and administration of supplementary oxygen. Convulsions are treated conveniently with intravenous sodium thiopental and conversion to general anaesthesia. When vital signs are stable, it may be feasible to continue with the proposed surgery under general anaesthesia in the knowledge that the patient needs continuing intensive support until the local anaesthetic action has terminated.

Prevention of central spread

Intraconal or extraconal injections should always be made with the patient looking straight ahead in the primary gaze position (see Fig. 32.9). The optic nerve is then slack (see Fig 32.8) and out of the way of the advancing needle. If the needle encounters the optic nerve in this position, it is unlikely to damage or perforate its sheath, as slackness in the structure allows the nerve to be pushed aside. If the eyeball is directed away from the primary gaze position in any other extreme direction, the optic nerve is stretched. When stretched, the nerve cannot be easily pushed aside. The most dangerous position is when the patient looks upwards and inwards, as this presents the stretched nerve to a needle directed from the inferotemporal quadrant. As in the prevention of haemorrhage, injections should not be made too deeply into the orbit, where the optic nerve is tethered to its sheaths as it emerges through the optic foramen. It is good practice to withdraw the needle by 1 mm from its maximum depth before injection is made. If the tip had been resting against the optic nerve sheath, this manoeuvre withdraws the tip to a safer position.

Puncture of the eyeball

Global puncture is a serious complication of local anaesthesia for eye surgery. It has been reported following both intraconal and extraconal injections and even following local anaesthesia for more minor procedures such as eyelid surgery. With appropriate care, it should be a very rare complication. The sclera is a tough structure and in most cases is not perforated easily.

Puncture of the eyeball is most likely to occur in patients with high myopia, previous retinal banding, posterior staphyloma or a deeply sunken eye with a narrow orbit (see Fig. 32.5).

Not all eyeballs are the same length and not all orbits are the same shape. In most patients who present for cataract surgery, an ultrasound measure is made of the axial length of the eyeball to calculate the power of the intraocular lens. Normal eyeballs have an axial length of 20–24 mm. High myopes have much longer axial lengths of 25–35 mm and extreme caution should be exercised in these patients. The axial length in patients for glaucoma surgery is not usually measured.

Global puncture is often a double puncture of the posterior segment of the eyeball; the tip of the needle is in the orbit at the time of injection and the local anaesthetic block may be good. Puncture is usually recognized at the time of surgery and presents as an exceptionally soft eye. In cataract surgery, if the block is good, the surgeon should be encouraged to proceed with the lensectomy but to stitch up the eye with twice as many sutures as normal. Without lensectomy, it may not be possible to observe the damage to the posterior segment of the eye. It can be expected that the needle track through the vitreous will form a band of scar tissue. If this is not excised, it contracts and detaches the retina, sometimes causing sudden total blindness in the affected eye.

Optic nerve damage

Fortunately, this is a rare complication which results usually from obstruction of the central retinal artery. This artery is the first and smallest branch of the ophthalmic artery, arising from that vessel as it lies below the optic nerve. It runs for a short distance within the dural sheath of the optic nerve and about 35 mm from the orbital margin, pierces the nerve and runs forward in the centre of the nerve to the retina. Damage to the artery may cause bleeding into the confined space of the optic nerve sheath, compressing and obstructing blood flow. If the complication is recognized soon enough, it may be possible to perform surgical decompression of the optic nerve.

Myopathy of the extraocular muscles

The inadvertent injection of a long-acting local anaesthetic into any extraocular muscle body may result in prolonged weakness, fibrosis or even necrosis of the muscle. The inferotemporal approach places the needle between the lateral and inferior rectus muscles and is the safest site for intraorbital injections. Recent evidence suggests that the addition of hualuronidase to the injectate will help to disperse the solution before lasting damage can be done. Persistent diplopia following local anaesthesia should be investigated with a suitable scan as urgent surgical intervention to the affected muscle may be required.

Vasovagal syncope

This is more likely to occur in young and anxious patients when eye blocks are administered. Painful injection with a blunt Atkinson needle may cause this response. It is important that a vein is cannulated before any block is given. Treatment is symptomatic and should include administration of oxygen, intravenous injection of an anticholinergic agent and appropriate positioning. Differentiation from central spread should be made by testing vision and extraocular movements in the opposite eye.

EXTRAOCULAR PROCEDURES

ANAESTHESIA FOR STRABISMUS SURGERY

The commonest procedure in paediatric ophthalmic surgery is correction of squint. The eye should be immobile with absent muscle tone. The use of a nondepolarizing muscle relaxant may be preferred as this prevents variation in muscle tone which may occur with an imbalance between the depth of anaesthesia and the applied surgical stimulus. Succinylcholine must be avoided. In patients who have had previous strabismus surgery or orbital trauma, the surgeon may need to differentiate between paretic and restricted eye movement by performing a forced duction test. Absence of muscle tone is necessary for this test to be performed accurately. If the surgeon is repairing the strabismus with an adjustable suture technique, it is also important that all traces of muscle relaxant have been eliminated by the time the suture is adjusted.

Squint and ptosis are presenting signs of the progressive external ophthalmoplegia (PEO) syndrome. Patients with this syndrome may have marked cardiac and respiratory decompensation and pose a significant hazard for anaesthesia. Preoperative pulmonary function testing is advisable. Muscular dystrophy and myasthenia gravis may also present with ptosis and strabismus.

Botulinum toxin is occasionally administered in the treatment of strabismus and blepharospasm. Ketamine is a suitable anaesthetic for children scheduled to undergo this procedure, as it does not reduce muscle power; the surgeon tests muscle power intraoperatively.

There is a rare association between malignant hyperthermia and strabismus.

Oculocardiac reflex

This reflex may be triggered by extraorbital muscle traction, causing severe bradycardia or even cardiac arrest. It is more pronounced in young people. Some anaesthetists give prophylactic atropine or glycopyrrolate at induction. When it occurs, the surgical stimulus must be suspended until the heart rate has recovered, and anticholinergic drugs given if necessary. A heart rate monitor which the surgeon can hear is useful.

Postoperative nausea and vomiting

The incidence of postoperative nausea and vomiting following squint surgery is high. Various antiemetic drugs and techniques are commonly used. As most of these operations are carried out as a day-surgery procedure under general anaesthesia, it is important to avoid preparations which cause excessive sedation.

EXAMINATION UNDER ANAESTHESIA

Children may require repeated examinations under anaesthesia (EUAs). If the purpose of the EUA is to measure IOP, as may be the case in neonates with congenital glaucoma, the method of anaesthesia must be discussed with the surgeon. Inhalational anaesthesia by mask is often satisfactory, but the surgeon may wish to measure IOP while the patient is still lightly anaesthetized, before IOP is reduced by the effects of anaesthetic drugs. Painless preoperative intravenous cannulation using EMLA local anaesthetic cream has made i.v. induction feasible for most children. The use of the laryngeal mask is ideal. Ketamine does not lower the IOP, but it is a long-acting anaesthetic and may cause hallucinations and nightmares postoperatively; it should be reserved for special cases.

DACROCYSTORHINOSTOMY

Open dacrocystorhinostomy (DCR) is carried out usually under general anaesthesia because the operation is frequently bilateral and may be complicated by haemorrhage. A laryngeal mask or a tracheal tube and throat pack may be necessary as blood may trickle down the nasopharynx. The nostril(s) may be packed with cocaine paste or another suitable vasoconstrictor before operation. Care must be taken not to exceed recommended dose levels of cocaine. The operation site may be infiltrated with epinephrine by the surgeon and caution is necessary with the use of halothane in this event.

The use of lasers for DCR has largely eliminated haemorrhage and local anaesthesia is preferable if open surgery is not planned.

DRUG INTERACTIONS

Patients with eye disease often use systemic or topical medications which may pose potential problems for the anaesthetist. Systemic absorption of potent eyedrops is reduced if the lacrimal puncta are occluded digitally while the drops are being inserted.

Cyclopentolate is an antimuscarinic with an action of up to 24 h; 1% drops are used to dilate the pupil and paralyse the ciliary muscle before surgery. Excessive systemic absorption causes toxic effects similar to those associated with an overdose of atropine. The young and the very old are particularly susceptible.

Phenylephrine is a direct-acting α-adrenergic stimulant and has weak β-effects; 2.5% or 10% drops are used to dilate the pupil. Systemic effects may cause an increase in myocardial irritability and hypertension. Dangerous interactions with monoamine oxidase inhibitors may occur.

Epinephrine is used intraoperatively in a dilute solution by the surgeon to reduce excessive bleeding.

Systemic absorption may be significant. Caution is necessary with halothane.

Timolol or other β-blocking agents are used topically to treat glaucoma. There may be significant systemic absorption, thereby exacerbating asthma and chronic obstructive airways disease. Precautions should be observed as for systemic β-adrenergic blocking drugs.

Ecothiopate iodide (phospholine iodide) is a potent anticholinesterase and is used rarely in the treatment of glaucoma. It depletes pseudocholinesterase and thus prolongs the action of succinylcholine.

Botulinum toxin A is an effective treatment in a variety of neuromuscular conditions including strabismus. It causes a decrease in skeletal muscle power by binding irreversibly to receptor sites on the cholinergic nerve terminal. Function does not return until new motor end-plates have formed. When injected locally into the extraocular muscle(s), the toxin binds rapidly and firmly to the tissue; in the doses used normally, it should not cause systemic side-effects.

Mannitol is an osmotic diuretic which reduces the volume of the vitreous humour. Infusions in doses of up to $1.5\,g\,kg^{-1}$ are given before surgery over a period of 30–45 min. There is an initial increase in circulating blood volume followed by a diuresis and decrease in blood volume. When combined with the induction of general anaesthesia, haemodynamic instability may occur. Particular caution must be exercised in patients with cardiovascular disease. A urinary catheter should be inserted preoperatively if patients are to receive mannitol in this way.

Acetazolamide, a carbonic anhydrase inhibitor, is used in the medical treatment of glaucoma. Its main actions are to reduce the production of aqueous humour and to facilitate drainage. It is of questionable value during surgery because it results in increased intrachoroidal vascular volume. Congenital glaucoma is treated with acetazolamide and repeated surgery. Metabolic acidosis may be a serious consequence of this treatment and the neonate presenting for anaesthesia for glaucoma surgery must be treated with special care. Any respiratory depression caused by sedatives, opioids or anaesthesia reduces the compensatory respiratory alkalosis. It may be advisable to perform blood gas analysis before anaesthesia.

FURTHER READING

Barry Smith G, Hamilton R C, Carr C A 1996 Ophthalmic anaesthesia: a practical handbook, 2nd edn. Arnold, London
Royal College of Anaesthetists and Royal College of Opthalmologists 2001. Local anaesthesia for intraocular surgery

33 Dental anaesthesia

Anaesthesia and dentistry have a long historical association. Some of the first anaesthetics given were for dental extractions and the use of anaesthesia was quickly taken into dental practice in the late nineteenth century. Dental anaesthetic techniques have evolved in parallel with the changes in practice in other aspects of anaesthesia. The days of the single-operator anaesthetist and the 'black gas' induction (100% nitrous oxide) are now long gone. For many years, dental anaesthesia was practised in a variety of sites varying from within dental schools to remote dental practices, with anaesthesia provided by anaesthetists, medical practitioners or indeed dentists. In the past 10–15 years a considerable change in routine dental practice has occurred.

Anaesthesia and dentistry cover three main types of surgery: first, outpatient anaesthesia for simple extractions of teeth, mainly in children ('dental chair anaesthesia'); secondly, day-case anaesthesia for straightforward extractions of molars or for minor oral surgery; and thirdly, inpatient emergency or elective treatment for more complicated extractions or oral surgical procedures. These three areas of anaesthetic practice are covered in this chapter. In addition, sedation techniques are described, as they are of increasing importance as a result of the changes in dental anaesthetic practice in the UK.

The provision of dental anaesthetic and sedation services was the subject of a major report by the Department of Health (1991). The recommendations of this report had far-reaching consequences on the provision of dental anaesthetic services and it has affected both anaesthetists and dentists. The recommendations within this report covered general anaesthesia, sedation and resuscitation. With regard to general anaesthesia, the report stated that its use should be avoided wherever possible and the same standards in respect of personnel, premises and equipment should apply wherever the anaesthetic is being administered. It further recommended that all anaesthetics should be administered by an accredited anaesthetist and that anaesthetic training should include specific experience in dental anaesthesia. It also made recommendations on the standard of equipment, techniques and facilities. In late 1998, the General Dental Council (GDC) amended its guidance to dentists in respect of general anaesthesia. It strengthened its previous statement that 'general anaesthesia is a procedure which is never without risk' to a clear statement that general anaesthesia should only be considered if there is an overriding clinical need and alternative methods have been explained. The guidance also put greater emphasis on the responsibilities of the dentist in providing the equipment and staff to a level similar to that found in hospital. The effect of this ruling and the publication of *Standards and guidelines for general anaesthesia in dentistry* by the Royal College of Anaesthetists (1999) and *A conscious decision: a review of the use of general anaesthesia and sedation in primary dental care* by the Department of Health (2000) have effectively concentrated the provision of anaesthesia for dental surgery to centralized facilities. Both reports stated that sedation should be used in preference to general anaesthesia wherever possible and made further recommendations on training in sedation techniques and on the drugs and techniques to be used. The Department of Health report placed strong emphasis on the teaching, training and assessment of resuscitation skills and resuscitation facilities within dental practices.

OUTPATIENT DENTAL ANAESTHESIA

The use of general anaesthesia for outpatient dental extractions (exodontia) has decreased steadily in England and Wales from a peak of over 2 million per year in the mid-1950s to around 1.2 million per year in 1970 and down to less than 200 000 per year in 1990. The current figure is less than 50 000. This steady decrease reflects several factors, including a general improvement in dental hygiene, a decreasing number of practices providing general anaesthetic services culminating in use of a hospital setting only from mid-2001, and the increased use of local anaesthetic and sedation techniques. The use of general anaesthesia for dental extractions has been much more common in the UK than elsewhere in Europe or North America. However, as noted in the Department of Health report, in the 35 years up to 2000 there were only 7 years in which there was not at least one death resulting from anaesthesia administered in a dental practice. General anaesthetic outpatient dental services are now provided only in centres such as DGHs, dental schools or medical centres.

PATIENT SELECTION

The selection of patients presenting for dental chair anaesthesia should be the same as for patients undergoing any outpatient procedure, i.e. only healthy ASA grade I and II patients are appropriate. The preoperative screening of patients may be particularly difficult as they are referred from a dental practice, but this is the situation in which careful selection of patients is of greatest importance. It is a requirement of the GDC that the dental practitioners involved have an understanding of the anaesthetic implications of common medical conditions and are able to exclude patients with significant cardiac or respiratory disease, renal or hepatic impairment, bleeding disorders or a potentially difficult airway at the time of referral. Patients who do not meet these criteria should be referred to a specialist centre for inpatient care.

The majority of patients are children between the ages of 4 and 10 years presenting for extraction of carious teeth. This group has a low incidence of systemic disease but a high incidence of respiratory tract infections. Dental problems requiring general anaesthesia are relatively uncommon under the age of 3 years, other than trauma to upper incisors ('A's and 'B's) resulting from a fall.

In adults, the indications for general anaesthesia are fewer and include situations where local analgesia is ineffective, such as dental abscess. Another indication for general anaesthesia is for patients who are unable to cooperate with treatment under local analgesia because of mental impairment or physical disability. It is important that this group receives full preoperative assessment in view of coexisting disease and concurrent medication which may influence anaesthesia. The use of general anaesthesia as an option in adults who do not like dental treatment under local analgesia should be abandoned in favour of the use of sedation techniques (see below).

It is important that the nature of the dental surgical procedure undertaken is appropriate for a day case. This implies that the surgery should be of short duration and not so extensive that it is difficult to provide adequate postoperative analgesia.

The patient's social circumstances must be taken into account when offering outpatient treatment. The patient must be accompanied before and after the surgery and supervised by an adult for 24 h. Some patients may need time to make appropriate domestic arrangements.

EQUIPMENT

The site at which outpatient dental anaesthesia is administered should be equipped to the standards required in the day-case anaesthesia report and the Department of Health report; i.e. the facilities for the anaesthetist and a surgeon should match those that would be provided in an inpatient theatre setting. For an anaesthetist, this is best dealt with under the areas of anaesthetic equipment, monitoring and resuscitation equipment.

The equipment necessary includes a modern anaesthetic machine which is capable of providing assisted ventilation if required. If the patients regularly include children, a low-resistance circuit is required. Some older anaesthetic machines included on-demand breathing circuits. These were developed to minimize anaesthetic gas use when the anaesthetist carried gas cylinders from practice to practice and there is no indication for their current use. Other equipment should include a variety of nasal and facial masks, oral and nasal airways, laryngoscopes with a variety of blades, including paediatric, and a range of oral and nasal tracheal tubes. A high-pressure suction unit should be available, preferably separate from the suction used by the dentist. The chair should be capable of head-down tilt and should be movable even in the event of power failure.

The minimum standards for monitoring during anaesthesia should be met (see Table 18.9). Although most of the procedures in dental practice are short, it is very important that monitoring is used in each case. There is a high potential for airway obstruction resulting in hypoxaemia and also a relatively high incidence of cardiac arrhythmias.

A full range of resuscitation equipment must be available; this should include a defibrillator, an emergency drug pack (Table 33.1), facilities for tracheal intubation and full delivery of high-flow oxygen with positive pressure if necessary, e.g. an Ambu or Laerdal bag. The GDC guidelines specify that the anaesthetist, dentist and dental nurse are trained in resuscitation

Table 33.1   List of emergency drugs to be available in sites used for dental anaesthesia

Oxygen
Epinephrine
Lidocaine 1%
Atropine
Calcium chloride
Sodium bicarbonate
Glyceryl trinitrate (tabs or spray)
Aminophylline
Salbutamol inhaler
Chlorphenamine (chlorpheniramine)
Dextrose 50%
Hydrocortisone
Midazolam
Dextrose/saline infusion bag
Colloid infusion bag
Flumazenil*
Naloxone*

* Only if site provides i.v. sedation.

and attend regular refresher courses. It is also recommended that they regularly practise resuscitation procedures as a team.

POTENTIAL PREOPERATIVE PROBLEMS

- Presentation of poorly prepared or inappropriate patients requiring dental treatment.
- High proportion of patients are children who may have upper respiratory tract infection.
- Dental abscesses may lead to a difficult airway.
- Site may have inadequate facilities or equipment.

INDUCTION OF ANAESTHESIA

Anaesthesia may be induced by the inhalational or intravenous route. Traditionally, the inhalational route has been used for young children and the intravenous

route for older children and adults. The introduction of EMLA cream and topical amethocaine has allowed the intravenous route to be used more frequently. However, EMLA cream should be applied 1 h before anticipated cannulation, which may be difficult for outpatients.

Inhalational induction has been described using all the agents in common use. Until recently, halothane was still the most widely used as it has advantages of ease of induction compared with enflurane and isoflurane which are more irritant. However, halothane is also associated with a high incidence of cardiovascular disturbances, in particular arrhythmias, which are more common in the presence of a raised P_aCO_2, a situation which may occur with respiratory depression or if the airway is compromised. Sevoflurane has replaced halothane as the agent of choice because of the ease of inhalational induction and limited cardiovascular and respiratory effects. It is important to note that induction of anaesthesia with sevoflurane leads to a quicker and smoother loss of consciousness than with halothane, but the time to achieve surgical anaesthesia is the same or even slightly longer with sevoflurane (Table 33.2). The use of high concentrations of sevoflurane after loss of consciousness may be accompanied by marked sinus tachycardia, particularly in young children.

Induction of anaesthesia in younger children may be difficult if they become frightened or uncooperative. The risk of this may be minimized by a friendly explanation of what is going to happen and the use of some visual aid such as a well-known cartoon character breathing into an anaesthetic mask. The induction may be made into a game such as blowing up a balloon (reservoir bag). It is often helpful to have one of the child's parents present during induction, having first explained to the parent the sequence of events and what is expected of the parent. The management of a screaming child who does not cooperate with either inhalational or i.v. induction is difficult. There is little to be gained and many potential problems in holding the child down with a mask on the face. This is very distressing for the child, the parents and all the staff involved. The potential for problems during induction is high in a child who has a blocked nose and secretions from crying and who is distressed and tachycardic before the procedure starts. It is best in this situation to delay anaesthesia until the child is calm. This may usually be done by allowing the parents and the child to sit quietly for half an hour to discuss the problem. In the worst cases, it may be better to bring the child back on another day, perhaps using oral premedication.

Following either intravenous or inhalational induction, anaesthesia is maintained usually by spontaneous respiration of an inhalational agent, nitrous

Table 33.2 Comparison of induction of anaesthesia, complications and recovery in children receiving sevoflurane or halothane (*n* = 50 in each group) for dental extractions

	Sevoflurane	Halothane
Time to loss of eyelash reflex (min)	1.5	1.9
Time to prop insertion (min)	3.9	3.5
Respiratory problem (*n*) (coughing, laryngospasm, etc.)	5	5
Arrhythmias		
Bigeminy (*n*)	0	15
Premature ventricular beats (*n*)	3	13
Time from end of operation to eye opening	7.3	7.8

Based on Paris et al (1997).

oxide and oxygen by nasal mask (Fig. 33.1). The use of incremental bolus doses of propofol to maintain anaesthesia during dental anaesthesia has been described and is the choice in some centres. Several studies have shown the benefits of using 50% inspired oxygen concentration in preference to 30%, as this has been shown to decrease the number and severity of hypoxaemic episodes.

THE OPERATION

The sequence of events is as follows:

1. Induction of anaesthesia.
2. Stabilization of the airway with a nasal mask.
3. Positioning of the gag or bite block by the dentist or anaesthetist.
4. Placement of a mouth pack to prevent debris from extracted teeth falling into the airway (Fig. 33.2).
5. Extraction of teeth (Fig. 33.3), if necessary changing sides with repositioning of the bite block and pack.
6. Finishing the operation.
7. Turning the patient on to the side for recovery of consciousness.

As the airway is shared by the dentist and anaesthetist, it is important that both know the requirements of the other. The dentist requires access to all four quadrants of the mouth and also some resistance to the pressure required for extraction of some teeth. In particular, for extraction of teeth from the lower jaw, the downward pressure required may potentially compromise the airway (see Fig. 33.3). The anaesthetist needs to maintain the airway throughout the procedure using the nasal mask. This implies that the anaesthetist needs access to the upper half of the face to place the thumb on the nasal mask, and the airway is maintained by forward lift of the lower jaw with the fingers (see Fig. 33.2). In placing the mouth gag, it is important not to use too large a size as this may make the airway more difficult to maintain. In placing the pack, it is also important that it is not sited too far posteriorly in the mouth such that it compromises the nasal airway (see Fig. 33.2). The responsibility for placing the pack and gag varies from centre to centre between the anaesthetist and the dentist. Whoever places it, it is important that a patent airway is re-established after placement of the pack and

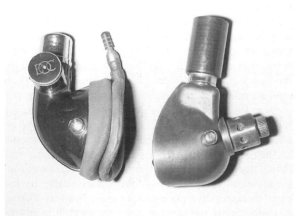

Fig. 33.1
Nasal masks used for dental anaesthesia.

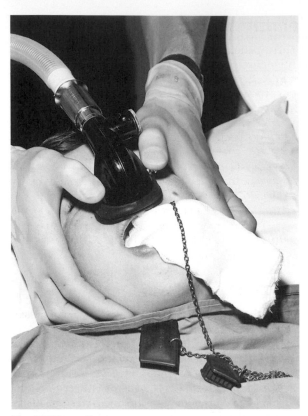

Fig. 33.2
The nasal mask has now been moved to cover the nose only and a gag and mouth pack inserted.

gag, before any operative procedure starts. If at any point throughout the procedure there is a problem with the airway it is important that the anaesthetist may interrupt surgery until the airway is restored.

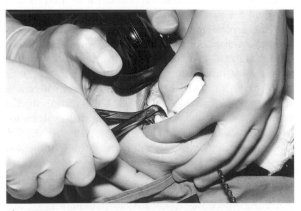

Fig. 33.3
Extraction of tooth from lower jaw. The dental pack is pushed to the left by the operator and the anaesthetist maintains the airway by upward lift of the lower jaw to counteract the downward pressure exerted by the dentist.

At the end of the procedure, the packs are usually placed across the sockets to absorb any continuing bleeding, the gag is removed and the patient is placed in the left lateral position and given 100% oxygen to breathe.

As in any general anaesthetic procedure, it is important that full resuscitative and support facilities are available immediately, in particular suction and facilities for oral tracheal intubation.

PERIOPERATIVE PROBLEMS

The potential problems associated with the perioperative period include:

- difficulty in induction of anaesthesia in an uncooperative child who will not tolerate a mask or insertion of an i.v. cannula
- airway problems during induction because of irritant gases or airway obstruction, during placement of the gag and pack, during extractions or during early recovery
- obstruction of the airway by bleeding or bits of broken tooth
- cardiac arrhythmias.

RECOVERY

At the end of the procedure, the patient continues to breathe 100% oxygen until return of consciousness. The recovery facilities must provide space for the patient to recover in the supine position. A nurse should be present to supervise the recovery of each patient.

POSTOPERATIVE ANALGESIA

It is usual to give postoperative analgesics during outpatient dental extraction procedures. The amount of pain experienced postoperatively varies with the number of teeth extracted and the difficulty encountered in extraction. If there has been a difficult extraction of a tooth that has produced trauma to the gums, there is considerably more pain than after simple extraction of, for example, a single upper incisor. Postoperative analgesia is provided usually with nonsteroidal anti-inflammatory drugs (NSAIDs) which are ideal for postoperative dental pain, as some of the pain originates from the tissue swelling and these agents act in part by decreasing swelling. Paracetamol and/or diclofenac given orally in the early postoperative period or as a suppository during anaesthesia are the most commonly used. It is appropriate to discuss the use of analgesic suppositories with the patient and/or the patient's parents preoperatively.

Alternatively, paracetamol or ibuprofen may be given orally in a liquid form in recovery. Inability to control postoperative pain is one reason for admitting the patient postoperatively. If it is anticipated that the surgery or extractions may produce considerable pain, the procedure may be deemed more appropriate for inpatient treatment.

FITNESS FOR DISCHARGE

There are several methods of assessing the patient's fitness for discharge from the recovery room. It is important that the patients are assessed by the medical practitioner and the dentist before discharge to identify any problems or potential problems which may arise. Assessment includes several clinical observations or the use of sophisticated tests of recovery. Clinical assessments include testing that the patient is alert and orientated, and able to stand and walk unassisted; simple scoring systems include the Steward's score and the Aldrete score.

POSTOPERATIVE PROBLEMS

The potential problems associated with the postoperative period may be classified under the headings of immediate or longer term:

Immediate

- hypoxaemia – secondary to diffusion hypoxaemia or airway problems
- airway problems – caused by laryngeal spasm, bleeding or debris in the airway
- vomiting.

Long term

- continued bleeding
- postoperative pain and swelling
- nausea and vomiting.

DAY-CASE ANAESTHESIA

Developments in provision of day-case facilities have allowed an increasing number of dental procedures to be undertaken on a day-case basis. This differs from outpatient, dental chair anaesthesia in that the patient goes through a formal admission to the hospital but is discharged home later in the day. The procedures for which this is appropriate are limited dental extractions, such as those of wisdom teeth, and minor oral surgical procedures including laser treatment.

PATIENT SELECTION

These patients are usually adults. They should be of ASA grade I or II and should comply with the standard criteria for selection of day-case patients. It is important to consider also the extent of the surgery involved and that a limitation may be the availability to provide adequate analgesia for the patient who is being discharged home. Therefore, caution should be exercised in undertaking extensive oral surgical procedures or difficult extractions of wisdom teeth. It is important that the patient is assessed formally by the anaesthetist before the induction of anaesthesia so that appropriate investigations may be undertaken. This avoids unnecessary delays or cancellation on the day of surgery. Ideally, the patients should be assessed at a preoperative anaesthetic clinic.

ANAESTHETIC TECHNIQUE

The patient should arrive early on the morning of surgery, fasted and accompanied. If appropriate, the patient may be given an oral premedicant, such as temazepam, to take at home before coming into hospital and this could be arranged at a preoperative assessment visit. The majority of patients, however, do not receive premedication. A full admission clerking of the patient should be made and the patient assessed by the anaesthetist.

The nature of the surgery involved dictates that the majority of these patients require nasotracheal intubation. As the majority of the patients involved are young, healthy and are mobilized early, the potential for post-succinylcholine muscle pains is high and the use of succinylcholine is best avoided. The advantages of succinylcholine in speed of intubation and in controlling the airway have to be weighed against the potential disadvantages. There are several methods of reducing the incidence of postoperative succinylcholine pains using pretreatment with a non-depolarizing relaxant, dantrolene or benzodiazepines. Many of these techniques have been shown to reduce the incidence of muscle pain but none completely abolishes it. The alternatives for achieving nasal tracheal intubation would be to use a non-depolarizing relaxant or, following intravenous or inhalational induction, to take the patient to a deep plane of anaesthesia breathing a volatile agent spontaneously. If the anaesthetist is satisfied that there is no preoperative indication of a difficult intubation, the use of a non-depolarizing relaxant is probably the easiest.

Following intravenous induction, the nasotracheal tube is inserted. There is a relatively high risk of causing nasal bleeding while inserting or removing a nasotracheal tube. Several measures have been described to minimize this, including the use of a soft rubber catheter pulled over the end of the tube to act as protection during passage through the nose. The catheter is removed through the mouth before the tube is placed in the trachea. The anaesthetist should then place the throat pack in the back of the mouth, around the tracheal tube to prevent any blood or debris falling into the back of the larynx. It is extremely important that the tail of the throat pack is brought out of the mouth and secured in some way to make sure that it is removed at the end of surgery. If for any reason the trachea cannot be intubated successfully using the nasal route, e.g. because of a deviated septum or previous nasal injury, orotracheal intubation may be used. While this is not ideal for allowing the dentist access to the operation site, it is an acceptable technique and a 'south-facing' orotracheal tube may be moved carefully to allow access to the appropriate quadrants. In addition, the use of a laryngeal mask and spontaneous ventilation has been described, but this also limits dental access.

At the end of surgery the patient should be turned to the left lateral, head-down position before tracheal extubation.

EXTUBATION

The trachea may be extubated while the patient is still quite deeply anaesthetized or when the patient is very lightly anaesthetized. In view of the potential for blood and secretions to drain into the larynx, it is recommended that the trachea is extubated during light anaesthesia and that the airway is maintained until that time using the nasotracheal tube.

Perioperatively, a small dose of a short-acting opioid may be used to provide analgesia for particularly painful procedures. It is also common practice to administer an NSAID perioperatively to produce postoperative analgesia. There are a number of options available for administration, including oral premedication, intravenous, intramuscular and suppositories. Many dental surgeons recommend the use of a dose of dexamethasone (8 mg) given perioperatively to help reduce the swelling and hence the pain. If the surgery is limited to one or two quadrants, it is appropriate to perform a local analgesic block during or at the end of surgery to help provide postoperative analgesia. However, it is not appropriate to produce local analgesic blocks in all four quadrants as this would create difficulties in swallowing secretions and in talking.

The patient should recover in a supine position and, when appropriate, be allowed to sit up and then gradually to mobilize. It is appropriate that discharge does not occur until the patient is fully recovered and should take place a minimum of 2 h postoperatively. Additional postoperative analgesia may be provided, if required, with regular oral medication such as a paracetamol/codeine mixture. It is important that the patient is assessed by a medical practitioner and dentist before discharge and that the patient has good pain control, has no evidence of continuing bleeding and is fully orientated. On discharge, the patient should be accompanied and should be given a set of written instructions for the postoperative period with regard to operating machinery, drinking alcohol and being accompanied. It is important that, should there be any problems, the patient has a contact telephone number to seek advice. As with all day-case procedures, should a problem arise peri- or postoperatively, such as continued bleeding or persistent uncontrolled pain, there must be an easily implemented procedure which would allow overnight admission of the patient to hospital.

INPATIENT DENTAL ANAESTHESIA

Elective surgical procedures of a more invasive nature are managed more appropriately on an inpatient basis, as are emergency procedures. These procedures include impacted wisdom teeth where considerable surgery is anticipated, oral surgical procedures on the gums and jaw and dental and submandibular abscesses requiring urgent treatment. In many of these patients, the anaesthetist must be particularly aware of the potential for difficulty in achieving tracheal intubation produced by limitation of jaw movement at the temporomandibular joint. It is very important in the preoperative assessment to make a full assessment of the airway. Limitation of jaw movement produced by pain or swelling cannot be relied upon to decrease after blockade with a muscle relaxant.

In general, inpatient dental cases are managed with nasotracheal intubation following intravenous induction. However, if difficulty is anticipated with the airway, an awake fibreoptic intubation or an inhalational induction should be considered. Following nasotracheal intubation, a throat pack is placed around the tracheal tube by the anaesthetist. It must be remembered that the swelling associated with intraoral infections will not resolve immediately, and may initially get worse. Thus, if the tracheal intubation has been difficult at induction, extreme care must be taken on extubation and there is a good argument, in severe cases, for leaving the tracheal tube in place for a few hours postoperatively to allow any swelling to decrease.

Some oral surgical procedures use laser therapy and a laser-protected tracheal tube may be required.

These operations may be painful and the perioperative use of a short-acting opioid and NSAID is recommended. Postoperatively, the patient may require i.m. or i.v. opioids with a PCA.

SEDATION

The move away from the use of general anaesthesia for dental procedures has been accompanied by increasing use of sedative techniques to permit dental procedures to be carried out under local analgesia in patients who are anxious or who are having more invasive procedures carried out. Although dentists receive training in the use of sedation, it is likely that, with its increasing use, anaesthetists may be called on to provide sedation for patients undergoing dental procedures. The Department of Health (1991) report defined sedation as:

> . . . a carefully controlled technique in which a single intravenous drug, or a combination of oxygen and nitrous oxide, is used to reinforce hypnotic suggestion and reassurance in a way which allows dental treatment to be performed with minimal physiological and psychological stress, but which allows verbal contact with the patient to be maintained at all times. The technique must carry a margin of safety wide enough to render unintended loss of consciousness unlikely. Any technique of sedation other than as defined above would be regarded as coming within the meaning of dental general anaesthesia.

The important aspects of this definition are that it states that a *single* i.v. drug is used, that it is only *part of an overall technique* of reassurance for the patient, that *verbal contact* is maintained throughout the procedure and that a *wide safety margin* from loss of consciousness is essential. This definition implies that the use of a benzodiazepine in combination with an opioid for a surgical procedure is regarded as general anaesthesia and not as sedation. Subsequent definitions essentially support this view, and, although a combination of midazolam and an opioid is used in some endoscopy practices, it is not used in dental sedation.

There are two techniques which are used: intravenous use of small doses of a benzodiazepine and, less commonly, inhalation of low concentrations of nitrous oxide in oxygen (termed *relative analgesia*).

INTRAVENOUS SEDATION

The aim of this technique is to have a patient who feels no anxiety, who is cooperative though drowsy, yet who is easily rousable. The procedure starts with intravenous cannulation and attachment of a pulse oximeter. Increments of midazolam are given, and the amount titrated to the patient's response. The endpoint for titration of midazolam may be the onset of Verrill's sign, which is drooping of the eyelids (ptosis). This is now thought to be too deep a level of sedation and an end-point at which the patient starts to have a delayed response to verbal command is thought to be more appropriate. It is important that verbal contact is not lost at any time.

The use of intravenous sedation with midazolam is occasionally associated with the occurrence of dreams which may be of a sexual nature. These may be very distressing to the patient and may lead to misunderstandings with the operator. There are two recommendations which should be followed to minimize this risk: first, the maximum dose of midazolam should be limited to 0.1 mg kg^{-1}; and secondly, the operator should always be accompanied throughout the procedure by another person, usually the practice nurse.

Midazolam should be administered slowly and it must be remembered that there is a lag time before the onset of its sedative effect. When the appropriate level of sedation has been reached, a local anaesthetic may be injected in the usual manner and the procedure may start. The initial dose of midazolam produces amnesia, which may persist for 10–15 min, and a longer period of anxiolysis. As the anxiolysis is the main reason for administering the drug, top-up doses should not be required too frequently. The patient should be monitored continuously using the pulse oximeter and it is important that the operator communicates regularly with the patient to assess the degree of awareness and comfort. At the end of the procedure, the patient should be given adequate time to recover before discharge. Flumazenil should be used only in the situation of accidental overdosage of benzodiazepine and not as a routine method of reversing sedation. The criteria for fitness for discharge that would apply to a patient receiving a general anaesthetic should also apply to those who receive intravenous sedation, i.e. they should be accompanied home and should not operate machinery or drive for the first 24 h.

INHALATIONAL SEDATION

Inhalational sedation involves the use of low inspired concentrations of nitrous oxide in oxygen and is also termed *relative analgesia*. The technique has been used in both adults and children but requires a degree of cooperation from the patient and significant input from the operator to make it work. The aim of the technique is to titrate a dose of inspired nitrous oxide which produces a light level of sedation and mild analgesia. This allows procedures to take place under subsequent local anaesthetic block. This technique may be useful in patients who have 'needle phobia' for local analgesic injections in the mouth. It is important for this procedure that the patient has been selected appropriately and understands what is involved. A nasal mask, which can be clipped round the head, is used and an initial concentration of 5–10% nitrous oxide in oxygen inhaled. This is stepped up in 5% increments to a maximum of 30% to provide an appropriate level of sedation and cooperation. The use of higher concentrations of nitrous oxide may lead to restlessness and occasionally to aggression in the patient. A Quantiflex flowmeter (Fig. 13.2) is very useful for administration of nitrous oxide in this technique, because when the initial flow has been set, the relative concentrations of nitrous oxide and oxygen may be varied using a single dial. During onset of sedation, it is important that the operator maintains verbal communication and assists in establishing anxiolysis to allow placement of the local block and commencement of the procedure. Recovery from this technique is rapid and it has the advantage compared with intravenous sedation that, following a short recovery period, the patient is ready for discharge early and there is less restriction on mobility in the first 24 h.

Relative contraindications to the use of relative analgesia include a blocked nose, deafness, inability to cooperate through either physical or mental disability, active neurological disease or severe respiratory disease.

FURTHER READING

Academy of Medical Royal Colleges 2001 Implementing safe sedation practice. Medical Academy of Royal Colleges, London

Department of Health 1991 Report on an expert working party on general anaesthesia, sedation and resuscitation in dentistry. Department of Health, Dental Division, London

Department of Health 2000 A conscious decision: a review of the use of general anaesthesia and conscious sedation in primary dental care. Department of Health, London

General Dental Council 1998 Maintaining standards: guidance to dentists on professional and personal conduct. Revised Nov 1998

Paris S T, Cafferkey M, Tarling M et al 1997 Comparison of sevoflurane and halothane for outpatient dental anaesthesia in children. British Journal of Anaesthesia 79: 280–284

Royal College of Anaesthetists 1999 Standards and guidelines for general anaesthesia in dentistry. Royal College of Anaesthetists, London

Anaesthesia outside the operating theatre environment

34

General anaesthesia outside the operating theatre suite is often challenging for the anaesthetist, as specialized environments pose unique problems. In hospital, the anaesthetist must attempt to provide a service for patients with standards, safety and comfort that are equal to those in the main operating department. Outside the hospital this level of service is more dependent on location and available resources.

ANAESTHESIA IN REMOTE HOSPITAL LOCATIONS

In-hospital remote locations include radiology, radiotherapy, accident and emergency departments and wards with areas designated for procedures such as ECT and assisted conception.

GENERAL CONSIDERATIONS AND PRINCIPLES

When anaesthetists ae required to use their skills (e.g. administer anaesthesia, analgesia, sedation, resuscitate, cannulate, etc.) outside the operating theatre, there are multiple considerations that apply equally to the different locations. These include:

1. Senior anaesthetists and not trainees should normally administer anaesthesia in remote locations. This is because skilled anaesthetic help may not be readily available (compared with an operating suite), patients are often challenging, e.g. paediatric or ITU, and the environment is unfamiliar.
2. The remote clinical area may not have been designed with anaesthetic requirements in mind. Anaesthetic apparatus often competes for space with bulky equipment (e.g. scanners) and, in general, conditions are less than optimal.
3. Monitoring capabilities and anaesthetic equipment should be of a standard similar to those used in the operating department. In reality, such equipment may not be readily available and the equipment used is often the oldest in the hospital. Nevertheless, the monitoring equipment should meet the minimum standards set by the Association of Anaesthetists of Great Britain and Ireland (AAGBI). The anaesthetist who is unfamiliar with the environment should spend time becoming accustomed to the layout and equipment. Compromised access to the patient and the type of monitors used during the procedure require careful consideration. Advanced planning helps prepare for unanticipated scenarios. Clinical observation may be limited by poor lighting.
4. Preparation of the patient may be inadequate because the patient is from a ward where staff are unfamiliar with preoperative protocols.
5. An anaesthetic assistant (e.g. operating department practitioner) should be present and this person may be unfamiliar with the environment. Maintenance of anaesthetic equipment may be less than ideal. Consequently, the anaesthetist must be particularly vigilant in checking the anaesthetic machine, especially as it may be disconnected and moved when not in use. Empty gas cylinders need to be replaced in older suites without piped gases, and also the anaesthetist must ensure the presence of drugs, spare laryngoscope and batteries, suction and other routine equipment.
6. Communication between staff of other specialities and the anaesthetist may be poor. This may lead to failure in recognizing each other's requirements. Education programmes for non-anaesthesia personnel regarding the care of anaesthetized patients may be of benefit.
7. Recovery facilities are often non-existent. Anaesthetists may have to recover their own patients in the suite. Consequently, they must be familiar with the location of recovery equipment, including suction, supplementary oxygen and

resuscitation equipment. Alternatively, patients may be transferred to the main hospital recovery area. This requires the use of routine transfer equipment, including monitoring and oxygen.

8. It may be useful to have a nominated lead anaesthetist responsible for remote anaesthetizing locations in a hospital. This individual should liaise with the relevant specialities (e.g. radiologists) to ensure that the environment, equipment and guidelines are suitable for safe, appropriate and efficient patient care.

ANAESTHESIA IN THE RADIOLOGY DEPARTMENT

In most hospitals, members of the anaesthetic department are called upon to anaesthetize or sedate patients for diagnostic and therapeutic radiological procedures. These procedures include ultrasound, angiography, computed tomography (CT) scanning and magnetic resonance imaging (MRI). The major requirement of all these imaging techniques is that the patient remains almost motionless. Thus, general anaesthesia may be necessary when these investigations and interventions are performed in children, the critically ill or the uncooperative patient. The presence of pain or prolonged procedures may also be an indication for anaesthesia.

Radiological studies may require administration of conscious sedation. This term describes the use of medication, often given by a non-anaesthetist, to alter perception of painful and anxiety-provoking stimuli while maintaining protective airway responses and the ability to respond appropriately to verbal command. Medical personnel responsible for the sedation should be familiar with the effects of the medication and skilled in resuscitation (including airway management). All the equipment and drugs required for resuscitation should be readily available and checked regularly. With a single operator for both the radiological procedure and administration of sedation there is the potential to be distracted from one responsibility and to allow side-effects to go untreated. Ideally, different individuals should be responsible for each of these tasks. Guidelines for prescribing, evaluating and monitoring sedation should be readily available. Chloral hydrate may be used in young children and benzodiazepines, opioids or propofol in adults. Patients should be starved before sedation and vital signs monitored and documented.

Intravascular contrast agents are used routinely during angiographic and other radiological investigations. The anaesthetist must always be aware of the risk of adverse reaction to contrast dyes. In recent years, low-osmolarity contrast media have been introduced, and these cause less pain and have fewer toxic effects than the older contrast agents, but are more expensive. Factors contributing to the development of adverse reactions include speed of injection, type and dose of contrast used and patient susceptibility.

Coronary and cerebral angiography are associated with a high risk of reaction. Other major risk factors include allergies, asthma, extremes of age (under 1 and over 60 years), cardiovascular disease and a history of previous contrast medium reaction. Fatal reactions are rare, occurring in about 1 in 100 000 procedures. Nausea and vomiting are common (and may demand prophylactic antiemetic), which may progress to urticaria, hypotension, arrhythmias, bronchospasm and cardiac arrest. Adequate hydration is important, as patients undergoing contrast dye procedures usually have an induced osmotic diuresis, which may exacerbate pre-existing renal dysfunction. A urinary catheter may be useful for patients undergoing long procedures.

Treatment of allergic reactions depends on the severity of the reaction. This usually consists of general supportive methods such as fluids, oxygen and careful monitoring. Drugs such as epinephrine (adrenaline), atropine, steroids and antihistamines should be readily available.

Healthcare workers are exposed to X-rays in the radiology and imaging suites. The greatest source is usually from fluoroscopy and digital subtraction angiography. Ionizing radiation from a CT scanner is relatively low because the X-rays are highly focused. Radiation intensity and exposure decrease with the square of the distance from the emitting source. The recommended distance is 2–3 m. This precaution, together with lead aprons, thyroid shields and movable lead-lined glass screens, keeps exposure at a safe level. A personal-dose monitor should be worn by personnel who work frequently in an X-ray environment.

Computed tomography

General principles

A CT scan provides a series of tomographic axial 'slices' of the body. It is used most frequently for intracranial imaging and for studies of the thorax and abdomen. Each image is produced by computer integration of the differences in the radiation absorption coefficients between different normal tissues and between normal and abnormal tissues. The image of the structure under investigation is generated by a cathode ray tube and the brightness of each area is proportional to the absorption value.

One rotation of the gantry produces an axial slice or 'cut'. A series of cuts is made, usually at intervals of

7 mm, but this may be larger or smaller depending on the diagnostic information sought. The first-generation scanners took 4.5 min per cut, but the newest scanners take only 2–4 s.

The circular scanning tunnel contains the X-ray tube and detectors with the patient lying stationary in the centre during the study. The procedure is noisy and patients occasionally are frightened or claustrophobic.

Anaesthetic management

Computed tomography is non-invasive and painless, requiring neither sedation nor anaesthesia for most adult patients. A few patients may require conscious sedation to relieve fears or anxieties. However, patients who cannot cooperate (most frequently paediatric and head trauma patients) may need general anaesthesia to prevent movement, which degrades the image. Anaesthetists may also be asked to assist in the transfer from the ITU and in the care of critically ill patients who require CT scans.

General anaesthesia is preferable to sedation when there are potential airway problems or when control of intracranial pressure (ICP) is critical. As the patient's head is inaccessible during the CT scan, the airway needs to be secured. In the majority of situations, tracheal intubation is more appropriate than the use of a laryngeal mask airway (e.g. full stomach). The scan itself requires only that the patient remains motionless and tolerates the tracheal tube. If ICP is high, controlled ventilation is essential to avoid hypercapnia.

A propofol/thiopental, nitrous oxide, oxygen, volatile and relaxant technique with tracheal intubation and mild hyperventilation is acceptable. Anaesthetic complications include kinking of the tracheal tube (especially during extreme degrees of head flexion required for examination of the posterior fossa; positioning and movement of the gantry during the procedure may cause kinking or disconnection of the anaesthetic circuit), hypothermia in paediatric patients and acute brainstem compression if the head is flexed excessively in the presence of an infratentorial tumour. If during the scan the anaesthetist is observing the patient from inside the control room, it is imperative that alarms/monitors have visual signals that may be easily seen.

Stereotactic-guided surgery is possible using CT scanners. Most procedures involve aspiration or biopsy of intracranial masses. This procedure is used because it minimizes injury to adjacent structures. Pins are used to hold a radiolucent frame around the head to ensure a motionless field inside the scanner. This allows precise localization. Access to the patient and airway with the frame attached inside the scanner is difficult.

Magnetic resonance imaging

General principles

Magnetic resonance imaging (MRI) is an imaging modality that does not use ionizing radiation, but depends on magnetic fields and radiofrequency pulses for the production of its images. The imaging capabilities of MRI are superior to those of CT for examining intracranial, spinal and soft tissue lesions. MRI differentiates clearly between white and grey matter in the brain, thus making possible the in vivo diagnosis of demyelination. It may display images in the sagittal, coronal, transverse or oblique planes and, unlike the CT scanner, is capable of detecting disease in the posterior fossa. It has the advantage that no ionizing radiation is produced.

An MRI imaging system requires a large magnet in the form of a tube, which is capable of accepting the entire length of the human body. A radiofrequency transmitter coil is incorporated in the tube that surrounds the patient; the coil also acts as a receiver to detect the energy waves from which the image is constructed. In the presence of the magnetic field, protons in the body align with the magnetic field in the longitudinal axis of the patient. Additional perpendicular magnetic pulses are applied by the radiofrequency coil; these cause the protons to rotate into the transverse plane. When the pulse is discontinued, the nuclei relax back to their original orientation and emit energy waves which are detected by the coil. The magnet is over 2 m in length and weighs approximately 500 kg. The magnetic field is applied constantly even in the absence of a patient. It may take several days to establish the magnetic field if it is removed and this is only done in an emergency as it is very expensive to shut down the field. The magnetic field strength is measured in tesla units. One tesla equals 10 000 gauss and the earth's surface strength is between 0.5 and 1.0 gauss. MRI strengths usually vary from 1 to 3 tesla. The force of the magnetic field decreases exponentially from the magnet and a safety line at a level of 5 gauss is usually specified. Higher exposure may result in pacemaker malfunction and unscreened personnel should not cross this level. At 50 gauss, ferromagnetic objects become dangerous projectiles.

The final MR image is made from very weak electromagnetic signals, which are subject to interference from other modulated radio signals. Therefore, the scanner is contained in a radiofrequency shield (Faraday cage). A hollow tube of brass is built into this cage to allow patient-monitoring cables and infusion lines to pass into the control room. This is termed the waveguide.

Anaesthetic management

The indications for general anaesthesia during MRI are similar to those for CT. In addition, the scanner is very noisy and the patient lies on a long thin table in a dark, confined space within the tube (typical diameter 50–65 cm). This may cause claustrophobia or anxiety-related problems which may require sedation or anaesthesia. Obese patients cannot be examined in this small magnetic bore. A complex scan may take up to 20 min and an entire examination more than 1 h.

Metal objects within or attached to the patient pose a risk. Jewellery, hearing aids or drug patches should be removed. Absolute contraindications include implanted surgical devices, e.g. cardiac pacemakers/defibrillators, cochlear implants, intraocular metallic objects and metal vascular clips. Patients fitted with a demand cardiac pacemaker should not be exposed to MRI because induced electrical currents may be mistaken for natural electrical activity of the heart and may inhibit pacemaker output. Metallic implants, e.g. intracranial vascular clips, may be dislodged from blood vessels. Joint prostheses, artificial heart valves and sternal wires are safe because of fibrous tissue fixation. Patients with large metal implants should be monitored for implant heating. Heating of the pulse oximeter probe may result in burns. A description of the safety of various devices is available on dedicated web sites. All patients should wear ear protection as noise levels may exceed 85 dB.

There are other unique problems presented by MRI. These include relative inaccessibility of the patient and the magnetic properties of the equipment. The body cylinder of the scanner surrounds the patient totally; manual control of the airway is impossible and tracheal intubation or use of a laryngeal mask airway is essential. The patient may be observed from both ends of the tunnel and may be extracted quickly if necessary. As there is no hazard from ionizing radiation, the anaesthetist may approach the patient in safety.

The magnetic effects of MRI impose some restrictions on the selection of anaesthetic equipment. Any ferromagnetic object distorts the magnetic field sufficiently to degrade the image. It is also likely to be propelled towards the scanner and may cause a significant accident if it makes contact with the patient or staff. Of relevance to anaesthetists is any equipment that needs to be used in the MRI room. The layout of the MRI room/suite determines if the majority of equipment needs to be inside the room and therefore MRI-compatible, or outside the room with long MRI-compatible circuits, leads and tubing to the patient. MRI-compatible anaesthetic machines and ventilators are manufactured and may be sited next to the magnetic bore to minimize breathing circuit length. They require piped gases or special aluminium oxygen/nitrous oxide cylinders. Consideration also needs to be given to intravenous fluid stands, infusion pumps and monitoring equipment, including stethoscopes and nerve stimulators. Laryngoscopes may be non-magnetic, but standard batteries should be replaced with non-magnetic lithium batteries. Laryngeal mask airways without a metal spring in the pilot tube valve should be available.

All monitoring equipment must be MRI compatible. Technical problems with non-compatible monitors include interference with imaging signals, resulting in distorted MRI pictures, and radiofrequency signals from the scanner inducing currents in the monitor which may give unreliable monitor readings. Special MRI-compatible monitors are available or unshielded ferromagnetic monitors may be installed just outside the MRI room and used with long shielded or non-ferromagnetic cables (e.g. leads may be fibreoptic or carbon fibre cable). Finger burns have resulted from current induction in non-compatible standard pulse oximeters. Ambient noise levels are such that visual alarms are essential. The AAGBI guidelines on services for MRI suggest monitoring equipment should be placed in the control room outside the magnetic area. A non-invasive automated arterial pressure monitor, in which metallic tubing connectors are replaced by nylon connectors, should be used. Distortion of the ECG may occur, which interferes with arrhythmia and ischaemia monitoring. Interference may be reduced by using short braided leads connected to compatible electrodes placed in a narrow triangle on the chest. Side-stream capnography requires a long sampling tube which leads to a time delay of the monitored parameters.

Anaesthesia is induced usually outside the MRI room in an adjacent dedicated anaesthetic area where it is safe to use ferromagnetic equipment (distal to the 5 gauss line). Most patients benefit from the use of short-acting drugs associated with rapid recovery and minimal side-effects. Sedation of children by organized, dedicated and multidisciplinary teams for MRI has been shown to be safe and successful. However, general anaesthesia allows more rapid and controlled onset with immobility guaranteed. All patients must be transported into the magnet area on MRI-compatible trolleys. During the scan the anaesthetist should ideally be in the control room but may remain in the scanning room in exceptional circumstances if wearing suitable ear protection. Should an emergency arise, the anaesthetist needs to be aware of the procedure for rapid removal of the patient to a safe area.

Occasionally, intensive care patients may require scanning. Careful planning is required. Essential infusion pumps require long extension tubing to reach the 30 gauss line. The tracheal tube pilot balloon valve spring should be secured away from the scan area. Pulmonary artery catheters with conductive wires and epicardial pacing catheters should be removed to prevent microshocks. Simple central venous catheters appear safe if disconnected from electrical connections, etc. All anaesthetized patients, especially infants, are at risk from hypothermia as the MRI room may be cold.

Staff precautions are essential. Screening questionnaires identify those at risk and training should be given. Long-term effects of repeated exposure to MRI fields are unknown. Pregnant staff should not work in the scanner. All potentially hazardous articles should be removed, e.g. watches, bleepers and stethoscopes. Bank cards, credit cards and other belongings containing electromagnetic strips become demagnetized within the vicinity of the scanner and personal computers, pagers and calculators may also be damaged.

MRI-guided surgery is a new, highly specialized form of surgery that may continue to be developed. It offers surgeons radiological images of the tissues immediately beyond their operative field. This is made possible by the development of an open-configuration scanner as opposed to the traditional closed tubular scanner. The open configuration consists of upright-paired coils between which the medical staff may access the patient. The absence of ionizing radiation places less restriction on the duration of staff presence. The anaesthetic considerations are similar to those of the traditional MRI scanner except that here the anaesthetist and all the related equipment are required to be in the vicinity of the scanner and therefore compatible with a magnetic field. Surgery that has been performed in this environment includes endoscopic sinus surgery and neurosurgery.

Intussusception

This condition occurs usually between the ages of 6 and 18 months. Commonly, the ileum invaginates into the caecum because of small bowel lymphadenopathy. General anaesthesia or sedation may be necessary in the radiology department during attempted reduction of the intussusception by instillation of rectal barium. Insufflation with air or oxygen is also possible.

The major problems are those of anaesthetizing any young child in an unfamiliar environment. Precautions should be taken to minimize a decrease in body temperature. Hypothermia may be exacerbated if the infant lies in cold barium that has been expelled. Fluid losses are always greater than expected and crystalloid or colloid may be needed to restore circulating blood volume.

Diagnostic and interventional angiography

General principles

Direct arteriography using percutaneous arterial catheters is used widely for the diagnosis of vascular lesions. Catheters are usually inserted by the Seldinger technique via the femoral artery in the groin. Injection of contrast medium provides images that are viewed by conventional cut film radiography or by digital subtraction angiography. New non-invasive angiographic techniques used with CT or MRI have reduced the need for direct arteriography for diagnosis of vascular lesions. CT may demonstrate major vascular lesions such as thoracic or abdominal aneurysms. The advent of spiral and double helical CT scanners allows whole vascular territories to be mapped within 30 s and produces superior images, including three-dimensional pictures. MRI is sensitive to the detection of flow and, together with more sophisticated scanning and data collection techniques, is increasingly used for assessment of vascular structures.

Anaesthetic management

Most angiographic procedures may be carried out under local anaesthesia or with sedation if necessary during more complex investigation. Sedation to augment local anaesthesia must be avoided in the presence of intracranial hypertension, as the increased $P_a\text{CO}_2$ leads to vasodilatation and a further increase in ICP; in addition, vasodilatation results in poor-quality angiography. General anaesthesia is usually necessary for children and may be required for nervous patients or those unable to cooperate. The drawbacks of general anaesthesia include prolonging the time taken for the investigation and increasing the cost and risks associated with anaesthesia. Moreover, the patient is unable to react to misplaced injections and untoward reactions. A conscious patient would describe symptoms, allowing the procedure to be stopped immediately. Interventional radiological procedures are more likely to require sedation or general anaesthesia because of patient discomfort and longer duration. General anaesthesia for angiography is more comfortable for the patient and ensures complete immobility during X-ray exposures.

Adequate hydration is essential for these patients, as they are often fasted and the contrast medium causes an osmotic diuresis. All i.v. cannulae and monitor leads may require extensions to enable the anaesthetist to remain an acceptable distance from the patient to minimize exposure. This also allows the anaesthetist to remain outside the range of movement of the imaging machine.

Complications of angiography

- *Local* – haematoma and haemorrhage, vessel wall dissection, thrombosis, perivascular contrast injection, adjacent nerve damage, loss and knotting of guide wires and catheters.
- *General* – contrast reactions of varying severity; emboli from catheter clots, cholesterol and air; and septicaemia and vagal inhibition.

Cerebral angiography

This may be performed to demonstrate tumours, arteriovenous malformations, aneurysms, subarachnoid haemorrhage and cerebrovascular disease. The risk of complications is generally increased in the elderly and those with pre-existing vascular disease, diabetes, stroke and transient ischaemic attacks. Many of these patients have intracranial hypertension. Therefore, control of arterial pressure and carbon dioxide tension is essential if these patients require general anaesthesia. Obtunding the pressor response to tracheal intubation and careful positioning to avoid increasing central venous pressure are necessary to prevent elevation of intracranial pressure. A relaxant/IPPV technique with moderate hyperventilation to induce hypocapnia (P_aCO_2 = 4.0–4.5 kPa) is often used. A moderate reduction in P_aCO_2 causes vasoconstriction of normal vessels, slows cerebral circulation and contrast medium transit times and improves delineation of small vascular lesions. The failure of autoregulation within tumours increases blood flow relative to that in other areas because of an intracerebral steal phenomenon and allows better visualization of their vascularity.

Transient hypotension and bradycardia or asystole may occur during cerebral angiography with contrast dye injection. This usually responds to volume replacement and atropine. Brain damage in the past was attributed to toxic contrast agents and local damage to carotid and vertebral arteries. Nowadays, complications during interventional neuroradiology include haemorrhage from rupture of the lesion or vessel and ischaemia as a result of thromboembolism (e.g. clot forming around the catheter tip), vasospasm, embolic material or hypoperfusion. All may occur rapidly with devastating results. Occasionally, urgent craniotomy may be required.

Embolization procedures

The use of angiographic embolization continues to grow and become more sophisticated. It is undertaken for vascular malformations and fistulae, aneurysms, tumours, acute haemorrhage and ablation of function of an organ. Venous embolization is used to treat gastro-oesophageal varices, testicular varices and ablation of adrenal gland function. It may be performed as an alternative to surgery, particularly if the patient is unhealthy or the operation carries a high risk, e.g. management of unclippable cerebral aneurysms or complex AV malformations. Its use before surgery may help to reduce intraoperative blood loss, e.g. reducing vascularity of central nervous system tumours, before surgery.

Embolization involves the injection of an embolic material to stimulate intravascular thrombosis, resulting in vessel occlusion. Embolic agents include gelatin sponge, polyvinyl alcohol particles, spiral metal coils, balloons and liquids such as ethyl alcohol. Patients must be watched carefully for disruption of flow in other vascular beds.

Anaesthetic management is similar to that for standard angiographic procedures. Sedation, local anaesthesia or general anaesthesia are administered according to the clinical situation. They may be long and painful procedures, in which case general anaesthesia would be the most pleasant option for the patient. In some cases, patient cooperation is required to help with the detection and avoidance of neurological or mechanical deficits that may arise from inadvertent occlusion of flow to vital tissues. These patients may be anaesthetized by intermittent propofol and short-acting opioids, or given midazolam sedation. Nausea and vomiting are common, so prophylactic antiemetics may be given. Often a high dose of contrast medium is used and, therefore, adequate hydration and a urinary catheter are important to minimize the development of renal failure. Increasing or decreasing arterial pressure may be needed as part of the treatment of the lesion or to treat complications.

Cardiac catheterization

General anaesthesia is required mainly for children (rarely in adults as sedation is usually adequate). In children (premature neonates to teenagers) congenital heart disease may cause abnormal circulations and intracardiac shunts, which often present with cyanosis, dyspnoea, failure to thrive and congestive heart failure. Patients may also have coexisting non-cardiac congenital abnormalities. Neonatal patients may be deeply cyanotic and critically ill. Initial echocardiography often gives a diagnosis but catheterization is required for treatment or determining the possibility of surgery. These radiological procedures include pressure and oxygen saturation measurements, balloon dilatation of stenotic lesions (e.g. pulmonary valve), balloon septostomy for transposition of the great arteries and ductal closure.

The ideal anaesthetic technique would not produce myocardial depression, would avoid hypertension and tachycardia, preserve normocapnia and maintain spontaneous respiration of air. All techniques have their limitations. Positive-pressure ventilation causes changes in pulmonary haemodynamics and therefore influences measurements of flow and pressure. Spontaneous respiration with volatile agents may not be suitable for patients with significant myocardial disease. The onset of action of anaesthetic drugs is affected by cardiac shunts and congestive failure. Contrast medium in the coronary circulation may cause profound transient changes in the ECG. Therefore, ECG and invasive arterial pressure monitoring should be used to allow rapid assessment of arrhythmias and hypotension. Children with cyanotic heart disease may be polycythaemic, thereby predisposing to thrombosis.

Pacemaker and cardioverter/defibrillator implantation

Pacemakers may be inserted in the cardiac catheter laboratory. These procedures may be performed under local or general anaesthesia depending on the circumstances. Implantation requires placing transvenous leads in the cardiac chambers and subcutaneous tunnelling to the device pocket. Testing of cardioverter/defibrillator units should be performed under general anaesthesia and the benefit of using direct arterial monitoring considered.

ANAESTHESIA FOR RADIOTHERAPY

Adults may require general anaesthesia for insertion of radioactive sources locally to treat some types of tumour. The commonest tumours to be treated in this way are carcinoma of the cervix, breast or tongue. These procedures are undertaken in the operating theatre and the anaesthetic management is similar to that for any type of surgery in these anatomical sites. These patients may require more than one anaesthetic for radiotherapy treatment. The anaesthetist may be exposed to radiation and appropriate precautions should be taken.

Radiotherapy is used increasingly in the management of a variety of malignant diseases which occur in childhood. These include the acute leukaemias,

Wilms' tumour, retinoblastoma and central nervous system tumours. High-dose X-rays are administered by a linear accelerator, while all staff must remain outside the room to be protected from radiation.

Anaesthesia in paediatric radiotherapy presents several problems:

1. Treatment is administered daily over a 4–6 week period and necessitates repeated doses of sedation or general anaesthesia.
2. The patient must remain alone and motionless for short periods during treatment, but immediate access to the patient is required in an emergency.
3. Monitoring is difficult as the child may be observed only on a closed-circuit television screen during treatment.
4. Recovery from anaesthesia must be rapid, as treatment is organized usually on an outpatient basis and disruption of normal activities should be minimized.

Before treatment begins, the fields to be irradiated are plotted and marked so that the X-rays may be focused on the tumour to avoid damaging the surrounding structures. This procedure requires the child to remain still for 20–40 min and takes place in semi-darkness. Radiotherapy treatment is of much shorter duration; two or three fields are irradiated for 30–90 s each. Anaesthesia or sedation may be required for both the focusing and the administration of radiation.

Anaesthetic management

A wide range of anaesthetic techniques has been used for radiotherapy. Ketamine may be given intravenously or intramuscularly but is not used widely by anaesthetists because of the following problems. It produces excessive salivation, even if an antisialagogue is prescribed, and there is a risk of airway obstruction or laryngospasm. Tachyphylaxis occurs with repeated use and sudden purposeless movements are not infrequent. The use of ketamine as a sole anaesthetic agent is often unsatisfactory.

Frequently, these children have a Hickman line in situ to ensure reliable iv. access for a range of medications and blood sampling. This makes induction of anaesthesia far simpler and avoids repeated i.v. cannulation, which may become technically difficult, but also increasingly distressing for the patient, parent and anaesthetist. The dead space volume of Hickman lines must always be remembered. Failure to flush these lines immediately after administering drugs may lead to disastrous consequences when the anaesthetic drugs are flushed into the bloodstream at a later time.

Inhalational induction with the child sitting on the parent's knee is an alternative technique.

When anaesthesia has been induced, the child is placed on a trolley and anaesthesia maintained with nitrous oxide, oxygen and volatile agent delivered via a laryngeal mask. No analgesia is required and tracheal intubation is generally not necessary. There is virtually no surgical stimulation and patients may be maintained at relatively light anaesthetic levels allowing for rapid emergence and recovery. Monitoring during the radiotherapy requires the patient, anaesthetic monitors and equipment to be observed continuously by closed-circuit television.

ANAESTHESIA FOR ELECTROCONVULSIVE THERAPY

Electroconvulsive therapy (ECT) is controlled electrical stimulation of the central nervous system to cause seizures. It is often administered in a dedicated ward area within a psychiatric hospital. Indications include severe depression and certain psychoses. The mechanism of the therapy remains unknown. The electrical stimulus applied transcutaneously to the brain results in a generalized tonic activity for about 10 s followed by a generalized clonic episode lasting up to 1 min or more. Seizure duration may be important for outcome and depends on age, stimulus site, stimulus energy and drugs, including anaesthetics. Seizure activity lasting 25–50 s is optimal for the antidepressant effect. Treatment may initially be 2 or 3 times per week for 3 weeks. Contraindications include increased intracranial pressure, recent cerebrovascular accident, phaeochromocytoma, cardiac conduction defects, and cerebral and aortic aneurysms. The risks from ECT and anaesthesia need to be balanced against potential benefits. Drug interactions with tricyclic antidepressants, monoamine oxidase inhibitors and lithium should be considered and managed appropriately. Seizures may cause sympathetic and parasympathetic discharge which precipitate cardiac arrhythmias and changes in blood pressure of variable magnitude and significance depending on the underlying medical conditions (e.g. hypertension, coronary artery disease, peripheral vascular disease). Emergence agitation, nausea, headache and fracture dislocations are other described complications.

Anaesthesia

The patient may be a poor historian because of the psychiatric condition, so a careful preoperative evaluation is essential. Anaesthesia with neuromuscular blockade is necessary to reduce physical and psychological trauma. The anaesthetic technique should allow a rapid recovery. Routine anaesthetic equipment and minimum standard of monitoring should be available. Pretreatment with glycopyrrolate is useful to reduce bradycardias and oral secretions. After preoxygenation, intravenous induction and a neuromuscular blocker are administered. A bite block is inserted when mask ventilation with oxygen is achieved and then the stimulus is applied to produce a seizure. Intubation of the trachea would be required in late pregnancy or other full-stomach situations. Ventilation should continue until the patient is breathing, as hypoxia and hypercapnia may shorten the seizure.

The intravenous anaesthetic agents commonly used include propofol and methohexital, which have similar ECT efficacy outcomes, but both cause pain on injection. Thiopental is associated with more hypertension and tachycardia than propofol and shortens the seizure duration compared with methohexital. Etomidate may prolong seizures and recovery and benzodiazepines result in short seizure duration. Larger than necessary doses shorten seizure activity. Sevoflurane has no advantages when compared with thiopental and is generally more time-consuming to administer.

Partial neuromuscular blockade is required to allow monitoring of the peripheral seizure duration and reduced physical symptoms help avoid trauma and minimize post-seizure muscle pain. Succinylcholine is often used in a dose of 0.5 mg kg^{-1} as this has a short duration. Subsequent doses for ECT may be modified as appropriate. Use of other neuromuscular blockers (e.g. mivacurium) may necessitate short postprocedural artificial ventilation and may not be as effective in preventing muscle contractions.

Cardiovascular drugs such as esmolol or labetalol may be required to minimize the acute haemodynamic changes of ECT in high-risk patients.

Anaesthetic drug administration and the patient's response should be accurately recorded as in other anaesthetic cases. This is particularly important with ECT because the therapy is repeated frequently over several weeks and consistent conditions are required to obtain the best ECT stimulus response.

ANAESTHESIA IN THE ACCIDENT AND EMERGENCY DEPARTMENT

Anaesthetists' involvement in Accident and Emergency (A&E) varies among hospitals depending on the skills of the resident A&E medical staff. The following clinical conditions usually require an anaesthetist to attend the A&E department:

- Preoperative assessment and resuscitation before emergency surgery, e.g. ruptured ectopic pregnancy or trauma victim.
- Specialist airway management for a patient with respiratory failure.
- Intensive care admission for a patient needing ventilatory and/or other organ support.
- Resuscitation as part of the cardiac arrest or trauma team.
- Patients requiring specialist cannulation skills.
- Anaesthesia for patients requiring procedures such as cardioversion or gastric lavage.

Ideally the anaesthetist attending A&E should be trained and experienced enough to manage these seriously ill patients. As in other remote locations, trained anaesthetic assistance is mandatory. Equipment and monitoring should be the minimum standard agreed for main operating theatres. Although the anaesthetist should ideally be available continuously (assuming the A&E department is admitting patients), there may be a delay if he or she is busy in theatre or ITU. Therefore, the emergency physician or A&E doctor may sometimes have provided the initial care of the patient. In these situations it is essential for the anaesthetist to obtain appropriate handover information and to check the patient/equipment carefully before accepting responsibility, e.g. before transferring the patient to CT scan and ITU.

ANAESTHESIA IN THE PRE-HOSPITAL ENVIRONMENT

The difficulties described in giving anaesthesia outside the operating theatre are compounded when working outside the hospital. Anaesthetists and other hospital staff may find themselves providing care in several situations:

- as a member of a hospital flying squad
- as an immediate care practitioner
- on duty (either paid or with the voluntary services) at an event such as a football match or festival
- Armed Forces medical staff in an incident response team.

Each of these situations has different clinical and logistic issues but there are some common areas. For this chapter the main example used is that of hospital staff attending a road accident. Working safely in the pre-hospital environment demands consideration of hazards at the scene and of the roles of the other emergency services.

For example, at a road accident, potential hazards include:

- broken glass
- spilt fuel
- fire and smoke
- jagged metal edges in damaged vehicles
- other traffic moving around the incident
- cutting and lifting equipment being used by the fire brigade.

PERSONAL PREPARATION FOR WORKING IN THE PRE-HOSPITAL ENVIRONMENT

It is unreasonable to expect hospital staff to get into an ambulance and attend a road accident and function effectively without training and preparation. The road accident is also a remote and unsupervised location and hospitals should only deploy staff with the correct clinical background to work in these situations.

Preparation includes having appropriate safety clothing and equipment such as:

- coveralls
- high-visibility jackets
- helmets
- eye and ear protection
- safety boots
- gloves.

For people attending ballistic incidents, this needs to include ballistic helmets and body armour.

Staff also need insurance to cover travelling to and from the incident and working at the incident. Advice on suitable equipment may be found on the British Association for Immediate Care (BASICS) website: *www.basics.org.uk*

Training in pre-hospital care

Several organizations provide training in pre-hospital care. These include:

- BASICS run courses in casualty extrication from vehicles and a pre-hospital emergency care certificate (PHEC, awarded jointly with the Royal College of Surgeons of Edinburgh). Information may be obtained from their website (see above).
- The Royal College of Surgeons of Edinburgh examines for a Diploma and Fellowship in Immediate Medical Care. Information may be obtained from the Faculty of Pre-hospital Care at the RCS, Edinburgh.

- The Royal College of Surgeons of England oversees the Pre Hospital Trauma Life Support Course, PHTLS.

Team working

Hospital personnel at an incident are there to support the Ambulance Service and they need to know whom to report to and how to work with ambulance staff and police. In addition, the Fire Service may be present to manage hazards and provide cutting equipment if needed for extrication. The police are present to coordinate the incident and the area around it, managing traffic flow and protecting evidence at the scene.

While everyone is concentrating their efforts on saving and treating the casualties, hospital staff need to understand that the other emergency services have their own roles, and the management of the incident continues after they and the casualties have left the scene.

Interservice working is addressed by the Major Incident Medical Management and Support (MIMMS) Course run by the Advanced Life Support Group: *www.alsg.org* and described in the MIMMS manual (see further reading).

WORKING AT THE SCENE

On arriving at an incident, the anaesthetist should report to the senior ambulance person, who has called the hospital flying squad or immediate care practitioner for a reason, such as

- multiple casualties
- trapped casualties.

They may also provide an explanation of what has happened, from which the mechanism of injury may be inferred and likely injuries anticipated.

Problems likely to be encountered are:

- *Access to the casualty.* The vehicle compartment around the casualty may be deformed and intruded. The vehicle may be on its side, upside down or in a ditch, making access to the casualty difficult.
- *Lighting.* The emergency services may provide portable lights, but in pre-hospital care the anaesthetist is often trying to assess and manage a casualty in poor light.
- *Noise.* Noise from generators and vehicles makes auscultation very difficult and interferes with communication with other team members and the other emergency services.

- *Environment.* Wet weather and cold conditions imply that casualties (and staff not wearing appropriate clothing) become hypothermic quickly.

Logistic considerations

The aim is to move the patient in the best clinical condition possible to the most appropriate hospital in the shortest time possible. In reality, a series of compromises is needed. Before carrying out any procedure, the clinician on scene needs to ask:

- *Is this essential?*
- Should it be carried out now, during the move to hospital or at the hospital?
- Am I helping the patient and the situation or causing undue delay?

For example, is it appropriate to struggle for 15 min to set up an intravenous infusion when the hospital is only 5 min travel time away?

- If the casualty is trapped and needs intravenous analgesia or anaesthesia to facilitate release, then probably yes, unless there are alternatives.
- If the casualty is ready to leave the scene except for this intervention, then probably no (unless there is no vehicle available to move the casualty).

Decisions such as these depend on many factors such as the overall situation, travel time to hospital, availability of ambulances and the needs of other casualties.

Clinical considerations

Airway

The main issue is oxygenation. As in hospital practice, simple methods should be tried first such as chin lift, jaw thrust, oral airway, nasopharyngeal airway and laryngeal mask.

Tracheal intubation may be desirable in a casualty at risk of aspiration but this may not be practical if access to the casualty is restricted. Simple methods should be used first and the situation reassessed as access to the casualty is improved (e.g. when the roof of the car has been cut off or when the casualty has been released from the vehicle).

A surgical cricothyroidotomy is an alternative definitive airway if tracheal intubation is not possible.

Cervical spine control

Many road accident casualties are at risk of cervical spine injury. Neck collars and other immobilization devices limit mouth opening and make airway management difficult. Paramedics may be asked to substitute manual in-line immobilization for the collar if the anaesthetist is having difficulty establishing a clear airway.

Breathing

As in hospital, inadequate ventilation is supported using a bag/valve mask. Life-threatening injuries such as tension pneumothorax may be difficult to diagnose. Some clinical signs, such as tracheal deviation, present late. Breath sounds may be difficult to hear because of the noisy environment. Clinical signs such as the presence of subcutaneous emphysema indicating an air leak should be sought. The decision to decompress a chest may have to be made on the basis of deteriorating ventilation and 'most likely' diagnosis.

Circulation

Control of bleeding with pressure dressings or tourniquet should be achieved before attempting intravenous access. Intravenous fluid resuscitation should be targeted at the injury being managed. Some injuries require hypotensive resuscitation until surgical control is achieved, others require normotension (for example, head injury to maintain cerebral perfusion). Blood loss may be very difficult to assess in the field. Blood can be difficult to see on soft muddy ground and may pool out of sight on the floor of vehicles.

Deficit

Casualties with a reduced Glasgow Coma Score (GCS) and at risk of pulmonary aspiration require airway protection (but see above).

Extremity

Fractures and dislocations may need to be reduced at the site of the accident, especially if this reduces bleeding or restores circulation to the distal limb. Analgesia is often needed (see below).

Anaesthetic and analgesic techniques

The principles of emergency anaesthesia are discussed in Chapter 28. In the pre-hospital environment, the same principles apply. Techniques that are familiar to the anaesthetist should be used. If the technique causes problems (e.g. apnoea or airway obstruction), the anaesthetist should have adequate access to the patient for appropriate management.

Local/regional anaesthesia

Ring blocks are effective for fingers trapped in machinery. Femoral block may help in the management of pain from a fractured femur.

Intravenous analgesia

The anaesthetist is limited to those drugs carried by the ambulance sevice and deployed by the flying squad. Intravenous morphine, nalbuphine and tramadol have all been used pre-hospital; they should be titrated to effect, and any complications arising from their use should be managed.

Low-dose intravenous ketamine is an effective analgesic. Small bolus doses of 10–20 mg, titrated to effect, are adequate in some casualties to allow fracture alignment or release of a trapped limb.

Inhalational analgesia

Many ambulances carry Entonox, which may be used alone or in combination with other drugs. The main concern with the nitrous oxide in Entonox is enlargement of a pneumothorax or other air-filled cavity.

Intravenous anaesthesia

Rapid-sequence induction using an i.v. anaesthetic agent may be the technique of choice to allow airway protection and control of ventilation in the injured casualty. Appropriate agents include etomidate, ketamine and propofol but with the dose moderated according to the casualty's haemodynamic status. Before embarking on general anaesthesia, the anaesthetist should consider such issues as:

- Is there suitable access to the casualty?
- Who is available to provide assistance?
- Is there appropriate monitoring?
- Is appropriate equipment available? Unlike the anaesthetic room where equipment is easily to hand, the pre-hospital practitioner works using a rucksack or other bag containing a very limited range of equipment.

Even with a supine casualty on the roadside, laryngoscopy and successful tracheal intubation is often more difficult than in the anaesthetic room. A bougie or introducer should always be immediately to hand. In bright sunlight, it is difficult to see the light from the laryngoscope bulb in a casualty's airway and an assistant may be posted between the sun light and the casualty.

TRANSFER TO HOSPITAL

The choice of hospital is decided usually by the medical and ambulance staff on scene and relayed to ambulance control. Ambulance control or the personnel on scene should contact the hospital so the receiving team is placed on standby and receives as much information about the casualty(s) as possible in advance.

A checklist for transfer includes:

- Is the airway secured for transport? A tracheal tube or laryngeal mask should to be tied or taped in place.
- Is oxygen being provided in adequate quantities?
- Is breathing adequate or is assistance required? If the patient's lungs are being ventilated using a mechanical ventilator, is the power capacity (gas, electricity or battery) adequate for the journey? Is there a back-up such as a self-inflating bag-valve mask?
- Is external bleeding controlled? Are i.v. cannulae/catheters taped securely in place? What variables have been selected (arterial pressure and/or pulse) as indicators of resuscitation requirements?
- If the patient has a reduced GCS, have remedial causes such as hypovolaemia or hypoglycaemia been considered?
- Are splints secured? Is spinal immobilization in place (where indicated)? Has a check been made that straps from splints and spinal immobilization devices are not interfering with respiration?
- Is the patient being kept warm with blankets?
- Is appropriate monitoring in place?

In some situations it is necessary to ignore much of this preparation and 'load and go' as fast as possible, e.g. some stabbing or gunshot incidents where the overriding need is surgical intervention.

Civilian helicopter ambulances provide a fast method of transporting a patient to hospital but these have some limitations. The attending staff may be unfamiliar with working in a helicopter, the space around the casualty is restricted compared with a ground ambulance and the environment is noisy; also, a second ambulance journey is often required at many UK hospitals to transport the patient from the helicopter landing site to the A&E department.

FURTHER READING

AAGBI 2000 Provision of anaesthetic services in magnetic resonance units. The Association of Anaesthetists of Great Britain and Ireland, May.

AAGBI 2006 Recommendations for standards of monitoring during anaesthesia and recovery. The Association of Anaesthetists of Great Britain and Ireland, December.

Advanced Life Support Group 2002 Major incident medical management and support, 2nd edn. BMJ Books, London

Ding Z, White P F 2002 Anesthesia for electroconvulsive therapy. Anesthesia and Analgesia 94: 1351–1364

Greaves I, Porter K (eds) 1999 Pre-hospital medicine: the principles and practice of immediate care. Arnold, London

Hashimoto T, Gupta D K, Young W L 2002 Interventional neuroradiology – anesthetic considerations. Anesthesiology Clinics of North America 20: 347–359

Holleran R S (ed) 2003 Air and surface patient transport: principles and practice, 3rd edn. Mosby, St Louis

Obstetric anaesthesia and analgesia 35

Obstetric anaesthesia and analgesia involve caring for women during childbirth in three situations:

- provision of analgesia for labour, usually by epidural or spinal analgesic techniques
- anaesthesia for instrumental (e.g. forceps or Ventouse) or caesarean delivery
- care of the critically ill parturient.

The obstetric anaesthetist is involved in the care of the parturient as part of a multidisciplinary team, including obstetricians, midwives, health visitors, physicians and intensive care specialists. There are few other areas of anaesthetic practice where communication skills and good record-keeping are so important. Successive reports from the Confidential Enquiries into Maternal Deaths (CEMD) have highlighted the problems of women with intercurrent medical disease and the importance of the obstetric anaesthetist in their care. This has led to the establishment of obstetric anaesthetic assessment clinics in many hospitals. The education of colleagues, patients and the public about the role of obstetric anaesthetists is essential so that patients are fully informed and hence feel more comfortable about consenting to regional anaesthesia and analgesia techniques when these may be indicated.

Many anaesthetists in training approach their obstetric module with trepidation for several possible reasons: all anaesthetists have heard that mothers may die, albeit rarely, as a result of general anaesthesia and that these were previously healthy young women. In addition, they may be aware of the challenge of performing regional blocks under the scrutiny of a partner in patients who are awake.

The Obstetric Anaesthetists' Association (OAA) recommendations for modular training in obstetric anaesthesia categorize the training modules into basic and advanced. In the obstetric anaesthetic module, trainees are expected to develop communication, organizational and technical skills. The OAA core curriculum provides the framework for this chapter and it is summarized under the following headings:

- anatomy and physiology of pregnancy
- basic obstetrics
- gastrointestinal physiology and antacid therapy
- pain and pain relief in labour
- epidural and subarachnoid analgesia
- regional anaesthesia for the parturient
- general anaesthesia for the parturient
- assessment of the pregnant woman presenting for anaesthesia and analgesia
- emergencies in obstetric anaesthesia:
  - major haemorrhage
  - failed intubation
  - pre-eclampsia and eclampsia
  - total spinal or epidural block
  - amniotic fluid embolus
  - maternal and neonatal resuscitation
- anaesthesia for interventions other than delivery
- audit
- pharmacology of relevant drugs.

ANATOMY AND PHYSIOLOGY OF PREGNANCY

An understanding of the physiological changes induced by pregnancy is vital to the clinician involved in the care of pregnant women. The obstetric anaesthetist must understand maternal adaptation to pregnancy in order to manipulate physiological changes following general anaesthesia or regional analgesia and anaesthesia in such a way that the condition of the neonate at delivery is optimized.

The physiological changes of pregnancy are exaggerated in multiple pregnancy. The success of assisted conception implies that obstetric anaesthetists care for more women with twins, triplets and quadruplets.

PROGESTERONE

The hormone progesterone may be considered the most important physiological substance in pregnancy. It is secreted initially in increasing amounts during the second half of the menstrual cycle to prepare the woman for pregnancy. Following conception, the corpus luteum ensures adequate blood concentrations until placental secretion is adequate. The most important physiological role of progesterone is its ability to relax smooth muscle. All other physiological changes stem from this pivotal function (Fig. 35.1).

HAEMATOLOGICAL AND HAEMODYNAMIC CHANGES

The increase in blood volume from 60–65 to 80–85 mL kg^{-1} is caused mainly by expansion of plasma volume, which starts shortly after conception and implantation and is maximal at 30–32 weeks (Fig. 35.2). Red cell volume increases linearly but not as much as plasma volume. Haemoglobin concentration decreases from 14 to 12 g dL^{-1} (Table 35.1). Thus, the haematocrit also

decreases. Cell-mediated immunity is depressed. Haematological changes return to normal by the sixth day after delivery.

The increase in blood volume is accompanied by an increase in cardiac output (Fig. 35.3) within the first 10–12 weeks by approximately 1.5 L min^{-1}. By the third trimester, cardiac output has increased by about 44% as a result of significant increases in heart rate (17%) and stroke volume (27%).

In normal pregnancy, despite the increased blood volume and hyperdynamic circulation, the pulmonary capillary wedge pressure (PCWP) and central venous pressure do not increase, because of the relaxant effect of progesterone on the smooth muscle of arterioles and veins. There are significant decreases in systemic (21%) and pulmonary vascular resistance (34%). These decreases permit the increased blood volume to be accommodated at normal vascular pressures. Although the stroke volume increases, the pulmonary cupillary wedge pressure (PCWP) does not increase, because the left ventricle dilates.

In essence, a large heart pumps a larger blood volume more quickly through an enlarged and expanding

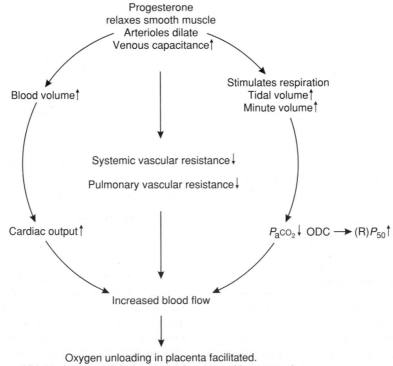

Fig. 35.1
Summary of the main actions of progesterone – it establishes the maternal physiological adaptation to pregnancy. $P_a\text{co}_2$, arterial carbon dioxide tension; ODC, oxyhaemoglobin dissociation curve; P_{50}, partial pressure of oxygen when haemoglobin is 50% saturated at pH 7.4 and temperature 37°C; HCO$_3^-$, bicarbonate.

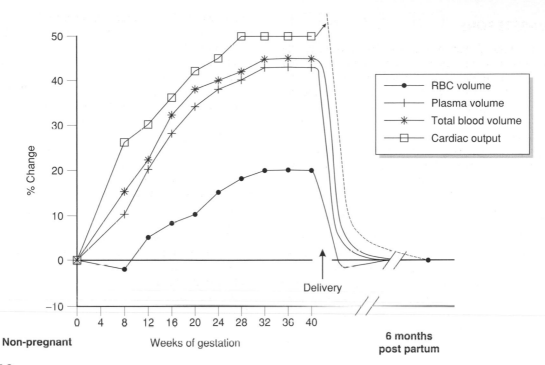

Fig. 35.2
Changes in blood, plasma and red cell volumes and cardiac output during pregnancy.

vascular bed which provides a low resistance to less viscous blood.

Despite the reductions in haemoglobin concentration and red cell mass, the physiological changes are geared to maximize oxygen transport to the placenta and eliminate carbon dioxide from the developing fetus.

Arterial and venous pressures

There is little change in systolic arterial pressure, but there is a marked decrease in diastolic pressure, which

is lowest at mid-pregnancy. Pregnant women who lie supine may suffer from aortocaval compression. Arterial pressure decreases because the gravid uterus compresses the inferior vena cava to reduce venous return and therefore cardiac output. The aorta is also frequently compressed, so that femoral arterial pressure may be lower than brachial arterial pressure. Compensation for aortocaval compression occurs through sympathetic stimulation.

Regional blood flow

There is an increased blood flow to various organs, especially the uterus and placenta, from 85 to 500 mL min^{-1} (see Fig. 35.3).

Renal blood flow is increased by about 400 mL min^{-1}. By 10–12 weeks, glomerular filtration rate (GFR) has increased by 50% and remains at that level until delivery. Twenty-four-hour creatinine clearance is increased; serum creatinine and urea concentrations decrease. Glycosuria often occurs because of decreased tubular reabsorption and the increased load. The renal pelvis, calyces and ureters dilate as a result of the action of progesterone and intermittent obstruction from the uterus, especially on the right.

Liver blood flow is *not* increased. Serum concentrations of total proteins, especially albumin, are reduced in

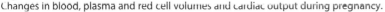

Table 35.1 Haematological changes associated with pregnancy

Variable	Non-pregnant	Pregnant
Haemoglobin	14 g dL^{-1}	12 g dL^{-1}
Haematocrit	0.40–0.42	0.31–0.34
Red cell count	4.2 x 10^{12} L^{-1}	3.8 x 10^{12} L^{-1}
White cell count	6.0 x 10^{9} L^{-1}	9.0 x 10^{9} L^{-1}
Erythrocyte sedimentation rate	10	58–68

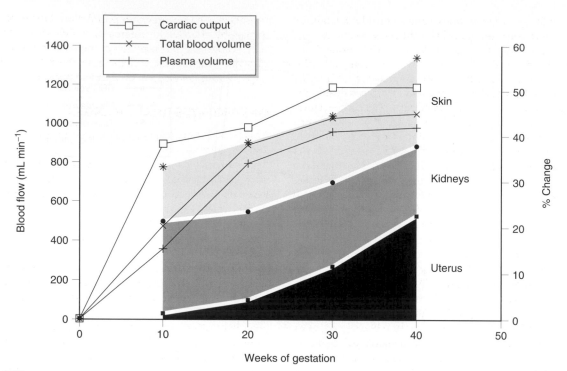

Fig. 35.3
Diagrammatic representation of changes in blood flow to various organs during pregnancy, together with percentage changes in cardiac output, and blood and plasma volumes.

blood, further reducing plasma oncotic pressure. Serum alkaline phosphatase concentration is increased by a factor of 2–4, but the major source of this enzyme is the placenta. Concentrations of aspartate aminotransferase (AST) and alanine aminotransferase (ALT) are altered only slightly in pregnancy; an increase in concentrations of these enzymes indicates liver dysfunction. Plasma cholinesterase concentration decreases by 30%. This is probably only clinically significant in women who are heterozygous for an abnormal gene or who have had plasmapheresis for Rhesus isoimmunization.

Blood flow to the nasal mucosa is increased. Nasal intubation may be associated with epistaxis.

There is a great increase in blood flow to the skin, resulting in warm, clammy hands and feet. The purpose of this vasodilatation, together with that in the nasal mucosa, is to dissipate heat from the metabolically active fetoplacental unit.

RESPIRATORY CHANGES

Respiratory function undergoes several important modifications (Table 35.2), also as a result of the action of progesterone. The larger airways dilate and airway resistance decreases. There are increases in tidal volume (from 10 to 12 weeks) and minute volume

Table 35.2   Changes in respiratory function in pregnancy

Variable	Non-pregnant	Term pregnancy
Tidal volume ↑	450 mL	650 mL
Respiratory rate	16 min^{-1}	16 min^{-1}
Vital capacity	3200 mL	3200 mL
Inspiratory reserve volume	2050 mL	2050 mL
Expiratory reserve volume ↓	700 mL	500 mL
Functional residual capacity ↓	1600 mL	1300 mL
Residual volume ↓	1000 mL	800 mL
P_aO_2 slight ↑	11.3 kPa	12.3 kPa
P_aCO_2 ↓	4.7–5.3 kPa	4 kPa
pH slightly ↑	7.40	7.44

P_aO_2, arterial oxygen tension; P_aCO_2, arterial carbon dioxide tension.

(up to 50%). Progesterone exerts a stimulant action on the respiratory centre and carotid body receptors.

Alveolar hyperventilation leads to a low arterial carbon dioxide tension (P_aCO_2) during the second and third trimesters. By the 12th week of pregnancy, P_aCO_2 may be as low as 4.1 kPa (P_aCO_2 gradually decreases during the premenstrual phase of the menstrual cycle). The respiratory alkalosis is accompanied by a decrease in plasma bicarbonate concentration resulting from renal excretion (base excess decreases from 0 to -3.5 mmol L^{-1}). Arterial pH does not change significantly. The oxyhaemoglobin dissociation curve is shifted to the right because the increase in red cell 2,3-diphosphoglycerate (2,3-DPG) concentration outweighs the effects of a low PCO_2 and high pH, both of which normally shift the curve to the left. The P_{50} increases from about 3.5 to 4.0 kPa. The oxyhaemoglobin dissociation curve (ODC) of HbF is to the left of that for HbA. As the oxygen tension decreases on the normal oxygen cascade, HbA unloads 4.7 mL of oxygen from each 100 mL of blood, whereas HbF unloads only 3.0 mL of oxygen. However, between an oxygen tension of 2.0 kPa (fetal tissue) and 4.5 kPa (placenta), HbF loads 10.3 mL of oxygen to each 100 mL of blood, compared with 8.8 mL for HbA. The loading–unloading advantages of HbF are at *low* oxygen tensions. Placental exchange of oxygen is regulated mainly by a change in oxygen affinities of HbA and HbF caused principally by altered hydrogen ion and carbon dioxide concentrations on both sides of the placenta.

Without the double Bohr and double Haldane effects, the diffusion gradients or placental blood flow would have to be increased considerably to maintain the same efficiency of gas transfer.

The functional residual capacity (FRC) is reduced by about 300 mL at term because of the enlarged uterus. The residual volume is also reduced by 20–30%. This substantial reduction, combined with the increase in tidal volume, results in large volumes of inspired air mixing with a smaller volume of air in the lungs. The composition of alveolar gas may be altered with unusual rapidity; inhalational induction of anaesthesia is rapid but alveolar and arterial hypoxia also develop more rapidly during apnoea or airway obstruction. In normal pregnancy, closing volume does not intrude into tidal volume.

Oxygen consumption ($\dot{V}O_2$) increases gradually from 200 to 250 mL min^{-1} at term (up to 500 mL min^{-1} in labour). Carbon dioxide production parallels oxygen consumption. Rapid desaturation occurs during apnoea at term. In the intervillous space, the diffusion gradient for oxygen is approximately 4.0 kPa, and for carbon dioxide is approximately 1.3 kPa.

The incidence of failed intubation in term parturients is approximately 1 in 300 cases, compared with 1 in 2200 in the non-pregnant population. This is caused in part by changes in pregnancy which affect the airway (Table 35.3). These factors increase the difficulty in seeing the larynx and increase the rate at which hypoxaemia develops in an apnoeic patient.

GASTROINTESTINAL CHANGES

These also stem from the effects of progesterone on smooth muscle.

A reduction in lower oesophageal sphincter pressure occurs before the enlarging uterus exerts its mechanical effects (an increase in intragastric pressure and a decrease in the gastro-oesophageal angle). These mechanical effects are greater when there is multiple pregnancy, hydramnios or morbid obesity. A history of heartburn denotes a lax gastro-oesophageal sphincter.

Placental gastrin increases gastric acidity. Together with the sphincter pressure changes, this makes regurgitation and inhalation of acid gastric contents more likely to occur during pregnancy.

Gastrointestinal motility decreases but gastric emptying is not delayed during pregnancy. However, it is delayed during labour but returns to normal by 18 h after delivery. Pain, anxiety and systemic opioids (including epidural and subarachnoid administration of opioids) aggravate gastric stasis. Small and large intestinal transit times are increased in pregnancy and may result in constipation.

The effects of labour on gastric emptying coupled with the mechanical changes cause the labouring woman to be at risk of regurgitation of gastric acid until approximately 18 h after delivery.

Changes in clotting factors

In the intrinsic pathway, factor VIII concentration doubles; in the extrinsic pathway, factor VII concentration

---

Table 35.3 Physiological changes of pregnancy which increase the risk of hypoxaemia

Interstitial oedema of the upper airway, especially in pre-eclampsia
Enlarged tongue and epiglottis
Enlarged, heavy breasts which may impede laryngoscope introduction
Increased oxygen consumption
Restricted diaphragmatic movement, reducing FRC

increases 10-fold. In the common pathway, factor X and fibrinogen concentrations increase. (This alters the negative surface charge on red cells which form rouleaux, and increases the ESR.) Concentrations of factors II and V increase in early pregnancy and then decrease steadily. Concentrations of antithrombin IIIa and factors XI and XIII decrease because of consumption at the placental site as a result of low-level coagulation with fibrin deposition (5–10% of total circulating fibrinogen). Bleeding time, prothrombin time and partial thromboplastin time remain within normal limits. See also Table 35.4.

Plasma fibrinogen concentration increases from the 12th week to twice that in the non-pregnant state. A progressive inhibition of fibrinolysis occurs from 11 to 12 weeks. Plasminogen remains unchanged, plasminogen activator activity decreases and the concentrations of the inhibitors (antiplasmin and macroglobulin) increase, leading to delayed fibrinolysis, especially in late pregnancy. The hypercoagulable state of the blood and the reduced fibrinolytic activity represent a compensatory response to local utilization of fibrin and are advantageous for haemostasis at placental separation.

Table 35.4 Coagulation changes in late pregnancy
Fibrinogen increased from 2.5 (non-pregnant value) to 4.6-6.0 g L^{-1}
Factor II slightly increased
Factor V slightly increased
Factor VII increased 10-fold
Factor VIII increased – twice non-pregnant state
Factor IX increased
Factor X increased
Factor XI decreased 60–70%
Factor XII increased 30–40%
Factor XIII decreased 40–50%
Antithrombin IIIa decreased slightly
Plasminogen activator reduced
Plasminogen inhibitor increased
Fibrinogen-stabilizing factor falls gradually to 50% of non-pregnant value

THE EPIDURAL AND SUBARACHNOID SPACES

Anatomy of the epidural space

The epidural space is the space between the periosteal lining of the vertebral canal and the spinal dura mater. It contains spinal nerve roots, lymphatics, blood vessels and a variable amount of fat (Figs 35.4, 35.5). Its boundaries are as follows:

- *superiorly* – the foramen magnum, where the dural layers fuse with the periosteum of the cranium; hence, local anaesthetic solution placed in the epidural space cannot extend higher than this
- *inferiorly* – the sacrococcygeal membrane
- *anteriorly* – the posterior longitudinal ligament
- *posteriorly* – the ligamentum flavum and vertebral laminae
- *laterally* – the pedicles of the vertebrae and the intervertebral foramina.

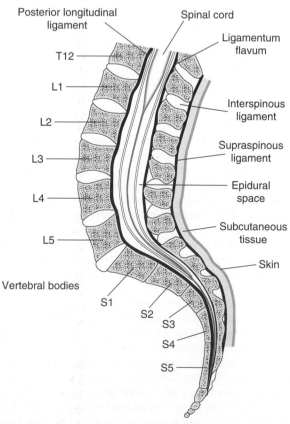

Fig. 35.4
The vertebral column. Note that the spinal cord ends at the level of L1 or L2 and that the dural sac extends to the level of S2 vertebra.

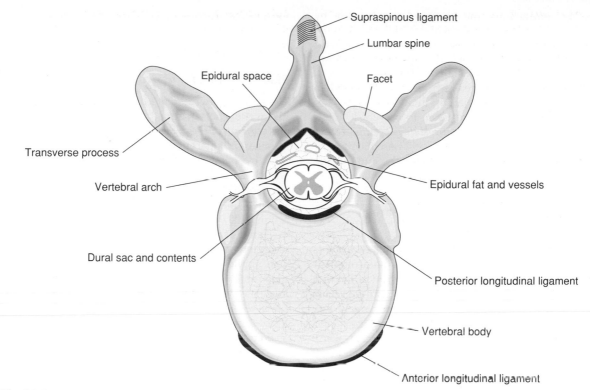

Fig. 35.5
Anatomical relations of the epidural space.

In the normal adult, the spinal cord begins at the foramen magnum and ends at the level of L1 or L2 (though it may end lower); here it becomes the cauda equina. The epidural space is a tube containing the spinal cord, the cerebrospinal fluid (CSF) and the meninges. It is crossed by 32 spinal nerves, each with a dural cuff: therefore it is a leaky tube. The subarachnoid space extends further than the cord, to the level of S2. Below this level, the dura blends with the periosteum of the coccyx. Between the dura and arachnoid is the subdural space, within which local anaesthetic solution may spread extensively

The volume of the vertebral canal is finite. An increase in volume of contents of one compartment reduces the compliance of the other compartments and increases the pressures throughout.

In pregnancy, the epidural veins are dilated by the action of progesterone. These valveless veins of Bateson form collaterals and become engorged as a result of aortocaval compression, during a uterine contraction or secondary to raised intrathoracic or intra-abdominal pressure, e.g. coughing, sneezing or expulsive efforts of parturition. The dose of local anaesthetic for epidural analgesia or epidural/sub-arachnoid anaesthesia is reduced by about one-third for the following reasons:

- Spread of local anaesthetic in either the subarachnoid or epidural space is more extensive as a result of the reduced volume.
- Progesterone-induced hyperventilation leads to a low P_aCO_2 and a reduced buffering capacity; thus, local anaesthetic drugs remain as free salts for longer periods.
- Pregnancy itself produces antinociceptive effects. The onset of nerve block is more rapid, and human peripheral nerves have been shown to be more sensitive to lidocaine during pregnancy. Increased plasma and CSF progesterone concentrations may contribute towards the reduced excitability of the nervous system.
- Increased pressure in the epidural space facilitates diffusion across the dura and produces higher concentrations of local anaesthetic in CSF.
- Venous congestion of the lateral foramina decreases loss of local anaesthetic along the dural sleeves.

In pregnancy, the epidural pressure is slightly positive and becomes negative a few hours after delivery.

During contractions, the pressure may increase by 0.2–0.8 kPa and become very high (2.0–5.9 kPa) in the second stage of labour. Because the spread of local anaesthetics is exaggerated during contractions, top-ups should not be administered at that time.

The CSF pressure increases from about 2.2 to 3.8 kPa during contractions and 6.9 kPa in the second stage.

Even if precautions are taken to prevent it, intermittent aortocaval compression always occurs in association with maternal movement. Consequently, the epidural veins become intermittently and unpredictably engorged

Pain pathways in labour and caesarean section

The afferent nerve supply of the uterus and cervix is via Aδ and C fibres that accompany the thoracolumbar and sacral sympathetic outflows. The pain of the first stage of labour is referred to the spinal cord segments associated with the uterus and the cervix, namely T10, 11, 12 and L1. Pain of distension of the birth canal and perineum is conveyed via S2–S4 nerves (Fig. 35.6). When anaesthesia is required for caesarean section, all the layers between the skin and the uterus must be anaesthetized. It is important to remember that the most sensitive layer is the peritoneum, and therefore the block should extend up to at least T4 and also include the sacral roots (S1–S5).

Placental transfer of drugs

The barrier between maternal and fetal blood is a single layer of chorion united with fetal endothelium. The surface area of this is vastly increased by the presence of microvilli. Placental transfer of drugs occurs, therefore, by passive diffusion through cell membranes which are lipophilic. However, this membrane appears to be punctuated by channels which allow transfer of hydrophilic molecules at a rate that is around 100 000 times lower.

Hence drugs cross the placenta by simple diffusion of un-ionized lipophilic molecules. Fick's law of diffusion applies. The rate is directly proportional to the maternofetal concentration gradient and the area of the placenta available for transfer, and inversely proportional to placental thickness. Lipid solubility, degree of ionization and protein binding affect placental transfer, as do the dose and route of administration and absorption, distribution and metabolism in the mother.

Lipid solubility

The placental membrane is freely permeable to lipid-soluble substances which undergo flow-dependent transfer. As the rate of transfer depends on the concentration gradient of the drug across the membrane and blood flow on each side, maternal hypotension reduces placental blood flow and, consequently, transfer of lipid-soluble drugs.

Hydrophilic substances

The placental membrane carries an electrical charge; ionized molecules with the same charge are repelled, while those with the opposite charge are retained within the membrane. The rate of this permeability-dependent transfer is inversely proportional to molecular size. Size limitation for polar substances begins at molecular weights between 50 and 100 Da. Ions diffuse much more slowly. Factors affecting the degree of ionization alter the rate of transfer.

Maternal pH

This alters ionization of a partially ionized drug. The maternal–fetal pH gradient also affects transfer. The degree of ionization of acidic drugs is greater on the maternal side and lower on the fetal side. The converse applies for basic drugs.

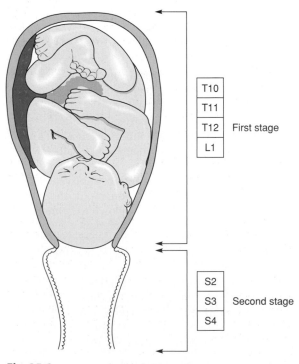

Fig. 35.6
Nerve supply to the uterus and birth canal.

T10
T11
T12   First stage
L1

S2
S3   Second stage
S4

Protein binding

A dynamic equilibrium exists between bound (unavailable) and unbound (available) drug. Protein binding is pH-dependent, e.g. acidosis reduces protein binding of local anaesthetics. Reduced albumin concentration increases the proportion of unbound drug. Many basic drugs are bound to α_1-glycoprotein, which is present in much lower concentrations in the fetus.

Effects of drugs on the fetus

Drugs may have a harmful effect on the fetus at any time during pregnancy. In the early stages of pregnancy (at a stage when the woman may be unaware that she is pregnant), the conceptus is a rapidly dividing group of cells and the effect of drugs at that stage tends to be an all-or-none phenomenon, either slowing cell division where no harm is done or causing death of the embryo. Drugs may produce congenital malformations (teratogenesis), and the period of greatest risk is from weeks 3 to 11. In the second and third trimesters, drugs may affect the functional development of the fetus or have toxic effects on fetal tissues. Drugs given in labour or near delivery may adversely affect the neonate after delivery. Hence, drugs should be prescribed in pregnancy only if the perceived benefit of the therapy to the mother outweighs the possible detrimental effects on the fetus. Drugs that have been extensively used should be prescribed in the lowest effective doses. These effects depend on fetal distribution, metabolism and excretion; for example, polar substances cross the placenta slowly, but when they reach the fetus, they are excreted rapidly into the amniotic fluid. Lipophilic substances are transferred quickly, but it may take up to 40 min for equilibration to occur.

Effects of drugs on the neonate

In many studies, the ratio of maternal vein to umbilical vein concentration is used; this indicates the situation at delivery only and gives little information on the effects or distribution of the drug in the neonate. The distribution differs because of the anatomical and physiological organization of the fetal circulation; for example, drugs accumulate in the liver because of the umbilical venous flow to the liver and are metabolized before distribution. The relatively high extracellular fluid volume explains the large volumes of distribution of local anaesthetics and relaxants. In addition, fetal plasma contains less α_1-glycoprotein and albumin at term, which affects protein binding of drugs,

particularly local anaesthetics. Many hepatic enzyme systems are immature; for example, the hydroxylating pathway is not developed. Renal function in the neonate is immature, and urinary elimination of drugs is reduced.

Inhalational anaesthetics diffuse readily, but provided that the induction–delivery interval is short, the fetus is minimally affected. Neonatal elimination is dependent on ventilation.

Neuromuscular blocking drugs, which are quaternary ammonium compounds and ionized fully, cross the placenta very slowly. Fetomaternal ratios at delivery are very low. Only prolonged administration of a relaxant, e.g. in the intensive care unit, might lead to neonatal paralysis. Bolus doses of succinylcholine are safe.

Thiopental is highly lipid-soluble, weakly acidic, 75% protein-bound and less than 50% ionized at physiological pH. It therefore crosses the placenta rapidly, with umbilical vein concentration closely following the relatively rapid decrease in maternal blood concentration. Fetal plasma concentration continues to increase for around 40 min after single exposure. However, because of the relatively large fetal volume of distribution, fetal and neonatal tissue concentrations are lower than maternal. The maintenance of high maternal thiopental concentration by repeated boluses maintains a high diffusion gradient, producing prolonged placental transfer and neonatal sedation. Doses of thiopental greater than 8 mg kg^{-1} produce neonatal depression, whereas doses of less than 4 mg kg^{-1} produce no significant neonatal effects providing induction to delivery time is less than 5 min. Thiopental in such doses does not affect Apgar score or umbilical cord gas tensions, but may produce subtle changes in the neuroadaptive (NACS) score, such as reduction in muscular tone, decreased excitability and a predominant sleep state in the first day of life. A dose of thiopental of 4–7 mg kg^{-1} is commonly advocated for induction of general anaesthesia because it ensures unconsciousness. Widespread clinical use testifies to the safety of thiopental.

Propofol is highly protein-bound, neutral and lipophilic. Propofol has been used for both induction and maintenance of anaesthesia for caesarean section. There is conflicting evidence concerning the effects of propofol on the neonate. Clearly, if propofol is administered by infusion and uterine blood concentrations are maintained, a high diffusion gradient is maintained across the placenta and therefore persistently high transfer of propofol. Induction doses as low as 2–3 mg kg^{-1} and maintenance doses as low as 5 mg kg^{-1} h^{-1} have been shown to cause significant neonatal depression. Neonatal elimination of propofol is slower than that in adults. Unless thiopental is contraindicated, there seems little advantage in using propofol for caesarean section.

Diazepam is a sinister agent. It is a non-polar compound which is bound to albumin, but the fetomaternal ratio may reach 2. The neonate may suffer from respiratory depression, hypotonia, poor thermoregulation and raised bilirubin concentrations. Prolonged maternal diazepam administration should be avoided, if possible.

Opioids are mainly weak bases bound to α_1-glycoprotein. Pethidine and its metabolite norpethidine depress all aspects of neurobehaviour in the neonate. Fetomaternal ratios increase to exceed 1 after 2–4 h. Neonatal elimination is slower, resulting in prolongation of the effects. Transfer of pethidine is increased in the presence of fetal acidosis. Depressant effects are maximum where administration to delivery time is 2–3 h. Fentanyl is highly lipid-soluble and albumin-bound, and rapidly crosses the placenta. Apgar scores are low after administration of intravenous fentanyl. Epidural administration of fentanyl in doses of less than 200 µg is not associated with any adverse effect on the fetus. Alfentanil is less lipophilic but more protein-bound to α_1-glycoprotein. Fetomaternal ratios are low and at caesarean section are more related to fetomaternal α_1-glycoprotein levels. Theoretically, Apgar and neurobehavioural scores should be less affected.

Sufentanil is principally bound to α_1-glycoprotein. Therefore, it should be a good opioid additive for epidural analgesia. However, a dose-related reduction in both Apgar and neurobehavioural scores has been observed. In doses of less than 30 µg, it appears not to affect the neonate adversely. It is not available or licensed for use in the UK.

Intrathecal doses of fentanyl and sufentanil have been associated with sudden fetal bradycardia occurring within 30 min of administration. In one study, there was associated uterine hypertonicity.

Remifentanil crosses the placenta rapidly but appears to have few adverse effects on neonatal blood gas tensions, Apgar or NACS scores. It is a promising agent for use in patient-controlled analgesia (PCA) in labour and as a continuous infusion for caesarean section. It may cause transient fetal bradycardia and loss of variability. However, its use outside clinical trials is not recommended. Its current preparation is unsuitable for spinal or epidural use.

Lactation and drugs in obstetric anaesthesia

Women are encouraged to breast-feed. Oestrogen and progesterone stimulate mammary development during pregnancy. These hormones inhibit prolactin. This inhibition ceases at delivery. Suckling triggers lactation and stimulates the release of more prolactin and oxytocin, both of which promote production of milk.

Many women wish to suckle their infant immediately after delivery and are encouraged to do so. The anaesthetist should know, therefore, if the drugs used for obstetric anaesthesia and analgesia are secreted in the milk and, if so, whether they are likely to have an adverse effect either on the process of lactation itself or on the neonate.

The effects of a drug administered to the mother on a breast-feeding neonate are determined by peak plasma concentration of the drug, its transfer into milk, composition of milk, volume ingested by the neonate, metabolism (including first-pass metabolism by the neonate), pharmacokinetics in the neonate and action in the neonate.

Many studies have relied on assessment of concentration of drug in milk with little consideration of resultant neonatal plasma concentration and the changing composition of breast milk.

Human breast milk consists of an isosmotic emulsion of fat in water, with lactose and protein in the aqueous phase. However, its composition varies with time. Colostrum (first milk) contains abundant protein and lactose but no fat. It has a high pH and specific gravity. Over the following 7–10 days, milk has less protein, less lactose and more fat. Colostrum is more likely to be contaminated by water-soluble drugs, whereas lipid-soluble drugs are secreted into mature milk. The volume of colostrum produced is around 10–120 mL, in contrast to ingestion of mature milk by the neonate of 130–180 mL kg^{-1} day^{-1} (600–1000 mL day^{-1}). Even in mature milk there is a significant diurnal variation in composition.

The maternal concentration of drug presented to the breast varies with dose, route of administration, volume of distribution, lipid solubility, ionization and protein binding.

The physicochemical properties of a drug which determine transfer into the milk are pK_a, the partition coefficient, degree of ionization and molecular weight. The pH of mature human milk is 7.09. Therefore, weak acids are less easily transferred than weak bases.

The total amount of drug contained in the milk depends on binding to milk protein, partition into milk lipid and the quantity which remains unbound in the aqueous phase, e.g. lipid-soluble drugs such as diazepam are concentrated in milk lipid. The dose of drug delivered to the neonate from the milk varies with the volume ingested. The higher gastric pH, different gastrointestinal flora and slow gastrointestinal transit of the neonate influence drug absorption.

The pharmacokinetics of drugs in the neonate may differ markedly from those in adults. Lipophilic and acidic drugs are bound to albumin and may displace unconjugated bilirubin. Metabolic pathways such as hydroxylation, conjugation and oxidation are immature. Immature renal function may delay excretion of drugs and active metabolites dependent on renal excretion.

Opioids. Morphine appears safe with conventional administration. PCA may increase maternal plasma concentration. It is transferred readily to breast milk but does not appear to cause neonatal depression, possibly because of first-pass metabolism. Codeine and dihydrocodeine are metabolized to morphine and are not associated with neonatal depression. Pethidine is associated with neurobehavioural depression of the neonate. Short-acting opioids such as fentanyl and alfentanil are safe, even by continuous epidural infusion.

Non-steroidal anti-inflammatory drugs. The non-steroidal antiinflammatory drugs (NSAIDs) ketorolac and diclofenac are safe. The neonate has immature biotransformation and excretory pathways. Aspirin should be avoided because high concentrations have been observed following a single oral dose. Neonates may be at risk of developing Reye's syndrome.

Paracetamol. Paracetamol is minimally secreted into breast milk. However, it is cleared by the liver more slowly than in adults. It is considered safe.

Thiopental and propofol. These drugs are detectable in milk and colostrum. However, the dose received by the neonate after a single induction dose is insignificant.

Diazepam. Diazepam and its metabolites are excreted in breast milk. As with placental transfer, there is the possibility of adverse effects on the neonate, especially with continuous administration.

Lidocaine and bupivacaine. The amounts excreted in breast milk are small or undetectable.

PHARMACOLOGY OF RELEVANT DRUGS

The detailed pharmacology of the drugs used during pregnancy is covered elsewhere in this textbook, but the following are of particular relevance.

SYNTOCINON (OXYTOCIN)

Oxytocin is the posterior pituitary hormone responsible for effective uterine muscle contraction. It is indicated in a labour where the rate of progress is slow and immediately after delivery (either normal vaginal, instrumental or caesarean section) in order to cause placental delivery and closure of uterine vasculature. For augmentation or induction of labour, Syntocinon is usually administered via a syringe pump using an increasing dose as set out in the delivery suite guidelines. The usual dose to prevent postpartum haemorrhage is 5 international units (IU), but up to 40 IU may be infused over several hours (via a syringe pump) to maintain myometrial contraction. It may also act on other types of vascular smooth muscle, resulting in hypertension. Syntocinon also has an antidiuretic hormone effect, so care should be taken if infused in dilute dextrose solution, as hyponatraemia may occur.

ERGOMETRINE

Ergometrine is also given to cause uterine contraction, usually in a dose of 500 µg. Ergometrine causes peripheral vasoconstriction, which may be severe, leading to hypertension and pulmonary oedema. It can cause nausea and vomiting as a result of its action on other types of smooth muscle and it is usually reserved for more severe cases of uterine atony. Ergometrine is contraindicated in pre-eclampsia.

SYNTOMETRINE

Syntometrine is a combination of ergometrine 500 µg and Syntocinon 5 units. It is administered routinely by i.m. injection at the delivery of the anterior shoulder to assist in placental separation and reduction in postpartum haemorrhage.

ATOSIBAN

Atosiban is an oxytocin antagonist used to decrease uterine contractions; it has few side-effects but it is expensive.

INDOMETACIN

Indometacin is a prostaglandin synthetase inhibitor. It may be given orally or rectally to inhibit contractions after cervical circlage. It can cause premature closure of the fetal ductus areteriosus and therefore should not be used after 32 weeks' gestation

RITODRINE

Ritodrine is occasionally given to arrest a premature labour. It is a β_2-adrenergic receptor agonist which relaxes uterine musculature and so prevents premature labour. The effect of ritodrine should be monitored carefully, as hypokalaemia, severe tachycardia, pulmonary oedema and hyperglycaemia may occur.

TERBUTALINE

Terbutaline is another β_2-agonist which may be given subcutaneously, intramuscularly or by slow intravenous infusion to treat overstimulated contractions associated with fetal distress. It is occasionally used as part of an in-utero fetal resuscitation regimen before emergency caesarean section.

PROSTAGLANDINS

Prostaglandins are a group of endogenous short polypeptides with a wide diversity of physiological functions. Prostaglandins may cause bronchospasm and also hypertension and are commonly used to 'ripen' the cervix in induction of labour.

Carboprost

Carboprost is prostaglandin $F_{2\alpha}$. It has an important role in the treatment of severe uterine atony unresponsive to Syntocinon or ergometrine. It is administered by i.m. injection or may be given into the myometrium at caesarean section. It should not be given intravenously. It may induce bronchospasm and hypertension.

Misoprostol

Misoprostol is a prostaglandin E_1 analogue. It may be used to induce labour for a non-viable fetus. It is usually given vaginally followed by oral doses. It may be given rectally to facilitate uterine contraction prior to delivery of the placenta (3rd stage) or to treat postpartum haemorrhage. It produces pyrexia, shivering, nausea and vomiting and diarrhoea.

Dinoprostone

Dinoprostone is prostaglandin E_2 which is given as a gel, tablets or pessary intravaginally to induce labour by 'ripening the cervix' prior to rupture of membranes and intravenous infusion of Syntocinon.

Mifepristone (RU486)

Mifepristone is a prostaglandin antagonist which causes luteolysis and trophoblastic separation. It is given orally with prostaglandins to induce labour after intrauterine death of the fetus and where labour is induced for a non-viable fetus. It is associated with headache, dizziness and gastrointestinal upset.

BASIC OBSTETRICS

NORMAL LABOUR

A large number of pregnant women are assessed as being 'low risk' and are predicted to have a normal labour, but the diagnosis of normal labour is retrospective. The descriptors of normal labour are:

- contractions occurring every 3 min and lasting 45 s
- progressive dilatation of the cervix (approximately $1 \, cm \, h^{-1}$)
- progressive descent of the presenting part
- vertex presenting with the head flexed and the occiput anterior
- labour not < 4 h (precipitate) or > 18 h (prolonged)
- delivery of a live healthy baby
- delivery of a complete placenta and membranes
- no complications.

The first stage of labour

Initially, the cervix effaces (i.e. becomes thin along its vertical axis and soft in consistency) and then cervical dilatation begins. The rate of cervical dilatation should be about $1 \, cm \, h^{-1}$ for a primiparous woman and $2 \, cm \, h^{-1}$ for a multigravid woman. It is standard practice to examine the woman every 4 h, or more frequently if there is cause for concern. Routine observations are made as follows and these are charted on the partogram which forms part of a standard National Maternity Record in the UK together with epidural record charts:

- fetal heart rate every 15 min
- maternal pulse rate half-hourly
- BP half-hourly
- temperature 4-hourly
- urinalysis at each emptying of the bladder.

The fetal heart may be monitored intermittently by auscultation using Pinard's stethoscope or by cardiotocographic monitoring. The cardiotocograph is recorded either intermittently or continuously depending on the conditions of the labour and fetus. The fetal heart may be recorded using either an abdominal transducer or a clip applied to the fetal head. Radiotelemetry is available in some units and this allows the woman to be mobile while her baby is monitored.

The second stage of labour

The second stage of labour commences at full dilatation of the cervix and terminates at the delivery of the baby. At full dilatation of the cervix, the character of the contractions changes and they become associated with a strong urge to push. In normal labour, Ferguson's reflex occurs, where there is an increase in circulating oxytocin secondary to distension of the vagina from the descending presenting part of the fetus, with consequent increased strength of uterine contractions at full dilatation. Epidural analgesia may attenuate the effect of this reflex. The second stage of labour may be classified into passive and active stages and this is particularly relevant when epidural analgesia is used. With epidural analgesia, the labouring woman does not have the normal sensation at the start of the second stage of labour produced by Ferguson's reflex, and therefore the active stage of pushing should commence only when the vertex is visible or the woman has a strong urge to push. A normal active second stage should not exceed 1 h of active pushing as the fetus may become acidotic.

The third stage of labour

The third stage of labour is the complete delivery of the placenta, membranes and the contraction of the uterus. It is usually managed 'actively' by administering an oxytocic (usually intramuscular oxytocin and ergometrine given at the delivery of the anterior shoulder to decrease the risk of a postpartum haemorrhage) but it may also be managed without an oxytocic. During the third stage of labour there is redistribution of the former placental blood flow (about 15% cardiac output). This results in an increase in circulating blood volume which is potentially dangerous to those women who have cardiac disease as it may precipitate heart failure immediately postpartum.

FETAL MONITORING

Recent developments have made it possible to assess fetal well-being in the antenatal period. An obstetric anaesthetist is often involved when a decision to deliver the baby early is made on the outcome of these assessments. The most commonly used tests are:

- serial ultrasonography
- serial Doppler flow studies
- cardiotocograph (CTG) monitoring.

It is important that the anaesthetist communicates with the obstetrician and understands how compromised the fetus is when asked to give analgesia or anaesthesia to these mothers. The degree of urgency for the delivery depends on the condition of the fetus.

Monitoring of the fetus is an important part of intrapartum care, as labour is a stressful event for the fetus. Fetal well-being may be monitored routinely using the following methods:

- fetal heart auscultation
- fetal heart cardiotocography

- colour of the liquor
- fetal blood sampling.

The ability of the fetus to maintain oxygenation is diminished with each uterine contraction. The normal fetus has a baseline heart rate of 110–150 beat min^{-1} and a variability of 5–20 beat min^{-1}. It may accelerate with contractions but should not decelerate. The normal CTG trace simultaneously records fetal heart and uterine contractions; it is therefore possible to monitor the effect of contractions on the fetal heart rate. Decelerations in fetal heart are classified as early, variable and late. Early decelerations are synchronous with contractions and are usually benign. Variable decelerations are variable in shape, extent and rate of occurrence and may or may not indicate hypoxaemia. Late decelerations persist after the end of the contraction and are usually pathological. Opioids or other sedative drugs may cause a flat trace with loss of beat-to-beat variability. Any trace that causes concern, especially in a high-risk pregnancy, is an indication for fetal blood sampling.

Colour of the liquor may be monitored when the membranes are ruptured. The liquor colour is observed for the presence of meconium. The appearance of new meconium may indicate fetal hypoxia, as hypoxaemia may cause the fetal anal sphincter to relax. The appearance of thick new meconium is an indication for urgent delivery. If meconium is aspirated into the lungs of the neonate, severe lung damage may ensue, and therefore a paediatrician should be present at delivery if meconium is present. When the fetus becomes hypoxic, there is an accumulation of lactic acid and a reduction in fetal pH. Fetal blood sampling allows more accurate assessment of fetal well-being than is afforded by the CTG and should be performed whenever there is anxiety about the CTG or when there is meconium in the liquor. When fetal blood sampling is performed, care must be taken to avoid maternal inferior vena caval compression, which may lead to impaired venous return from the mass of the gravid uterus on the inferior vena cava (IVC), with resultant hypotension and syncope. This is most likely to happen if the woman lies supine, and hence it is often termed the 'supine hypotension syndrome'. Parturients at or near term should always lie on the side or at a 15° tilt from horizontal.

Values for fetal pH are as follows:

- pH > 7.25: normal
- pH 7.20–7.25: borderline abnormality and sampling should be repeated 30 min later
- pH < 7.20: significant acidosis requiring urgent delivery of the baby.

Urgency of delivery is guided by the results of fetal monitoring and does not fall into the Confidential Enquiry into Perioperative Deaths (CEPOD) categorization for urgency.

Urgency of caesarean section delivery is classified into the following four grades:

Grade 1. Emergency: immediate threat to life of woman or fetus.

Grade 2. Urgent: maternal or fetal compromise which is not immediately life-threatening.

Grade 3. Scheduled: needing early delivery but no maternal or fetal compromise.

Grade 4. Elective: at a time to suit the patient and the maternity team.

This should be clearer than the present three-point classification of emergency, urgent and elective. The classification applies at the time of decision to operate, e.g. an episode of fetal compromise caused by aortocaval compression responding to therapy, followed some hours later by caesarean section for failure to progress, would be graded as 3, not 2. Similarly, a case booked as an elective procedure for malpresentation could eventually be classified as Grade 3 if the woman goes into labour before the chosen date of surgery.

MATERNAL ANTACID THERAPY

Mendelson first described the syndrome of aspiration of gastric contents in 1946. He described the pathological changes seen when solid food or liquid gastric contents are inhaled during anaesthesia in pregnancy. The chemical pneumonitis that resulted from inhalation of the acid gastric contents in pregnancy prompted the following recommendations:

- Withhold oral feeding during labour and substitute parenteral administration where necessary.
- Wider use of local anaesthesia where indicated and feasible.
- Alkalinization and emptying of stomach contents before general anaesthesia.
- Competent administration of general anaesthesia, with appreciation of the dangers of aspiration during induction and recovery.
- Adequate delivery room equipment, including transparent masks, suction, laryngoscope and tilting table.
- Anaesthetist to remain with the patient until return of laryngeal reflexes.

These recommendations still hold true today and have been reiterated in successive reports of CEMD. There are still no clear guidelines for oral intake in labour, although most units allow free access to clear fluids (solid food and milk prohibited). There has been progress towards the increasing use of regional anaesthesia and there has also been an improvement in the standard of obstetric anaesthesia.

As it has been shown that acid aspiration causes chemical pneumonitis, various methods are used routinely to reduce the acidity of the stomach contents. Particulate antacids, e.g. magnesium trisilicate, were used until they themselves were implicated in causing a chemical reaction in the lungs of animals. This led to the use of non-particulate antacids of which the most popular is 0.3 mol sodium citrate 30 mL administered orally less than 30 min before general anaesthesia. In addition, H_2-antagonists have now become standard gastric acid prophylaxis. Ranitidine 150 mg may be administered orally 6-hourly throughout labour. Whether or not it should be administered to all labouring women or only those perceived to be at risk of anaesthetic intervention is controversial. It is routine practice to administer oral ranitidine before elective caesarean section, e.g. in two doses – one the night before and the second on the morning of operation. Metoclopramide 10 mg may be administered before anaesthesia to hasten gastric emptying. It may be given either orally or intravenously depending on the urgency of the situation.

PAIN AND PAIN RELIEF IN LABOUR

It is only in the last 150 years that effective methods of pain relief have been available. Queen Victoria was given chloroform by John Snow for the birth of her eighth child and this did much to popularize the use of pain relief in labour. Many women go into labour unaware that they may need pain relief, although 75% of first-time mothers experience sufficient pain for them to request pain relief. Melzack, using the McGill pain questionnaire, found that the pain of labour is amongst the most severe in the human experience of pain, equivalent to the pain of the amputation of a digit. Several studies have tried to assess the pain of labour. Melzack found the following for primigravidae: 9.2% very mild, 29.5% mild, 37.9% moderate and 23.4% severe.

THE EFFECT OF PAIN AND ANALGESIA ON THE MOTHER AND FETUS

A long, painful labour may lead to an exhausted, frightened and hysterical mother incapable of decision-making. A traumatic labour may, in extreme circumstances, lead to a post-traumatic stress syndrome.

Figure 35.7 summarizes the effects of pain. Pain compromises placental blood flow and renders uterine contractions less effective. Increased catecholamine secretion results in increased myocardial work and arterial pressure and may also compromise blood flow to the placenta by peripheral vasoconstriction. Activation of the adrenocortical hormones may adversely affect electrolyte, carbohydrate and protein metabolism.

The ideal analgesic

The ideal analgesic for labour should provide excellent rapid-onset pain relief in both first and second stages without risk or side-effects to mother or fetus and should also retain the mother's ability to mobilize and be independent during labour. Many women do not wish complete pain relief, and therefore the analgesic should be easy to control. There is no ideal analgesic at the present time, but it is perhaps most closely approached by low-dose central neuraxial (spinal or epidural) techniques which provide effective analgesia in over 90% cases while preserving motor function to a large degree. Effective epidural (or spinal) analgesia reverses the adverse physiological effects of labour pain listed above by blocking the psychological and biochemical stress response, resulting in improved maternal well-being and placental perfusion.

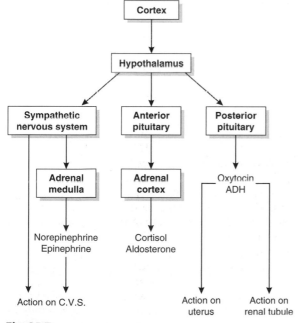

Fig. 35.7
The adverse effects of pain in labour on mother and fetus.

LABOUR ANALGESIA

Labour analgesia may be classified broadly into the following areas:

- non-pharmacological
- parenteral
- inhalational
- regional.

Non-pharmacological analgesia

Birth preparation classes

In the 1930s, Grantly Dick-Read proposed that childbirth may be painless, as it is a normal life-event, and that society had conditioned women to believe that childbirth was painful. He proposed that education of women about the process of labour and delivery and training them in relaxation therapy would obviate any need for analgesics. Active partner participation was encouraged.

The goals of childbirth preparation are to fully inform women about what to expect in labour and to enhance their ability to cope without analgesia. Fernand Lamaze popularized the technique in North America and Frederick Leboyer modified the technique to suggest birth in quiet conditions with gentle initial handling of the newborn. Although there are few controlled studies on outcome, published observations do not indicate any benefits in terms of outcome of labour and reduced maternal morbidity from childbirth preparation.

Environment and the management of labour

Continuous support in labour is associated with shorter labours and reduced requirement for analgesia. Traditional cultures have always had the support of experienced women to be with the woman in labour. Midwifery (literally 'with woman') has its roots in this role of emotional support. Mobility in labour is helpful in maintaining the dignity and independence of the woman in labour, and while it is thought to be helpful, there are no randomized, controlled trials to support the view that pain is easier to cope with when ambulant. Most would accept that a bath or shower is relaxing, although whether this should be extended to water birth is controversial.

Transcutaneous electrical nerve stimulation

The transcutaneous electrical nerve stimulation (TENS) technique is based on Melzack and Wall's 'gate control' theory of pain. It involves passage of a small electrical current through skin to reach the peripheral nervous system. Myelinated, larger-diameter nerve fibres (Aβ) have a lower threshold for stimulation by external electrical impulses than myelinated Aδ and unmyelinated C fibres, which transmit pain impulses. Selective stimulation of large-diameter fibres, transmitting touch and vibration sense, inhibits painful stimuli transmission to the substantia gelatinosa of the dorsal horn of the spinal cord. The TENS electrodes should be applied at the appropriate dermatomal levels involved with the transmission of pain in labour (see Fig. 35.6). The TENS machine then emits a low background stimulus that may be boosted with each contraction. There is little evidence that use of TENS reduces the need for analgesics, duration of labour or incidence of instrumental delivery.

Hypnosis

First used by James Braid in 1843, hypnosis involves the patient being in a state of intense concentration, where positive feelings are suggested and reinforced and negative ones played down. Clearly, this requires the continuous presence of a skilled hypnotist throughout the labour, preceded by several training sessions with that therapist before labour. While this method may provide reliable analgesia for a small number of women, it has not proved suitable on a large scale for labour analgesia.

Acupuncture

Acupuncture has only recently received attention for labouring women. In volunteer parturients, it was found to be ineffective in almost 80% of cases.

Parenteral (systemic) analgesia

Many opioids have been used to provide obstetric analgesia, but the most popular have been pethidine, morphine and diamorphine. Pethidine has become established in obstetric practice without good scientific data to support its use, and in the UK two doses of 100 mg may be prescribed for a labouring woman by a midwife. Pethidine is given by intramuscular injection and the maximum effect is seen about 1 h after administration. The analgesic effects are variable and pethidine may also cause significant side-effects, such as maternal sedation, nausea and vomiting, dysphoria and inhibition of gastric emptying. It may also have adverse effects on the fetus (see above) as it freely crosses the placenta, potentially causing CTG abnormalities and respiratory and neurobehavioural depression of the newborn. It is stan-

dard practice for paediatric staff to be available at delivery of an infant whose mother has received pethidine within 3h of delivery. These problems are not obviated by the use of PCA with pethidine. The use of remifentanil PCA for labour pain has been the subject of a number of relatively small-scale studies and it may be useful for women in whom regional analgesia is contraindicated

Inhalational analgesia

The ideal inhalational agent should be a good analgesic in subanaesthetic doses, have a rapid onset of action and recovery, and not accumulate. Nitrous oxide is relatively insoluble in blood and has these properties. Other anaesthetic agents have been investigated, but so far only isoflurane has shown promise and it has been used as Isonox (50% nitrous oxide and 50% oxygen with 0.2% isoflurane) with some success. In the UK, nitrous oxide is supplied as Entonox, which is 50% nitrous oxide and 50% oxygen under pressure in a cylinder (see Chs 11 and 13). Entonox is administered usually via an on-demand valve with a face mask or mouthpiece. Administration needs to be timed for the maximum analgesic effect to coincide with the peak of the contraction. Most women tend to hyperventilate while breathing Entonox, and therefore there are often alternating phases of hyperventilation and then hypoventilation, especially if the Entonox is administered after pethidine. Although Entonox is a reasonably effective analgesic, many women feel faint and nauseated and may vomit or become out of control.

Regional analgesia for labour

This is described below.

EPIDURAL AND SUBARACHNOID ANALGESIA

This is the most effective form of analgesia in labour, with up to 90% of women reporting complete or near-complete pain relief. However, it is invasive and patients require careful monitoring.

INDICATIONS FOR EPIDURAL ANALGESIA

In addition to relief of pain and distress, there are several indications for which epidural analgesia may be helpful in securing a good outcome from labour. These are summarized in Table 35.5.

Table 35.5 Indications for epidural analgesia

Maternal request
Occipitoposterior presentation
Pregnancy-induced hypertension or pre-eclampsia
Prematurity or IUGR
Intrauterine death
Induction or oxytocin augmentation of labour
Instrumental or caesarean delivery likely
Previous caesarean delivery
Presence of significant concurrent disease (e.g. heart disease, diabetes, hypertension)
Twin pregnancy

CONTRAINDICATIONS TO EPIDURAL ANALGESIA IN LABOUR

Maternal refusal

There is a small number of women who, after a careful explanation of the risks and benefits of regional analgesia, refuse consent, possibly because of medical problems, e.g. complex back surgery. Ideally, discussions should take place in the antenatal period and clear notes should be made in the medical record.

Bleeding disorders

These may be acquired or congenital. The potential to cause bleeding in the epidural space varies widely. Epidural haematoma is a serious complication of an epidural and may cause spinal cord compression with resultant paraplegia. Each case needs careful assessment as to the risks and benefits of administering the regional anaesthetic. This assessment may need team planning with haematology and obstetric staff. Most units have delivery suite guidelines for the common problems, e.g. pre-eclampsia, prophylactic heparin, etc.

Sepsis in the lumbar area and systemic sepsis

Local infection in the area adjacent to the epidural site may introduce infection into the epidural space, potentially leading to the formation of an epidural abscess. The presence of systemic infection or systemic inflammatory response syndrome (SIRS) may cause the instrumentation involved in siting the epidural to become itself a focus for development of a local infection. An expert assessment of the risk–benefit ratio for using an epidural analgesia must be made in these circumstances.

TECHNIQUE OF EPIDURAL ANALGESIA

Preparation

Consent. Information should be given to the woman about regional analgesia and anaesthesia in the antenatal period. Leaflets, videos and parentcraft classes are important in ensuring that women are well informed before labour. It is often difficult to explain the risks and benefits of epidural analgesia to a woman who is distressed and under the effects of pethidine and Entonox; under these circumstances, misunderstandings may arise.

Intravenous cannulation. A continuous infusion of crystalloid (at about 500 mL h^{-1} initially) should always be commenced before embarking on the block.

Arterial pressure. A baseline arterial pressure value is recorded.

Bladder contents. The patient should have recently emptied her bladder.

Clothing. The patient should be wearing suitable clothing.

Positioning. The position of the patient is the same for epidural, spinal or combined spinal-epidural (CSE) block: either the lateral or the sitting position. There is no evidence that any position is superior, but the lateral position minimizes the risk of aortocaval compression, while the sitting position may enable bony landmarks to be palpated more easily and may be more comfortable for the patient. There is evidence that the lateral position is associated with less hypotension than the sitting position during induction of spinal and CSE blocks. These positions are compared in Table 35.6.

Normal labour

In the lateral position, the knees and hips are fully flexed and the neck is flexed onto the chest in order to maximize the intervertebral distance. In both positions, the iliac crests are palpated and a line drawn between them bisects either the spinous process of L4 or the L4–5 intervertebral space (Fig. 35.8).

Conduct of the epidural

1. Epidural, spinal and CSE blocks are performed in a strictly aseptic manner. After cleaning the area

Table 35.6   Comparison of sitting and lateral positions for performing spinal or epidural procedures

Sitting	Lying (left lateral)
Advantages	
Midline easier to identify in obese women	Can be left unattended without risk of fainting
Obese patients may find this position more comfortable	No orthostatic hypotension
	Uteroplacental blood flow not reduced (particularly important in the stressed fetus)
Disadvantages	
Uteroplacental blood flow decreased	May be more difficult to find the midline in obese patient
Orthostatic hypotension may occur	
Increased risk of orthostatic hypotension if Entonox and pethidine have been administered	
Patient sitting on edge of bed may be too far away from a small anaesthetist for good manual dexterity	
Assistant (or partner) needed to support patient	

with iodine or chlorhexidine, it is important to ensure that there is no contamination of the epidural equipment by the skin preparation fluid and that the skin is dry before the epidural is sited.

2. Cover the back with sterile drapes.
3. Identify the bony landmarks. For labour analgesia, intervertebral spaces L2–5 are the positions of choice. The L4 spinous process is palpated and the desired space identified (see Fig. 35.8). Tuffier's line, which joins the iliac crests, passes through the spinous process of L4 or the L4–5 interspace.
4. A skin wheal of local anaesthetic (1% lidocaine) is raised at the intended point of insertion of the Tuohy needle and the superficial ligaments in the path of the epidural needle are infiltrated.
5. With the bevel cephalad, the Tuohy needle is advanced firmly through the skin and subcutaneous tissue until it becomes anchored in the superficial ligaments (supraspinous and infraspinous).
6. The methods of identifying the epidural space are:
   –tactile, with loss of resistance to either air or saline
   –visual, using a hanging-drop technique.
   With the loss-of-resistance technique, the stilette is removed and a loss-of-resistance syringe containing saline or air is attached to the Tuohy needle. This is a tactile technique, whereby there is a loss of

resistance to injection through the gradually advancing needle as it passes through the ligamentum flavum (Table 35.7).

7. As the anaesthetist advances the Tuohy needle with the fingers and thumb of the left hand on the Tuohy needle wings, the dorsum of the hand

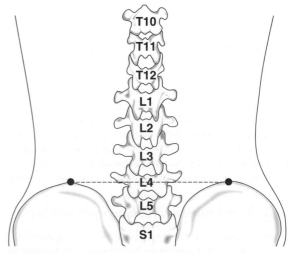

Fig. 35.8
The lumbar spine. A line drawn between the iliac crests crosses either the spinous process of the L4 vertebra or the L4–L5 intervertebral space.

Table 35.7 Comparison of air and saline for loss-of-resistance technique

Saline	Air
Advantages	
May give a better end point for loss of resistance	If fluid appears during insertion it can be assumed to be CSF until proved otherwise
May push the dura away from the point of the needle, thus reducing the chances of dural puncture	No filter is required
	No dilutional effect; the small amount of air used does not usually distort the tissues
	No possibility of confusion with other substances
Disadvantages	
May be confused with CSF	More difficult to define the point of loss of resistance with air than with saline
Must be filtered to avoid introduction of minute glass particles	
Dilutes the local anaesthetic which is put into the epidural space	
Another ampoule is opened, thus providing a possibility for user error	
Preservative-free saline must be used	

should be resting on the patient's back in order to control the advance of the needle using either intermittent or continuous pressure on the piston of the loss-of-resistance syringe. The epidural space is identified by loss of resistance. The advantages and disadvantages of air or saline use for loss of resistance are summarized in Table 35.7. Loss of resistance to saline has become the standard technique.

8. When loss of resistance is confirmed, the distance from the skin at which the epidural space lies is noted.
9. The plastic catheter introducer is placed on the end of the Tuohy needle and the catheter is advanced to 15–20 cm, at the same time warning the patient that she may feel pins and needles in one of her legs or her back. The catheter should never be withdrawn back through the Tuohy needle, as a part of it may be sheared off and left inside the patient's epidural space. If withdrawal of the catheter is necessary, the needle and catheter are removed together.
10. The Tuohy needle is withdrawn, having first noted the distance from skin to epidural space, ensuring the catheter stays in position. Ensure that 3–4 cm of catheter is within the epidural space.

11. The filter is attached and the catheter is checked to ensure that no blood or CSF flows back using gravity. A test dose may now be given.
12. The epidural catheter is fixed.

Test dose

This classically involves administration of a small dose of local anaesthetic (e.g. 2 mL 2% lidocaine or 3 mL 0.5% bupivacaine) to check for inadvertent intrathecal or vascular placement. Hypotension or marked motor block within 5 min of such a test dose suggests intrathecal placement. If an inadvertent intravascular injection occurs, the early signs are circumoral tingling and pallor and possibly a metallic taste in the mouth. The current use of dilute concentrations of local anaesthetics with the opioid fentanyl has led to a change of practice in some centres regarding the test dose. With ambulatory or 'walking' epidurals, a CSE technique or an epidural with 0.1% bupivacaine/fentanyl 2 µg mL^{-1} may be used. A 15 mL bolus is commonly given to commence ambulatory epidural analgesia, amounting to 15 mg bupivacaine in total. This dose is increasingly being given without a preceding test dose in order to spare the amount of bupivacaine given and hence minimize motor block.

This 15 mg dose is equivalent to a test dose of 3 mL 0.5% bupivacaine; hence, even if it were given intrathecally, it would not cause a higher spinal than the standard test dose.

Combined spinal-epidural for labour and the 'walking' epidural

In 1993, anaesthetists in Queen Charlotte's Hospital in London described the CSE technique for labour analgesia; this minimized motor block to the extent that a large proportion of their patients walked around the delivery suite.

Technique

The Tuohy needle is advanced to identify loss of resistance in the lumbar region (as for an epidural). Then, a 24–27 gauge 120 mm-long pencil-point (e.g. Whitacre or Sprotte) needle is advanced through the Tuohy to puncture the dura, and an intrathecal injection of 1 mL 0.25% bupivacaine with 25 µg fentanyl is given. The spinal needle is withdrawn and the epidural catheter is passed and left in place as before. The intrathecal injection usually produces rapid-onset analgesia (< 5 min) and approximately 70% of patients have normal or near-normal leg power such that they may walk. The intrathecal injection has an analgesic duration of the order of 90 min, after which the epidural component of the CSE is used, usually commencing with a 15 mL bolus of bupivacaine 0.1% with fentanyl 2 µg mL^{-1}, without a test dose, as described above. Similar degrees of mobility have been achieved using epidural boluses or infusions of low-concentration bupivacaine and fentanyl mixtures without the need for the initial intrathecal injection.

Assessment

The preservation of motor function and reduced need for bladder catheterization have increased maternal satisfaction with epidural analgesia, although there have been concerns that proprioception may be affected even with this low dose of local anaesthetic, potentially making walking hazardous. The medico-legal position of the anaesthetist in the event of a fall of a parturient during a walking epidural is unclear. Nonetheless, if visual and vestibular function is intact, proprioceptive impairment seems to have a minimal effect on walking. Many parturients do not wish to walk and, moreover, clinical trials to date have not shown that walking significantly alters outcome of labour.

MANAGEMENT OF THE LABOURING WOMAN WITH EPIDURAL ANALGESIA

Posture

A labouring woman should be positioned with at least a 15° left-lateral tilt to prevent aortocaval compression (supine hypotension syndrome). The weight of the gravid uterus compresses the vena cava and aorta against the vertebral bodies, thereby restricting blood flow. The reduction in systemic vascular resistance in women with epidural analgesia decreases the ability of the woman to maintain her arterial pressure, and therefore she is more likely to faint. In addition, the lumbosacral spine should be supported, as the epidural may allow unnatural positions to be adopted, which would usually produce back discomfort. Prolonged abnormal posture may contribute to low back pain after the epidural has worn off; in the past this has been ascribed incorrectly to the epidural itself.

Monitoring of mother and baby

A partogram is a chart upon which the progress of mother and baby is documented. It records arterial pressure, temperature, uterine contractions, fetal heart rate, cervical dilatation in relation to time in labour, intravenous fluids, urinary output and drugs given (Fig. 35.9).

Analgesia for the first stage of labour requires a sensory block extending from T10 to L1, while for the second stage, S2–S5 block is desirable. The aim is to provide effective analgesia with minimal side-effects. Local anaesthetics injected into the epidural space affect all nerves to some degree in the following order: sympathetic fibres, pain fibres, proprioception fibres and finally motor fibres. The volume of local anaesthetic solution governs the spread of the block, whereas the concentration of local anaesthetic governs the density of block with an increased risk of motor block.

Maintenance of analgesia

Epidural analgesia for labour may be maintained by the following:

Repeated bolus administration. After the first dose has been given by the anaesthetist, boluses are usually administered as required by a midwife trained in the use of epidural analgesia. The volume and concentration need to be great enough to provide adequate analgesia, but large volumes may cause too great a spread of block, with attendant toxicity and

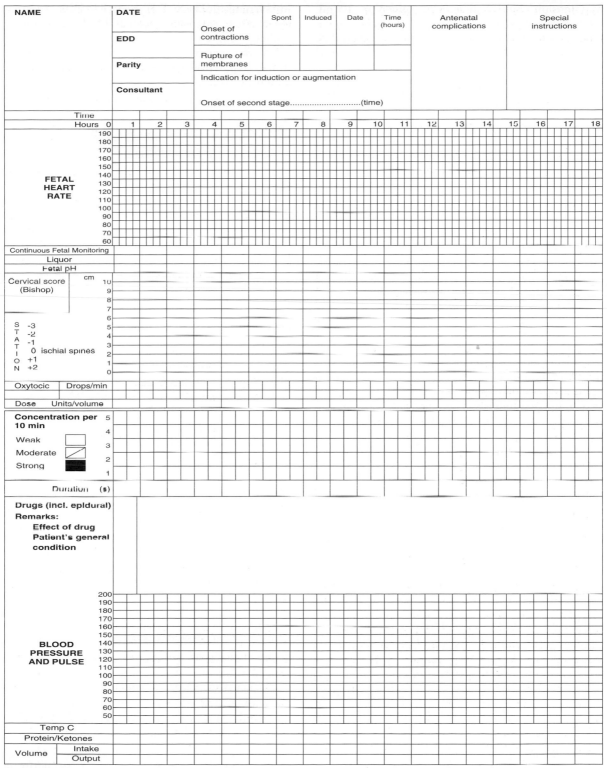

Fig. 35.9
Example of partogram.

hypotension. Bupivacaine 0.25% given in 10 mL boluses was standard practice until relatively recently but in most units has been replaced by more dilute mixtures using 0.1% bupivacaine and 2 µg mL^{-1} fentanyl in 10–15 mL boluses. The lower concentration of local anaesthetic reduces the incidence of hypotension and increases the ability of the woman to mobilize. The disadvantage of boluses is the possibility of intermittent pain if top-ups are not administered at appropriate intervals and the legal requirement for two midwives to check and administer each top-up can cause problems on busy delivery suites.

Continuous infusion by syringe pump. Local anaesthetic/fentanyl mixture is infused epidurally at a constant rate (e.g. 0.1% bupivacaine containing 2 µg mL^{-1} of fentanyl infused at a rate of 10 mL h^{-1}). The sensory level and the analgesia should be checked regularly to maintain good pain relief. The infusion method is particularly indicated when there is a need for cardiovascular stability (e.g. the patient with cardiac disease or pre-eclampsia). It is associated with the administration of greater amounts of local anaesthetic solution and increasing motor block as labour progresses.

Patient-controlled epidural analgesia (PCEA). This involves establishing analgesia with an initial bolus dose and maintaining analgesia by allowing the patient to self-administer boluses of analgesic solution as required by depressing a button on a special computer-controlled volumetric syringe. There may or may not be a low-dose background infusion, although background infusion does not improve the effectiveness of the epidural. The advantage of this method is that it gives more control to the patient.

Problems maintaining epidural analgesia:

Epidural is not effective. If the epidural is not providing good analgesia within 15–20 min with 15 mL 0.1% bupivacaine/fentanyl 2 µg mL^{-1} or 10 mL of 0.25% bupivacaine, the catheter is probably not in the epidural space and it should be withdrawn and re-sited.

Missed segment or unilateral block. Groin pain is the most common manifestation of a missed segment, i.e. L1, and it is important to ensure that the bladder is empty and the block is not unilateral. A bolus of dilute bupivacaine and fentanyl or a small bolus, e.g. 5 mL of 0.25% bupivacaine, often gives analgesia. If there is persistent groin pain present between contractions, the possibility of uterine dehiscence should be excluded.

Hypotension. If the patient feels faint or her arterial pressure decreases, she should be turned onto her side to exclude aortocaval compression.

Intravenous fluids and oxygen should be administered while extensive regional block is excluded. Catheter migration may occur and an accidental spinal may manifest itself at any stage of the epidural. If the hypotension persists, ephedrine should be administered.

REGIONAL ANAESTHESIA FOR THE PARTURIENT

The common indications for anaesthesia for parturients are caesarean section, forceps delivery, retained placenta and suturing of trauma to the birth canal. Regional anaesthesia is the technique of choice. Anaesthesia is discussed under the following headings:

- elective caesarean section
- emergency caesarean section
- forceps and Ventouse delivery
- retained placenta
- trauma to the birth canal
- post-delivery analgesia
- complications of regional anaesthesia and analgesia in obstetrics.

ELECTIVE CAESAREAN SECTION

Regional anaesthesia is the technique of choice for elective caesarean section. Although most women presenting for elective caesarean section expect to be awake for the delivery of their baby, they still need careful preoperative explanation of the procedure with explanation of the risks. As many hospitals admit women on the day of surgery, it may be difficult to give sufficient time to the preoperative visit, and therefore it is advisable to have an information sheet for the woman before admission to hospital. The woman should be warned about hypotension (and associated nausea and vomiting), post-dural puncture headache and the possibility of an imperfect block. The techniques available are as follows:

- spinal anaesthesia
- epidural anaesthesia
- combined spinal-epidural anaesthesia.

Spinal anaesthesia is the most popular choice for elective caesarean section, with increasing popularity of the CSE technique.

Spinal anaesthesia

Most spinal anaesthetics are performed with the patient on the operating table as this reduces the need to move. The following points are mandatory:

- routine pre-anaesthetic equipment check
- monitoring of arterial pressure, ECG and oximetry
- intravenous infusion of crystalloid, initially at a rate of 500 mL h^{-1}
- vasopressor available, e.g. ephedrine or phenylephrine
- aseptic technique.

Ensure that drugs are available for the administration of general anaesthesia.

Spinal anaesthesia may be performed with the patient in either the sitting or the lateral position, curled up as for siting an epidural. The choice of needle is important so as to minimize the incidence of post-dural puncture headache; it is generally accepted that the conical tip or pencil-point needle is best, although a small Quincke tip needle may be used if the others are unavailable. It is important to remember that the spinal cord ends around L2 in a normal adult, so the spinal needle should be inserted at L3/4 or below. It has been shown that anaesthetists commonly misjudge the level at which they insert the spinal needle and are more often cephalad of the desired space. Spinal cord trauma and associated chronic neurological deficit may result from inadvertently cephalad insertion of a spinal needle. Therefore, the appropriate interspace should be chosen with care. After infiltration with local anaesthetic the spinal needle introducer is then inserted, followed by the spinal needle, and the chosen local anaesthetic is injected when free flow of CSF is identified. If a spinal nerve is touched, the patient experiences excruciating pain radiating along the route of that nerve. The spinal needle must be removed and the patient reassured. Local anaesthetic must not be injected if there is any possibility of it being given into a nerve as this may cause permanent neurological damage.

Hyperbaric bupivacaine 0.5% is the drug of choice and 2.5 mL (12.5 mg) is usually sufficient. An opioid should be added to the local anaesthetic as this improves the quality of anaesthesia and provides postoperative analgesia. Fentanyl 25–50 µg, morphine 0.1–0.3 mg or diamorphine 0.1–0.3 mg may be used. Epidural and spinal opioids may cause delayed respiratory depression and therefore their use is dependent on the availability of appropriate postoperative care. All drugs injected into the epidural space or the CSF should be in preservative-free solution. Arterial pressure should be measured at 1-min intervals and the patient placed horizontal, ensuring that aortocaval compression is prevented by lateral tilt. The block should be tested for loss of sensation to a combination of cold, pinprick and touch. It is good practice to test the block from the sacral roots to the thoracic dermatomes, even though it is unusual for a spinal block to be patchy or to miss the sacral roots. The height of the block should be T4 bilaterally. Hypotension is conventionally treated with ephedrine in boluses of 3 mg or as an infusion, although there is increasing popularity for the use of prophylactic ephedrine to avoid the development of hypotension. Phenylephrine is increasingly used as an alternative to ephedrine either as a boluses of 0.05–0.1 mg or as a decreasing infusion starting at 0.1 mg min^{-1} with an aim of maintaining normotension. The patient should be carefully observed at all times.

Surgery may start when the anaesthetist is happy that there is good anaesthesia. Peritoneal traction and the swabbing of the paracolic gutters are the most stimulating parts of the operation and the times when pain or discomfort is most likely to be experienced. Exteriorization of the uterus is to be discouraged as this is challenging even to the most perfect block. Pain or discomfort should be treated promptly. Nitrous oxide and/or small doses of intravenous opioids, e.g. fentanyl or alfentanil, are useful. If the pain is severe, general anaesthesia should be offered and administered if appropriate. Syntocinon 5 units are normally administered intravenously after the delivery of the baby to assist myometrial contraction. Routine postoperative care should take place in a well-equipped recovery area.

Epidural anaesthesia

Epidural anaesthesia was the regional anaesthetic of choice until pencil-point spinal needles were introduced. The disadvantages of epidural anaesthesia are that the onset of the block is longer than that for spinal anaesthesia and that the spread of the block may be patchy, often giving poor anaesthesia of the sacral roots. The cardiovascular stability that can be achieved with an epidural is excellent and this implies that the technique may be considered the anaesthetic of choice in some patients with heart disease or pre-eclampsia. When the epidural catheter is in place, anaesthesia can be achieved by local anaesthetic, often combined with an opioid.

The following are standard prescriptions for an epidural anaesthetic:

- bupivacaine 0.5% 15–20 mL with 1 in 200 000 adrenaline (freshly added) – this should be given in divided doses
- lidocaine 2% 15–20 mL with 1 in 200 000 adrenaline (freshly added) – this should be given in divided doses
- fentanyl 50 µg or diamorphine 2.5 mg – this should be administered in addition to the local anaesthetic and has been shown to improve the quality of the anaesthesia.

The use of stereoisomers such as levobupivacaine and ropivacaine which are less cardio- and neurotoxic than equivalent racemic mixtures is controversial. Some systemic absorption occurs when large boluses of local anaesthetic are given and the effects of this may be diminished by the use of the same volume of an appropriate stereoisomer such as levobupivacaine. It is essential to test the block by testing each dermatome in a systematic way from the thoracic level down to the sacral roots to ensure that good anaesthesia has been produced before surgery starts.

Combined spinal-epidural anaesthesia

There are various techniques for CSE, although the 'needle through needle' technique described above is probably the most popular. A full description of the other techniques is outside the remit of this chapter. The CSE allows increased flexibility by combining an epidural and a spinal. The spinal anaesthetic is a single-shot technique and while most of the time this is no problem, delay in starting surgery, a difficult, long operation or failure of the block may occur. The epidural may not achieve such profound or rapid anaesthesia, although it has the advantages of flexibility and cardiovascular stability.

In the CSE technique, the spinal is usually conducted using the same dose of drugs as listed in the spinal section and the epidural, although placed as an 'insurance', is often used only for postoperative pain relief. The CSE may also be used as a sequential block, with a smaller intrathecal dose of local anaesthetic being given (e.g. 5–7.5 mg), followed by an epidural top-up to achieve full anaesthesia. This method provides greater cardiovascular stability as the onset of the block is slower, while an excellent sacral block is achieved with the spinal anaesthetic. This technique has extended the use of regional anaesthesia in pre-eclampsia.

EMERGENCY CAESAREAN SECTION

Regional anaesthesia has increased in frequency for emergency caesarean section partly because of the increased use of spinal anaesthesia and also because of the increase in use of epidural analgesia in labour.

Topping up an existing epidural

A labour epidural may be topped up to achieve anaesthesia within 10–20 min using either lidocaine 2% with 1 in 200 000 adrenaline (5 µg mL^{-1}) or bupivacaine 0.5% with 1 in 200 000 adrenaline. Sodium bicarbonate may be added to each of these solutions (e.g. 1–2 mL of 8.4% sodium bicarbonate) to increase the pH and thus the speed of onset of anaesthesia. A lipophilic opioid such as fentanyl 50–100 µg should be added to this mixture. The epidural should be topped up incrementally while the patient is monitored continuously. Between 10 and 20 mL of local anaesthetic solution are usually needed. While the epidural is being topped up, it is important to explain what is going to happen and to ensure that the woman understands what she is likely to feel and that help is available if pain or discomfort is experienced.

Spinal anaesthesia for an emergency

Spinal anaesthesia is to be encouraged for the woman who has no epidural in situ and who requires an emergency caesarean section. There are times when general anaesthesia is indicated, but these decrease as experience with spinal anaesthesia increases. Spinal anaesthesia may be used in the same manner as for an elective caesarean section; however, it is important to explain the procedure to the woman as fully as possible in the time available and to be present after the caesarean section to describe events slowly. Follow-up is particularly important in the emergency situation.

FORCEPS AND VENTOUSE DELIVERY

Surgical anaesthesia is required for any operative delivery, except for a simple 'lift-out' by forceps or Ventouse. For a simple lift-out, the labour epidural should be well topped up. Ideally, time to achieve good perineal anaesthesia should be allowed before the woman is placed in the lithotomy position for the assisted delivery. Bupivacaine 0.5% or lidocaine 2% with adrenaline 1 in 200 000 in a dose of around 10 mL is appropriate. If the delivery is more complex than a simple lift-out, surgical anaesthesia is required. It is preferable to deliver such patients in the operating theatre where caesarean section may be performed if there is any doubt about the ability to deliver the baby vaginally. Severe fetal distress may occur during attempted instrumental delivery, requiring immediate caesarean section. Therefore, the anaesthetist should prepare (and assess) the anaesthetic as if for caesarean section using any of the prescriptions for caesarean delivery mentioned above.

RETAINED PLACENTA

Regional anaesthesia may be used for manual removal of retained placenta after a careful assessment of blood loss. It is easy to underestimate the blood loss if there has been a continuous trickle of blood for some time. If the woman is not significantly hypovolaemic, the anaesthetic of choice is a spinal, unless there is an epidural in situ. Both techniques should provide good surgical anaesthesia with a block extending from at least T10 to the sacral roots.

TRAUMA TO THE BIRTH CANAL

The anaesthetist is often asked to provide anaesthesia for the repair of birth trauma. The full extent of the damage may not be known as it may not be possible to examine the woman without anaesthesia. The trauma may be extensive and involve disruption of the anal sphincter, which is classified as a third-degree tear. There may be considerable blood loss and it is important to assess this before performing regional anaesthesia. If there is an epidural in situ, this may be topped up for the repair. If there is no epidural, then a spinal anaesthetic is the technique of choice. Hyperbaric bupivacaine 0.5% in a volume of 1.5 mL provides good sacral analgesia.

POST-DELIVERY ANALGESIA

The anaesthetist is usually involved in the continuing care of the woman post-delivery and this includes the provision of pain relief for:

- normal delivery
- tears
- forceps and Ventouse
- caesarean section.

Normal delivery

The pain experienced after a normal delivery is caused mainly by uterine contractions and also bruising of the perineum. Simple analgesia in the form of paracetamol is usually adequate, although if there is severe bruising of the perineum, NSAIDs are helpful, e.g. diclofenac suppositories.

Tears and episiotomy

After the repair of an episiotomy or tear there may be considerable pain which needs more than simple analgesia. NSAIDs provide excellent analgesia for most women. If the woman has had a third-degree tear repaired, she may often have had a regional anaesthetic for the repair, and the use of epidural or intrathecal opioids provides good postoperative analgesia, particularly if combined with rectal diclofenac.

Forceps and Ventouse delivery

An episiotomy is usually performed to facilitate the forceps or Ventouse delivery and this may be extensive; therefore, pain management as above is appropriate.

Caesarean section

The extensive use of regional anaesthesia for caesarean section has led to intrathecal and epidural opioid analgesia being routine practice in most units. Combined with NSAIDs, paracetamol and other simple analgesics, this enables women to mobilize early after caesarean section. It is prudent to have clear postoperative guidelines for the care of women in the postoperative period and these should include sedation scores. Those women who are unable to have NSAIDs do not have such good pain control and continuing epidural opioid analgesia may be needed. Those women who have had their caesarean section under general anaesthesia may be managed with PCA using morphine in the same way as other postoperative patients. This is combined with NSAIDs where appropriate.

COMPLICATIONS OF REGIONAL ANAESTHESIA AND ANALGESIA IN OBSTETRICS

Although regional anaesthesia is now very safe and effective, all procedures have potential complications.

Shearing of the epidural catheter

An epidural catheter should not be withdrawn through a needle as this may damage or shear the catheter. Any sheared portion of catheter is inert and sterile and thus unlikely to cause a problem, but a full account should be made in the medical record.

Post-dural puncture headache

The incidence of post-dural puncture headache (PDPH) is 0.5–1% and is often higher in teaching hospitals. It may occur at the time of epidural insertion or be caused later by catheter migration into the intrathecal space (usually because of a defect in the dura caused during epidural insertion). The clinical presentation is of an occipital headache which may radiate anteriorly, aggravated by sitting and possibly associated with nausea, distorted hearing, photophobia and, rarely, diplopia resulting from stretching of the sixth cranial nerve as it passes through the dura. The differential diagnoses of meningitis, subarachnoid haemorrhage, sagittal sinus thrombosis or even cerebral space-occupying lesions should be considered and excluded by history and simple clinical examination.

Management of post-dural puncture headache

Approximately 75% of women who receive a dural puncture with a 16–18G Tuohy needle will suffer from PDPH. Classically, treatment is to re-site the epidural in an adjacent interspace and, following delivery, wait to see whether a headache will appear and then persists (conservative treatment) before offering definitive treatment. It is possible that threading the epidural catheter into the CSF at the time of dural puncture and using intermittent intrathecal top-ups may reduce the eventual incidence of PDPH. However, the use of an intrathecal catheter in labour produces significant risks of infection and confusion with an epidural catheter.

- Bed rest is still recommended, although it is worthless in terms of reducing eventual onset of PDPH.
- Infusion of epidural normal saline 60 mL before the epidural catheter is removed may reduce the incidence of PDPH, as may infusion, under gravity, of normal saline for 12–24h postpartum.
- Give i.v. and oral fluids to prevent dehydration.
- Give simple analgesics, e.g. paracetamol, 500 mg 4-hourly.

If conservative management fails to prevent the appearance of PDPH, then:

- Caffeine 0.5% infusion may produce cerebral vasoconstriction. It is used in around 6% of UK centres.
- Antidiuretic hormone may also relieve symptoms by an unknown mechanism.
- Corticotrophin and sumatriptan have both been used but are probably ineffective.
- Blood patch: a sample of the patient's own venous blood is collected under aseptic conditions and injected into the same or an adjacent epidural space

to seal the CSF leak. It is around 75% effective (although the quoted range is 70–98%). The procedure may be repeated. It is not usually recommended as a first-line treatment because it carries complications such as infection, arachnoiditis and potential problems with subsequent epidurals. In some centres a prophylactic blood patch is performed using the re-sited epidural catheter at the end of labour in an effort to reduce the risk and duration of PDPH.

Backache

Backache is common after childbirth, 50% of women suffering at some stage in pregnancy. An anaesthetist is often called to assess patients with backache if they have received an epidural. Certainly, insertion of epidural anaesthesia may contribute to short-term acute back pain if it causes:

- an epidural haematoma
- an epidural infection causing abscess or meningitis
- mild local bruising from poor technique.

However, long-term backache is not caused by epidural anaesthesia, as has been clearly shown in two prospective studies of over 1000 women giving birth, followed up the day after delivery and 3 months later. The incidence of new-onset backache was of the order of 40–50%, but there was no difference in the incidence of backache at 3 months between those who had received an epidural and those who had not. There was a trend towards a slightly higher chance of back pain on day 1, explained by minor local trauma.

Epidural haematoma

This is a very rare but potentially disastrous complication. The signs of an epidural haematoma are:

- new-onset, severe back pain
- prolonged, profound motor weakness > 6h after the last top-up or cessation of an infusion
- sudden onset of incontinence.

Immediate CT or MRI scan is warranted to confirm the diagnosis, and neurosurgical evacuation of the haematoma within 8h of the onset of symptoms usually results in a good outcome.

Epidural abscess or meningitis

These conditions are rare. An abscess, as with a haematoma, may give rise to a space-occupying lesion in the epidural space, resulting in compression of the spinal cord and its nutrient arteries, leading to paraplegia. Meningitis may occur as a complication of regional techniques and may be bacterial, viral or chemical. It is essential that a good aseptic technique is used when regional blocks are sited and that meningitis is excluded in the differential diagnosis of headache.

Systemic toxic reaction

This is a result of high blood concentration of local anaesthetic, caused either by a total dose greater than the body's ability to metabolize it or by too rapid administration (bolus or infusion). Local anaesthetic toxicity is described in Chapters 4 and 19.

Hypotension

Hypotension is usually defined as a 25% decrease in systolic or mean arterial pressure or an absolute decrease of 40 mmHg. Small decreases in pressure are insignificant and may be associated with improved uteroplacental blood flow, if due to vasodilatation. Rapidly developing hypotension after spinal anaesthesia may cause unpleasant dizziness and nausea in about 50% of patients, if no prophylaxis is given, and should be treated with vasopressors, e.g. ephedrine or phenylephrine, until arterial pressure is restored, while at the same time maintaining normovolaemia and ensuring that there is no aortocaval compression.

Neurological deficit

Neurological deficit may be caused by the drugs used for the procedure or by trauma from the needles or catheter. The incidence of dysaesthesiae and persistent numbness or weakness of more than 1 week's duration resulting from an epidural is approximately 1:150 000. Where a particular nerve root has been bruised by the epidural needle or catheter, reassurance may be given that these symptoms resolve over 3–6 months, but patients should be followed up on an outpatient basis. Several peripheral nerves may be injured during delivery and falsely attributed to the epidural:

- lateral popliteal nerve – by stirrups, causing foot drop
- lateral cutaneous nerve of the thigh – by groin pressure from the lithotomy position, causing anterolateral thigh numbness
- femoral nerve or sciatic nerve – by the lithotomy position, causing weak quadriceps with loss of

knee reflex or pain in the back of the leg with loss of ankle reflex, respectively
- sacral plexus and obturator nerves – these cross the pelvic rim and rarely may be damaged by occipital presentation or forceps delivery.

Arachnoiditis

Inflammation of the arachnoid membrane, caused by chemical toxins (wrong substance injected) or infection, usually presents as intractable back pain, potentially leading to permanent neurological damage. It is extremely rare.

As any complications may have medicolegal implications, it is important to:

- document the problem at the time
- explain the problem to the patient and relatives
- ensure consultant involvement.

GENERAL ANAESTHESIA FOR THE PARTURIENT

Since the 1960s, a triennial report termed the Confidential Enquiry into Maternal Deaths (CEMD) has provided an audit of obstetric and anaesthetic practice. Recent reports have demonstrated decreasing numbers of deaths from anaesthesia. The increasing safety of anaesthesia in obstetrics is the result of many factors:

- increasing use of epidural analgesia in labour
- increasing use of regional anaesthesia for operative delivery
- increase in dedicated consultant obstetric anaesthetic sessions
- improved teaching of obstetric anaesthesia
- improved assistance for the anaesthetist.

Deaths caused by anaesthesia generally result from hypoxaemia and/or acid aspiration associated with a failure to intubate the trachea and difficulty in maintaining the airway during general anaesthesia (GA). The most recent report (2000–2002) detailed increasing numbers of deaths due to anaesthesia (six deaths and one late death), all of which were general anaesthetics. Deaths were due to oesophageal intubation (three deaths), aspiration, inadequate supervision, isolated sites and anaphylaxis. General anaesthesia in the parturient is more than 16 times more likely to result in death than a regional anaesthetic. The decreasing use of general anaesthesia in obstetric anaesthesia further exacerbates this problem by decreasing experience of a technique that may be required in an emergency.

However, general anaesthesia continues to be required in the following situations:

- in an extreme emergency, e.g. severe fetal distress or maternal haemorrhage
- where there is a contraindication to regional anaesthesia
- where the patient refuses to have a regional anaesthetic; this may be because of a previous bad experience with regional anaesthesia.

Currently, about 10–20% of caesarean sections in the UK are performed under GA. The main anaesthetic considerations are the risk of aspiration of acidic gastric contents (as little as 25 mL with pH < 2.5 may lead to a 50% mortality rate) and hypoxaemia resulting from airway difficulties. The previous sections on physiology of pregnancy, anatomy and antacid therapy have highlighted many of the problems that should be considered when a pregnant woman presents for a general anaesthetic. It is essential that a thorough pre-anaesthetic check is performed, with particular attention to the difficulties that may be encountered with tracheal intubation (Table 35.8). It is mandatory that anaesthetists familiarize themselves with the operating theatre and the anaesthetic equipment (Table 35.9), in addition to the guidelines and equipment that are available for difficult and failed intubation. Drugs and equipment should be checked at the beginning of each period of duty on the delivery suite so that an emergency can be dealt with in a calm and ordered manner.

CAESAREAN SECTION

Preparation

1. Check the equipment again. Ensure that the suction equipment is working and that the table tilts head-down.
2. Perform a pre-anaesthetic check on the patient with particular attention to the airway and gastric contents.
3. Ensure that the assistant is ready.
4. Ensure that the patient is well positioned, paying particular attention to aortocaval compression and position for tracheal intubation.
5. Insert a 16-gauge i.v cannula and ensure that an infusion flows well.
6. Check that full routine monitoring is in use.
7. Preoxygenate the patient's lungs for 3 min using a well-applied face mask.
8. Check that the assistant knows how to apply cricoid pressure.
9. Start the anaesthetic using a rapid-sequence induction.

Technique

It is standard practice to use thiopental to induce anaesthesia in a dose of at least 4 mg kg^{-1}. This should be followed rapidly by succinylcholine 1–1.5 mg kg^{-1}. Cricoid pressure should be applied as consciousness begins to be lost and continued until the tracheal tube is confirmed to be in the trachea. Anaesthesia should be continued using nitrous oxide 50% and volatile agent in oxygen and positive-pressure ventilation.

Table 35.8 Clinical methods to assess the airway
Mouth opening (5 cm interincisor gap, equivalent to two fingers' breadth)
Mallampatti grade
Temporomandibular joint mobility (should be able to protrude lower incisors in front of upper incisors)
Neck mobility (90° flexion of head on neck)
Weight > 100 kg increases risk
Risk of airway oedema (increased by pre-eclampsia, stridor, URTI)

Table 35.9 Equipment that should be available for general anaesthesia in a maternity unit
Two Macintosh laryngoscopes (one standard, one long blade)
Short-handled Macintosh laryngoscope (or 'Polio-blade' laryngoscope)
McCoy laryngoscope
Bougie
Wide selection of tracheal tubes
Selection of oral and nasal airways
Laryngeal mask airway size 3
Percutaneous cricothyroidotomy kit

Isoflurane is commonly used and should be administered in a concentration of at least 0.5 MAC with nitrous oxide. High concentrations cause excessive uterine relaxation, while lower concentrations predispose the patient to awareness. The historical use of techniques where anaesthetic concentrations were employed that caused an excessive risk of awareness is now unacceptable. When using a circle breathing system, care is needed to prime the system with an adequate fresh gas flow and concentrations of the volatile agent, so that the desired 0.5 MAC level is reached quickly. If the fetus is compromised, there is evidence that the use of 100% oxygen with a volatile agent may be beneficial to the fetus by increasing oxygen transfer across the placenta (with a concomitant increase in inspired vapour concentration). There is also increasing use of conventional gas ratios of nitrous oxide and oxygen (i.e. 66:33) from the beginning of the anaesthetic. This has become more common since the introduction of oximetry and continuous analysis of expired gas concentrations. After the delivery of the baby, an opioid, e.g. morphine, may be given with oxytocin, and an antibiotic to prevent wound infection. At this stage the concentrations of nitrous oxide and inspired volatile agent may be altered to more conventional ratios. Additional non-depolarizing muscle relaxant (e.g. atracurium 25 mg) may be administered after the effect of the succinylcholine has worn off, as confirmed by a nerve stimulator. Residual neuromuscular block should be antagonized before tracheal extubation, with the patient in the lateral position and with a slight head-down tilt. Routine postoperative care in an appropriately staffed, fully equipped recovery area is essential. At this time, postoperative pain relief should be optimized and the baby should be given to the mother whenever possible.

ASSESSMENT OF THE PREGNANT WOMAN PRESENTING FOR ANAESTHESIA AND ANALGESIA

Successive CEMD reports highlight the problems of women with intercurrent medical disease and the fact they are at increased risk in pregnancy and labour. There are many more women with a coincident significant medical problem becoming pregnant and it is important that these problems are recognized in the antenatal period. A good history should be taken. Recent developments in the national maternity record should facilitate significant medical problems being highlighted as the proposed record incorporates an extensive health questionnaire to be filled in by the woman and her midwife. The effect of the physiological changes of pregnancy on the disease must be recognized and appropriate investigations instigated.

Women with cardiac or respiratory disease require careful assessment, as the physiological changes of pregnancy and delivery may have a profound effect on the disease. Many of these women have good reserves for normal day-to-day activities but are unable to cope with the added stress of labour. Antenatal assessment often includes echocardiography, ECG and pulmonary function tests. Assessment of the medical record is particularly relevant where the woman has undergone surgery. Clear plans for labour and delivery need to be written in the record by all the medical team, including the anaesthetist.

The other more common medical conditions occurring in women of child-bearing age are neurological disease, significant back problems including major surgery, drug allergies, previous anaesthetic problems and difficulties with tracheal intubation. Obesity, maternal age and smoking are also risk factors that should not be overlooked.

EMERGENCIES IN OBSTETRIC ANAESTHESIA

Emergencies in obstetric anaesthesia may be classified as follows:

- haemorrhage
- failed intubation
- pre-eclampsia and eclampsia
- total spinal or epidural block
- amniotic fluid embolus
- maternal and neonatal resuscitation.

HAEMORRHAGE

Significant bleeding occurs in 3% of all pregnancies and it may occur in either the antepartum or postpartum period.

Antepartum haemorrhage

Seventy per cent of all cases of antepartum haemorrhage result from placenta praevia and abruptio placentae.

Placenta praevia occurs when the placenta implants on the lower uterine segment and overlies the cervical os. It is assessed as being either anterior or posterior and the grade depends on the extent to which the placenta covers the os. In a grade 4 placenta praevia, the placenta covers the os, and in a grade 1 placenta praevia the placenta extends to the os. Significant bleeding may occur which may necessitate blood transfusion or urgent delivery. The potential extent of the haemorrhage depends on the position of the placenta and this may be assessed by ultrasound scan. There are four factors that increase the potential for significant bleeding:

- In placenta praevia the veins on the anterior wall of the uterus are distended.
- If the placenta is anterior then the surgical incision extends through the placenta, causing significant haemorrhage.
- If the placenta covers the os then a raw area is left after its delivery. This area of the os does not have the same ability to contract as the normal myometrium, and may thus continue to bleed.
- The presence of uterine scarring, e.g. from a previous caesarean section, may predispose to pathological invasion of the uterine wall to produce a placenta accreta or percreta. This may mean that separation of the placenta and uterus is impossible and profuse bleeding occurs which may require hysterectomy.

Women with diagnosed placenta praevia are usually delivered by elective caesarean section. As the condition may be associated with severe haemorrhage, which may be life-threatening, it is advisable that senior obstetric and anaesthetic staff are involved with the delivery of these patients. Blood should always be cross-matched and equipment should be available to administer large volumes (i.e. 1 L min^{-1}) of warmed fluids. Both general and regional anaesthesia may be used. Regional anaesthesia is associated with a reduced blood loss but may be associated with blood pressure changes that are difficult to manage, and a potentially distressed patient.

Abruptio placentae is defined as the premature separation of the placenta after the 20th week of gestation. It is associated with a perinatal mortality rate of up to 60%. Placental abruption may result in concealed or revealed haemorrhage. Typically, the woman presents with abdominal pain, which may be severe, together with signs indicative of acute blood loss in proportion to the amount of blood lost. A trap for the unwary is that placental abruption may be associated with pre-eclampsia; therefore, if the pre-abruption arterial pressure was markedly elevated, the post-abruption BP may still appear normal, and so mask hypovolaemia. A large amount of blood loss is often associated with a consumptive coagulopathy and this occurs particularly with concealed haemorrhage.

Postpartum haemorrhage

Postpartum haemorrhage is the most frequent reason for surgery in the immediate postpartum period. Causes include:

- Retained placental tissue, including:
  - placenta accreta: the placenta is abnormally adherent to the uterus but is normally placed (80% of cases)
  - placenta increta: the adherence includes the myometrial muscle (15% of cases)
  - placenta percreta: the adherence of the placental tissue extends right through to the peritoneal surface of the uterus (5% of cases), the commonest indication for caesarean hysterectomy.
- Uterine atony – the failure of the uterus to contract at the site of placental separation. The risk of uterine atony may be increased by:
  - overdistension of the uterus (e.g. polyhydramnios, multiple gestation)
  - prolonged (> 18 h) or precipitous (< 4 h) labour
  - multiparity
  - hypotension
  - uterine infection.
- Laceration of the birth canal – predisposing factors include instrumental delivery and a large infant.

Anaesthetic management of haemorrhage

Although regional anaesthesia has a role in the management of acute postpartum haemorrhage, the associated sympathetic block interferes with physiological compensatory mechanisms, potentially aggravating acute hypovolaemia. For this reason, GA is the preferred option in this situation.

Preoperative assessment

Estimation of the degree of blood loss is notoriously unreliable in the obstetric setting, and hence clinical estimation of the following signs of hypovolaemia should be undertaken:

- hypotension
- tachycardia > 120 beat min^{-1}
- urinary output < 0.5 mL kg^{-1}h^{-1}
- capillary refill time > 5 s
- anxiety, agitation or confusion
- transient or minimal response to 1–2 L crystalloid or 500 mL colloid fluid challenge.

The most recent triennial CEMD in the UK (2000–2002) noted that deaths caused by haemorrhage continued to be a problem, with rising numbers of deaths caused by postpartum haemorrhage. Substandard management was identified in 15 of the 17 deaths caused by haemorrhage. Successive reports of the CEMD have highlighted the problems of haemorrhage and the need for each unit to have clear guidelines for major haemorrhage. Anaesthetists should be involved early in the management of such patients so that appropriate resuscitation, monitoring and planning for delivery may be developed. 'Fire drills', regular multidisciplinary practice sessions for haemorrhage and other emergencies, should be a routine of modern obstetric anaesthetic practice.

The delivery suite team, including the anaesthetist, would:

- involve senior medical staff early
- request baseline haemoglobin and haematocrit
- place two large-gauge peripheral venous cannulae
- maintain circulating fluid volume
- administer group-compatible blood if possible or O-negative blood in a life-threatening situation
- consider insertion of invasive monitoring such as CVP or arterial monitoring
- involve the haematologist early for blood products and advice
- arrange postoperative admission to intensive care.

Intraoperative management

Attempts to restore circulating blood volume should precede, but not delay definitive treatment. Rapid-sequence induction of GA is mandatory. Care with induction agents such as thiopental and propofol is required in hypovolaemic patients, as profound hypotension may ensue, leading to cardiovascular collapse. Ketamine $0.5–1$ mg kg^{-1} stimulates the sympathetic nervous system and helps to preserve arterial pressure during induction of anaesthesia.

Anaesthesia may be maintained with N_2O/O_2 mixtures and an opioid such as fentanyl $1–2$ μg kg^{-1} with cautious administration of a volatile anaesthetic agent. Ultimately, hysterectomy may be a life-saving procedure and should be discussed before anaesthesia with a patient at high risk of haemorrhage. Techniques to conserve the uterus include circumferential uterine suture, intrauterine balloon, internal iliac balloon insertion or emboilization of uterine vessels using interventional radiological techniques.

FAILED INTUBATION

Failed intubation of the trachea reflects the relatively high incidence of airway difficulties in obstetric patients (approximately 1 in 300 compared with 1 in 2220 in non-pregnant patients). The increased incidence of difficult intubation in parturients is caused by changes in the soft tissues of the airway resulting in swollen upper airway mucosa, swollen and engorged breasts and full dentition. The decreasing use of general anaesthesia in obstetrics may lead to a relative lack of experience in this technique, with increased anxiety for both junior and senior anaesthetists.

The modified failed laryngoscopy/intubation drill is an essential algorithm and should be displayed prominently in all obstetric theatres (Fig. 35.10). The essential points to take from the algorithm are to call for help when unexpected difficulty with laryngoscopy or intubation arises and to avoid repeated attempts at intubation without maintaining oxygenation. The insertion of a laryngeal mask airway (LMA) may facilitate ventilation and, if used, cricoid pressure should be applied continuously.

PRE-ECLAMPSIA AND ECLAMPSIA

Hypertensive disorders (approximately 1 in 100 000 pregnancies) are among the leading causes of maternal mortality. Pre-eclampsia is defined as hypertension with proteinuria and pathological oedema after week 20. Eclampsia is defined as the occurrence of convulsions and/or coma during pregnancy not resulting from neurological disease.

Aetiology of eclampsia and pre-eclampsia

The aetiology is unknown, but current knowledge may be summarized as follows.

Immunological factors. In the normal placenta, the vascular bed is of low resistance. In pre-eclampsia, there is abnormal migration of the trophoblast into the myometrial tissue and this leads to constriction of the spiral arteries, which increases the resistance in the vascular bed. Prostacyclin and nitric oxide may be involved in this process.

Endothelial factors. Normotensive pregnant women demonstrate an increase in the activity of the renin–angiotensin–aldosterone system (RAAS) and a reduced response to exogenous angiotensin II. In pre-eclamptic women this does not occur and this has been linked to a lack of nitric oxide production by endothelial cells.

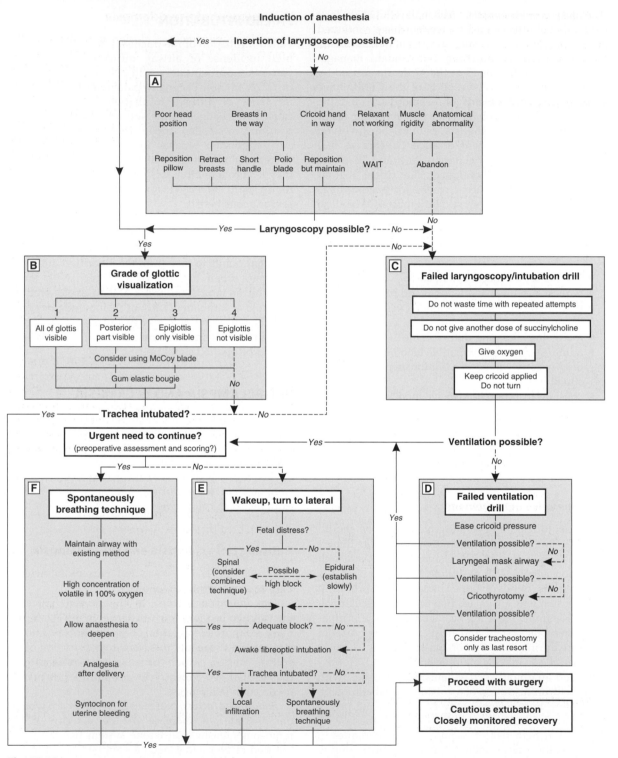

Fig. 35.10
Failed laryngoscopy/intubation drill.

Platelet and coagulation factors. Endothelial dysfunction may lead to a lack of nitric oxide and prostacyclin, altering the balance of platelet function in favour of platelet aggregation.

Clinical presentation of pre-eclampsia

Clinically, pre-eclampsia is a multisystem disorder, and the predominant features in each system are as described below.

Cardiovascular system. Hypertension is defined as systolic arterial pressure >140 mmHg or diastolic arterial pressure >90 mmHg. Cardiac output and systemic vascular resistance are usually increased. Blood volume is decreased by up to 30% in severe cases, but with a normal CVP and pulmonary capillary wedge pressure (PCWP) unless there is pulmonary oedema. This may be attributable to vasoconstriction, and therefore the patient is at risk of volume overload. Patients with pre-eclampsia may not have a raised arterial pressure, although it is significantly raised above baseline pressure at the beginning of pregnancy.

Central nervous system. Classically, this disease is accompanied by severe headache, visual disturbances and hyperreflexia. Seizures may occur without warning.

Renal system. Glomerular filtration rate is reduced by 25% compared with normal pregnant women, as a result of glomerular oedema, reducing the filtration efficiency such that proteinuria may occur. Although serum creatinine concentration rarely increases above normal, increased blood urea concentrations may be an early marker of deterioration.

Haematological system. Platelet and coagulation disorders may occur as discussed above. A rapidly decreasing platelet count is indicative of a worsening of pre-eclampsia, and low platelets may be associated with HELLP syndrome (haemolysis, elevated liver enzymes and low platelets). In general, a platelet count of 100×10^9 L^{-1} (taken within the last 12 h) and above is safe for insertion of an epidural catheter. At levels below this, a clotting screen is advised and the risks and benefits of regional block should be assessed.

Respiratory system. Pre-eclampsia increases the risk of airway oedema, which may make tracheal intubation hazardous. Pulmonary oedema may occur at any time, including up to 24 h after delivery, as a result of increased capillary permeability and decreased plasma oncotic pressure.

Management of pre-eclampsia

Obstetric management is designed to stabilize the mother and deliver the baby. It is essential that the mother is assessed and monitored carefully; this includes full biochemical and haematological screen, monitoring of arterial pressure, heart rate, fluid balance and oxygen saturation. High-dependency care is essential. Treatment of hypertension is essential and in the acute situation the drugs of choice are hydralazine, labetalol or nifedipine. Magnesium sulphate should be used in moderate to severe cases as prophylaxis against eclampsia. Magnesium inhibits synaptic transmission at the neuromuscular junction, causes vasodilatation, and has a central anticonvulsant effect at the NMDA receptor. A loading dose of 4 g (in 100 mL saline) is given over 30 min, followed by a maintenance dose of 1 g h^{-1}. Serum concentrations may be monitored, with hourly assessment of peripheral limb reflexes. As serum concentrations increase above 10 mmol L^{-1}, there is progressive reduction in reflexes, respiratory arrest and asystole. The therapeutic range is 4–7 mmol L^{-1}.

Pre-eclamptic patients are classically vasoconstricted and hypovolaemic, so careful fluid administration is advisable during treatment of hypertension. There is continued debate concerning the suitability of crystalloid or colloid in these patients and a discussion of this is outside the remit of this chapter. It is important to remember that the woman may already be receiving antihypertensive therapy, e.g. methyldopa or nifedipine.

The role of epidural analgesia and anaesthesia in pre-eclampsia

Epidural analgesia is specifically indicated for labour analgesia in pre-eclampsia because:

- It provides excellent pain relief.
- It attenuates the hypertensive response to pain.
- It reduces circulating stress-related hormones and hence assists in controlling arterial pressure.
- It improves uteroplacental blood flow.
- These women have a higher incidence of caesarean section, and the presence of an epidural allows extension of the block.

If hypotension occurs, a crystalloid bolus (500 mL) may be administered, with the patient in a lateral tilt and receiving O_2. If this is not adequate, a bolus of ephedrine 3 mg or phenylephrine 50–100 µg may be given; however, because of increased sensitivity of the circulation to exogenous vasopressors, caution is essential. Regional anaesthesia is the anaesthetic of choice if the woman is to be delivered by caesarean section, and although epidural anaesthesia has been the routine technique, there is increasing evidence to show that spinal anaesthesia or CSE may be the anaesthetic of choice for these women.

Eclampsia

If the woman has an eclamptic fit, the ABC of basic resuscitation should be commenced and it is essential that there is no compression of the aorta or vena cava during resuscitation. The treatment of eclampsia is 4 g magnesium sulphate by slow intravenous bolus as recommended in 1995 by the Eclampsia Trial Collaborative Group.

TOTAL SPINAL OR EPIDURAL BLOCK

Too large a volume of local anaesthetic or its inadvertent deposition in the subarachnoid space may lead to profound, extensive block. The time from injection of the anaesthetic solution to onset of symptoms depends upon the exact location of the injection:

- The effects of an epidural overdose are seen 20–30 min after the bolus.
- The effects of a subdural injection are seen 10–20 min after the bolus.
- The effects of a subarachnoid injection are seen within 2–5 min.

Local anaesthetic reaching the fourth ventricle results in respiratory arrest and may cause profound hypotension. Full resuscitation, including tracheal intubation and ventilation, external cardiac massage and vasopressors and inotropes are given as necessary. Spontaneous brainstem function returns as the excessively high block regresses over a period of 30 min to 4 h. However, when the mother has been stabilized, the baby is usually delivered by emergency caesarean section.

AMNIOTIC FLUID EMBOLISM

Amniotic fluid embolism (AFE) has been estimated to occur in 1:20 000 to 1:30 000 live births and has been associated with a mortality of 26–86%. Amniotic fluid embolus is difficult to diagnose definitively and this may result in under- and overreporting of cases. It does not seem to result from the systemic effects of

amniotic fluid per se. There were five deaths caused by AFE in the 2000–2002 CEMD. Amniotic fluid embolus has been described as a postmortem diagnosis depending on the pathological finding of fetal squames in the lung tissue. More recently, a clinical diagnosis has been used rather than a postmortem diagnosis. The woman presents with sudden collapse, usually after a rapid labour, but may present following an obstetric intervention, during labour or even during caesarean section. There may be preceding cyanosis, a confusional state, respiratory distress, left ventricular failure with hypotension and acute pulmonary oedema. This is followed rapidly by development of a consumptive coagulopathy and resultant haemorrhage. Management of this emergency involves resuscitation, with administration of oxygen and maintenance of the airway, including tracheal intubation and cardiopulmonary resuscitation, if necessary. If the fetus is undelivered, immediate caesarean section may be necessary to facilitate maternal resuscitation. Volume support with inotropes may be indicated. Treatment of the coagulopathy and intravenous fluids may be required. A protracted period of intensive care treatment may be necessary. All suspected cases of AFE in the UK should be reported to the National Amniotic Fluid Embolism Register

MATERNAL AND NEONATAL RESUSCITATION

Severe haemorrhage, amniotic fluid embolism, pulmonary embolus or other even more uncommon causes may result in an acutely collapsed mother. In these circumstances, immediate resuscitation is required, in the standard manner, but aortocaval compression should be avoided. Unsuccessful resuscitation is often caused by profound hypovolaemia. Caesarean section may be considered as part of the resuscitation in extreme situations; immediate delivery may dramatically improve the mother's condition and the success of emergency resuscitation. The best chance of fetal survival in such circumstances is emergency delivery.

Neonatal resuscitation

The condition of the infant at birth may be assessed by:

- Apgar score – a clinical scale based on colour, heart rate, respiratory rate, capillary perfusion and tone of the limbs. It is obtained at 1 and 10 min after delivery, with maximum score being 10.

- Umbilical cord vein pH, which is normally 7.25–7.35.

The process of resuscitation of the infant begins with gentle physical stimulation, suction of oral secretions and drying the baby. If there is little response and the heart rate is less than 80 beat min^{-1}, oxygen 100% is given by face mask. If respiration is inadequate and the heart rate is still less than 80 beat min^{-1}, ventilation is assisted at a rate of up to 60 breath min^{-1} for 1 min by bag and mask. If the heart rate is still less than 80 beat min^{-1}, cardiopulmonary resuscitation is started, taking care not to cause damage to the delicate thoracic cage. This is continued with oxygenation and ventilation. Only if all of these measures fail to increase heart rate above 80 beat min^{-1} should the administration of adrenaline be considered. The newborn must be kept warm throughout.

More detailed neurobehavioural testing includes the NACS and Scanlon scoring systems.

ANAESTHESIA FOR INTERVENTIONS OTHER THAN DELIVERY

EXTRACTION OF RETAINED PRODUCTS OF CONCEPTION

Up to 20% of all confirmed pregnancies end in spontaneous abortion within the first trimester, and extraction of retained products of conception (ERPC) is indicated where there are retained placental products. These women are often very distressed and need sympathetic care. They should be assessed for blood loss, and although there is usually no problem, there is a significant risk of severe haemorrhage that may necessitate resuscitation, including blood transfusion. In the first trimester, anaesthesia is similar to that required for cervical dilatation and hysteroscopy. Anaesthesia may be induced with an i.v. induction agent, with or without a short-acting opioid such as fentanyl (1–2 µg kg^{-1}), and maintained via a face mask or LMA (as the procedure usually lasts 5–7 min) with the patient spontaneously breathing N_2O/O_2 and 1–2 MAC of volatile agent. Adequate depth of anaesthesia is required before cervical dilatation, as vagal stimulation in an inadequately anaesthetized patient may lead to bradycardia and laryngospasm. After cervical dilatation, the level of anaesthesia may be reduced to 0.5–1.0 MAC.

Cervical circlage

This is a surgical procedure required occasionally for women with a history or active clinical features of an incompetent cervix, usually presenting as premature, precipitate labour. To reduce the risk of this occurring, a suture (Shirodkar suture) is placed around the cervix, in a procedure lasting 20–30 min. As this is usually performed in the second trimester or later, the anaesthetic considerations for any pregnant woman apply. Regional (spinal) anaesthesia is the technique of choice, with the required block height of T10–S5 being achieved using 1.5 mL hyperbaric bupivacaine with or without fentanyl 25 µg. If general anaesthesia must be undertaken, use of rapid-sequence induction is mandatory if the patient is at more than 12 weeks' gestation.

The pregnant patient with a surgical (non-obstetric) emergency

The incidence of general surgical emergencies is undiminished in pregnancy, and thus pregnant patients may require anaesthesia for laparotomy or any other procedure. If delivery is not anticipated, the anaesthetic technique should ensure good delivery of oxygen to the placenta. Use of depressant drugs such as opioids is not contraindicated. After the 13th week of gestation, the risk of regurgitation of gastric contents increases, so rapid-sequence induction should always be performed.

FURTHER READING

Chestnut D H (ed) 1999 Obstetric anesthesia, 2nd edn. Mosby, St Louis

Collis R, Plaat F, Urquhart J (eds) 2002 Textbook of obstetric anaesthesia. Greenwich Medical, London

Harmer M 1997 Difficult and failed intubation in obstetrics. International Journal of Obstetric Anesthesia 6: 25–31

Holdcroft A, Thomas T 2000 Principles and practice of obstetric anaesthesia and analgesia. Blackwell Science, Oxford

Guidelines for obstetric anaesthetic services 2005 Association of Anaesthetists of Great Britain and Ireland and Obstetric Anaesthetists' Association

MacEvilly E, Buggy D 1996 Back pain and pregnancy (review). Pain 64: 405–414

Reynolds F (ed) 2000 Regional anaesthesia in obstetrics. A millennium update. Springer, London

RCOG 2004 Why mothers die: a report of the triennial Confidential Enquiry into Maternal Death 2000–2002.

Royal College of Obstetricians and Gynaecologists, London

Van Zundert A, Ostheimer GW 1996 Pain relief and anesthesia in obstetrics. Churchill Livingstone, Edinburgh

Yentis S M, Bridhouse A M, May A et al 2000 Analgesia, anaesthesia and pregnancy. A practical guide. WB Saunders, London

http://www.oaa-anaes.ac.uk/

Paediatric anaesthesia

36

The differences in anatomy and physiology between children, especially infants, and adults have important consequences in many aspects of anaesthesia. The differences also account for the different patterns of disease seen in intensive care units (ICUs). Although major psychological differences persist throughout adolescence, a 10- to 12-year-old child may be thought of, anatomically and physiologically, as a small adult.

PHYSIOLOGY IN THE NEONATE

RESPIRATION

Control of respiration in newborn infants, especially premature neonates, is poorly developed. The incidence of central apnoea (defined as a cessation of respiration for 15 s or longer) is not uncommon in this group. The likelihood of this increases if the patient is given a drug with a sedative effect. Potentially life-threatening apnoea may occur. The incidence is reduced by postoperative administration of xanthine derivatives such as caffeine and theophylline which act as central respiratory stimulants. Because of this problem, it is wise to admit for overnight oximetry and apnoea monitoring all children under 60 weeks' postconceptual age who have had surgical procedures, no matter how minor. Hypoxaemia in the neonate and small child appears to inhibit rather than stimulate respiration and this is contrary to what one might expect.

The newborn has between 20 and 50 million terminal air spaces. At 18 months of age, the adult level of 300 million is reached by a process of alveolar multiplication. This explains why infants who suffer with respiratory distress of the newborn improve as they grow older. Subsequent lung growth occurs by an increase in alveolar size. The lung volume in infants is disproportionately small in relation to body size. Their metabolic rate is nearly twice that of the adult, and therefore ventilatory requirement per unit lung volume is increased. Thus, they have far less reserve for gas exchange.

Before the age of 8 years, the calibre of the airways is relatively narrow. Airway resistance is therefore relatively high. Small decreases in the diameter of the airways as a result of oedema formation or respiratory secretions significantly increase the work of breathing. Elastic tissue in the lungs of small children is poorly developed. As a result of this, compliance is decreased. This has important consequences in that airway closure may occur during normal tidal ventilation, thereby bringing about an increase in alveolar–arterial oxygen tension difference ($P_{A-a}O_2$). This explains why P_aO_2 is lower in the infant than in the child. The decreased compliance results in ventilatory units with short time constants. Consequently, the infant is able to achieve adequate alveolar ventilation whilst maintaining a high respiratory rate. However, because of the increased resistance and decreased compliance, the work of breathing may represent up to 15% of total oxygen consumption (Table 36.1). The high respiratory rate is necessary because the metabolic rate of the infant is nearly twice that of the adult. The high alveolar minute ventilation explains why induction and emergence from inhalational anaesthesia are relatively rapid in small children. The high metabolic rate also explains why desaturation occurs very rapidly in children.

The ratio of physiological dead space to tidal volume V_D/V_T is similar to that of the adult at about 0.3. However, because the volumes are smaller, modest increases in V_D produced by equipment such as humidification filters may have a disproportionately greater effect (Table 36.2).

Ventilation in small children is almost entirely diaphragmatic. Because the ribs are horizontal, there is no 'bucket handle' movement of the ribs as occurs in the adult. It is therefore important to appreciate that normal minute ventilation is respiratory rate-dependent. The infant's diaphragm is made of fast twitch fibres. This type of muscle fibre exhausts easily if it has to work against a load. This implies that in infancy, when

Table 36.1   Lung mechanics of the neonate compared with the adult

	Neonate	Adult
Compliance (mL cmH$_2$O^{-1})	5	100
Resistance (cmH$_2$O L^{-1} S^{-1})	30	2
Time constant (s)	0.5	1.3
Respiratory rate (breath min^{-1})	32	15

Table 36.3   Variation in arterial pressure (mmHg) and heart rate (beat min^{-1}) with age

Age	Systolic BP	Diastolic BP	Heart rate
Neonate	70–80	40–50	100–180
1 year	90–100	60–80	80–130
6 years	95–100	50–80	70–120
12 years	110–120	60–70	60–100

Table 36.2   Respiratory variables in the neonate

Tidal volume (V_T)	7 mL kg^{-1}
Dead space (V_D)	(V_T) × 0.3 mL
Respiratory rate	32 breath min^{-1}

lung compliance is low, the work of breathing is reduced by breathing rapidly. Consequently, if the work of breathing is increased by an increase in airway resistance, respiratory failure may easily ensue.

It is important to appreciate that the infant's response to hypoxaemia may be bradypnoea and not tachypnoea as occurs in the adult.

CARDIOVASCULAR SYSTEM

The process of growth demands a high metabolic rate. It is, therefore, not surprising that infants and children have a higher cardiac index (compared with the adult) so that oxygen and nutrients may be delivered to actively growing tissues. The ventricles of neonates and infants are poorly compliant, so even though the ventricles of infants demonstrate the Frank–Starling mechanism, the main determinant of cardiac output is heart rate. Infants tolerate heart rates of 200 beat min^{-1} with ease (Table 36.3). Bradycardia may occur readily in response to hypoxaemia and vagal stimulation and it represents a decrease in cardiac output. Immediate cessation of the stimulus, and treatment with oxygen and atropine, are absolutely crucial. A heart rate of 60 beat min^{-1} in an infant is considered a cardiac arrest and requires cardiac massage. Arrhythmias are rare in the absence of cardiac disease. The usual cardiac arrest scenarios are electromechanical dissociation and asystole, not ventricular fibrillation.

Even though infants and children have a higher cardiac index, arterial pressure tends to be lower than in adults because of a reduced systemic vascular resistance associated with an abundance of vessel-rich tissues in the infant. The pressure increases from approximately 80/50 mmHg at birth to the normal adult value of 120/70 mmHg by the age of 16 years. Children under the age of 8 years who are normo-volaemic at the start of anaesthesia tend not to exhibit a decrease in arterial pressure when central neural blockade such as spinal anaesthesia is administered. They do not require fluid preloading as an adult would to avoid hypotension, because venous pooling tends not to occur as venous capacitance cannot increase. The reasons for this are that the sympathetic nervous system is less well developed and so infants tend to be venodilated at rest. Secondly, they have a lower extremity:body surface ratio and as a consequence have a smaller venous capacitance.

As in all patients, the cardiovascular system must be carefully monitored. Pulse oximeter probes placed on the extremities provide a good index of peripheral perfusion. Auscultation of heart sounds, especially by an oesophageal stethoscope, is useful as the volume of heart sounds tends to be diminished as cardiac output decreases. Non-invasive measurement of arterial pressure is undertaken easily using an appropriately sized cuff. Complications preclude the use of invasive monitoring of arterial and central venous pressures for all but major cases.

Blood volume

The stage at which the umbilical cord is clamped determines the circulating blood volume of the neonate. Variations of up to ±20% may occur. The average blood volume at birth is 90 mL kg^{-1}, and this decreases in the infant and young child to 80 mL kg^{-1}, attaining the adult level of 75 mL kg^{-1} at the age of 6–8 years. Blood losses of greater than 10% of the red cell mass should be replaced by blood, especially if additional losses are expected. However, most children who have a normal haemoglobin concentration at the start of surgery can tolerate losses of up to 20% of their red cell mass. Children may tolerate a haematocrit of 25% and the decision to transfuse blood must be balanced against the risks, which include transmitted infection and antibody formation. The latter may cause problems in later life, especially in female children during child-bearing years.

Haemoglobin

At birth, 75–80% of the neonate's haemoglobin is fetal haemoglobin (HbF). By the age of 6 months, adult haemoglobin (HbA) haemopoiesis is fully established. HbF has a higher affinity for oxygen than HbA. This is demonstrated by the leftward shift of the oxygen haemoglobin dissociation curve (Fig. 36.1). Low tissue PO_2 and metabolic acidosis in the tissues result in the avidity of HbF for oxygen being reduced, thereby aiding delivery of oxygen. Alkalosis produced by hyperventilation results in less oxygen being available and it is therefore sensible to maintain normocapnia.

If blood transfusion is required, it is crucial that blood is filtered and warmed – the smaller the child, the more important is this precaution. A syringe used via a tap in the intravenous giving set is probably the safest way of avoiding inadvertent overtransfusion. The circulating volume of a 1 kg neonate is of the order of 80 mL. Common sense dictates that blood loss should be monitored carefully, so swabs should be weighed and, if possible, all suction losses collected in a graduated container.

RENAL FUNCTION AND FLUID BALANCE

Body fluids constitute a greater proportion of body weight in the infant, particularly the premature infant, compared with the adult (Table 36.4). In an adult, most of the total body water is in the intracellular compartment. In a newborn infant, most of the total body water is in the extracellular compartment. With increasing age, the ratio reverses. Plasma volume remains constant throughout life at about 5% of body weight.

The kidneys are immature at birth. Both glomerular filtration rate (GFR) and subsequent reabsorption by the renal tubules are reduced. The GFR at birth is of the order of 45 mL min^{-1} 1.7 m^{-2}. This increases rapidly to about 65 mL min^{-1} 1.7 m^{-2} and then gradually approaches the adult value of 125 mL min^{-1} 1.7 m^{-2} by the age of 8 years. Thus, there is inability to handle excessive water and sodium loads. Overtransfusion may lead to pulmonary oedema and cardiac failure. The maturation in renal function is produced by hyperplasia in the first 6 months of life and then by a

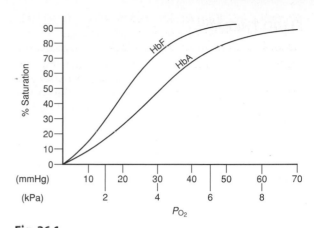

Fig. 36.1
Effects of fetal haemoglobin (HbF) on oxygen dissociation curve. HbA, adult haemoglobin; PO_2, partial pressure of oxygen.

process of hypertrophy in the first year. Care must also be exercised when drugs eliminated by the renal route are used in infants; either reduced doses or an increased dosage interval should be employed. Renal maturation is not just an increase in size but also of function. The ability to modify the ultrafiltrate produced at the glomerulus increases with age. It follows that sodium bicarbonate and glucose homeostasis mechanisms are not fully developed. Medical intervention may be required to ensure that biochemical values are kept within normal ranges.

Poorly developed mechanisms exist for conserving water in the kidneys and gastrointestinal tract. Increased cutaneous water loss because of a large surface area:volume ratio through poorly keratinized skin may lead to a turnover of fluid in the infant of about 15% of total body water per day. Dehydration ensues very rapidly in an infant who is kept fasted.

Table 36.4 Distribution of water as a percentage of body weight

Compartment	Premature	Neonate	Infant	Adult
ECF	50	35	30	20
ICF	30	40	40	40
Plasma	5	5	5	5
Total	85	80	75	65

ECF, extracellular fluid; ICF, intracellular fluid.

FLUID THERAPY

An intravenous infusion delivering maintenance fluids should be in place for all neonates requiring surgery. Maintenance fluid requirements increase over the first few days of life (Tables 36.5, 36.6). The normal infant requires of the order of 3–5 mmol kg^{-1} of sodium and an equivalent amount of potassium per day to maintain normal serum electrolyte concentrations. The ability of the infant's kidneys to eliminate excess sodium is limited. Exceeding this amount in the absence of loss results in hypernatraemia and its sequelae. Infants undergoing any procedure more than the briefest should also have their calorific needs addressed. This may be achieved by including glucose-containing fluids in the regimen; failure to do so results in hypoglycaemia and ketosis. This may occur rapidly because of the limited glycogen stores and high metabolic rate of the infant.

It is imperative that the anaesthetist recognizes and resuscitates the dehydrated infant appropriately before surgery. Clinical examination of skin turgor, capillary refill, tension of fontanelles, arterial pressure and venous filling may aid estimation of hydration, but electrolyte and haemoglobin concentrations and haematocrit, urine volumes and plasma and urine osmolalities should be monitored if problems of fluid balance exist (Table 36.7).

Table 36.5 Fluid requirements in the first week of life

Day	Rate (mL kg^{-1} day^{-1})
1	0
2, 3	50
4, 5	75
6	100
7	120

Table 36.6 Maintenance fluid requirements

Weight (kg)	Rate (mL kg^{-1} day^{-1})
Up to 10 kg	100
10–20 kg	1000 + 50 × [weight (kg) − 10] mL
20–30 kg	1500 + 25 × [weight (kg) − 20] mL

Intravenous fluids should be administered using a system that allows small volumes to be given accurately. This may vary from the anaesthetist injecting fluid using a syringe to microprocessor-controlled syringe driver pumps. The latter are preferable, as fluid is given at a steady rate and the anaesthetist's hands are free to tend to other tasks. During surgery, fluid administration should be increased to account for increased losses occurring through evaporation from exposed viscera and third-space losses.

The intraosseous route may be used to carry out fluid resuscitation and drug therapy in shocked children. The needle should be inserted in an aseptic fashion to minimize the risk of osteomyelitis. Although various sites have been described for needle insertion, the proximal end of the tibia below the tuberosity is probably the easiest to perform. The intraosseous route is safer than attempting central venous cannulation in the shocked child in whom veins are difficult to discern. The usual fluid administered in this situation is human albumin solution. This is given as a 10 mL kg^{-1} bolus and repeated until clinical improvement occurs.

TEMPERATURE REGULATION AND MAINTENANCE

Homeothermic animals possess the ability to produce and dissipate heat. Heat loss occurs by one of four processes: radiation, convection, evaporation and conduction. The environment in which the patient is situated governs the relative contribution of each. The neutral thermal environment is defined as the range of ambient temperatures at which temperature regulation is achieved by non-evaporative physical processes alone.

The metabolic rate at this temperature is minimal. The temperature of such an environment is 34°C for the premature neonate, 32°C for the neonate at term and 28°C for the adult.

Heat may be produced by one of three processes: voluntary muscle activity, involuntary muscle activity and non-shivering thermogenesis. Infants under the age of 3 months do not shiver. The only method available to increase their temperature in the perioperative period is non-shivering thermogenesis. The process is mediated by specialized tissue termed brown fat. It differentiates in the human fetus between 26 and 30 weeks of gestation. It comprises between 2% and 6% of total body weight in the human fetus and is located mainly between the scapulae and in the axillae. It is also found around blood vessels in the neck, in the mediastinum and in the loins. Brown fat is made of multinucleated cells with numerous mitochondria and

Table 36.7   Effects of dehydration in the young infant

	Mild	Moderate	Severe
Percentage loss of body weight	5	10	15
Clinical signs	Dry skin and mucous membranes	Mottled cold periphery Depressed fontanelles Oliguria ++	Shocked Moribund Unresponsive to pain
Replacement	50 mL kg^{-1}	100 mL kg^{-1}	150 mL kg^{-1}

has an abundant blood and nerve supply. Its metabolism is mediated by catecholamines. The substrate used for heat production is mainly fatty acids.

Radiation accounts for about 60% of the heat loss from a neonate in a 34°C incubator placed in a room at 21°C. If the infant were in a thermoneutral environment of 34°C, the percentage loss by radiation would decrease to about 40% of the total heat loss, and, in addition, the total heat loss in this environment would be lower. The reason for this is that heat loss by radiation is a function of skin surface area and the difference in temperature between the skin and the room. The second major source of heat loss in the neonate is convection. This is a function of skin temperature and ambient temperature. The neonate possesses minimal subcutaneous fat that may act as thermal insulation and as a barrier to evaporative loss. A neonate has a body surface area:volume ratio about 2.5 times greater than the adult; thus, a neonate may become hypothermic very rapidly.

If neonates are allowed to become hypothermic during anaesthesia, unlike adults they attempt to correct this by non-shivering thermogenesis. Metabolic rate increases and oxygen consumption may double. The increase in metabolic rate puts an additional burden on the cardiorespiratory system and this may be critical in neonates with limited reserve. The release of noradrenaline in response to hypothermia causes vasoconstriction, which in turn causes a lactic acidosis. The acidosis in turn favours an increase in right-to-left shunt, which causes hypoxaemia. As a result, a vicious positive feedback loop of hypoxaemia and acidosis is set up. The protective airway reflexes of a hypothermic neonate are obtunded, thereby increasing the risks of regurgitation and aspiration of gastric contents. The action of most anaesthetic drugs is potentiated by hypothermia. This effect is particularly important with regard to neuromuscular blocking drugs. The combination of hypothermia and pro-

longed action of these drugs increases the chances of the neonate hypoventilating after surgery.

Many precautions should be taken to ensure that the neonate's body temperature is maintained. First, the child must be transported to theatre wrapped up and in an incubator set at the thermoneutral temperature. The theatre should be warmed up to the thermoneutral temperature, ideally a few hours before the planned start of surgery. This interval allows the walls of the theatre to warm up and this reduces the net heat loss by radiation. One must appreciate that heat loss by radiation is a two-way process. The child loses heat by radiation to the walls and also gains heat from the walls. All body parts that are not needed for insertion of cannulae and for monitoring should remain covered until the child has been draped with surgical towels. If the child has to be exposed, overhead radiant heaters may be used. During surgery, the child should lie on a thermostatically controlled heated blanket. Forced air warming systems are effective in maintaining the child's temperature during surgery; these work on the principle of blowing filtered, warmed air into quilted blankets with perforations. This allows warmed air to come into direct contact with the patient. Simple measures such as using a bonnet to reduce heat loss from the head are very effective. Intravenous fluids and fluids used to perform lavage of body cavities must be warmed. Anaesthetic gases should be humidified and warmed in order to preserve ciliary function and to reduce heat loss from the respiratory tract.

MONITORING

It is important in all procedures to measure temperature. For short procedures, an axillary temperature probe may be sufficient. In longer operations, core temperature should be measured at one of a variety of sites, such as rectal, bladder, nasopharyngeal and oesophageal. The oesophageal probe is often the preferred method, as most modern oesophageal probes may be connected to a stethoscope. The anaesthetist is therefore able to listen to heart sounds in addition to recording the patient's temperature. When active heating methods such as cascade humidifiers and heated blankets are used, it is important that temperature gradients between the patient and the warming device are kept to less than 10°C. Failure to observe this may result in burns to the skin and the respiratory tract. In the ICU, simultaneous measurement of core and peripheral temperatures, though not often used in theatre, may serve as a useful guide to adequacy of the cardiac output. Decreases in cardiac output result in a reduction of blood flow to the peripheries and this is reflected in a core–peripheral temperature gradient greater than 3–4°C.

PHARMACOLOGY IN THE NEONATE

DEVELOPMENTAL PHARMACOLOGY

Drugs given via the oral or rectal route are absorbed by a process of passive absorption. This process is dependent on the physicochemical properties of the drug and the surface area available for absorption. Most drugs are either weak bases or weak acids. The un-ionized portion of the drug therefore depends on the pH of the fluid in the gut. The gastric pH of the neonate is higher than that of the older child and adult. The consequence is that drugs inactivated by a low pH undergo greater absorption. Examples of these include antibiotics such as penicillin G.

Factors which determine the distribution of intravenously administered drugs include protein and red cell binding, tissue volumes, tissue solubility coefficients and blood flow to tissues. Neonates, in particular preterm infants, have lower plasma concentrations of albumin. In addition, the albumin is qualitatively different in that its ability to bind drugs is lower than that of adult albumin. The concentration of α_1-acid glycoprotein is also lower in this group of patients; this protein is the major binding protein for alkaline drugs, which include opioid analgesics and local anaesthetics.

The blood–brain barrier is immature at birth; thus, it is more permeable to drugs. In addition, the neonate's brain receives a larger proportion of the cardiac output than does the adult brain. Consequently, brain concentrations of drugs are higher in neonates than in adults. For example, administration of morphine, which has low lipid solubility, results in high concentrations in the neonate's brain and therefore it should be used with caution and in reduced amounts in this age group.

In a neonate, total body water, extracellular fluid and blood volume are proportionally larger in comparison with an adult. This results in a larger apparent volume of distribution for a parenterally administered drug. This explains in part why neonates appear to require larger amounts of some drugs on a weight basis to produce a given effect. However, plasma concentrations tend to remain high for longer because they have smaller muscle mass and fat stores to which drugs redistribute.

The action of most drugs is terminated by metabolism or excretion through the liver and kidney. In the liver, phase I reactions convert the original drug to a more polar metabolite by the addition or unmasking of a functional group such as -OH, -NH$_2$ or -SH. These reduction/oxidation reactions are a function of liver size and the metabolizing ability of the appropriate microsomal enzyme system. The volume of the liver relative to body weight is largest in the first year of life. The enzyme systems in the liver responsible for the metabolism of drugs are incompletely developed in the neonate. Their activity appears to be a function of postnatal rather than post-conceptual age, because premature and full-term infants develop the ability to metabolize drugs to the same degree in the same period after birth. Adult levels of activity are achieved within a few days of birth. Phase II reactions that involve conjugation with moieties such as sulphate, acetate, glucuronic acid, etc., are severely limited at birth. Most of these conjugation reactions are in place by the age of 3 months. The kidney ultimately eliminates most drugs. As mentioned above, GFR is lower in young children than in adults. However, by the age of 3 months the clearance of most drugs approaches adult values.

SPECIFIC DRUGS IN PAEDIATRIC ANAESTHESIA

Inhalational agents

Alveolar and brain concentrations of inhalational anaesthetic agents increase rapidly in children, because they have a greater alveolar ventilation rate in relation to functional residual capacity (FRC) and because of the preponderance of vessel-rich tissues. Induction and excretion of the agent at the termination of anaesthesia are more rapid.

The minimum alveolar concentration (MAC) value of anaesthetic agents changes with age, because of age-related differences in blood/gas solubility coefficients. From birth, MAC increases to a peak at the age of 6 months and then declines gradually until the adult value is reached. It is worth stating at this juncture that malignant hyperthermia has been reported or is possible with all the presently available volatile anaesthetic agents and that all potentiate the duration of neuromuscular blocking drugs.

Nitrous oxide

Nitrous oxide is used as a carrier gas for most inhalational anaesthetic agents. It is also used for its MAC-sparing effect. The effect is most marked with halothane, with which a 60% reduction can be achieved. However, with the newer agents such as sevoflurane, only a 25% reduction may be produced. Thus, there would appear to be little to be gained by adding nitrous oxide to a sevoflurane anaesthetic. A major problem with nitrous oxide is its greater solubility compared with nitrogen. It diffuses into closed nitrogen-containing spaces at a greater rate than nitrogen leaves, thereby causing expansion. This effect is particularly important in lung lesions such as pneumothorax and congenital lobar emphysema. Expansion of the bowel in exomphalos or gastroschisis may make surgical reduction into the peritoneal cavity difficult.

Halothane

This agent has been the gold standard for induction of anaesthesia in children, because until recently its odour was one of the least pungent. It shares with all anaesthetic agents the ability to depress the myocardium. However, it also slows heart rate, causing a decrease in cardiac output. It is therefore prudent to give an anticholinergic before its administration. Induction with halothane is smooth, and because most vaporizers allow 5 × MAC to be administered, it may be given in almost 100% oxygen. This is a useful feature when anaesthetizing a child with an airway problem. Another property which makes halothane useful in this situation is its prolonged action compared with the newer volatile agents, as it is undesirable that anaesthesia 'lightens' during instrumentation of the airway. In adult anaesthetic practice, repeat administrations of halothane within a period of less than 3 months may be associated with hepatic dysfunction and occasionally with fulminant hepatic failure. The exact mechanism of this toxic effect is not clear, but some have speculated that a reductive metabolite of halothane is responsible. Reductive hepatic metabolism of drugs is developed poorly in children and this may explain why this problem is extremely rare in children. However, if a child needs a second anaesthetic within 3 months of a first halothane anaesthetic, a risk–benefit assessment has to be undertaken. Economic considerations dictate that this is the most widely used inhalational agent for induction and maintenance of anaesthesia in children

worldwide. As one might predict from its physical characteristics, emergence from halothane anaesthesia tends to take longer compared with the newer agents. It is acceptable to induce anaesthesia with halothane and then to use a less lipid-soluble agent for maintenance.

Isoflurane

Cardiac output tends to be well maintained when less than 1 MAC of this agent is used for maintenance of anaesthesia. However, because of its pungency, it is not a suitable agent for induction. In spite of the fact that it has a low blood/gas partition coefficient, induction tends to be slow because of breath-holding. It may be used for maintenance of anaesthesia after halothane or intravenous induction.

Sevoflurane

The blood/gas partition coefficient of 0.68 results in rapid induction of anaesthesia with this agent and also a quick recovery. It is the least pungent of the currently available agents. It is possible to turn the vaporizer to its maximum output of 8% without experiencing significant problems of coughing, breath-holding or laryngeal spasm. There is little to be gained by including nitrous oxide during induction, as the MAC-sparing effect on sevoflurane is not as great as with other agents. It is not unusual to observe slowing of the heart rate during induction, but it is not usually necessary to give an anticholinergic. Cardiac arrhythmias do not commonly occur during induction or maintenance with this agent. Economic considerations dictate that the agent is used mainly for induction, followed by a cheaper agent such as isoflurane for maintenance. Sevoflurane is an excellent choice for induction in children with upper airway obstruction, but it is probably wise to change over to halothane before instrumentation of the airway. The reason for doing this is so that the child does not 'lighten' during the procedure. The agent is partly degraded by soda lime to compound A, which is nephrotoxic in rats because they possess the enzyme beta-lyase. This hazard would appear to be theoretical in humans.

Desflurane

The blood/gas partition coefficient of 0.42 suggests that induction should be rapid, but this is not so because desflurane is very irritant to the upper airway. It may be used for maintenance of anaesthesia with the benefit that emergence is very rapid. This may be particularly desirable in the ex-premature infant. Cost and the fact that the agent has to be delivered using a special vaporizer limit the use of this agent in paediatric practice.

Intravenous agents

The availability of topical local anaesthetic creams has resulted in venepuncture and cannulation being relatively atraumatic for children. As a consequence, intravenous induction has become more common.

Barbiturates

Thiopental is the most widely used in this class of agents. A dose of 5–6 mg kg^{-1} of a 2.5% solution is required in the healthy child. The main advantage of this agent is that injection into a small vein is pain-free. The agent can be given rectally using a 10% solution at a dose of 30 mg kg^{-1}, but induction and recovery tend to be slow with this technique.

Propofol

This agent may be used for both induction and maintenance of anaesthesia as part of a total intravenous technique. Although not common in paediatric anaesthetic practice, the technique of total intravenous anaesthesia using propofol is very useful in the child prone to malignant hyperthermia or the child with porphyria. Induction and maintenance doses tend to be larger in the younger healthy patient. The reasons for this are because of a larger central volume of distribution and because the clearance of the agent is higher compared with the adult. Pain on injection is a problem and this may be lessened by the addition of 0.2 mg kg^{-1} of lidocaine. Propofol stabilized in a medium-chain triglyceride emulsion appears to cause less pain on injection.

Ketamine

The current formulation of this drug is a racemic mixture of the S(+) and R(−) enantiomers. It is possible to separate the two enantiomers, although at present this does not appear to be a commercially viable proposition. The reason for doing this is that the S(+) enantiomer is twice as potent, recovery is quicker and the incidence of emergence psychic reactions is lower. One of the major advantages of ketamine is the intense analgesia it provides. The analgesia has both spinal and supraspinal components. Epidural administration of the drug in combination with local anaesthetic significantly prolongs the duration of analgesia compared with local anaesthetic alone. The lack of cardiovascular depression in vivo is a feature that allows the drug to be used for inducing anaesthesia in children with congenital heart disease. Occasionally, pulmonary vascular resistance may increase, and as a consequence pulmonary pressures also increase. Even though upper airway reflexes are relatively well preserved, aspiration of gastric contents may still occur. The drug has bronchodilator properties and may be used for sedating the child with status asthmaticus to allow artificial ventilation in the ICU. It is prudent to administer an anticholinergic when the drug is used for maintenance of anaesthesia, because increased salivation and bronchial secretions are potential problems. Emergence from ketamine anaesthesia is slower than with other agents. It may be accompanied by emergence phenomena such as hallucinations and unpleasant dreams. The incidence of these can be reduced by concurrent administration of a benzodiazepine.

Opioids

These may be used in large doses as the sole agent to provide stable haemodynamic conditions for children with cardiac disease. The major disadvantage of using this technique is that drug effects persist into the postoperative period, causing respiratory depression. As a result, postoperative mechanical ventilation is mandatory. Morphine is the drug used most commonly for the management of severe pain in children. Hepatic glucuronidation is the process by which it is eliminated. Morphine is converted to morphine-3- and morphine-6-glucuronide. These metabolites are active. Morphine-3-glucuronide antagonizes the analgesic effects of morphine-6-glucuronide. The very young suffer from respiratory depression at lower morphine infusion rates. This is probably because of sensitivity of the brainstem and also because the ratio of morphine-3- to morphine-6-glucuronide is lower. Remifentanil is the newest of the synthetic opioids. This drug is unique in that its metabolism to a virtually inactive metabolite is by non-specific esterases in blood and tissue. The half-life of the drug is independent of the duration of infusion. There are few data on the use of this drug in infants and children, and at present it is unlicensed for use in children under the age of 2 years. However, it is likely to be valuable in infants because of its lack of accumulation and short half-life. Opioid-induced respiratory depression may be reversed by naloxone. The reversal is short-lived and it is probably wise to mechanically ventilate the lungs of children in this state.

Neuromuscular blocking drugs and their antagonists

The neuromuscular junction in infants is not mature. Electrophysiological studies demonstrate that the response of the junction is similar to what one might observe in a patient with myasthenia gravis. In other words, the junction is very sensitive to the effects of neuromuscular blockers. These drugs are polar and as a result distribute mainly to the extracellular space. Because this space is larger in the infant, the dose of drug required to depress twitch tension is similar or slightly larger than that required for adults on a dose/unit weight basis. The larger volume of distribution explains why drugs that depend on the kidneys or liver for elimination have a longer duration of action. Conversely, drugs such as atracurium which are degraded by a combination of ester hydrolysis and Hoffman elimination act for a shorter time because of the larger extracellular space.

Anticholinesterases are used to antagonize residual neuromuscular blockade. The appropriate anticholinergic to match the duration and onset should be combined with the anticholinesterase in order to minimize muscarinic side-effects. Atropine with edrophonium and glycopyrronium with neostigmine are the recommended combinations. The dose requirements are similar to those of adults and reversal should not be attempted in the presence of profound blockade. The edrophonium/atropine combination has a quicker onset of action and a shorter duration of action. This combination, although not readily available, might be more appropriate for reversing the currently widely used intermediate-duration drugs.

Succinylcholine

This depolarizing neuromuscular blocking drug has the most rapid onset of action of any currently readily available agent. It is therefore the drug of choice for the patient with a full stomach and also for the treatment of laryngeal spasm. In the infant, it has the ability to cause bradycardia after only a single dose. It is wise to administer an anticholinergic before administration. A hyperkalaemic response is not seen after administration to children with myelomeningocele or cerebral palsy. It is one of the most potent triggers for malignant hyperthermia. The incidence of this increases if succinylcholine is preceded by induction with halothane. Fatal cardiac arrest has occurred in a small number of patients. It is presumed that these patients had unsuspected muscular dystrophies and that the drug caused massive muscle breakdown. As it is not possible to predict which patients might exhibit this response, it would be wise to limit the use of the drug to patients with a full stomach and for the relief of laryngospasm.

Non-depolarizing agents

Onset and duration of action and the response in patients with renal and hepatic disease are probably the most important considerations when choosing one of these agents. Rocuronium has the most rapid onset of all the currently available agents. The onset of all these drugs may be increased by giving larger doses, but this is counterbalanced by a correspondingly longer duration of action. Recently, a new amino-steroid, rapacuronium, was evaluated in paediatric practice. Data suggested that its onset of action was similar to that of succinylcholine and that its duration of action was comparable to that of mivacurium. Mivacurium has the shortest duration of action of the currently available drugs. However, there were several reports of bronchospasm and hypoxaemia, especially in small children, and the drug was withdrawn. Mivacurium is best suited for the short surgical procedure, which usually matches its duration of action. Very occasionally, a patient may be cholinesterase-deficient, in which case its duration is long. Atracurium, rocuronium and vecuronium have an intermediate duration of action, making them the most commonly used, as the duration of most paediatric operations falls into this category. Cisatracurium and pancuronium are best reserved for the long procedure. Pancuronium is excreted renally and should be used with caution in the patient with renal failure. In spite of the fact that vecuronium and rocuronium are excreted by the liver, their duration of action is minimally affected by hepatic disease. Atracurium or cis-atracurium is the most obvious choice for patients with renal or hepatic disease, as elimination is altered minimally by organ failure.

ANAESTHETIC MANAGEMENT

PREOPERATIVE PREPARATION

For all elective surgery, it should be possible to prepare the child and family for what is to be expected in the perioperative period. This may be done in a wide variety of ways, including hospital tours, educational videotapes and pamphlets. The optimum choice depends on the age and intellectual ability of the child. Children possess great insight, and to attempt to keep forthcoming events secret is only likely to lead to mistrust and fear. All children should be visited preoperatively by the anaesthetist responsible for caring for them in the perioperative period. This is the opportunity not only to assess fitness for anaesthesia and surgery but also, when appropriate, to allay anxiety, answer questions and to find out what the child's preferences are for mode of induction, pain relief, etc.

Children who are systemically unwell should not have elective surgery. It is not unusual for a child to present with coryzal symptoms alone. There is an increased incidence of airway problems during anaesthesia; these children are more at risk of laryngeal spasm, breath-holding and bronchospasm, and in the postoperative period the chance of post-intubation croup is increased. The decision to proceed should be made only by a senior anaesthetist. Occasionally, these symptoms precede a more serious upper or lower respiratory tract infection. In very rare cases, the viraemic phase of the illness may be associated with a myocarditis. Each case should be dealt with on its merits. Children who have active viral illnesses such as chickenpox should not have elective surgery, nor should children who have recently been immunized using live vaccines, for two reasons: first, there is an associated myocarditis or pneumonitis; and, secondly, to protect others on the ward who may be immunocompromised.

It is extremely important that the child is weighed before arrival in theatre, because body weight is the simplest and most reliable guide to drug dosage. Veins suitable for placement of cannulae should be identified and, if possible, local anaesthetic cream applied and covered with an occlusive dressing. If it has not been possible to weigh the child, the weight may be estimated from the child's age (Table 36.8).

PREOPERATIVE FASTING

Morbidity and mortality caused by aspiration of gastric contents are extremely rare in children undergoing elective surgery. What is becoming increasingly clear is that prolonged periods of starvation in children, especially the very young infant, are harmful. These children, who have a rapid turnover of fluids and a high metabolic rate, are at risk of developing hypoglycaemia and hypovolaemia. Research has shown that children allowed unrestricted clear fluids up to 2 h before elective surgery have a gastric residual volume equal to or less than that of children who have been fasted overnight. The essential message is that children should, rather than could, be given clear fluids up to 2 h before induction. Solids (including breast and formula milk) should not be given for at least 4 h

before the anticipated start of induction. In the emergency setting, e.g. the child who has sustained trauma shortly after ingesting food, it is probably best (if possible) to wait 4 h before inducing anaesthesia. Clearly, in this situation risk–benefit judgements have to be made. If it is surgically possible to wait 4 h, an i.v. infusion of a glucose-containing solution must be commenced and, if necessary, appropriate fluid resuscitation undertaken.

PREMEDICATION

The advent of local anaesthetic creams has reduced the necessity for sedative premedication. Currently, two formulations are available:

- *EMLA* has been available for more than a decade. Venepuncuture is usually painless if it has been applied and an occlusive dressing placed over the site at least 1 h before the planned procedure. It is wise to apply it over at least two locations marked by the anaesthetist in case the first attempt fails. It should not be used in the very small child or on mucous membranes because of the danger of systemic absorption of prilocaine that results in methaemoglobinaemia. It should not be left on the skin for more than 5 h. A major disadvantage of EMLA is that it causes some venoconstriction and this obscures the vein.
- *Tetracaine gel* is the other agent available for this purpose. It has the advantage of a quicker onset of action and also provides analgesia for a considerable period of time after the occlusive dressing has been removed (4 h). This is an advantage in the day-care unit, because it may be applied as part of the admission procedure for all the children, left on for about 45 min and then removed, as small children often object to the presence of the occlusive dressing.

Occasionally, a sedative premedicant drug is required. This is particularly useful for the child who, in spite of good preoperative preparation, remains apprehensive. Currently, the injectable form of midazolam given orally is gaining widespread popularity. The dose used is $0.5 \, mg \, kg^{-1}$. An effect occurs within 10 min, with the peak at 20–30 min after administration. It may be used for day-case patients without a significant effect on discharge time. The bitter taste is a disadvantage. This should be eliminated when an oral formulation becomes available. One should err on reducing the dose if the patient is concurrently taking drugs that inhibit hepatic enzymes, because the duration of action of midazolam may be significantly prolonged.

Table 36.8 Estimates of children's weight	
Age	*Approximate body weight (kg)*
Neonate	3
4 months	6
1–8 years	2 × age + 9
9–13 years	3 × age

An alternative to midazolam is oral ketamine in a dose 3–10 mg kg^{-1}. An antisialagogue (e.g. atropine 0.02 mg kg^{-1}) should be added to prevent excess salivation. The larger the dose, the more likely it is that the child may experience postoperative nausea and vomiting. If profound degrees of sedation are required, it is possible to combine midazolam and ketamine. The incidences of nausea and vomiting and of excess sedation in the postoperative period are increased.

Intramuscular premedication is generally not tolerated well by children. Often, it is the event in their hospital stay that they dislike the most. Rectal administration of induction agents has been used, such as thiopental in doses of 25–30 mg kg^{-1}. This form of premedication may be used only under the direct supervision of the anaesthetist, as respiratory depression is a distinct possibility. A relatively new route for premedication administration is the intranasal route. This is particularly useful for the child who refuses to swallow an oral premedication. Drugs that have been used by this route include ketamine and midazolam in the doses mentioned above. At this stage it is not known how much of the drug goes through the cribriform plate directly into the central nervous system. Until this issue is clarified, it is best not to use this route routinely, because midazolam or its preservative and the preservative used with ketamine are neurotoxic when applied directly to neural tissue.

INDUCTION

It is important that children are accompanied into the anaesthetic room by someone with whom they are familiar. This person is usually a parent but may be a ward play specialist with whom the child feels comfortable. It is equally important that whoever accompanies the child is not coerced into doing so. Children usually detect anxiety in their parents and this tends to have an adverse effect on their behaviour.

The person accompanying the child should be informed on the ward of what to expect in the anaesthetic room. For example, if an inhalational induction is planned, he or she should be made aware of some of the signs of the excitation phase that the child might exhibit. If an i.v induction is planned, the person should be made aware of how to assist the anaesthetist by distracting the child.

Unlike adult practice, it is not possible to have all the necessary monitoring devices placed on the child before induction. In most cases, it should be possible to place an appropriately sized pulse oximeter probe on a digit. Most children also allow the placement of a precordial stethoscope. The appropriate monitoring should be placed as soon as possible after the start of

anaesthesia. The anaesthetist must always have present an assistant who is used to paediatric anaesthesia.

When inhalational induction is planned, clear, scented plastic masks are much more acceptable to little children than the traditional Rendell–Baker rubber masks. Clear masks allow respiration and the presence of vomitus to be observed. An alternative to using a mask is cupping one's hand over the face of the child while holding the T-piece. It is important to ensure that the flow of fresh gas is directed away from the child's eyes as anaesthetic gases may be irritant.

Airway management

The ratio of dead space to tidal volume tends to remain constant at about 0.3 throughout life in the healthy person. Anaesthetic apparatus such as connectors and humidification devices significantly increase dead space and should be kept to the minimum. This is especially important if the child breathes spontaneously during anaesthesia.

The Rendell–Baker masks were developed to fit around the facial anatomy of the child in an attempt to minimize equipment dead space. In fact, the flow of gas in a clear mask is such that the advantage of using Rendell–Baker masks is minimal. These masks are much more difficult to use than the clear ones with a pneumatic cushion. When using a face mask, it is important that the soft tissue behind the chin is not pushed backwards by the fingers, thereby obstructing the airway. The anaesthetist's fingers should rest only on the mandible.

The Jackson–Rees modification of the Ayre's T-piece is the breathing system used traditionally for children under 20 kg in weight. It has been designed to be lightweight with a minimal apparatus dead space. The apparatus may be used for both spontaneous and controlled ventilation. The open-ended reservoir bag is used for manually controlled ventilation. This mode of ventilation is especially useful in the neonate and infant, as one is able to detect changes in compliance produced by tube displacement. The reservoir bag also allows the application of continuous positive airway pressure for both the spontaneously breathing child and one undergoing ventilation. This may be helpful in improving oxygenation. The bag may be removed and an appropriate ventilator such as the Penlon 200 attached to the expiratory limb. A minimum gas flow rate of 3 L min^{-1} is required to operate this apparatus satisfactorily. Fresh gas flows of 300 mL kg^{-1} for spontaneous respiration and flows of 1000 mL plus 100 mL kg^{-1} for controlled ventilation usually result in normocapnia. It is difficult to scavenge the T-piece system. For the older child, it is satisfactory to use a Bain,

Humphrey ADE or circle absorber system. It is easy to scavenge the waste gases from these systems with the resultant benefit of reducing pollution of the theatre environment. In addition, the circle system offers economic advantages because of the low fresh gas flows required.

The Guedel airway is a useful adjunct in maintaining the airway of a child undergoing anaesthesia. It is important that the appropriate size of airway is used. If an airway is too small or too large, it may obstruct the child's airway completely. A reliable way of selecting the correct size is to place the flange of the airway at the angle of the mouth. The correctly sized airway should reach the angle of the mandible. The tongue should be depressed using a depressor or even the blade of the laryngoscope and the airway inserted. The method used in adults of rotating the airway through 180° during insertion is not recommended for small children because of the possibility of damaging the pharynx and subsequently compromising the airway. It is important that all procedures involving the airway of a child, including suction of the pharynx, are performed under direct vision.

The laryngeal mask airway is a major advance in anaesthetic airway management. It does not protect the airway against aspiration of refluxed gastric contents. It should be used only when it is planned that the child is to breathe spontaneously during surgery. It follows that it is unwise to use the device when neuromuscular blocking drugs are used. The mask may be displaced easily, which may result in airway obstruction and gastric insufflation. With these provisos, it may be used for a variety of operations where in the past tracheal intubation would have been mandatory, such as squint correction and tonsillectomy. Because of the large cross-sectional area of the mask tube, airway resistance increases only a small amount, if at all. Masks are available to fit all children, including neonates. The neonatal (size 1) mask is not popular for several reasons: it is relatively difficult to insert; it may be displaced very easily; and it increases apparatus dead space, resulting in rebreathing and hypercapnia.

It is mandatory to intubate the trachea during artificial ventilation. Intubation of the trachea confers many advantages. The lungs are protected against aspiration of gastric contents, ventilation is controlled and bronchoalveolar toilet may be performed. Operations in the oral cavity of a small child are not possible without tracheal intubation. It is very difficult to maintain the airway of a neonate using an airway and a face mask for any but the shortest surgical procedure requiring general anaesthesia. It is usually wise to intubate the trachea electively in most situations. Insertion of a tracheal tube results in a reduction of the cross-sectional area of the airway. A 3.5 mm tube in a neonate causes an increase in resistance by a factor of 16. Neonates with a tracheal tube must undergo artificial ventilation in order to reduce the work of breathing.

The vocal cords should be visible in order to be certain of intubating the trachea. In order to be able to do this, the anaesthetist has to align three imaginary axes: one through the trachea, one through the pharynx and one through the mouth. In the older child and adult, this is usually achieved by placing a pillow under the head – the familiar 'sniffing the morning air' position. A layrngoscope blade is then put into the vallecula in front of the epiglottis and the laryngeal structures lifted. Because of anatomical differences, the technique needs to be modified for the infant. Infants have a head which is large and a neck which is short relative to the size of the body. Instead of placing a pillow under the head, it is usually necessary to place a small pad or pillow under the torso. An alternative is to ask the assistant to gently raise the torso off the surface on which the child is lying. The larynx of a child under the age of 2 years tends to sit higher in the neck opposite the vertebral bodies of C3–4, whereas in the older child it is opposite C5–6. This results in the larynx being more anterior during laryngoscopy. The epiglottis of the infant is relatively large and, because the cartilaginous support is not fully developed, tends to be floppy. The anaesthetist cannot usually elevate the epiglottis sufficiently in order to be able to see the vocal cords if a curved blade such as the Macintosh is used. Instead, the anaesthetist has to use a straight blade and place it on the posterior surface of the epiglottis whilst lifting. In addition to the above, gentle cricoid pressure helps to bring the three axes into alignment. This may be performed with the little finger of the left hand.

In the adult, the narrowest part of the airway is the glottic opening. In the child, the narrowest part is the cricoid ring, which cannot be seen during laryngoscopy. It is very important that the correct size of tube is selected. If too large a tube is selected, the tracheal mucosa is damaged and the child may develop post-intubation croup; if it is too small, excessive leak makes effective positive pressure ventilation impossible. The ring forms a natural cuff around the tube, thereby eliminating the need for a pneumatic cuff. Generally, cuffed tubes are used only in children above the age of 10 years. The reason for this is that the pressure may render the underlying trachea ischaemic and subsequently lead to post-intubation croup. If possible, tracheal intubation should not be performed in children having day-case procedures. The laryngeal mask has eliminated the need for this.

The following formula is used to calculate the internal diameter of the appropriate size of tube:

$$(age/4) + 4\,mm$$

An alternative is to use a tube with an external diameter similar to that of the child's little finger. It is important that tubes with internal diameters 0.5 mm larger and smaller than the predicted size are readily available.

The tip of the tracheal tube should lie at the mid-trachea. For oral intubation, the measurement from the alveolar ridge to the mid-trachea is about $(age/2) + 12$ cm. An alternative is three times the internal diameter of the tube. For nasal intubation, the measurement is $(age/2) + 15\,cm$.

For neonates, the best guide is related to weight (Table 36.9).

After tracheal intubation has been performed, the lung fields and epigastrium should be auscultated to confirm correct placement. Additional confirmation of correct placement using a capnograph is essential. If intubation has been preceded by a period of difficult mask ventilation, it is not unusual for the stomach to become inflated. The inflated stomach decreases excursion of the lungs and results in arterial desaturation. If this has occurred, the stomach should be deflated by passing an orogastric tube, which is removed as soon as the task is complete.

Because children have a relatively short trachea, it is easy for the tube to become displaced and enter a main bronchus or for the trachea to become extubated. It is vital that the tube is well secured. It is best to use adhesive tape and secure the tube to the immobile maxilla rather than to the mandible. Preformed tubes such as the RAE are not recommended for the infant because inadvertent bronchial intubation easily occurs.

MONITORING

There is no substitute for an experienced, vigilant anaesthetist directly observing the child. Changes in colour, inappropriate movement, respiratory obstruc-tion and changes in respiratory pattern may be observed quickly and treated. A precordial stethoscope and pulse oximeter should always be attached before induction. The precordial stethoscope should be changed to an oesophageal one after the trachea has been intubated. The stethoscope is used as a qualitative measure of cardiac output. A volume-depleted infant has quiet heart sounds. The increase in intensity of the sounds after volume boluses may be discerned easily. Most oesophageal stethoscopes have a built-in temperature probe. If it is not possible to use this method to monitor temperature, then an alternative site such as the rectum must be used. It is unwise to even consider extubating the trachea of a hypothermic infant. Ideally, ECG and arterial pressure monitoring should be in place before induction. In practice this is not always possible. Usually these devices are put in place as soon as the child is asleep. Capnography is mandatory for the child who has a tracheal tube or laryngeal mask.

DAY SURGERY

Day-case surgery confers many advantages in children. Children who are admitted to hospital often develop behavioural problems, perhaps as a result of separation from parents and disruption of family life. These problems may manifest as an alteration of sleep pattern, bedwetting and regression of developmental milestones.

Most children make excellent candidates for day-case surgery. They are usually healthy and the procedures performed are usually of short to intermediate duration. Only experienced surgeons and anaesthetists should undertake day-case surgery. Because this form of surgery is performed by experienced personnel, even ASA III patients may be considered. Children who are under 60 weeks' post-conceptual age, those who have diseases that are not well controlled (e.g. poorly controlled epilepsy) and those with metabolic disease (e.g. insulin-dependent diabetes) that may result in hypoglycaemia should always be admitted electively for overnight stay.

Parents must be given clear written instructions well before the planned date of surgery. They should be told how long their child should be fasted before surgery. They should also be asked to make arrangements so that two responsible adults with their own transport accompany the child home.

Sedative premedication is rarely required for a child who has been well prepared. Children accompanied to the anaesthetic room by their parents usually remain calm. It makes sense to use agents with the shortest half-life. Regional anaesthesia performed

Table 36.9	Estimates of tracheal tube size in neonates	
Weight (kg)	Internal diameter (mm)	Length from alveolar ridge (cm)
1	2.5	7
2	3	8
3	3.5	9

after induction is useful in reducing the amount of anaesthetic needed intraoperatively and also provides excellent postoperative analgesia, especially when long-acting agents such as bupivacaine or ropivacaine are used. Paracetamol or diclofenac given as suppositories at the end of surgery ensure that the child remains comfortable when the local anaesthetic has regressed. It is essential to seek the parent's informed consent for regional anaesthesia and rectal analgesics.

After surgery, the child should be allowed to recover in a fully equipped and staffed recovery ward. The child is returned to the day ward only when protective reflexes have returned. The child is discharged home when oral fluids are tolerated, but if the child has received intraoperative hydration, it is possible to ignore this criterion. Another yardstick used is whether the child has passed urine or not; this is particularly important if the child has been given a caudal block. Occasionally, caudal blocks and inguinal blocks result in weakness of the leg. In this case, it is advisable to wait for the block to regress before discharging the child; clearly, this applies only to children who are walking. Ondansetron is useful in the treatment of postoperative nausea and vomiting, as the lack of any sedative effect is conducive to an early discharge. Children who have undergone tracheal intubation should remain on the day ward for at least 2 h to ensure that post-intubation croup does not occur.

Parents should be given an adequate supply of postoperative analgesics. It is crucial to emphasize the importance of giving analgesics pre-emptively 'by the clock' instead of waiting for the child to complain of pain.

PAEDIATRIC REGIONAL ANAESTHESIA

Most children admitted to hospital experience regional anaesthesia. The commonest use is probably the application of topical preparations of lidocaine/prilocaine or tetracaine before venesection or intravenous cannulation. Topical anaesthesia is not limited to these uses. It may be used as the sole anaesthetic, in suitable children, for procedures such as division of preputial adhesions and removal of simple skin lesions adhesions. Procedures performed in this way often do not involve an anaesthetist.

Whenever possible, regional anaesthesia is combined with general anaesthesia. Children who are anaesthetized in this way wake up quickly and appear to be less troubled by nausea and vomiting than when general anaesthesia is used without a regional block. In the day-case surgery setting, this leads to earlier discharge and a more pleasant experience for the child and the family.

Wound infiltration is a technique which is not usually performed by, but which is supervised by, the anaesthetist. Examples include wound infiltration after pyloromyotomy or herniotomy. The anaesthetist advises the surgeon as to the volume of anaesthetic that may be used safely. This technique is mostly used at the end of surgery because of the distortion of anatomy that the infiltration of local anaesthetic might cause. Occasionally, the surgeon may be persuaded to inject at the beginning, especially if local anaesthetic with a vasoconstrictor is used, as this provides the surgeon with a 'dry' field. A good example of this would be for removal of accessory auricles or encapsulated subcutaneous lesions.

Central neuraxial and peripheral nerve blocks are almost always performed on anaesthetized children. The anaesthetist must therefore be experienced in identifying fascial planes with needles and must also be confident with the use of the nerve stimulator. Generally speaking, a peripheral block is preferred to a neuraxial block because of a lower complication rate. Complications associated with neuraxial blocks include inadvertent intravascular or intrathecal injection and permanent nerve injury. The risk–benefit ratio and surgical/patient considerations have to be taken into account before selecting a block. For example, a penile ring block, while safe and simple, might make it difficult for the surgeon to perform a circumcision.

The ilioinguinal/iliohypogastric block is used for surgery in the groin area. It provides excellent analgesia for inguinal herniotomy. This block may be combined with infiltration anaesthesia if the child needs orchidopexy. Local anaesthetic is deposited under the aponeurosis of the external oblique muscle at a point a finger's breadth medial to the anterior superior iliac spine. Very occasionally, the local anaesthetic may block the femoral nerve. The parents should be warned about this beforehand so that they can assist their child when taking the first steps after anaesthesia.

The dorsal nerves of the penis are blocked by injection of local anaesthetic, each side of the midline, into the subpubic space. If more than $0.1\,mL\,kg^{-1}$ is injected, the anatomy may be distorted. The block is appropriate for circumcision but for hypospadias surgery a caudal epidural is probably a better choice. The dorsal penile arteries, which run alongside the nerves, are end arteries. The local anaesthetic solution should not contain vasoconstrictor.

The paediatric equivalent of the 3-in-1 femoral nerve block is the fascia iliaca block. The femoral, obturator and lateral cutaneous nerves of the thigh are blocked reliably using this approach. The block has the advantage of being distant from neurovascular structures, thereby reducing the opportunity for complications.

The injection point is as follows. A line is drawn from the anterior superior iliac spine to the pubic tubercle. The needle is inserted 0.5 cm below this line at the junction of the medial two-thirds and lateral one-third. The regional block needle is advanced until two 'pops' have been felt and the local anaesthetic is then deposited. The two 'pops' represent the needle traversing the fascia lata and fascia iliaca, respectively. The block may be used to reduce femoral fractures in the A&E department. An elegant technique is to apply topical local anaesthetic to the injection site before performing the block. The block may also be used to obtain muscle biopsies. Metatarsal and metacarpal blocks are usually the only blocks required for surgery on the extremities. It is unusual to require a brachial plexus block.

The combination of auriculotemporal and great auricular nerve blocks is useful for pinnaplasty. Operation on the ears is associated with nausea and vomiting and it is probable that these blocks help in reducing the incidence of this side-effect. The great auricular nerve is a branch of the superficial cervical plexus. It is blocked by infiltrating about 3 mL of local anaesthetic anterior to the tip of the mastoid process. This anaesthetizes the posterior aspect and the lower third of the anterior surface of the ear. The auriculotemporal nerve is a branch of the mandibular division of the trigeminal nerve and it supplies the superior two-thirds of the anterior surface of the ear. An additional 1–2 mL of local anaesthetic deposited subcutaneously immediately anterior to the external auditory meatus blocks this nerve.

Caudal epidural blockade is probably the most commonly used block in children. The sacrococcygeal membrane (otherwise known as the sacral hiatus) is the unfused laminae of the S5 vertebral body. If one were to imagine an equilateral triangle, the base of which is a line joining the posterior iliac spines, the sacral hiatus would be the apex of this triangle. In children this point is higher than one would first imagine and it is always above the natal cleft. The epidural space in children is devoid of fat. This implies that by increasing the volume of solution injected, a predictable higher dermatomal level may be reached. The Armitage formula is the most commonly used to calculate the volume of local anaesthetic. Analgesia over the sacral dematomes is achieved by injecting 0.5 mL kg^{-1} volume of solution. It is necessary to inject 1 mL kg^{-1} to reach the lower thoracic dermatomes and 1.25 mL kg^{-1} to reach the mid-thoracic dermatomes. Another benefit derived from the absence of epidural fat is that it is possible to advance a catheter from the sacral region to the mid-thoracic region. This is used to provide analgesia after laparotomy in neonates. In small babies, the epidural space may be found at a depth of 1 mm kg^{-1} from skin. In older children, the thoracic dermatomes may be blocked by threading the catheter from the lumbar epidural space to the thoracic. It is safer to avoid a direct thoracic approach because the tributaries to the anterior spinal artery may be damaged easily. Sometimes, preservative-free clonidine or ketamine is added to the local anaesthetic mixture to prolong the duration of a single-shot caudal. The dural sac in babies usually ends opposite the S3–S4 intervertebral space and because of differential growth rises to end opposite the S1–S2 intervertebral space. Therefore, there is a potential for a total spinal block after caudal injection. The chances of this complication occurring may be reduced significantly by careful attention to how far one advances the needle or cannula into the space. One should also wait a short while with the hub of the needle or cannula open to air so that blood or CSF may drip out; if this happens, the technique has to be abandoned.

In babies, the spinal cord ends opposite the body of L3. Because of differential growth, the spinal cord 'ascends' in the spinal canal so that by the time the child is 1 year old it is at the adult level opposite the L1–2 intervertebral space. In the UK, spinal anaesthesia is used exclusively to provide anaesthesia for infra-umbilical surgery in the ex-premature infant who is less than 60 weeks post-conceptual age. At any age, damage to the spinal cord is avoided by injecting below an imaginary line joining the iliac crests.

SPECIFIC OPERATIONS IN THE NEONATE

INGUINAL HERNIA REPAIR

This is one of the commonest operations in the neonatal period. The incidence in this age group is highest amongst preterm infants. General anaesthesia is avoided because of the risk of postoperative apnoea. The choice is between spinal and caudal epidural anaesthesia. Spinal anaesthesia offers the advantage of a quick onset with profound muscle relaxation in less than 2 min. Unfortunately, the duration of action is very short – of the order of about 40 min; the reason for this is probably a higher cardiac index than in adults. Addition of α_1-agonists such as phenylephrine and adrenaline may prolong the block to about 1 h. Caudal anaesthesia is also possible in this situation, the main disadvantages being a slower onset time and the potential complications of injecting large quantities of local anaesthetic. However, the block lasts a long time so that bilateral hernia repair is easily possible. The child should have an intravenous cannula in situ, but unlike adult practice there is no need for volume preloading, nor is there a need to administer vasoactive drugs such as ephedrine.

PYLOROMYOTOMY

Pyloric stenosis usually presents in weeks 4–8 of life. A previously well male child develops projectile vomiting. Untreated, the child becomes severely dehydrated with a hypokalaemic, hypochloraemic metabolic alkalosis. As the obstruction is at the level of the pylorus, the body loses hydrogen and chloride ions but none of the alkaline small bowel secretions. The kidney is thus presented with a large bicarbonate load, which exceeds its absorptive threshold and this results initially in alkaline urine. As further fluid depletion occurs, the renin–angiotensin–aldosterone axis is activated in an attempt to preserve circulating volume. This results in an exchange of sodium ions for hydrogen and potassium ions, which leads to a paradoxical aciduria with a worsening hypokalaemia and metabolic alkalosis.

The initial management is insertion of a nasogastric tube and an intravenous cannula. A solution of 5% glucose in 0.45% saline to which 40 mmol L^{-1} of potassium chloride has been added is given at a rate of 6 mL kg^{-1} h^{-1}. The nasogastric tube is aspirated and the aspirate replace with 0.9% saline. The child is ready for surgery between 24 and 48 h after commencing this regimen. A normal serum potassium concentration and a bicarbonate concentration of 25 mmol L^{-1} are used to indicate that sufficient volume replacement has taken place.

In theatre, the child's stomach should be washed with warm saline until the aspirated fluid is clear. Induction should be smooth, by either the inhalational or intravenous route according to the experience of the anaesthetist. Postoperative analgesia is provided by wound infiltration followed by either rectal or oral paracetamol, depending on when the surgeon decides that the child may be fed.

TRACHEO-OESOPHAGEAL FISTULA AND OESOPHAGEAL ATRESIA

Six types of this condition (A–F) have been described. The commonest is C in which the proximal oesophagus ends as a diverticulum and the lower part exists as a fistula off the trachea just above the carina. Cardiovascular anomalies such as septal defects and coarctation of the aorta often coexist with this condition. An echocardiogram should always be performed before surgery. The corrective surgery should be performed as a matter of urgency as a one-stage repair, as delay results in soiling of the lungs and pneumonitis. Preoperatively, the child

should be nursed in an upright position to prevent soiling of the lungs by gastric fluid. It is important that a tube is placed in the diverticulum and continuous suction applied to aspirate the saliva that the child cannot swallow. If the lungs should become soiled, then antibiotics and physiotherapy are required and the operation should be performed as soon as the child's condition has been optimized.

An inhalational induction is the preferred method for induction. Positive-pressure ventilation results in distension of the stomach and subsequent impairment of oxygenation. The tracheal tube should be inserted with the bevel facing up so that the posterior wall of the tube occludes the fistula. Initially, the tube should be inserted further than predicted and then withdrawn gently until both lungs are being ventilated. Manual ventilation is recommended as surgical traction may easily occlude the neonate's soft trachea.

The lungs should be ventilated postoperatively in order that adequate amounts of analgesia may be given and also to prevent traction on the oesophageal anastomosis by movement of the head.

DIAPHRAGMATIC HERNIA

In this condition, the abdominal contents herniate through a defect in the diaphragm, usually on the left side. The abdominal contents exert pressure on the developing lung and, if the defect is large enough, the mediastinum is shifted to the right and the growth of the contralateral lung is also impaired. Repair of the hernia is not an emergency and the child should be managed medically. Problems that have to be managed include ventilation, acidosis and pulmonary hypertension. Surgery is considered when the child's condition has been optimized medically. Positive-pressure ventilation by bag and mask may expand the abdominal viscera and should be avoided. Nitrous oxide should also be avoided for the same reason. The defect is usually repaired through an abdominal incision. It is not always possible to fit the viscera in the peritoneal cavity, in which case a silastic silo may be used and the contents introduced gradually. It is wise to avoid cannulation of veins in the lower extremity as the return of abdominal viscera increases the pressure in the inferior vena cava. Infants who present soon after birth with severe symptoms do not usually survive as they have inadequate amounts of lung tissue to sustain life.

EXOMPHALOS AND GASTROSCHISIS

Embryologically, these are two separate conditions. However, both present similar challenges to the anaesthetist. The abdominal contents, which have herniated through the abdominal wall, offer a large surface area from which heat and fluid may be lost. It is imperative that the abdominal contents are placed into a clear sterile polythene bag as soon as possible after birth. The defects should be corrected as a matter of urgency. Nitrous oxide should be avoided to facilitate surgery and a nasogastric tube must be in place to decompress the stomach. If it is not possible to return all the viscera into the peritoneal cavity, a silastic silo may be used. It is usual to ventilate the child's lungs postoperatively because of the reduction in compliance caused by return of the viscera to the peritoneum. As with all congenital anomalies, associated abnormalities are described with these conditions, particularly with exomphalos.

POSTOPERATIVE CARE

Unless they are being admitted to an ICU, all children should be nursed in a properly equipped and staffed recovery unit. Oxygen should be administered until the child has good oxygen saturation breathing room air. The cardiovascular and respiratory systems should be monitored and interventions carried out appropriately. It is becoming increasingly popular to have a step-down area attached to the recovery unit. This is an area where the child may be accompanied by the parents but may still be monitored closely. The child is returned to the ward when warm, pain-free and haemodynamically stable. It is the anaesthetist's responsibility to ensure

Table 36.10   Paediatric resuscitation chart

	Age and weight						
	Neonate 3.5 kg	3 months 5 kg	1 year 10 kg	3 years 15 kg	6 years 20 kg	8 years 25 kg	12 years 40 kg
Tracheal tube							
Size (4 + age/4); cm	3.0	3.5	4.0	5.0	5.5	6.0	7.0
Length (oral); cm	9	10	11	13	14	15	17
Length (nasal); cm	11	13	14	16	19	20	22
Epinephrine 1:10 000							
i.v./i.o./t.[a] $0.1\,mL\,kg^{-1}$ repeated as necessary	0.5 mL	0.5 mL	1 mL	1.5 mL	2 mL	2.5 mL	4 mL
Sodium bicarbonate 8.4%							
$1\,mL\,kg^{-1}$ i.v.	3 mL	5 mL	10 mL	15 mL	20 mL	25 mL	40 mL
Atropine 500 μg in 5 mL							
$0.2\,mL\,kg^{-1}$ i.v./t.	1 mL	1 mL	2 mL	3 mL	4 mL	5 mL	8 mL
Calcium chloride 10%							
$0.1\,mL\,kg^{-1}$ i.v.	0.5 mL	0.5 mL	1 mL	1.5 mL	2 mL	2.5 mL	4 mL
Defibrillation (J)							
$4\,J\,kg^{-1}$	10	20	40	60	80	100	160
Colloid volume (mL)							
$10\,mL\,kg^{-1} \times 2$–3 as necessary	35	50	100	150	200	250	400

i.v., intravenous; i.o., intraosseous; t., tracheal.
[a] For tracheal administration, give 10 times i.v. dose.
N.B. All drugs and fluids may be administered via the intraosseous route.

Drug infusions
Epinephrine: $0.03\,mg\,kg^{-1}$ in 50 mL glucose 5%; start at $2\,mL\,h^{-1}$.
Dopamine: $3\,mg\,kg^{-1}$ in 50 mL glucose 5%; 3–20 mL h^{-1}.
Dobutamine: $3\,mg\,kg^{-1}$ in 50 mL glucose 5%; 5–20 mL h^{-1}.
Isoproterenol: $0.25\,mg\,kg^{-1}$ in 50 mL glucose 5%; 1–4 mL h^{-1}.

that appropriate analgesia and intravenous fluids have been prescribed.

Useful information for dealing with paedratic emergencies is shown in Table 36.10.

FURTHER READING

Baum V 1999 Anesthesia for genetic, metabolic and dysmorphic syndromes of childhood. Williams & Wilkins, Baltimore

British Journal of Anaesthesia 1999 Postgraduate educational issue: the paediatric patient. Br J Anaesthesia 83

Dalens B 2001 Regional anesthesia for infants, children and adolescents, 2nd edn. Williams & Wilkins, Baltimore

McKenzie I et al 1997 Manual of acute pain management in children. Churchill Livingstone, Edinburgh

Motoyama E K, Davis P J 2006 Smith's anesthesia for infants and children. Mosby, St Louis

Peutrell J M, Mather S J 1997 Regional anaesthesia for babies and children. Oxford University Press, Oxford

Rowney D A, Doyle E 1998 Epidural and subarachnoid blockade in children. Anaesthesia 53: 980–1001

Anaesthesia for vascular, endocrine and plastic surgery

37

MAJOR VASCULAR SURGERY

Many aspects of vascular surgery have changed during the last two decades largely as a result of advances in radiological and cardiological practice. Examples include improvements in the treatment of myocardial infarction and the development of endovascular aortic surgery, lower limb and carotid angioplasty; such progress is likely to continue. However, vascular anaesthesia remains a challenging area of practice. Anaesthesia for major vascular surgery involves several general considerations. Specific features of the commoner vascular procedures are described in this chapter: elective and emergency repair of abdominal aortic aneurysm, lower limb revascularization and carotid endarterectomy.

GENERAL CONSIDERATIONS

Peripheral vascular disease is a manifestation of generalized cardiovascular disease, and therefore coronary artery disease is present in the majority of patients presenting for major vascular surgery. Most patients are elderly and have a high incidence of other coexisting medical disease, in particular:

- ischaemic heart disease
- hypertension
- congestive cardiac failure
- pulmonary disease
- renal disease
- diabetes mellitus.

Vascular surgery is associated with a high morbidity and mortality, mostly resulting from cardiac complications (myocardial infarction, arrhythmias and cardiac failure) (see Chs 19 and 23). It is therefore vital that cardiac function is assessed preoperatively and the risks of surgery evaluated and discussed with the patient. Although the outcome of subsequent vascular surgery is improved in those who have previously undergone coronary revascularization by coronary artery bypass grafting (CABG), this is associated with additional risks. Percutaneous coronary angioplasty with or without insertion of intracoronary stents is increasingly being used as an alternative to CABG in suitable patients, although its role and optimal timing before planned noncardiac surgery are not established. Elective surgery should be postponed for at least 4–6 weeks after coronary stent insertion and a delay of 3 months may be better unless surgery is more urgent. However, coronary revascularization should be performed only if indicated because of the severity of coronary disease and is not justified simply to improve outcome from subsequent vascular surgery.

The institution of perioperative beta-blockade reduces perioperative myocardial ischaemia, morbidity and mortality in the highest-risk patients undergoing major vascular surgery (i.e. those with documented inducible myocardial ischaemia or multiple cardiac risk factors). Chronic beta-blockade does not protect higher-risk patients from perioperative cardiac morbidity, the reasons for which are unclear. The optimum duration, dose and role of individual regimens for beta-blockade are not established, especially in lower risk patients, but the anaesthetist should consider commencement of beta-blockade (e.g. atenolol 25–100 mg or bisoprolol 2.5–10 mg o.d.). 1–2 weeks preoperatively, titrated towards a heart rate of 60–70 min^{-1} in patients at risk of myocardial ischaemia (see Ch. 23).

Minimum investigations before major vascular surgery should include ECG, chest X-ray, full blood count and serum urea and electrolyte concentrations, but more invasive or specialized tests may be required. (see Ch. 15) Some assessment of exercise tolerance should be made, as it is a useful indicator of functional cardiac status. However, many vascular patients are limited by intermittent claudication or old age and may have a sedentary lifestyle. In this case, a patient with severe coronary artery disease may have no symptoms of angina and a normal resting ECG. In some patients (e.g. those with limited functional capacity or life expectancy because of severe intractable coexistent

671

medical conditions), the risks of elective vascular surgery may outweigh the overall potential benefits and invasive surgery may not be appropriate.

Preoperative evaluation should therefore aim to:

- assist risk assessment and the decision to perform surgery
- establish the best surgical options (e.g. noninvasive or endovascular surgery) for an individual
- allow optimization of coexisting medical conditions including coronary revascularization if indicated
- permit consideration and institution of perioperative beta-blockade
- allow timing of surgery and required facilities (e.g. ICU) to be organized.

ABDOMINAL AORTIC ANEURYSM

Abdominal aortic aneurysms (AAAs) occur in 2–4% of the population over the age of 65 years, predominantly in males. Most are situated below the origin of the renal arteries and they tend to expand over time. The risk of rupture increases markedly when the aneurysm exceeds 5.5 cm in diameter and elective surgery is then indicated. The mortality from elective AAA repair is decreasing and is now 5–8%, but mortality from a ruptured AAA is up to 90% overall, and 50% in those who survive until emergency surgery can be performed. Consequently, screening programmes are in place to identify patients with a small asymptomatic aneurysm. Surgery involves replacing the aneurysmal segment with a tube or bifurcated prosthetic graft, depending on the extent of iliac artery involvement. In all cases, the aorta must be cross-clamped (see below) and a large abdominal incision is required. Surgery is prolonged and blood loss may be substantial. Patients are elderly with a high incidence of coexisting disease. These factors contribute to the high morbidity and mortality of this procedure. Endovascular aortic aneurysm surgery avoids some of these problems (see below).

Elective open AAA repair

Preoperative evaluation and risk assessment is paramount. All vasoactive medication (except perhaps ACE inhibitors and angiotensin-II receptor antagonists) must be continued up to the time of surgery and an anxiolytic premedication is advantageous. Preoperative addition of a beta-blocker may be indicated. The patient may have recently undergone arteriography and the injection of large volumes of radiopaque dye may cause

renal dysfunction. Maintenance of hydration with intravenous crystalloids is advisable the night before surgery.

An arterial and two large intravenous cannulae should be inserted before induction of anaesthesia, with monitoring of ECG and pulse oximetry. Cardiovascular changes at induction may be diminished by preoperative hydration and careful titration of the intravenous induction agent. After neuromuscular blockade, the trachea is intubated (see below) and anaesthesia continued using a balanced volatile/opioid technique. Perioperative epidural analgesia is favoured by many anaesthetists and may be undertaken before or after induction of anaesthesia (see below).

Several important considerations apply to patients undergoing aortic surgery (Table 37.1). The following are required:

- two large (14-gauge) cannulae for infusion of warmed fluids
- arterial catheter for intra-arterial pressure monitoring and blood sampling for acid–base and blood gas analysis
- central venous catheter for measurement of right atrial pressure
- continuous ECG monitoring for ischaemia (CM5 position) ± ST-segment analysis
- oesophageal or nasopharyngeal temperature probe
- urinary catheter
- nasogastric tube.

In the more compromised patient, e.g. with ischaemic heart disease and poor left ventricular function, a pulmonary artery catheter should be used to measure cardiac output and monitor fluid manage-

Table 37.1 Major anaesthetic considerations for patients undergoing aortic surgery

High incidence of coexisting cardiovascular and respiratory disease
Cardiovascular instability during induction of anaesthesia, aortic cross-clamping and declamping
Large blood loss and fluid shifts during and after surgery
Prolonged major surgery in high-risk patients
Marked heat and evaporative fluid losses from exposed bowel
Potential postoperative impairment of respiratory, cardiac, renal and gastrointestinal function

ment and left ventricular preload. Transoesophageal echocardiography or oesophageal Doppler monitoring may also be helpful. All possible measures should be undertaken to maintain body temperature, including heated mattress and overblanket, warmed intravenous fluids, and warmed and humidified inspired gases. The ambient temperature should be warm and the bowel may be wrapped in clear plastic to minimize evaporative losses.

Three specific stimuli may give rise to cardiovascular instability during surgery:

- *Tracheal intubation.* Laryngoscopy and tracheal intubation may be accompanied by marked increases in arterial pressure and heart rate which may precipitate myocardial ischaemia in susceptible individuals. This response may be attenuated by the i.v. administration of a beta-blocker (e.g. esmolol 1.5 mg kg^{-1}) or a rapidly-acting opioid (e.g. alfentanil 10 µg kg^{-1}) before intubation.
- *Cross-clamping of the aorta.* Clamping of the aorta causes a sudden increase in afterload which increases cardiac work and may result in myocardial ischaemia, arrhythmias and left ventricular failure. The effect on preload is variable. The degree of overall cardiovascular disturbance depends on the site of aortic cross-clamping and is greater at the supracoeliac compared with the infrarenal level. Vasodilators – e.g. sodium nitroprusside (SNP) or glyceryl trinitrate (GTN) – are often infused just before clamping (and continued up to clamp release) to obviate these problems. While the aorta is clamped, distal blood flow is dependent on the collateral circulation. The lower limbs, large bowel and kidneys suffer variable degrees of ischaemia during which inflammatory mediators are released from white blood cells, platelets and capillary endothelium. These mediators include oxygen-free radicals, neutrophil proteases, platelet-activating factor, cyclo-oxygenase products and cytokines, including interleukins.
- *Aortic declamping.* Declamping of the aorta causes a sudden decrease in afterload with reperfusion of the bowel, pelvis and lower limbs. Inflammatory mediators are swept into the systemic circulation causing vasodilatation, metabolic acidosis, increased capillary permeability and sequestration of blood cells in the lungs. This is a critical period of anaesthesia and surgery because hypotension after aortic declamping may be severe and refractory unless circulating volume has been well maintained. If relative hypervolaemia is produced during the period of clamping by infusion of fluids to produce a CVP of greater than 12–14 mmHg

(and perhaps administration of GTN or SNP until shortly before clamp release), declamping hypotension is less of a problem and metabolic acidosis may be diminished. Declamping hypotension usually resolves within a few minutes but vasopressors or inotropes are frequently required. Prophylactic mannitol 0.5–1.0 g kg^{-1} i.v., or slow or sequential clamp release, may be beneficial in countering some of these effects. Renal blood flow decreases even when an infrarenal cross-clamp is used, and steps to maintain renal function are often required. The single most important measure is the maintenance of extracellular fluid volume (i.e. CVP >12–14 mmHg). Mannitol, low-dose dopamine or furosemide may also be administered, although the evidence for their efficacy is conflicting.

Bleeding is a problem throughout the operation but may be particularly severe at aortic declamping as the adequacy of vascular anastomoses is tested. The role of cell salvage is established in aortic surgery but other modes of autologous blood transfusion (predonation, normovolaemic haemodilution) may be valuable. In addition to red cells, specific clotting factors are often required. It is often preferable to reserve the use of clotting factors until the anastomoses are complete and most of the anticipated blood loss has occurred. Many surgeons request the administration of heparin 2000–5000 units i.v. before graft insertion and it may be appropriate to reverse its effects with protamine (0.5 mg per 100 units of heparin).

Most patients are elderly and are unable to tolerate the large heat loss occurring through the extensive surgical exposure, which necessitates displacement of the bowel outside the abdominal cavity. Hypothermia causes vasoconstriction, which may cause myocardial ischaemia, delayed recovery and difficulties with fluid management during rewarming, as large volumes of intravenous fluid may be required. Therefore, all measures should be taken to prevent hypothermia.

The postoperative period

Postoperatively, the patient should be transferred to a high-dependency or intensive care unit. Artificial ventilation is continued until body temperature has increased to normal levels, the consequent vasodilatation has been treated with i.v. fluids and any continued blood loss from oozing has subsided. Provision of effective analgesia is very important. Patients have a high incidence of postoperative cardiovascular and respiratory complications; renal dysfunction and ileus are also common and close monitoring is required for several days.

Emergency open repair

The principles of management are similar to those discussed above. However, the patient may be grossly hypovolaemic and arterial pressure is often maintained only by marked systemic vasoconstriction and the action of abdominal muscle tone acting on intra-abdominal capacitance vessels. Resuscitation with intravenous fluids before the patient reaches the operating theatre should be judicious; permissive hypotension has been shown to limit the extent of haemorrhage and improve outcome. The patient is prepared and anaesthesia induced on the operating table. While 100% oxygen is administered by mask, an arterial and two large-gauge i.v. cannulae are inserted under local anaesthesia. The surgeon then prepares and towels the patient ready for surgery and it is only at this point that anaesthesia is induced using a rapid-sequence technique. When muscle relaxation occurs, systemic arterial pressure may decrease precipitously and immediate laparotomy and aortic clamping may be required. Thereafter, the procedure is similar to that for elective repair.

The prognosis is poor for several reasons. There has been no preoperative preparation and most patients have concurrent disease. There may have been a period of severe hypotension, resulting in impairment of renal, cerebral or myocardial function. Blood loss is often substantial and massive transfusion of red cells and clotting factors is usually required. Postoperative jaundice is common because of haemolysis of damaged red cells in the circulation and in the large retroperitoneal haematoma which usually develops after aortic rupture. In addition, postoperative renal impairment and prolonged ileus often occur. Artificial ventilation and organ support are required for several days and the cause of death is usually multiorgan failure.

Endovascular aortic aneurysm repair

Endovascular aortic aneurysm repair (EVAR) has emerged recently as an alternative to open surgery. A balloon-expandable stent-graft is inserted under radiological guidance via the femoral or iliac arteries into the aneurysm to exclude it from the circulation. It is performed via groin incisions and the aortic lumen is temporarily occluded from within, rather than being cross-clamped. The cardiovascular, metabolic and respiratory consequences are reduced in comparison with conventional surgery. Graft technology and expertise have improved considerably over the last decade:

blood loss and postoperative pain are less, ambulation occurs earlier and short-term mortality may be reduced compared with open surgery. However, 40% of patients have an aneurysm which is morphologically unsuitable for EVAR, repeated radiological procedures (e.g. angioplasty) are required in up to 20% of patients and the long-term outcome compared with open surgery is not established. The procedure usually takes 1–2 h and may be performed by radiologists and/or surgeons but many of the anaesthetic considerations are the same, as the patients have the same incidence of coexisting disease. In some cases, EVAR may be preferred as a less invasive technique in patients judged unfit for open surgery. In many centres, EVAR is performed in the radiology suite, in which case the anaesthetist must ensure that anaesthetic facilities for high-risk patients are adequate.

EVAR may be performed under general, regional or local anaesthesia with or without sedative adjuncts. In all cases, direct arterial pressure monitoring is mandatory because rapid fluctuations in arterial pressure may occur during stent-graft deployment. In awake patients, hyoscine 20 mg i.v. may be useful to decrease bowel motility during stent-graft placement. CVP monitoring is not usually necessary unless dictated by the patient's medical condition (e.g. moderate/severe cardiac disease). However, large-diameter cannulae should be inserted and vasoactive drugs readily available because if endovascular repair is not technically feasible, conversion to open surgery may be required. At this point, the patient may be already anaemic, hypovolaemic and hypothermic, and consequently mortality is appreciable. EVAR has also been used to repair contained ruptured or leaking AAAs or thoracic aortic aneurysms.

SURGERY FOR OCCLUSIVE PERIPHERAL VASCULAR DISEASE

Peripheral reconstructive surgery is performed in patients with severe atherosclerotic arterial disease, causing ischaemic rest pain, tissue loss (ulceration or gangrene), severe claudication with disease at specific anatomical sites (aortoiliac, femoropopliteal, popliteal or distal), or failure of nonsurgical procedures. Most are heavy smokers, suffer from chronic pulmonary disease and have widespread arterial disease. Exercise tolerance is limited by claudication, so patients may have severe coronary artery disease despite few symptoms. Surgical revascularization is performed to salvage the ischaemic limb, but arterial angioplasty is a less invasive alternative and is increasingly performed as a first-line procedure in suitable patients. Patients presenting for surgical reconstruction are often those in whom angioplasties have failed and may have more severe vascular disease. Short-term mortality after lower limb revascularization is comparable to that following AAA repair and long-term outcome is worse as a consequence of associated cardiovascular disease. Acute limb ischaemia which threatens limb viability requires rapid intervention comprising full anticoagulation, intrathrombus thrombolysis after arteriography, analgesia, and revascularization via embolectomy, angioplasty or bypass surgery as indicated. The clinical findings of sensory loss and muscle weakness necessitate intervention within 6 h and therefore preoperative evaluation and correction of risk factors may be limited.

Bypass of aortoiliac occlusion

Aortic bifurcation grafting is performed to overcome occlusion in the aorta and iliac arteries and to restore flow to the lower limbs. Because the disease evolves gradually, a considerable collateral circulation usually develops. Normal surgical practice is to side-clamp the aorta, maintaining some peripheral flow, and to declamp the arteries supplying the legs in sequence. Thus, the cardiovascular and metabolic changes are less severe than those seen during open AAA surgery, but the anaesthetic considerations and management are similar.

Peripheral arterial reconstruction

The commonest procedures involve the insertion of an autologous vein or synthetic vascular graft between axillary and femoral, or femoral and popliteal arteries. Axillofemoral bypass surgery is performed in those not considered fit for open aortic surgery, and these patients are often particularly frail. All these operations are prolonged and an IPPV/relaxant balanced anaesthetic technique is suitable. A meticulous anaesthetic technique is paramount with particular attention to the maintenance of normothermia and administration of i.v. fluids. Hypothermia or hypovolaemia may cause peripheral vasoconstriction, compromising distal perfusion and postoperative graft function. Blood loss through the walls of open-weave grafts may continue for several hours after surgery and cardiovascular status should be monitored closely during this time. Epidural analgesia may be used alone or as an adjunct to general anaesthesia for lower limb procedures. Despite theoretical advantages, epidural anaesthesia has no effect on graft function per se but it does provide effective postoperative analgesia. However, i.v. heparin is usually administered during and after surgery (see below) and the risks of

epidural haematoma should be considered. Oxygen therapy should be continued for at least 24 h after surgery, and monitoring in a high-dependency unit is often required.

CAROTID ARTERY SURGERY

Approximately 30% of cases of acute stroke are fatal, and another 30% result in significant disability. Carotid endarterectomy is performed to prevent disabling embolic stroke in patients with atheromatous plaques in the common carotid bifurcation, or internal or external carotid arteries. Most patients are elderly, with generalized vascular disease. Cerebral autoregulation may be impaired and cerebral blood flow is therefore proportional to systemic arterial pressure. The main risk of surgery is the production of a new neurological deficit (which may be fatal or cause permanent disability), although cardiovascular complications account for 50% of the overall morbidity and mortality.

Carotid endarterectomy is unusual in that it is a preventative operation with well-defined indications based on the results of large-scale, randomized studies performed in Europe and the USA. In patients with a previous stroke and a carotid stenosis >70%, the benefits of surgery outweigh the risks, whereas in those with mild stenosis (< 30%), the risks outweigh the benefits and medical treatment with antiplatelet drugs is preferred. Therefore, the patients presenting for surgery are those with the most severe disease, and the potential benefits are only realized if the overall perioperative mortality and morbidity are low (< 5%). Specific perioperative risk factors are age >75 years, female sex, systolic hypertension, peripheral vascular disease (probably as a marker for coronary artery disease), experience of the surgeon and ipsilateral cerebral symptoms. Longer-term outcome is also worse in smokers and those with diabetes or hyperlipidaemia. As with other aspects of vascular surgery, carotid artery angioplasty is receiving some interest as an alternative to surgical endarterectomy, although its place is yet to be established.

During surgery, the carotid artery is clamped, after which cerebral perfusion is dependent on collateral circulation via the circle of Willis. A temporary shunt is usually inserted to bypass the site of obstruction, minimizing clamping time and the period of potential cerebral ischaemia. Several methods are available to assess cerebral blood flow during clamping, before proceeding with the endarterectomy; if flow is adequate, some surgeons prefer not to use a temporary shunt. Monitoring of neurological status in an awake patient is considered by many to be the 'gold standard', but other methods include:

- transcranial Doppler ultrasonography of the middle cerebral artery
- measurement of arterial pressure in the occluded distal carotid segment (the 'stump' pressure)
- EEG monitoring
- recording somatosensory evoked potentials
- measurement of jugular venous oxygen tension.

Although most strokes related to surgery are associated with thromboembolism rather than hypo- or hypertension, and the majority of these are caused by inadvertent technical surgical error, the anaesthetist has a crucial role in the maintenance of cardiovascular stability before, during and after surgery. Rapid swings in arterial pressure are common because of the effects of surgical manipulation, clamping on carotid sinus baroreceptors and vagal reflexes in patients with cardiovascular disease. The aims of anaesthesia for carotid endarterectomy also include airway protection and provision of neurological protection as required. Most intraoperative strokes are apparent on recovery from anaesthesia and early postoperative neurological assessment is important. Any residual postoperative effects of anaesthesia may confuse the diagnosis of intraoperative embolism or ischaemic change, so a technique that permits rapid return of function is required. These aims may be achieved using general, local or regional anaesthetic techniques, with or without sedative or analgesic adjuncts. Local infiltration of the surgical field may be used alone or in combination with superficial or deep cervical plexus blockade. The advantages of locoregional techniques include definitive neurological monitoring (therefore allowing selective use of shunts), preservation of cerebral and coronary autoregulation, and the maintenance of higher cerebral perfusion pressures during the procedure (Table 37.2). However, these techniques rely on good cooperation between the patient, the surgeon and the anaesthetist. Many patients find it difficult to lie still and supine for the duration of the procedure, particularly those with cardiac failure or respiratory disease; this may be compounded by diaphragmatic compromise as phrenic nerve paralysis may accompany deep cervical plexus blockade. Sudden loss of consciousness or seizures may occur if cerebral perfusion is inadequate after clamping, and subsequent airway control may be very difficult because access is limited. General anaesthesia avoids these problems, allows manipulation of P_aCO_2 and both volatile agents and propofol reduce cerebral oxygen requirements, but hypotension may be more common compared with regional anaesthesia. Cerebral and coronary autoregulation are also preserved using low doses of volatile agents. Overall, there is currently no good evidence that cardiac or neurological outcome is better with any specific anaesthetic technique.

The primary aim of anaesthesia is to maintain cerebral perfusion during carotid clamping, using a technique which provides cardiovascular stability and

Table 37.2 Suggested advantages and disadvantages of local or general anaesthesia for carotid surgery

Advantages	Disadvantages
Local anaesthesia	
Definitive CNS monitoring	Technical difficulties
Maintenance of higher cerebral perfusion pressure	Patient discomfort lying supine during prolonged procedure
Maintenance of cerebral autoregulation	Sedative or analgesic supplementation usually required
Allows selective shunting	Lack of airway protection
Arterial pressure usually higher so less vasopressors required compared with GA	Difficult access to patient if intraoperative neurological or cardiac complications occur
Avoids 'minor' complications of general anaesthesia	
General anaesthesia	
Patient comfort	Some method of monitoring of cerebral blood flow required
Airway protection	'Minor' complications of general anaesthesia (e.g. sore throat, sedation, nausea, vomiting)
Reduced CMRO$_2$	
Cerebral autoregulation maintained using low doses of volatile agents	
Therapeutic manipulation of arterial CO$_2$ possible	

allows rapid recovery. An intra-arterial cannula is mandatory for monitoring of arterial pressure, which should be maintained particularly during carotid clamping. The airway is not accessible during surgery, and tracheal intubation with a well-secured reinforced tracheal tube is advisable. Anaesthesia should be induced cautiously using an i.v. agent and maintained with a balanced technique using an inspired oxygen concentration of 50% in air or nitrous oxide (100% inspired oxygen produces cerebral vasoconstriction) with isoflurane, sevoflurane or desflurane. All anaesthetic agents should be short-acting, and remifentanil, alfentanil or low-dose fentanyl (100–200 µg) are useful adjuncts. Hypotension may potentially occur after induction and during the placement of cerebral monitoring, but it should be treated promptly. Vasopressors (e.g. ephedrine 3–6 mg, or phenylephrine 25–50 µg increments) are frequently required and should be drawn up before induction of anaesthesia. A high P_aO_2, normocapnia and normothermia should be maintained. Blood loss and fluid requirements are usually modest. Postoperatively, pain is unusual and the combination of wound infiltration with local anaesthetic with a nonsteroidal anti-inflammatory analgesic during surgery is effective.

Patients should be monitored in a high-dependency environment for several hours postoperatively. Hypertension is common in the early postoperative period because of impaired circulatory reflexes; pain from the wound or from bladder distension may contribute. Hypertension is associated with adverse neurological outcomes because it may compromise the graft or cause intracranial haemorrhage. Arterial pressure should be controlled to achieve systolic pressures < 165 mmHg and diastolic pressures < 95 mmHg, accounting for the range of individual preoperative values. Intravenous alpha- or beta-blockers or an infusion of a vasodilator (e.g. GTN, hydralazine or SNP) may be required as prophylaxis or treatment.

The other main postoperative complication is the development of a haematoma. Initial treatment involves local pressure and reversal of heparin with protamine. However, local oedema and the presence of a large haematoma may cause airway compromise and hypoxaemia requiring urgent surgical exploration. Induction of general anaesthesia in these circumstances is particularly hazardous and evacuation of the haematoma under local infiltration is usually preferable. Recurrent laryngeal nerve damage is a recognized complication of carotid endarterectomy. In most cases this simply causes a hoarse voice but in patients who have had a previous contralateral carotid endarterectomy, specific preoperative evaluation of vocal cord function should be performed before surgery.

CARDIOVERSION

Direct current (DC) cardioversion is an effective treatment for some re-entrant tachyarrhythmias, which may produce haemodynamic instability and myocardial ischaemia and which do not respond to other measures. Atrial fibrillation of less than 6 months' duration, atrial flutter, supraventricular tachycardia and ventricular tachycardia may be converted to sinus rhythm, although maintenance of sinus rhythm depends usually on subsequent antiarrhythmic drugs. Cardioversion has little effect on contractility, conductivity or excitability of the myocardium, and has a low incidence of side-effects or complications.

Pre-anaesthetic assessment

Patients may present with a chronic arrhythmia for elective cardioversion or as an emergency in extremis with a life-threatening arrhythmia. They may have other serious cardiovascular pathology such as rheumatic disease, ischaemic heart disease, recent myocardial infarction or cardiac failure. Digoxin therapy predisposes to postcardioversion arrhythmias; in some centres, it is withheld for 48h before cardioversion. If DC cardioversion is required in a patient receiving digoxin, the initial DC dose should be low (e.g. 10–25 J) and increased if necessary. In some patients there is a significant risk of embolic phenomena, e.g. those with:

- mitral stenosis and atrial fibrillation of recent onset
- atrial fibrillation and a dilated cardiomyopathy
- a prosthetic mitral valve
- a history of embolic phenomena.

These patients should receive prophylactic anticoagulants for 2–3 weeks before cardioversion, and anticoagulation should be continued afterwards. Accurate knowledge of the medical and drug history and thorough clinical examination are essential before anaesthesia.

Cardioversion

Direct current (DC) electrical discharge passed through the heart depolarizes all excitable myocardial cells and interrupts abnormal pathways and foci. The electrodes are usually positioned on the anterolateral chest with the patient supine, but the anteroposterior arrangement, with the patient in the lateral position, is sometimes used. The paddles should not be sited over the scapula, sternum or vertebrae and the skin must be protected with electrolyte jelly, saline-soaked gauze or any type of conducting pad.

The ECG monitoring lead chosen should demonstrate a clear R wave in order to synchronize the discharge away from the T wave and thus reduce the risk of development of ventricular fibrillation. If the arrhythmia does not convert after the first 50 J discharge, further shocks are given, using an increased energy discharge of up to 200 J.

Despite the use of synchronized discharge, ventricular fibrillation may be produced in the presence of hypokalaemia, ischaemia, digoxin toxicity and QT prolongation (e.g. caused by quinidine or tricyclic antidepressants).

Anaesthesia

Treatment should be carried out only in areas specifically designed for the purpose and with a full range of drugs, resuscitation and monitoring equipment available. These must be checked by the anaesthetist, and patients prepared as for a surgical procedure.

ECG monitoring, oximetry and measurement of arterial pressure are instituted. A vein is cannulated and the patient's lungs are preoxygenated before i.v. induction of anaesthesia. The choice of drug is determined by the cardiovascular stability and recovery period required. If the patient is shocked, precautions to prevent aspiration of gastric contents should be taken and a rapid-sequence induction with cricoid pressure and tracheal intubation should be performed. However, many patients are admitted for elective cardioversion on a day-case basis, and a technique using i.v. propofol and spontaneous ventilation is suitable.

As soon as the patient is unconscious, the airway is secured and oxygenation maintained with a suitable breathing system. Before activation of the defibrillator, it is important to check that the patient is not in contact with any person or metal object. If repeated shocks are required, incremental doses of the anaesthetic may be given. The patient should be monitored carefully both during anaesthesia and after recovery of consciousness, in particular for evidence of recurrent arrhythmia, hypotension, pulmonary oedema, or systemic or pulmonary embolism.

SURGERY FOR TUMOURS OF THE ENDOCRINE SYSTEM

Amine precursor uptake and decarboxylation (APUD) cells originate from neuroectoderm and are distributed widely throughout the body. They synthesize and store neurotransmitter substances, including serotonin, ACTH, calcitonin, melanocyte-stimulating hormone (MSH), glucagon, gastrin and vasoactive intestinal polypeptide. Neoplastic change within these cells produces the group of tumours termed apudomas, e.g. carcinoid, pancreatic islet cell tumour, pituitary and thyroid adenoma, medullary carcinoma of thyroid and small cell carcinoma of the lung. These may be orthoendocrine or paraendocrine – the former produce amines and polypeptides associated normally with the constituent cells, while the latter secrete substances produced usually by other organs. Two orthoendocrine apudomas in particular may produce significant problems for the anaesthetist.

CARCINOID TUMOUR

Carcinoid tumours are rare tumours derived from enterochromaffin cells of the intestinal tract, most commonly the small bowel or appendix. However, they may arise at any site in the gut and rarely in the gallbladder, pancreas or bronchus. They are usually benign. Malignant change occurs in 4% and may produce hepatic metastases. Carcinoid tumours secrete a variety of vasoactive peptides and amines (e.g. kinins, serotonin, histamine and prostaglandins) which have a variety of effects on vascular, bronchial and gastrointestinal smooth muscle activity. These compounds are normally metabolized in the liver and carcinoid tumours are often asymptomatic unless the mediators reach the systemic circulation from hepatic metastases or an extra-abdominal primary, e.g. bronchus, producing the clinical symptoms of carcinoid syndrome.

Kallikrein acts on circulating plasma kininogen to produce bradykinin and tachykinins. Bradykinin is a potent vasodilator which causes flushing, bronchospasm and increased intestinal motility and contributes to hypotension and oedema. Adrenergic stimulation and alcohol ingestion increase the production of bradykinin. Serotonin (5-hydroxytryptamine, 5-HT) causes abnormal gut motility, diarrhoea and bronchospasm. It has positive inotropic and chronotropic effects and produces vasoconstriction. It may cause endocardial fibrosis, leading to pulmonary and tricuspid stenosis or regurgitation (though bronchial carcinoid tumours may lead to left-sided cardiac valvular lesions). Histamine secretion may cause bronchoconstriction and flushing. Acute attacks of carcinoid syndrome may also be precipitated by fear or hypotension.

Diagnosis is confirmed by high urinary excretion of 5-hydroxyindoleacetic acid (5-HIAA), a metabolite of 5-HT. Urinary 5-HIAA concentrations correlate with tumour activity and perioperative complications.

Primary and secondary tumours are localized by CT, MRI and ultrasound scans. Although medication may alleviate some symptoms the definitive treatment of carcinoid tumours is surgery, including excision of the primary tumour and resection or radiofrequency ablation of hepatic metastases. The main anaesthetic considerations are perioperative prevention of mediator release, and preparation for control of carcinoid crises. Systemic release of carcinoid mediators can be exacerbated or precipitated by anxiety, tracheal intubation, inadequate analgesia, tumour manipulation or the administration of catecholamines or drugs which cause histamine release. In severe cases, acute intraoperative cardiovascular instability (arrhythmias and extreme fluctuations in arterial pressure) and resistant bronchospasm may occur.

Management

Patients may receive drugs to diminish symptoms of diarrhoea, flushing and bronchospasm, but specific agents are used to inhibit synthesis, prevent release or block the actions of the mediators released by the tumour. The most important drug is the somatostatin analogue octreotide, which improves both symptoms and biochemical indices, and is useful in the prevention and management of perioperative hypotension and carcinoid crisis. Somatostatin (half-life 1–3 min) is secreted naturally by the pancreas and regulates gastrointestinal peptide production by inhibiting the secretion of growth hormone, thyroid-stimulating hormone (TSH), prolactin and other exocrine and endocrine hormones. Octreotide, the octapeptide analogue of somatostatin, has a longer half-life, high potency and low clearance, and may be given i.v. or s.c. The usual s.c. dose is 50–200 µg every 8–12 h. It is useful for symptom relief in other conditions, notably acromegaly, VIPoma and glucagonoma. It may cause gastrointestinal side-effects, gallstones and impaired glucose tolerance.

5-HT antagonists (ketanserin, methysergide) and antihistamines, e.g. ranitidine, chlorphenamine (chlorpheniramine), are also used. Cyproheptadine has both antihistamine and anti 5-HT actions.

Conduct of anaesthesia

Perioperative management should be in close cooperation with both physician and surgeon, and the patient's regular medication should be continued up to the time of surgery. The possibility of cardiac valvular lesions should be considered. Hypovolaemia and electrolyte disturbance should be corrected before operation. Anxiolytic premedication with minimal cardiovascular disturbance is desirable; an oral benzo-diazepine is often used alone or together with an antihistamine, although oversedation should be avoided. Octreotide must be continued as premedication 50–100 µg s.c. 1 h preoperatively. It may also be administered during surgery as an i.v. infusion at 50–100 µg h^{-1}. A smooth anaesthetic technique is essential, and techniques which may cause hypotension, including epidural and subarachnoid block, should be used with extreme caution. Drugs which release histamine (e.g. thiopental, morphine, meperidine (pethidine), atracurium, mivacurium) should be avoided.

Careful intravenous induction of anaesthesia with etomidate or propofol should be accompanied by measures to obtund the potentially exaggerated pressor response to tracheal intubation. Succinylcholine is best avoided as it may cause peptide release and non-depolarizing muscle relaxants with minimal histamine release and cardiovascular stability (e.g. rocuronium or vecuronium) are preferable. Anaesthesia should be maintained with opioids (e.g. fentanyl or remifentanil), inhaled nitrous oxide and a volatile agent. Bronchospasm may be severe and should be treated with octreotide or aminophylline rather than adrenaline, and a flow-generator type of ventilator capable of delivering the inspired gases at high pressure should be used. Continuous monitoring of ECG and direct arterial pressure should be commenced before induction of anaesthesia. Major fluid shifts may occur during surgery, and the effects of circulating peptides may distort the physiological response to hypovolaemia. Central venous pressure measurement is advisable when large blood loss is likely, and pulmonary artery catheterization may be required in patients with cardiac complications. Intraoperative hypotension may be severe and should be treated with intravenous fluids and octreotide 100 µg i.v. Sympathomimetic drugs may cause alpha-mediated peptide release and are not recommended for the treatment of bronchospasm or hypotension. Hypertension is usually less severe and usually responds to increased depth of anaesthesia, beta-blockade or ketanserin.

Close cardiovascular monitoring and good analgesia are required postoperatively and the patient should be observed in a high-dependency or intensive therapy unit. The use of epidural analgesia is controversial, but an epidural infusion of fentanyl alone or with bupivacaine 0.1% has been used successfully.

PHAEOCHROMOCYTOMA

Phaeochromocytomas are derived from chromaffin cells that secrete catecholamines (predominantly noradrenaline, but also adrenaline and occasionally dopamine), which occur in less than 0.1% of hypertensive

Table 37.3 Associations of phaeochromocytoma with other syndromes
Von Hippel–Lindau disease (retinocerebral haemangioblastoma)

MEN IIa (Sipple's syndrome)
   Phaeochromocytoma
   Medullary cell thyroid carcinoma
   Hyperparathyroidism

MEN IIb (mucosal neuroma syndrome)
   Phaeochromocytoma
   Medullary cell thyroid carcinoma
   Mucosal neuromata
   Marfanoid habitus

Phaeochromocytoma-paraganglionoma syndrome
Von Recklinghausen's disease (multiple neurofibromatosis)

Table 37.4 Anaesthetic considerations in patients with phaeochromocytoma

Preoperative
Hypertension
Hypovolaemia (vasoconstriction with reduced circulating volume)
Pharmacological stabilization
   α-blockade
   β-blockade
   Control of catecholamine synthesis
End-organ damage
Anxiolytic/sedative premedication

Intraoperative
Severe cardiovascular instability, particularly:
   at induction of anaesthesia and tracheal intubation
   during pneumoperitoneum (laparascopic procedures)
   during tumour handling
   following ligation of venous drainage
Hypoglycaemia after tumour removal

Postoperative Hypotension Hypoglycaemia Somnolence, opioid sensitivity Hypoadrenalism LV dysfunction

patients. The majority present in middle-aged adults but may be found in childhood. Most are found as a single benign tumour of the adrenal medulla, but 10% occur in ectopic sites, e.g. paravertebral sympathetic ganglia. Approximately 10% of phaeochromocytomas are malignant, and 10% are bilateral. Genetic factors are frequently involved and they may be associated with multiple endocrine neoplasia (MEN) and other syndromes (Table 37.3).

The clinical features depend on the quantity of hormones secreted and on which is predominant, though episodes may be paroxysmal and clinical findings may be normal between attacks. Noradrenaline-secreting tumours tend to cause severe refractory hypertension, headaches and glucose intolerance; circulating blood volume is reduced and vasoconstriction occurs. Adrenaline-secreting tumours trigger palpitations, anxiety and panic attacks, sweating, hypoglycaemia, tachycardia, tachyarrhythmias and occasionally high-output cardiac failure. Malaise, weight loss, pallor and psychological disturbances may occur, and end-organ damage (e.g. retinopathy, nephropathy, dilated cardiomyopathy) may arise as a consequence of hypertension. They present several problems to the anaesthetist (Table 37.4).

Diagnosis

Diagnosis is important as the mortality of patients undergoing unrelated surgery with an unsuspected phaeochromocytoma is up to 50%. Diagnosis is confirmed by measurement of high plasma and urine concentrations of free catecholamines. Random 1-h or 24-h urinary excretion of catecholamine metabolites (metanephrines and 3-methoxy-4-hydroxymandelic acid (HMMA; also known as vanillylmandelic acid [VMA])), are a less sensitive alternative. In some cases a clonidine suppression test may be required to distinguish between hypertensive patients and those with phaeochromocytoma. Magnetic resonance imaging (MRI) of the abdomen is probably the investigation of choice to localize tumours greater than 1 cm in diameter. Computed tomography (performed without intravenous contrast media, which may precipitate release of hormone) is an alternative. Confirmation of the identity and position of an adrenal mass is by uptake of [^{131}I] m-iodolbenzylguanidine (MIBG) monitored by gamma camera.

Preoperative preparation

Medical treatment of the effects of the tumour must be achieved before surgery. Alpha-adrenergic antagonists counteract the increased peripheral vascular resistance and reduced circulating volume, and phenoxybenzamine (noncompetitive, nonselective), prazosin and doxazosin (α_1-selective, competitive antagonists) have been used successfully. Noncompetitive alpha-antagonists are preferable, as surges of catecholamine concentrations, occurring particularly during tumour handling, do not overwhelm the effects of a noncompetitive drug. Phenoxybenzamine is given in increasing titrated doses over 2–3 weeks before surgery, starting from 10 mg b.d. up to a usual dose of 40–50 mg b.d. In this way, the circulating volume expands gradually with normal oral intake of fluid. Adverse effects include initial postural hypotension, tachycardia, blurred vision and nasal congestion. A beta-adrenergic antagonist may be required later to control tachycardia, but acute hypertension, cardiac failure and acute pulmonary oedema may occur if beta-blockade is introduced first because of unopposed alpha-mediated vasoconstriction. Propranolol, metoprolol and atenolol are useful agents if beta-blockade is required. Labetalol is favoured by some physicians, but its beta-effect predominates and alpha-antagonists should be administered first. Occasionally, phenoxybenzamine or phentolamine may be given by i.v. infusion (e.g. for 48–72 h preceding surgery). In this event, intravascular volume must be monitored by measurement of CVP, and i.v. colloids are often required to maintain a normal circulating volume. Alternatively, catecholamine synthesis may be suppressed actively by administration of alpha-methyl-p-tyrosine, a tyrosine hydroxylase inhibitor. This drug may be very successful in controlling catecholamine effects but may cause severe side-effects, including diarrhoea, fatigue and depression and is usually reserved for long-term medical treatment in patients considered unsuitable for surgery.

Preoperative investigations depend on the patient's physical condition; the presence of end-organ damage should be determined. Nephrectomy may be required to completely remove the tumour and renal function should be assessed preoperatively. Echocardiography may also be useful.

Conduct of anaesthesia

Sudden, severe hypertension (due to systemic release of catecholamines) may occur during tumour mobilization and handling, particularly if preoperative preparation has been inadequate. Severe hypotension may occur after ligation of the venous drainage of the tumour (when catecholamine concentrations decrease acutely). Marked fluctuations in arterial pressure may also occur during induction of anaesthesia and tracheal intubation.

Sedative and anxiolytic premedication is useful and both alpha- and beta-adrenergic antagonists should be continued up to the day of surgery. Monitoring of ECG, CVP and direct arterial pressure must be commenced before induction of anaesthesia. Intraoperative monitoring should include temperature, blood gas tensions and glucose concentration; transoesophageal echocardiography or pulmonary artery catheterization may be required if significant cardiomyopathy is present. Anaesthetic drugs should be selected on the basis of cardiovascular stability, and agents which have the ability to provoke histamine (and hence catecholamine) release are best avoided (Table 37.5). The exact choice of individual anaesthetic drugs is less important than careful conduct of anaesthesia, which may be induced by slow administration of thiopental, etomidate or propofol and maintained with nitrous oxide in oxygen, supplemented by sevoflurane or isoflurane. Desflurane has the theoretical disadvantage of causing sympathetic stimulation if concentrations are increased too rapidly. The use of moderate doses of opioids (e.g. fentanyl $7–10\,\mu g\,kg^{-1}$) may aid cardiovascular stability. Drugs should be immediately available to treat acute hypertension (e.g. SNP, phentolamine or nicardipine), tachycardia or arrhythmias (e.g. esmolol). Hypotension is treated with fluids initially but vasopressors (e.g. ephedrine, phenylephrine or noradrenaline) may be required. Intravenous magnesium sulphate may be useful: it suppresses catecholamine release from the tumour and adrenergic nerve endings, is a direct-acting vasodilator and has antiarrhythmic effects but has a narrow therapeutic window and plasma Mg^{2+} concentration should be monitored. Perioperative epidural analgesia may attenuate some of the cardiovascular responses, except during tumour handling, and is use-

Table 37.5   Drugs which should be avoided in patients with phaeochromocytoma

Atropine
Succinylcholine
d-Tubocurarine
Atracurium
Pancuronium
Droperidol
Morphine
Halothane

ful for postoperative analgesia. However, it should be used judiciously to avoid hypotension. Postoperative problems may include hypoglycaemia, somnolence, opioid sensitivity, hypotension and hypoadrenalism. Invasive monitoring should be continued for 12–24 h after surgery and the patient must be nursed in a high-dependency or intensive care unit.

Recent improvements in imaging, preoperative tumour localization and surgical technique have increased the popularity of laparoscopic adrenalectomy for phaeochromocytoma via transperitoneal or retroperitoneal routes. These are associated with less postoperative pain and earlier mobilization and recovery compared with open surgery. Overall, cardiovascular disturbance may be less, but the creation of a pneumoperitoneum during transperitoneal laparoscopy may cause large surges in catecholamine concentrations in addition to those occurring during tumour mobilization. Similar anaesthetic considerations apply, therefore, as for open surgery.

PLASTIC SURGERY

Plastic surgery includes the reconstitution of damaged or deformed tissues (congenital abnormalities or resulting from trauma, burns or infection), removal of cutaneous tumours or cosmetic alteration of body features. Division or removal of the abnormality often necessitates skin grafting. Major plastic surgery includes the formation and repositioning of free and pedicle grafts and the movement of skin flaps.

GENERAL CONSIDERATIONS

Many of these procedures have important common features. Patients may be physically deformed and attention should be directed to their psychological state. This is influenced by long periods of confinement and rehabilitation, concern over disfigurement or loss of limb function and occasionally chronic pain. The presence of local or generalized infection and the patient's state of nutrition are important factors in postoperative outcome and should be considered. Conversely, cosmetic surgery of the face, tattoo removal, breast augmentation and removal of unwanted adipose tissue are usually performed on healthy patients. Surgery is often prolonged, requiring special attention to blood and fluid replacement therapy, and maintenance of body temperature. Pain is usually peripheral in origin but may be severe,

particularly from donor skin graft sites; local anaesthetic techniques (nerve or plexus blockade, or local infiltration) are very effective.

Anaesthesia for prolonged procedures should be administered using humidified gases in a warmed theatre environment using a technique which minimizes protracted recovery from anaesthesia. A remifentanil-based technique supplemented by a relatively insoluble volatile agent (e.g. isoflurane, desflurane or sevoflurane) is effective. Alternatively, a total intravenous technique may be employed, although the vasodilatation produced by volatile agents may be beneficial to surgical outcome. Nitrous oxide may produce bone marrow depression with exposure of more than 8 h duration and an oxygen/air mix should be substituted. Fluid balance should be maintained scrupulously. Significant haemorrhage is common during plastic surgery. Blood transfusion is frequently required, though microvascular flow is optimal with a haematocrit of approximately 0.3 and overtransfusion should be avoided. The outcome of microvascular surgery depends on adequate blood flow through a patent graft. Volatile anaesthetic agents and regional or sympathetic blockade cause vasodilatation, which may be helpful. However, graft blood flow may be impaired by hypotension, venous congestion, or vasoconstriction caused by hypovolaemia, hypothermia, hypocapnia or pain. Therefore, maintenance of normal arterial pressure, circulating volume and cardiac output, normothermia, and provision of good analgesia are important to maximize peri- and postoperative perfusion of the surgical site. Vascular spasm may be diminished by the use of local vasodilators.

The patient must be positioned to avoid ligament strain, and lumbar support is useful during long procedures. Pressure areas should be protected with soft padding to prevent pressure injury, particularly over bony prominences, and a ripple mattress used. Measures should be taken to prevent DVT formation. When surgery has been completed, wound dressing and bandaging may be lengthy procedures. Bandages may be applied around the trunk and the patient must be lifted carefully to avoid injury.

HEAD AND NECK

Tracheal intubation using a reinforced tube is recommended for surgery in this area. Tumours or scarring of the neck, deformity of facial bones and cleft palate can make tracheal intubation particularly difficult. The airway should be assessed carefully before anaesthesia, any difficulties anticipated and a complete range of equipment should be available. The administration of muscle relaxants in such patients may be unwise before the airway is secured by intubation; awake fibre-optic intubation under local anaesthesia or an inhalational technique should be considered. The method of maintenance is determined by the condition of the patient, the type and duration of surgery (frequently prolonged) and the experience and preference of the anaesthetist. Venous drainage is improved and bleeding reduced in head or neck surgery if the patient is positioned in a 10–15° head-up tilt. Hypotensive techniques may also be indicated, in which case an arterial cannula is advisable for measurement of arterial pressure. It is important to protect the eyes from pressure, the ears from blood and other fluids and the tracheal tube and anaesthetic tubing from dislodgement. It may be difficult to monitor chest movement, and access to the arms may be impossible. An i.v. infusion with extension tubing is essential; there should be access to a three-way tap for injection of drugs.

TRUNK

Surgery performed on the trunk may be prolonged and require unusual patient positioning, e.g. hip flexion during and after abdominoplasty. Specific considerations include potential haemorrhage during breast reduction surgery, and the use of restrictive dressings applied after surgery.

LIMBS

Local anaesthesia (e.g. by blockade of nerve plexuses in the neck, axilla or groin) may be an advantage in terms of analgesia and vasodilatation for surgery on upper or lower limbs. The duration of some plastic surgical operations and the use of a surgical tourniquet to provide a bloodless field may preclude some techniques, but prolonged neural blockade may be achieved using a catheter technique and by using an agent with a prolonged action (e.g. bupivacaine or ropivacaine). Intravenous sedative drugs or light general anaesthesia are useful adjuncts to help the patient tolerate a prolonged procedure. Specific nerve blocks may be useful; for example, blockade of the femoral and lateral cutaneous nerve of the thigh provides good analgesia for skin graft donor sites during and after operation. Bier's block is of limited value because of tourniquet pain, and cuff deflation may be required by the surgeon to identify bleeding points.

Surgical techniques of reimplantation and microsurgical repair of the limbs are well established and make specific demands upon the anaesthetist. These include maintenance of general anaesthesia for up to 24 h, control of vascular spasm and provision of optimum conditions for postoperative recovery.

BURNS

Thermal burn injuries are common, and despite improvements in outcome over the last few decades can result in significant morbidity and mortality. Factors associated with death include increased age, the size and depth of the burn and the presence of inhalational injury. The anaesthetist may be involved with victims of thermal burns at an early stage during basic resuscitation and airway management, during transfer to or management in a critical care or specialized burns unit, or for the provision of general anaesthesia for:

- excision of damaged tissue and escharotomies
- excision of granulation tissue and subsequent grafting
- changes of dressing
- reparative plastic procedures to relieve contractures, permit limb function or correct deformities.

Surgeons now perform debridement of burns with escharotomies at an earlier stage as infection and sepsis are reduced, and cosmetic results better.

Burns are classified according to the depth of burn and percentage of body surface area (BSA) involved. Partial-thickness burns may be confined to the epidermis (superficial epidermal or first-degree burns), extend to the superficial or deeper layers of the dermis (superficial or deep dermal, second-degree burns). Full-thickness (third-degree) burns extend through the dermis into the subcutaneous tissues. Both deep dermal and full-thickness burns require excision and grafting. The Wallace rule of nines may be used to assess the area of burns in order to guide fluid management but is inaccurate in children. Lunn and Browder charts are more accurate and are widely available.

PATHOPHYSIOLOGY

Early death in victims of fire is usually caused by hypoxaemia, resulting either from a reduction in inspired oxygen concentration in a smoke-filled atmosphere or from poisoning by products of combustion, e.g. carbon monoxide, hydrogen cyanide, hydrogen sulphide and ammonia. The affinity of carbon monoxide for haemoglobin is 200-fold greater than that of oxygen, so in the presence of high carboxyhaemoglobin concentrations arterial oxygen content is reduced. The oxygen dissociation curve is also distorted and shifted to the left, resulting in reduced oxygen delivery to the tissues. Inhalation of hot gases causes direct thermal upper airway burns with supraglottic oedema which may lead to airway obstruction within a few hours. Inhalation of smoke particles and toxic products of combustion can cause an inhalational injury comprising mucosal oedema, mucociliary damage, bronchospasm and loss of surfactant with the development of pneumonitis over the next 1–4 days. In addition to the local inflammatory response at the site of the burn, major burns also cause the widespread systemic release of cytokines, notably TNFα interleukin-1 (IL-1) and IL-6. These may mediate the development of the systemic inflammatory response syndrome and contribute to the acute lung injury. Persistently elevated IL-6 concentrations are associated with a poor prognosis. Cardiovascular changes after burn injuries include increased microvascular permeability with extravasation of plasma proteins, reduced plasma oncotic pressure and interstitial oedema. This is most marked at the site of the burn but also occurs throughout the vasculature, leading to marked hypovolaemia within hours. Myocardial contractility and cardiac output decrease independently of the reduction in circulating volume because of circulating depressant factors and diastolic dysfunction. Systemic vascular resistance is increased. If resuscitation is adequate, cardiac output may increase markedly after the first 24 h. Plasma potassium and urea concentrations increase initially because of cell tissue necrosis and haemolysis; muscle breakdown results in rhabdomyolysis. Renal failure may occur early after major burns primarily because of inadequate fluid resuscitation, but haemolysis or rhabdomyolysis may contribute. The sympatho-adrenal response to burns includes enormous increases in plasma concentrations of catecholamines, aldosterone, ACTH, and AVP. These result in marked retention of sodium and water with increased excretion of potassium, calcium and magnesium so that hypokalaemia and anaemia are common after the first 48 h post-burn. There is also a hypercatabolic state with tachycardia, hyperpnoea and hyperpyrexia which may persist for several weeks or months. Muscle breakdown occurs in association with decreased protein synthesis, increased lipolysis and glycogenolysis so that nutritional and calorie requirements are increased markedly. Sepsis frequently develops following severe burns, often leading to widespread metabolic derangement, multiorgan failure and death.

Recovery from burns trauma may be protracted. The anaesthetist must be aware of the probable requirement for multiple administrations of general anaesthesia, frequent use of opioid analgesics in the early stages and the importance of psychological support throughout the patient's stay in hospital.

INITIAL MANAGEMENT

The initial assessment and management of acute burn injuries are similar to those applied to other victims of trauma and are summarized in Table 37.6. The aim of immediate treatment is to secure the airway and administer high-flow humidified oxygen through a non-rebreathing system; tracheal intubation and IPPV with 100% oxygen may be required to maintain an adequate P_aO_2. Fluid resuscitation should be commenced. Intravenous fluids guided by a formal protocol are required if the burn exceeds 10–15% of body surface area. Early warning signs of upper airway

Table 37.6 Initial management of patients with severe burns

1. History – time, extent and mechanism of burn, age and weight of patient, brief medical history
2. Airway assessment
3. Breathing – administer 100% humidified oxygen via a non-rebreathing mask
4. Circulation – establish two large-bore i.v. cannulae and commence fluid resuscitation
5. Assess neurological status
6. Exposure with environmental control
7. Analgesia – i.v. opioids
8. Formally assess burn area and re-evaluate fluid requirements
9. Monitoring – vital signs, urine output
10. Investigations – ABG, COHb, U&E, FBC, clotting screen, cross-match blood, ECG, CXR
11. Secondary survey to exclude other injuries
12. Burns dressings

burns include facial or intraoral burns, singed facial or nasal hair, carbonaceous sputum, hypoxaemia, dyspnoea, cough or wheeze, though these are not universally present in the early stages and airway obstruction may develop later. A history of burns in an enclosed space is highly suggestive. A high index of suspicion for airway burns should be maintained in all cases and prophylactic tracheal intubation is often justified, particularly in children or if interhospital transfer is required. However, the decision to secure the airway by tracheal intubation may be difficult and a senior anaesthetist should be involved. Hoarseness or stridor may indicate impending airway obstruction and tracheal intubation in these cases is mandatory. Pulse oximeters are unreliable in the presence of carboxyhaemoglobin as they cannot distinguish between oxyhaemoglobin and carboxyhaemoglobin and therefore overestimate true oxygen saturation; arterial blood gas analysis is required. Burns are extremely painful and carefully titrated intravenous opioids should be administered. Indications for ICU admission include potential airway problems, burns involving >20% BSA, and the presence of other injuries.

Tissue burns produce rapid fluid shifts and oedema formation, particularly during the first 36 h. The resulting depletion of intravascular volume is greatest in the first few hours and it is essential that a fluid replacement regimen is started as early as possible to avoid hypovolaemic shock and acute renal failure. Crystalloid-based regimens such as the Parkland formula, are used commonly (Table 37.7) although mixed colloid–crystalloid regimens based on that of Muir and Barclay are sometimes used. Many advocate administration of crystalloid solutions only in the first 24 h, with colloids added thereafter. However, the pathophysiology of fluid shifts is complex and these formulae should be used only as a guide to fluid therapy. The type of resuscitation fluid used initially is less important than the early commencement of therapy. Vital signs, urine output and body temperature should be observed closely, and volume replacement titrated to achieve a urine output of 0.5–1.0 mL kg^{-1} h^{-1} (1.0–1.5 mL kg^{-1} h^{-1} in children). In some patients CVP monitoring may be necessary. Haematocrit, base deficit and serum lactate and urea and electrolyte concentrations should be monitored.

ANAESTHETIC PROBLEMS

Airway

Securing the airway in a patient with head and neck burns is vital but may be extremely challenging.

Table 37.7   Fluid regimens for burned patients
1. Estimate/measure weight
2. Estimate percentage area of burn using 'rule of nines' for adults and 'rule of tens' for children
3. Proceed with regimen if > 15% burns in adults or > 10% in children
4. Parkland formula: Requirements in first 24 h (mL) = body weight × % burn × 4 Fluids given as Ringer's lactate alone, 50% within first 8 h, 50% between 8 and 24 h Colloids administered only after first 24 h
5. Muir & Barclay formula: Requirements in each time period (mL) = body weight (kg) × % burns × 0.5 Fluids (human albumin solution 4.5%) according to formula in *each* of the following periods: 0–4 h 4–8 h 8–12 h 12–18 h 18–24 h 24–36 h In addition, water as 5% dextrose is required at 1–2 mL kg^{-1}h^{-1}.

N.B. These formulae should only be used as a guide to fluid requirements and individual prescriptions should be adjusted according to response.

In the initial stages, airway obstruction may occur. Many anaesthetists would use an inhalational induction in the conscious patient, although raw, painful tissues may render proper application of a face mask difficult. Awake fibre-optic intubation may be preferable in adults. A rapid-sequence induction using succinylcholine may be inadvisable (see below). In all cases, facilities and expertise for emergency cricothyroidotomy or tracheostomy should be available, although elective tracheostomy is generally undesirable because of the risk of subsequent pulmonary sepsis and local infection in damaged skin. Later, as soft tissues fibrose and distort, the range of movement in the neck and temporomandibular joints may become grossly restricted and render laryngoscopic intubation impossible.

It may be difficult to secure the tracheal tube in patients with facial burns. Several ingenious methods have been devised, such as suspension of the anaesthetic breathing system from the ceiling, the use of umbilical tape to tie the tube in place and wiring the tube to the upper teeth. Tracheal intubation is often necessary for several days until airway oedema subsides. In this situation, or after prolonged surgery, the pharynx should be examined closely before tracheal extubation, as laryngopharyngeal oedema may cause respiratory obstruction when the tracheal tube is removed.

Ventilation

Mechanical ventilation should be used in the severely burned patient and careful monitoring of ventilation is required. Humidification of inspired gas, physiotherapy and bronchial toilet are mandatory; bronchodilators and PEEP may be necessary. Acute lung injury developing over the first 4 days after burns causes alveolar oedema and hypoxaemia. This may be exacerbated by the administration of large volumes of fluid during resuscitation, but fluid restriction is associated with a worse outcome. Newer techniques include bronchial lavage, nebulized heparin and acetyl cysteine. The hypermetabolic state in large burns results in large increases in oxygen consumption and carbon dioxide production; i.v. nutrition increases the latter. The principles of artificial ventilation in burns patients are identical to those in acute lung injury from other causes and may involve the delivery of low tidal volumes, minimal airway pressures and permissive hypercapnia, so that a sophisticated ventilator may be required for patients undergoing relatively simple surgical procedures.

Fluid balance

Enteral feeding is established as soon as possible. The modern practice of early tissue excision is accompanied by extensive and rapid blood loss, and it is essential to establish adequate venous access with facilities for warming infused fluids; cross-matched blood must be available before surgery. Surgeons frequently use adrenaline during burn debridement to minimize blood loss and the anaesthetist should take measures to counteract any cardiovascular effects. Blood loss is particularly difficult to monitor during burns surgery, and should be measured as accurately as possible. Vascular access may be difficult and it is often necessary to utilize veins in less conventional sites that have escaped injury (e.g. axilla or scalp).

MONITORING

Cutaneous burns may make conventional monitoring (e.g. ECG electrode or blood pressure cuff placement)

difficult. Invasive arterial pressure monitoring is indicated during early-phase surgery where there is potential for rapid blood loss. Urine output and body temperature should be monitored. Central venous catheterization may be required in the presence of extensive burns, although catheter-related sepsis is a hazard.

PATIENT POSITIONING

Burns surgery may require the patient to be positioned in unusual postures (e.g. prone or lateral), and the anaesthetist should be prepared because changes of position may be required during a procedure.

TEMPERATURE LOSS

Heat loss is increased from a burned area by evaporation and inability of cutaneous vessels to constrict and prevent radiation. The anaesthetist should minimize heat loss during anaesthesia and surgery by use of a warming blanket, foil blanket, blood warmer, gas humidifier and an ambient theatre-temperature and humidity of 27°C and 50%, respectively.

ANAESTHETIC DRUGS

Personal preference and the problems of repeated administration of anaesthesia govern the choice of anaesthetic agent. An inhaled nitrous oxide/oxygen mixture (Entonox) and i.v. ketamine are useful for analgesia during burns dressings. However, it is not safe to assume that the airway is preserved during ketamine anaesthesia and antisialagogue premedication is useful to diminish salivation. Diazepam may control the emergence hallucinations suffered by some patients who receive ketamine. Intravenous opioids (by infusion, boluses or patient-controlled analgesia) are effective alternatives. Supplementary analgesics are required in the short and long term, e.g. acetaminophen, non-steroidal anti-inflammatory drugs. Adjunctive therapies include clonidine, tricyclic antidepressants, topical and systemic local anaesthetics or transcutaneous electrical nerve stimulation. For surgical procedures, a balanced technique using a volatile agent and opioid is indicated. The disposition and action of many drugs are affected following burns, e.g. there is marked resistance to the effects of nondepolarizing muscle relaxants from 1 week after major burns.

Succinylcholine should be not be administered from 24 to 48 h after the burn. In the presence of muscle damage, it may cause acute hyperkalaemia in concentrations sufficient to cause cardiac arrest. The mechanism involves upregulation of cholinergic receptors with the proliferation of immature receptor isoforms and extrajunctional receptors. The most dangerous period in this regard is probably between 4 days and 10 weeks after thermal injury.

FURTHER READING

Kaplan JA, Lake CL, Murray MJ 2004 Vascular anesthesia, 2nd edn. Elsevier, New York

MacLennan A, Heimbach D M, Cullen B F 1998 Anesthesia for major thermal injury. Anesthesiology 89: 749–770

Stoelting R K, Dierdorf S F 2002 Anesthesia and co-existing disease, 4th edn. Churchill Livingstone, New York

Wildsmith A J, Bannister J (eds) 1999 Anaesthesia for major vascular surgery. Arnold, London

38 Neurosurgical anaesthesia

Neurosurgical procedures include elective and emergency surgery of the central nervous system, its vasculature and the cerebrospinal fluid (CSF), together with the surrounding bony structures, the skull and spine. Almost all require general anaesthesia. Apart from a conventional anaesthetic technique which pays meticulous attention to detail, the essential factors are the maintenance of cerebral perfusion pressure and the facilitation of surgical access by minimizing blood loss and preventing increases in central nervous tissue volume and oedema.

APPLIED ANATOMY AND PHYSIOLOGY

ANATOMY

Brain

The brain comprises the brainstem, the cerebellum, the midbrain and the paired cerebral hemispheres. The brainstem is formed from the medulla and the pons with the medulla connected to the spinal cord below and with the cerebellum posteriorly. The medulla contains the ascending and descending nerve tracts, the lower cranial nerve nuclei and the respiratory and vasomotor (or vital) centres. Running through the brainstem is the reticular system which is associated with consciousness. A lesion or compression of the brainstem secondary to raised intracranial pressure produces abnormal function of the vital centres that is rapidly fatal (coning). The cerebellum coordinates balance, posture and muscular tone. The midbrain connects the brainstem and cerebellum to the hypothalamus, the thalamus and the cerebral hemispheres. The cerebrum consists of the diencephalon containing the thalamus, hypothalamus and the two cerebral hemispheres. The thalamus contains the nuclei of the main sensory pathways. The hypothalamus coordinates the autonomic nervous system and the endocrine systems of the body. Below the hypothalamus is the pituitary gland. Pituitary tumours may produce the signs of a space-occupying lesion, restrict the visual fields by compressing the optic chiasma or give rise to an endocrine disturbance. The cerebral hemispheres comprise the cerebral cortex, the basal ganglia and the lateral ventricles. A central sulcus or cleft separates the main motor gyrus (or fold) anteriorly from the main sensory gyrus posteriorly. Each hemisphere is divided into four areas or lobes. The function of the different lobes is incompletely understood. However, the frontal lobe contains the motor cortex and areas concerned with intellect and behaviour. The parietal lobe contains the sensory cortex, the temporal lobe is concerned with auditory sensation and the integration of other stimuli, and the occipital lobe contains the visual cortex. Lesions of the cerebral hemispheres give rise to sensory and motor deficits on the opposite side of the body.

Spinal cord

The spinal cord is 45 cm long and passes from the foramen magnum, where it is continuous with the medulla, to a tapered end termed the conus medullaris at the level of the first or second lumbar vertebrae. At each spinal level, paired anterior (motor) and posterior (sensory) spinal roots emerge on each side of the cord. Each posterior root has a ganglion containing the cell bodies of the sensory nerves. The roots join at each intervertebral foramen to form a mixed spinal nerve.

Cerebrospinal fluid

Cerebrospinal fluid (CSF) fills the cerebral ventricles and the subarachnoid space around the brain and the spinal cord. The CSF acts as a buffer, separating the brain and spinal cord from the hard bony projections inside the skull and the vertebral canal. It is produced by the choroid plexus in the lateral, third and fourth ventricles by a combination of filtration and secretion

(Fig. 38.1). The total volume of CSF is 150–200 mL. CSF passes back into the venous blood through arachnoid villi. Blockages which obstruct the normal flow of CSF through the ventricular system or prevent its reabsorption lead to a build-up in CSF pressure, dilatation of the ventricles and hydrocephalus.

Meninges

Three meninges or membranes surround the brain and the spinal cord. These are the dura mater, the arachnoid mater and the pia mater. Around the brain, the dura mater is a thick, strong, double membrane which separates into its two layers in parts to form the cerebral venous sinuses. The outer or endosteal layer is strongly adherent to the skull bones and is the equivalent of the periosteum. The inner layer is continuous with the dura which surrounds the spinal cord. The major artery supplying the dura mater is the middle meningeal artery, which may be damaged in a head injury and skull fracture, leading to the formation of an extradural haematoma. The arachnoid mater is a thin membrane normally adjacent to the dura mater. Cortical veins from the surface of the brain pass through the arachnoid mater to reach dural venous sinuses and may be damaged by relatively minor trauma, leading to the formation of a subdural haematoma. The pia mater is a vascular membrane closely adherent to the surface of the brain and follows the contours of the gyri and sulci. The space between the pia and arachnoid maters is the subarachnoid space and contains CSF.

The dura mater forms a sac which ends below the cord, usually at the level of the second sacral segment. The dura extends along each nerve root and is continuous with the epineurium of each spinal nerve. There is an extensive subarachnoid space between the arachnoid mater and the pia mater. The space between the dura and the bony part of the spinal canal (the extradural or epidural space) is filled with fat, lymphatics, arteries and an extensive venous plexus.

Vascular supply

The arterial blood supply to the brain is derived from the two internal carotid arteries and the two vertebral arteries. The vertebral arteries are branches of the subclavian arteries and pass through foramina in the transverse processes of the upper six cervical vertebrae. They join together anterior to the brainstem to form the single basilar artery, which then divides again to form the two posterior cerebral arteries. These vessels and the two internal carotid arteries form an anastomotic system known as the circle of Willis at the base of the brain. The main arteries supplying the cerebral hemispheres are the anterior, middle and posterior

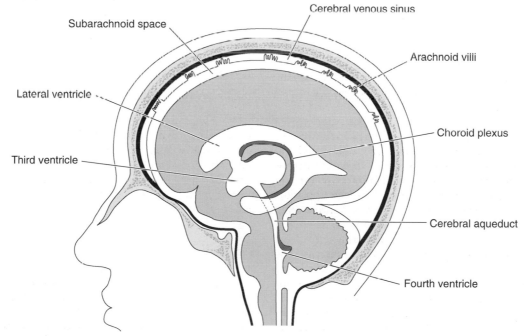

Fig. 38.1
The ventricular system and subarachnoid space.

cerebral artery for each hemisphere. The majority of cerebral aneurysms are of vessels that are part of, or very close to, the circle of Willis. Other important vessels supplying the brainstem and the cerebellum branch from the basilar artery. Venous blood drains into the cerebral venous sinuses, whose walls are formed from the dura mater. These sinuses join and empty into the internal jugular veins.

The blood supply to the spinal cord comes from the single anterior spinal artery formed at the foramen magnum from a branch from each of the vertebral arteries, and from the paired posterior spinal arteries derived from the posterior inferior cerebellar arteries. The anterior artery supplies the anterior two-thirds of the cord. There are additional supplies from segmental arteries and also a direct supply from the aorta, usually at the level of the eleventh thoracic intervertebral space. The blood supply to the spinal cord is fragile, and infarction of the cord may result from even minor disruption of the normal arterial supply.

Autonomic nervous system

The autonomic nervous system is classified on anatomical and physiological grounds into the functionally opposing sympathetic and parasympathetic nervous systems. The central areas responsible for coordinating the autonomic nervous system are mostly in the hypothalamus and its surrounding structures, and in the frontal lobes. The sympathetic nervous system cells arise from the lateral horn of the thoracic and first two lumbar segments of the spinal cord. The neurones of the parasympathetic nervous system exit the central nervous system with the third, seventh, ninth and tenth cranial nerves and from the second to the fourth sacral segments of the spinal cord.

INTRACRANIAL PRESSURE

With normal cerebral compliance, the intracranial pressure (ICP) is 7–15 cmH_2O (5–11 mmHg) in the horizontal position. When moving to the erect position, the ICP decreases initially, but then, because of a decrease in reabsorption, the pressure returns to normal. ICP is related directly to intrathoracic pressure and has a normal respiratory swing. It is increased by coughing, straining and positive end-expiratory pressure. In cases of reduced cerebral compliance, small changes in cerebral volume produce large changes in ICP and such critical changes may be induced by drugs used during anaesthesia (e.g. halothane, isoflurane and vasodilators), elevations in P_aCO_2 and posture, as well as by surgery and trauma (Fig. 38.2).

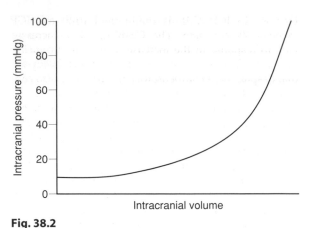

Fig. 38.2
The intracranial pressure/volume relationship.

CEREBRAL BLOOD FLOW

Under normal conditions, the brain receives about 15% of the cardiac output, which corresponds to a cerebral blood flow (CBF) of 50 mL per 100 g tissue or 600–700 mL min^{-1}. The cerebral circulation is able to maintain a constant blood flow between mean arterial pressures of 60 and 140 mmHg by the process of autoregulation. This is mediated by a primary myogenic response involving local alteration in the diameter of blood vessels in response to changes in transmural pressure. Above and below these limits, or in the traumatized brain, autoregulation is impaired or absent, so that cerebral blood flow is related directly to cerebral perfusion pressure (CPP) (Fig. 38.3). This effect is also seen in association with cerebral hypoxia and hypercapnia, in addition to acute intracranial disease and trauma. As CPP decreases as a result of systemic hypotension or an

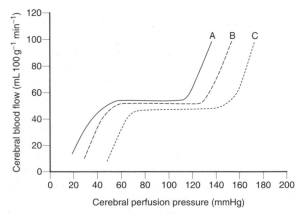

Fig. 38.3
Autoregulation of cerebral blood flow. **(A)** Drug-induced vasodilatation. **(B)** Normal. **(C)** Hypertension or haemorrhagic hypotension.

increase in ICP, CBF is maintained until the ICP exceeds 30–40 mmHg. The Cushing reflex increases CPP in response to the increase in ICP by producing first a reflex systemic hypertension and then bradycardia, despite these compensatory mechanisms also contributing to an increase in ICP. In the treatment of closed head injuries, where both ICP and mean arterial pressure are being monitored, it is essential to maintain the resultant CPP with vasopressor therapy where cerebral perfusion is borderline, because even transient absence of flow to the brain may produce focal or global ischaemia with infarction. Figure 38.3 also demonstrates that haemorrhagic hypotension associated with excess sympathetic nervous activity results in a loss of autoregulation at a higher CPP than normal, while the use of vasodilators to induce hypotension shifts the curve to the left, maintaining flow at lower levels of perfusion pressure. Vasodilators also differ in their effect, so that autoregulation is preserved at a lower CPP with sodium nitroprusside than with autonomic ganglionic blockade (e.g. trimetaphan). Cerebral metabolic rate also affects CBF; the increased electrical activity associated with convulsions produces an increase in lactic acid and other vasodilator metabolites. This, together with an increase in CO_2 production mediated possibly by changes in CSF pH, produces an increase in CBF. Conversely, cerebral metabolic depression, in association with either deliberate or accidental hypothermia or induced by drugs, reduces CBF.

CEREBRAL METABOLISM

The energy consumption of the brain is relatively constant, whether during sleep or in the awake state, and represents approximately 20% of total oxygen consumption at rest, or 50 mL min^{-1}. Cerebral metabolism relies on glucose supplied by the cerebral circulation as there are no stores of metabolic substrate. The brain can tolerate only short periods of hypoperfusion or circulatory arrest before irreversible neuronal damage occurs. The brain also metabolizes amino acids, including glutamate, aspartate and γ-aminobutyric acid (GABA), together with release and subsequent inactivation of neurotransmitters.

The energy production of the brain is related directly to its rate of oxygen consumption, and the cerebral metabolic rate for oxygen (CMRO$_2$) is used to measure this index of cerebral activity. By the Fick principle, CMRO$_2$ is equal to the CBF multiplied by the arteriovenous oxygen difference. Although barbiturates have been used to reduce cerebral metabolic rate, propofol and benzodiazepines have a similar, although less profound, effect. All are used in the sedation of patients with head injury and postoperative

neurosurgical patients, and the choice is related more to the anticipated duration of sedation than to differences in the effects of the drugs, with the exception of prolonged barbiturate coma induced by infusion of thiopental.

EFFECTS OF OXYGEN AND CARBON DIOXIDE ON CEREBRAL BLOOD FLOW

Physiologically, carbon dioxide is the most important cerebral vasodilator. Even small increases in P_aCO_2 produce significant increases in CBF and therefore ICP. There is an almost linear relationship between P_aCO_2 and CBF (Fig. 38.4). Over the normal range, an increase of P_aCO_2 by 1 kPa increases CBF by 30%. Conversely, hyperventilation to produce a P_aCO_2 of 4 kPa produces cerebral vasoconstriction and a decrease in ICP, although this is compensated for by an increase in CSF production over a more prolonged period of hyperventilation, such as that used in the treatment of head injuries. This is why there is no advantage in aggressive hyperventilation regimens in head injury management. Hypocapnia below a P_aCO_2 of 4 kPa has little acute effect on ICP, and hyperventilation beyond this point to lower ICP should be avoided except as a last resort, because the vasoconstriction induced may be associated with a reduction in jugular bulb oxygen saturation, suggesting hypoperfusion and ischaemia. At a P_aCO_2 above 10 kPa, the increase in CBF becomes less marked.

Unlike the acute effects of carbon dioxide, alterations in P_aO_2 have little effect on CBF over the normal range. It is only when P_aO_2 decreases below about 7 kPa that cerebral vasodilatation occurs, and further reductions are associated with dramatic increases in CBF.

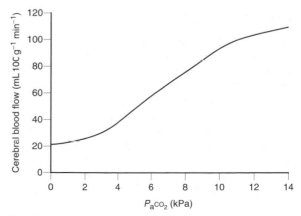

Fig. 38.4
The effect of increasing P_aCO_2 on cerebral blood flow.

GENERAL PRINCIPLES OF ANAESTHESIA FOR INTRACRANIAL SURGERY

Most intracranial operations involve a craniotomy, i.e. removal of a piece or flap of bone to gain access to the meninges and brain substance beneath. A smooth anaesthetic technique is essential, avoiding increases in arterial and venous pressures and changes in carbon dioxide concentration while at the same time avoiding a decrease in cerebral oxygenation.

Most anaesthetists maintain hypnosis with either an inhalational anaesthetic agent, usually sevoflurane, or with a continuous infusion of propofol. Intraoperative analgesia is provided by a short-acting opioid such as fentanyl or remifentanil. Neuromuscular blockade and IPPV are usually used. It is extremely important to ensure adequate fixation of the tracheal tube and intravascular cannulae and to protect the eyes, because access to the head and limbs is severely restricted during the operation. Continuous monitoring of the electrocardiograph and arterial pressure is essential; direct arterial pressure and temperature monitoring are normally used, together with continuous measurement of oxygen saturation, and end-tidal carbon dioxide and inspired anaesthetic agent concentrations. Central venous pressure monitoring is used in some instances. At the end of the procedure, the patient must be transferred to the recovery room with no residual neuromuscular blockade or opioid-induced respiratory depression, as both may produce critical increases in ICP related to hypercapnia and hypoxaemia. Long-acting drugs with a marked sedative action are used cautiously perioperatively so that a pathological failure of return to consciousness is not masked.

INDUCTION OF ANAESTHESIA

An intravenous infusion of an isotonic electrolyte solution should be started through a large-gauge intravenous cannula before induction. Intravenous induction should be used whenever possible. However, inhalational induction in children may be appropriate if the risk of a crying, distressed child is more likely to increase ICP than the vasodilator effects of high inspired concentrations of volatile anaesthetic agents. Both thiopental and propofol reduce ICP and are suitable induction agents. Etomidate may be used for induction in the elderly. The intravenous anaesthetic should be given with an appropriate dose of short-acting opioid and a neuromuscular blocking agent to facilitate a smooth induction and tracheal intubation, avoiding hypoxaemia and hypercapnia. A nerve stimulator should be used to ensure complete muscle paralysis before attempting direct laryngoscopy, to prevent any coughing or straining. It is important to remember that cerebral perfusion may be reduced when the ICP is raised, and an induction technique which produces significant hypotension may critically reduce cerebral perfusion in patients with a space-occupying lesion (SOL) or intracranial and subarachnoid haemorrhage associated with vasospasm.

The most commonly used techniques to reduce the hypertensive response to laryngoscopy and tracheal intubation are supplementary short-acting opioids (fentanyl, alfentanil) or short-acting β-adrenoceptor blockade (e.g. esmolol). If remifentanil is given as a coinduction agent, an infusion is usually started immediately after the induction dose and acts to control the hypertensive response. A reinforced disposable tracheal tube is used. Careful positioning of the tube is vital because any intraoperative flexion of the neck may result in intubation of the right main bronchus if the tip of the tube is initially placed too close to the carina. After the tube has been secured, the neck should be flexed gently while listening for the presence of breath sounds in both axillae. The tube should be secured in place with several layers of sticky tape to prevent it peeling away after application of surgical 'prep' solution to the scalp. Cotton ties should not be used as they may compress the internal jugular veins, increasing venous pressure leading to a reduction in cerebral perfusion pressure, and increased intraoperative haemorrhage. A pharyngeal throat pack is often placed. A pack is essential if transnasal surgery (e.g. trans-sphenoidal hypophysectomy) is planned. Many anaesthetists use a throat pack routinely to help stabilize the tracheal tube in the mouth. A nasogastric tube is placed in patients who are going to be prone for prolonged periods, or if surgery around the brainstem is planned that might lead to postoperative bulbar palsy.

The eyes are protected by covering with paraffin gauze, padding with a folded swab and then covering with a waterproof tape. Skin cleaning ('prep') solutions must be prevented from entering the eyes. Low molecular weight heparin is not used to prevent deep venous thrombosis (DVT), despite the significant risk of DVT in this group of patients. The risks of perioperative haemorrhage tend to outweigh the advantages in the majority of patients. Thromboembolism (TED) stockings are used pre- and postoperatively and the intraoperative use of pneumatic compression leggings is a useful compromise.

POSITIONING

Many neurosurgical operations are long and positioning of the patient to facilitate optimum access, while preventing hypothermia, pressure sores and peripheral nerve injury, is important. Supratentorial cranial surgery involving the frontal or frontotemporal areas is performed with the patient supine, while parietal and occipital craniotomies are carried out in the lateral or three-quarters prone ('park bench') position. In all cases, care must be taken to avoid neck positions which impede venous drainage. The fully prone position is used for surgery in the posterior fossa, around the foramen magnum, and the cervical spine. The patient is supported on chest and iliac crest blocks or a purpose-built frame, both of which allow unimpeded respiratory movements and avoid abdominal compression. The use of 'jelly packs' on top of the support blocks reduces the incidence of pressure damage, which may be serious in the frail and elderly. In the prone position, pressure areas may develop over the facial bones, particularly around the eyes; again, careful padding is vital. The neck should be kept in a neutral position, if possible, to avoid stretching the brachial plexus and if it is necessary to have the arms up, they should not be excessively abducted nor should there be anything pressing into the axillae.

HEAT LOSS

Temperature should be monitored. It is important to prevent heat loss during prolonged surgery. However, there are theoretical benefits of allowing the body to cool intraoperatively (to around 35°C) if cerebral ischaemia is likely (for example during temporary clipping in aneurysm surgery). This can be achieved usually by passive cooling, and it is imperative to re-warm the patient before the end of surgery. Temperature is maintained by warming intravenous fluids and using forced warm air blankets.

MAINTENANCE OF ANAESTHESIA

The basis of anaesthesia for neurosurgery is mild hyperventilation with or without nitrous oxide in oxygen to produce a $P_a CO_2$ of around 4.0 kPa, supplemented with an opioid analgesic (fentanyl boluses, or a remifentanil infusion) and either a volatile anaesthetic agent or a propofol infusion. For elective neurosurgery, the evidence for or against the use of nitrous oxide is mixed. If nitrous oxide is omitted, it is usually replaced by remifentanil, a substitution that has its own problems – remifentanil, unless used carefully, may produce hypotension. When remifentanil is stopped, there may be rebound hypertension and the sudden onset of pain or agitation. For the brain 'at risk' of ischaemia, the evidence against the use of nitrous oxide is more clear. When nitrous oxide is used, care must be taken in very

long operations because of the risk of inducing a vitamin B_{12} deficiency. Sevoflurane is the volatile agent of choice, given that its effects on the cerebral vasculature are much less than those of isoflurane. At clinical concentrations, sevoflurane has no effect on cerebral autoregulation and causes only a minimal increase in ICP. Some anaesthetists use total intravenous anaesthesia with propofol by TCI for neuroanaesthesia. There is no evidence that one technique is associated with an improved outcome compared with any other.

The choice of neuromuscular blocking agent depends usually on personal preference. In most cases, these drugs should be given by infusion. A peripheral nerve stimulator should be used, and the infusion rate titrated to maintain an adequate degree of block (one twitch of the train-of-four stimulus pattern should be present), while preventing overdosage so that the block may be reversed completely shortly (10–15 min) after stopping the infusion and administering an anticholinesterase.

The initial part of a craniotomy is painful, but after the bone flap has been reflected and the dura incised, pain is not a significant feature again until closure of the wound. For this reason, supplementary intraoperative opioids in large doses are unnecessary and the use of a low concentration of hypnotic agent is sufficient to maintain anaesthesia. Use of opioids during maintenance does allow use of less hypnotic agent. Reflex vagal stimulation can occur, particularly following stimulation of the cranial nerve roots or during vascular surgery around the circle of Willis and the internal carotid artery. This may necessitate immediate administration of atropine to avoid severe bradycardia or even asystole.

Maintenance of normal arterial pressure is important in all patients, but may be a particular problem during induction in very sick or elderly patients. Hypotension, with the consequent reduction in cerebral perfusion, should be treated by infusion of a moderate volume of fluid, but it is advisable to administer a vasopressor such as ephedrine at an early stage.

Use of techniques permitting rapid recovery (for example sevoflurane, propofol, remifentanil) are particularly valuable in situations where the patient is required to wake up and move to command intraoperatively, e.g. during spinal surgery or trigeminal nerve radiofrequency lesion generation.

FLUID REPLACEMENT THERAPY

Most patients who present for elective intracranial operations are satisfactorily hydrated preoperatively. The main exceptions are those with a high ICP associated with nausea and vomiting, and patients with general debility and cachexia. The main intraoperative distinctions between patients are related to the underlying pathology. Cerebral tumours are associated with oedema and raised ICP, and therefore such patients may be fluid restricted preoperatively. However, intraoperative hypotension must be avoided and careful fluid administration pre- and intraoperatively is essential. Cerebrovascular surgery is associated with vasospasm and therefore blood flow is the prime prerequisite. A normal circulating blood volume is essential if the perfusion pressure is to be maintained, and although a slight reduction in haematocrit to about 0.30 is optimal for perfusion, adequate fluid replacement must be given.

SUPPLEMENTARY DRUG THERAPY

Patients with a tumour or some other lesions may already be receiving an antiepileptic (usually phenytoin or carbamazepine), and others may require intravenous phenytoin perioperatively, depending on the site of surgery. Patients receiving high-dose steroids need peri- and postoperative dexamethasone; the normal dose is 4 mg 6-hourly with 8–16 mg as an intraoperative bolus. Perioperative antibiotics are administered to all patients; a common choice is cefuroxime 1.5 g, which may need to be repeated during long operations.

MONITORING DURING NEUROSURGICAL ANAESTHESIA

Standard monitoring should be commenced before induction. In patients in whom cardiovascular instability may be a problem, including the very elderly and frail and following subarachnoid haemorrhage, this should include direct arterial pressure monitoring started before induction. Arterial cannulation is now used routinely in all intracranial operations, for surgery of the cervical spine, and in other situations in which rapid fluctuations in arterial pressure may occur. It also facilitates arterial sampling for blood gas analysis. Central venous pressure measurement should be used where major blood loss is expected, such as surgery for vascular tumours and meningiomas, or clipping of cerebral aneurysms, and should be considered for posterior fossa or cervical spine surgery, in which air embolism can occur. Accurate placement of the tip of the catheter in the right atrium is important if aspiration of air is to be attempted. Oxygen saturation and end-tidal carbon dioxide concentration are monitored continuously in all patients. A precordial or oesophageal stethoscope may be used to auscultate cardiac and respiratory sounds and also abnormal flow murmurs produced by air embolism. An oesophageal stethoscope is used more frequently in children.

Cerebral oximetry, transcranial Doppler, electroencephalography and evoked potentials are used in specific situations.

MECHANISMS FOR REDUCING INTRACRANIAL PRESSURE

The methods used commonly to reduce ICP (or to limit increases) are drugs, ventilation, posture and drainage. Diuretics such as mannitol 10% or 20% or furosemide deplete the intravascular fluid volume and subsequently reduce CSF production. A bolus of an intravenous anaesthetic agent such as propofol or thiopental may be used to reduce the cerebral metabolic rate, causing a reduction in cerebral blood flow and therefore cerebral blood volume and ICP. Direct drainage of CSF may be accomplished either by lumbar puncture or by direct puncture of the cisterna magna or lateral ventricles. A move to an increased head-up position reduces venous congestion and ICP, but arterial hypotension must be avoided. Hypercapnia must be prevented by the use of IPPV, while moderate hyperventilation produces cerebral vasoconstriction and a reduction in cerebral blood volume.

ELECTIVE HYPOTENSION

Although elective hypotension was formerly one of the mainstays of cerebrovascular surgery, its use has diminished considerably in recent years, because of the increasing appreciation that cerebral perfusion is all-important. Most aneurysm surgery in now carried out at normotension; indeed, if the patient has an element of cerebral vasospasm, any reflex hypertension should be maintained. Hypotension is now a therapy of last resort if bleeding is torrential and it is otherwise impossible for the surgeon to regain control. If hypotension is required, the choice of technique is determined by the anticipated duration of induced hypotension. The alternatives are a short-acting β-adrenoreceptor blocker such as esmolol, or increasing the depth of anaesthesia with a volatile agent. Direct vasodilators are rarely used because of the risk of steal away from areas of poor perfusion, and the possibility of increasing cerebral blood volume and affecting the ICP. Hypotensive anaesthesia is used more frequently in spinal surgery, although the risks of inducing ischaemia in the cord substance are the same as in the brain. In this situation, evoked potentials may be used to assess cord function during periods of hypotension.

ANAESTHESIA FOR ELECTIVE INTRACRANIAL SURGERY

Operative treatment may range from the removal of either an intracerebral or an extracerebral tumour to the clipping of an arterial aneurysm in the region of the circle of Willis. The preoperative condition of patients who present for craniotomy varies enormously. The level of consciousness ranges from completely awake and orientated to comatose; some patients are confused, disorientated, euphoric or aggressive.

INTRACRANIAL TUMOURS

Gliomas usually grow quickly and the history may be short; meningiomas are slow-growing and the history may be slow and insidious. Unlike gliomas, the volume effect of a meningioma is usually minimal because a reduction in the volume of the other intracranial contents compensates. However, the volume effects may eventually become apparent, especially if there is bleeding into the meningioma.

Patients with an intracranial tumour are usually taking steroids (normally dexamethasone 4 mg every 6–8 h), which may precipitate a latent diabetic state, requiring insulin during the acute episode. Most patients have some symptoms of raised ICP, such as headache, nausea, vomiting or visual disturbances. Anticonvulsant therapy may have been prescribed to patients who have presented with fitting or who are thought to be at risk. Some patients may be frankly dehydrated, and while it is important to avoid aggressive preoperative fluid therapy, as this may elevate ICP further, hypovolaemia must be treated before induction of anaesthesia.

Attempts at total excision of all the macroscopically identifiable glioma tissue is now considered futile for the majority of fast-growing lesions. Large portions of tumours are excised if pressure symptoms are the main presenting feature. For most tumours, the greatest need is for a tissue diagnosis. If lesions are small, deep-seated or near critical areas, a radiologically-guided biopsy is appropriate. Stereotactic biopsy involves a CT scan with a rigid metal frame firmly attached to the skull. Trigonometry is then used to find coordinates, relative to the frame, that describe the exact site of the lesion (to within 1 mm). A biopsy needle is then passed through the brain to sample tissue from this site. The frame is applied after induction of anaesthesia and, because the small shifts in brain volumes cause the lesion to move, the P_aCO_2 should be maintained at a constant level for both the CT scan and the biopsy. Frameless biopsy surgery may now be performed using image-guidance techniques where a scan of the brain (and skull) is compared with topographical features of the head in theatre to guide a biopsy needle.

CEREBROVASCULAR LESIONS

Patients with vascular lesions including intracranial aneurysms and arteriovenous malformations may present acutely. Congenital lesions are seen frequently in young and previously healthy patients. Intracranial aneurysms occur in the older age group and may be associated with other, more widespread cardiovascular disease. Subarachnoid haemorrhage is now graded using the WFNS scale (Table 38.1). Although clipping should prevent the risk of further bleeding, significant perioperative morbidity and mortality result from vasospasm, which may occur pre- or postoperatively. The current trend is to undertake emergency cerebral angiography and clipping of aneurysms in good-grade patients, but to delay surgery in the poor-grade patients until their condition improves. The calcium channel blocker nimodipine is used to reduce or prevent vasospasm. By preference, it is given orally as the hypotensive effects are less.

An alternative method of treating intracranial aneurysms is by interventional radiological 'coiling' (see below). It was used initially for inaccessible posterior circulation aneurysms; it has now become the technique of choice for most aneurysms in some centres. As many of the risks of open aneurysm surgery apply equally in this situation, a full, conventional neurosurgical anaesthetic technique should be used, including direct arterial pressure monitoring. If technical problems or aneurysm rupture occur, immediate

Table 38.1 World Federations of Neurosurgeons (WFNS) grading of subarachnoid haemorrhage

WFNS grade	GCS	Motor deficit
1	15	Absent
2	13–14	Absent
3	13–14	Present
4	7–12	Present or absent
5	3–6	Present or absent

GCS, Glasgow Coma Scale.

transfer to theatre for emergency craniotomy may be necessary.

Patients with intracerebral haemorrhage range from completely lucid to confused, and the preoperative assessment must take this into account. Those in the older age group may be receiving drugs with cardiovascular effects and are also frequently receiving aspirin or warfarin, which may be a contraindication to urgent craniotomy.

As flow is more pressure-dependent in areas with vasospasm, it is necessary to avoid both hypotension and hypertension. Similarly, excessive hypocapnia should be avoided. A normal cerebral perfusion pressure should be maintained. Although fluid replacement therapy may be all that is required, the careful use of a vasoconstrictor such as ephedrine may be necessary in the interval between induction and incision. Nimodipine therapy interacts with inhalational anaesthetic agents to enhance their hypotensive effects. Postoperatively, nimodipine therapy is continued for several days until the risk of vasospasm has passed. Blood entering the CSF either as a result of the initial haemorrhage or during operation is an extreme irritant. Its presence may cause large increases in plasma catecholamine concentrations with corresponding hypertension and vasospasm. Blood which clots in the aqueduct of Sylvius causes obstruction to CSF flow and noncommunicating hydrocephalus, necessitating temporary ventricular drainage or ventriculoperitoneal shunt.

Temporary clipping of feeding vessels (or to prevent anastomotic backflow from tributaries) may be required to allow safe application of the permanent clip to the neck of the aneurysm. Temporary clips may also be required if the aneurysm bursts intraoperatively, to allow the surgeon to stop the haemorrhage. These clips cause temporary ischaemia in the territory supplied by that vessel. Attempts are usually made to reduce the risk of permanent ischaemic damage. Metabolic suppression with intravenous anaesthetic agents and mild hypothermia have been used. There is, however, no evidence that these techniques have any effect on outcome.

ANAESTHESIA FOR INTERVENTIONAL NEURORADIOLOGY

In addition to coiling of intracranial aneurysms, radiologists treat a variety of other lesions including AVMs and carotid-cavernous sinus fistulae. These procedures use several techniques including detachable coils and glue placed within vessels to interrupt blood supply. The blood vessels supplying some tumours, such as meningiomas, may also be occluded before surgical excision. Most of these procedures are not painful, although headaches may occur. However, to allow precise localization of the lesion and accurate placement of the intravascular catheters, the patients have to lie very still, sometimes for several hours. General anaesthesia is usually necessary and the same precautions about changes in arterial pressure and ICP apply as for intracranial vascular surgery. Arterial cannulation is performed, both to monitor arterial pressure and to enable blood sampling for coagulation studies. Heparin is used during the procedure. If thrombus starts to form in the feeding vessels, antiplatelet treatment is started. Aneurysm rupture necessitates immediate craniotomy, clot evacuation and open clipping of the aneurysm neck. It is important not to underestimate the need for a full neuroanaesthetic technique, simply because a craniotomy is not being performed.

PITUITARY SURGERY (HYPOPHYSECTOMY)

The pituitary fossa is approached either through a frontotemporal craniotomy for large suprasellar tumours, or through the nose or ethmoid sinus for smaller lesions. The importance of pituitary surgery lies in the endocrine abnormalities such as acromegaly, which may be caused by an adenoma, or those which result from surgical hypophysectomy, such as diabetes insipidus. Glucocorticoid replacement is required in the immediate perioperative period; mineralocorticoid requirements increase only slowly over the subsequent days. Diabetes insipidus may present in the immediate postoperative period and requires stabilization with vasopressin until the degree of the imbalance is known.

Acromegalic patients who present for pituitary surgery may pose considerable difficulties in tracheal intubation and venous access. If the transoral, nasal or ethmoidal approaches are used for surgery, a pharyngeal pack must be inserted and the airway protected to prevent aspiration of blood and CSF.

CSF SHUNT INSERTION AND REVISION

The majority of patients who present for insertion or revision of a ventriculoperitoneal shunt are children with congenital hydrocephalus, often resulting from spina bifida or from intraventricular haemorrhage after premature birth. Older patients may require a permanent shunt after intracranial haemorrhage or head injury. The major anaesthetic considerations lie in the presentation of a patient with severely raised ICP who may be drowsy, nauseated and vomiting, with resultant dehydration. Compensatory systemic hypertension to maintain cerebral perfusion may also be present. Rapid-sequence induction may be indicated to avoid aspiration; the increase in ICP caused by succinylcholine is of secondary importance. Artificial ventilation to control P_aCO_2 is essential to prevent further increases in ICP, and volatile anaesthetic agents should be used with care for the same reason. When the ventricle is first drained, a rapid decrease in CSF pressure may result in an equally rapid reduction in arterial pressure, which no longer needs to be elevated to maintain cerebral perfusion. Adequate venous access is important to allow rapid resuscitation in response to this severe but temporary hypotension. Shunt surgery may be painful, particularly at the site of insertion into the peritoneum or from the tunnelling of the catheter under the skin. Use of long-acting opioids has to be balanced against the need to have the patient achieve at least the preoperative level of consciousness.

An endoscopic technique may be used to create a new passage for the flow of CSF. The sudden changes in ICP from the use of irrigating fluid and the passage of the neuroendoscope near to vital structures may result in dramatic changes in heart rate and arterial pressure.

FUNCTIONAL SURGERY

Surgery for Parkinson's disease and epilepsy is performed in an awake patient. The initial exposure may be made under general anaesthesia, but the mapping of the brain, and the surgery itself (e.g. inducing a lesion in the basal ganglia), are performed awake under local anaesthesia only. Surgery to remove slow-growing or benign tumours from the 'eloquent' areas near the main motor and sensory gyri may also be performed this way, to guide the surgeon and help avoid damage to these areas.

TREATMENT OF TRIGEMINAL NEURALGIA

This extremely debilitating condition is usually treated medically with large doses of antiepileptic drugs. However, surgical lesions of the trigeminal ganglion are performed when the side-effects of medical treatment become unacceptable. Lesions of the ganglion are induced by radiofrequency ablation or injection of either phenol or alcohol. All these techniques are very painful and require general anaesthesia. The patient is anaesthetized while the ganglion is identified radiologically, awakened to allow identification of correct placement of the needle, and then re-anaesthetized for generation of the lesion or neurolytic injection. If the

CSF is entered during localization of the ganglion, nausea frequently occurs and vomiting with the patient in the supine position should be anticipated. Some cases of trigeminal neuralgia are caused by an abnormal vascular loop compressing the trigeminal nerve in the posterior cranial fossa. A small craniotomy and decompression of the nerve is then extremely successful in curing the symptoms; the problems of anaesthesia and surgery in this area are highlighted below.

POSTERIOR FOSSA CRANIOTOMY

Surgery in the posterior cranial fossa involves lesions of the cerebellum and fourth ventricle. In addition, the prone position facilitates operations on the foramen magnum and upper cervical spine. Bone is usually removed as a craniectomy in the posterior fossa rather than by raising a bone flap.

In the past, some surgeons favoured the sitting position because this produced superb venous drainage, relative hypotension and excellent operating conditions. The patients were frequently allowed to breathe a volatile anaesthetic agent (usually trichloroethylene) spontaneously so that changes in their respiratory pattern could be used to monitor the progress of fourth ventricular surgery in the region of the respiratory centre. This posed several major anaesthetic problems. Patients in the sitting position are prone to hypotension, which results inevitably in poor cerebral perfusion. Air embolism is also a severe potential problem because when the skull is opened many of the veins within the bone are held open and, if the venous pressure at this point is subatmospheric, air may enter the veins, leading to systemic air embolism. For these reasons, the sitting position is no longer used other than in exceptional circumstances and posterior fossa surgery is carried out in the 'park bench' position; operations on the cervical spine are performed with the patient prone and supported on blocks. Although this change has diminished the risks of cerebral hypoperfusion and consequent hypoxia, air embolism is still a potential problem. The operative site, particularly with a moderate head-up tilt, is still above the level of the heart and the veins are still held open by the surrounding structures.

Detection and treatment of air embolism

The mainstay of detection is vigilance and a high index of suspicion. The main period of risk during surgery in the prone position is when the posterior cervical muscles are cut and the craniectomy is being performed. Air embolism may occur in the supine position as the patient is often placed slightly head-up to encourage venous drainage. Surgery near the dural venous sinuses may result in a sinus being opened. This may lead to torrential bleeding, but if the head is raised it may alternatively lead to air entrainment as the walls of the sinuses, formed by the dura, are held apart. The severity of the effects of air embolism depend upon the volume of air entrained, and the time course of the accumulation of the air in the central circulation.

The main practical method of detection is by end-tidal carbon dioxide monitoring, because the 'airlock' produced in the pulmonary circulation results in a rapid reduction in CO_2 excretion (usually together with a reduction in oxygen saturation). Arterial pressure decreases and cardiac arrhythmias are frequently seen. The use of an oesophageal stethoscope permits auscultation of the classic 'mill-wheel' murmur with large quantities of air, but requires continuous listening. Doppler ultrasonography is probably the most accurate method of early detection before the embolus leaves the heart, but frequently suffers from interference. Unfortunately, there are many false positives with more sensitive techniques such as Doppler ultrasonography. In practice, provided that the sitting position is not used, large air emboli are uncommon. Treatment consists of preventing further entry of air by telling the surgeon, who immediately floods the operative field with saline, lowering the level of the head and increasing the venous pressure by jugular compression. Nitrous oxide, if used, should be stopped. Ideally, the air should be trapped in the right atrium by placing the patient in the left lateral position; it is then occasionally possible to aspirate air through a central venous catheter, which is commonly inserted for posterior fossa explorations. Vasopressors are sometimes required until the circulation is restored; occasionally, full cardiopulmonary resuscitation is necessary.

RECOVERY FROM ANAESTHESIA FOR ELECTIVE SURGERY AND POSTOPERATIVE ANALGESIA

The majority of patients are allowed to wake up as usual at the end of operation, preferably in a dedicated neurosurgical recovery room. Cerebral compliance following surgical intervention is often critical, particularly following removal of a space-occupying lesion or traumatic haematoma, and it is essential to avoid hypercapnia or hypoxaemia, both of which may increase ICP. The Glasgow Coma Scale (Table 38.2) or an equivalent for children is recorded. Patients should return rapidly to at least their preoperative level of consciousness. A failure to achieve this, or a deterioration after an initial awakening, should alert carers to possible ischaemia or raised ICP. Re-imaging or immediate wound exploration is then required. Seizures after elective intracranial neurosurgery are surprisingly rare and, if they occur, should be treated immediately and the cause identified.

Complete reversal of nondepolarizing neuromuscular blockade must be achieved and judicious use of intraoperative opioids should remove the need for administration of naloxone. Nonopioid analgesics may be used, but nonsteroidal anti-inflammatories are avoided because of the risk of inhibiting platelet function and precipitating a postoperative intracranial bleed. Temperature should be returned to normal by passive or active techniques. Ideally, all patients who have undergone intracranial surgery should be cared for in a high-dependency unit environment. After prolonged major procedures or when severe oedema is likely, elective postoperative sedation and lung ventilation may be necessary.

Table 38.2   The Glasgow Coma Scale

Clinical sign	Response	Score
Eyes open	Spontaneously	4
	To verbal command	3
	To pain	2
	No response	1
Best motor response to verbal command or to painful stimulus	Obeys	6
	Localizes pain	5
	Flexion withdrawal	4
	Abnormal flexion (decorticate rigidity)	3
	Extension (decerebrate rigidity)	2
	No response	1
Best verbal response	Orientated, converses	5
	Disorientated, converses	4
	Inappropriate words	3
	Incomprehensible sounds	2
	No response	1
	Total (minimum 3, maximum 15)	

ANAESTHESIA FOR EMERGENCY INTRACRANIAL SURGERY

The main indication for emergency intracranial surgery is bleeding as a result of trauma, which may be exacerbated in patients treated with anticoagulant drugs, including aspirin and clopidogrel. Intracranial haematomata may arise either epidurally (extradurally), subdurally or intracerebrally and may accumulate either rapidly or slowly. Patients receiving warfarin may develop a subdural haematoma after a very minor head injury. Many patients who present for anaesthesia and surgery are unconscious or semiconscious and irritable as a result of raised ICP and cerebral compression. Virtually all patients with head injury have had an emergency CT scan as part of their initial management. Many have undergone tracheal intubation and ventilation of the lungs for this procedure and are subsequently kept anaesthetized and taken straight to the operating theatre for surgery to decompress the brain. It is important to remember that with an expanding intracranial haematoma speed is of the essence if cerebral damage is to be minimized or avoided. While adequate anaesthetic time must be taken to ensure safety, excessive delays may seriously affect the overall result of decompression and make the difference between a good and merely a moderate recovery.

The anaesthetic maintenance technique is similar to that used for elective intracranial surgery, consisting of careful use of a hypnotic, a short-acting intravenous opioid, neuromuscular blockade and IPPV to a P_aCO_2 of 4 kPa. Tracheal intubation in patients at risk of regurgitation and aspiration of stomach contents should be facilitated with succinylcholine. If the patient is unconscious, the initial anaesthetic requirements may be small. Most acute haematomas are evacuated through a full craniotomy, because, if necessary, the bone flap may be left out or allowed to 'float' free, providing a method of decompression in the case of severe oedema. Chronic subdural collections may be evacuated via burr holes. These are usually performed under general anaesthesia, but may be undertaken with local anaesthesia alone in very frail, elderly patients. Many chronic subdural haematomas recur and underlying brain substance injury is not uncommon. As the patient's brain is decompressed, the level of consciousness may lighten considerably and it may be necessary to deepen anaesthesia to prevent the patient becoming aware. It is important to avoid long-acting opioid analgesics because these may mask the eye signs and the level of consciousness, which are used to follow the progress of cerebral trauma post-operatively.

MANAGEMENT OF THE HEAD-INJURED PATIENT

Head-injured patients, their subsequent treatment and rehabilitation represent a considerable proportion of neurosurgical practice. The immediate management requires meticulous attention to the prevention of any secondary brain injury from ischaemia; little can be done about the primary insult to the brain or spinal cord. In recent years, the awareness of both the medical profession and the general public has had a profound effect on general resuscitation simply by improving airway management in the unconscious patient. The resuscitation and immediate care of all head-injured patients uses the same A-B-C principles taught on ATLS and ALS courses for care of all trauma victims and other seriously ill patients. Particular points to note for head injury care are as follows:

1. *Initial airway maintenance*, remembering that patients with craniofacial injuries often have associated damage to the cervical spine. Tracheal intubation is usually necessary, must be accomplished without excessive neck manipulation and should be performed by an experienced person. It is important to make intubation as atraumatic as possible; consequently, sedation and neuromuscular blockade should be used irrespective of the level of consciousness, except in the most severe situation. The benefits of succinylcholine often outweigh the potential risks. Nasotracheal intubation is contraindicated.
2. *Maintenance of adequate ventilation* with oxygen-enriched air. Avoidance of hypoxaemia and hypercapnia is essential.
3. *Maintenance of an adequate circulating volume and arterial pressure*. Hypotension after head injury greatly worsens outcome. Other injuries which may affect the circulatory state must be identified while resuscitation is being performed.
4. *Sedation and analgesia, and neuromuscular blockade*, are usually continued to allow management of other injuries, CT scanning and possible inter-hospital transfer
5. *Detailed assessment of thoracic, abdominal and limb injuries* and appropriate therapy to stabilize the patient's cardiovascular and respiratory systems before transfer to the CT scanner and X-ray room. Other life-threatening injuries must be dealt with

to prevent secondary brain injury caused by hypoxia or hypotension.

6. *Invasive arterial pressure monitoring*, together with ECG, end-tidal CO_2 and pulse oximetry. All of these are important in the early detection of deterioration in ICP, cardiovascular stability or respiratory function. A contused, oedematous and noncompliant brain tolerates only minimal changes in oxygen supply or carbon dioxide tension before ICP increases still further.

7. *After the CT scan*, many patients are transferred directly to the neurosurgical operating theatre for evacuation of haematoma or insertion of an intraventricular catheter or pressure transducer. Some patients who are scanned in peripheral hospitals have their scans relayed to the main neurosurgical centre. The patient is then transferred directly by ambulance to the neurosurgical operating theatre, but both cardiovascular and neurological stability must be achieved before the journey. Realistically, this involves the transfer of a sedated, intubated and ventilated patient, pretreated with mannitol to minimize acute increases in ICP.

INTENSIVE CARE OF HEAD-INJURED PATIENTS

The main benefits of intensive care are in the provision of optimal conditions to allow recovery from the primary cerebral injury while minimizing any secondary damage. In practice this means:

Sedation. This is usually achieved with an infusion of either propofol or midazolam together with an opioid (usually morphine or alfentanil). Thiopental may be beneficial in cases of severely compromised cerebral blood flow and metabolism.

Ventilation. It is particularly important in patients suffering from multiple trauma, especially with the combination of head and chest injuries, to ensure optimal oxygenation in the face of pulmonary contusion. This is normally achieved by the use of IPPV and may involve the use of positive end-expiratory pressure, the effects of which on the noncompliant brain are probably not as severe as in the normal situation, whereas the damage caused by hypoxaemia could be fatal. There is evidence to suggest that marked hyperventilation worsens outcome, and the main benefits of mechanical ventilation are the prevention of hypercapnia and the provision of adequate cerebral oxygenation.

Detailed neurological assessment. This centres on the Glasgow Coma Scale, which is based upon eye opening, and verbal and motor responses (see Table 38.2). Each response on the scale is assessed numerically; the lower the number, the more impaired is the response. The numbers are summed to produce a score. The lowest score is 3 and the highest 15. Brain function may also be assessed by use of the electroencephalogram (or a processed EEG monitor such as the cerebral function analyzing monitor [CFAM]), transcranial Doppler, near-infrared spectroscopy and other techniques used primarily for research.

ICP monitoring. It is very helpful to be able to monitor the effectiveness of therapy used to manage a raised ICP, and in particular to demonstrate an effective cerebral perfusion pressure. The ICP is monitored using a transducer inserted either extradurally, subdurally or into the brain parenchyma. This may be undertaken in the ICU or in the operating theatre. ICP often increases in response to stimulation, physiotherapy, tracheal suction, etc., but should return to the pre-stimulation value within 5–10 min. Frequent and prolonged increases in ICP demonstrate a low cerebral compliance and the need for further sedation and ventilation. If weaning from mechanical ventilation is started and the ICP increases and remains elevated, the patient should be re-sedated and the lungs ventilated for a further 24-h period. It is beneficial to nurse head-injured patients in a 15° head-up tilt to assist in ICP reduction, provided that coexisting conditions permit.

Adequate fluid therapy and nutrition. Although otherwise healthy patients with an isolated head injury have very low metabolic requirements, many fail to absorb from the gastrointestinal tract because of the effects of sedative and opioid drugs or simply secondary to head trauma; associated hypoxaemia exacerbates the problem. It is sometimes necessary to introduce parenteral nutrition, particularly in patients who are catabolic from coexisting injuries. As in elective patients at risk from elevated ICP caused by cerebral oedema, head-injured patients are also at risk from excessive intravenous fluid therapy, particularly if hypotonic solutions are used. Fluid restriction may be appropriate, and if large amounts of fluid have been given during initial resuscitation, a gentle drug-induced diuresis with furosemide to create an overall negative fluid balance (or at least to prevent a positive balance) may be appropriate. Fluid overload also impairs oxygenation further in potentially hypoxaemic patients with combined head and chest injuries, or following aspiration at the time of head injury. The use of mannitol 20% tends to be reserved for the emergency treatment of raised ICP rather than the treatment of simple fluid overload.

High-dependency nursing care. Provision of appropriate care for the unconscious patient, even when breathing spontaneously, is difficult, and demands a high intensity of nursing care. Intensive or high-dependency care centralizes nursing, medical and monitoring resources to provide optimal care of the head-injured patient.

ANAESTHESIA FOR CT AND MRI SCANNING

This is discussed in detail in Chapter 34.

SURGERY OF THE SPINE AND SPINAL CORD

Many neurosurgical procedures involve surgery around or on the spinal cord, usually either for the decompression of nerves as a result of a prolapsed intervertebral disc or degenerative arthritis, or for the decompression of the cord when the spinal canal is occupied by tumour (see also Ch. 30).

ANAESTHESIA FOR CERVICAL SPINE SURGERY

The cervical spine may be approached from either the anterior or the posterior route, depending largely upon the site of cord compression. Although the posterior approach is less likely to damage vital structures, the patient must lie prone, and hypotension, blood loss and access, particularly in a large individual, may cause problems.

Preoperative assessment is perhaps one of the most important factors in neurosurgical anaesthetic practice, because an unstable cervical spine is a major reason for the proposed surgery. In many patients, the neck may be relatively unstable and the patient may be in a cervical collar or even neck traction. Bony degeneration from rheumatoid or osteoarthritis produces severe cord compression. However, with regard to tracheal intubation, the neck tends to be unstable in flexion and relatively stable in extension in most patients. It is essential to assess the range of neck movement fully with the collar removed, either in the ward or in the anaesthetic room, in addition to the

assessment of the ease of tracheal intubation. It is doubly unlucky to have a difficult intubation in a patient with an unstable neck! If problems are anticipated, the normal 'difficult intubation' drill should be followed, using the methods with which the anaesthetist is most familiar. Severe ankylosing spondylitis involving the neck probably presents the most awkward problem related to the rigid immobility of the cervical spine. Additional factors which apply particularly in rheumatoid patients include anaemia, steroid therapy, fragile skin, and renal and pulmonary problems (see Ch. 23).

Anterior cervical decompression

This technique involves exposing the anterior aspect of the cervical vertebral bodies and their interposing discs through a collar incision, removing the intervertebral disc and drilling out a cylinder of bone down to the posterior longitudinal ligament, or mechanically distracting the disc space. The cord is decompressed microscopically through this hole, which is then filled with a bone graft taken from the iliac crest to produce a fusion. Single or multiple levels are involved, but the neck may be quite rigid for future intubation if several adjacent fusions are carried out.

Apart from the potential problems of tracheal intubation, anaesthesia is relatively straightforward, although pneumothorax is a potential problem with operations at the C7–T1 level. Retraction of the oesophagus and, more particularly, the carotid sheath and sinus may produce severe temporary cardiovascular disturbance (usually sinus bradycardia). Postoperative haemorrhage may lead to acute airway obstruction.

Posterior cervical laminectomy

Patients are usually placed prone, with the neck flexed, and in a slightly head-up posture to reduce haemorrhage. Bleeding from the nuchal muscles is often a problem and air embolism remains a potential risk. The main difficulties, as in all spinal surgery in the prone position, arise from epidural venous bleeding, and the changes in intrathoracic pressure from IPPV can have a significant effect. In addition, prolonged cord compression can result in an autonomic neuropathy which may produce significant hypotension both at induction and when the patient is turned into the prone position. Cervical laminectomy may be accompanied by posterior fusion with either bone or metal, which results in immediate postoperative stability.

ANAESTHESIA FOR THORACOLUMBAR DECOMPRESSIVE SURGERY

In most instances, patients are placed in the prone position, either supported on chest and iliac crest blocks or in the 'jack-knife' position. As the spine is an extremely vascular area, hypotensive anaesthesia is used occasionally to decrease bleeding, and particularly the venous ooze in the operative field. This is also reduced considerably if it is possible to place the operative site above the level of the heart – another advantage of the patient lying prone. Lumbar microdiscectomy for sciatica and one-level laminectomy are usually quite minor. However, multiple-level laminectomies, surgery to correct spinal deformities such as scoliosis and surgery to stabilize vertebrae destroyed by metastatic tumours are often associated with torrential bleeding and the need for massive blood transfusion. Thoracic discs and tumours such as neurofibromata are approached occasionally by the transthoracic route, involving thoracotomy and a combined approach with the patient in the lateral position. Bronchial intubation and one-lung anaesthesia may be needed to facilitate access in this situation.

Spinal cord monitoring using somatosensory- or motor-evoked potentials allows identification of spinal cord ischaemia during surgery. These potentials are affected by many anaesthetic agents, particularly the volatile anaesthetic agents, and a TIVA-based technique is preferred.

POSTOPERATIVE CARE

Although many patients who have undergone spinal or intracranial surgery are awake and conscious in the immediate postoperative period, some still require active, intensive treatment. This is important particularly in patients who have raised ICP (or when ICP is liable to rise) and in those who have undergone cerebral aneurysm surgery, when postoperative vasospasm may be a problem. Elective postoperative ventilation to control cerebral oxygenation and to produce a mild decrease in ICP is occasionally used, with continuous monitoring of both arterial and intracranial pressures. If vasospasm is present, specific vasodilator therapy with nimodipine is continued, together with a hyperperfusion regimen as described earlier, to prevent local areas of cerebral ischaemia which may result in hemiplegia. In general, postoperative opioids are avoided following craniotomy or upper cervical spine surgery; simple analgesics and codeine phosphate are most commonly used to provide analgesia. Long-acting opioids may be used with great care, and may be necessary after cessation of a remifentanil infusion.

Surgery of the thoracic and lumbar spine, particularly involving fusion with an autologous bone graft, is associated with significant postoperative pain. Intramuscular opioids, nonsteroidal anti-inflammatory drugs and patient-controlled analgesia have all been used to good effect. Systemic rather than regional analgesia is preferable because the graft donor site is often the most painful area. Urinary retention is a frequent problem, and temporary or intermittent catheterization may be required.

FURTHER READING

Matta B F, Menon D K, Turner J M (eds) 2000 Textbook of neuroanaesthesia and critical care. Greenwich Medical Media, London

Van Aken H (ed) 2002 Neuroanaesthetic practice, 2nd edn. BMJ Publishing Group, London

Anaesthesia for thoracic surgery

39

Thoracic anaesthesia offers particular anaesthetic challenges:

- control of the airway during bronchoscopy
- protection of the airway in patients with oesophageal disease, lung abscess, bronchopleural fistula or haemoptysis
- positioning a double-lumen tracheal tube to maintain anaesthesia in the lateral position with the chest opened and one lung collapsed
- postoperative care of a patient after lung tissue resection.

In common with major surgery at other sites, thoracic patients frequently have:

- parenchymal lung disease in addition to their presenting complaint
- a painful wound after surgery
- the potential for substantial haemorrhage
- the need for intravenous fluids after surgery.

Diagnosis, staging and resection of intrathoracic malignant disease occupy a large part of thoracic surgical practice. There is also a need for drainage and obliteration of an expanded pleural space to remove infection, or prevent lung collapse and re-accumulation of air or liquid in the pleural space. Resection of bullous lung disease may improve the respiratory mechanics of the chest where there is parenchymal lung disease elsewhere.

PREOPERATIVE ASSESSMENT

HISTORY AND EXAMINATION

Thoracic patients often exhibit the respiratory symptoms of cough, sputum, haemoptysis, breathlessness, wheeze and chest pain, or oesophageal symptoms of dysphagia, pain and weight loss. Other common chest features include hoarseness, superior vena cava obstruction, pain in the chest wall or arm, Horner's syndrome,

cyanosis and pleural effusion. Lung tumours may cause extrathoracic symptoms by metastatic spread, principally to brain, bone, liver, adrenals and kidneys, or by endocrine effects such as finger clubbing, hypertrophic pulmonary osteoarthropathy, Cushing's syndrome, hypercalcaemia, myopathies (e.g. Eaton–Lambert syndrome), scleroderma, acanthosis and thrombophlebitis.

Anaemia, cardiac disease and lung disease may cause breathlessness. To distinguish between loss of lung tissue and reversible airways disease, the patient's own history of daily activity may reveal diurnal variation in breathlessness and associated symptoms of sputum, stridor and wheeze. Symptoms may conflict with the results of pulmonary function tests which require voluntary effort, if the tests have been performed ineffectively. Wheeze during expiration and stridor during inspiration are likely to result from airway obstruction below and above the thoracic inlet, respectively.

Production of sputum is the most common stimulus to cough, which is therefore almost universal in cigarette smokers. A dry cough may result from tumour or external compression of the upper airways.

Oesophageal tumours are associated with dysphagia. The restriction on ingestion of food exacerbates the cachexia of malignant disease. At induction of anaesthesia, patients are at risk of regurgitation of food and secretions from above the oesophageal obstruction.

Preoperative features of weight loss and protein-calorie malnutrition, and hypoalbuminaemia make postoperative pulmonary infection, multiorgan failure and delayed wound healing more likely. Patients with pre-existing chronic lung disease are more likely to suffer postoperative pulmonary complications.

Cyanosis may result centrally from intrapulmonary shunting caused directly by diseased tissue or because of lung collapse consequent to proximal airway obstruction. Peripheral cyanosis is possible in the face and arms if the superior vena cava becomes obstructed by mediastinal spread.

Many major thoracic surgical procedures are preceded by rigid bronchoscopy, which requires clinical assessment of upper airway patency at the preoperative visit. Forced ventilatory effort by the patient may elicit stridor or wheeze, and palpation of the neck and inspection of the airway demonstrated on chest radiograph may reveal tracheal abnormality.

DIFFERENTIAL DIAGNOSIS

Preoperative investigations are required to confirm a diagnosis and stage the disease, in order to assess if the disease is resectable. Tumours are staged by assessing the spread of the primary tumour, presence of local lymph node spread and distant metastases (TNM staging). Further tests to assess physiological reserve are required to determine if the patient is operable.

INVESTIGATIONS

A variety of preoperative investigations are performed to determine resectability. The chest radiograph may reveal changes months before symptoms are manifest. Of symptomatic patients, 98% have chest radiograph abnormalities. Lung tumours are central in 70% of patients and may show collapse or cavitation more peripherally in the lung. Tumours are commonly 3–4 cm in size by the time of presentation. Other features include tracheal deviation, superior vena cava obstruction, pleural effusions and air-filled cavities.

Tumour diagnosis and staging involves sputum cytology, bronchoscopy, needle biopsy, mediastinoscopy and mediastinotomy. Computed tomography (CT) and magnetic resonance imaging (MRI) of the chest may reveal the spread of disease. Biochemistry, bone scans and ultrasound scans of the abdomen may detect metastatic disease. Barium studies and oesophageal ultrasound are similarly able to diagnose and stage carcinoma of the oesophagus.

Investigations are used to quantify physiological reserve by measuring mechanical and parenchymal function, and cardiopulmonary interaction. Rather than to deny surgery to patients, this is done to allocate resources to borderline patients to minimize their postoperative complications. Investigations to diagnose lung collapse, oedema, infection and bronchospasm allow patients to be presented in their best possible state on the day of surgery.

Whole-lung testing

Spirometry using voluntary effort, pulse oximetry and arterial blood gas tensions breathing air are influenced by the function of the whole lung.

Mechanical testing. Spirometry tests only the mechanical bellows function of the lung. Testing relies on voluntary effort and effective technique by the patient. From total lung capacity, the patient exhales to residual volume to measure the forced vital capacity (FVC). This is reduced in restrictive lung disease, such as cryptogenic alveolar fibrosis. The volume of gas exhaled forcibly in the first second gives the forced expiratory volume in 1 s (FEV_1). By definition, FEV_1 measures function when the lung is expanded well. In health, patients can exhale 70–80% of their vital capacity in 1 s, the FEV_1%. The remainder of the vital capacity may take another 2 s to exhale. With obstructive lung disease, the FEV_1% is reduced below 70% and the time taken to exhale the vital capacity is prolonged. The FEV_1% of patients with restrictive lung disease is preserved, although the absolute value of FVC, and therefore the volume exhaled in 1 s, is reduced. Values of 2 L for FVC and 1.5 L for FEV_1 offer a lower limit when screening for pneumonectomy. An FEV_1 of 1.0 L is cautionary for single lobectomy, because a whole-lung $FEV_1 > 800$ mL after surgery is about the amount a patient requires to avoid being dependent on mechanical ventilation.

Predicted postoperative (ppo) lung function may be calculated using lung segments. From a total of 19 segments, 3 in the upper lobes, 2 in both the middle lobe and lingual and 4 in the left and 5 in the right lower lobes (Fig 39.2), the fraction of lung remaining is multiplied by the preoperative spirometry measurement to give the predicted postoperative measurement of spirometry (ppo FEV_1 = preoperative FEV_1*(1−(resected segments/19)).

Using whole-lung spirometry to predict postoperative lung function may be invalidated if the regional function of the lung is not known. For example, a patient with an FEV_1 of 1.5 L may have the same or better FEV_1 after lobectomy if the main bronchus of the affected lobe was occluded completely at the time of testing before surgery. The oxygenation of blood of such a patient may be improved by the removal of a nonfunctioning lung or lobe through which considerable right-to-left shunt existed.

Parenchymal lung function. Arterial oxygen tensions < 8 kPa or carbon dioxide tensions > 6 kPa indicate increased risk for lung resection. The diffusing capacity of carbon monoxide (D_{LCO}) correlates with the total functioning area of the alveolar capillary membrane. Predictive postoperative values may be calculated in the same way as for mechanical function. Ppo D_{LCO} values < 40% predicted in health – normal range 100–150 mL min^{-1} mmHg^{-1} – correlate with increased postoperative respiratory complications.

Cardiopulmonary interaction. Cardiopulmonary exercise testing requires a patient to be able to pedal a bicycle ergometer and breathe through a mouthpiece. Increasing exercise to a peak allows calculation of maximum oxygen uptake expressed in $mL\,kg^{-1}\,min^{-1}$. Patients with $V_{O_2}max > 15\,mL\,kg^{-1}\,min^{-1}$ have been able to withstand lobectomy, whereas a ppo $V_{O_2}max > 10\,mL\,kg^{-1}\,min^{-1}$ is required to contemplate pneumonectomy.

Regional lung function

Ventilation/perfusion lung scans offer an indication of regional lung function. The relative contribution of the two separate lungs may be determined horizontally, but vertically within a lung, regions are indicated as upper, middle and lower zones rather than individual lobes or lung units.

Invasive assessment

For patients with borderline lung function for whom surgical resection offers great prognostic advantage, the risks and discomfort of invasive assessment of regional lung function may be worth the information obtained on likely residual function after surgery. Balloon occlusion of a main pulmonary artery before surgery or clamping a pulmonary artery during surgery allows some assessment of pulmonary artery pressures and oxygenation after resection. Inadequate blood oxygenation, arterial carbon dioxide tensions greater than $6.0\,kPa$ and mean pulmonary artery pressures greater than $25\,mmHg$ at rest, or greater than $35\,mmHg$ with exercise, indicate inadequate function and increased operative risk.

Any intrathoracic operative procedure places an immediate burden on the right ventricle. Diagnosis of a failing right ventricle or coexisting pulmonary artery hypertension may render a patient's chest pathology inoperable.

TREATMENT

Before surgery, patients should be motivated to stop smoking and lose excess weight. Reversible airway narrowing should be treated with bronchodilators such as salbutamol, terbutaline, theophylline, inhaled steroids or sodium cromoglycate. By giving antibiotics to treat chest infection, and loosening and removing bronchial secretions with inhaled nebulized water aerosols, chest physiotherapy and postural drainage, the incidence of pulmonary complications is reduced. Collapse in lung not intended for resection should be expanded, and pulmonary oedema treated by improving heart failure. Overnight, stopping smoking improves bronchial reactiv-

ity and reduces carboxyhaemoglobin concentrations. Eight weeks after cessation of smoking, the excessive production of mucus is reduced. This makes tracheobronchial clearance easier and improves small airway function.

ANATOMY

The bronchial tree and the views obtained when facing the patient are illustrated in Figure 39.1 and the bronchopulmonary segments are shown in Figure 39.2. The trachea leads from the cricoid cartilage below the larynx at the level of the sixth cervical vertebra (C6) and passes $10–12\,cm$ in the superior mediastinum to its bifurcation at the carina into left and right main bronchi at the sternal angle, T4/5. During inspiration, the lower border of the trachea moves inferiorly and anteriorly. The trachea lies principally in the midline, but is deviated to the right inferiorly by the arch of the aorta. The oesophagus is immediately posterior to the trachea and behind it is the vertebral column. The wall of the trachea is held patent by 15–20 cartilaginous rings deficient posteriorly where the trachealis membrane, a collection of fibroelastic fibres and smooth muscle, lies. It is wider in transverse diameter (20 mm) than anteroposteriorly (15 mm). The trachea passes from neck to thorax via the thoracic inlet at T2.

The right main bronchus is larger and less deviated from the midline than the left. The origin of the right upper lobe bronchus arises laterally 2.5 cm from the carina, whereas the origin of the left upper lobe arises laterally after 5 cm. These dimensions determine the relative ease of isolating each lung and ventilating them independently using double-lumen bronchial tubes.

The oesophagus is a continuation of the pharynx at the level of the lower border of the cricoid cartilage (C6) 15 cm from the incisor teeth. It passes immediately anterior to the thoracic spine and aorta and descends through the oesophageal hiatus of the diaphragm at T10, to the left of the midline at the level of the seventh rib. There are four slight constrictions, at its origin, as it is crossed by the aorta and left main bronchus and at the diaphragm, at 15, 25, 27 and 38 cm from the incisors.

RADIOGRAPHIC SURFACE MARKINGS

The apices of the lungs extend 2.5 cm above where the middle and inner thirds of the clavicle meet. Lung borders descend behind the medial end of the clavicle to the middle of the manubrium. The lung border is behind the body of the sternum and xiphisternum before sweeping

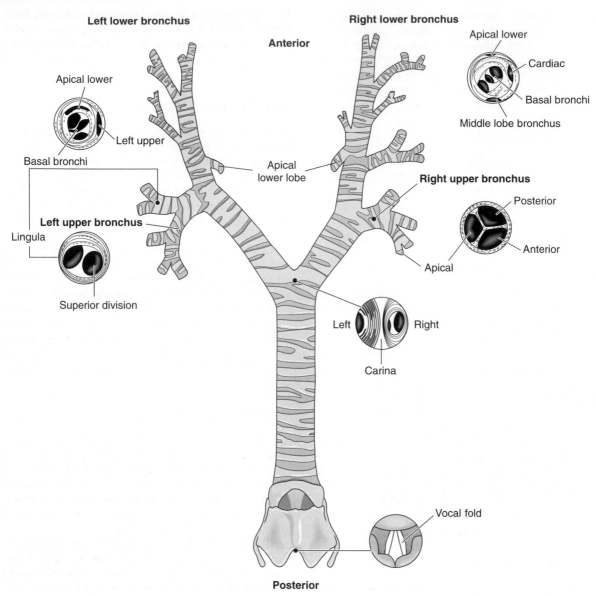

Fig. 39.1
Larynx, trachea, main and lobar bronchi.

inferiorly and laterally down to the level of the eleventh thoracic vertebra. On the left at the level of the horizontal fissure at the fourth costal cartilage (T7), the medial border of the lung is displaced to the left of the sternal edge in the cardiac notch. The oblique fissure descends from 3 cm lateral to the midline at T4, inferiorly and anteriorly to the sixth costal cartilage 7 cm from the midline. The diaphragmatic reflection of the pleura extrudes below the lung to the lower border of T12.

INDUCTION AND MAINTENANCE OF ANAESTHESIA

All currently available anaesthetic agents may be, and have been, used in anaesthesia for thoracic surgery. They are used in a way that is compatible with a strategy to maintain anaesthesia and haemodynamic stability during the procedure, while allowing the patient

A

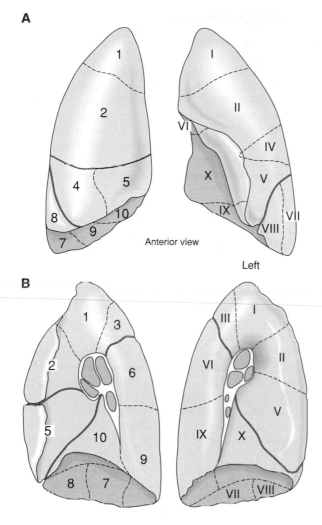

Anterior view

Left

B

Medial view

Fig. 39.2
Bronchopulmonary segments.

to drugs used in anaesthesia because of debility from the extent of their disease or from systemic effects, such as prolonged effects of neuromuscular blocking drugs in patients with Eaton–Lambert syndrome associated with carcinoma of the bronchus.

LATERAL THORACOTOMY

Many thoracic procedures are performed through a posterolateral thoracotomy incision between the fifth and eighth ribs. Patients have to be positioned on their side with the neck flexed, dependent shoulder brought forward and the arm raised under the pillow to protect shoulder and brachial plexus. The upper shoulder is flexed to 90° and the arm supported. Hips and knees are flexed together with a pillow between the legs. Padding, strapping, lower leg compression devices and diathermy pad complete the preparation for surgery (Fig. 39.3). Positioning with the chest flexed laterally away from the operative side on a beanbag which is then aspirated of air, or breaking the operating table, may improve surgical access. The upper wrist has a tendency to flex, so radial artery cannulae cause less trouble when on the dependent side. Peripheral and jugular vein cannulae are more accessible on the operative side.

THE LATERAL POSITION

In health, with the chest erect, the right lung takes 55% of the pulmonary blood flow and the left lung 45%. In the right lateral position, the right lung takes 65% and the left lung 35% because of the influence of gravity. In the left lateral position, differences are reversed; the right lung takes 45% and left lung 55%. These changes persist under anaesthesia.

However, anaesthesia does affect the changes to ventilation of the two lungs in the lateral position. Awake, there is more ventilation to the dependent lung; similarly, the bases receive proportionately more ventilation than the apices when the chest is erect. The dependent lung has a less negative intrapleural pressure than the upper lung and is on a more favourable

to breathe spontaneously in relative comfort immediately after surgery is complete. Large doses of i.v. opioid drugs are unlikely to achieve all these aims. Thoracic surgery patients may demonstrate sensitivity

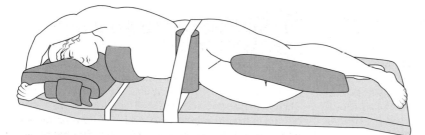

Fig. 39.3
Patient in right lateral position for thoracic surgery.

part of the pressure–volume curve. A change in pressure produces a greater change in volume in the dependent lung than the upper lung. Under anaesthesia, conditions for ventilation between the two lungs are reversed. Functional residual capacity is reduced. With paralysis of the diaphragm, the mechanical advantage of the greater curve of the lower diaphragm is lost and the lower lung is compressed by the mediastinum and abdominal contents. Awkward positioning on the operating table may further impede the lower lung. The lower lung is now in a less favourable position on the pressure–volume curve and any change in pressure produces greater change in the volume of the upper lung than the dependent lung. Anaesthesia therefore produces much worse ventilation/perfusion mismatch in the lateral position, with more blood going to the dependent lung and more ventilation going to the upper lung. Application of positive end-expiratory pressure up to $10\,cmH_2O$ improves the changes in ventilation and tends to restore ventilation to the dependent lung.

ONE-LUNG ANAESTHESIA

The principal indications for one-lung anaesthesia are:

- isolation of the lungs
- ventilation of one lung alone
- bronchopulmonary alveolar lavage
- collapse of one lung to allow surgical access to other structures.

Isolation of a diseased lung with sepsis or haemorrhage may be necessary to protect the healthy lung. When there is inadequate ventilation of both lungs because of a large bronchopleural or bronchocutaneous fistula, a large unilateral bulla or because the compliance of two lungs is so different that they require independent ventilation, satisfactory oxygenation may be obtained by ventilation of one lung alone. Pulmonary alveolar proteinosis may be treated by bronchoalveolar lavage. This requires that only one lung be lavaged with liquid at a time, whilst the other is protected. Video-assisted pulmonary and pleural surgery, and intrathoracic, nonpulmonary surgery such as oesophageal, aortic and spinal surgery may require the lung to be collapsed to allow access to the operative structures.

Ventilation of one lung alone may require either a double-lumen tracheal tube (Fig. 39.4), a bronchial blocker (Fig. 39.5) or a bronchial tube. The double-lumen tube has greatest flexibility to allow changes from ventilation of two lungs to one lung then back to two lungs during or at the end of surgery. It allows aspiration of the main bronchi independently, and insufflation of oxygen to the nonventilated lung. It has a larger external diameter than the bronchial blocker or bronchial tube and may be difficult to position correctly where tracheal and bronchial anatomy is distorted. The two separate lumens are narrow and present a high resistance to spontaneous ventilation. This is overcome by positive-pressure ventilation, but a single-lumen tube may have to be substituted at the end of surgery if resumption of spontaneous ventilation is not immediate. A bronchial blocker with a hollow lumen allows insufflation of oxygen, some suctioning and may be used with a jet ventilator, which overcomes some of the disadvantages of the technique. The Rüsch bronchial blocker illustrated in Figure 39.5 has a 170 cm long, 2 mm stem (outside diameter) with a central lumen to a 2.75 mm diameter balloon, which accepts 5 mL air. It may be passed down a bronchoscope with a lumen greater

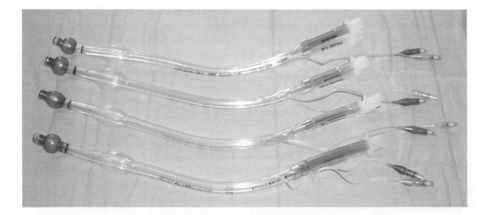

Fig. 39.4
Four left-sided Bronchocath double-lumen endobronchial tubes with balloons inflated, from 35 FG (uppermost) to 41 FG (lowest).

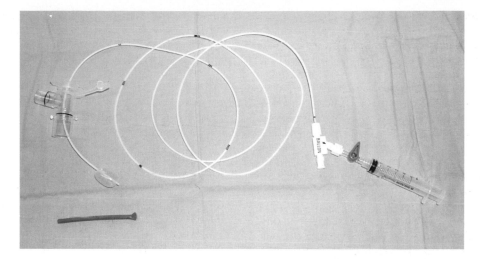

Fig. 39.5
A Rüsch 6 FG bronchial blocker (360601) – balloon is inflated with 5 mL air. The balloon guard is below the balloon and the stem passes through the 1.8 mm seal in the connector for the anaesthetic circuit. Luer-lock fittings (labelled 'balloon') to inflate the balloon and aspirate/inflate down the central lumen are on the right.

than 2.8 mm diameter or the 15 mm tapered connector with a 1.8 mm seal shown.

POSITIONING DOUBLE-LUMEN BRONCHIAL TUBES

Double-lumen bronchial tubes provide an effective means of isolating each lung to protect the other from blood and secretions. They allow ventilation of one lung only, or both lungs independently. Being longer and with lumens more narrow than single-lumen tracheal tubes, they have a greater resistance to air flow. They are therefore not usually suitable for spontaneous ventilation. Disposable polyvinyl chloride tubes (Fig. 39.6) have substantially replaced the re-usable red rubber Robertshaw double-lumen tubes. Sizes of tube in common use in adult practice range from 35 to 41 French gauge (FG). Sizes 37–39 are usually suitable for men and 37 for women, but sizes 41 and 35 are available for individuals at extremes of the range of adult build. Left- and right-sided versions of double-lumen bronchial tubes are necessary (Fig. 39.6) as they are curved anteroposteriorly and the balloon of the right bronchial tube is fenestrated to conduct gases down the right upper lobe bronchus, which would otherwise be occluded by the cuff of the tube (Fig. 39.7). The left upper lobe bronchus arises 2.5 cm further down the main bronchus than the right, so it is less likely to be occluded by the balloon of the bronchial tube.

Positioning double-lumen bronchial tubes correctly is a skill learned quickly with practice. The task is usu-ally straightforward, but however experienced the anaesthetist, great difficulties may be encountered with some patients. An incorrectly positioned double-lumen bronchial tube may rapidly compromise the supply of oxygen to the lungs during thoracic surgery, with disastrous results. The correct position of double-lumen bronchial tubes may be confirmed by clinical technique or by using an intubating fibreoptic laryngoscope.

Clinical technique

The patient lies supine on a level operating table with the head supported on a single pillow pulled clear of the shoulders to flex the neck and extend the head. After induction of anaesthesia and muscle relaxation, the larynx is identified by laryngoscopy. The double-lumen bronchial tube is held at 90° to its eventual anatomical position, to align the curve of the bronchial lumen anteroposteriorly. The bronchial lumen is passed between the cords until it rests within the trachea. The double-lumen bronchial tube is then rotated 90° back to point the bronchial lumen towards its intended bronchus. The head is turned away from the side of the bronchial lumen and the double-lumen bronchial tube advanced gently until resistance is encountered and the bronchial tube is thought to be in the correct position. The tracheal cuff is then inflated and the lungs ventilated manually through both lumens of the tube. Visible movement of both sides of the chest, detection of a recognizable trace of exhaled carbon dioxide, breath sounds auscultated in both

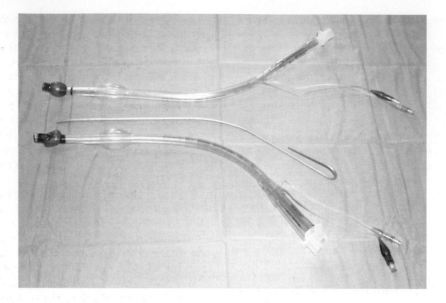

Fig. 39.6
Left (upper) and right (lower) 39 FG double-lumen bronchial tubes are shown with a flexible introducer, which may be used to shape the tube to enable insertion.

axillae and an unchanging pulse oximetry reading reassure the anaesthetist that the airway is controlled. Difficulties encountered whilst isolating individual lungs may be addressed after returning to this position of control.

The tracheal lumen of the breathing circuit is then clamped and the breathing system distal to the clamp opened to air. Breath sounds are confirmed on the bronchial side. Two or more millilitres of air are then injected into the bronchial cuff until the leak of air from the tracheal tube is no longer audible or palpable, and breath sounds auscultated over the side opposite to the bronchial lumen cease. The tracheal lumen is then closed, and the clamp is released and applied to the bronchial system; the circuit is opened and the procedure is repeated to confirm that chest movement and air entry occur to the tracheal side and not the bronchial side and that there are no air leaks from the anaesthetic system. The double-lumen bronchial tube is then secured with a tube tie at the teeth by a clove hitch, and the tube tie is knotted round the neck by a bow to enable its quick release at the end of the procedure.

When each lumen of the double-lumen tube (DLT) is clamped, there should be a detectable increase in airway pressure during the breathing cycle when the tidal volume is directed down one lung. The peak airway pressure may then be controlled below $30\,cmH_2O$ by reducing the tidal volume and increasing the ventilatory rate whilst maintaining the minute volume of ventilation. If there is no change on the ventilator or airway pressure gauges when one lumen of the tube is clamped, the bronchial lumen is likely to end in the trachea or else there is a substantial leak past the bronchial cuff. The position of the DLT should always be re-checked after the patient has been subjected to any changes in position, e.g. from supine to lateral, etc.

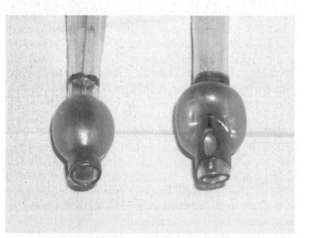

Fig. 39.7
Bronchial balloons inflated on left-sided (left) and right-sided (right) bronchial double-lumen tubes. The right tube is eccentric and shows the side lumen to allow inflation of the right upper lobe.

Using the fibreoptic intubating laryngoscope

Confirming the correct position of a double-lumen bronchial tube using a fibreoptic intubating laryngoscope should avoid many problems encountered with ventilation of the lungs during thoracic surgery. However, if parenchymal lung disease is so extensive that one lung is insufficient to keep tissues oxygenated, if pneumothorax develops on the side of the ventilated lung, or if the double-lumen tube is subsequently dislodged, problems with ventilation may still be encountered. A practical solution to the conflict between the costs and time for each use and cleaning of the fibreoptic intubating laryngoscope and the benefits of positioning the double-lumen bronchial tube correctly may be reached by:

- using left-sided double-lumen bronchial tubes for all operations except left lung resections
- confirming correct position of left-sided double-lumen bronchial tubes clinically
- using the fibreoptic intubating laryngoscope to confirm the correct position of left-sided double-lumen bronchial tubes where clinical testing does not demonstrate correct position conclusively, and correct position of all right-sided double-lumen bronchial tubes.

Vascular cannulae and epidural catheters may be inserted before or after induction of anaesthesia depending on clinical need. If bronchoscopy precedes thoracotomy then one sequence of events might be as follows:

- Anaesthesia is induced for bronchoscopy, followed by insertion of a double-lumen bronchial tube into the trachea. The tracheal cuff is inflated and ventilation of both lungs confirmed as anaesthesia is maintained.
- Peripheral venous, arterial, central venous and urinary catheters are inserted as required, if not already in place before induction of anaesthesia.
- The patient is turned onto the side with the operative side uppermost. The neck and hips are flexed to insert the epidural catheter; otherwise the patient is positioned for surgery.
- The fibreoptic intubating laryngoscope is passed down the bronchial lumen of the double-lumen bronchial tube until the carina is identified.
- Both lungs are ventilated if the bronchial lumen connector makes a seal around the laryngoscope; otherwise the bronchial lumen is clamped.
- When the patient is lying on the side, the anaesthetist manipulates the laryngoscope tip in a vertical plane (i.e. horizontal section in the patient). For a right-sided double-lumen tube, the tip of the laryngoscope is directed downwards (to the right main bronchus) and advanced until the orifice of the right upper lobe bronchus is identified.

Positioning the double-lumen tube often leaves the orifice of the right upper lobe bronchus covered by the tip of the bronchial tube (Fig. 39.8).

- The tracheal cuff is then deflated, the laryngoscope is held fixed relative to the patient and the double-lumen tube advanced. The blue bronchial cuff then occludes sight of the orifice of the right upper lobe bronchus until the side hole in the bronchial cuff lies over it. Sight of bronchial rings of the right upper lobe bronchus confirms the correct position of the double-lumen bronchial tube (Fig. 39.9).
- The double-lumen tube is then held firm and the bronchial cuff inflated with 2 mL of air. Uninterrupted sight of the right upper lobe bronchus confirms that this manoeuvre has not moved the side hole of the bronchial tube relative to the bronchus. The bronchi to the right middle and lower lobes may be seen through the distal lumen of the bronchial tube (Fig. 39.10). Withdrawing the intubating laryngoscope may give a view of the origins of all three lobar bronchi (Fig. 39.11).
- The double-lumen tube is then held against the teeth or gums of the maxilla, the mark on the tube there is noted and the laryngoscope is removed from the bronchial lumen. Without moving it, the tube is tied with a clove hitch over this mark and the tube tie tied round the neck with a bow.

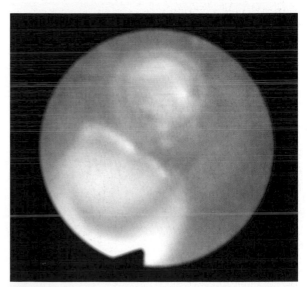

Fig. 39.8
Distal opening of bronchial lumen at 12 o'clock shows right middle and lower bronchi. The side opening of the bronchial lumen at 7 o'clock is against the wall of the right main bronchus and is not over the right upper lobe bronchus. The patient is lying on the right. Orientation: left, cephalad; upper, left; right, caudad; lower, right.

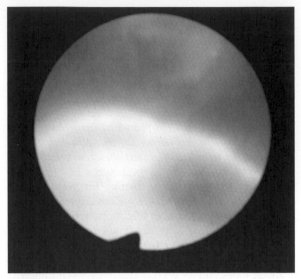

Fig. 39.9
The double-lumen tube has been repositioned so that the side opening of the bronchial lumen at 6 o'clock is now over the right upper lobe bronchus. The patient is lying on the right. Orientation: left, cephalad; upper, left; right, caudad; lower, right.

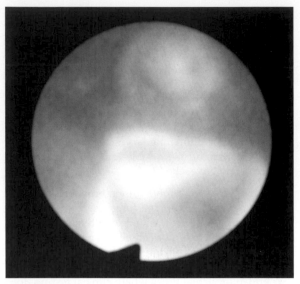

Fig. 39.11
The intubating laryngoscope is withdrawn to show the right middle and lower lobe bronchi through the distal opening at 12 o'clock and the right upper lobe bronchus through the side opening at 6 o'clock. The patient is lying on the right. Orientation: left, cephalad; upper, left; right, caudad; lower, right.

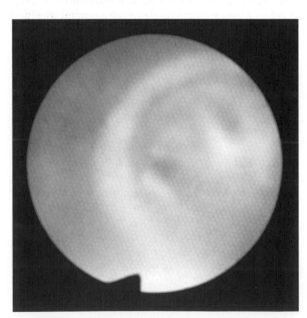

Fig. 39.10
Distal opening of bronchial lumen at 3 o'clock shows right lower and middle lobe bronchi. The dark colour at 9 o'clock is the bronchial lumen cuff. The patient is lying on the right. Orientation: left, cephalad; upper, left; right, caudad; lower, right.

- The tracheal cuff is then inflated with 5 mL of air and the fibreoptic laryngoscope is then passed down the tracheal lumen until the carina is identified again. The bronchial lumen is seen to pass down the correct main bronchus and the bronchial cuff in its main bronchus is seen to be inflated, but not herniating to impinge over the lumen of the other main bronchus (Fig. 39.12).
- The laryngoscope is removed from the tracheal lumen and both lungs are ventilated.
- Bronchial and tracheal lumens are clamped in turn, observing airway pressures, leaks and the extent of ventilation of each lung.

Passing a suction catheter down the bronchial lumen before starting removes secretions faster than is possible through the suction port of the fibreoptic intubating laryngoscope. Lubrication of the laryngoscope with water-soluble jelly aids its passage down both lumens and prevents the tube being dislodged when the laryngoscope is withdrawn. A receiver of warm water with detergent aspirated through the suction port reduces fogging of the tip of the laryngoscope. Warm soapy water provides a ready supply of fluid to unblock the suction port during the procedure and flush it through at the end, so that the suction port

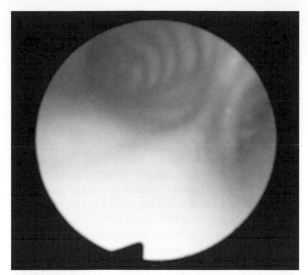

Fig. 39.12
The intubating laryngoscope has been passed down the tracheal lumen. The carina passes from 2 o'clock anteriorly to 6 o'clock posteriorly. The left main bronchus is to the left at 10–12 o'clock. On the other side of the carina, the dark crescent confirms that the inflated bronchial cuff is not herniating over the left main bronchus and the bronchial tube to the right of the cuff passes down the right main bronchus. The patient is lying on the right. Orientation: left, cephalad; upper, left; right, caudad; lower, right.

does not block with encrusted aspirate before there is an opportunity to clean the laryngoscope.

Clinical testing is specific – a problem detected with the position of the bronchial double-lumen tube is likely to predict a real problem if left uncorrected before surgery begins. However, it is not very sensitive. Inadequate isolation of one lung and excessive airway pressures may be encountered after apparently successful positioning of the tube. Correct alignment of the fenestration in the bronchial cuff over the origin of the right upper lobe bronchus is particularly difficult to predict by clinical means alone.

MODE OF VENTILATION

Surgery through a thoracotomy wound with the patient breathing spontaneously causes the same problem as trauma patients experience with large open chest wounds. The pleural space with the chest open is at atmospheric pressure. During inspiration, gas flows from trachea and lung in the open chest into the dependent lung. During expiration, the flow is reversed, causing the lung in the open chest to inflate. Gas is transferred from lung to lung during the paradoxical ventilation of the lung in the open chest, preventing excretion of carbon dioxide and rendering gas

inspired into the dependent lung hypoxic. Packing the chest or isolating the lung in the open chest with a blocker or bronchial double-lumen tube may stop paradoxical ventilation of the lung in the open chest. Both devices increase the resistance to gas flow to the dependent lung, and so mechanical one-lung ventilation is usual during thoracic surgery.

PHYSIOLOGICAL CHANGES

With one lung perfused but not ventilated, a substantial right-to-left shunt should produce significant hypoxaemia. Because of the greater solubility of carbon dioxide and its more linear dissociation curve, the gradient from arterial to alveolar partial pressure of carbon dioxide is smaller than that for oxygen. Increasing alveolar ventilation of the ventilated lung reduces arterial carbon dioxide tension without substantially increasing arterial oxygen tension. Because of the flat portion of the oxygen dissociation curve, when haemoglobin is saturated fully, a further increase in alveolar oxygen tension has only a small effect on oxygen content in solution and has no effect on the oxygenation of the blood in the nonventilated lung. Hence this does not improve hypoxaemia caused by right-to-left shunt.

The severity of hypoxaemia observed is much less than that expected were regional perfusion to remain unaltered. As observed above, the lateral position directs more blood to the dependent lung because of gravity. In the nonventilated lung, alveolar hypoxia results in increased vascular resistance, which directs more blood to the dependent ventilated lung, further reducing shunt and hypoxaemia. This protective change is termed hypoxic pulmonary vasoconstriction (HPV) and it is impaired by anaesthetic agents. However, in clinical practice, other compensatory mechanisms in the intact human lung reduce shunt.

HPV has no effect if the alveolar oxygen tension is either 100% or 0%, or if the alveolar oxygen tension is the same throughout all lung units. It is more likely to have an effect with the 20–30% of cardiac output that shunts through the nonventilated lung during one-lung anaesthesia. HPV effects are also maximal when pulmonary artery pressures and mixed venous oxygen saturation tensions are normal. The results of excessively high or low pulmonary artery pressures exceed the marginal changes in pulmonary artery pressures obtained by HPV. Similarly, an abnormally low mixed venous oxygen tension caused by low cardiac output or high oxygen consumption, for example by hyperthermia or shivering, has greater influence than any changes possible with HPV. High peak and end-expiratory ventilation pressures in the dependent lung increase its pulmonary vascular resistance and overcome any benefits of HPV in the nonventilated lung. Excessive alveolar pressures may increase dead space by producing a region of lung that is ventilated but not perfused.

Volatile anaesthetic agents and pulmonary vasodilators such as glyceryl trinitrate, sodium nitroprusside, isoprenaline, dobutamine and nitric oxide have been demonstrated to inhibit HPV. However, clinically there are far more variables than in the controlled conditions of the experimental laboratory bench. Poor positioning of the patient which compromises blood flow to the dependent lung, malposition of a double-lumen bronchial tube, low cardiac output caused by inadequate blood volume replacement or impediment to blood flow by surgical manipulation may have a greater influence on hypoxaemia than the effects of changes in HPV.

Hypoxaemia during one-lung anaesthesia may be minimized by:

- correct positioning of the bronchial tube
- increasing inspired oxygen concentration to 50%
- a tidal volume of 10 mL kg^{-1} or less to avoid increasing dead space
- positive end-expired pressure of no more than 5–10 cmH$_2$O to minimize dependent lung collapse without increasing vascular resistance
- maintaining cardiac output and pulmonary artery pressures near the normal range.

Insufflation of oxygen to the nonventilated lung either at atmospheric pressure or with continuous positive alveolar pressure of 5 cmH$_2$O should avoid the need for pharmacological intervention such as inhaled nitric oxide to the ventilated lung. During lung resection, when the pulmonary artery is clamped, the adequacy of gas exchange should be reassessed. The loss of shunt through diseased lung tissue may limit the loss of lung function expected after removal of lung tissue.

ANAESTHESIA FOR THORACIC SURGERY PROCEDURES

RIGID BRONCHOSCOPY

Rigid bronchoscopy in thoracic surgery is performed most often to obtain tissue diagnosis and determine if a lesion may be resected. Other indications include removal of foreign bodies and secretions, and control of haemorrhage. Therapeutic procedures such as laser therapy, tracheal or bronchial stenting and alveolar lavage may be performed through a rigid bronchoscope.

Anaesthesia should permit the passage of a straight rigid bronchoscope of up to 9 mm external diameter, allow oxygenation and removal of carbon dioxide, avoid awareness, and control movement, coughing and reflex haemodynamic responses to mechanical stimulation of the tracheobronchial tree. This may be achieved by spontaneous ventilation, apnoeic oxygenation or, more usually, positive-pressure jet ventilation. Spontaneous ventilation avoids inhaled foreign bodies being propelled more distally into the bronchial tree. However, it offers much less control than when neuromuscular blockade is used, and anaesthesia sufficient to cause respiratory depression is required to control reflex responses to bronchoscopy. Apnoeic oxygenation may be achieved by delivering oxygen into the conducting airways by a catheter and relying on diffusion down a concentration gradient from oxygenated airways to alveoli, where oxygen is absorbed continuously. Although effective in maintaining oxygenation measured by pulse oximetry, arterial carbon dioxide tension increases by about 0.5 kPa min^{-1}. Using apnoeic oxygenation, enough time may be available to complete the surgical procedure, but eventually, assisted or spontaneous ventilation has to resume to ventilate the alveoli.

Positive-pressure ventilation may be performed by intermittent occlusion of the bronchoscope or, more conveniently, by high-pressure jet ventilation using a Sanders Venturi technique. Oxygen at 400 kPa is released by a trigger held by the anaesthetist through a narrow orifice of 18–14G. The gas is directed through the jet at the operator end of the bronchoscope towards the patient end. The high-pressure jet entrains atmospheric air and inflates the chest. Care must be taken to avoid pulmonary barotrauma by limiting delivery of oxygen under pressure to short intermittent bursts according to the chest movement observed and ensuring that there is a large unobstructed opening at the observer end of the bronchoscope to allow gas under pressure to escape from the conducting airways. Oxygenation may be monitored by pulse oximetry. Intermittent ventilation may usually be restricted to times when the operator is not looking down the bronchoscope.

With the patient supine, removal of the pillow or extension of the neck by lowering the head of the operating table may be necessary to allow the bronchoscope to pass down the trachea. Antisialagogue premedication dries oropharyngeal secretions and aids visibility. Induction of anaesthesia by inhalation of volatile anaesthetic agents may be necessary occasionally to confirm that adequate ventilation may be achieved under anaesthesia where there is some obstruction to the upper airways. Depolarizing or competitive neuromuscular blocking agents may be used according to the needs of the patient or intended procedure. Topical local anaesthetic and a systemic opioid with a rapid onset of action help to obtund the haemodynamic response to bronchoscopy. Intermittent positive pressure ventilation with a Venturi device requires a total intravenous anaesthetic technique.

Local trauma and bleeding are the most common complications. Ventilation after bronchoscopy may be impaired by persisting effects of anaesthetic drugs, or compromise to the upper airway. A chest radiograph in the recovery room may provide early detection of pneumothorax or air in the mediastinum.

RIGID OESOPHAGOSCOPY

Fibreoptic oesophagogastroduodenoscopy is performed usually as an outpatient procedure under sedation, without demands for anaesthetic assistance. Rigid oesophagoscopy under general anaesthesia presents the anaesthetist with patients who are at risk of aspirating gastric contents. Patients with achalasia may have large volumes of fetid fluid accumulated in their oesophagus. All oesophagoscopy patients should undergo rapid-sequence induction with the suction catheter to hand and suction switched on. In patients with achalasia, there should be an attempt to drain the oesophagus before anaesthesia, which should be induced in a steep head-up tilt or in the left lateral position.

When anaesthesia has been induced and the cuff of the tracheal tube inflated to protect the airway, the tracheal tube should be passed to the left-hand side of the tongue to allow the oesophagoscope to be inserted behind where the tracheal tube usually lies. The tracheal tube is taped or tied securely, and then held at all times by the anaesthetist. This prevents the tracheal tube being dislodged by the operator on the withdrawal of the oesophagoscope on most occasions, and makes the anaesthetist aware immediately of dislodgement of the tracheal tube, regurgitation of fluid into the oropharynx or requests for the tracheal cuff to be deflated as the oesophagoscope is passed through the cricopharyngeal sphincter.

Manipulations to the head or neck may be required to pass the oesophagoscope. Damage to the teeth or mucosal surfaces may occur. When the oesophagoscope has passed down the oesophagus, anaesthesia may be maintained with the patient breathing spontaneously. At the end of the procedure, patients should be awake and able to cough and protect the airway before tracheal extubation, which takes place with the patient lying on the left side with suction apparatus and trained assistance ready to hand as at induction of anaesthesia.

Perforation of the oesophagus is an unusual but serious complication. Patients should have been awake for 1 h after oesophagoscopy without complaint of chest discomfort and have an unchanged chest radiograph before ingestion of oral fluids resumes.

CERVICAL MEDIASTINOSCOPY AND ANTERIOR MEDIASTINOTOMY

Both procedures are used to stage the extent of spread of intrathoracic malignancy or obtain a tissue diagnosis. Ventilation of both lungs through a single-lumen tracheal tube is usually adequate and surgical access may be improved by resting the shoulders on a sandbag and the head on a head ring.

Analgesia after surgery may be helped by infiltration of the wound by local anaesthetic, or transverse superficial cervical plexus and intercostal nerve blocks. Whilst the procedures are usually straightforward, there is always the potential for significant haemorrhage, damage to surrounding structures and compromise to the airway from haematoma after surgery.

VIDEO-ASSISTED THORACOSCOPIC SURGERY

Improvements in imaging and thoracoscopic instruments have allowed more elaborate procedures than biopsy, such as lung resection, lung reduction surgery, pleurectomy and sympathectomy. The video image is magnified on monitors, but so too is movement and there is little space within the chest for instruments and camera lenses. A collapsed motionless lung may be essential, thereby requiring one-lung anaesthesia.

Pain after video-assisted thoracoscopic surgery (VATS) procedures is less intense and prolonged than after posterolateral thoracotomy. Patients are much more comfortable after the chest drain is removed than thoracotomy patients at the same stage after surgery. A single paravertebral block at the level of the chest drain and intercostal incisions with bupivacaine 0.5% 20 mL followed by oral analgesia may be sufficient to allow patients to take deep breaths and cough after thoracoscopic surgery.

PULMONARY LOBECTOMY

One-lung anaesthesia allows dissection in a field disturbed only by the movement of the mediastinum. Inflation of the lung temporarily may help to identify the lung fissures. Passive insufflation of the collapsed lung either through a suction catheter or with 5 cm continuous positive airway pressure may augment oxygenation achieved by one-lung anaesthesia. Surgical traction on mediastinal structures and disturbance to the mediastinum by surgeons' hands, instruments or retractors may cause bradycardia, interruption of the venous return to the heart or compression of the chambers of the heart.

When the bronchial stump is closed and haemostasis secured, the chest may be filled with warm saline and the airway pressure held at $40\,cmH_2O$ to test the integrity of the stump.

When chest drains are in position, reinflation of the remaining lobe(s) is achieved by applying gentle positive pressure to the anaesthetic breathing system. Observing the pleural surface confirms if all superficial lung tissue is reinflated. As the chest is closed, a subatmospheric pressure of $5\,kPa$ is applied to the chest drains via an underwater seal. A significant air leak through damaged lung becomes apparent immediately if the ventilator reservoir collapses or if a reduction in the expired minute volume is detected by the ventilator alarm. The suction is then disconnected from the chest drains and reapplied when the patient resumes spontaneous breathing. Chest drains are then left without being clamped until the remaining lung has re-expanded fully, drainage has ceased and there is no air leak, when the chest drains are removed.

PNEUMONECTOMY

The operative lung should be collapsed as soon as skin disinfection and draping begin. Problems with oxygenation may then be apparent early in the procedure. Borderline oxygenation may improve when the pulmonary artery is clamped and shunt through the lung to be resected is interrupted. Intrapericardial dissections for tumours that have extensive local spread pose a risk of sudden, substantial haemorrhage. The integrity of the stump of the main bronchus may be tested when the lung has been removed (as after lobectomy).

When the chest is closed at the end of surgery, the remaining lung is fully inflated and the chest drain to the pneumonectomy space is clamped. Clamps are released for 5 min every hour to ensure that no air, blood or excess fluid accumulates in the pneumonectomy space. Leaving the chest drains open continuously may lead to a reduction in the pneumonectomy space and the mediastinum being shifted to the operative side as the remaining lung becomes hyperinflated, with consequent respiratory embarrassment. The pleural space fills with serosanguinous fluid after pneumonectomy and fibroses subsequently, reducing the size of the space.

PLEURECTOMY AND PLEURODESIS

Recurrent pneumothorax or pneumothorax which fails to respond to conservative measures may require pleurectomy to re-expand the lung and prevent recurrence. Pleurectomy and talc pleurodesis are usually possible by thoracoscopy. Pain after pleurectomy is much greater than after diagnostic thoracoscopic procedures even with the same number of intercostal wounds. Patients may require the same analgesia as if the procedure had been performed via a thoracotomy wound.

EMPYEMA

Patients may remain remarkably well despite a large collection of purulent material in the pleural space. Collections may arise after pulmonary infection, oesophageal rupture, and following thoracoscopy and thoracotomy. Chest drainage before surgery may reduce the volume of pleural fluid, but organized infection has to be removed by open surgery. There may be considerable blood loss during decortication of an empyema.

LUNG CYSTS AND BULLAE

Bullae are thin-walled, air-filled cavities within the lung which communicate slowly with the bronchial tree. In the presence of bullae, there is always the potential for tension pneumothorax under positive-pressure ventilation, and the creation of a bronchopleurocutaneous fistula after insertion of a chest drain.

Similar changes in size may occur during anaesthesia with liquid-filled cysts. There is the added risk of soiling parenchymal lung tissue elsewhere with the liquid should the cyst rupture.

BRONCHOPLEURAL FISTULA

Although most common after lung resection surgery, bronchopleural fistulae may occur after acute respiratory distress syndrome (ARDS) and any intrathoracic sepsis. The chest should be drained before induction of anaesthesia to reduce the amount of purulent fluid in the chest cavity and avoid the prospect of tension pneumothorax. Anaesthesia should be induced with the affected side dependent, followed by prompt bronchial intubation of the main bronchus on the unaffected side, in order to isolate the healthy lung from contamination by purulent secretions from the affected side. One-lung ventilation allows surgery on the affected side. Should there still be lung tissue on the affected side, high-frequency jet ventilation offers a means of keeping lung tissue inflated and ventilated in the presence of a large air leak, with mean intrathoracic pressures lower than with conventional intermittent positive-pressure ventilation.

TRACHEAL SURGERY

Unless cardiopulmonary bypass is used, there must be a changing sequence of means of ventilating the lungs during surgery, and measures to keep the neck flexed after surgery to avoid tension on the tracheal repair before it heals.

Until the tracheal lesion is resected, airway obstruction must be overcome during the early stages of anaesthesia. Maintaining spontaneous ventilation initially allows assessment of the adequacy of assisted ventilation under anaesthesia. With the lesion exposed, ventilation of one or both lungs through an incision in the trachea distal to the lesion allows resection of the lesion and repair of the posterior wall of the trachea. A narrow tracheal or bronchial tube is passed through the larynx beyond the anastomotic site, and this allows space for repair of the anterior wall of the trachea. Suturing the chin to the skin over the sternum keeps the neck in flexion until the tracheal anastomosis heals.

TRACHEOSTOMY

The neck is extended by placing a sandbag under the shoulders and securing the head on a head ring. The pharynx should be aspirated when surgical dissection of the trachea is complete, because incision of the second and third tracheal rings frequently bursts the cuff on the tracheal tube. The tracheal tube is then withdrawn sufficiently far to allow insertion of the tracheostomy tube, but is not withdrawn from the trachea. This retains a means of ventilating the lung and a conduit into the trachea to replace the tracheal tube over a bougie should initial attempts to introduce the tracheostomy tube be unsuccessful. When the tracheostomy tube is positioned correctly, it is connected to a sterile catheter mount within the draped area and then to the anaesthetic system, which may be draped subsequently. The sandbag is removed before the neck wound is sutured.

Pneumomediastinum and pneumothorax may occur intraoperatively because of damage to the posterior tracheal wall. Haemorrhage and damage to other structures may occur immediately, or later as a result of the effects of pressure from a malpositioned tracheostomy tube.

OESOPHAGEAL SURGERY

Oesophagectomy is often preceded by oesophagoscopy with all the attendant risks of pulmonary aspiration. Thoracic approaches to the oesophagus may require one-lung ventilation to provide access for surgery. Oesophagectomy may take some hours and be associated with considerable fluid loss into the wound and surrounding tissues.

After surgery, effective analgesia is necessary to enable the patient to expand the chest and cough effectively. Patients should be nursed sitting or supported on pillows to avoid regurgitation of gastrointestinal fluid and subsequent aspiration. Total parenteral nutrition is not required as a routine, but may be necessary in the presence of postoperative complications such as mediastinitis from an anastomotic leak.

POSTOPERATIVE CARE

Pulmonary function is impaired after thoracic surgery beyond any changes expected after lung resection. There is a 35% reduction in functional residual capacity after lung resection, which takes 6–8 weeks to recover to preoperative values. However, thoracic surgery patients should be able to breathe spontaneously immediately after anaesthesia and surgery. A need for mechanical ventilation after surgery is likely to result from problems in patient selection, or during surgery and anaesthesia intraoperatively. The advantages of mechanical ventilation may be obtained during surgery. The lungs may be expanded under direct vision of the pleural surface and the bronchial tree aspirated. A mini-tracheostomy tube may be inserted through the cricothyroid membrane at the end of surgery, with the trachea extubated and the lungs ventilated through a laryngeal mask, to help aspiration of the trachea of patients unable to cough effectively. Prolonged mechanical ventilation exposes thoracic patients to regional lung collapse and nosocomial pulmonary infection.

A high inspired oxygen concentration to overcome hypoxaemia is usually required for the first 24 h after surgery and during sleep at night until chest drains are removed (assessed by pulse oximetry). Patients breathing air with a $P_a\text{CO}_2$ greater than 6.0 kPa before surgery are at increased risk of ventilatory failure after surgery and require oxygen therapy tailored to response. Most other patients benefit from oxygen 40–60% by plastic face mask or nasal prongs.

The posterolateral thoracotomy wound is exceedingly painful. Untreated, each breath provokes pain.

To minimize pain, respiration is rapid and shallow. Analgesia sufficient to permit deep inspiration and productive coughing without respiratory depression is necessary to restore adequate spontaneous ventilation after thoracic surgery. Continuous epidural analgesia or (if that is contraindicated) paravertebral nerve blockade is more likely to achieve these aims than systemic opioid analgesia. Epidural local anaesthetic or opioids, or mixtures of the two, may be infused through a catheter introduced between the fifth and eighth thoracic vertebrae, depending on the sites of wound and chest drains, and the size and alignment of the intervertebral spaces. Bupivacaine $0-15\,mg\,h^{-1}$, or fentanyl $0-50\,\mu g\,h^{-1}$, alone or in combination, may be given as continuous infusions or background infusions with additional patient-controlled demands.

After oesophageal surgery, oral fluids are withheld for some days whilst a nasogastric tube drains the stomach. After lung resection in the morning, patients may be able to manage some food in the evening. Fluids i.v. are required for the first 24 h, although less is given than after other forms of major surgery. Maintenance fluids are restricted to avoid pulmonary oedema in remaining lung tissue that has been handled or through which there is a relatively increased pulmonary artery flow after lung resection. Ringer lactate solution $10\,mL\,kg^{-1}\,h^{-1}$ in theatre and dextrose/saline $1\,mL\,kg^{-1}\,h^{-1}$ thereafter, with the equivalent of saline 0.9% 500 mL in 24 h, provide maintenance fluids; blood and colloid may be added to replace further losses and support the circulation.

Patients are likely to be cold after thoracic surgery as a result of lying in theatre covered only by sterile drapes and with the chest open during surgery. Simple means to conserve heat during surgery by warming i.v. fluids and humidification of inspired gases, followed by convective warming blankets in the recovery room, may restore body temperature to normal soon after surgery is finished.

Arrhythmias are common after thoracotomy, especially atrial tachyarrhythmias, which may affect 9–33% of patients over 60 years of age. They occur often 2–3 days after surgery and increase the risk of hypotension and stroke. Prophylaxis has proved ineffective and 85% resolve during hospital stay. Of the remainder, almost all resolve within 2 months.

FURTHER READING

Bastin R, Moraine J-T, Bardocsky G et al 1997 Incentive spirometry performance. Chest 111: 559–563

Benumof J L 1995 Anaesthesia for thoracic surgery, 2nd edn. WB Saunders, Philadelphia

Benumof J L, Alfery D D 2000 Anesthesia for thoracic surgery. In: Miller R D (ed) Anesthesia, 5th edn. Churchill Livingstone, Philadelphia, pp 1665–1752

Schroeder D 1999 The preoperative period summary. Chest 115: 44S–46S

Sherry K 1996 Management of patients undergoing oesophagectomy. The report of the National Confidential Enquiry into Perioperative Deaths 1996/1997. Nuffield Provincial Hospitals Trust, London, p 57–61

Shimizu T, Kinouchi K, Yoshiya I 1997 Arterial oxygenation during one lung ventilation. Canadian Journal of Anaesthesia 44: 1162–1166

Slinger PD (ed) 2004 Progress in thoracic anaesthesia. Lippincott, Williams & Wilkins, New York, pp 1–357

Youngberg J A, Lake C L, Roizen M F, Wilson R S 2000 Cardiac, vascular and thoracic anaesthesia. Churchill Livingstone, Philadelphia

Zibrak J D, O'Donnell C R, Marton K 1990 Indications for pulmonary function testing. Annals of Internal Medicine 112: 763–771

Anaesthesia for cardiac surgery

40

The cardiac surgical theatre, with its profusion of personnel and equipment, is often intimidating to the trainee anaesthetist. However, the principles of anaesthetic care are similar to those elsewhere, the main difference being that essential organ perfusion is usually achieved artificially when the heart itself is the object of surgery. Operations are termed 'open heart' or 'on-pump' when the functions of the heart and lungs are assumed by an extracorporeal pump and gas exchange unit (cardiopulmonary bypass, CPB). Coronary artery surgery can also be performed without CPB, known as off-pump coronary artery surgery or OPCAB. A small number of cardiac operations are performed through a thoracotomy incision and are termed 'closed' procedures.

Excluding the insertion of pacemakers, more than 39 000 cardiac operations are undertaken each year in the UK in NHS hospitals. Approximately 30 000 are for ischaemic heart disease and the remainder are for congenital abnormalities and acquired valvular disease.

CONGENITAL CARDIAC ABNORMALITIES

These occur at a rate of 6–8 per 1000 live births. Correction of a third may be undertaken without CPB, but the remainder, including septal defects, valve abnormalities and cyanotic lesions such as Fallot's tetralogy, require cardiopulmonary bypass.

ACQUIRED VALVULAR DISEASE

Stenosis or incompetence most commonly involves the mitral and aortic valves. Surgery usually comprises replacement with an artificial valve or repair, guided by intraoperative transoesophageal echocardiography. Artificial valves may be mechanical prostheses with a tilting disc or tissue valves (usually a pig valve) specially mounted and prepared (heterograft). Mechanical valves are reliable but necessitate the patient receiving anticoagulants for life. This is not usually necessary when porcine heterografts are used,

but re-operation is common because of valve failure after about 10 years.

ISCHAEMIC HEART DISEASE

The concept of revascularizing ischaemic myocardium was introduced in the 1960s with the insertion of a portion of saphenous vein from aorta to coronary artery distal to a stenosis (Fig. 40.1). Since then, coronary artery bypass grafting (CABG) has become the most commonly performed cardiac operation. The internal mammary artery is used routinely as a graft conduit. Complete arterial revascularization is possible using arteries such as the radial and epigastric arteries. Improved surgical techniques have increased the popularity of off-pump coronary artery surgery but its precise role remains uncertain.

Angina is relieved in 80–90% of patients, but life expectancy is not increased in all groups when compared with medical treatment. Prognosis is improved by surgery in patients with disease of the left main coronary artery or its two principal branches, triple-vessel disease or impaired left ventricular function.

CARDIOPULMONARY BYPASS

The essential components of a cardiopulmonary bypass circuit are:

- pumps
- an oxygenator
- connecting tubes and filters
- fluid prime of these components.

These are normally arranged as shown in Figure 40.2. Blood from the venous side of the circulation, the venae cavae or right atrium, is drained by gravity to a venous reservoir and thence to a gas exchange unit (oxygenator) where oxygen is delivered to, and carbon dioxide removed from, the blood. The 'arterialized' blood is pumped into the arterial side of the circulation, usually into the ascending aorta. The

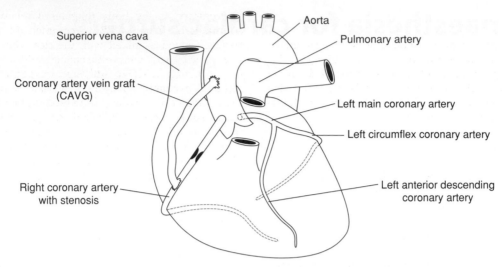

Fig. 40.1
Diagrammatic representation of coronary arteries and CAVG. 'Triple' vessel disease includes right, left circumflex and left anterior descending arteries.

heart and lungs are thus 'bypassed' or isolated and their function maintained temporarily by mechanical equipment remote from the body. A heat exchanger in the oxygenator varies the temperature of blood rap-

idly and redundant or spilled blood in or around the bypassed heart may be drained and returned to the venous reservoir for oxygenation and subsequent return to the circulation.

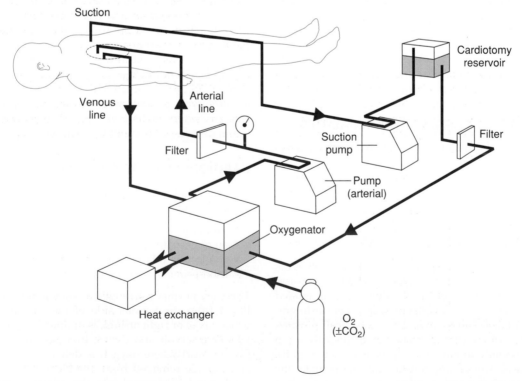

Fig. 40.2
Components of a cardiopulmonary bypass circuit.

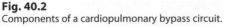

Pumps

Roller pumps displace blood around the circuit by intermittent compression of the circuit tubing during each sweep. By intermittent acceleration of the roller head, a 'pulsatile' waveform may be achieved, but there is no evidence that this slightly more physiological flow improves outcome.

Oxygenator

Membrane oxygenators (Fig. 40.3) comprise a semi-permeable membrane which separates gas and blood phases and through which gas exchange occurs.

Connecting tubes, filters, manometer, suction

These must be sterile and nontoxic and should damage blood as little as possible. They may be coated with heparin. A filter should also be incorporated in the arterial tubes to remove gas emboli which would pass directly to the aorta. Suction pumps are supplied to vent blood collecting in the pulmonary circulation or left ventricle during bypass and also to remove spilled blood from the pericardial sac. The blood is collected in the 'cardiotomy' reservoir, filtered and returned to the main circuit. This suction also causes damage to blood components.

Fluid prime

Originally, it was anticipated that connection of the circulation to an external circuit would necessitate the bypass circuit being filled with anticoagulated whole blood. This increases exposure to donor blood and may lead to incompatibility reactions. However, this is unnecessary as the body tolerates a relatively low haematocrit. When CPB is commenced and the patient's blood is mixed with the clear fluids which prime the bypass circuit, the haematocrit decreases to approximately 20–25%. Although oxygen content is reduced, availability may be increased by improved organ blood flow resulting from reduced blood viscosity. In some patients (low body weight, children or those with a low preoperative haemoglobin in whom dilution would reduce the haematocrit to below 20%), blood may be added to the prime. In the normal adult, 'clear' primes are used almost exclusively (usually a crystalloid/colloid mixture). Most units have individual recipes for addition to the prime (e.g. mannitol, sodium bicarbonate and potassium) to achieve an isosmolar solution of physiological pH.

PREOPERATIVE ASSESSMENT

Most patients presenting for cardiac surgery have undergone comprehensive cardiological investigation and are taking medications. In addition to the routine investigations undertaken before any operation, specialized techniques are used to assess the cardiac lesion and degree of resultant dysfunction. The results of these investigations permit the anaesthetist to identify patients at particular risk where extra care and monitoring are required.

EXERCISE ELECTROCARDIOGRAPHY

Various stress protocols are used whereby a standard exercise test provokes ischaemic changes and symptoms. Changes in rhythm, rate, arterial pressure

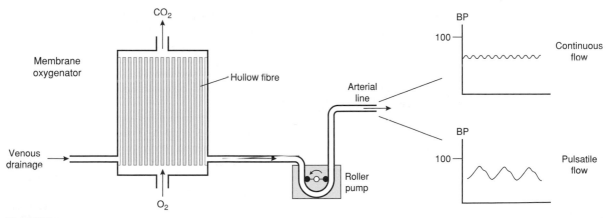

Fig. 40.3
Diagrammatic representation of a membrane oxygenator.

and conduction are recorded. The anaesthetist identifies the most useful ECG leads to monitor during surgery and may note the rate–pressure product (heart rate × systolic arterial pressure) at which ischaemia occurs, although this is unreliable under anaesthesia.

CARDIAC CATHETERIZATION

Considerable information may be obtained from catheterization:

- Evidence of failing function or of gradients across stenosed valves may be identified by pressure monitoring.
- Oximetry of blood at different sites indicates if shunts are present (Fig. 40.4).
- Cardiac output may be measured.
- The injection of radiopaque dye into aorta or ventricles assesses incompetence of valves and the efficiency of ventricular contraction (ejection fraction) and wall motion:

$$\text{Ejection fraction (EF)} = \frac{\text{end-diastolic volume} - \text{end-systolic volume}}{\text{end-diastolic volume}}$$

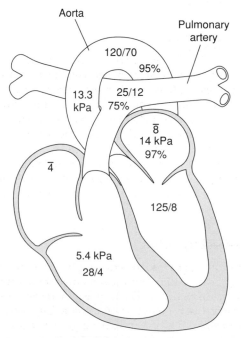

Fig. 40.4
Diagram of catherization values in a normal adult: pressures (mmHg), oxygen saturations (%) and tensions (kPa).

- Injection of dye into coronary arteries defines the anatomy of the coronary circulation and the degree of patency or sites of stenosis.

ECHOCARDIOGRAPHY

Ultrasound is used to identify myocardial motion and valvular function. Preoperatively, this may be performed using a transthoracic or transoesophageal approach. The latter involves passing an ultrasound probe into the oesophagus under sedation. The proximity of the heart and oesophagus allows high-quality 'real-time' images of the anatomy and function of the heart. Doppler techniques allow recognition of the direction and velocity of blood flow and are valuable in the diagnosis of valvular disease.

RADIONUCLIDE IMAGING

By imaging the activity of an appropriate radioisotope as it passes through the heart or into the myocardium, ventricular function and myocardial perfusion may be assessed. Technetium images blood volume and may be used to demonstrate abnormal wall motion and EF. Thallium, which is taken up by the myocardium, may be used to assess regional blood flow. These techniques may be used before and after exercise and/or therapy, e.g. dobutamine infusion.

PREOPERATIVE DRUG THERAPY

Beta-blocking agents. Continued administration of these drugs up to the time of surgery is desirable, as discontinuation may increase the risk of perioperative infarction.

Calcium antagonists have a negative inotropic effect but, as with the β-blockers, it is preferable to continue therapy throughout the perioperative period.

Nitrates should be continued and may be included in the premedication if indicated.

Digitalis. In most centres, digoxin is discontinued 24–48 h before surgery to diminish digoxin-associated arrhythmias after surgery.

Diuretics should be continued until the day before surgery.

Anticoagulants, including aspirin and clopidogrel, are usually stopped up to 1 week before surgery to permit coagulation to return towards normal. If there is a high risk of embolism, anticoagulants should be continued and coagulation defects treated postoperatively with transfusion of blood products.

Angiotensin-converting enzyme (ACE) inhibitors are prescribed for hypertension and cardiac failure. They may produce significant vasodilatation and hypotension intraoperatively and postoperatively. Perioperative use varies from unit to unit – they may be stopped up to 1 week before surgery or continued until the day of operation.

Potassium-channel activators may be continued up to the day of operation.

OTHER INVESTIGATIONS REQUIRED BEFORE SURGERY

Haemoglobin. Haemoglobin should be adequate ($> 11 \text{ g dL}^{-1}$) to prevent excessive haemodilution during bypass.

Coagulation. Clotting studies should be performed before surgery. Specific defects require correction before surgery, or alternatively the appropriate blood products should be made available.

Electrolytes. Serum potassium concentration should be within normal limits.

Urea and creatinine. Raised concentrations indicate an increased risk of renal failure postoperatively. Adequate urine output should be ensured after operation.

Liver function tests. Abnormal values may indicate congestive cardiac failure.

ASSESSMENT OF RISK

The mortality rate associated with cardiac surgery has decreased in the last 2–3 decades but is still significant. Operative mortality for coronary artery surgery is relatively constant at 2–3% even though patients are older and sicker. Valve surgery is usually associated with a mortality of 3–10%. When more extensive surgery is undertaken, e.g. multiple valve replacement or coronary artery vein graft (CAVG) plus valve replacement, mortality rate increases.

Patients with an increased risk of perioperative complications may be identified during preoperative assessment. Increased risk is associated with the following factors:

- age > 65 years
- female sex
- recent unstable angina or myocardial infarction
- emergency surgery or re-operation
- poor left ventricular function as shown by:
  left ventricular end-diastolic pressure > 18 mmHg
  ejection fraction < 30%
  dyskinetic wall motion
- increasing number of vessels affected
- other system disease, e.g. diabetes mellitus, cerebrovascular or peripheral vascular disease, renal failure and obesity.

MONITORING

Extensive and accurate monitoring is essential throughout the perioperative period for the safe practice of cardiac surgery.

ECG

ECG should be monitored throughout the perioperative period. The ideal system is one which allows simultaneous multiple-lead monitoring or at least switching between leads II and V5, for accurate identification of ischaemia. Rate and rhythm should also be observed.

Systemic arterial pressure

Arterial cannulation is mandatory: this permits not only direct measurement but also facilitates sampling of arterial blood for analysis.

Central venous pressure

Right-sided filling pressure should be monitored by a catheter placed into a central vein. In selected cases, a flow-directed pulmonary artery catheter (PAC) may be inserted at or before induction to monitor left-heart filling pressure.

Cardiac output

Cardiac output (CO) may be measured by thermodilution using a PAC. This, together with the derivatives of stroke work, pulmonary and systemic vascular resistances and tissue oxygen flux, allows accurate titration of vasoactive infusions. Modified PACs allow real-time measurement of CO, mixed venous oxygen saturation and right ventricular function.

CO may also be measured by techniques such as oesophageal Doppler and pulse contour analysis but these have not replaced thermodilution in routine practice.

Echocardiography

Transoesophageal echocardiography is very useful during anaesthesia. Abnormal motion of the ventricular wall detected in this way is a reliable index of myocardial ischaemia and may guide drug therapy or indicate the need for further surgical revascularization. When repair of an abnormal valve is attempted, it guides the surgeon's choice of operation and indicates the adequacy of the repair. Similarly, problems with a replaced valve are immediately obvious and may be corrected before chest closure.

EEG

A simple guide to cerebral activity and perfusion may be obtained from the various forms of processed EEG monitor. The value of this technique and of the monitoring of evoked potentials is uncertain.

Temperature

Core temperature should be monitored from the nasopharynx, which approximates to brain temperature.

Biochemical and haematological analysis

Facilities should be available for immediate analysis of blood gas tensions, acid–base balance, and serum potassium and blood glucose concentrations.

Measurement of packed cell volume and coagulation status should also be available. Activated clotting time (ACT) can be measured quickly in the operating theatre using the Haemochron apparatus (normal = 100–120 s), but access to the haematology laboratory should be rapid for assessment of a full clotting screen. Thromboelastography – the assessment of viscoelastic changes in blood during clotting – may usefully assess haemostatic function in theatre.

Display

ECG, pressure waveforms and a digital output of heart rate and pressures should be displayed clearly on screens visible to surgeon, anaesthetist and perfusionist.

PATHOPHYSIOLOGICAL CONSIDERATIONS

The anaesthetist should have a clear understanding of the fundamental principles of cardiac physiology. Accurate monitoring reveals alterations in cardiac function and permits the anaesthetist to manipulate factors which ensure adequate pump output (Fig. 40.5) and myocardial blood supply.

Preload and contractility determine the amount of work that the heart performs. In the failing heart, the afterload determines how much work is expended in overcoming pressure compared with that used to provide forward flow. Thus, cardiac output may be increased either by increasing preload or contractility, or by reducing afterload. However, oxygen consumption is raised by increasing heart rate, contractility, preload or afterload. Augmentation of cardiac output by increasing preload or contractility may thus have a detrimental effect on oxygen balance. However, reduction of afterload may increase

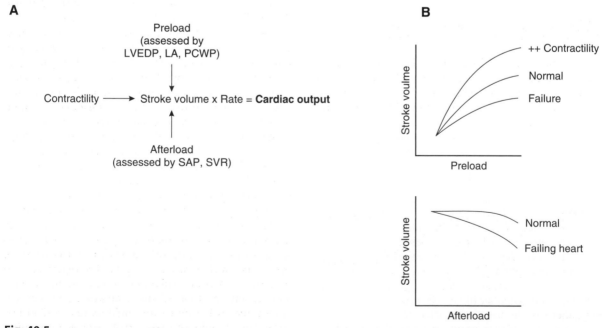

A

Preload
(assessed by
LVEDP, LA, PCWP)
↓
Contractility ⟶ Stroke volume x Rate = **Cardiac output**
↑
Afterload
(assessed by SAP, SVR)

B

Stroke voulme vs Preload:
++ Contractility
Normal
Failure

Stroke volume vs Afterload:
Normal
Failing heart

Fig. 40.5
Important aspects of mechanical function.

cardiac output while simultaneously reducing oxygen demand.

Adequate coronary perfusion demands maintenance of diastolic aortic pressure at adequate levels. Oxygen supply to the myocardium occurs predominantly in diastole and is dependent on the gradient between diastolic aortic pressure and intraventricular pressure, and on the diastolic time. The portion of myocardium most at risk of developing ischaemia is the left ventricular endocardium. Figure 40.6 illustrates how these variables affect oxygen supply and demand in the myocardium and how a satisfactory supply/demand ratio may be preserved.

Care of the patient with valvular heart disease depends on the valvular lesion. Abnormal heart rates are not tolerated well by a heart with a diseased valve. Incompetent valves tend to perform better if afterload is maintained at a low level, as this reduces the regurgitant fraction and increases forward flow. Patients with valvular stenosis require adequate preload and do not tolerate rapid reduction in peripheral resistance. This is especially true of patients with aortic stenosis where most of the afterload to left ventricular ejection is caused by the stenosed valve itself. This afterload is fixed and cannot be reduced by lowering peripheral resistance. Vasodilatation in these patients produces marked hypotension and results in failure of perfusion of the hypertrophied myocardium with no increase in forward flow through the stenosed valve.

ANAESTHETIC TECHNIQUE

There is no single preferred anaesthetic technique for cardiac surgery. The choice of a specific agent is less important than the care with which the drug is administered and its effects monitored. The techniques

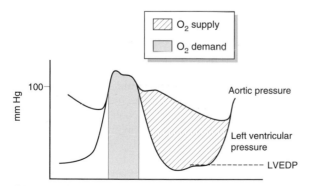

Fig. 40.6
The factors which determine myocardial oxygen supply and demand.

described here are suitable for standard CABG, i.e. with cardiopulmonary bypass. Anaesthesia for off-pump coronary surgery is complicated by severe haemodynamic alterations when the heart is positioned by the surgeon and by intraoperative myocardial ischaemia when coronary arteries are cross-clamped during anastomosis of the grafts. Readers are referred to more specialized texts for details of management.

PREMEDICATION

The most important preoperative preparation comprises a full explanation to patients of what is about to occur and their development of rapport with, and confidence in, the nursing and medical staff.

Most patients may be sedated preoperatively with an oral benzodiazepine (lorazepam 2–4 mg or temazepam 20–50 mg). In the particularly anxious patient, heavy sedation may be required to prevent increases in heart rate and arterial pressure before operation. A combination of an oral benzodiazepine and an intramuscular opioid is also satisfactory.

INDUCTION

All drugs and equipment should be ready and the theatre and bypass circuit available for immediate use before the patient arrives in the anaesthetic room.

Before induction, ECG electrodes should be applied and the ECG trace displayed. Arterial and large-gauge venous cannulae should be inserted under local anaesthesia. The lungs should be preoxygenated.

Induction may be achieved in a variety of ways. The standard agents may be given in small doses (e.g. thiopental 1–3 mg kg⁻¹, etomidate 0.05–0.2 mg kg⁻¹), or large doses of an opioid (e.g. morphine 1–4 mg kg⁻¹, fentanyl 10–100 μg kg⁻¹) may be administered with a benzodiazepine to obtain unconsciousness. A combination of these techniques may be used; consciousness is obtunded by an opioid in moderate dose and hypnosis is then produced by a small dose of an induction agent. An alternative is a target-controlled infusion of propofol with the target concentration increased in small steps, perhaps accompanied by an infusion of a short-acting opioid such as alfentanil or remifentanil.

As consciousness is lost, a muscle relaxant is administered and ventilation supported when necessary. Almost all currently available relaxants have been used during cardiac surgery. The objective is to undertake tracheal intubation without cardiovascular stimulation and thus adequate analgesia/anaesthesia is required. A low-pressure, high-volume, cuffed tracheal tube should be used. Positive-pressure ventilation is continued, usually with an oxygen/air mixture.

Percutaneous cannulation of a subclavian or internal jugular vein is performed using a multilumen catheter to allow monitoring and infusion. Nasopharyngeal and peripheral temperature probes are applied and a urinary catheter inserted. Mechanical ventilation is continued with a breathing system containing a humidifier and bacterial filter.

Previously identified 'poor-risk' patients may require more extensive monitoring of pressures and cardiac output before induction and catheters may be inserted under local anaesthesia. Induction may be undertaken in theatre with the full team ready for immediate surgery. Adequate sedation must be provided during insertion of invasive monitoring catheters.

MAINTENANCE – PRE-BYPASS

During this period, surgical procedure involves preparation of the patient, skin incision and sternotomy. Harvesting of arterial and venous grafts follows and then insertion of arterial and venous bypass cannulae.

Anaesthetic management is designed to maintain stability of heart rate and arterial pressure, particularly at moments of profound stimulation, notably skin incision and sternotomy. If a technique based on i.v. opioids or volatile anaesthetics has been chosen, then additional i.v. analgesic drug or inhalational anaesthetic should be given before stimulation. Alternatively, opiate infusion rates may be increased temporarily as necessary, perhaps accompanied by increased target concentrations of propofol. The tendency of isoflurane to produce a 'coronary steal' (the diversion of blood *away from* ischaemic muscle) is not of clinical importance. There is evidence that it improves the ability of the heart to tolerate myocardial ischaemia by a mechanism involving ATP-dependent potassium channels.

Arterial blood gas tensions, serum potassium concentration, haematocrit and the activated clotting time (ACT) should be measured when surgery is under way and conditions are stable. Before cannulation for bypass, heparin ($300\,units\,kg^{-1}$; $3\,mg\,kg^{-1}$) should be injected into a secure central catheter of proven patency. ACT measurement should be repeated 3 min after injection of heparin; the value should exceed four times normal. Cardioplegia should be prepared and stored at 4°C.

When preparations are complete, the bypass pump commences and circulation is assumed by the bypass circuit.

MAINTENANCE – ON BYPASS

Two factors complicate the provision of anaesthesia during cardiopulmonary bypass. Firstly, haemodilution, hypotension, nonpulsatile flow and hypothermia may alter the pharmacokinetics of drugs administered previously. Secondly, by short-circuiting the lungs, bypass prevents conventional inhalational anaesthesia. Techniques therefore include administration of bolus doses of an opioid or benzodiazepine, administration of a volatile agent into the gas flow of the oxygenator or continuous intravenous infusion of propofol. Additional doses of muscle relaxant may also be given. When full-pump oxygenator flow is reached and ventricular ejection ceases, ventilation is suspended.

Surgery is preceded usually by cross-clamping the aorta to isolate the heart and prevent backflow. In the case of valvular surgery, the appropriate valve is exposed, excised and a new valve sutured in place. During coronary artery vein grafting, the distal anastomoses are usually completed first and, following release of the cross-clamp to permit restoration of myocardial perfusion, the proximal anastomoses are constructed using a portion of the aorta isolated by a side-clamp (Fig. 40.7).

Myocardial preservation

Most surgical techniques on the heart require it to be immobile. On bypass, the aorta is cross-clamped between the aortic cannula and the aortic valve, thus isolating the heart from the flow of oxygenated blood. During aortic cross-clamping, ischaemic damage to the myocardium may be minimized by attempts to reduce myocardial oxygen consumption. Techniques of myocardial preservation include hypothermia to reduce basal metabolic rate and cardiac arrest to reduce oxygen requirements to a minimum, the latter usually achieved by injecting 500–1000 mL of crystalloid cardioplegic solution around the coronary arteries. Many cardioplegic solutions are available; the majority contain potassium and a membrane-stabilizing agent, e.g. procaine. In some centres, warm blood-based cardioplegic and reperfusate solutions are infused continuously to minimize ischaemic and reperfusion injuries and improve delivery of oxygen and other substrates to the myocardium.

Cooling is achieved by the use of ice-cold cardioplegia and by pouring cold fluid (4°C) into the pericardial sac and into the heart chambers if they have been opened. If the heart is cooled to 15°C, it withstands total ischaemia for approximately 1 h. The technique used most commonly involves moderate hypothermia of the whole body to 32°C and local cooling of the myocardium to a temperature of 15–18°C. If cross-clamping times are prolonged, cardioplegic cooling must be repeated if spontaneous cardiac contraction resumes.

A

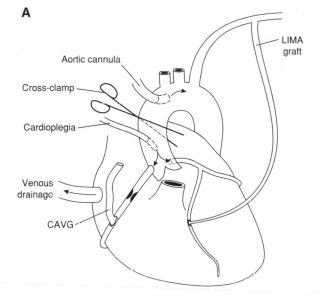

B

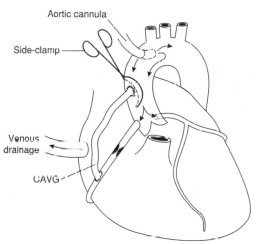

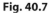

Fig. 40.7
Arrangement of cross-clamp, cardioplegia and anastomoses.
(A) A left internal mammary artery (LIMA) graft. **(B)** Vein graft
with side clamp on aorta.

A modification to this traditional technique has
been the combination of local cooling of the heart with
body temperatures of 33–37°C during CPB in an
attempt to limit postoperative hypothermia.

Perfusion on bypass

At normothermia, a pump flow of $2.4\,L\,min^{-1}\,m^{-2}$ of
body surface area is required to prevent inadequate
perfusion of the tissues. The pressure achieved within
the vascular system is dependent on pump output

and systemic vascular resistance. Controversy exists
regarding optimum perfusion pressure, as essential
organs, particularly the brain, may be damaged if
mean arterial pressure is < 45 mmHg. Unfortunately,
perfusion is difficult to assess clinically, especially in
the hypothermic patient.

Following the onset of bypass, haemodilution
causes marked decreases in peripheral resistance and
arterial pressure, which in most instances resolve spontaneously in 5–10 min. If this does not occur, arterial
pressure may be increased by raising systemic resistance with a sympathomimetic agent, e.g. metaraminol
or phenylephrine. Frequently, peripheral resistance
and arterial pressure increase during the hypothermic
period of bypass as a result of increasing concentrations of catecholamines and then decrease as active
rewarming results in profound vasodilatation.

Coagulation control

Adequate anticoagulation must be maintained during
CPB; ACT should be measured every 30 min and extra
heparin administered as necessary.

Oxygen delivery

Arterial blood samples should be obtained regularly
and blood gas tensions and haematocrit measured.
Continuous blood gas analysis is increasingly common. Oxygen carriage is dependent on haemoglobin
concentration in addition to adequate oxygen tension.
Haematocrit may be permitted to decrease to 20% but
further reduction should be prevented by the addition
of packed cells or blood to the bypass circuit.

Acid–base balance

The development of metabolic acidosis suggests
that perfusion is inadequate and, if necessary (base
deficit > $6–8\,mmol\,L^{-1}$), sodium bicarbonate may be
administered.

Serum potassium

Serum potassium concentration should be maintained
at approximately $4.5\,mmol\,L^{-1}$ by the administration of
potassium chloride (10–20 mmol) as required.

RESTORATION OF SPONTANEOUS HEARTBEAT

When the cross-clamp has been removed, oxygenated
blood again flows into the coronary arteries, washing
out cardioplegia and repaying the oxygen debt.

Usually, the heart regains activity spontaneously. In a minority of patients, it starts to beat in sinus rhythm but reverts usually to ventricular fibrillation; internal defibrillation is required to convert fibrillation to sinus rhythm and is successful only if pH, serum potassium concentration, oxygenation and temperature are approaching normal values. The heat exchanger in the oxygenator is used to raise the temperature of blood, but peripheral temperature is often depressed for some time. If a spontaneous heartbeat cannot be maintained, pacing wires should be attached to the epicardium to initiate activity artificially.

TERMINATION OF BYPASS

When body temperature exceeds 36°C, metabolic indices are normal and a regular heartbeat is present, the establishment of spontaneous cardiac output is attempted. An increasing volume of venous return is diverted into the right atrium past the extracorporeal cannulae by constricting the venous return catheter to the pump. Blood is now passing again through the pulmonary circulation and mechanical ventilation should be restarted; 100% oxygen is given, as the gas-exchanging efficiency of the lung is unknown at this stage and any air bubbles which have not been vented enlarge in volume if nitrous oxide is introduced.

Any output or ejection from the left ventricle gives a 'blip' on the arterial pressure trace after a QRS complex. If the myocardium is contracting satisfactorily, pump flow is reduced cautiously and the heart, now receiving all the venous return, achieves normal output.

Arterial pressure is the most easily measured index of successful termination of bypass but is a derivative of cardiac output and peripheral resistance. If there is doubt regarding pump efficiency, cardiac output should be measured and peripheral resistance derived.

If CPB is discontinued successfully, preload should be optimized by infusion of as much as possible of the residual fluid contained in the pump circuit. This is facilitated by the administration of vasodilators such as GTN. If cardiac output is inadequate, the circulation is reassumed by the bypass pump and the heart allowed more time to recover.

Low output

If the heart is unable to generate sufficient output to maintain body perfusion after preload has been optimized, further action is required. An increase in contractility is produced by inotropic drugs. The simplest is a bolus of dilute adrenaline, but the most commonly used drugs are dobutamine, dopamine (both 2–20 µg kg^{-1} min^{-1}) or adrenaline (0.05–0.2 µg kg^{-1} min^{-1}) by infusion.

All these drugs tend to precipitate tachyarrhythmias; adrenaline and dopamine also cause vasoconstriction in high doses. They all increase myocardial oxygen demand and may precipitate infarction in patients with ischaemic heart disease.

Alternatively, a phosphodiesterase inhibitor such as milrinone or enoximone may be given. These drugs act by inhibiting phosphodiesterase type III found in cardiac muscle, thus reducing the breakdown of cyclic AMP. They improve myocardial performance and are potent arterial and venous dilators. By reducing afterload, they not only reduce myocardial oxygen demand but also, in the failing ventricle, augment forward flow into the aorta. Administration is by bolus dose during CPB after aortic cross-clamp removal and subsequently by intravenous infusion.

If these pharmacological methods fail to produce an adequate cardiac output, the intra-aortic balloon pump (IABP) may be used.

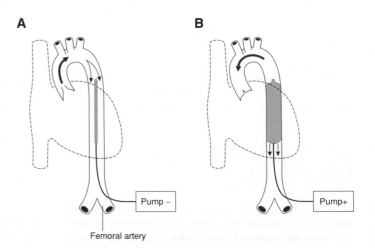

Fig. 40.8
Intra-aortic balloon pump. **(A)** Systole. **(B)** Diastole.

Intra-aortic balloon pump

The principle of the IABP is illustrated in Figure 40.8. If the balloon in the aorta is inflated immediately after systole, diastolic filling pressure is augmented and myocardial oxygen balance improved. Inflation also displaces blood from the aorta and increases peripheral flow. The balloon is deflated immediately before systole and this creates a low pressure in the aorta as ventricular output commences, reducing afterload (and thus oxygen consumption) and at the same time augmenting output.

COAGULATION CONTROL

When the bypass cannulae have been removed, residual effects of heparin are antagonized with protamine. Protamine 1 mg (or less) is given for each 100 units of heparin; the dosage may be titrated using the ACT. The drug should be given slowly, especially if there is residual hypovolaemia or raised pulmonary vascular resistance. Protamine may produce systemic hypotension rapidly, as a result of peripheral vasodilatation, but may also cause pulmonary vasoconstriction. In excessive dosage, it has anticoagulant effects.

Heparin is not the only factor which may cause bleeding during and after bypass. Contact of blood with foreign surfaces in the bypass circuit and suction tubing causes consumption of clotting factors and of platelets. Thus, if heparin appears to have been reversed satisfactorily and unexplained bleeding persists, thromboelastography or a full clotting screen should be performed. Platelet concentrate should be infused if the platelet count is low or platelet function unsatisfactory and clotting factors may be replaced by the infusion of fresh frozen plasma and/or cryoprecipitate.

Surgically, the period following termination of bypass is concerned with prevention of haemorrhage and closure of the chest with drains in situ. In addition to the maintenance of unconsciousness, the anaesthetist must ensure the efficiency of myocardial performance, oxygen balance and peripheral perfusion together with correction of metabolic, biochemical, haematological or temperature abnormalities.

CONTROL OF THE CIRCULATION AFTER BYPASS

Despite measures to protect the myocardium during bypass, the heart suffers some deterioration in function and its contractility is reduced postoperatively.

Thus, it operates on a lower Frank-Starling curve (see Fig. 40.5) and requires a higher preload to produce the same output. The contractility of the myocardium later improves and this increased efficiency permits a reduction in preload.

In addition, the peripheral circulation usually remains vasoconstricted for several hours postoperatively. In patients with reasonable ventricular function, hypertension may thus occur after bypass, especially in operations involving the aortic valve. The increased afterload results in additional myocardial oxygen consumption and tends to reduce cardiac output.

Reduction of peripheral resistance and systemic arterial pressure by a vasodilator such as sodium nitroprusside protects suture lines from damage, decreases oxygen demand, increases cardiac output if preload is not reduced excessively, improves peripheral perfusion and accelerates warming.

Conversely, some patients are very vasodilated after CPB, with cardiac output normal or even increased. This reflects a whole-body inflammatory response to CPB with the release of numerous vasoactive mediators. Treatment is with an infusion of norepinephrine or perhaps vasopressin, which is a very potent vasoconstrictor.

OTHER ASPECTS OF MAINTENANCE AFTER BYPASS

In addition to maintaining cardiac function and oxygen supply to the tissues during this period, the anaesthetist should ensure that normality is regained as soon as possible, and maintained, in respect of the following.

Temperature

Core temperature is raised easily on bypass via the oxygenator. However, the efficiency of rewarming the peripheral tissues depends on the patient's weight, total flow rate and peripheral perfusion. After bypass, there is often a decrease in core temperature (after-drop).

Biochemical monitoring

Essential monitoring includes blood gas tensions, acid–base balance, serum potassium concentration and haematocrit.

Cardiac rhythm

Heart block

Epicardial pacing wires should be inserted if AV dissociation occurs, traditionally to allow ventricular pacing. Atrial pacing (for bradycardia) or AV sequential pacing (for heart block) ensures that the atrial contribution to ventricular filling is not lost. This is particularly important if ventricular compliance or function is poor.

Supraventricular arrhythmias

Direct current cardioversion is the most convenient treatment when the chest is open. After chest closure, options include amiodarone, β-blockade, verapamil or adenosine.

Ventricular arrhythmias

The threshold for arrhythmias is reduced by hypokalaemia and serum potassium concentration should be maintained above 4.5 mmol L^{-1}. If ventricular arrhythmias persist, lidocaine is the drug of first choice.

TRANSFER TO POSTOPERATIVE ITU

It is normal to prolong the same level of support and monitoring undertaken during surgery into the postoperative period. The duration of this care depends on the individual patient's response to surgery and speed of recovery.

Transfer of the patient from theatre to the intensive care unit may involve journeys along corridors and into lifts. It is essential that controlled ventilation is continued and ECG, arterial oxygen saturation and arterial pressure monitored during transfer. Battery-powered infusion pumps are essential to allow uninterrupted vasoactive drug infusions during transfer.

POSTOPERATIVE INTENSIVE THERAPY

The facilities and staff used to treat patients after cardiac surgery vary considerably. Some hospitals nurse these patients in a general ITU or specialist cardiac ITU, while others have cardiac surgery recovery areas where early tracheal extubation is normal.

Regardless of location, there should be a well-practised routine for the care of patients after surgery. Usually, ventilation of the lungs and full cardiovascular monitoring are recommended immediately. The principles of care in this phase are similar to those described for the period of anaesthesia after termination of bypass.

HAEMODYNAMIC CARE

On return to the ITU, attention is directed usually towards achieving vasodilatation, reduction of afterload and maintenance of preload. Blood transfusion may be required. Urine output may be maintained with diuretics, but usually spontaneous diuresis occurs in response to the fluid load received in theatre. Serum potassium concentration must be monitored carefully and abnormalities corrected.

The majority of patients stabilize and regain adequate peripheral perfusion over the succeeding 3–4 h, permitting the level of cardiovascular support to be reduced.

In a minority of patients, low cardiac output requires the continued use of inotropic agents, vasodilators and, if necessary, IABP for some time.

BLOOD LOSS

This should be measured accurately. If excessive (300–400 mL h^{-1}), it may be necessary to re-operate on the patient. Attention to the coagulation system is required and additional protamine or coagulation factors prescribed as necessary. The most sinister complication of excessive bleeding is cardiac tamponade, which requires rapid thoracotomy and evacuation of blood from the chest. If deterioration occurs rapidly, thoracotomy must be undertaken in the ITU.

VENTILATION

In the 1960s, morphine anaesthesia for valve surgery in patients with poor ventricular function dictated that postoperative mechanical ventilation was required for 18–24 h. Later, the aims of postoperative ventilation were to avoid shivering following hypothermic bypass and to prevent hypoxaemia and hypercapnia during the period of haemodynamic instability which is common in the first few postoperative hours. These aims were generally achieved by assisting ventilation for 4–8 h and this remains current practice in most units. Thus, when the patient's arterial pressure, peripheral perfusion and core and peripheral temperatures are satisfactory, urine output is good, blood loss is less than 100 mL h^{-1}, and the patient is conscious and maintaining satisfactory blood gas tensions with an inspired oxygen concentration of 50% or less, a trial of spontaneous ventilation is indicated. If respiratory volumes are adequate and the patient is not distressed, the trachea may be extubated.

In some centres, earlier extubation is undertaken. The trachea is extubated either in the operating theatre or within 2 h of surgery, provided that the criteria for extubation detailed above are met. This is possible only if cross-clamp and bypass times are brief and an effort is made to minimize temperature after-drop following cardiopulmonary bypass.

Unfortunately, some patients still require prolonged mechanical ventilation after cardiac surgery. The principles of their care are as detailed in Chapter 41.

ANALGESIA AND SEDATION

The anaesthetic technique used determines the timing of administration of postoperative analgesia. Even after high-dose opioid techniques, patients usually show some response in the first 2–3 h after surgery and it is useful to assess cerebral function at this stage in case damage has occurred. Pain relief is produced most commonly with i.v. opioids either by bolus dose or by continuous infusion supplemented by a propofol infusion for sedation. Recovery is rapid after the propofol infusion is stopped and this may facilitate early extubation.

An alternative is epidural infusion analgesia if a catheter has been inserted preoperatively. Concerns over the risk of epidural haematoma in patients who are fully anticoagulated after catheter insertion have prevented the widespread use of this technique.

As important as pharmacological support is the human rapport which should be achieved between staff and patient.

FURTHER READING

Hensley F A, Martin D E, Gravlee G P 2002 A practical approach to cardiac anesthesia, 3rd edn. Lippincott, Williams & Wilkins, Philadelphia

Kaplan H A, Reich D L, Konstadt S N (eds) 2006 Cardiac anesthesia, 5th edn. WB Saunders, Philadelphia

Wasnick J D 1998 Handbook of cardiac anesthesia and perioperative care: a demythologized approach. Butterworth-Heinemann, Boston

41 The intensive care unit

The intensive care unit (ICU) is the hospital facility within which the highest levels of continuous patient care and treatment are provided. The Department of Health NHS Executive defines intensive care as 'a service for patients with potentially recoverable conditions who can benefit from more detailed observation and treatment than can safely be provided in general ward or high dependency areas'.

The optimal size of an ICU in terms of bed numbers relates to the number of acute beds in the hospital. In the UK, this is generally 1–2% of the total number of acute beds. The design of ICUs varies from hospital to hospital but they are characterized by being designated areas in which there is a minimum nurse:patient ratio of 1:1 in addition to a nurse in charge at all times, 24 h cover by resident medical staff and the facilities to support organ system failures. High-dependency units (HDUs) are designated areas with a nurse:patient ratio of 1:2 in addition to a nurse in charge at all times, continuous *availability* of medical staff either from the admitting speciality or from the ICU, and an appropriate level of monitoring and other equipment. ICUs and HDUs may be either separate geographical entities or may be combined, with the beds occupied and staffed according to the prevailing need for ICU or HDU levels of care. Care on ICU, HDU and ordinary wards is generally referred to as Level 3, Level 2 and Level 1 care respectively.

The physical space for each bed in an ICU is greater than on an ordinary ward because several nurses may need to treat a patient simultaneously and bulky items of equipment often need to be accommodated. Each bed area is supplied with piped oxygen, vacuum suction, medical compressed air and sometimes nitric oxide. The plethora of electronic monitors requires at least 12 electric power sockets (with emergency back-up electrical supply) at each bed. Sufficient bedside storage space is needed for drugs and disposable equipment. Each bed area should be equipped with a self-inflating resuscitation bag to enable staff to maintain artificial ventilation if the mechanical ventilator or gas supply fails.

WHO SHOULD BE ADMITTED?

The cost of providing ICU services is very high, and the resource is finite. ICU care must be directed towards patients who are most likely to benefit. It is equally important to identify patients who are not ill enough to benefit, and those who will die despite ICU treatment. ICU admission is indicated for:

- patients requiring, or likely to require, advanced respiratory support (see below) alone
- patients requiring support of two or more organ systems
- patients with comorbidity who require support for an acute reversible failure of another organ system.

CATEGORIES OF ORGAN SYSTEM SUPPORT

Advanced respiratory support

- Mechanical ventilatory support (excluding mask continuous positive-airways pressure, CPAP) or noninvasive ventilation.
- The possibility of sudden deterioration in respiratory function requiring immediate tracheal intubation and mechanical ventilation.

Basic respiratory monitoring and support

- The need for an inspired oxygen concentration of more than 40%.
- The possibility of progressive deterioration to the point of needing advanced respiratory support.
- The need for physiotherapy to clear secretions at least 2-hourly.
- Patients in whom the tracheal tube has been removed recently after a prolonged period of intubation and mechanical ventilation.
- The need for mask CPAP or noninvasive ventilation.

- Patients whose trachea is intubated to protect the airway but who do not need mechanical ventilation.

Circulatory support

- The need for vasoactive drugs.
- Support for circulatory instability caused by hypovolaemia from any cause unresponsive to modest volume replacement.
- Patients resuscitated after cardiac arrest where ICU or HDU care is considered clinically appropriate.

Neurological monitoring or support

- Central nervous system depression sufficient to compromise the airway and impair protective reflexes.
- Invasive neurological monitoring.

Renal support

- The need for acute renal replacement therapy.

ADMISSION TO ICU

The decision to admit a patient to an ICU must take other factors into account. The referral should ideally be on a consultant-to-consultant basis and no patient should be admitted or refused admission without discussion with the ICU consultant. The reversibility of the patient's illness must be considered; if it is not reversible, and incompatible with life, then the patient should not be admitted. Such decisions are not made easily and occasionally it is necessary to admit the patient and to provide active treatment for a period of time to assess the response. Intensive care cannot reverse chronic ill health, and admission may be inappropriate for a patient who has significant comorbidity which severely limits quality and length of life. However, some patients adapt to comorbidity to the extent that they accept a quality of life which others would regard as unendurable; denying such patients admission based on the presence of comorbidity alone is difficult to justify, and the patient's views must be respected. If possible, the consultant should discuss with the patient and the relatives the range of treatment options and possible outcomes. However, acutely ill patients can rarely discuss details of their care, and relatives may find it difficult to make an objective judgement. If a patient has made an Advance Decision ('Living Will') then its contents must be respected.

DISCHARGE FROM ICU

The patient should be discharged when the condition(s) that necessitated admission have been treated successfully and when organ failure has resolved. Discharge should be to an area which provides an appropriate level of care. It is unusual for an ICU patient to be discharged directly to the ward without receiving a period of 'step-down' high-dependency care within the ICU to determine that the clinical course is evolving satisfactorily. Thereafter, discharge may take place to either an HDU or the ward as determined by the patient's clinical condition. Many ICUs offer a 'critical care outreach team'; one of its functions is to follow up recently discharged ICU patients.

Approximately 25% of ICU patients die in the ICU, often as a result of treatment limitation in the face of continued deterioration despite maximal appropriate supportive therapy. In such patients, palliative and compassionate care should be continued in the ICU if death is imminent, although if death is inevitable but likely to be delayed, it may be appropriate to transfer the patient to a non-ICU/HDU area for terminal care.

STAFFING CONSIDERATIONS

THE ICU CONSULTANT

Difficult therapeutic and ethical policy decisions may be required at any time in the ICU. It is essential that they are taken by an individual whose previous experience allows a reasonable assessment of the likely outcome and whose therapeutic expertise is likely to give the patient the optimal chance of recovery. The ICU consultant, if not physically present in the unit, must always be available by telephone and should not be involved in any activity which precludes his or her attendance there within 30 min. Because of the critical nature of ICU patients' illnesses, the ICU consultant expects to be informed immediately of any significant change in their condition. The consultant's base speciality is relatively unimportant, but appropriate training and experience are crucial.

THE ROLES OF THE ICU RESIDENT

Communication

Although medical involvement with therapy in the ICU is greater than anywhere else in the hospital except the operating theatre, it should be appreciated that the major proportion of the care which patients receive in the ICU is provided by nursing staff, who have greatly extended roles, experience and responsibility. ICU nursing staff have undertaken specific training to enable them to perform titration of fluid replacement, analgesia, inotropic drug therapy and weaning from mechanical ventilation. The route by which complex instructions and information are transmitted between medical and nursing staff is of vital importance. A system in which a relatively junior clinician serves as a 'final common pathway' for all instructions works well in practice provided that the doctor involved is present within the unit at all times so that the nurses may obtain clarification of instructions, report changes in status and receive immediate help in emergencies. When the patient, relatives or friends are spoken to, it is vital that the nurse is present and takes part in the discussions. The content of such discussion must be recorded accurately in the patient's notes.

Confusion is minimized if the nursing staff take orders only from the unit staff and not directly from visiting clinicians, however eminent, even if they are nominally in charge of the patient. This is to ensure that the nurses who execute orders are able to confer with the person who gave them in case of difficulties. In addition, many patients may be under the care of several clinical teams (e.g. multiply injured patients may be treated by a selection from the orthopaedic, general, neuro-, dental, plastic or urological surgeons), so that it is essential that one individual is available to draw attention to, and when necessary harmonize, often conflicting therapeutic regimens. The ICU resident, because of his or her continuous presence in the unit, should be better informed about the patient's recent diagnostic results, physiological status and therapeutic responses than any visiting clinician and should attempt to use current knowledge to guide treatment along rational lines. The ICU consultant must be available to support the resident if conflict occurs, and also to deal with clinical problems.

The department which provides the unit staff differs from hospital to hospital; units serving primarily a single speciality (e.g. cardiac surgery or neurosurgery units) are usually staffed by the speciality involved, whereas most general ICUs are staffed by the anaesthetic department, which is well used to providing round-the-clock emergency services.

Therapeutic functions

The resident is the first doctor consulted by the nursing staff. It is necessary to decide rapidly whether the problem is within the resident's expertise or if more experienced help should be obtained. The number of

occasions when immediate emergency action is required should be relatively small for patients already under the care of experienced ICU nurses (e.g. unforeseen circulatory collapse, accidental tracheal extubation), but resuscitative measures are often required for patients at the time of admission to the unit. The ICU consultant must be informed of any impending admission so that the therapeutic plan may be discussed. Decisions to exclude patients from the ICU should not be taken by the junior resident alone.

Most calls from the unit to the resident are the result of alterations in measurements or observations rather than a major catastrophe. Tracheal intubation and obtunded consciousness make direct communication with many patients extremely difficult, so that assessment of their problems is based primarily on clinical observation and interpretation of patterns of change in physiological status. The resident should remember that the majority of intensive care nurses (and especially the sisters and charge nurses) have an enormous amount of 'bedside' experience with critically ill patients and considerable reliance should be placed on their observations.

Assessment of patients

ICU patients often have multiple pathologies which interact with each other and with any comorbidity. When dealing with a newly admitted emergency patient, assessment and resuscitation often take place simultaneously and follow the standard pattern of recognizing and dealing with problems in the order of airway, breathing and circulation. The resident should heed *all* the patient's problems and the responses to the treatments instigated. When called to a patient, the resident should begin to assess the patient's condition by thorough clinical examination in a systematic manner to ensure that nothing is missed. An example of such a system and some of the matters that the resident should consider under each heading are shown in Table 41.1.

Full assessment and examination of each patient, even if stable, should be carried out at least daily. The physiological status of critically ill patients can change very quickly and the majority of the parameters measured in ICU are displayed on large paper charts on an hourly basis. Modern electronic data capture systems collect information much more frequently, and allow staff to identify both acute changes and slower trends.

The ICU resident must be familiar with the equipment and documentation used within the unit. Accurate chart review is an essential part of assessment and treatment planning. Any changes to treatment must be recorded accurately and contemporaneously so that the effects of the changes may be observed.

Table 41.1   An example of a system for assessment of ICU patients

A. *Airway:* Is the airway patent or at risk? What do I need to do to secure it? Is the cervical spine at risk? Type of tracheal tube? Position? How long has it been in place? Time for tracheostomy? Type of tracheostomy tube? Security of tube? What is coming up the tube? Cuff pressure?

B. *Breathing:* Spontaneous ventilation – rate, depth, character, etc.? Mode of ventilation? Mechanical ventilation parameters? Inspired oxygen concentration? PEEP or CPAP level? Position of patient? Nitric oxide or other adjuncts? Clinical examination findings? Arterial blood gas analysis? Chest X-ray or other imaging?

C. *Circulation:* ECG, pulse, blood pressure, CVP? Haemodynamic data, e.g. cardiac index, SVRI, PVRI, PCWP, etc.? Inotropic or other vasoactive drugs? Heart sounds? Fluid balance, plasma osmolality? Peripheral circulation/oedema?

D. *Disability/ depth of sedation:* Sedation score or Glasgow Coma Score? Focal neurology? Pupils? Fitting? Cerebral function monitors? Other specialized neurological monitors, e.g. ICP, jugular bulb saturation or transcranial Doppler?

E. *Equipment:* Is it all working, calibrated and accurate? Is there any other monitoring that would safely give useful information?

F. *Fluids:* How much and what fluid to give? Fluid balance 24 h/cumulative? Fluid output from where? Fistulae, drains, wounds? What is it – quality and quantity?

G. *Gut:* Is it working? Can I use it to feed the patient? Prokinetic drugs? Dietary supplements/stress ulcer prophylaxis? Nasogastric tube aspirate/drainage? Wounds healing or not? Stomas – viable working or not? Bowel activity?

H. *Haematology:* Check *all* blood results, haematology, clotting, biochemistry, serology. Is there any additional blood test that can help? Is transfusion required?

I. *Imaging:* X-rays? Ultrasound? CT scanning? MRI? Echocardiography? Doppler? Nuclear medicine?

J. *Joints and limbs:* Fractures, dislocations, other trauma? DVT and appropriate prophylaxis?

K. *Kelvin:* Temperature and temperature chart?

L. *Lines:* Examine all catheters/cannulae (intravenous, intra-arterial and others) and ask yourself: When placed? Where placed? Are they necessary? Replacement or removal? Signs of sepsis?

M. *Microbiology:* Aggressive microbiological surveillance: swabs, blood cultures, sputum, bronchoalveolar lavage, drain fluid, urine, removed line tips. Strict asepsis and cross-infection avoidance – touch a patient, wash your hands. Check results daily. Directed antimicrobial therapy only. Antibiotic levels, doses and course duration. Make friends with your microbiologist: joint daily ward rounds.

N. *Nutrition:* All patients need feeding. Enteral nutrition is best. Nasogastric feeding, oral, percutaneous gastrostomy, jejunal feeding, intravenous feeding?

O. *Other consultants:* Nobody knows everything – arrange appropriate specialist opinions. Let the patient's general practitioner and hospital consultant know one of their patients is in the ICU

P. *Pain relief and psychological support:* Prescribe analgesia by appropriate routes, intervals and doses. Talk to your patient always, even if there is a depressed level of consciousness. Explain procedures simply and carefully. Give sedation and psychotropic drugs if indicated.

Q. *Question:* If you are unsure of what to do, ask your consultant. You should never undertake a task for which you have been inadequately trained.

R. *Relatives:* Keep relatives fully informed, be honest when discussing prognosis, ask for information on past medical history and daily activity if appropriate. Always hold discussions away from the bedside unless the patient is fully aware/autonomous and can participate. Always hold discussions with the patient's nurse present and document your comments.

S. *Skin:* Examine skin for perfusion, wounds, signs of systemic disease or infection. Pressure area care, mouth care etc.

Table 41.1   An example of a system for assessment of ICU patients—Cont'd

T. *Trauma and transport:* Multiple trauma patients require multidisciplinary management. Trauma patients may not have had a complete secondary survey; late diagnosis of unrecognized problems may cause significant morbidity and mortality. Transport of ICU patients within or between hospital requires the same level of care and monitoring that they receive in the ICU itself.

U. *Universal precautions:* Owing to the plethora of infectious diseases transmitted by blood and other bodily fluids, all staff should be aware of the necessity of wearing gloves, aprons and occasionally face guards when performing invasive procedures.

V. *Visitors:* These may be the patient's relatives or other medical personnel involved in the patient's care. Visiting colleagues should be treated with respect and courtesy, but ultimately all changes to therapy *must* be discussed with the ICU consultant.

W. *What to do:* When the patient has been fully assessed, you must formulate a plan to deal with the problems. This plan must be documented clearly in the notes and discussed with the bedside nurse. Parameters must be agreed within which the nurse is able to vary the components of the therapeutic regimen according to the patient's response and outside which you need to reassess the patient. Time is an important part of your plan and regular reassessment is essential.

Y. *Why?:* Every time you review the patient, ask yourself why the patient was admitted and what the active problems are now. Keep on track and forget nothing!

CLINICAL GUIDELINES

It is impossible to provide a comprehensive review of all the conditions requiring ICU care and full treatment regimens for such conditions in one chapter. The following sections present a set of guidelines designed to help the resident in the fundamental processes of managing respiratory and cardiovascular failure, which are the two commonest reasons for admission to ICU.

RESPIRATORY PROBLEMS

Who should receive artificial ventilation?

Patients who are unable to maintain adequate levels of oxygenation or who develop hypercapnia may be candidates for mechanically assisted ventilation, provided that their pulmonary pathology is potentially reversible. Ventilatory failure may have developed already (in which case arterial blood gas values are abnormal) or may be judged as likely to occur (when blood gas values may be normal but the patient is 'exhausted').

Hypoxaemia

The commonest indication for artificial ventilation of a patient's lungs in the ICU is inability to maintain a satisfactory P_aO_2. There are many pathological conditions which produce hypoxaemia, but all have the same basic problem – an area (or areas) of lung with greater pulmonary blood flow than alveolar ventilation. Blood flow through areas of lung from which ventilation is completely absent is said to be 'shunted' and hypoxaemia caused by this mechanism shows little improvement when the inspired oxygen concentration is increased. Some clinical conditions which are associated frequently with hypoxaemia, and common responses to therapy, are listed in Table 41.2. Central cyanosis (seen best in the lips) shows that significant hypoxaemia is present, but if moderate anaemia (Hb < $10\,g\,dL^{-1}$) is present, as it is in many ICU patients, severe hypoxaemia (P_aO_2 < 6 kPa) may occur without obvious cyanosis.

The initial treatment of hypoxaemia is the administration of oxygen by face mask. At least 40% oxygen should be given, either by means of a fixed-performance mask (e.g. 40, 50 or 60% Ventimask) or by supplying at least $6\,L\,min^{-1}$ of oxygen to a variable-performance mask (e.g. Hudson). Low-concentration, fixed-performance masks and other devices which deliver 24–35% oxygen should be reserved for use in patients with chronic lung conditions in whom hypoxic drive may be maintaining ventilation. The effect of oxygen therapy should be assessed continuously by pulse oximetry and blood gas analysis should be carried out after 30 min. This gives a more reliable measure of oxygenation in addition to providing information regarding the P_aCO_2 and acid–base status.

If P_aO_2 remains below 7 kPa in a patient with previously healthy lungs, the inspired oxygen concentration should be increased and blood gas values measured again after 20 min. In addition, measures to combat infection, pulmonary oedema or bronchospasm should

Table 41.2   Some causes of hypoxaemia and usual responses to therapy

| Clinical condition | O₂ by mask | Response to therapy | |
		IPPV	Need for PEEP
1. Pulmonary oedema			
(a) Cardiac	Fair	Good	Uncommon
(b) Permeability	Poor	Fair	Often needed
2. Asthma (bronchodilators may make worse)	Good	Good but technically very difficult	Uncommon
3. Chronic bronchitis	Fair (Ventimask)	Good	Uncommon
4. Emphysema	Good (Ventimask)	Good	Rare, beware pneumothorax
5. Pneumonia			
(a) Lobar	Poor	Poor	Try, often disappointing
(b) Bronchial	Fair	Good	Useful
6. Pulmonary contusion	Fair	Fair	Often needed, beware pneumothorax
7. Right-to-left intracardiac shunts	Poor	Disastrous	Never
8. Retained secretions	Poor	Good, access for suction important	Helpful
9. 'Exhaustion'	Not accepted	Good	Uncommon

be introduced as appropriate, analgesia given if indicated and chest physiotherapy started. Mechanical ventilation is indicated if P_aO_2 does not remain above 7–8 kPa. A decreased level of consciousness and/or airway compromise may mandate early tracheal intubation and mechanical ventilation. If these are absent, administration of oxygen by mask CPAP should be tried if there are no contraindications.

Mask CPAP. A tightly applied face mask with a high-volume, low-pressure soft plastic rim held in place by a special harness is connected to a circuit delivering an air/oxygen mixture of the required F_IO_2. The flow rate of fresh gas into the circuit must be sufficient to keep the positive pressure set by the expiratory valve (2.5–10 cmH₂O) almost constant throughout the respiratory cycle with only a minimal pressure decrease during inspiration. Various commercial systems using Venturi or bellows systems are available but they consume large amounts of fresh gas. For CPAP to be successful, the patient must receive adequate analgesia, be alert and cooperative, and have no facial injuries (including a basal skull fracture).

Patients often find the tight-fitting mask uncomfortable and require short periods of respite with an ordinary fixed F_IO_2 mask. At higher levels of CPAP (> 7.5 cmH₂O), the work of breathing against the expiratory valve may result in an elevation of P_aCO_2, and CPAP alone is generally not effective in most cases of respiratory failure associated with hypercapnia.

If the patient does not have a functioning nasogastric tube, then air swallowing and gastric dilatation may be a problem and hinder diaphragmatic excursion or provoke regurgitation.

Patients who are unable to maintain adequate oxygenation often have a pulmonary problem which is associated with other pathology. Persisting inability to cough effectively because of pain and/or weakness leads to retention of secretions and progressive alveolar collapse. The prophylactic use of tracheal intubation and intermittent positive-pressure ventilation (IPPV) has become common in patients who normally produce significant quantities of bronchial secretions and whose ability to cough has been impaired by injury or operation to the chest and/or upper abdomen. Patients in whom pain rather than weakness is the major defect may often be managed more conservatively if first-class pain relief is provided (e.g. by epidural or i.v. infusion of opioid), together with physiotherapy, and the use of nasal airways or selective use of minitracheotomy to facilitate suction.

Hypercapnia

Carbon dioxide clearance is related directly to alveolar ventilation. Causes of inadequate ventilation, together with the likely duration of the disability, are listed in Table 41.3. It may be inappropriate to start IPPV in clinical situations where ventilatory insufficiency cannot be reversed by therapy. For some patients, noninvasive (i.e. nonintubational) forms of respiratory support (NIRS) are applicable. The types of NIRS used most widely are noninvasive positive-pressure ventilation (NIPPV) by mask and negative-pressure ventilation (NPV). NIPPV and NPV have been used successfully in the management of patients with non-

traumatic causes of ventilatory failure, particularly for home ventilation of patients who chronically retain carbon dioxide or who have high spinal injury, and who do not have a permanent tracheostomy but require nocturnal ventilation. NIPPV uses a portable electrically powered volume- or pressure-cycled ventilator to deliver synchronized positive-pressure breaths via a tight-fitting nasal or full face mask held in place by a harness. NPV requires a made-to-measure 'cuirass' which is worn over the chest and sealed at the neck and waist. This is connected to a pump which cyclically produces negative pressure within the cuirass; the intrathoracic pressure is exceeded by atmospheric pressure and air flows into the chest. The pump then cycles to atmospheric pressure and expiration occurs as a result of the normal elastic recoil of the lungs and chest wall. The device is essentially a miniature version of the old cylindrical 'iron lung'.

Patients whose dysfunction is described in the lower part of Table 41.3 are likely to make vigorous efforts to maintain normocapnia, while those in whom the

Table 41.3   Some causes of inadequate spontaneous ventilation

Site of dysfunction	Common causes	Probable duration of inadequacy
A. Patients usually unable to increase ventilation (appear passive)		
1. Respiratory centre	Brain injury (coning)	Permanent
	Pharmacological depression (e.g. opioids, barbiturates)	Hours (depends on drug)
2. Upper motor neurones	High spinal damage (above C4)	Permanent
3. Lower motor neurones	Poliomyelitis	Weeks but may be permanent
	Polyneuritis	Months
	Tetanus	Weeks
4. Neuromuscular junction	Myasthenia gravis	Weeks or months
	Neuromuscular blockers	Minutes or hours
5. Respiratory muscles	Myopathies, dystrophies	Permanent
B. Patients who attempt to increase ventilation (appear dyspnoeic)		
6. Chest wall		
(a) Deformity	Kyphoscoliosis	Permanent
	Burn eschars	Until incised
(b) Damage	Rib fractures	Days or weeks
7. Lungs – reduced compliance	Pulmonary fibrosis	Permanent
	ARDS	Days or weeks
8. Airways – increased resistance	Upper airway obstruction: croup, epiglottitis	Until relieved
	Lower airway obstruction: asthma	Days
	Bronchitis and emphysema	Permanent

dysfunction may be described broadly as 'neurological' are usually unable to make any significant improvement in minute volume despite a progressive increase in P_aCO_2. Mechanical ventilation is required usually if P_aCO_2 exceeds 7 kPa in patients who habitually maintain a P_aCO_2 in the normal range (4.7–5.3 kPa), or if P_aCO_2 increases by more than 2 kPa above the patient's usual level.

Exhaustion is indicated by a pattern of laboured, rapid, shallow breathing which is often accompanied by deterioration in the level of consciousness. This situation may occur in a wide range of clinical conditions, including cardiac failure and severe septicaemia, when the institution of artificial ventilation may be followed by an improvement in oxygenation, a reduction in pulse rate and reversal of a trend towards metabolic acidosis. When it occurs in conjunction with myocardial failure, a disproportionate amount of the limited cardiac output is used to maintain ventilation, and artificial ventilation may allow adequate perfusion of vital organs to be resumed. Mechanical ventilation is probably required if the respiratory rate remains at or above 45 breath min^{-1} for more than 1 h.

Mechanical ventilation

Tracheal intubation

To enable IPPV to be carried out effectively, a cuffed tube must be placed in the trachea either via the mouth or nose, or directly through a tracheostomy. In the emergency situation, an orotracheal tube is usually inserted. If the patient is conscious, anaesthesia should be induced carefully with an appropriate dose of i.v. induction agent and muscular relaxation produced, usually with succinylcholine. The full range of adjuncts for difficult intubation should be available.

The critically ill patient is often exquisitely sensitive to i.v. anaesthesia, and cardiovascular collapse may occur; consequently, full resuscitation equipment must be immediately available.

If the patient is unconscious, a muscle relaxant alone may be necessary (but not obligatory) to facilitate the passage of the tube; however, an i.v. induction agent and muscle relaxant should always be used in patients with severe head injury to prevent an increase in intracranial pressure (ICP) during laryngoscopy and tracheal intubation.

Many patients are hypoxaemic, and it is essential that 100% oxygen is administered before tracheal intubation.

After muscle relaxation has been induced, the tube should be inserted by the route which is associated with the least delay.

If the patient is unconscious and the victim of blunt trauma, when cervical spine injury is a possibility, the cervical spine should be immobilized during intubation using manual in-line immobilization (MILI). Using this technique, oral intubation is safe even in the presence of biomechanical instability of the cervical spine. If the patient has a rigid neck collar in place before intubation, MILI should be applied and the collar removed to facilitate laryngoscopy, and then replaced before discontinuing MILI.

Cricoid pressure should be applied to minimize the risk of aspirating gastric contents. A sterile, disposable plastic tube with a low-pressure cuff should be used. The tube should be inserted such that the top of the cuff lies not more than 3 cm below the vocal cords. The proximal end of the tube should then be cut so that the incompressible plastic connector lies between the incisor teeth if an oral tube is used, or in the external nares if nasal intubation is selected.

Nasotracheal intubation is less popular than formerly in the ICU because of increased recognition of the risk of sepsis from sinusitis.

The head should be placed in a neutral or slightly flexed position (on one pillow) after tracheal intubation and a chest X-ray taken to ensure that the tip of the tube lies at least 5 cm above the carina.

Bronchial intubation is the commonest dangerous complication during mechanical ventilation as the tracheal tube may migrate down the trachea when the patient is moved during normal nursing procedures. Intubation of the right main bronchus cannot be detected reliably by observation of chest movements or by auscultation of the chest because of the exaggerated transmission of breath sounds during IPPV, although absent or asynchronous chest movement may occur when pulmonary collapse has taken place. Bronchial intubation is one of the causes of a sudden decrease in compliance, and restlessness and coughing often occur if the end of the tube irritates the carina. If this is suspected, the tube should be withdrawn gradually by up to 5 cm while lung compliance and chest expansion are observed carefully. The position of the tube should always be confirmed by a chest radiograph.

When the upper airway or larynx is obstructed and conventional tracheal intubation is not possible (e.g. occasional cases of epiglottitis or laryngeal trauma), the emergency airway of choice is cricothyroidotomy. Tracheostomy is used more commonly as a planned procedure to make management easier and more comfortable in patients who require ventilation for prolonged periods (e.g. tetanus, poliomyelitis, Guillain–Barré syndrome) or to aid weaning. In such cases, it is performed as a formal operation under general anaesthesia after the airway has been secured using a tracheal tube. In most ICUs, percutaneous dilatational tracheostomy is employed. This technique can be performed at the bedside, often using broncho-scopic control. It should be undertaken only by fully trained staff.

Management of patients undergoing ventilation

The aims of IPPV are to maintain adequate oxygena-tion of the tissues with an inspired oxygen concentra-tion of less than 50% and to maintain the $P_a\text{CO}_2$ at a satisfactory level without causing iatrogenic lung injury or cardiovascular compromise.

Arterial oxygenation

This is controlled by manipulating the inspired oxygen concentration and by varying the end-expiratory pres-sure. Figure 41.1 describes measures that may be used to maintain arterial oxygenation within the desired limits ($P_a\text{O}_2$ = 10–15 kPa and $S_a\text{O}_2$ > 95%). Pulse oxime-try is a useful continuous monitor, but does not reli-ably reflect small but significant changes in $P_a\text{O}_2$. Inspired concentrations of oxygen exceeding 50–60% should be avoided for more than a few hours if possi-ble because of the risk of oxygen-induced pulmonary damage. However, in severe hypoxaemia, it may be necessary to ignore this risk.

ARTERIAL OXYGENATION

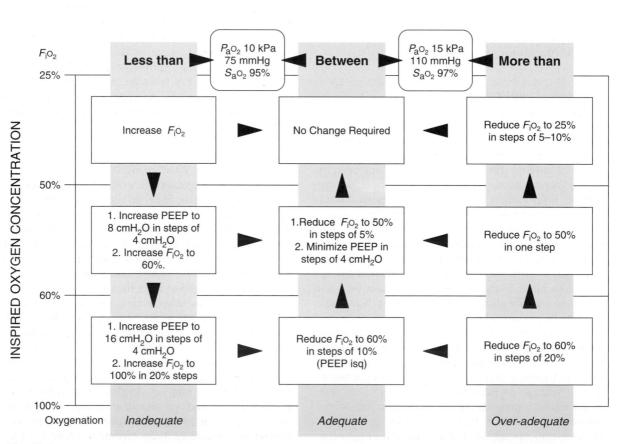

Fig. 41.1
Control of arterial oxygenation. To use this diagram: 1. Measure the inspired oxygen concentration ($F_i\text{O}_2$) and arterial blood gases and find appropriate box on diagram. 2. Adjust $F_i\text{O}_2$ and/or positive end-expiratory pressure (PEEP) as suggested. Where more than one action is proposed, proceed in the order described. In general, the greater the deviation from adequacy, the larger the steps required. 3. Repeat measurements after 20–30 min and readjust if necessary. NB: If $P\text{O}_2$ is measured on samples of mixed (or central venous) blood before and after adding or increasing PEEP, effect of PEEP on cardiac output and oxygen flux may be assessed (see text).

Carbon dioxide tension

This is controlled during conventional ventilation by changing the respiratory rate and/or tidal volume. It is desirable to minimize the changes in $P_a\text{CO}_2$ (especially if initially elevated), because too rapid a reduction may lead to decreases in cerebral blood flow, cardiac output and arterial pressure. In patients with normal or low $P_a\text{CO}_2$ before IPPV, minute volume should be adjusted to produce a $P_a\text{CO}_2$ of 4.5–5 kPa, a value at which spontaneous ventilatory efforts should be minimal. If the initial $P_a\text{CO}_2$ is high, its value should not be reduced by more than 1 kPa h^{-1} and, if raised chronically (e.g. in chronic bronchitis), it should not be reduced below the patient's own 'normal' level when well. If the $P_a\text{CO}_2$ is below 4 kPa, minute volume should be reduced by decreasing the respiratory rate. Because $P_a\text{CO}_2$ increases relatively slowly, at least 1 h should elapse before contemplating further changes in minute volume.

Mode of ventilation

Intermittent positive-pressure ventilation (IPPV), or controlled mandatory ventilation (CMV), is the basic mode of mechanical ventilation used during balanced anaesthesia, but it is rarely used in its simplest form in the ICU. When CMV is used, the ventilator is set to deliver a fixed tidal volume at a fixed rate to produce a fixed minute ventilation sufficient to ensure adequate CO_2 elimination. Any attempt by the patient to take a spontaneous breath during any part of the respiratory cycle is unsuccessful. In addition, the ventilator continues to deliver mandatory breaths, even if the patient is attempting to breathe; consequently, very high inflation pressures may be generated if the ventilator cycles to inspiration while the patient is coughing or attempting to breathe out, resulting in impaired gas exchange, a risk of barotrauma to the lungs and depression of cardiac output. To enable patients to tolerate CMV, it is often necessary to provide deep sedation and, in some cases, to administer a neuromuscular blocking drug. Oversedation of critically ill patients tends to decrease cardiac output by depressing myocardial function or by vasodilatation; this is a risk particularly in patients who have received inadequate fluid resuscitation, in the elderly, and in other patients with myocardial dysfunction. Drug-induced paralysis in ICU patients can result in very unpleasant memories and, if used for a long period, may result in prolonged impairment of neuromuscular function, with muscle wasting, weakness and increased difficulty in weaning from mechanical ventilation.

Modes of ventilation have been developed which allow preservation of the patient's own respiratory efforts by detecting an attempt by the patient to breathe in and synchronizing the mechanical breath with spontaneous inspiration; this technique is termed synchronized intermittent mandatory ventilation (SIMV). If no attempt at inspiration is detected over a period of some seconds then a mandatory breath is delivered to ensure that a safe total minute volume is provided. Another technique is termed pressure support ventilation (PSV). When PSV is employed, each spontaneous breath is detected and then assisted by delivering gas until a preset level of positive pressure is achieved. The technique is, in essence, patient-triggered, pressure-limited ventilation and may be used only if the patient has a normal intrinsic respiratory rate.

These more advanced techniques allow satisfactory levels of ventilation without the need to provide deep sedation, and with a lower mean intrathoracic pressure than occurs using CMV. Consequently, less sedation is required, respiratory muscle tone is preserved, there is greater cardiovascular stability and the risk of barotrauma is reduced.

The choice of the best mode of ventilation for an individual patient often changes at different periods in the disease process, and the technique which provides the best gas exchange is often found only by trial and error.

Ventilator-induced lung injury

When pulmonary pathology has resulted in the development of acute lung injury (ALI) or acute respiratory distress syndrome (ARDS), either directly or indirectly as a result of a cytokine-mediated systemic inflammatory response, then the lung is particularly at risk of secondary injury as a result of injudiciously aggressive ventilatory strategies using conventional modes of ventilation. Attempts to achieve 'normal' arterial blood gas tensions often require the use of very high tidal volumes, high respiratory rates and high peak inflation pressures. Many ventilators are capable of delivering these preset variables regardless of the compliance or resistance of the lungs. If all the alveolar subunits of the lungs had normal and equal compliance, the tidal volume would be distributed equally. However, diseased lung is nonhomogeneous; some units have normal compliance and others have poor compliance with long time constants. Some alveolar subunits are available to be ventilated and others are not. As a result of the inhomogeneity, the more normal alveolar subunits are ventilated preferentially and subjected to pressures which cause overdistension; both high tidal volumes and high pressure can cause overdistension. Overdistension injury resulting from excessively high tidal volumes is termed 'volutrauma' and overdistension injury resulting from excessive pressures is termed 'barotrauma'.

In extreme cases of barotrauma, gas from overdistended, ruptured alveoli forms interstitial pulmonary emphysema and tracks along the adventitia of intrapulmonary blood vessels. Eventually, the gas bubbles coalesce as they migrate centrally and mediastinal emphysema occurs.

If the process persists, gas bursts through the mediastinal pleura to cause a pneumothorax. Unrecognized pneumothorax is a serious complication during positive-pressure ventilation because the volume of the pneumothorax enlarges with each breath and tension pneumothorax may occur rapidly.

Even if pneumothorax does not develop, repeated overdistension of alveoli by high tidal volumes may contribute to a deterioration of the underlying lung problem. The cyclical opening and closing of the alveoli result in a shearing injury. Exudative pulmonary oedema may form as a result of increased alveolar permeability; compliance decreases further, and the tidal volume is displaced to more normal alveoli so that the injury is propagated. The insult is probably increased by concurrent oxygen toxicity as a result of the use of high F_IO_2 in an attempt to preserve an adequate arterial oxygen tension.

Lung protective ventilatory strategies

The end-points of the pathophysiology of ventilator-induced lung injury (VILI) and the pathophysiology of diseased lung injury are identical and it seems reasonable to prevent exacerbation of lung injury by the adoption of a lung protective ventilatory strategy. The mechanism of VILI suggests that the avoidance of overdistension, shear stress injury and oxygen toxicity should be the main strategy of such a technique.

Pressure and volume limitation strategy

A reduction in volutrauma may be achieved theoretically by the use of low tidal volumes during ventilation. Classically, relatively large tidal volumes (10–12 mL kg^{-1}) have been used to ensure normocapnia in the range of 4.5–5.5 kPa, but in the presence of lung inhomogeneity, this leads to overdistension, high peak inspiratory pressures and the production of VILI. Reducing the tidal volume to 6–8 mL kg^{-1} and limiting peak inspiratory pressure in the presence of poorly compliant lung result in a decreased incidence of overdistension and a reduction in transalveolar pressure. Overdistension does not seem to occur if the transalveolar pressure is kept below 35 cmH$_2$O, which equates to a plateau airway pressure of 35–45 cmH$_2$O. The main disadvantage of pressure limitation (also called pressure-controlled ventilation, PCV) is that minute ventilation is decreased and hypercapnia occurs; however, this may be acceptable if the probability of survival is improved ('permissive hypercapnia'). The low lung volumes generated during PCV increase the tendency of alveoli to collapse and this must be countered by a concurrent lung recruitment strategy.

Lung recruitment strategy

Shear forces induce alveolar damage because of the cyclical opening and subsequent closure of alveoli. Collapse of alveoli at end-expiration at low or zero PEEP produces the maximum degree of alveolar injury. The use of higher levels of PEEP tends to hold alveoli open, stops them collapsing totally at end-expiration and limits the shear forces applied. The level of PEEP required to prevent collapse and to recruit unopened alveoli is difficult to calculate on an individual basis, although an estimate may be made from the patient's pressure/volume static compliance curve by choosing the lower inflection point on the ascending limb or the upper inflection point on the descending limb. However, constructing such curves by the application of successively increasing tidal volumes and measuring the pressure that each volume generates is not very physiological and the PEEP level produced is probably not appropriate to all of the various alveolar time constants present in an inhomogeneous diseased lung. Arbitrary incremental levels of PEEP may be applied at, say, 4, 8, 12 and 16 cmH$_2$O to determine the level which produces the best oxygenation for a given F_IO_2 with the least cardiovascular compromise. Alternative strategies for recruiting closed or semi-closed alveolar subunits involve giving an occasional single large tidal breath and holding end-inspiration for 20 s.

The effects of PEEP on the circulation should be monitored by observing trends in arterial pressure and by measuring changes in the oxygen concentration in mixed (or central) venous blood. The supply of oxygen available to the body (the oxygen flux) is the product of the cardiac output and the arterial oxygen content. PEEP often increases the arterial oxygen content but may depress cardiac output so that oxygen flux is reduced. If this happens and total body oxygen consumption remains unchanged, less oxygen is returned to the heart and the oxygen content in the mixed (or central) venous blood decreases. If venous oxygen saturation does decrease after the application of (or an increase in the level of) PEEP, then:

- PEEP should be reduced by $5\,cmH_2O$
- inspired oxygen concentration should be increased by 10%
- measurements of arterial and venous P_{O_2} should be repeated after 20 min.

Alternative modes of ventilation

For simple elective postoperative ventilation in patients with non-diseased lungs, the modes described above are usually adequate, but occasionally, as the lungs become more diseased, alternative modes of ventilation must be used. Taking into account the mechanism of VILI and the theoretical advantages of avoiding overdistension and shear injury while promoting lung recruitment, it is possible to formulate alternative strategies for ventilating injured lungs. The aim should be to use a ventilatory mode that opens underventilated alveolar units, keeps them open for as long as possible to allow optimal gas exchange at volumes and transalveolar pressures which do not induce secondary lung injury or produce haemodynamic instability, and then allows exhalation to a lung volume and positive end-expiratory pressure which prevent alveolar collapse and allow adequate carbon dioxide excretion.

Pressure-controlled inverse ratio ventilation

For an alveolar subunit of a given compliance, a high pressure applied for a short time produces volume expansion which may be equal to that produced by a lower pressure applied for a longer period. PCV may be used with a range of I:E ratios, from the 'normal' 1.2 to the equal ratio 1:1 or inverse ratios of 2:1 or even 3:1. Pressure-controlled inverse ratio ventilation (PCIRV) offers theoretical advantages in terms of lung protection and recruitment, particularly when combined with PEEP in some patients with poor lung compliance and alveoli with long time constants. The improvement in oxygenation which often occurs may be the result of reduced arteriovenous shunt, decreased ventilation–perfusion mismatch or increased functional residual capacity as a result of intrinsic PEEP developing due to the short expiratory phase. While the development of intrinsic PEEP has some advantages in terms of alveolar recruitment, too much, particularly in the presence of bronchospasm or other obstruction to expiration, may promote volutrauma. Where evidence of increasing intrinsic PEEP is found, the expiratory time should be increased.

The use of PCIRV is not tolerated by unsedated patients because the inverse I:E ratio is a very uncomfortable pattern of ventilation. High doses of sedative drugs and occasionally neuromuscular blocking drugs are required to facilitate the optimal pattern of ventilation.

In chest trauma with coexisting blunt myocardial injury, sedation to the required depth often requires inotropic support to maintain cardiac output. Hypovolaemic patients may suffer a decrease in cardiac output particularly at inverse ratios of 3:1 as a result of the prolonged positive intrathoracic pressure. Trauma patients with a head injury and raised ICP in combination with lung contusion form a not infrequent group of patients where a lung protective ventilatory strategy with permissive hypercapnia is at odds with the need to control P_aCO_2 to low normocapnia for ICP control.

Tracheal gas insufflation and PCIRV

In some patients with very poor lung compliance, the short inspiratory time associated with the use of PCIRV may result in a tidal volume so small that the anatomical and equipment dead spaces come to represent a large proportion of the tidal volume, resulting in a progressive increase in P_aCO_2. The dead space may be washed out by placing a catheter coaxially in the tracheal tube to lie with its tip just above the level of the carina. Tracheal gas insufflation (TGI) flushes out the dead space, so that gas rebreathed from the dead space contains no CO_2. Correct positioning of the catheter is vital, because movement of the catheter may cause damage to the tracheal mucosa. The catheter gas must be humidified and the inspired oxygen concentration should be the same as that of the gas delivered by the ventilator.

High-frequency ventilation

High-frequency oscillation (HFO) uses a tidal volume lower than dead space volume. Small tidal volumes are generated by pistons or electromagnetic diaphragms to produce oscillatory gas flows at rates of between 150 and 3000 breath min^{-1}. HFO combined with recruitment manoeuvres is currently under investigation in both adults and children. The concept has potential advantages in patients with established barotrauma or a bronchopleural fistula where very low mean airway pressures may be advantageous.

Prone positioning

Despite the use of high F_IO_2, PEEP and optimal PCIRV, some patients become progressively more difficult to oxygenate. Another strategy to improve ventilation is to place the patient in the prone position. The improved gas exchange was thought to occur as gravity redistributed blood from the dorsal regions of the lungs, where atelectasis had developed, to the anterior segments where alveoli were more recruitable. Recent work has suggested that the improvement is related to changes in regional pleural pressure. This may result partly from the decreased volume of lung compressed by the mediastinal structures in the prone position. In the prone position, pleural pressure becomes more uniform and reduces ventilation–perfusion mismatch. The technique is not popular with nursing staff because it is very labour-intensive; four people are needed to turn the patient and great care is required to ensure that the airway and vascular catheters/cannulae are not dislodged. A recent multicentre trial in Europe has shown that although oxygenation is improved in responders, the effect does not result in improved survival to discharge.

Inhaled nitric oxide

Nitric oxide (NO) is an ultra-short-acting pulmonary vasodilator which improves oxygenation by dilating pulmonary vessels adjacent to the best ventilated alveolar units. When given by inhalation, it is delivered preferentially to the more recruited alveoli of the inhomogeneous lung and diffuses rapidly out of the alveoli to the pulmonary capillaries, causing relaxation of vascular smooth muscle and dilatation of the blood vessel. It is bound rapidly and inactivated by haemoglobin (in 110–130 ms) and its vasodilator effects are therefore limited to the pulmonary circulation.

The blood flow past underventilated alveoli is normally reduced as a result of the hypoxic vasoconstrictor response, but the improved blood flow induced by NO in the vessels adjacent to open alveoli reduces the resistance of vessels in areas of the lung which are well ventilated, increasing the proportion of blood which perfuses these areas. This results in a net reduction in intrapulmonary shunt and an increased P_aO_2. Patients with very severe hypoxaemia may be saved from a hypoxic death, while in moderate hypoxaemia, it may be possible to reduce F_IO_2, thereby reducing the risk of oxygen toxicity.

NO is administered in concentrations of 5–20 parts per million (ppm) in patients whose oxygenation has failed to improve despite optimization of PCIRV, PEEP and prone positioning; the dose used should be the lowest which is effective in achieving a 20% improvement in P_aO_2:F_IO_2 ratio. In high concentrations (> 100 ppm), NO is highly reactive and toxic, and the delivery system used must conform to rigid safety standards. During the use of NO, the concentration of methaemoglobin in the blood and the inspired nitrogen dioxide concentration must be measured. NO therapy is expensive and potentially dangerous. It improves oxygenation in the short term in about 50% of patients but the effect is often transient. A similar pulmonary vasodilator effect may be achieved by the use of nebulized prostacyclin. A recent multicentre controlled trial demonstrated an improvement in oxygenation in responders but this was not reflected in an improved survival rate. The manufacture of medical-quality NO in the UK has now been discontinued and most adult units have abandoned its use via pipeline systems. A small portable system is available for paediatric use in the treatment of persistent pulmonary hypertension.

Extracorporeal gas exchange

Extracorporeal gas exchange (ECGE), also termed extracorporeal membrane oxygenation (ECMO), represents the final option if all other avenues of providing ventilatory support have failed. Partial cardiopulmonary venovenous bypass is initiated using heparin-bonded vascular catheters, and extracorporeal oxygenation and carbon dioxide removal are achieved using a membrane oxygenator. A low-volume, low-pressure, low-frequency regimen of ventilation is continued to contribute to respiration. The concept is that by providing adequate oxygenation and carbon dioxide removal with minimal ventilation, the lungs are 'rested' and lung healing is more likely to occur. Its use in trauma patients is particularly difficult as any active bleeding is worsened because the extracorporeal circulation system requires anticoagulation. Currently, in the UK, the availability of ECGE in adults is limited to a few centres carrying out evaluative research.

Assessment of ventilated patients

A checklist for 'troubleshooting' the patient undergoing artificial ventilation is shown in Figure 41.2.

Attempts to breathe out of phase with the ventilator may cause significant problems with oxygenation and carbon dioxide clearance, and may generate very high peak airway pressures. The first priorities are to exclude and, if necessary, correct hypoxaemia or hypercapnia (see Figs 41.1, 41.2) and to detect any adverse effects or complications of ventilation. When these problems have been excluded, a change in sedation, analgesia or mode of ventilation, or rarely the use of neuromuscular blockade, may be indicated.

Reassurance, analgesia and sedation

All but a few patients require some sedation or analgesia while receiving IPPV through a tracheal tube. Ideally, patients should require only light sedation,

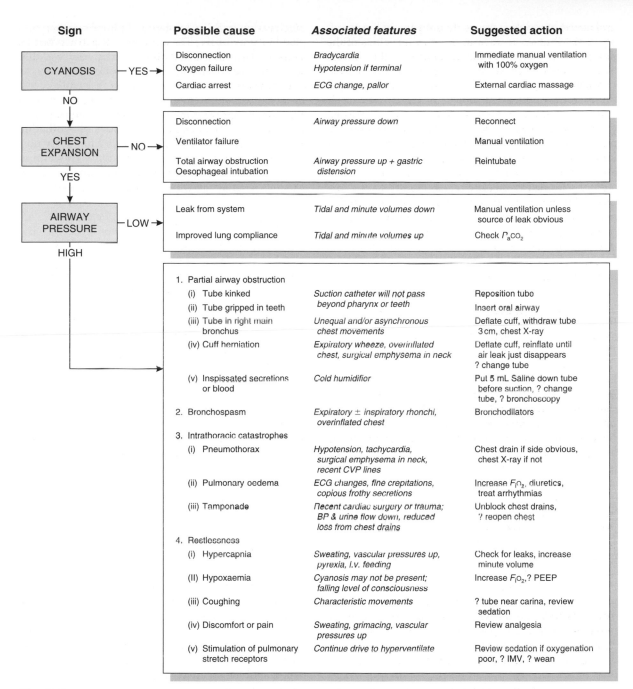

Sign	Possible cause	Associated features	Suggested action
CYANOSIS — YES →	Disconnection Oxygen failure Cardiac arrest	*Bradycardia* *Hypotension if terminal* *ECG change, pallor*	Immediate manual ventilation with 100% oxygen External cardiac massage
NO ↓			
CHEST EXPANSION — NO →	Disconnection Ventilator failure Total airway obstruction Oesophageal intubation	*Airway pressure down* *Airway pressure up + gastric distension*	Reconnect Manual ventilation Reintubate
YES ↓			
AIRWAY PRESSURE — LOW →	Leak from system Improved lung compliance	*Tidal and minute volumes down* *Tidal and minute volumes up*	Manual ventilation unless source of leak obvious Check P_aCO_2
HIGH ↓			

1. Partial airway obstruction		
(i) Tube kinked	*Suction catheter will not pass beyond pharynx or teeth*	Reposition tube
(ii) Tube gripped in teeth		Insert oral airway
(iii) Tube in right main bronchus	*Unequal and/or asynchronous chest movements*	Deflate cuff, withdraw tube 3 cm, chest X-ray
(iv) Cuff herniation	*Expiratory wheeze, overinflated chest, surgical emphysema in neck*	Deflate cuff, reinflate until air leak just disappears ? change tube
(v) Inspissated secretions or blood	*Cold humidifier*	Put 5 mL Saline down tube before suction, ? change tube, ? bronchoscopy
2. Bronchospasm	*Expiratory ± inspiratory rhonchi, overinflated chest*	Bronchodilators
3. Intrathoracic catastrophes		
(i) Pneumothorax	*Hypotension, tachycardia, surgical emphysema in neck, recent CVP lines*	Chest drain if side obvious, chest X-ray if not
(ii) Pulmonary oedema	*ECG changes, fine crepitations, copious frothy secretions*	Increase F_iO_2, diuretics, treat arrhythmias
(iii) Tamponade	*Recent cardiac surgery or trauma; BP & urine flow down, reduced loss from chest drains*	Unblock chest drains, ? reopen chest
4. Restlessness		
(i) Hypercapnia	*Sweating, vascular pressures up, pyrexia, i.v. feeding*	Check for leaks, increase minute volume
(ii) Hypoxaemia	*Cyanosis may not be present; falling level of consciousness*	Increase F_iO_2, ? PEEP
(iii) Coughing	*Characteristic movements*	? tube near carina, review sedation
(iv) Discomfort or pain	*Sweating, grimacing, vascular pressures up*	Review analgesia
(v) Stimulation of pulmonary stretch receptors	*Continue drive to hyperventilate*	Review sedation if oxygenation poor, ? IMV, ? wean

Fig. 41.2
Checklist for the patient undergoing ventilation.

except when unpleasant or painful procedures are performed, so that they can understand and cooperate with therapy. The experienced ICU nurse explains exactly what is happening, reassures and develops methods of communication that do not distress the patient. Such explanations should be brief, as attention span is short in the sick, and should be repeated frequently because memory is impaired. Regular assessment and formal sedation scoring (Table 41.4) should be carried out to avoid oversedation and the associated risks of cardiovascular depression and delayed recovery of consciousness.

The use of sedative drugs to treat pain, or the use of analgesic drugs to produce sedation, almost invariably results in an overdose and in prolongation of recovery. Sedative and analgesic drugs should be given in a ratio appropriate to the needs of the individual patient for anxiolysis and the treatment of pain. Midazolam and propofol are the drugs used most commonly to produce sedation; midazolam is cheaper, but propofol results in more rapid recovery, particularly after prolonged periods of infusion. Morphine and alfentanil are used widely to provide analgesia; alfentanil has a shorter elimination half-life and is useful if weaning from mechanical ventilation is anticipated within the next few hours. Continuous infusions of remifentanil (an ultra-short-acting opioid analgesic) or dexmedetomidine (an α_2-agonist) are under investigation. Metabolism of sedative drugs and accumulation of metabolites normally excreted in the urine result in wide variability in the effects of these drugs not only among individuals but also at different stages of illness in each patient.

Weaning from mechanical ventilation

Weaning is the process by which the patient's dependence on mechanical ventilation is gradually reduced to the point where spontaneous breathing sufficient to meet metabolic needs may be sustained. Because of the adverse effects of mechanical ventilation, weaning should be undertaken at the earliest opportunity.

Pressure support modes

The newer modes of ventilation such as pressure support ventilation or assisted spontaneous breathing with modern microprocessor-controlled ventilators allow the patient to participate actively in ventilation

Table 41.4   An example of a sedation scoring system for use with intensive care patients

Inadequate	Anxious and agitated or restless, or both
Desired	Cooperative, orientated and tranquil
	Responds to command only
	Brisk response to light glabellar tap or loud auditory stimulus
Too deep	Sluggish response to light glabellar tap or loud auditory stimulus
	No response to light glabellar tap or loud auditory stimulus

much earlier in the resolution of lung failure than was possible previously. These modes detect a patient's attempt to breathe spontaneously, synchronize with it and support it to a preset level of positive pressure. At low levels, this compensates for the resistance of the tracheal tube and breathing system; at higher levels, it allows the patient to generate an adequate tidal volume with minimal effort. These modes of ventilation are appropriate only for patients with a relatively normal respiratory rate and normal I:E ratio. The level of pressure support can be reduced gradually as the patient's ventilatory capabilities improve, and when the level of pressure support has been reduced to the value of PEEP, the patient has been weaned to CPAP. The use of such systems allows lower levels of sedation and avoidance of neuromuscular blocking drugs, and reduces disuse atrophy of the respiratory muscles. Weaning is thus a dynamic process in which the mode of ventilation changes from one which necessitates no participation by the patient to one in which mechanical assistance is reduced by titration against the patient's capability to sustain adequate gas exchange.

T-piece methods

Not all ICUs use these 'step-down' modes of ventilation routinely. An alternative is to use trials of spontaneous breathing with CPAP using a simple T-piece system. Periods of spontaneous breathing are allowed without any mechanical support and mechanical ventilation is restarted if the patient shows objective signs of diminished respiratory function. The periods of spontaneous breathing are increased progressively until tracheal extubation is possible.

There is conflicting evidence regarding the superiority of one method over the other and it seems likely that the mode of weaning needs to be individualized in the same manner as the mode of ventilation by taking into account the needs of the patient and the stage of the underlying disease.

If the need for mechanical support is likely to be prolonged, tracheostomy is often performed to prevent the adverse effects of prolonged orotracheal intubation and to facilitate weaning by reducing dead space, work of breathing and the need for sedation, while improving clearance of secretions and rendering re-ventilation easy if necessary.

Optimizing weaning

Although weaning is undertaken as early as possible in all patients, the chances of success are greatly increased if some preconditions are met:

- The original requirement for mechanical ventilation has resolved.
- Sedative and analgesic drugs have been reduced to doses which do not depress ventilation.
- Inspired oxygen concentration is less than 50%.
- CO_2 elimination is not a problem and there is no respiratory acidosis.
- There is no metabolic acidosis.
- Nutritional status, trace elements, minerals, etc., are normal.
- Sputum production is minimal or sputum clearance good.
- Neuromuscular function is adequate.
- The patient is calm, cooperative and pain free.
- There is no high-grade fever.

Monitoring during weaning

Respiratory rate, tidal volume, oxygen saturation, P_aCO_2 and P_aO_2 should be monitored and variables should be set beyond which weaning should be discontinued. When setting such variables, it is important to remember that the levels of P_aO_2 and P_aCO_2 should reflect the premorbid 'normal' values, which are often higher than the physiological norm. Although these vital signs offer objective criteria, the appearance of restlessness, tiredness, confusion, sweatiness, use of accessory muscles and generally abnormal respiratory patterns often occur before changes in vital signs and should be heeded as a warning sign that weaning has been unsuccessful.

CARDIOVASCULAR FAILURE

Although actual or expected ventilatory failure is the commonest reason for admission to the general ICU, cardiovascular failure is a frequent finding in the critically ill patient. When associated with pulmonary problems, the effects of cardiovascular insufficiency may be exacerbated because of reduced oxygenation of blood. Cardiovascular failure may be acute or chronic. When it develops rapidly (e.g. heart failure after myocardial infarction or peripheral circulatory failure after haemorrhage), it is termed 'shock' and, unless the condition is corrected rapidly, admission to an ICU is necessary. Shock is a state in which the circulation is unable to provide adequate perfusion to meet the metabolic needs of the tissues. Unchecked, shock leads to generalized tissue hypoxia and multiple organ dysfunction. When reperfusion occurs, a secondary insult can worsen the initial injury. Cardiovascular monitoring and support in the ICU are designed to pre-empt the development, or provide early recognition, of circulatory shock followed by rapid and effective support of the circulation to prevent the downward spiral into multiple organ failure.

Cardiovascular monitoring

It is possible to monitor the cardiovascular system clinically by the volume of the pulse, skin temperature, capillary refill, detection of tachycardia and sweating, or by identifying surrogate markers of cardiac output such as urine output. Biochemical evidence of established tissue hypoxia, such as metabolic acidosis with a raised blood lactate concentration, is another indicator of shock but may also occur in other forms of metabolic derangement. These are all late, insensitive signs of shock, and significant delays in treatment, with an adverse effect on prognosis, occur if reliance is placed on them.

In critically ill patients, alterations in preload, cardiac function and afterload may occur very quickly and unpredictably, so that real-time measurement of these changes is vital to ensure early intervention and assessment of the effect of therapeutic interventions.

ECG

The ECG is monitored routinely in ICU patients although the presence of a bedside nurse has reduced the requirement for automatic arrhythmia detection systems of the type found in coronary care units.

Systemic arterial pressure

This may be measured intermittently by a conventional or automated sphygmomanometer or continuously by direct intra-arterial recording from the radial, brachial, dorsalis pedis or femoral arteries. Percutaneous arterial cannulation is used widely to monitor arterial pressure and to give ready access to arterial blood samples. Enormous technical efforts are being made to design noninvasive systems which may make invasive procedures less necessary, but at present their accuracy and dependability are inadequate in critical situations. Direct intra-arterial measurement is vital if inotropic or other vasoactive drugs are being used.

Central venous pressure

Central venous pressure (CVP) may be measured from a catheter introduced into the superior vena cava and connected to an electronic manometer. Multilumen catheters allow secure access for infusions of various drugs which may be incompatible with each other and for administration of intermittent sedatives without fear of inadvertent flushing in of inotropic or other

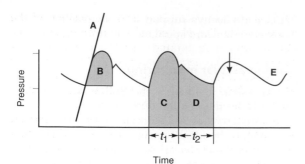

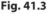

Visible sign	Physiological effect
A - rate of pressure increase	Myocardial contractility
B - area under pressure	Stroke volume
C - systolic pressure x time(t_1)	Myocardial oxygen consumption
D - diastolic pressure x time(t_2)	Myocardial oxygen supply
E - loss of waveform detail	Catheter occlusion (flush it!)

Fig. 41.3
Information to be gained from the arterial pressure signal.

drugs; they also provide a dedicated route for temporary intravenous nutrition. The pressure transduced from the catheter is not usually useful as an absolute value; trends over a period of time are much more important, although rapid changes in response to administration of vasoactive or inotropic drugs, or fluid challenges, may also be significant. CVP readings must be interpreted in the knowledge that a high reading may be caused by high pulmonary artery pressure, high intrathoracic pressure or some other pulmonary abnormality, and not necessarily by cardiac abnormality or volume overload.

Pulmonary artery pressure

Pulmonary artery pressure (PAP) is measured by insertion of a flow-directed pulmonary artery catheter (PAC). The information gained from measurement of pulmonary capillary wedge pressure (PCWP) permits a distinction to be drawn between pulmonary oedema from high left atrial pressure (when PCWP is high) and that caused by increased permeability of pulmonary capillaries (when PCWP is not elevated). This may be helpful particularly in patients with multiple injuries and pulmonary problems, severe septicaemia or actual or incipient left ventricular failure.

PACs are used also to provide information relating to other haemodynamic variables such as cardiac output measured by thermodilution or continuous methods. Some types of PAC also give a continuous reading of mixed venous oxygen saturation. Computerized monitoring systems use these measurements to pro-

vide a wide range of derived parameters which may assist in resuscitation and treatment.

The indications for insertion of a PAC include:

- patients who require inotropic/vasoactive drug therapy
- assessment of fluid loading in SIRS/sepsis, after massive blood loss or other situations in which balancing preload and afterload is difficult, e.g. severe eclampsia with hypertension, pulmonary oedema and oliguria
- diagnosis of noncardiogenic pulmonary oedema in ARDS
- pre-optimization of high-risk patients before surgery.

Complications of PAC insertion include those of central venous cannulation, but in addition they include arrhythmias during insertion, valve erosion causing a sterile or infective vegetation, pulmonary infarction, rupture of pulmonary artery and massive haemorrhage.

Before acting on the values measured using a PAC, its position must be checked on a chest X-ray. The tip of the catheter should lie in a zone in the pulmonary vasculature where pulmonary capillary pressure should exceed alveolar pressure. In addition, PCWP should be less than the mean pulmonary artery pressure, and the Po_2 of a sample of blood in the wedged position should be greater than mixed venous Po_2. Other pitfalls in practice are that high intrathoracic pressures falsely elevate PCWP – 5 cm of PEEP increases PCWP by 1 mmHg. This change is exaggerated further if the tip of the PAC is in a zone of low pulmonary blood flow or if the patient is hypovolaemic. Mitral regurgitation gives a falsely high value of PCWP as a result of the large v-wave; measuring the pressure at the top of the a-wave is more accurate. As the catheter warms and becomes thermolabile, it tends to migrate distally even when the balloon is deflated; if this occurs, it must be withdrawn until a pulmonary artery trace is identified, because prolonged wedging may cause pulmonary infarction. The balloon should always be deflated passively after measuring PCWP and the catheter must never be withdrawn with the balloon inflated as this may cause vascular rupture.

A recent retrospective analysis of a large US database has suggested that there may be increased mortality in patients with PACs as compared with controls. This may reflect the now abandoned practice of 'goal-directed therapy' and further prospective randomized trials are under way. A PAC should not be inserted unless the potential benefits to the patient exceed the risks.

Pulse contour analysis

The peripheral arterial pulse waveform is a function of the cardiac output, the peripheral vascular resistance, peripheral vascular compliance and the arterial pressure (Fig. 41.3). If the cardiac output is measured for a given peripheral arterial waveform, then after calibration, changes in the peripheral pulse waveform can be used to calculate changes in the cardiac output. The two most popular systems available are the LiDCO and PiCCO systems. Both systems use intermittent cardiac output determination using a specific indicator to calibrate the continuous pulse waveform analysis. The lithium indicator dilution (LiDCO) method involves a small bolus of lithium chloride being given into a central venous vein, and as this circulates around the body, the lithium level is determined by a lithium-sensitive electrode connected to an arterial line. The cardiac output is then calculated using standard indicator dilution techniques and used to calibrate subsequent changes in pulse wave contour analysis. A similar system, the PiCCO, uses a thermodilution technique using an injection of cold fluid, which is detected by changes in output from a thermistor placed in a femoral arterial catheter. A recent advance of this technique is to use smaller radial artery-placed catheters. Both techniques seem to give reliable indications of changes in cardiac output once the devices have been correctly calibrated. The disadvantage of the techniques is the requirement for relatively expensive disposable circuits.

Transoesophageal echocardiography (TOE)

A Doppler ultrasound probe passed into the oesophagus to lie alongside the descending arch of the aorta allows continuous measurement of velocity waveforms. The waveform produced by transoesophageal echocardiography is triangular, consisting of a measurement of time and velocity. The peak velocity is at the apex of the triangle and is an index of left ventricular contractility. The flow time is determined by the width of the base of the triangle and is corrected for heart rate to give an index of left ventricular filling. The area under the curve is proportional to the stroke volume passing the probe behind the aorta. The machine uses an internal nomogram based on height, weight, age and sex to determine the normal width of the aorta, and this allows the velocity measurements to be converted to flow and cardiac output. The accuracy of the technique is sensitive to the experience of the user as the position of the probe, determined by the sound made by the waveform, and the contours of the waveform, are dependent on precise placement.

Any patient movement displaces the position of the probe and the Doppler signal will alter significantly. The technique is limited usually to unconscious patients with an intubated trachea. When correctly positioned, the probe is useful in determining the effects of fluid challenges on the flow time constant and the indexed stroke volume.

The data may be improved if the ejection fraction is measured simultaneously. The 'flow time' (the duration of the systolic flow) is related to circulating volume and peripheral resistance. Information may also be obtained relating to global left ventricular function and the presence of any structural abnormality if the probe has M-mode capability. The response to fluid challenges is readily seen in real time without exposing the patient to the risks of a PAC; this may be useful in high-risk surgical patients who require optimization of cardiovascular function before surgery.

Gastric tonometry

The gut functions at relatively low levels of perfusion and oxygenation compared with other tissues and is at risk of ischaemia when the body attempts to compensate for a low cardiac output from any cause by vasoconstriction of the splanchnic circulation. Mucosal acidosis may be used as an early marker of shock. A gastric tonometer consists of a catheter with a silastic balloon at its tip which is inserted into the stomach or colon to lie against the wall. The balloon is filled with saline, and over a period of time CO_2 from the gut wall dissolves in the saline. The P_{CO_2} in the saline is assumed to be the same as the P_{CO_2} in the gut mucosa. The P_{CO_2} in the saline and the arterial bicarbonate concentration are entered into the Henderson–Hasselbalch equation to calculate intramucosal pH (pHi). The lower the pHi, the greater is the degree of ischaemia.

Cardiovascular support

Whatever the cause of cardiovascular failure, the aim of treatment is to restore organ perfusion and oxygenation to their premorbid levels. This may be achieved only by manipulating preload, myocardial contractility, heart rate and afterload. Therapy must be rapid if irreversible organ damage is to be avoided.

The first step is to ensure that there are no airway or breathing problems before adjusting preload with optimization of fluid therapy monitored using the methods described above. When preload has been optimized, persisting evidence of shock is treated with appropriate inotropic or other vasoactive drugs;

careful monitoring is essential because each patient's response varies.

The choice of drug is determined by the patient's underlying pathophysiology; where low cardiac output persists, dobutamine or adrenaline may be used, while cardiac failure with pulmonary oedema may require vasodilators or intra-aortic balloon counterpulsation. Blood flow may need to be redirected (e.g. by use of dopexamine to promote splanchnic blood flow). If a high-output, vasodilated state exists after fluid loading (e.g. in SIRS/sepsis), a vasoconstrictor such as noradrenaline should be used. The drugs and doses must be titrated against the patient's response with the aim of achieving a normal haemodynamic state.

In the general ICU population, the pursuit of supranormal values of oxygen delivery and cardiac output confers no survival benefit and increases mortality in some groups of patients. Stimulating a diseased myocardium with increasing doses of inotropes merely leads to tachycardia, arrhythmias, myocardial ischaemia and decreased survival. The use of inotropic and other vasoactive substances must be coupled with simultaneous optimization of preload and afterload.

If metabolic acidosis is severe (base deficit >15 mmol L^{-1}), the response to inotropes is often reduced; metabolic acidosis which persists after fluid resuscitation and correction of tissue hypoxia may require treatment with sodium bicarbonate and renal support.

SUPPORT OF OTHER SYSTEMS

Renal support

Primary renal disease is a rare cause of admission to the ICU, whereas secondary renal disease causing oliguria is very common in ICU patients. This stems from the extreme sensitivity to oxygen deprivation of those portions of the renal tubules that lie in the medulla. These normally work at the lowest level of the oxygen cascade and suffer early if tissue perfusion is reduced. Prevention of dysfunction progressing to established renal failure depends upon preservation of perfusion and avoidance of hypoxia. Cardiac output, perfusion pressure and intravascular volume should be optimized before considering any other renal support, such as a diuretic. The use of low-dose dopamine has been abandoned; it merely acts as a diuretic and is subject to the same restrictions.

Sudden cessation of urinary output should be regarded as being caused by obstruction until proved otherwise. All drugs should be reviewed for possible nephrotoxic effects and their doses adjusted if cumu-

lation is a problem. Any life-threatening complication such as hyperkalaemia should be treated appropriately until definitive renal support can be arranged. In patients with rhabdomyolysis from any cause, aggressive fluid loading combined with alkalinization of urine and administration of mannitol may protect the kidney from further damage. Other renal protection regimens are unproven. Infusion of a loop diuretic is used in some ICUs to reduce distal tubular oxygen consumption in patients with nonoliguric renal failure.

Renal replacement therapy

The absolute indications for renal replacement therapy (RRT) are uncontrollable hyperkalaemia, acidaemia, severe salt and water overload unresponsive to diuretics in the presence of good urine volume, and severe uraemia or anuria unrelated to obstruction. In most ICUs, continuous venovenous haemofiltration (CVVH) is used with a pump and filter in an extracorporeal circuit connected via a double-lumen vascular catheter placed in a central vein. These systems rely on the production of large volumes of what is essentially 'glomerular filtrate' by ultrafiltration of water and small solutes through the filter's semipermeable tubules. Accurate i.v. replacement with an equal volume of specific replacement fluid is required to maintain fluid balance; replacing slightly less allows the equivalent amount of water to be removed from the patient. In very catabolic septic patients, the ultrafiltration effect may be enhanced by passing dialysis fluid through the filter via a separate channel in a counter-current manner (continuous venovenous haemodiafiltration, CVVHD). The use of continuous slow techniques is tolerated better than intermittent haemodialysis in unstable ICU patients.

Neurological support

Despite the wide range of pathologies that require patients to be admitted to the ICU for specialized neurological support, some specific treatment regimens are common to them all.

Irrespective of the primary cause of neurological damage, secondary injury may be caused by hypoxaemia, hypotension, hypercapnia and metabolic disturbances. Consequently, the airway should be secured, the lungs ventilated to achieve a $P_{a}CO_2$ of 4–5 kPa, the inspired oxygen concentration adjusted to sustain a $P_{a}O_2$ in excess of 12 kPa and appropriate steps taken to maintain blood pressure within the normal range. Intravenous administration of glucose should be avoided and insulin should be administered intravenously if the blood glucose concentration exceeds 11 mmol L^{-1} because hyperglycaemia increases the risk of secondary brain injury. The plasma osmolality and serum sodium concentration should be monitored carefully because hypo-osmolality of the plasma creates an osmotic gradient across the blood–brain barrier and may provoke cerebral oedema.

In patients with raised ICP, it may be appropriate to monitor cerebral perfusion pressure (CPP) by direct measurement of ICP and mean arterial pressure. ICP should be maintained within the normal range if possible; sudden increases may occur in patients who are restless or hypertensive, and adequate sedation and analgesia are usually important components of therapy. CPP may be increased by judicious fluid loading and the use of pressor agents. However, high arterial pressure should be avoided, because many patients with brain injury have impaired cerebral autoregulation and a high CPP may result in increased cerebral oedema.

Administration of neuromuscular blockers is rarely required except to prevent shivering if surface cooling has been used in an attempt to decrease cerebral metabolic rate.

Cerebral blood flow may be monitored using radioisotope methods, or estimated using transcranial Doppler techniques, jugular venous bulb oxygen saturation or tissue oxygen electrodes placed within the skull.

Electrical activity of the brain may be monitored using techniques such as compressed spectral array or the cerebral function analysing monitor.

In modern neurosurgical ICUs, a combination of these techniques is often used to produce multimodal analysis of brain function, and therapy is adjusted to maximize oxygen delivery, minimize oxygen consumption, preserve cerebral blood flow and normalize ICP.

CARE BUNDLES

There is an increasing interest in the development of 'care bundles' for specific ICU illnesses. The concept is that published data showing a survival advantage for one type of treatment may be combined with other successful types of treatment in an attempt to produce a 'bundle' of evidence-based treatments, all of which have been shown to improve outcome. The hope is that if all these treatments are combined, the bundle of care may confer a greater probability of survival than the components of the bundle if applied singly. The

ranking of evidence-based recommendations is based on the type of investigation:

- Type I: large-scale randomized prospective controlled trials with clear results and low alpha or beta error
- Type II: small randomized prospective controlled trials with uncertain results and moderate to high alpha/beta error
- Type III: nonrandomized trials with contemporaneous controls
- Type IV: nonrandomized trials, historical controls and expert opinion
- Type V: nonrandomized trials, uncontrolled studies and expert opinion.

A grading system may then be applied:

- Grade A: supported by at least 2 level I investigations
- Grade B: supported by 1 level I investigation
- Grade C: supported by level II investigations only
- Grade D: supported by at least 1 level III investigation
- Grade E: supported by level IV or V evidence.

The most widely adopted bundle of care relates to mechanical ventilation for the treatment of acute lung injury (ALI) and ARDS:

- *low tidal volumes* (6mL per kg predicted body weight) *and capped plateau airway pressure* (30cmH$_2$O) – Grade B
- *sedation holidays and use of sedation scores* when continuous sedative infusions are interrupted on a daily basis to allow intermittent decreased sedation score reduces length of ICU stay – Grade B
- *permissive hypercapnia* (accepting a P_aCO$_2$ above normal to allow pressure limitation and low plateau airway pressures) – Grade C
- *semi-recumbent positioning* (head up by 45° unless contraindicated) during ventilation to reduce the incidence of ventilator-induced pneumonia – Grade C
- *lung recruitment by PEEP* to prevent alveolar collapse at end-expiration – Grade E
- *avoidance of neuromuscular blocking drugs* reduces the incidence of skeletal muscle weakness associated with critical illness
- *protocol driven weaning* – still under study in ALI/ARDS; Grade A in other causes of respiratory failure.

Other care bundles have been developed, most notably for the treatment of sepsis and septic shock. This core bundle was developed by the Surviving Sepsis Campaign and includes lung protective ventilatory strategy, tight glycaemic control, low dose steroid therapy and resuscitation to achieve a central venous oxygen saturation of above 70%. The problem with care bundles is that they are developed by amalgamating individual treatments which, although evidence-based individually, have not been investigated in combination. Another risk is involved when the bundle components have been investigated for a specific illness but are then applied to a different disease with some similar pathophysiological features.

GENERAL INTENSIVE CARE

Visitors to ICUs often focus on the technology and fail to appreciate the intensity of the nursing and paramedical support needed for each patient. Skin care, tracheal suction, stress ulcer prophylaxis, DVT prophylaxis, turning, washing, eye, mouth and bowel care, mobilization and passive movement, and psychological support to the patient (and relatives) take considerable patience and skill and are important contributors to good outcome.

All ICU patients need nutrition as soon as possible, regardless of the reason for admission. Very few ICU patients are able to take a normal diet. There is increasing evidence that early enteral nutrition improves outcome and some evidence that specific diet supplements such as glutamine may improve immune function and survival. With the exception of patients with gastrointestinal obstruction, prolonged paralytic ileus, short bowel syndrome or enterocutaneous fistula, the majority of ICU patients may be fed via the enteral route within 48 h. A fine-bore nasogastric tube may be inadequate in some patients and a nasojejunal tube, feeding jejunostomy or percutaneous gastrostomy may be used. Parenteral feeding is the route of last resort but is better than nothing.

Of all ICU patients who die after spending more than 5 days in the ICU, 80% die in a manner which involves sepsis. Cross-infection is a particular risk and strict asepsis and personal hygiene are vital. The emergence of multiresistant microorganisms is an increasing problem and is conquered best by control of cross-infection, good aseptic techniques and regular microbiological surveillance, with swabs, blood cultures and other samples being taken at every opportunity. The widespread use of prophylactic or broad-spectrum antibiotics is to be avoided.

OUTCOME AFTER INTENSIVE CARE

Intensive care has developed without much research into its efficacy in terms of improved survival and quality of life after discharge. Very few of the procedures performed commonly in the ICU have been subjected to scientific scrutiny, but it would be impossible ethically to allocate critically ill patients randomly to receive either ward or ICU care in an attempt to conduct a prospective controlled trial of the ICU process as a whole. Consequently, observational audit methods have been developed to compare actual outcome with predicted outcome in terms of survival. In the near future, all ICUs in the UK will be required to gather data to assess their performance. These methods require an objective scoring system which can assess severity of illness reproducibly and which takes into account the case mix of the ICU. Survival or death after ICU is influenced not only by the quality, timing and type of care but also by the age of the patient, the severity of illness, the presence of comorbidity, the illness which precipitates admission and the presence of any emergency or elective treatment given before admission.

The Intensive Care National Audit Research Centre (ICNARC) used the acute physiology and chronic health evaluation (APACHE) score developed by Knauss to compare ICU mortality and total hospital mortality among 22 057 ICU patients between 1995 and 1998 in 62 ICUs in England and Wales. The data showed an average mortality of 20.6% in ICUs and a total hospital mortality of 30.9%, but the mortality in different hospitals varied threefold. Because of the problems of case mix variability, these scoring systems are best used for comparative audit so that deviations from the norm may be identified and investigated, or for evaluative research; for example, severity of illness could be used to stratify patient groups into those with similar predicted outcomes of death so that the success or failure of a specific intervention may be evaluated within a homogeneous group of patients.

Scoring systems should not be used to individualize treatment decisions within the ICU. The higher the APACHE score, the less likely a patient is to survive. For example, a 71-year-old man admitted to ICU after emergency abdominal aortic aneurysm repair may have physiological abnormality and comorbidity which gives him an APACHE score of 22. For this *condition*, with this score, the probability of death is 60.5%, but the probability of death for this *patient* cannot be predicted; he may be one of the 39.5% who survive! Thus, at their present level of accuracy, scoring systems cannot be used alone to identify patients in whom continued treatment is futile.

ICU care is supportive rather than curative and has the ability to prolong the process of dying. This is not in the best interests of a patient who continues to deteriorate despite maximal supportive therapy. In such patients, the continuation of treatment is both futile and unethical. About 70% of deaths in ICUs occur after limitation of treatment. This is not euthanasia; the patient dies of the underlying disease process when the supporting therapies are withdrawn. The identification of patients in whom there should be a change from aggressive supportive therapy to compassionate, palliative care is difficult. Opinions may vary as to what constitutes futility, the timing of the change to palliative care and the nature of the treatments to be withdrawn. There is variability among countries, and among ICUs within the same country.

In terms of predicting which patients are unlikely to survive, those who are comatose and unresponsive after severe brain damage are amongst the easier to distinguish. The signs of 'brainstem death' are well recognized and a scheme of assessment is shown in Table 41.5. If brainstem death is a likely diagnosis, the possibility of organ donation should always be considered and discussed with the patient's family. It is best if these discussions are initiated by ICU staff who are experienced in dealing with bereaved relatives.

Assessments of functional disability, quality of life and return to work among patients who have survived an admission to the ICU are more difficult to quantify than death, but the small numbers of studies which have been undertaken suggest that mortality is significantly higher than would be expected in matched individuals for several years, that a significant proportion of patients report impaired quality of life and that many remain unable to work for prolonged periods after discharge. However, the majority of patients survive and return to a reasonable quality of life.

Improving outcome

Many patients who undergo elective or, more commonly, emergency surgery receive inadequate preoperative preparation in respect of volume resuscitation or cardiovascular support. These patients are particularly at risk from hypovolaemia and myocardial ischaemia in the perioperative period, and suffer an exaggerated stress response. These factors amplify postoperative SIRS because of decreased organ perfusion. There is increasing evidence that outcome may be improved in

---

Table 41.5 Recognition of brainstem death. Brainstem death may be assumed if: (a) the answer to each of the 10 questions is 'no'; and (b) the assessment is repeated with the same results after at least 4 h. If the answer to any of the questions is 'yes' or 'don't know', active treatment must be continued

1. Is there any doubt as to the cause of the coma and brain damage (e.g. trauma, cerebrovascular accident, drowning)?

2. Has the patient received (or taken) any drugs which could have either depressed the central nervous system (e.g. alcohol, sedatives, hypnotics, analgesics) or impaired muscular capabilities (e.g. muscle relaxants)?

3. Are there any metabolic or endocrine disturbances which could affect neural function (e.g. blood glucose changes, uraemia, hepatic dysfunction)?

4. Is the patient's temperature less than 35°C? (Midbrain failure is often followed by a rapid decrease in temperature, but hypothermia itself may induce coma. If the temperature is below 35°C, active warming must be started and further cooling minimized with 'space blankets'.)

5. Do the pupils react to light?

6. Are there corneal reflexes?

7. Do the eyes move during or after caloric testing?

8. Are there motor responses in the cranial nerve distribution in response to painful stimulation of the face, trunk or limbs?

9. Does the patient gag, cough or otherwise move following the passage of a suction catheter into the nose, mouth or bronchial tree?

10. Does the patient show any respiratory activity at all when the arterial carbon dioxide tension exceeds 7 kPa (checked on an arterial sample)?

high-risk surgical patients if blood volume and cardio-vascular function are optimized preoperatively.

The fact that the most seriously ill patients are now nursed in specialized areas has resulted in 'deskilling' of ward-based nursing and medical staff. The increased throughput of surgical patients, together with the reduction in the working hours of trainee medical staff, has resulted in a risk that patients may deteriorate in the ward unnoticed, or that their deterioration may be treated inadequately, so that there may be great difficulty in resuscitation when the true severity of the patient's condition is recognized. The total hospital mortality of patients admitted to the ICU from other hospital wards (45%) is significantly greater than the mortality among patients admitted from the accident and emergency department (30%) or from the operating theatre (20%).

There is therefore a need for an area within the hospital which can provide an intermediate level of care. These areas are usually called high-dependency units (HDUs). The development of HDUs should proceed in tandem with education of ward-based medical and nursing staff and with the development of 'critical care outreach' teams. Increasingly, the barriers between ICU, HDU and the postanaesthesia care unit (PACU) are becoming blurred so that critically ill patients may receive the level of care most appropriate for the severity of their illness and the progress of their disease at all times during their stay in hospital.

PAEDIATRIC INTENSIVE CARE

It is important to realize that neonates, infants and children are not simply 'small adults'. In addition to the range of adult diseases, they may suffer from additional problems because of developmental abnormalities, inborn errors of metabolism, increased susceptibility to infection, immature brain, immune function, renal function and thermoregulatory mechanisms, and these all add to the complexity of critical illness in neonates and infants. The provision of paediatric intensive care ideally requires a designated unit staffed by paediatrically trained intensive care doctors, nurses and supporting subspecialities. The general requirements for the paediatric intensive care unit in terms of medical cover, nursing cover and equipment are remarkably similar.

Monitoring of cardiorespiratory function in paediatric patients requires the use of much smaller pieces of equipment and the alarm settings must be set to reflect the normal parameters found for a child of that age. Continuous monitoring of arterial blood pressure and central venous pressure, and even pulmonary artery pressure, is possible providing appropriately sized catheters and sites are used. In addition to the complications associated with arterial cannulation in adults, small infants are susceptible to retrograde embolization during flushing of the arterial cannula and it should be remembered that disconnection and haemorrhage, if unrecognized, may result in the loss of a large proportion of an infant's blood volume very quickly. Pulmonary artery pressure monitoring is rarely performed in paediatric intensive care except following surgery for congenital heart disease, and often the PA catheter is inserted directly at the time of surgery; alternatively, a directly placed left atrial catheter may be used. Noninvasive monitoring of P_{O_2} and P_{CO_2} is possible in small children because of the thinness of their epidermis. In transcutaneous monitoring, the electrodes are heated to around 40–45°C, which arterializes the capillary blood and maximizes capillary blood flow. These electrodes allow continuous changes in P_{O_2} or P_{CO_2} to be monitored but the electrodes have to be moved around to prevent burns occurring.

SPECIFIC PROBLEMS IN PAEDIATRIC ICU

Persisting fetal circulation

The change in circulation from the feto-placental pattern to the neonatal pattern provides a major challenge to the newborn. In the normal fetal circulation, 60% of the blood returning to the right atrium passes through the foramen ovale into the left ventricle and ascending aorta. At birth, closure of the umbilical vessels results in increased systemic vascular resistance and lung expansion leads to a reduction in pulmonary vascular resistance. Pulmonary blood flow therefore increases, leading to a rise in left atrial pressure. Functional closure of the foramen ovale occurs and the ductus arteriosis becomes constricted and eventually thrombosed. If high pulmonary blood flow still occurs, for example as the result of congenital heart lesions such as ventricular septal defect or patent ductus arteriosus, these changes may be arrested and pulmonary hypertension occurs. Persistent pulmonary hypertension results in preservation of the normal fetal circulation with right to left shunting occurring through the foramen ovale and ductus arteriosus. This results in increasing hypoxaemia and acidosis, which in turn increases the pulmonary vascular resistance, setting up a vicious circle. There are numerous causes of persistent fetal circulation, including primary pulmonary hypoplasia, diaphragmatic hernia, meconium aspiration, chronic placental insufficiency, severe sepsis or severe lung disease due to hyaline membrane disease of the premature infant. Treatment must be aimed at relieving the underlying cause and correction of hypoxaemia. Treatment aimed at reducing pulmonary vascular resistance includes maintaining a high oxygen saturation, the use of CPAP or positive end-expiratory pressure to prevent lung collapse, hyperventilation to generate a respiratory alkalosis and support of the cardiovascular system with fluids and inotropes. In very severe cases, selective treatment with pulmonary vasodilators such as inhaled nitric oxide, nebulized protaglandins or intravenous tolazoline may be used. In the most extreme cases, extracorporeal membrane oxygenation has been proven to be effective.

Hypothermia

Neonates have a high surface area to body weight ratio and do not have a thick layer of subcutaneous fat. Thus, they are more at risk of losing heat than older children or adults. In addition, their thermoregulatory mechanisms are less efficient and they are unable to generate heat by shivering or lose heat by sweating. Thermogenesis in the newborn is largely derived as a result of oxidation of the brown fat found in the intrascapular and perirenal areas. Brown fat reserves are greatly reduced in premature infants, who are particularly at risk of becoming cold very quickly. The mere loss of body temperature can greatly increase cardiovascular or respiratory dysfunction. Body temperature should be maintained by appropriate use of incubators and radiant heaters.

Birth asphyxia

Birth asphyxia may be caused by chronic placental failure, depression of maternal cardiorespiratory function from any cause immediately before or during delivery, obstetric complications such as prolapsed umbilical cord, multiple births or prematurity, or from postnatal problems such as acute respiratory distress syndrome from any cause. Asphyxia at birth is recognized by the process of Apgar scoring. Newborn babies with Apgar scores of between 5 and 7 generally are treated by stimulation and suction of the nose, mouth and pharynx with oxygen by mask. Moderate birth asphyxia (Apgar 3–4) is treated generally with bag-valve mask ventilation with oxygen and correction of any metabolic acidosis. Babies with severe asphyxia (Apgar 0–2) require cardiopulmonary resuscitation including tracheal intubation and positive-pressure ventilation with oxygen. After correction of acidosis and volume resuscitation, with or without the use of inotropes, the baby should be transferred to the neonatal intensive care unit. In general terms, oral tracheal tubes are used for resuscitation, and tubes are moved to the nasotracheal site when prolonged ventilation is required. Vascular access may be very difficult in a newborn child, particularly if the child is hypovolaemic or hypothermic, and umbilical veins or the external jugular vein may be used.

RESPIRATORY FAILURE

Respiratory failure is a very common cause of admission to the paediatric intensive care unit. Oxygen consumption is much higher in the infant than in the older child or adult and this may be increased by the presence of either systemic illness, fever or agitation. The increased metabolic rate also implies that carbon dioxide levels increase twice as fast as those in older children and adults. Infants and neonates have a much greater susceptibility to respiratory disease than adults for several reasons. The thoracic cage is less well developed and the chest wall softer. Increased respiratory effort leads to retraction of bony and soft tissues rather than increased minute ventilation. Chest wall/rib cage recession causes a tendency towards increased small airways collapse and intrapulmonary shunting. The lungs are relatively immature, particularly in premature infants, and there may be surfactant deficiency which also promotes increased alveolar collapse.

Respiratory distress in the newborn is recognized by the combination of tachypnoea and distortion of the chest wall to include sternum and rib retraction, use of the accessory muscles of the neck and flaring of the alae nasi. If these signs are not recognized early, then slowing of the respiratory rate and apnoea may follow as a result of respiratory fatigue. Respiratory failure may be caused by upper or lower airway obstruction, pulmonary disease per se, such as hyaline membrane disease or bronchopulmonary dysplasia, pneumonia, aspiration of meconium, pulmonary oedema or pulmonary hyperplasia, or from compression of the lungs due to diaphragmatic hernia, pneumothorax or secondary to raised intra-abdominal pressure following repair of exomphalos or gastroschisis. In addition, respiratory failure may occur as a result of either acquired or inherited neurological or muscular disease. Immaturity of the immune system, which persists for the first 6 months of life, may lead to an increased susceptibility to infection.

The mode of oxygen therapy is often dictated by the size of the patient. Neonates may be nursed in an incubator if inspired oxygen concentrations of less than 40% are required. Where higher oxygen concentrations are required, a plastic headbox may be used. Older children may tolerate a face mask but their variable peak inspiratory flow rates and tendency to remove the mask makes calculation of inspired O_2 concentrations difficult. In the past, the use of high inspired oxygen concentrations led to the development of retrolental fibroplasia and subsequent blindness. The safe maximum level of oxygenation is unknown but an endpoint of between 6 and 10 kPa is generally recommended. Intubation of the trachea may be required if oxygenation is not achievable by incubator, headbox or face mask therapy, or if hypercapnia occurs. Nasal intubation is the safest by allowing firm tube fixation, which lessens the chance of inadvertent extubation, or migration of the tube endobronchially, decreases sedation requirements and allows a T-piece system to be applied to provide CPAP. In general terms, in neonates who are intubated, CPAP should be used routinely at physiological levels of around 2 cmH$_2$O to prevent airway collapse. Where mechanical ventilation is used, then the risk of volutrauma and barotrauma are always present and peak inspiratory pressure, PEEP, CPAP and inspiratory flow rates must be controlled carefully and set to an appropriate level for the patient's size and age. All the complications found in adult continuous positive-pressure ventilation may be found in children. High-frequency ventilation, or high-frequency oscillatory ventilation, is used more commonly in paediatric patients than in adults.

CARDIOVASCULAR FAILURE

Support of the cardiovascular system in children is most often required in patients with hypovolaemia or sepsis. Hypovolaemia may be caused by bleeding, but a much more frequent cause is fluid losses from the gastrointestinal tract by vomiting, diarrhoea, ileus or repeated nasogastric suction. Sepsis produces a distributive pattern of shock, as in adults. Cardiogenic shock is an important problem when congenital heart disease is present. During hypovolaemia, small children initially compensate by vasoconstriction and tachycardia. Bradycardia is a sign of impending decompensation. Treatment of shock should follow an ABC pattern and fluid should be given in repeated boluses of 20 mL kg^{-1} of 0.9% saline or Hartmann's solution, or 10 mL kg^{-1} of blood or colloid every 5 or 10 min until blood pressure, heart rate and peripheral perfusion have returned to normal. If more than 40 mL kg^{-1} of colloid has been given, then some would suggest that central venous monitoring should be commenced, an arterial cannula inserted and inotropic support instigated.

NEUROLOGICAL PROBLEMS

Brain injury may occur as a result of trauma, ischaemia, infection or metabolic derangement and is a common cause of death in children. In the Western world, trauma is the most common cause of death in children after the first year of life. The pattern of mechanism of injury is related to age and age-related behaviour. Falls and nonaccidental injury are commoner in younger children, whereas cycle and motor vehicle accidents become more common in older children. Significant head injury occurs in 75% of children admitted with blunt trauma, and the death rate is very high. Treatment algorithms are essentially identical to those in adults, following the standard primary survey/secondary survey system, and paying strict attention to correction of problems with airway, breathing or circulation. Structural injury to the brain may occur as a result of haemorrhage from an arteriovenous malformation, aneurysm or tumour, or either primary or secondary hydrocephalus. Infections such as meningitis and encephalitis are frequent causes of coma in children, but other biochemical problems such as hypoglycaemia, electrolyte disorders or severe dehydration should be considered. Children in coma should undergo tracheal intubation and mechanical ventilation of the lungs if there is evidence of upper airway obstruction or loss of airway reflexes, abnormal respiratory pattern, apnoea, deepening coma or signs of progressive elevation of intracranial pressure such as bradycardia, hypertension, abnormal capillary reflexes or localizing signs. Computed tomography is the initial investigation of choice. In the absence of evidence of hydrocephalus, lumbar puncture should be performed to exclude meningitis or encephalitis. Under the age of 4 years, a modified Glasgow Coma Score should be used.

DEHYDRATION AND SHOCK

Classically, the signs of moderate dehydration in children are described as decreased peripheral perfusion as shown by poor or decreased capillary refill, deep breathing and decreasing skin turgor. However, these signs are not specific and may develop after only a small amount of volume loss (about 5%). Intravenous access may be very difficult in severely shocked children and the interosseous route may be used. The most commonly chosen site is at the junction of the upper and middle thirds of the tibia (0–12 months of age), the medial malleolus (1–5 years) and the iliac crest (over 5 years). A 20-gauge interosseous needle is held perpendicular to the bone and inserted by gentle rotation about its long access after a small skin incision has been made. Fluid may be administered under pressure from a syringe but pain is a common problem.

OUTCOME OF PAEDIATRIC INTENSIVE CARE

Mortality in paediatric intensive care units has been quoted as ranging from 5% to 15%. If patients who have been admitted with severe pre-existing disease or disability are excluded, then the majority are reported to make a normal or nearly normal recovery and to have a normal life expectancy. Prediction of mortality on intensive care units in a manner analogous to APACHE scoring is carried out using the Paediatric Risk of Mortality Score – PRISM. PRISM scoring may be used to calculate standardized mortality ratios and compare outcome between paediatric intensive care units. In general terms, paediatric patients with the same degree of severity of illness generally do better than adults. For example, while multiple organ failure increases mortality, the prognosis is better than for adults. There is evidence that mortality is reduced if children are looked after in specialist paediatric intensive care units rather than mixed intensive care units, i.e. treating both adults and children. General intensive care units should have the facility to stabilize and treat small children for around 24 h before arranging for safe transfer to a specialist paediatric intensive care unit.

ETHICAL CONSIDERATIONS

The availability of advanced methods of life support in the ICU may generate numerous ethical dilemmas. The majority of the patients treated are noncompetent in that they are unconscious or rendered unconscious by either the disease process or by the use of sedative drugs. Treatment in intensive care is governed by the same four basic principles as those that govern general medical practice. *Autonomy* is the right of all individuals to exercise self-determination. To do this they must be able to understand and believe the information given. *Beneficence* is the concept that any action that is performed on the patient should be in that patient's best interest. The corollary of that is that any action carried out on a patient must not harm that patient, which is the concept of *non-maleficence*. Finally, the concept of *justice* in terms of the maximum benefit for the majority of the patients must be applied. The majority of intensive care patients are not autonomous because they are not *competent*, as a result of the effects of disease or drugs administered. This leads to the potential for *paternalism* to occur – the attitude that 'doctor knows best'. The ethical practice of critical care medicine must apply these principles to each individual patient.

Autonomy and competence

The key issue in decisions based on autonomy is one of capacity, in that the patients must be able to make an informed choice, i.e. they are competent. For example, if a patient refuses a treatment, understands that the refusal of that treatment will lead to death, believes that this is the definite result and has the ability to weigh the information and make this decision, then the patient is fully mentally competent and the decision must be obeyed. The most frequent example of this in anaesthesia relates to the practice of Jehovah's Witnesses refusing to receive blood transfusion even if a blood transfusion were necessary to prevent their death. Providing this decision has been made and documented in advance, perhaps in the form of an advanced directive, then doctors may not interfere with this decision. Patients who do not have the capacity to think, retain, understand and believe the information required to make a valid treatment decision are incompetent. In such situations, the medical and nursing staff looking after them should act in the patient's best interest and the decisions of the attending medical team should be in accordance with that of a responsible body of medical opinion.

Beneficence versus maleficence

The concept of beneficence and non-maleficence is best understood by the statement that we must always do our patients some good and never do them any harm. The treatment we offer must therefore have a positive risk:benefit ratio. Beneficence and non-maleficence must be individual patient-based. Consider the example of a patient who has developed a massive intracerebral haemorrhage. That patient may be deeply unconscious and for the moment still breathing spontaneously, but if the disease process is left to develop, the patient may become apnoeic and die. If one were to intubate the trachea and ventilate the lungs of such a patient then perhaps apnoea would still develop but life would be maintained. The patient may develop brainstem death and become suitable for organ donation. Some would argue that such interventions would increase the number of organs available for donation and that consequently one would be doing a good deed for other patients. However, the action of electively intubating the trachea and ventilating the lungs of such patients can have no possible benefit for the individual patient concerned, even though such an action might benefit other patients requiring organ donation. The treatment is *futile*, is of no benefit to the individual patient and should not be carried out.

The most frequent example of beneficence and non-maleficence related to individual patients occurs when the intensive care unit is full and another patient needs admission. Who should be transferred: the most stable patient already in a bed to another intensive care unit, or a very unstable patient from the accident and emergency ward? Some would say that it is unethical to transfer a patient who is already in an intensive care bed to another unit as the transfer is not in that patient's best interest and would expose that patient to risk, even though this action would benefit the treatment of the unstable patient. The stable patient is therefore exposed to maleficence for the benefit of another patient. The beneficence versus non-maleficence argument is countered in this case by acknowledging that all the patients concerned require an intensive care bed and that intensive care staff owe a duty of care to all patients requiring intensive care and not just to those patients who are already in a bed. The risk of transfer of a stable patient may well be much smaller than the risk of transfer of an unstable patient and consequently the beneficence–non-maleficence balance rests in favour of transferring the most stable patient.

Futility

The principle of justice in treatment of intensive care patients is based on the fact that all patients have an equal right to all treatments. The problem here is that some patients who may have extensive comorbidity or very advanced disease have no prospect whatsoever of responding to such treatment and therefore to offer them such treatment is unjust. Where a treatment has no possible chance of being successful then that treatment is futile and should not be carried out. Hippocrates stated that doctors should not treat patients who were 'overmastered by their disease'. In other words, we should not treat patients in whom there is no possibility of recovery. Treatment should be limited on the basis of futility. There is no legal distinction between the withdrawal of life-sustaining treatment or limiting or withholding treatment. If death is felt to be inevitable then providing treatment merely prolongs that process and is consequently of no benefit, i.e. maleficent, and provides no beneficence to the patient. Therefore, it would seem ethically reasonable to discontinue such treatment.

The majority of patients who die in intensive care units die as a consequence of treatment withdrawal in the face of continued deterioration despite maximal appropriate supportive therapy. This is termed *imminent demise futility*. The concept of futility may be further classified into physiological futility, i.e. where the degree of injury is such that no treatment could possibly succeed. An example of this would be performing a thoracotomy for someone who had sustained a car-

diac arrest following blunt chest trauma. *Interactive futility* occurs where a medical intervention preserves life in terms of physiological function but would not restore that individual's ability to interact with his surroundings, for example a person in a persistent vegetative state. Because the withdrawal of basic treatment – feeding and hydration – may be involved in such cases, the opinion of the courts is necessary.

The remaining and most difficult area is *qualitative futility*. In these patients, the treatment could well sustain life but at a cost that a reasonable body of medical opinion would believe to be unacceptable. This may relate to someone who was treated and would remain permanently undergoing ventilation, unconscious and quadriplegic. Decisions such as these are inevitably subjective and based upon the opinions formed by the medical and attending staff.

Withdrawal of life-sustaining treatment

When the decision to withdraw life-sustaining treatment has been made, the decision should be discussed with a noncompetent patient's relatives. Legally, in England and Wales, they cannot give consent but may give their assent. The method of treatment withdrawal varies from country to country. In the USA it is very common to undergo a process of 'terminal weaning' whereby the trachea is extubated in the knowledge that patients cannot sustain their own ventilation effectively. This is less frequently practised in the United Kingdom as the time from the treatment withdrawal to time of death is often very short. Withdrawal of artificial ventilation would allow death to occur much more quickly than withdrawal of renal support, but there is no ethical or logical distinction between the withdrawal of one or the other as both may be regarded as futile treatments in the face of an inevitable death. The majority of units withdraw all supportive therapy, e.g. inotropes, PEEP, high F_IO_2, antibiotics or renal support, but may well continue baseline ventilation if the patient has no possibility of breathing spontaneously. If patients can breathe spontaneously, then they are allowed to do so. If the patient shows signs of distress, then it is ethically acceptable to prescribe morphine and sedatives to relieve that distress, even though the side-effects of such drugs may hasten death secondarily. In patients who have received large doses of sedatives/analgesics for some time, the doses required to relieve pain may be large. The intention of the prescription is not to hasten death but to relieve pain and suffering. This is known as the doctrine of double effect. It is neither legal nor ethical to administer a drug with the sole intention of causing death.

Guidance to medical staff has been published by both the General Medical Council and the BMA. These stated 'developments in technology have led to a misconception in society that death can almost always be postponed. There needs to be a recognition that there comes a point in all lives where no more can reasonably or helpfully be done to benefit patients other than keeping them comfortable and free from pain.' Neither organization has published specific guidance for intensive care patients but the principles are transferable. Recent court decisions have re-emphasized the right of a competent patient both to refuse treatment or to receive the basic treatment of hydration and nutrition. When treatment withdrawal/limitation decisions are made, the reasoning behind them should be discussed with all the medical and nursing team, a full explanation given to the relatives and their assent obtained. Palliative or compassionate care should be continued on the intensive care unit if the death is imminent, but where death is likely to be prolonged or delayed, then the patient may be discharged to a more suitable area for terminal care.

FURTHER READING

Brooks A, Girling K, Riley B et al. (eds) 2005 *Critical Care for Postgraduate Trainees*. Hodder Arnold, London

Craft T, Nolan J, Parr M 1999 Key topics in critical care. BIOS Scientific Publishers, Oxford

Hillman K, Bishop G 2004 Clinical intensive care, 2nd edn. Cambridge University Press, Cambridge

Singer M, Grant I S 1999 ABC of intensive care. BMJ Publications, London

Webb A R, Shapiro M, Singer M, Suter P 1999 Oxford textbook of critical care. Oxford University Press, Oxford

42 Management of chronic pain

Recent advances in the understanding of the fundamental mechanisms involved in the transmission and modulation of noxious impulses have significantly extended the range of assessment tools and treatments clinicians offer to patients with pain. The majority of medical pain specialists in the UK are anaesthetists. Historically, anaesthetists have been responsible for the relief of pain in the perioperative period and have developed skills in percutaneous neural blockade. This expertise, developed originally with local anaesthetics, was then extended to neurolytic agents. Initially, pain clinics started as nerve-blocking clinics and most pain management clinics continue to be directed by anaesthetists. However, with increasing awareness of the complexity of the pain experience, there has been recognition that other healthcare professionals have a significant role in the management of patients with chronic pain. A multidisciplinary approach involving anaesthetists, other healthcare professionals, such as psychologists, physiotherapists, occupational therapists, nurse specialists and other medical practitioners, is being offered increasingly to patients with pain. Pain management clinics are available in most hospitals in the United Kingdom, although there is variation in the services offered. However, changes in the way that healthcare is delivered may lead to pain management services being offered increasingly in primary care in addition to the secondary care setting.

DEFINITIONS OF PAIN AND RELATED TERMS

Pain: 'an unpleasant sensory and emotional experience associated with actual or potential tissue damage, or described in terms of such damage' (The International Association for the Study of Pain (IASP), 1986).

This definition emphasizes that pain is not only a physical sensation but also, ultimately, a subjective psychological event. It accepts that pain may occur in spite of negative physical findings and investigations. Pain has sensory, cognitive and motivational-affective dimensions and has been described as a biopsychosocial experience, as illustrated in Figure 42.1. This must be taken into account when assessing and planning a treatment strategy for the patient with pain.

Acute pain: pain associated with acute injury (including surgery) or disease.

Chronic pain: pain that either occurs in disease processes in which healing does not take place or persists beyond the expected time of healing – arbitrarily 3 months.

Pain management: a multidisciplinary approach to the assessment and treatment of patients with (acute and chronic) pain.

Pain management programme: a cognitive-behavioural programme for patients with persistent pain and disability.

Pain medicine: the diagnostic and therapeutic activities of medical practitioners.

Pain medicine is often used interchangeably with pain management to describe the work done by medical practitioners and is the term favoured in countries such as the USA and Australia.

THE PARADIGM OF PAIN

Pain management concerns postoperative, acute and chronic pain and cancer-related symptom control in children and adults. A joint report of the (then) College of Anaesthetists and the Royal College of Surgeons of England highlighted the need to improve standards of postoperative pain management and many hospitals have established acute pain teams. However, many hospitalized patients suffer from acute non-postoperative pain. This may be caused by trauma, burns or acutely painful medical conditions (e.g. cardiac pain, osteoporotic vertebral collapse). Some medical conditions may cause recurrent acute painful episodes such as sickle-cell crisis or acute exacerbations of chronic pancreatitis. Unrelieved acute pain may lead to chronic pain. Chronic pain is a complex biopsychosocial phenomenon and a single pathophysiological

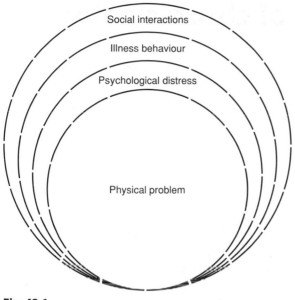

Fig. 42.1
An illustration of pain as a biopsychosocial phenomenon.

Labels (outer to inner):
Social interactions
Illness behaviour
Psychological distress
Physical problem

explanation is not available for many chronic nonmalignant pain states. Palliative care services may refer cancer-related pain problems to the anaesthetist for management as a hospital inpatient, an outpatient, in a hospice or in the home. There are many common areas within the management of acute and chronic pain, and pain is increasingly viewed as a continuum rather than two separate entities, with subsequent merging of management techniques and staff.

Postoperative, recurrent, chronic persistent and cancer-related pain occurs also in children. Difficulties in pain assessment and unsubstantiated fears and myths regarding pain in children and its treatment have led to less than optimal management. Recommendations for the management of pain in children have been published recently and are detailed in the further reading section.

EPIDEMIOLOGY OF CHRONIC PAIN

The prevalence of chronic pain within the general population has proved difficult to estimate because of variations in the populations studied, the methods used to collect data and the criteria used to define chronic pain. Recent data have suggested that the prevalence of chronic pain in the UK is 13%, i.e. 1 in 7 of the population.

Pain is the single biggest cause of disability in the UK and has a significant economic impact through those affected being unable to work. It is the second most common cause of days off work through sickness, accounting for 206 million working days lost in the UK in 1999–2000. In 2001–2002, the total cost of persistent pain in terms of benefit claimed in the UK was £6.7 billion, with musculoskeletal pain costing £1.46 billion.

Untreated pain may reduce quality of life for sufferers and carers, resulting in helplessness, isolation, depression and family breakdown.

Pain is experienced by 20–50% of patients with cancer at the time of diagnosis and by up to 75% of patients with advanced disease.

CLASSIFICATION OF PAIN

Pain may be classified according to its aetiology.

NOCICEPTIVE PAIN

Nociceptive pain results from tissue damage causing continuous nociceptor stimulation. It may be either somatic or visceral in origin.

Somatic pain

Somatic pain results from activation of nociceptors in cutaneous and deep tissues, such as skin, muscle and subcutaneous soft tissue. Typically, it is well localized and described as aching, throbbing or gnawing. Somatic pain is usually sensitive to opioids.

Visceral pain

Visceral pain arises from internal organs. It is characteristically vague in distribution and quality and is often described as deep, dull or dragging. It may be associated with nausea, vomiting and alterations in arterial pressure and heart rate. Stimuli such as crushing or burning, which are painful in somatic structures, often evoke no pain in visceral organs. Mechanisms of visceral pain include abnormal distension or contraction of smooth muscle, stretching of the capsule of solid organs, hypoxaemia or necrosis and irritation by algesic substances. Visceral pain is often referred to cutaneous sites distant from the visceral lesion. One example of this is shoulder pain resulting from diaphragmatic irritation.

NEUROPATHIC PAIN

Neuropathic pain is caused by a primary lesion or dysfunction in the peripheral and/or central nervous system. It is characteristically dysaesthetic in nature and patients complain of unpleasant abnormal sensations. There may be marked allodynia, i.e. a normally nonpainful stimulus, such as light touch, evokes pain. Pain may be described as shooting or burning and may occur in areas of numbness. Neuropathic pain may develop immediately after nerve injury or after a variable interval. It is often persistent and relatively resistant to opioids. There is a tendency for a favourable response to centrally modulating medication, such as anticonvulsants and tricyclic antidepressants.

There are many causes of neuropathic pain. Lesions in the peripheral nervous system include peripheral nerve injuries, peripheral neuropathies, HIV infection, certain drugs and tumour infiltration. Central neuropathic pain is associated with lesions of the central nervous system, such as infarction, trauma and demyelination and is very resistant to treatment.

Sympathetically maintained pain

Pain that is maintained by sympathetic efferent innervation or by circulating catecholamines is termed sympathetically maintained pain (SMP). It may be a feature of several pain complaints. Sympathetic nerve block provides at least temporary reduction of pain, but current thinking is that this does not imply a mechanism for the pain. Thus, the condition previously termed 'reflex sympathetic dystrophy' has now been renamed 'complex regional pain syndrome type I', as not all patients with this clinical diagnosis have relief of pain following sympathetic nerve block.

Complex regional pain syndrome (CRPS) type I is a syndrome that can develop in a limb after mild soft tissue trauma or a fracture (Fig. 42.2). The pain is characteristically burning in nature and associated with allodynia (abnormal sensitivity of the skin). It is associated at some point with swelling, abnormal sweating and changes in skin blood flow. Atrophy of the skin, nails and muscles can occur and localized osteoporosis may be demonstrated on X-ray or bone scan. Movement of the limb is usually restricted as a result of the pain, and contractures may result. Treatment is directed at providing adequate analgesia to encourage active physiotherapy and improvement of function. In cases with sympathetically maintained pain, sympathetic nerve block may be part of this treatment strategy.

Complex regional pain syndrome type II is a condition that has the features described above, but which occurs after partial injury of a nerve or one of its branches.

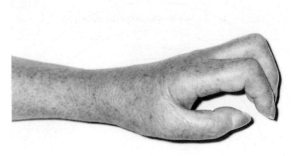

Fig. 42.2
Complex regional pain syndrome type I following Colles' fracture.

MANAGEMENT OF CHRONIC PAIN

Patients present with pain resulting from many different pathological processes and some examples of common painful conditions are listed in Table 42.1.

ASSESSMENT

Comprehensive assessment of patients with pain is a vital first step. Pain is generally thought of as a symptom rather than a disease in its own right. Efforts should be made to investigate, diagnose and, if possible, treat the underlying cause of the pain before using empirical pain-relieving techniques. However, there is now a growing body of animal and human evidence that chronic pain may involve increased sensitivity of spinal cord neurones and changes in the spinal cord and the brain, which are responsible for the symptoms.

The key elements of a pain history should be ascertained using a structured interview. The interview includes assessment of the pain, the effect of pain on the patient's mood and also the impact of the pain on quality of life and functioning. Many patients with pain become relatively deconditioned and this in itself may contribute to the pain. Assessment may be recorded and audited using certain scales such as the Brief Pain Inventory.

The key elements in taking a pain history include:

- location, either verbally or graphically using a pain diagram
- mode of onset and frequency
- aggravating factors
- relieving factors
- quality, e.g. burning, shooting – e.g. use McGill Pain Questionnaire

Table 42.1   Some common painful conditions

Malignant aetiology

Primary tumours

Metastases

Treatment-related, e.g. post-surgery, post-chemotherapy pain

Nonmalignant aetiology

Musculoskeletal

   Back pain

   Osteoarthritis

   Rheumatoid arthritis

   Osteoporotic fracture

Neuropathic

   Trigeminal neuralgia

   Postherpetic neuralgia

   Brachial plexus avulsion

   Radicular pain of spinal origin

   Peripheral neuropathy

   Chronic regional pain syndrome (CRPS)

Visceral

   Urogenital pain

   Pancreatitis

Post-surgery

   Phantom pain

   Stump pain

   Scar pain

   Post-laminectomy

Ischaemic

   Peripheral vascular disease

   Raynaud's phenomenon/disease

   Intractable angina

Headaches

- intensity, e.g. verbal rating scale, visual analogue scale, faces pain scale (children)
- previous treatments
- current medication (analgesics and others)
- basic psychological assessment
- patient's own ideas as to causation
- impairment and disability
- concurrent medical illnesses.

Many patients, especially those with malignancy, have more than one site of pain and separate histories should be taken for each complaint as their aetiology may differ. Particular care and skill are needed when taking a pain history from children and the elderly. An appropriate physical examination relevant to the pain complaint should be performed. Special reference might be made to tender points and trigger points in muscles and scars, neurological deficit and signs implicating involvement of the sympathetic nervous system including vasomotor, sudomotor and trophic changes. Physiotherapy assessment may be part of the initial screening interview. Occasionally, additional laboratory, radiological and electrophysiological tests may be needed for full evaluation. Basic psychological assessment may be made by the clinician, sometimes aided by questionnaires (e.g. Hospital Anxiety and Depression Scale). If full psychological evaluation is indicated, it should be performed either by a psychiatrist or by a clinical psychologist, preferably one who is an integral member of the pain management team.

Chronic pain affects not only the patient, but also the family. Patients with chronic pain become depressed, anxious and medication-dependent. They lose their job, financial security and social status. Their relationships deteriorate. Interviewing of the patient's relatives or significant others may be important in assessing the impact of the pain on family dynamics and lifestyle.

EXPLANATION

Chronic pain is a complex phenomenon and often multifactorial in aetiology. From the history, examination and investigations the pain complaint should be diagnosed, if possible. Then the pain should be classified according to whether it appears to be nociceptive (somatic or visceral), neuropathic or mixed. Full explanation of the pain complaint and the results of investigations should be discussed with the patient. This may involve admitting that there is no structural explanation for the pain, but impressing upon the patient that this is a reflection of our currently inadequate methods for imaging pain and does not imply that the pain is imagined. A patient-led problem list should be formulated and patient expectations for treatment should be explored and, if necessary, rationalized. The limitations of the medical model of disease for some chronic pain complaints should be explained. Total relief of chronic pain is often not possible. A treatment plan should be formulated jointly with the patient after discussion of the available treatments and the potential benefits and side-effects of those options. Several methods of treatment may be used in the same patient, either concomitantly or sequentially. Pain management techniques may be offered at any stage during the treatment programme, if resources allow.

In chronic pain management, there are often many ways to tackle a particular problem. There may be more or less evidence of benefit for each alternative treatment and each may possess a side-effect profile that needs to be considered. It is essential to explain fully to patients the probable efficacy of the treatments offered, the potential hazards and the option not to treat.

The range of interventions for chronic pain is shown in Figure 42.3.

MEDICATION

Many patients in pain are prescribed analgesic drugs. The pharmacology of these agents is discussed fully elsewhere (see Ch. 5) and only aspects of particular relevance to their use in chronic pain are mentioned below.

Paracetamol

Paracetamol 4000 mg daily is a better analgesic than placebo, but probably not as effective as NSAIDs. However, in the elderly patient, paracetamol may be useful because of its low side-effect profile.

Non-steroidal anti-inflammatory drugs

NSAIDs possess analgesic and anti-inflammatory action and are used widely in the management of mild to moderate pain. They are effective analgesics for pain from osteoarthritis, rheumatoid arthritis, dysmenorrhoea and bony metastases. Topical NSAIDs also provide effective pain relief.

Opioid analgesics

Cancer pain

Approximately 75% of patients with advanced cancer develop significant pain before death. Most cancer pain responds to pharmacological measures and successful treatment is based on simple principles that have been promoted by the World Health Organization and are extensively validated. Analgesic drugs should be taken 'by mouth', 'by the clock' (i.e. regularly) and 'by the analgesic ladder' (Fig. 42.4). Cancer pain is continuous and medication must be taken regularly. It is given orally unless intractable nausea and vomiting occur or unless there is a physical impediment to swallowing. The first step on the 'analgesic ladder' is a non-opioid, such as paracetamol, aspirin or an NSAID. If this is inadequate, a weak opioid such as codeine is added. The third step is substitution of the weak opioid by a strong opioid. Inadequate pain control at one level requires progression to a drug on the next level, rather than to an alternative of similar efficacy. Adjuvant analgesics, such as tricyclic antidepressants or anticonvulsants, may be used at any stage.

Using these strategies, pain may be controlled successfully in about 90% of patients with cancer pain without resorting to other interventions.

Morphine is the strong oral opioid of choice. Immediate-release oral morphine, either in liquid or tablet form, is given as often as necessary in increasing dosage, until pain is controlled. When the required daily dose has been established, it is usual to convert to sustained-release morphine tablets, which need to be taken only once or twice daily. In addition, immediate-release morphine elixir or tablets should be

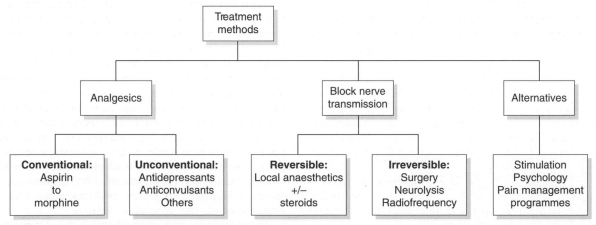

Fig 42.3
Treatment methods (adapted from Moore A, Edwards J, Barden J, McQuay H 2003 Bandolier's little book of pain. Oxford University Press).

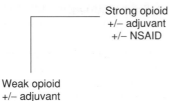

Fig. 42.4
The WHO analgesic ladder.

prescribed for breakthrough pain. The dose of morphine necessary to treat breakthrough pain is one-sixth of the total daily morphine requirement.

Education of the medical and nursing professions, and also the patient and family, is still necessary to ensure that adequate doses of opioids are prescribed and taken. Healthcare professionals often overestimate the side-effects of morphine. Respiratory depression is uncommon when morphine is prescribed for cancer pain. Surveys have shown that patients are concerned about side-effects of morphine, especially tolerance, addiction, constipation and drowsiness. Tolerance does not appear to be a problem clinically. Many patients with stable disease take the same dose of morphine for prolonged periods of time. Disease progression may necessitate an increase in dose, but there is no upper limit to the dose of morphine and pain control is usually regained without difficulty. Addiction (psychological dependence) does not occur in patients with cancer pain, and if the pain is relieved by other means, such as radiotherapy or a nerve block, many patients will stop their opioids. Physical dependence always occurs and patients should be warned not to stop opioids precipitously. Nausea and vomiting may occur when morphine is first commenced and an antiemetic may be prescribed for the first week after commencing this medication, but often it may then be stopped. Sedation and cognitive impairment may occur as the dose is increased but these usually resolve. However, there is no tolerance to the constipating effect of morphine and laxatives need to be taken regularly.

Efforts should be made to reassure both patients and relatives of the efficacy and safety of morphine analgesia in both short and long term to ensure that medication is taken regularly.

Alternative opioids and alternative routes of administration. Oxycodone hydrochloride is a semisynthetic congener of morphine. It is available as an immediate-release and a sustained-release preparation. It is approximately twice as potent as morphine (i.e. 10 mg oral morphine is equivalent to 5 mg oxycodone). Its advantage in renal failure is the lack of detectable clinically relevant active metabolites, therefore avoiding cumulation. Oxycodone may also be helpful in neuropathic pain, possibly because of putative kappa-agonistic properties.

Hydromorphone is a semisynthetic opioid with a rapid onset and a shorter duration of action than morphine. It is more potent than morphine, with 1.3 mg of hydromorphone being equivalent to 10 mg of morphine. Immediate-release, sustained-release preparations and parenteral preparations are available.

Methadone is a potent opioid analgesic and also an N-methyl-D-aspartate (NMDA) receptor antagonist. Methadone is absorbed rapidly by the oral route and has a long half-life that may range from 13 to 51 h. Initial dosing must be monitored carefully as relatively small doses of methadone may be needed in comparison with the previous opioid dose. When repeated doses are given, the drug accumulates and after the first few days, the frequency of administration may need to be reduced to two or three times daily. Methadone should be considered a third-line drug indicated for cancer pain that appears poorly responsive to morphine, diamorphine, fentanyl, oxycodone or hydromorphone in spite of dose escalation and the use of adjuvant drugs. Methadone is available as tablets, linctus and injection.

Transdermal drug delivery. If a patient is unable to take medication by mouth, there are various alternative routes for opioid administration. A transdermal drug delivery system has been developed for fentanyl and buprenorphine. Fentanyl patches are applied to the skin and drug from the reservoir diffuses through the rate-controlling membrane and forms a subcutaneous depot from which the drug is taken up into the circulation. There is wide variation in absorption rates and time to steady-state serum concentrations of fentanyl. After removal of the patch, the terminal half-life has been shown to be 17 ± 2.3 h, indicative of the time taken for the drug to clear from the subcutaneous depot. Transdermal fentanyl is available in patches that deliver 25, 50, 75 and $100 \mu g \, h^{-1}$ of fentanyl. They should be placed on unbroken skin usually on the upper body and need to be changed every 72 h. An appropriate dose of immediate-release morphine or oral transmucosal fentanyl lozenges should be prescribed for breakthrough pain.

Buprenorphine patches are matrix patches in which buprenorphine is incorporated within an adhesive matrix, allowing constant release of buprenorphine into the systemic circulation at a predetermined rate over a minimum of 72 hours. The dose of buprenorphine delivered is dependent upon the amount of drug held in the matrix and the area of the patch. Three patch strengths are available: 35, 52.5 and 70 µg h^{-1}. For all three patch strengths, elimination half-time is about 25 h.

The pharmacokinetic data are of the utmost importance when considering changing medication from an opioid delivered by patch technology to an oral or parenteral opioid or vice-versa. Both are suitable for patients who cannot or prefer not to take oral medication or who are intolerant of morphine. However, the delay in onset of analgesia makes them unsuitable for treatment of acute pain.

Subcutaneous administration. Continuous subcutaneous administration is another alternative method of administration if oral medication cannot be taken. A small portable battery-operated syringe driver fitted with a 20 mL syringe containing the total daily opioid dose is usually used. Because of its greater solubility, diamorphine is the drug of choice in the UK for this route of administration. A conversion ratio of 3 mg oral morphine to 1 mg subcutaneous diamorphine is used.

Morphine suppositories are available for rectal administration.

Spinal administration. Opioids may be administered spinally, either epidurally or intrathecally, for:

- patients whose pain is controlled effectively by oral opioids but who suffer intolerable unacceptable side-effects, such as drowsiness or vomiting
- patients whose pain cannot be controlled by the use of oral or systemic opioids.

Only a small proportion (less than 2%) of patients with cancer pain are candidates for spinal opioids. Much smaller doses of drug are required when given spinally and thus side-effects are minimized. The daily dose of morphine via the epidural route is 1/10 of the oral 24-h dose and the intrathecal dose is 1/10 of the epidural dose. Contraindications to the insertion of a spinal catheter are similar to those in the acute situation. Side-effects, such as respiratory depression, itching and urinary retention, that cause such concern in the opioid-naive patient are rare in cancer patients who have been chronically exposed to systemic opioids.

The field of spinal opioid therapy is sufficiently new that guidelines for selection of route (intrathecal or epidural), choice of drug (opioid or opioid/local anaesthetic combination), administration protocol (intermittent bolus or continuous infusion) and equipment (tunnelled or totally implanted catheter and reservoir) are still being formulated.

Before introducing this technique, it is essential to devise formal protocols and an education programme for hospital, hospice and primary care nurses and doctors to facilitate management of the patient in any of these settings.

Non-cancer pain

Weak opioid drugs, e.g. dihydrocodeine, are useful for moderate pain. However, they may be taken in excess, and often with only little benefit, by the patient with chronic nonmalignant pain. Treatment in the pain management clinic may involve weaning the patient off such medication.

The use of strong opioids in nonmalignant pain is controversial. There is a lack of good-quality research about the long-term risks and benefits of opioids in chronic pain. There is some evidence that opioids relieve pain and improve function in patients with non-cancer pain. However, there are other studies which conclude that chronic opioid therapy exacerbates psychological distress, impairs cognition and worsens outcome. There is also concern about opioid-induced hyperalgesia, immune function and fertility. The controversy is also compounded by the perceived risk of psychological dependence (addiction) and the poorly understood phenomenon of tolerance. The British Pain Society has published recommendations for the appropriate use of opioids for persistent non-cancer pain and also specific information for patients on this subject.

Adjuvant analgesics

These are drugs that have primary indications other than pain but are analgesic in some painful conditions. Full explanation regarding this must be given to the patient.

Oral corticosteroids

The mechanism by which corticosteroids produce analgesia is unknown. They reduce inflammatory mediators, specifically prostaglandins. They reduce peritumour oedema, thus relieving pain by reducing pressure on adjacent pain-sensitive structures. They are administered for cerebral metastases, spinal cord compression, superior vena caval compression and neural infiltration or compression. In cancer patients, they are also prescribed for their euphoric effect and to stimulate appetite.

Anticonvulsants

Anticonvulsants are used in the treatment of neuropathic pain. The precise mechanism of action is unclear and does vary among different anticonvulsants. For example, it is thought that carbamazepine blocks sodium channels and that gabapentin acts on the alpha-2-delta subunit of the calcium channel. Anticonvulsants may also act on NMDA receptors. Therefore, if one anticonvulsant at maximum dosage is ineffective then it is worthwhile trying another. Gabapentin, pregabalin, carbamazepine and phenytoin have product licences for use in neuropathic pain and trigeminal neuralgia.

In a variety of neuropathic pains, anticonvulsants have an NNT for at least 50% relief of 2.9, indicating that they are effective. Data from studies show that for every patient who benefited, one had a minor adverse effect, but continued with the treatment. Sedation and ataxia are common side-effects of these drugs and may limit dose escalation, especially in the elderly.

Tricyclic antidepressants

Tricyclic antidepressants have an important role in the management of pain, independent of their effect on mood. Tricyclic drugs are postulated to act as analgesics by reducing the reuptake of the amine neurotransmitters norepinephrine and serotonin into the presynaptic terminal, increasing the concentration and duration of action of these substances at the synapse and thereby enhancing activity in the descending inhibitory pain pathway. Tricyclics also block sodium channels and suppress ectopic neuroma discharge.

Animal models of acute pain have consistently demonstrated the antinociceptive effect of tricyclic drugs. Controlled clinical trials have shown beneficial results in postherpetic neuralgia, diabetic neuropathy, atypical facial pain and central pain. The NNT for effectiveness for antidepressants in neuropathic pain is 2.9. The effective dose of a tricyclic drug for analgesia is usually lower than that required for depression (although a dose response for analgesia has been demonstrated) and analgesia is apparent in 3–4 days compared with 3–4 weeks for antidepressant effects. Amitriptyline is the commonest tricyclic drug prescribed as an analgesic and the normal starting dose is 10–25 mg nocte. Side-effects include sedation (which can be beneficial), constipation and a dry mouth. Other tricyclic drugs used as analgesics include imipramine and Prothiaden (dosulepin). Selective serotonin reuptake inhibitors, such as fluoxetine, appear to be less effective analgesics. There has been a recent suggestion that the serotonin-noradrenergic reuptake inhibitors (SNRIs) may help in neuropathic pain, but further work on this is needed.

Antiarrhythmic drugs

Sodium channel blockers may be used to reduce pain caused by nerve damage. Both intraveneous lidocaine (up to 5 mg kg^{-1}) and oral mexiletine reduce neuropathic pain. Intravenous lidocaine is also effective in fibromyalgia (based on small patient numbers), but not in cancer-related pain. Unfortunately, the benefits of lidocaine are short-lived and the studies are generally small.

Ketamine

Ketamine is an NMDA receptor antagonist; it has been used successfully as an analgesic via intravenous, subcutaneous and oral routes. Psychometric side-effects may be a problem.

Capsaicin cream

Capsaicin is an alkaloid derived from chillies. It depletes substance P in local sensory nerve terminals. Local application may alleviate pain in painful diabetic peripheral neuropathy, osteoarthritis, postherpetic neuralgia, intercostobrachial neuralgia and psoriasis.

Cannabis

Animal studies suggest that cannabinoids reduce hyperalgesia and allodynia in neuropathic, inflammatory and cancer pain. Human trials have also reported modest benefit in neuropathic pain. Cannabinoids act on CB1 receptors which are located in the brain and their CB2 counterparts found peripherally. Further research is needed to identify which cannabinoids may produce analgesia without psychotropic side-effects.

NEURAL BLOCKADE IN PAIN MANAGEMENT

Nerve blocks have been performed for many years in the management of pain. A nerve block comprises an injection of a local anaesthetic (sometimes combined with steroid) or a neurolytic agent around a peripheral or central sensory nerve, a sympathetic plexus or a trigger point. Correct use of nerve blocks in the treatment of chronic pain requires an experienced practitioner with a thorough knowledge of anatomy and an understanding of pain syndromes. Neural blockade should be undertaken in appropriate locations by clinicians who are fully acquainted with the techniques involved and who are competent to manage the complications that may arise. The use of radiological control and contrast media is strongly advocated to confirm accurate needle placement.

Potential sites for neural blockade are demonstrated in Figure 42.5, and indications for neural blockade are listed in Table 42.2. Some comments about commonly performed nerve blocks are made in the section below. For a full description of the techniques of neural blockade, the reader should consult suggested texts in the further reading section.

Local anaesthetics

Local anaesthetics have been injected into muscle trigger points for the relief of myofascial pain and it has been shown that prolonged relief of pain may result from a series of local anaesthetic blocks to peripheral nerves. It is unclear why pain relief may persist after the duration of pharmacological action.

Corticosteroids

Corticosteroids have been shown to block transmission in normal unmyelinated C fibres and to suppress ectopic neural discharges in experimental neuromas.

They are sometimes added to local anaesthetics when injected into painful scars.

Epidural steroids

Epidural steroids have been used since 1962 for nerve root pain. A recent meta-analysis of all randomized, controlled trials has concluded that epidural administration of corticosteroids is more effective in reducing lumbosacral radicular pain (in both the short and long term) than placebo. In addition, McQuay and Moore (1998) have addressed the question 'How well do they work?' by investigating the short-term (1–60 days) and long-term (12 weeks–1 year) efficacy of epidural steroids for sciatica. They used the NNT as a measure of clinical benefit. The NNT for short-term, greater than 75% pain relief was just under 7.3. This implies that for seven patients treated with epidural steroids, one will obtain more than 75% pain relief in the short term who would not have done so had he or she received the control treatment (placebo or local anaesthetic). The NNT for long-term (12 weeks–1 year) improvement was 13 for 50% pain relief.

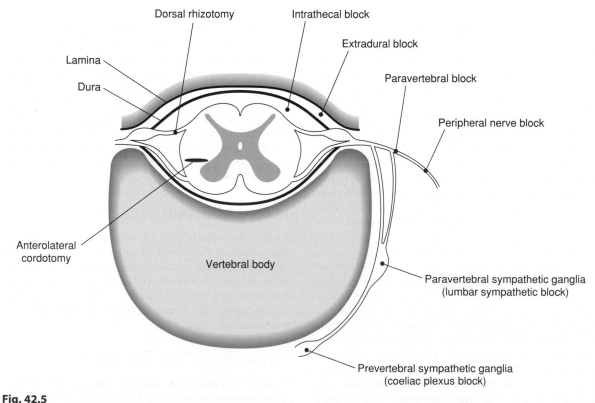

Fig. 42.5
Potential sites for neural blockade.

Table 42.2   Indications for neural blockade

Nerve block	Indications
Trigger point injections	Myofascial pain, scar pain
Somatic nerve block	Nerve root pain, scar pain
Trigeminal nerve block and branches	Trigeminal neuralgia
Stellate ganglion block	SMP, CRPS
Coeliac plexus block	Intra-abdominal malignancy, especially pancreas
Superior hypogastric plexus block	Malignant pelvic pain
Lumbar sympathetic block	Ischaemic rest pain SMP, CRPS Phantom and stump pain
Epidural steroids/root canal injections	Nerve root pain, benign or malignant
Intrathecal neurolytics	Malignant pain
Percutaneous cervical cordotomy	Unilateral somatic malignant pain, short life expectancy

SMP, sympathetically maintained pain; CRPS, complex regional pain syndrome.

However, the use of epidural steroids is not without potential hazards and controversy. The most common side-effects relate not to the steroid but to technical aspects of the technique. There have been reports of dural tap (2.5%), transient headache (2.3%) and transient increase in pain (1.9%). As with any spinal technique, an aseptic technique must be used and the usual contraindications observed. Methylprednisolone acetate and triamcinolone are the steroids most commonly used. It has been shown that neither of these preparations is deleterious when injected into the epidural space. However, they may have harmful effects if injected inadvertently into the subarachnoid or subdural spaces.

Before an epidural steroid injection is undertaken, the patient should receive a consultation during which the perceived merits, expectations, risks and possible complications are fully explained. This should include an explanation that the steroid preparation is being used outside of its product licence. The doctor should be satisfied that the procedure is indicated, that appropriate neurological examination and investigations have been performed and that there is no contraindication to the procedure. Written consent should be obtained. Arrangements should be made for the outcome to be formally monitored by the doctor who prescribed the procedure or the one who performed it. Provision should be made for an earlier consultation if necessary.

Spinal endoscopy is a minimally invasive procedure developed to enable the physician to visualize the epidural space and nerve roots. The epidural space can be accessed with a spinal endoscope and a steerable catheter via the sacral hiatus. This technique allows for a direct visual examination of a specific nerve root and any associated pathology. The catheter is used as a blunt dissector to lyse adhesions that may encapsulate the affected nerve root. In addition, irrigation of the nerve root with saline may 'wash away' inflammatory mediators.

Nerve root injection

Steroids may also be injected around a nerve root as it emerges from the intervertebral foramen. This is an alternative to an epidural steroid injection and may be useful when the level of nerve compression is demonstrated by an MRI scan. X-ray screening is essential. This technique may be used in the cervical, thoracic and lumbar regions.

Lumbar and cervical facet blocks

Chronic back and neck pain are common complaints in pain management clinics. Lumbar and cervical facet joints have been considered to be potential sources.

Injections of steroid into both lumbar and cervical facet joints are commonly performed procedures, although there is controversy about long-term benefit. Radiofrequency lesions of the facet nerves have been reported to give long-term relief in some patients.

Sympathetic nerve blocks

Visceral nociceptive afferents travel in the sympathetic nervous system to the spinal cord. Visceral pain tends to be less opioid sensitive than somatic pain. Percutaneous sympathetic blocks may therefore be useful in the management of severe cancer-related visceral pain that is poorly controlled with opioids or controlled only with intolerable side-effects.

Percutaneous coeliac plexus block using 50% alcohol is one of the most commonly used and effective blocks performed for cancer pain. It is used for pain resulting from upper gastrointestinal neoplasms, in particular carcinoma of the pancreas. Radiological screening, either X-ray or CT, is mandatory, although this in itself does not ensure absence of complications. Hypotension, especially postural hypotension, should be anticipated and managed appropriately. Serious complications are rare, but include paraplegia.

The superior hypogastric plexus innervates the pelvic viscera. Superior hypogastric plexus block with phenol has been used for pelvic pain from cervical, prostatic, colonic, rectal, bladder, uterine and ovarian malignancy and rectal tenesmus.

Chemical lumbar sympathectomy using phenol is performed for inoperable ischaemic leg pain. Radiological screening using contrast medium is necessary to ensure correct needle placement. The complication rate is low, the most common complication being genitofemoral neuralgia, with the reported incidence varying from 4% to 15%.

Stellate ganglion and lumbar sympathetic block with local anaesthetic is sometimes helpful in the treatment of sympathetically mediated pain, CRPS types I and II, amputation stump and phantom pain.

Intravenous regional sympathetic block with guanethidine

The intravenous regional guanethidine technique was reported in 1974 and it became a popular method of treating CRPS. The technique is the same as intravenous regional analgesia (IVRA), but with the addition of guanethidine 10–20 mg. However, a recent systematic review of the randomized, controlled studies of intravenous regional guanethidine block in the treatment of CRPS failed to show evidence of effectiveness.

Neurolytic techniques

Neural destruction can be produced with alcohol, phenol, heat or cold. In general, the use of neurolytic techniques has diminished in the last two decades. There are many reasons for this, including the improved use of analgesic drugs, the recognition that the effect of neuroablative procedures is often transient, the development of neurostimulatory techniques and appreciation of the cognitive and behavioural elements of pain. The clinical indications for neurolytic techniques are now limited to patients with cancer pain and a few selected non-cancer conditions. Careful thought with regard to the potential benefits and risks of the procedure, appropriate patient selection and fully informed consent are essential before performing a neurolytic procedure.

Chemical neurolysis

The commonest neurolytic agents used are phenol and ethyl alcohol. Phenol acts by coagulating proteins and destroys all types of nerves, both motor and sensory. It is available in water or in glycerol. Its most frequent indication is for lumbar sympathetic block for peripheral vascular disease. Large systemic doses cause convulsions followed by central nervous system depression and cardiovascular collapse. Alcohol is the neurolytic agent of choice for coeliac plexus block when the large volume required prohibits the use of phenol. It produces a higher incidence of neuritis than phenol and is not used for other blocks.

Radiofrequency lesions

A destructive heat lesion may be produced using a radiofrequency current. The radiofrequency electrode comprises an insulated needle with a small exposed tip. A high-frequency alternating current flows from the electrode tip to the tissues, producing ionic agitation and a heating effect in tissue adjacent to the tip of the probe. The magnitude of this heating effect is monitored by a thermistor in the electrode tip. Damage to nerve fibres sufficient to block conduction occurs at temperatures above 45°C, although in practice most lesions are made with a probe tip temperature of 60–80°C. An integral nerve stimulator is used to ensure accurate placement of the probe. Whereas the spread of neurolytic solutions is unpredictable, radiofrequency lesions are more precise. The size of the lesion depends on the tip temperature, the duration of the current and the length of the exposed needle tip. Lower-temperature lesions are now being used in an attempt to produce analgesia without nerve destruction in pulsed radiofrequency lesioning.

Radiofrequency lesions of the trigeminal nerve may be used to treat trigeminal neuralgia in the elderly patient whose pain is uncontrolled by anticonvulsant drugs and who is unsuitable for microvascular decompression.

Cryotherapy

A cryopobe can produce lesions in the nervous system using the Joule–Thompson effect (with nitrous oxide as the refrigerant gas) to produce cooling. The probe tip may reach a temperature of −75°C. There is complete functional loss after a cryolesion; however, recovery may be expected after several weeks. Painful neuritis has been reported and has led to this technique being used infrequently.

STIMULATION-INDUCED ANALGESIA

Transcutaneous electrical nerve stimulation, spinal cord stimulation, deep brain stimulation and acupuncture may produce stimulation-induced analgesia.

Transcutaneous electrical nerve stimulation

Transcutaneous electrical nerve stimulation (TENS) has been used widely since Melzack and Wall proposed the gate control theory in 1965. They postulated that large-diameter primary afferents exert a specific inhibitory effect on dorsal horn nociceptive neurones and that stimulation of these fibres would alleviate pain. Conventional TENS produces high-frequency, low intensity stimulation which relieves pain in the area in which it produces paraesthesia. Stimulation variables of TENS may be altered to produce low-frequency acupuncture-like TENS, which, unlike conventional TENS, produces analgesia, which is antagonized by naloxone.

A small battery-powered unit is used to apply the electrical stimulus to the skin via electrodes (Fig. 42.6). These are placed over the painful area, on either side of it or over nerves supplying the region, and stimulation is applied at an intensity that the patient finds comfortable. Adverse effects are minimal, with allergy to the electrodes being the commonest problem encountered. TENS is used for a variety of musculoskeletal and neuropathic pains and has been advocated recently for refractory angina. Tolerance to TENS does occur sometimes. It may be possible to overcome this by changing stimulation variables.

TENS has been used also for acute postoperative pain and for analgesia for the first stage of labour. However, there is evidence of lack of analgesic effect in

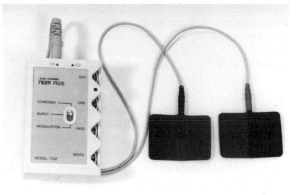

Fig. 42.6
A transcutaneous electrical nerve stimulator.

both these areas, although women using it as a method of pain relief tend to favour it for future births. Whilst studies have shown clear benefit from the use of TENS in chronic pain, there is a general lack of evidence for effectiveness of TENS rather than evidence of lack of effect.

Spinal cord stimulation

Spinal cord stimulation (SCS) has been advocated as a reversible method for the management of intractable pain, especially that of neuropathic origin. Electrical stimulation may be applied to the spinal cord via electrodes implanted surgically or positioned percutaneously in the epidural space under X-ray control. To be effective, the stimulating electrode must be positioned to produce artificial paraesthesia in the distribution of the pain. It is usual practice for the patient to undergo a period of trial stimulation. Patients showing substantial improvement in pain relief and other outcome measures may be considered for permanent implantation of a battery-driven stimulus generator. The patient uses a magnet to activate the stimulator. The equipment is expensive and a proportion of patients obtain good relief initially only to have their pain return after some months.

SCS has also been demonstrated to promote local blood flow and ischaemic ulcer healing in patients with peripheral vascular disease. More recently, spinal cord stimulators have been implanted for angina. Studies have confirmed fewer ischaemic episodes, reduced frequency of hospital admissions and improved quality of life. Concern has been raised that SCS may mask the pain of myocardial infarction, but this is not the case and mortality rates in patients with stimulators are similar to those of the general population with coronary artery disease.

Acupuncture

The Chinese have believed for 4000 years that inserting needles at specific points in the body produces analgesia. According to Chinese philosophy, *chi*, the life force, circulates around the body in pathways termed meridians. Injury and illness can block the flow of *chi*, causing pain and disease. Acupuncture is believed to release these blocks and balance the energy of the patient. Traditionally, acupuncture points are stimulated by the insertion of fine needles, which are then rotated manually or stimulated by heat (moxibustion) or electrically.

Acupuncture is widely used for treating chronic pain and yet there is little evidence that it is effective in the long term. There are good studies which show that acupuncture is ineffective for fibromyalgia, osteoarthiris, neck and back pain. Acupuncture may also cause harm, such as infection or pneumothorax.

PSYCHOLOGICAL TECHNIQUES

Pain is not merely a sensation of tissue damage, but a complex interaction of biochemical, behavioural, cognitive and emotional factors. Chronic pain patients become anxious, depressed, distressed, functionally impaired and lose self-esteem. These important aspects should be addressed in the pain management clinic. A clinical psychologist is an essential member of the pain management team. A cognitive and behavioural approach investigates how thoughts (often negative) and behaviours (often maladaptive) reinforce the chronic pain state. Cognitive and behavioural techniques can be used to reduce the helplessness and hopelessness of the pain patient and to increase the level of functioning and emotional well-being in spite of the pain.

Pain management programme

A pain management programme is a psychologically based rehabilitative treatment for patients with chronic pain which remains unresolved by currently available medical or other physically based treatments.

The aim of a pain management programme is to reduce the disability and distress caused by chronic pain by teaching sufferers physical, psychological and practical techniques to improve their quality of life. It aims to enable patients to be self-reliant in managing their pain. It differs from other treatment provided in the pain clinic in that pain relief is not the primary goal.

A pain management programme is facilitated by a multidisciplinary healthcare team. Key clinical staff include a doctor with experience in pain management, a clinical psychologist, a physiotherapist and an occupational therapist, all trained in pain management. Information and education about the nature of pain and its management, medication review and advice, psychological assessment and intervention, physical reconditioning, advice on posture and graded return to the activities of daily living are components of pain management programmes.

EVIDENCE-BASED PRACTICE

There is an increasing drive for evidence-based medicine and for offering to patients only those interventions that are known to be effective. For many of the procedures that are commonly used in the pain management clinic, the evidence is not available and further work is required to gather this evidence. However, the effectiveness of some of the interventions used for chronic pain has been studied and the results are summarized in Table 42.3.

Table 42.3 Effectiveness of some of the interventions used for chronic pain
Effective interventions (of those studied)
Minor analgesics
Anticonvulsant drugs
Antidepressant drugs
Systemic local anaesthetic-type drugs for neuropathic pain
Topical NSAIDs in rheumatological conditions
Topical capsaicin in diabetic neuropathy
Epidural corticosteroids for back pain and sciatica
Psychological interventions
Interventions studied where evidence is lacking
TENS in chronic pain
Relaxation
Spinal cord stimulation
Ineffective interventions (of those studied)
Intravenous regional sympathetic block with guanethidine
Injections of steroids in or around shoulder joint

COSTS OF PAIN MANAGEMENT SERVICES

There is little information on the costs of pain management services. A detailed study of the costs incurred by users of specialty pain clinic services in Canada has shown that users incur less direct healthcare costs than nonusers with similar conditions. Similar results were shown by a small study of NHS pain clinic attendees. This showed that the pain clinic covered its costs by reducing consumption elsewhere and by reducing GP consultations and private treatments.

Advances in knowledge of pain pathophysiology by scientists and increasingly close cooperation between them and clinicians have led to a better understanding of mechanisms sustaining chronic pain and an increase in therapeutic options. In addition, the increasing acceptance by the medical profession and the general public of the importance of psychological factors in chronic pain has opened up new treatment opportunities. There is evidence of the effectiveness of many of the treatments used in the management of chronic pain, but further work is needed on those interventions where information is lacking and in identifying which patients may benefit most from specific treatments.

FURTHER READING

Cousins M J, Bridenbaugh P O (eds) 1998 Neural blockade in clinical anesthesia and management of pain. Lippincott, Philadelphia

Dolin S J, Padfield N L (eds) 2004 Pain medicine, 2nd edn. Butterworth-Heinemann, Oxford

Grady K M, Severn A M, Eldrige P R (eds) 2002 Key topics in chronic pain. BIOS Scientific Publishers, Oxford

McQuay H J, Moore R A 1998 An evidence-based resource for pain relief. Oxford University Press, Oxford

McMahon S, Koltzenburg M (eds) 2005 Wall and Melzack's textbook of pain, 5th edn. Elsevier, London

Moore A, Edwards J, Barden J, McQuay H 2003 Bandolier's little book of pain. Oxford University Press, Oxford

Regnard C F, Tempest S 1998 A guide to symptom relief in advanced disease. Hochland and Hochland, Hale, Cheshire, UK

Southall D (ed) 1997 Prevention and control of pain in children. A manual for health care professionals. BMJ Publishing Group, London

Stannard C F, Booth S 2005 Churchill's pocketbook of pain, 2nd edn. Churchill Livingstone, Edinburgh

Twycross R, Wilcock A 2001 Symptom management in advanced cancer. Radcliffe Medical Press, Oxon

Waldman S D, Winnie A P 1996 Interventional pain management. W B Saunders, Philadelphia

Wedley J R, Gauci C A. 1994 Handbook of clinical techniques in the management of pain. Martin Dunitz, London.

Appendix A
Clinical trials and statistics

'A clinical trial is a carefully and ethically designed experiment with the aim of answering some precisely framed question.' This definition by Sir Austin Bradford Hill, a pioneer of clinical trials, is worth remembering: careful, ethical, precisely framed. There are many types of research that provide information on which medical practice is based. The clinical trial is one of these types, but the one known to most practising anaesthetists. Statistics are important in the interpretation of clinical trials and pragmatically candidates for examinations in anaesthesia know they must 'learn some statistics'. But it is a knowledge of good study design, not of statistics, that is the key to good clinical research.

TERMINOLOGY

There is some confusion and overlap of terms. Scientific research may be observational or experimental. Although a clinical trial is, as Bradford Hill defines, an experiment, there are undercurrents to the word that make 'experiment' better avoided. A clinical trial is better described as a series of experiments: each patient is the subject of an experiment, providing a set of observations. If those observations are numerical, they are often termed *data*. The noun 'data' is in the plural ('the data are shown in the table . . . '), although many now accept that modern usage allows the singular ('the data is shown in the table . . . '). *Measurements* and *findings* are other words applied to the *outcomes* of a clinical trial.

The words *trial* and *study* may be synonymous – a 'clinical trial' or a 'clinical study' – and synonymous also with 'research project'. This meaning is implied in 'study design' and 'study protocol'. 'Study' is the better word here: 'trial' is applicable only to some types of experimental clinical research, whereas design and protocol are important in all scientific research. But a term is needed for each episode (i.e. each patient) in a

clinical trial, and 'study' is often used in that sense ('the study period started at induction of anaesthesia and lasted until the patient left the recovery ward . . . ').

STUDY DESIGN

The study design is the framework ensuring that, as far as possible, difficulties have been sorted out before the study starts. Formally, for any research involving humans or human material or patient records, a study design is needed for submission to an ethics or grant-awarding committee. Informally, there should be a design for any research, even if only a loose one, otherwise the research is likely to lack discipline.

Because this Appendix is largely about clinical trials, it is helpful to use simple, practical examples: a study of a new antiemetic in the treatment of postoperative nausea and vomiting; the effect of an intravenous induction agent on systolic arterial pressure; a comparison of the effect of two intravenous induction agents on arterial pressure; and a study of the effect of duration of surgery on patients' body temperature. These examples are used to illustrate principles and tests. Because the purpose of clinical trials is in some way to improve the management of patients, underlying most aspects of study design is the need to be as sure as possible that the improvement was indeed due to the investigators' intervention, and not to confounding factors. The purpose of good study design is the avoidance of bias.

BACKGROUND

Good study design starts long before the first patient is recruited, with a comprehensive survey of previous similar studies. Even in these days of electronic databases, the best starting place is a recent textbook or review. There are several reasons why investigators need to know what has been done before: to know

775

what remains unknown; to frame their question precisely; to improve the chances of the study providing valid answers; and to prevent needless repetition. Even after their study has started, investigators must remain aware of new relevant work, but any alteration to study design at that stage may affect the validity of the findings.

SPECIFIC OBJECTIVES

After the initial survey, the specific objectives of the study should be clear: postoperative nausea after laparoscopic cholecystectomy in women; arterial pressure on induction in patients already taking a β-blocking drug for hypertension; temperature changes during elective aortobifemoral reconstruction.

PATIENT SELECTION CRITERIA

For some studies, any patient presenting for the chosen operation is suitable, but that is unusual. Almost always, some unsuitable patients have to be excluded, if only on grounds of extremes of age. A study of postoperative nausea might exclude patients with a history of hiatus hernia; one of arterial pressure changes might exclude patients with a defined degree of hypertension; and one of temperature changes might exclude patients who have had amputations of the lower limb. Exclusions must be defined in the study design; some study designs contain long lists of both inclusion and exclusion criteria. Exclusions (patients predetermined as ineligible) differ from eligible patients refusing consent and differ again from withdrawals (eligible patients who failed to complete the study). All three categories of patients not included in the study must be admitted in the final report, and remembered when drawing conclusions from the findings. Generalization of the findings may be unsafe if only women aged less than 65 years are studied, if half the patients refuse consent, or if equipment failure forces withdrawal of patents.

TREATMENT SCHEDULES

The only difference between the groups in a clinical trial should be the study treatment. Everything else should be standardized: premedicant drugs, induction agents, neuromuscular blocking agents, infusion fluids and use of techniques such as epidurals. Clearly, the degree of standardization depends on the trial: in almost all anaesthetic studies, the induction of anaesthesia is standardized; but the size and site of an intravenous cannula is not important if it can have no influence on the outcome of the study.

Study treatment is best given so that neither clinician nor patient is aware of which treatment the patient is receiving: a *double-blind trial*. Sometimes the clinician knows but not the patient, which is termed a *single-blind trial*. If different anaesthetists are giving the anaesthetics and making the observations in a study, all those involved should remain unaware. If it is not possible to blind all those involved, care should be taken to avoid implicit or explicit clues being leaked to the supposedly blinded investigators. Many simple drug trials are easy to make blind, but blinding is less easy if the interventions are more complex. Sometimes, investigators get clues even though technically the study is blind; it is easy to prepare and inject from masked syringes that may contain either thiopental or propofol, but patients complaining of pain during the injection may be presumed to be receiving propofol. Study design might include a questionnaire for the investigators, to determine to what extent blinding was successful.

A non-blinded study is not invalid; some studies are impossible to blind. But non-blinded studies tend to overestimate treatment effects – in other words, these studies are inevitably biased. Put simply, investigators find what they want to find; patients feel how they expect to feel. This is part of human nature.

Other terms to mention under this heading are *placebo*, *control* and *baseline*. In a comparison of a new treatment with the accepted standard treatment, the control group receives the standard treatment. If there is not yet an effective treatment for a condition – prophylaxis of postoperative nausea and vomiting is a good example – there is a place for a placebo group; the best study design would be for three groups: placebo, established drug and new drug. A placebo does not contain active drug but should otherwise be the same, e.g. in appearance and taste, as the test treatments. Placebos are a way of trying to negate the effect of simply doing something: the non-specific effect of medical treatment. Placebos are an obvious ethical issue (see below). Prophylaxis for postoperative nausea and vomiting is in general ineffective and not everyone prescribes it, so it can be argued that giving a placebo does not deprive patients of effective treatment. However, treatment of established nausea and vomiting is more effective and a placebo may be considered unethical.

The terms control and baseline are sometimes confused. A placebo group is a control group; in a two-group study of standard and new antiemetics, the standard group is the control group. In the study of the effect of anaesthetic induction on arterial pressure, readings taken before induction are not control readings but baseline readings with which post-induction readings are compared.

Patients *act as their own controls* if they receive both treatments in a trial. In practice, this is rarely feasible in a study of antiemetics, and uncommon in anaesthetic studies. In a *crossover* trial, patients receive first one and then the other drug, blinded and in random order. These trials may be complicated, including placebo periods and also periods of receiving one or other test drug. There may also be *wash-in periods* to establish drug effect and *wash-out periods* to remove that effect before the next drug is given. These trials are expensive, and unlikely without the backing of the pharmaceutical industry.

PATIENT EVALUATION

In a clinical trial, investigators measure variables (such as arterial pressure and temperature) and seek outcomes (such as postoperative nausea). The techniques and scales must be standardized as rigorously as the treatments, even for variables and outcomes that may be measured objectively, such as arterial pressure (but see measurement bias below). In a study of postoperative nausea, investigators need to decide, for example, whether to record nausea and vomiting separately, whether to record vomiting as yes/no or as number of vomits, whether to use a visual analogue score and for how long and over what periods to record observations from each patient. The best way to decide how to evaluate patients is from reports of previous similar studies, because using similar methods makes comparison with those studies easier. But it is wise first to check that those methods are feasible in the investigators' own circumstances.

When there are few patients to study and research is difficult, such as in the ICU, the temptation is to record as much as possible from each patient. The danger is of ending up with a welter of figures and over-complicated analyses, which obscure rather than clarify. Investigators should refine and simplify their question to define a *primary outcome variable*, and not become distracted by collecting data.

TRIAL DESIGN

The examples of the antiemetic and induction arterial pressure studies are both *experimental* studies in which the investigators are looking for the effect of interventions; that of operative temperature is an *observational* study, although that term is reserved more correctly for epidemiological research in which the investigators study factors outside their control, such as the effects of smoking. All are *prospective* studies: the investigators define the conditions and the observations come after the question. In a *retrospective* study,

observations are sought from pre-existing records, such as patients' notes; the investigators cannot define the conditions. In general, the greatest value of retrospective studies is in defining rather than in answering questions.

Studies may be *longitudinal*, in which patients are studied over time, or *cross-sectional*, of which a simple example is a snapshot postoperative survey of satisfaction. A *cohort* study is a long-term, longitudinal, prospective study, e.g. of a group of patients who all have the same disease. A cohort is a special type of sample (see below). A *case-control* study is a retrospective study in which patients with a disease are compared for pre-existing risk markers with people who do not have the disease. These definitions are sometimes used rather loosely, and studies may use more than one form of design.

RANDOMIZATION

Allocation to treatments by randomization is an important way of avoiding bias. *Randomized double-blind controlled trials* (RCTs) are probably the best way of determining which of two treatments, on average, gives the better outcome. It must be stressed, however, that just because a trial is randomized and double-blind does not, of itself, mean that the conclusions are justified or generalizable.

Randomization ensures that neither investigators nor patients know which treatment they receive until the time comes to give that treatment: there is no preselection. Randomization makes it less likely that, in an anaesthetic study, preoperative factors determine which treatment is given. Another important reason for randomization is that much of medical statistics is based on the assumption that the samples are random and that differences between them therefore behave similarly to the differences between truly random samples.

Randomization by flipping a coin is random but is open to the manipulation, sometimes subconscious, of saying that the coin 'wasn't flipped properly'. Random number tables or a computer's random number generator (all statistical computer programs include these) are better methods of true randomization: an odd number denotes treatment A, an even number treatment B. Clearly, the investigators must not see the next number in the table until the next patient is ready for treatment. This is usually managed by putting codes into sealed envelopes, taken sequentially by the investigators.

Simply using a coin or random numbers causes problems in small studies because of the likelihood of generating unequal groups, which cause statistical difficulties. The usual remedy is *block randomization*. In an intended study of 40 patients, which is probably an average-sized clinical study but in statistical terms is small, block randomization ensures two groups of 20 receive each treatment. If there are known important preoperative factors that affect outcome, e.g. smoking in a study of postoperative chest infections, randomization can be *stratified*, so that smokers and non-smokers are allocated by separate randomization.

Investigators should always describe their method of randomization, or, if they have not randomized treatments, they should explain why. Randomization is difficult when patients or investigators have clear views about which treatment they think is better.

PATIENT CONSENT

Patients must be given all the information necessary to make the decision as to whether to give freely their fully *informed consent* to enter the study. The information must be given in a non-coercive way, in words they understand. For all except the simplest of studies, patients are given a written information sheet. Discussion of possible risks of the study include far smaller risks than customarily discussed before non-research clinical procedures (although customs and attitudes change, and informed consent to treatment and to research are converging as informed consent to treatment demands more and more detail). Patients sign a consent sheet: one copy is kept with the study paperwork, and another is given to the patient. Ideally, a copy should also be filed in the clinical notes.

Much of the work of ethics committees (see below) is concerned with the what and how of information provided to patients.

REQUIRED SIZE OF STUDY

The size of the study (i.e. the number of patients that need to be recruited) determines the power of the study (i.e. the likelihood of obtaining an answer). This is discussed in some detail below (see type II error), but is mentioned now because these *power calculations* are part of study design and are an important ethical issue. The notation for size of study group is n.

DESIGN DEVIATIONS

Sometimes investigators discover faults with the collection of information in a trial which mean that the patient can no longer be included. There are serious risks of introducing bias if patients are withdrawn from a study after randomization. Data from withdrawn patients must always be admitted, but it may not be possible to include those data in the general cal-

culations. It is always best, before the trial begins, to think very carefully about how protocol violations may arise, and to have some plans for what to do in that eventuality. If it is important that a particular number of patients is recruited; one plan is to have some extra randomized envelopes available to replace patients who have dropped out. It infringes randomization and blinding simply to replace patients who drop out of one treatment group with additional patients having the same treatment. It is better to include enough patients in the original design, so that a few withdrawals do not matter.

Patients sometimes start in one group and, for clinical reasons, are transferred to a different treatment. A patient whose epidural is ineffective and who is prescribed intramuscular analgesia must, for the purposes of analysis, remain in the epidural group; this is known as analysis by *intention-to-treat*.

PLANS FOR STATISTICAL ANALYSIS

A medical statistician should be contacted early. The more complex the analysis – the more treatments being compared, the more groups of patients, the less well known the intended statistical test – the more important is good statistical advice. It is not a good idea to make casual inquiries of non-specialized statisticians. A statistician will advise about randomization and n, as well as plans for analysis, which must be drawn up before the data are generated.

The fewer measurements that are made, and the fewer comparisons that are made between them, the easier is the statistical analysis. Investigators must be especially wary of making *subgroup analyses* not set out in the original design. An example would be looking for different nausea scores between men and women, or in people above or below a certain weight, when all that was originally intended was to compare the two treatments. Subgroup analyses after the event ('post hoc') risk type I errors (see below).

ADMINISTRATION

Each investigator's job during the study must be defined: who gives the anaesthesia, who makes the measurements or observations, who undertakes the analysis. In a simple study, one investigator may do everything, but there are few clinical trials in which this is possible. There must be plans for monitoring the progress of the trial; forms must be filled in and stored properly, with efficient indexing so that any patient's records can be found quickly if needed. Any supporting institution – drug company, grant-giving body or government agency – can come at any time and demand to see the records. Workbooks and original records from clinical studies of medicinal products must be kept for 15 years.

In the United Kingdom (UK), the Data Protection Act must be complied with if personal information from any patient is stored in a computer file.

ETHICAL ISSUES

Any research study that involves patients or healthy volunteers, human tissue, the recently deceased, or healthcare staff must be reviewed by a research ethics committee. Following European directives, and the setting up of Research Governance in the UK, applying for ethical approval for research has become highly formalized.

EXPERIMENTAL DATA AND SOME TYPES OF BIAS

EXPERIMENTAL DATA

Data are either *categorical* or *numerical*; categorical data are often referred to as *lower-order* data. Categorical data may be nominal or ordinal. The simplest type of *nominal categorical data* allocates observations to one of two possibilities, e.g. yes or no, male or female, general anaesthesia or local anaesthesia. Nominal data may be of more than two categories, e.g. the categorizing of diabetes as diet-controlled, tablet-controlled, or insulin-controlled.

In *ordinal categorical data,* the categories are ranked, e.g. when pain is assessed as none, mild, moderate, or severe. These categories can be ranked by number, as 0, 1, 2, or 3. The common method of measuring pain in millimetres along a *visual analogue scale* (VAS) still produces ordinal categorical data. The essence of this type of data is that, whereas within one patient at one time, mild is less than moderate, or 1 is less than 2, there is no certainty that, even for that patient, mild today is the same as mild tomorrow, or that 1 is less than 2 by the same degree as 2 is less than 3; and there is no way of knowing whether one patient's mild is the same as another patient's. Without the need for statistical theory, this is the reason why it is illogical to deal with numbers measured on an ordinal scale arithmetically in the same way as higher-order data.

Numerical data are either discrete or continuous. An example of *discrete numerical data* is number of children: one child is less than two children by the same degree that two is less than three. Whereas no family can have 2.4 children, it is now logical to speak of an average-sized family as having 2.4 children: discrete numerical data can be dealt with arithmetically.

Examples of continuous numerical data are arterial pressure and serum sodium concentrations; an increase or decrease of 10 mmHg or 3 mmol L^{-1} is the same, whatever level the change occurs from. In practice, we treat most continuous data as discrete data in the sense that we usually measure to the nearest unit. Clearly, this depends on the precision of our instruments, the units and whether or not it makes clinical sense to measure to greater precision. Measuring arterial pressure in mmHg, it makes little sense in anaesthetic practice to record with more precision than to the nearest 5 mmHg; measuring arterial gas tensions, it does make sense to measure to fractions of a kilopascal (kPa). Whatever precision is chosen, if the data are theoretically continuous, they may be analysed arithmetically.

Continuous data may be treated as if they were categorical: patients can be categorized as normotensive or hypertensive. This is sometimes a reasonable approach for input variables (i.e. baseline characteristics) to a study, when it is useful to stratify randomization (see above) according to entry baseline arterial pressure. If applied to outcome variables, it causes statistical problems, one of which is the serious loss of information that occurs when all arterial pressures are lumped together above whatever arbitrary cut-off is chosen.

BIAS

Table A1.1 lists some types of bias, and some examples of how they arise. Bias has already been discussed (see study design, above) but it is appropriate to discuss it further here.

It is a common problem that patients studied in clinical trials are unrepresentative of the population from which they are drawn (selection bias) and to which it is hoped to apply the conclusions of the trials. This problem has two causes, both of which are difficult to circumvent. First, most clinical trials are performed in large centres, but most patients are treated in more peripheral units. For many reasons, it is likely that neither the patients nor the treatments they receive are the same in these different settings. The best example of this effect is the two- to threefold difference in mortality among patients included in trials of treatments of myocardial infarction (commonly 7–10% mortality) and patients treated in the community (commonly 15–20%). Patients in trials are often the most favourable patients treated in the most favourable conditions. To a lesser extent, this probably

Table A1.1   Types of bias in clinical trials

Type of bias	Stage of bias	Example of how bias can occur
Selection	Entering patients into the trial	Sample unrepresentative of population
		Controls not comparable with study group
		Exaggeration of a factor
Intervention	Applying treatments	Patients receiving more attention because of their treatment group, e.g. epidural trials
Follow-up	Assessing treatments	Subjects 'lost' to follow-up
Measurement or information	Collecting data	Investigators' conscious or subconscious action
	Making measurements	Inaccurate or uncalibrated instruments
	Making observations	Patients' mistaken recollection
Analysis	Collating data	Withdrawals or design violations
	Statistical analysis	'Massaging' data
Interpretation	Putting results into context	Prejudices of the investigator

happens in most trials. The second cause is the well-known phenomenon that, even in the same institution, patients included in trials do better than patients who are not included.

A good example of intervention bias might occur in an unblinded comparison of epidural and intramuscular analgesia. Patients know epidural analgesia is more complicated, and might expect it to be better; anaesthetists are likely to spend more time optimizing epidural analgesia.

Follow-up bias, when patients are lost to the study for whatever reason, causes the same statistical difficulties as other withdrawals after randomization. There is the added difficulty that the patients cannot be analysed by intention-to-treat (see above), because the data are not available for analysis.

Examples of causes of measurement or information bias are investigators transcribing readings incorrectly, inaccurate instruments, or patients' mistaken recollections. Instruments and monitors used for research must always be calibrated before use, and researchers should know the limits of measurement of any apparatus they use. For some instruments, e.g. noninvasive arterial pressure monitors, it is adequate to read the technical parts of the manual, but it is sensible to use a recently serviced machine. Better, although probably not practical in most hospitals, is to use dedicated research machines. However, many pieces of equipment that we take for granted in clinical practice, e.g. blood gas analysers, must be cali-

brated specially if they are used for research. If a blood sample is analysed by the hospital's laboratory, the technicians should be asked for the limits of accuracy; for any special analyses, e.g. those used in pharmacokinetic studies, the investigators may have to construct their own *standard curves* when measuring plasma concentrations of drugs.

When considering the accuracy of a measurement, there are two indices: *precision* (an indication of the variability when the same measurement is made repeatedly, e.g. the concentration of a drug in a single blood sample) and *offset* (the difference between the measured value and the true value). Confusingly, offset is often termed bias. Precision and offset need to be measured over the full range of expected values. Precision may be assessed for any instrument (and is often given as the *coefficient of variation*; see below), but offset may be assessed only when there is some way of knowing the true value. The accuracy of noninvasive arterial pressure may be measured against invasive intra-arterial measurement, which is taken as the true arterial pressure.

It is at the analysis stage that investigators must be especially careful not to introduce bias. The unexpected and the peculiar must be reported together with the expected and routine, even though sometimes there are valid reasons for rejecting a measurement, e.g. accidental contamination of a sample.

As long as humans are involved in research, investigators will be biased when they interpret their findings. At this stage of a research project, the caution passes from the investigators to the readers.

STATISTICS

Even when doing research, clinicians need not know any calculations, because they are now performed by computer programs. Clinicians do need to know the principles underlying the calculations, or risk applying an incorrect statistical test.

There are two types of statistics: *descriptive statistics* describe data, and include the mean and standard deviation; *inferential statistics* allow conclusions to be drawn from observations, and include the standard error of the mean, confidence limits, correlation coefficients and the special statistics of the Student's *t*-test and the chi-squared test. (Student was the pseudonym of the statistician who described the *t*-distribution.)

PROBABILITY

A correct understanding of probability is essential to understanding statistics.

A coin, when flipped, may land heads or tails. This is a random event. We can work out the expected probabilities for any sequence of heads or tails in a given number of flips. In an exactly analogous way, we make the assumption that when we draw samples of patients from the population for our clinical trials, and when we make measurements from those patients, the patients and measurements will behave with random variability. We can therefore compare our measurement from the real world of clinical trials with the expected behaviour of random numbers, derived from statistical theory that we need know nothing about.

Probability is denoted by P: a 50% probability, such as obtaining a head from flipping a coin, is written as $P = 0.5$. The convention for statistical significance is $P < 0.05$. If the likelihood is less than 1 in 20 that the findings of a clinical trial occurred by chance, then by convention we are prepared to accept that the finding did not occur by chance, but occurred because of whatever intervention we made in the clinical trial.

It is stressed here and later that $P < 0.05$ does not ensure that the findings did not occur by chance. In fact, one in 20 times that is precisely what will have happened (a type I error; see below). One in 20 is taken as the cut-off of statistical significance only as a convention, although it is regarded by many investigators – mistakenly – as the magic figure of respectability.

To help appreciate this, consider what happens if a coin is flipped five times: what is the chance of a run of five heads? There is a one in two chance for each flip, and probabilities are multiplied. The chance of two heads in a row is one in two times two ($1/4$ or $P = 0.25$), and thus of five heads is one in two × two × two × two × two ($1/32$ or $P = 0.031$). This probability is less than the magic figure. The logic of declaring the outcome of a clinical trial on a probability of $P < 0.05$ is thus the same as declaring that a coin is biased from observing just five flips. The correct logic is that the coin *might be* biased and the more times the coin is flipped the more certain one becomes, analogous to clinical trials in which the larger the number of patients studied the more certain one is about the treatment.

Increasingly, journals are asking for results to be presented as *confidence intervals* (see below). Probabilities are dimensionless and difficult to interpret clinically. Confidence intervals are expressed in the same units as the measurements and are thus readily understood by clinicians. Confidence intervals of 95% and a probability of 0.05 are equivalent, and the underlying mathematical calculations are the same (and in these days of computers there is no need to know them).

A SIMPLE OUTLINE

Table A1.2 appears here for reference while reading the remainder of the chapter. It shows how to handle the data from the four simple example studies. For each question, there are measurements, a representation of those measurements (by descriptive statistics) and an analysis (by inferential statistics). At the end of this process, the investigators know the probability of their findings having occurred by chance, and the 95% confidence intervals on those findings.

DESCRIPTIVE STATISTICS

When an experimental sample is small, e.g. fewer than six, all the data should be shown. Information is lost as soon as any summary statistics are used, but there are too many data in most clinical trials for it to be practical to show them all. Data are described by an *index of central tendency* – the *median* or the *mean*; and an *index of dispersion* – the *range*, the *interquartile range*, or the *standard deviation*. Both these indices are needed; giving the index of central tendency of a measurement without any indication of its dispersion (i.e. of its variability) is misleading. It is not unusual for investigators to omit variability to make results look less messy, but science, especially clinical science, is often messy.

Although the discussion of types of data (above) went from lower-order to higher-order, it is more

Table A1.2   Four simple clinical questions: type of data, the measurements, representation and analysis (see text for details)

Question	Type of data	Measurement	Representation and graph	Analysis
Two drugs for postoperative sickness	Categorical Nominal	Yes/no	Proportions	Chi-squared (χ^2) → P
Two drugs for postoperative sickness	Categorical Ordinal	Score 0–10	Medians Interquartile ranges Ranges Box-and-whisker plot	Mann–Whitney U → P
Induction of anaesthesia and arterial pressure	Numerical Continuous	Arterial pressures before and after	Means Standard deviations Dots and error (SD) bars	Student's t → P
Two anaesthetic agents and arterial pressure	Numerical Continuous	Arterial pressures at various times	Means Standard deviations Dots and error (SD) bars	ANOVA Student's t → P
Duration of surgery and change of body temperature	Numerical Continuous	Times and temperatures	Scatter plot	Correlation (r) Regression (m) → P

convenient to deal with mean and standard deviation first, because most people are already familiar with them. It is also useful to understand them before trying to explain why they are sometimes inappropriate.

There is another index of central tendency: the *mode*. This is the most commonly occurring value. It is not useful statistically and is not discussed in detail.

The mean

The mean is the average value: it is the sum of the values divided by the number of values. Thus for a sample of five observations (x_1 to x_5) – 24, 27, 28, 31 and 34 – the sum (notation: Σx) is 144, and the mean (notation: $\bar{x}$) is 28.8. It is reasonable to present the mean and other statistics to one significant figure more than the data; here that is to one decimal place. Computer packages present data to as many significant figures as requested, but too many is spurious precision. (Note that presenting the mean of a sample of only five could be criticized as unnecessary statistics but is used here for ease of calculation.)

The standard deviation

The simplest index of dispersion is the full range (24 to 34 for our sample of five), but full range is easily distorted by outliers, which exaggerate the range of values likely to be seen. The most familiar index of

dispersion is the standard deviation (SD). Clinicians need know only a few statistical calculations, but it is worth reading how to calculate the SD.

If we take our sample, calculate how each observation varies from the mean (–4.8, –1.8, –0.8, 2.2, 5.2), and sum these deviations, the sum is zero. (The sum of deviations from the mean is always bound to be zero: readers who cannot see intuitively that this is so are likely to have some difficulties with the mathematical aspects of anaesthesia and should seek help to improve their understanding.) The mathematical trick is then to square the deviations, which removes the minus values (23.04, 3.24, 0.64, 4.84, 27.04). The sum of these squared deviations is 58.8, and the mean squared deviation is 58.8 divided by 5, which is 11.76. The mean squared deviation is a statistic known as the *variance*, which is central to much statistical theory (it is the variance referred to in the ANOVA, see below), but is not much used practically in an obvious way.

The last step is to take the square root of the variance (3.43), and this is the standard deviation; it is the square root of the average squared deviation from the mean.

There is one refinement. Because small samples (small here implies less than 30) tend to underestimate the true SD, the summed squared deviation is divided not by the number in the sample (n), but by one less ($n–1$), which gives a value of SD of 3.83.

So our sample has a mean of 28.8 with a standard deviation of 3.8 (the SD should have the same number of decimal places as the mean). This is usually printed as 28.8 ± 3.8, but it is better to put the SD in brackets: 28.8 (3.8). The implication of this description is that we would expect to find 95% of the observations within two standard deviations of the mean. Most anaesthetists are familiar with this idea, although it needs discussion of the normal distribution to understand it more fully (see below).

The *coefficient of variation* is the standard deviation divided into the mean. It is a useful comparator, e.g. for instruments used in chemical analyses, because scaling the standard deviation to the mean gives a relative idea of an instrument's precision (see above).

The median

The median is the middlemost value: for our sample it is 28. As there cannot be a true middlemost value of an even-numbered sample, the median is then taken as the average of the two values bracketing the middle of the sample. Note that if one peripheral value were different (say, 24, 27, 28, 31 and 44), the median would still be 28 but the mean would be 30.8 and the SD 7.8.

The interquartile range

This is the index of dispersion that goes with the median. It is not sensible to describe an interquartile range for a sample of only five (in fact, a mean and SD are scarcely more sensible, but this number was chosen only for convenience). The interquartile range is described most easily for a sample of 100. If the observations, e.g. 100 nausea scores, are ranked in order from 1 to 100, the quartiles are the 1st to 25th scores (which will be the lowest scores), 26th to 50th, 51st to 75th, and 76th to 100th (which will be the highest scores). The interquartile range is the 26th to 75th score. For $n \neq 100$, the quartiles are the equivalent proportions of the sample.

Which descriptive statistics are appropriate?

Taking a sample of 12 nausea scores – 0, 0, 0, 0, 1, 1, 1, 4, 4, 10, 10, 10 – the mean and SD can be calculated; they are 3.4 (4.2). These statistics can be calculated from any sample consisting of numerical values, but what meaning do these calculations have? They imply that 95% of the observations are within 2 SDs of the mean: but that implies that 95% of the nausea scores are expected within the range −5 to 11.8. Both these values are off the scale and are clinically meaningless, which is why mean and SD should not be used for these data. Certainly, the data are far from normally distributed, which is the technical reason for not using

mean and SD; but these 12 nausea scores give the commonplace, clinically evident reason. On the other hand, the median is 1, and the interquartile range is 0–7; these numbers make clinical sense and can be sensibly compared with another sample.

THE NORMAL DISTRIBUTION

Further consideration of which descriptions to use requires some understanding of the normal distribution, which is the behaviour of many of the variables measured in anaesthesia research. That a variable follows the normal distribution does not imply that the variable is normal in the everyday sense; nor is a variable abnormal just because it does not follow the distribution. The distribution is sometimes known as the Gaussian distribution (after the mathematician Gauss).

The familiar smooth, bell-shaped curve of the normal distribution is an example of a *frequency histogram*. These diagrams, in which the value of the variable is put on the x-axis and the number of observations with that value on the y-axis, are useful when first surveying research data. Systolic arterial pressure is normally distributed: the upper part of Figure A1.1 could be the frequency histogram of arterial pressure in a healthy, young population. The notation for the population mean is μ, and for the population SD is σ. Two-thirds of the observed arterial pressures are within 1 SD (σ is the mathematical symbol; SD is the conventional abbreviation) of the mean, 95% within 2 SDs and 99% within 3 SDs (these numbers are accepted approximations). The conventional acceptance of $P < 0.05$, the 95% confidence intervals of the observations, is thus the range covered by two standard deviations each side of the mean: this does not imply that any measurement or patient outside this range is necessarily abnormal. Note that in the normal distribution, the mean and median (and the mode) are the same.

These proportions have to be remembered, and the question why they should be what they are is not easy to answer. The curve is described by a mathematical equation, from which the proportions are worked out, and from which can also be worked out how many observations are expected in whatever part of the curve is under consideration. Clinicians need not know the equation, except to know that this mathematical description of the normal distribution depends on the mean and the standard deviation: if these are known, then the distribution is completely described. Thus, the mean and standard deviation are the *parameters* of the normal distribution. This is where the terms parameter and parametric in statistics come from; they imply that the variable in question behaves according to a mathematically described distribution.

783

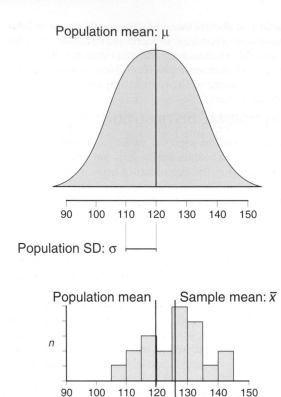

Fig. A1.1
The normal distribution. Frequency histograms of arterial pressure measurements from the population and from a sample. The known values are the sample mean ($\bar{x}$) and the sample standard deviation (s). The standard error of the mean (SEM) is calculated from s, and the confidence limits around the mean of the measured sample from the SEM. This allows an estimate of the population mean from the sample mean or, if the population mean is known, indicates the likelihood that the sample came from the population. See text for more details.

It need not be the normal distribution. Variables can follow the Poisson distribution, for which the only parameter is the mean. An example is bed occupancy in intensive care units. Knowing the mean bed occupancy allows inferences to be made about how many beds will be occupied for how many days, and what the likelihood is of any number of beds being occupied on any one day. (For a near guarantee of an available bed in a six-bedded unit, mean occupancy should be no more than 2.7 patients. The Poisson distribution tells us that most units in the UK have too few beds!)

The values of t and χ^2 (see Table A1.2 and below) are also parametric, although familiarity with the shape of the distributions is not necessary. One other distribution clinicians may encounter is the *binomial distribution*, which describes the frequency of occur-

rence of coin flips, dice rolls and hands of playing cards. The binomial distribution is non-parametric.

As a further explanation of the word 'parameter', pharmacokinetic parameters determine the concentration of a drug in the body compartments with respect to time. Another way of thinking of parameters is via the equation of a straight line: $y = mx + c$ (see regression, below). Here, y and x are the variables; m and c are the constants in the equation and may be thought of as the parameters that control the relationship between y and x. To avoid confusion, the distinction between variables (which are measured directly in clinical trials) and parameters (which are not) is important.

More on the representation of data

We know from previous research that arterial pressure is normally distributed. Sometimes, investigators do not know what distribution a variable follows, and this is determined in a pilot study before the main study. There are formal tests for normality, but looking at the frequency histogram is often enough. Another check is that the mean and median are the same, and that the range of observations is approximately five standard deviations.

Parametric data, described by the mean and SD, are shown in diagrams by the familiar dot and error bars. (This is not an error in the sense of mistake; they would be better termed variability bars.) The bars must always be defined, in case they are not one standard deviation but some other index. Data that are known not to be parametric are best shown by *box-and-whisker plots* (Fig. A1.2). If there is any doubt, it is better to assume the data do not conform to a particular distribution, and to use a non-parametric description. This is also probably the best way to deal with small samples (e.g. less than 10) of parametric data.

Skewed distributions and transforming data

Some distributions, although smooth, are *skewed*: they have a tail. A good example is wake-up times after anaesthesia. Most patients wake up in a few minutes, but some take longer, and a few take much longer. The effect of this is that the longer times 'drag' the mean towards the tail (as in the simple calculation above), and the mean wake-up time is longer than the median (a *positive skew*). Such data can be analysed using non-parametrically based statistics, but parametrically based statistics are more *powerful* (see below). Skewed data can sometimes be *transformed*, by taking logarithms or by other mathematical manipulations, so that they assume the normal distribution. The decision to transform data should ideally be taken before the study is done.

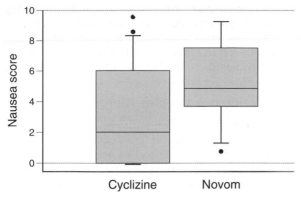

Fig. A1.2
Box-and-whisker plots are shown for an imaginary clinical trial of the antiemetics cyclizine and novom. The central horizontal line of the box is the median, the lower line the 25th centile and the upper line the 75th centile. The 'whiskers' usually represent the 10th–90th centile range. The dots beyond the whiskers are outliers, beyond the 10th–90th centiles. If outliers are not shown in this way, the whiskers should represent the full range.

INFERENTIAL STATISTICS

From sample to population

It is unusual that we know the population mean and standard deviation, and they are usually *inferred* from a sample. The inferential statistic is the *standard error of the mean* (SEM), which is used to estimate the mean of the population or, if the population mean is known, to decide whether or not the sample is likely to be drawn from that population. The SEM is one of the least understood and most misused statistics; it is not an index of dispersion, although it is often used as such because it is smaller than the SD and looks better on graphs. The SEM is also the key to understanding much of inferential statistics and the comparing of samples that underlies most clinical trials. If the explanation here is too abbreviated, readers are advised to look at Rowntree (1991).

Stating first an extended definition:

> *The standard error of the mean is the standard deviation of all possible sample means of a given size, and from it can be calculated the confidence limits around the mean of the measured sample. These limits indicate, to the chosen probability, the likely mean of the population.*

If the measured sample is the whole, large, population, then the sample mean *will be* the population mean. If the sample is half the population, the sample mean will still be extremely close to the population mean. However, the smaller the sample, the less likely it is that its mean will be exactly the population mean, and sometimes it will be substantially different. It should be intuitively obvious that the mean of a smaller sample – even if selected in a correctly random fashion – is more likely to misrepresent the mean of the population.

There is another way of expressing this. If many samples of the same size are taken (instead of the usual single sample of that size) the *means of those samples* are more similar to one another if the samples are large than if they are small. The means of these samples can themselves be treated as data, and a frequency histogram constructed: the sample means follow the normal distribution; and the larger the samples, the narrower is the distribution. In exactly the same way that the SD of the distribution of data is calculated, so may the SD of the sample means be calculated. The larger the value of n, the smaller the SD of the sample means. This SD of the sample means is the SEM (see definition, above). Thus, 95% of sample means (of a given n) will be within ±2 SEMs of the population mean (and 99% within ±3 SEMs), in exactly the same way that 95% of observations are within ±2 SDs (and 99% within ±3 SDs) of the population mean.

This logic is applied to a single trial sample, because statistical theory allows calculation of the SEM from the sample standard deviation (notation s): SEM = $s/\sqrt{n}$. Then the 95% confidence intervals of the sample mean are 2 SEMs and there is 95% confidence that the population mean lies within that range.

(The *central limit theorem* of statistics states that the distribution of samples is normal whatever the distribution of the original data. This theorem is often used to justify applying parametrically based statistics to non-parametric data, but the clinical nonsense of parametric descriptions of these data is more important than statistical theory. The central limit theorem is beyond basic statistical knowledge.)

Probability and samples

An important implication of 95% of sample means lying within ±2 SEMs of the population mean is that 5%, i.e. 1 in 20, do not. If 20 samples are drawn at random from a normally distributed population, on average one of them will be statistically significantly different from the population mean. This effect of pure chance is a type 1 error (see below). The size of the sample does not matter: at a probability of 0.05, on average one of 20 samples drawn at random from a normally distributed population will be statistically significantly different. However, the larger the sample, the smaller the absolute difference will be. It is thus less likely that a difference due to chance will be clinically important and warrant being noticed.

Comparing samples: the null hypothesis

Although the research question may be 'Is novom better than cyclizine?' or 'Does propofol cause greater hypotension than thiopental at induction?', the statistical approach is via the *null hypothesis*. A hypothesis must be grounded (i.e. based on previous knowledge) and testable (otherwise it is not a hypothesis but a speculation), and the essence of the test is that the hypothesis is falsifiable. The philosophy of this (due to Popper) is that we can never know the truth, but progression in knowledge takes us further towards the truth. Thus, we start with the null hypothesis that novom and cyclizine have the same effect. If we show a difference, then we reject the null hypothesis and accept that one of the drugs is a better antiemetic – *at our chosen level of probability* (but we can be wrong: see type I error). If we fail to show a difference, we support the null hypothesis (but we can be wrong: see type II error).

Comparing proportions: a new drug for postoperative sickness by 'yes/no'

If 17 patients of 40 given cyclizine and 11 of 40 given novom vomit, the data are represented as *proportions* (17/40 and 11/40) (data should not be represented as percentages). These two proportions are then tested by the chi-squared test for the probability that the proportions happened by chance. As with all statistical tests, it is not necessary to know the details of the test; the essential knowledge is knowing which test to apply. The principle of the chi-squared test is a comparison of the proportions that actually occurred in the study with the proportions that would have occurred if there had been no difference between the groups. For the calculations, for each cell in the 2×2 *table* the expected occurrences are subtracted from the observed occurrences; the null hypothesis states that there is no difference between the two proportions, so the expected value is $(17 + 11)/2 = 14$ for both drugs. (Here there are two groups, but the test can be applied to any number of groups. There is also no requirement that the groups be the same size.) The calculation gives chi-squared (notation: χ^2), and the value is looked up in statistical tables (or provided by the computer program) to give the probability. The larger the number of tested groups, the larger χ^2 needs to be to reach the chosen P. The tables account for this; χ^2 is checked against the number of *degrees of freedom* in the data (degrees of freedom is a difficult statistical idea, and not necessary to a simple knowledge of statistics).

The chi-squared test is not suitable if any of the expected values is less than 5. A simple solution is to apply Yates' correction; but it may be better to use Fisher's exact test. These details are beyond the scope of this Appendix.

Comparing two samples of ordinal data: a new drug for postoperative sickness by nausea score

Comparisons of two samples of non-parametric data such as these (or of numerical data whose distribution is unknown or uncertain) is by a *ranking test*. When the two groups are of different patients, the data are *unpaired*, and the *Mann–Whitney U-test* is appropriate. Before computers, such tests were tedious. The calculations for the *t*-test (see below) are easy with pencil and paper by substituting in equations. There are no equations for ranking tests, and no alternative to the laborious listing and ranking of all the data.

The data are ranked from lowest to highest to determine the median and interquartile ranges (see above); the procedure is the same for the statistical test, but the rankings are summed and compared between the two groups (imagine doing that for two samples of 100 patients). This is best explained by example.

The first few nausea scores in a trial of cyclizine (group C) and novom (group N) using a 100 mm visual analogue scale are:

Group C	0	5	12	13	15 . . .
Group N	3	6	9	10	12 . . .

These scores are ranked and the scores from novom are identified by underlining:

Rank order: 0 $\underline{3}$ 5 $\underline{6}$ $\underline{9}$ $\underline{10}$ 12 $\underline{12}$ 13 15 . . .

Ranking: 1 $\underline{2}$ 3 $\underline{4}$ $\underline{5}$ $\underline{6}$ 7.5 $\underline{7.5}$ 9 10 . . .

The rankings are then summed for each group. Shared scores rank equal, which is why the scores of 12 each rank 7.5:

Group sum of ranks:

Group C $= 1 + 3 + 7.5 + 9 + 10 = 30.5$

Group N $= \underline{2} + \underline{4} + \underline{5} + \underline{6} + \underline{7.5} = \underline{24.5}$

If the null hypothesis is true, the rank sums are equal; the more unequal they are, the less support there is for the null hypothesis. P is read from a table of expected rank sums against n. The whole procedure is now done by computer, with no need to read from tables.

A paired test, the *Wilcoxon signed rank test*, is appropriate when a study is done within-patient, each patient being his or her own control. The pair differences are ranked and the rank sums calculated for the positive and negative differences. Again, the less equal these sums are, the more likely it is that the null hypothesis will be rejected. This is the paired equivalent of the Mann–Whitney. Some confusion arises because the Mann–Whitney test is also known as the *Wilcoxon two-sample test*.

Comparing two samples of numerical, normal, data: the effect of an induction agent on arterial pressure

When samples are very large, i.e. more than 120, they can be compared simply by referring to the normal distribution. It follows from the description above that two samples, the means of which are separated by more than 2 SEMs, are statistically significantly different at $P < 0.05$. The familiar Student's t-test extends this idea to small samples, when direct reference to the normal distribution becomes inaccurate (the reasons for this do not matter). Assumptions of the t-test are that the data are drawn from normally distributed populations (although the samples themselves do not have to be rigidly normal) and that the variances (and hence the SEMs) of the two samples are not too different.

Analogous to the Mann–Whitney and the Wilcoxon tests, the *unpaired t-test* is for data from two different groups of patients and the *paired t-test* is for two groups of data from the same patients (e.g. before and after induction). The paired test is more powerful because the calculations are on the differences between the paired readings, which gives a smaller SEM and, as alluded to above, t is the ratio of the difference between the means and the SEM. For samples of about 30, t is about 2.05 at $P = 0.05$; for samples of 10, t is 2.26 (i.e. the difference between the means is 2.26 SEMs). Thus, if t is larger than this value, we reject the null hypothesis at $P = 0.05$.

The basic question asked by the t-test is whether the samples could come from the same population, or whether they are better described as coming from two different populations.

The t-test can be one- or two-tailed. This commonly causes confusion. The safe option is always to do a two-tailed test. A one-tailed test is appropriate only when a comparison can move only in one direction (i.e. the two outcomes comparing groups A and B are A = B or A > B, but A < B is impossible). This is almost never true in clinical trials, and the commonest reason that investigators use a one-tailed test is that $P < 0.05$ is more easily achieved.

Comparing more than two samples: a comparison of the effects of two induction agents on arterial pressure

A graph from this type of trial is likely to show means and standard deviations for each drug before induction and at intervals after induction. The obvious way to analyse these data is by repeated t testing, comparing arterial pressures with baseline arterial pressure and between the two groups at each time of measurement.

This *multiple testing* is incorrect because of the additive risk of a difference occurring by chance: 10 comparisons each at $P < 0.05$ gives an overall $P < 0.5$. One approach is first to do an ANOVA. This is the acronym for *analysis of variance*, which is a way of assessing the probability that there are measurements within the data that are statistically different from the rest. If ANOVA gives $P < 0.05$, then Student's t can be used to tease out the precise differences. The non-parametric equivalent of ANOVA is the *Kruskal–Wallis test*, which would be suitable for nausea scores measured at intervals postoperatively.

Another approach to the problem is to use a so-called *summary statistic*, so that for each patient the change in arterial pressure is represented by a single number such as the area enclosed by the graph of arterial pressure against time. (The most familiar way that anaesthetists might compare areas under curves, although this has nothing to do with multiple testing, is probably in the measurement of bioavailability, see page 8).

Multiple testing is a recurring problem and statistical advice should be sought. A common simple adjustment is the *Bonferroni correction*, by which P is adjusted to a higher level of probability to offset the risk of spurious significance.

Relating variables to one another: correlation and regression – the relationship between duration of surgery and body temperature

Analysis aiming to link two variables should start with a *scatter plot* – a graph in which the *independent variable*, e.g. time, is plotted on the x-axis and the *dependent variable*, e.g. temperature, on the y-axis (Fig. A1.3). If the relationship is linear, *least-squares statistics* are applied. The *correlation coefficient* (r), sometimes termed the Pearson correlation coefficient, describes the amount of scatter: it is the degree of agreement between the two variables. The *regression coefficient* (m) describes how y depends on x: it is the slope, or gradient, of *the line of best fit* (as in the equation for a straight line, see above). Whether correlation

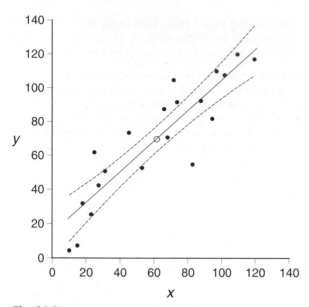

Fig. A1.3
A scatter plot of two variables: x is the independent (or 'known') variable; y is the dependent (or 'unknown') variable. Using least-squares statistics, the correlation coefficient (r) is 0.90 and the line of best fit (shown by the solid line) is $y = 0.90x + 14.6$. All three coefficients (of correlation, gradient and intercept) are only best estimates, and their confidence intervals should be reported. The 95% confidence 'envelope' is shown by the dotted lines: with the restraint that the line must pass through the means of x and y (marked by the open circle), there is 95% confidence that the true relation between y and x is defined by this envelope. Note that the lines should not extend horizontally beyond the measured values of x.

or regression is appropriate depends on whether it is sensible to *predict y from x*.

Thus, if weight is plotted against height for a sample of men, taller men are, on average, heavier, but the relationship does not allow sensible prediction of the weight of an individual man who is 1.83 m tall. Calculating r is sensible, but not m. On the other hand, if a subject breathes carbon dioxide mixtures, the resulting alveolar ventilation in that subject is predictable from the arterial tension, and m is a sensible measurement. As m is a constant in an equation, clearly it can have any value at all, can be positive or negative, and its units depend on x and y. However, r is a dimensionless measure of scatter. It is +1 for a perfect line of positive gradient, −1 for a perfect negative line, and zero if there is no correlation.

The statistics r and m are only best estimates of the true relationship between x and y, in the same way that $\bar{x}$ is an estimate of the true mean. Their probabilities and, better, confidence intervals must be given. Confidence intervals are shown graphically as an

'envelope' showing the 95% (or 99%) range around the line of best fit.

The relationship between two variables need not be linear. Least-squares statistics are used to fit any line, e.g. for the well-known exponential relation between drug concentration and time after injection (see Ch. 1). Or y may depend on several variables, so the data fit an equation of the form $y = m_1x_1 + m_2x_2 + m_3x_3 \ldots$. This is *multiple regression*. Sometimes the variables are nominal data. For example, if y is the likelihood of postoperative nausea, one of the terms may be for sex, which is represented in the equation as 0 or 1, and the coefficient applied to each term is often termed the 'weighting'. This is *logistic regression*. Regression using more than one term is not for amateurs in statistics.

Regression is inappropriate for ordinal data because the relationship between the variables cannot be described by equation. There are non-parametrically based estimates of r, e.g. Spearman's rank correlation.

Clinicians must beware of confusing *association* between variables, whether correlation or regression, with *causation*. For example, alcohol consumption and incidence of lung cancer are correlated, but alcohol does not cause lung cancer. The *confounding variable* is tobacco use. A common cause of false association is both variables changing with time.

Type I and type II errors

Type I error is best thought of as a *false positive*. A difference is found (or a gradient is described, etc.) when there is not one: the null hypothesis is rejected when it is in fact true. It is impossible to avoid type I error, but it is less likely if P is smaller or, as explained above, n is larger. Type I errors occur despite the best study design. They come to light only if a study is repeated, or a follow-on study uncovers an illogicality in the chain of inference.

Type II error is a *false negative*. A difference is not found but there is one: the null hypothesis is not rejected when it should have been. The commonest cause of type II error is that n is too small. Type II error is linked with the *power* of a study, and power calculations are important in study design; the convention is that n should be large enough to give at least an 85–90% chance of finding a difference that exists. Underpowered studies risk rejecting treatments that are actually effective. Investigators need to know the variability of the data (which for normal data is the SD), to choose P and to decide what clinically important difference they are seeking. For simple, two-sample studies, n is then read from tables or nomograms. The sample will need to be larger if P is smaller, the SD is larger, or the sought difference is smaller. For a study to have 90% power at $P < 0.05$ when the sought difference is equal to the SD of the data, there should be two samples of 20. For more complicated studies, investigators should seek statistical advice.

Tests of prediction

As screening for diseases becomes more common, clinicians need to know the language of prediction. Examples from anaesthesia are the prediction of postoperative cardiac complications, and of death on the intensive care unit; a test is done or a score is applied on a sample of patients and the result is correlated with the outcome. The test may predict the outcome (true positive or true negative) or may fail to predict (false positive or false negative). There is the risk of patients testing as false positives becoming the 'worried well', who may undergo unpleasant investigations to rule out the diagnosis. Patients testing as false negatives miss out on treatment and may sue their doctors when the diagnosis becomes apparent. False positives and false negatives are inevitable in screening, although too often they are taken as evidence of faults in the screening service.

Sensitivity is the proportion of true positives correctly identified by the test, and *specificity* is the proportion of true negatives correctly identified (Table A1.3). Confusingly, specificity is also termed *selectivity*. (These are not synonymous terms for false-positive rate and false-negative rate, which are ambiguous and should be avoided.) *Positive predictive value* is the proportion of patients testing positive who are correctly diagnosed. There are no agreed 'acceptable' proportions for these indices, because they depend on the nature of the disease and the investigations or treatments made necessary by diagnosis. It is arguable that incurable diseases should not be screened for at all.

One important factor in screening is the *prevalence* of the disease in the population (cases per unit number), in other words how common the disease is (note that *incidence* is occurrence per unit number in a given time). The less common the disease, the more likely are false negatives. A test that is 95% specific (which is extremely high for any screening test) for a disease that occurs in only one person per 1000 will turn up 50 false positives if all 1000 people are screened.

Presenting the results of clinical trials

The results of most clinical trials are presented as percentage changes in outcome ('15% less vomiting with novom'). Increasingly, more clearly defined indices are presented, especially when results are pooled from single trials for *meta-analysis*, a statistical pooling technique used in *systematic review*, which is the basis of *evidence-based medicine*. There are a number of indices, and each has its place. *Absolute risk reduction* is the actual percentage change in outcome; *relative risk reduction* is the percentage change in outcome related to the prevalence or incidence of the condition. *Odds ratio* is a comparison of outcomes with two treatments, or of treatment with control, but is not an easy number for clinicians to deal with. The clearest way of presenting numerical results from a clinical trial is by *numbers-needed-to-treat* (NNT). This describes the number of

Table A1.3 Prediction and screening. A two-by-two table showing the results of a screening test, and the definitions of sensitivity and specificity (which are usually expressed as percentages)

Test says	Patient has disease		Patient does not have disease		Number of patients
'Yes, patient has disease'	True positive SENSITIVITY: proportion with disease correctly forecast	a $= a/(a + c)$	False positive	b	$= a + b$
'No, patient does not have disease'	False negative	c	True negative SPECIFICITY: proportion without disease correctly forecast	d $= d/(b + d)$	$= c + d$
		$a + c$		$b + d$	$a + b + c + d = n$

Letters a, b, c and d represent the numbers of patients in each box.

patients who have to be treated for one patient to have a favourable outcome. As with prediction, the acceptable NNT depends on the seriousness of the disease and the possible complications (and cost) of the treatment. All these indices should be presented with their confidence intervals. A good explanation of these indices, and other important aspects of the design and interpretation of clinical studies can be found at the *Bandolier* website (*http://www.jr2.ox.ac.uk/bandolier/*). For the application of the techniques of evidence-based medicine, and some of its problems, see Tramèr (2003).

INTERPRETATION OF CLINICAL TRIALS

It is unfortunately true that the standard of clinical trials (in the whole of medicine) is generally poor. A continuing problem is that many trials are too small, risking both type I and type II errors. Because investigators are understandably more enthusiastic when things go well, trials with positive results are more likely to be published than those with negative results, so-called *publication bias*. Other common problems are overcomplexity and data dredging (looking at different subgroups and with different statistical tests in an effort to find 'significant' results). Evidence-based medicine pools results from clinical trials and, if the numbers are large, the standard errors and resulting confidence limits are small. But all that does is to risk compounding the uncertainty of the poor original research.

Whatever the statistical calculations produce, only clinicians are capable of interpreting whether a treatment is worth applying: statistical significance does not of itself imply clinical significance. Always remember that statistics, unlike mathematics, cannot prove or disprove anything. All statistics do is to present probabilities, and the clinician must then decide what action to take, based on these probabilities.

FURTHER READING

Altman D G 1991 Practical statistics for medical research. Chapman & Hall, London

Browner W S 1994 A simple recipe for doing it well. Anesthesiology 80: 923

Cruikshank S 1998 Mathematics and statistics in anaesthesia. Oxford Medical Publications, Oxford

Greenhalgh T 2000 How to read a paper, 2nd edn. BMJ Publishing Group, London

Rowntree D 1991 Statistics without tears. Penguin, London

Tramèr MR (ed) 2003 Evidence-based-resource in anaesthesia and analgesia, 2nd edn. BMJ Publishing Group, London

Appendix B
Clinical data

Appendix B (Ia) Abbreviations used in text and appendices

α	adrenoceptor type (after Ahlquist)
ABO	nomenclature for blood groups (after Landsteiner)
ACD	acid citrate dextrose
ACE	angiotensin-converting enzyme
ACh	acetylcholine
ACT	activated clotting time
ACTH	adrenocorticotrophic hormone
ADH	antidiuretic hormone
ADP	adenosine diphosphate
AER	auditory evoked response
AHF	antihaemophilic factor (factor VIII)
AIDS	acquired immunodeficiency syndrome
AIP	acute intermittent porphyria
ALS	advanced life support
ALT	alanine aminotransferase
AMP	adenosine monophosphate
AMPA	γ-amino-3-hydroxy-5-methyl-4-isoxazole propionate
ANP	atrial natriuretic peptide
ANS	autonomic nervous system
APACHE	acute physiological and chronic health evaluation
APTT	activated partial thromboplastin time
ARDS	acute respiratory distress syndrome
ASA	American Society of Anesthesiologists
Asp	L-aspartate
AST	aspartate aminotransferase
AT	antithrombin
ATP	adenosine triphosphate
AUC	area under curve
AV	atrioventricular
β	adrenoceptor type (after Ahlquist)
B	bone marrow-dependent (as in B cells)
BM	Boehringer Mannheim (makers of BM Stix blood glucose testing strips)
BP	boiling point
BP	*British Pharmacopoeia*
BSA	body surface area
BW	body weight
BZ	benzodiazepine
C	cervical or coccygeal vertebra
C	compliance
C	content
°C	degrees Celsius
C_3F_8	perfluoropropane
Ca	calcium
$CaCO_3$	calcium carbonate
cAMP	cyclic adenosine monophosphate
CaO	calcium oxide
CAVG	coronary artery vein graft
CBF	cerebral blood flow
CC	closing capacity
CCT	central conduction time
CCU	coronary care unit
CDH	Christiansen Douglas Haldane (effect)
CEPOD	Confidential Enquiry into Perioperative Deaths (UK)
CFAM	cerebral function analyzing monitor
CFM	cerebral function monitor
CGRP	calcitonin gene-related peptide
CHO	carbohydrate
CI	cardiac index (cardiac output/body surface area)
CK	creatine kinase
Cl	clearance (of drug)
cm	centimetre (10^{-2} m; not a unit in the SI system)
cmH_2O	centimetres of water
$CMRO_2$	cerebral metabolic rate for oxygen
CMV	cytomegalovirus
CNS	central nervous system
C_0	concentration at time = 0
CO	cardiac output
CO_2	carbon dioxide
cp	centipoise

CPAP	continuous positive airways pressure	EF	ejection fraction
CPB	cardiopulmonary bypass	EMD	electromechanical dissociation (PEA)
CPD	citrate phosphate dextrose	EMG	electromyogram
CPD-A	citrate phosphate dextrose with adenine	EMLA®	eutectic mixture of local anaesthetic
CPK	creatine phosphokinase	EMMV	extended mandatory minute ventilation (or volume)
CPP	cerebral perfusion pressure	EMO	enzyme modified porcine (insulin)
CPPV	continuous positive pressure ventilation	EMP	Epstein and Macintosh (of Oxford)
CPR	cardiopulmonary resuscitation	ENNS	early neonatal neurobehavioural score
^{51}Cr	chromium atom – isotope weight 51 Da (radiolabelled)	ENT	ear, nose and throat
		EP	evoked potential
CRB	chain recombinant technology using bacteria (insulin)	EPI	Eysenck personality inventory
		EPP	end-plate potential
CSF	cerebrospinal fluid	ERPOC	evacuation of retained products of conception
C_{ss}	concentration at steady state		
C_t	concentration at time t	ESWL	extracorporeal shock wave lithotripsy
CT	computed tomography		
CTM	cricothyroid membrane	EUA	examination under anaesthesia
CV	closing volume	EVR	endocardial viability ratio
CVP	central venous pressure	F	Faraday's constant
C_x	clearance of x	FDP	fibrin degradation products
Δ	delta – minimal increment (of)	$Fe^{2+(3+)}$	iron ionized – ferrous (ferric) ion
δ	delta opioid receptor	FEV_1	forced expiratory volume (in 1 s)
D	dose (of drug)	FF	filtration fraction
d	density	FFA	free fatty acid
d	deci (one-tenth part)	FFP	fresh frozen plasma
Da	dalton (measure of atomic weight)	FGF	fresh gas flow
D&C	dilatation and curettage (of uterus)	F_IO_2	fractional inspired oxygen concentration
DAP	diastolic arterial pressure		
DBS	double burst stimulation	FRC	functional residual capacity
DC	direct current	FSH	follicle-stimulating hormone
DCR	dacrocystorhinostomy	FVC	forced vital capacity
DDAVP	desmopressin	g	gram
DFP	di-isopropyl fluorophosphonate	G6PD	glucose-6-phosphate dehydrogenase
DIC	disseminated intravascular coagulation		
		GABA	γ-aminobutyric acid
DNA	deoxyribonucleic acid	GFR	glomerular filtration rate
DoH	Department of Health	GH	growth hormone
Dopa	Deoxyphenylalanine	GI	gastrointestinal
2,3-DPG	2,3-diphosphoglycerate	Glu	L-glutamate
dTC	dextrotubocurarine	Gly	glycine
DVT	deep vein thrombosis	GMP	glutamate monophosphate
EC	European Community	GTN	glyceryl trinitrate
ECC	extracorporeal circulation (heart bypass)	η	viscosity
		h	hour
ECF(V)	extracellular fluid (volume)	H^+	hydrogen ion
ECG	electrocardiogram	H_1	histamine – type 1 receptor
ECM	external cardiac massage	H_2	histamine – type 2 receptor
ECT	electroconvulsive therapy	HAFOE	high air flow oxygen enrichment
EDTA	ethylenediaminetetra-acetic acid	Hb	haemoglobin
ED_x	effective dose for x% of population	HbA	adult haemoglobin
EEG	electroencephalogram	HbF	fetal haemoglobin

HbNH	carbamino haemoglobin	IVC	inferior vena cava
HBsAg	hepatitis B surface antigen	IVF	in vitro fertilization
hCG	human chorionic gonadotrophin	IVRA	intravenous regional anaesthesia
HCO_3^-	bicarbonate ion	J	joule
H_2CO_3	carbonic acid	κ	kappa – opioid receptor type
Hct	haematocrit	K	kelvin
HDU	high-dependency unit	K^+	potassium ion
He	helium	K^+_i	potassium ion (inside cell)
HFFDV	high-frequency forced diffusion ventilation	K^+_o	potassium ion (outside cell)
		KCCT	kaolin cephalin clotting time
HFJV	high-frequency jet ventilation	kg	kilogram
HFOV	high-frequency oscillatory ventilation	kPa	kilopascal
		l	length
HFPPV	high-frequency positive-pressure ventilation	L (n)	lumbar vertebra (number n)
		LAP	left atrial pressure
HFV	high-frequency ventilation	LATS	long-acting thyroid stimulator
Hg	mercury	lb in^{-2}	pounds per square inch
5-HIAA	5-hydroxyindoleacetic acid	LDH	lactate dehydrogenase
HIV	human immunodeficiency virus	LH	luteinizing hormone
HLA	human leucocyte antigen	LISS	low ionic strength saline
HOCM	hypertrophic obstructive cardiomyopathy	lm	lumen
		LMA	laryngeal mask airway
HPA	hypothalamopituitary axis	LMN	lower motor neuron
hPL	human placental lactogen	ln	natural logarithm (to base e)
HPV	hypoxic pulmonary vasoconstriction	log	logarithm (to base 10)
		LOS	lower oesophageal sphincter
HR	heart rate	LSCS	lower-segment caesarean section
5-HT	5-hydroxytryptamine (serotonin)	LVEDP	left ventricular end-diastolic pressure
HTLV	human T cell leukaemia virus		
Hz	hertz (cycles per second)	μ	micro (10^{-6}); mu opioid receptor type
I	infusion rate		
IABP	intra-aortic balloon pump	μV	microvolts
ICF(V)	intracellular fluid (volume)	m	metre
ICP	isometric contraction period; intracranial pressure	mA	milliampere
		MAC	minimum alveolar concentration (for anaesthesia)
ID	internal diameter		
I/E	inspiratory/expiratory	MAO	monoamine oxidase
IgA	immunoglobulin type A (γ-globulin A)	MAOI	monoamine oxidase inhibitor
		MAP	mean arterial pressure
IgE	immunoglobulin type E (γ-globulin E, reagin)	MC	Mary Caterill (name of proprietary mask)
IgG	immunoglobulin type G (γ-globulin G)	MC	monocomponent – 'free of impurities' (as in insulin)
ILM	intubating laryngeal mask (airway)	MCV	mean corpuscular volume
i.m.	intramuscular	MEAC	minimum effective analgesic concentration
IMV	intermittent mandatory ventilation		
INR	international normalized ratio	MEPP	miniature end-plate potential
IOP	intraocular pressure	mg	milligram
IPPV	intermittent positive-pressure ventilation	Mg^{2+}	magnesium ion
		MH	malignant hyperthermia
IRP	isometric relaxation period	MI	myocardial infarction
ISA	intrinsic sympathomimetic activity	min	minute
ITU	intensive therapy unit	mL	millilitre
i.v.	intravenous	mm	millimetre

mmHg	millimetres of mercury	P_{BC}	hydrostatic pressure in Bowman's capsule
MMPI	Minnesota multiphasic personality inventory	PCA	patient-controlled analgesia
MMV	mandatory minute ventilation	P_{CAP}	hydrostatic pressure in capillary
mN	millinewton	PCWP	pulmonary capillary wedge pressure
mol	mole		
mosmol	milliosmole	PDPH	post-dural puncture headache
MRI	magnetic resonance imaging	PE	pulmonary embolus
ms	millisecond	$P_{\bar{E}}$	mean expired partial pressure
MSH	melanocyte-stimulating hormone	$P_{E'}$	end-expired partial pressure
mV	millivolt	PEA	pulseless electrical activity (EMD)
MVP	mean venous pressure	PEEP	positive end-expiratory pressure
MW	molecular weight	PEFR	peak expiratory flow rate
N	newton (unit of force)	PF	pathological fibrinolysis
N/A	not available; not applicable	PG(X)	prostaglandin type (X)
Na	sodium	pH	hydrogen ion activity (negative logarithm to base 10 of the measured hydrogen ion concentration)
Na^+	sodium ion		
NACS	neurological & adaptive capacity score		
Na/K-ATPase	sodium- and potassium-dependent adenosine triphosphatase	P_I	inspired partial pressure
		PIFR	peak inspiratory flow rate
NEEP	negative end-expiratory pressure	pK_a	expression of dissociation constant in an equilibrium (negative logarithm to base 10 of the dissociation constant)
NH_3	ammonia		
NH_4^+	ammonium ion		
NHS	National Health Service (UK)		
NMDA	N-methyl-D-aspartate	PMGV	piped medical gases and vacuum systems
NMR	nuclear magnetic resonance		
NO	nitric oxide	PONV	postoperative nausea and vomiting
N_2O	nitrous oxide	ppm	parts per million
NSAID	non-steroidal anti-inflammatory drug	PRN	pro re nata (as needed)
		PRP	platelet-rich plasma
NTD	neural tube defect	PTA	plasma thromboplastin antecedent (factor IX)
O_2	oxygen		
ODC	oxyhaemoglobin dissociation curve	PTF	post-tetanic facilitation
ODP	operating department practitioner	PTP	post-tetanic potentiation
osmol	osmole	P_tCO_2	transcutaneous oxygen partial pressure
π	pi (= 3.14159)		
π_{BC}	oncotic pressure in Bowman's capsule	PTT(K)	partial thromboplastin time (kaolin)
		PVC	polyvinyl chloride; premature ventricular contraction
π_{CAP}	oncotic pressure in capillary		
P	electrocardiographic nomenclature	PVR	pulmonary vascular resistance
P_{50}	oxygen tension which results in a haemoglobin saturation of 50%	$\dot{Q}_t$	total liquid flow in unit time
		QRS	electrocardiographic nomenclature
Pa	pascal (unit of pressure)	ρ	rho (= density)
P_A	alveolar partial pressure (of gas)	r	radius (of circle or sphere)
P_a	arterial partial pressure (of gas)	R	universal gas constant
PAFC	pulmonary artery flotation catheter	RA_x	renal artery concentration of x
PAH	*para*-aminohippuric acid	RAP	right atrial pressure
PAP	pulmonary artery pressure	RAST	radioallergosorbent test
PAOP	pulmonary artery occlusion pressure (= PCWP)	RBF	renal blood flow
		RDS	respiratory distress syndrome
		Re	Reynolds number (dimensionless)
P_B	barometric pressure	REM	rapid eye movement
		RH	relative humidity

Rh(x)	Rhesus blood group (major phenotype x)	TBG	thyroxine-binding globulin
		TBW	total body water
RLF	retrolental fibroplasia	TEC®	temperature controlled (vaporizer)
RNA	ribonucleic acid	TENS	transcutaneous electrical nerve stimulation
RPF	renal plasma flow		
RPP	rate–pressure product	TEPP	tetraethyl pyrophosphate
RQ	respiratory quotient	TFA	trifluoroacetyl
RSD	reflex sympathetic dystrophy	TISS	therapeutic intervention severity score
RV	residual volume		
RV_x	renal vein concentration of x	TIVA	total intravenous anaesthesia
s	second	TLA	translumbar aortography
S	saturation (of haemoglobin)	TLC	total lung capacity
SA	sinoatrial	Tm	tubular maximal reabsorption
SAB	subarachnoid block	TMJ	temporomandibular joint
SAGM	saline adenine glucose mannitol	TMP	trimetaphan camsylate
SAP	systolic arterial pressure	TNS	transcutaneous nerve stimulation
s.c.	subcutaneous	TOF	train of four
SDP	subdural pressure	TPR	total (systemic) peripheral resistance
SF_6	sulphur hexafluoride	TSH	thyroid-stimulating hormone
SG	specific gravity	TURP	transurethral resection of prostate
SH	sulphydryl group	TWC	total water content
SI	*Système International d'Unités*	TXA_2	thromboxane A_2
SIADHS	syndrome of inappropriate antidiuretic hormone secretion	U	urine concentration
		UK	United Kingdom
SIIFT	syndrome of inappropriate intravenous fluid therapy	URT(I)	upper respiratory tract (infection)
		USA	United States of America
SIMV	synchronized intermittent mandatory ventilation	V	volt
		V	volume
SNP	sodium nitroprusside	$\dot{V}_t$	volume per unit time (gas flow)
SOL	space-occupying lesion	v	velocity
SR	slow release	V4R	mobile chest lead in electrocardiography (position 4 reversed)
SRS-A	slow-reacting substance of anaphylaxis		
SSRI	selective serotonin reuptake inhibitor	VC	vital capacity
		V_d	dead space (ventilation); volume of distribution
STOP	surgical termination of pregnancy		
STP	standard temperature and pressure	$V_{d(ANAT)}$	anatomical dead space
		$V_{d(PHYS)}$	physiological dead space
SV	stroke volume	VF	ventricular fibrillation
SVC	superior vena cava	VFP	ventricular fluid pressure
SVP	saturated vapour pressure	VIC	vaporizer in circuit
SVT	supraventricular tachycardia	VIE	vacuum insulated evaporator
T	thymus-dependent (T cells)	VIP	vasoactive intestinal peptide
T	temperature	VOC	vaporizer out of circuit
$t_{1/2\alpha}$	α half-life (distribution half-life)	VT	ventricular tachycardia
$t_{1/2\beta}$	β half-life (elimination half-life)	V_t	tidal volume
T_3	tri-iodothyronine	vWF	von Willebrand factor
T_4	thyroxine	W	watt
TA	titratable acid		

Appendix B (Ib)
SI system

The **Système International d'Unités** (SI system) has been developed to reduce the large number of units in everyday physical use to a much smaller number, with standard symbols.

The seven base units are derivatives of the MKS system of physical measurement:

Length	metre	m
Mass	kilogram	kg
Time	second	s
Electric current	amp	A
Thermodynamic temperature	kelvin	K
Amount of substance	mole	mol
Luminous intensity	candela	cd

Any other units are derived units and may be expressed by multiplication or division of base units:

Volume   cubic metre m^3

Force newton N $kg\,m\,s^{-2}$ = $J\,m^{-1}$ (J/m)

Work joule J $kg\,m^2\,s^{-2}$ = $N\,m$

Power (rate of work) watt W $kg\,m^2\,s^{-3}$ = $J\,s^{-1}$ (J/s)

Pressure (force/area) pascal Pa $kg\,m^{-1}\,s^{-2}$ = $N\,m^{-2}$ (N/m²)

X^{-1} has been used in preference to the solidus (/), either of which is specified in the standard.

Non-standard units such as the litre (L), day, hour and minute may be used with SI but are not part of the standard.

VOLUME

The SI unit of volume is the cubic metre, but for medical purposes the litre (L or dm^3) is retained.

TEMPERATURE

A temperature difference of 1 kelvin (1 K) is numerically equivalent to 1 degree Celsius (1°C). In everyday use the degree Celsius is retained. The Fahrenheit scale is no longer used medically. It is being phased out of use with the general public.

Fraction	SI prefix	Symbol	Multiple	SI prefix	Symbol
10^{-1}	deci	d	10	deca	da
10^{-2}	centi	c	10^2	hecto	h
10^{-3}	milli	m	10^3	kilo	k
10^{-6}	micro	μ	10^6	mega	M
10^{-9}	nano	n	10^9	giga	G
10^{-12}	pico	p	10^{12}	tera	T
10^{-15}	femto	f			
10^{-18}	atto	a			

The magnitude of a unit is expressed by the addition of standard prefixes and symbolic prefixes. The magnitude of SI units usually changes by 10^3 per step.

It can be seen that the SI handling of 'kilogram' is non-standard; the name of the base unit already contains a preficacial multiple. Names of decimal multiples and submultiples of the unit of mass are formed by attaching prefixes to the word 'gram'.

PRESSURE MEASUREMENTS – CONVERSION FACTORS

Old units	SI units	Old to SI (conversion factor)	SI to old (conversion factor)
mmHg	kPa	0.133	7.5
bar	kPa	101.3	0.01
cmH_2O	kPa	0.0981	10
lb/sq in	kPa	6.894	0.145

MOLES

Moles = weight in g / molecular weight
Thus 1 mol H_2O = 18 g / 18
18g H_2O = 1 mol

For univalent ions, moles and equivalents are numerically equal, but for multivalent ions the number of equivalents must be divided by the valency to obtain the molar value. Thus 10 mEq Ca^{2+} = 5 mmol Ca^{2+}.

MOLES/OSMOLES

Strictly, the SI unit of osmolality should be the mole, this representing the calculated number of particles/molecules in solution. However, the osmole is also used; this is the measured osmolality (the number of osmotically active particles per kilogram of solution). Thus, the molar value for osmolality is theoretical, while the osmolar value is empirical.

Appendix B (II)
Inhalational anaesthetic agents – physical properties

Name	Formula	MW (Da)	BP (°C)	SVP (kPa, 20°C)	MAC (%)	Flammable in O_2	Ostwald solubility coefficients at 37°C			
							Blood/ gas	Fat/ blood	Oil/ gas	Oil/ H_2O
Nitrous oxide	N_2O	44	−88	(5300)	105	0	0.47	2.3	1.4	3.2
Halothane	$CF_3CHClBr$	197	50	32	0.75		2.5	51	224	220
Enflurane	$CHFClCF_2OCF_2H$	184.5	56	23	1.7	6	1.9	36	98	120
Isoflurane	$CF_3CHClOCF_2H$	184.5	49	32	1.15	6	1.4	45	91	174
Desflurane	$CF_2HOCFHCF_3$	168	23.5	89	7.3	18–21	0.42	27	18.7	
Sevoflurane	$CH(CF_3)_2OCH_2F$	200	58.5	21	2.0		0.59	48	54	
Chloroform	$CHCl_3$	119	61	21.3	0.5		10		260	100
Cyclopropane	$CH_2CH_2CH_2$	42	−33	638	9.2	2–60	0.45		11.5	34.4
Diethyl ether	$C_2H_5OC_2H_5$	74	35	56.5	1.9	2–82	12	5	62	3.2
Ethyl chloride	C_2H_5Cl	64.5	13	131	2.0	4–67	3.0			
Fluroxene	$CF_3CH_2OCHCH_2$	126	43	38	3.5	4	1.4		48	90
Methoxyflurane	$CHCl_2CF_2OCH_3$	165	105	3	0.2	5–28	13	38	950	400
Trichloroethylene	$CHClCCl_2$	131	87	8	0.17	9–65	9		960	400

MW, molecular weight; BP, boiling point; SVP, saturated vapour pressure; MAC, minimum alveolar concentration.
Drugs listed below the bold line have no product licence in the UK. They are of historical interest only. MAC values are for young adults; MAC is higher in children, and decreases in older adults.

Appendix B (III)
Cardiovascular system

Appendix III: Cardiovascular system

Blood flows	Normal values	
	% of cardiac output	Flow (mL min⁻¹) (70 kg man)
Heart	4	200
Brain	14	700
Liver	25	1250
Kidneys	24	1200
Lung	3	150
Muscle	19	950
Skin	5	250
Fat	5	250
Remainder	1	50
Total	**100**	**5000**

ECG times	
P wave	< 0.10 s
PR interval	0.12–0.20 s
QRS time	0.05–0.08 s
QT time	0.35–0.40 s
T wave	< 0.22 s

	Pressures (mmHg)	
	Range	Mean
Central venous pressure (CVP)	0–8	4
Right atrial (RA)	0–8	4
Right ventricular (RV)		
Systolic	14–30	25
End-diastolic (RVEDP)	0–8	4
Pulmonary arterial (PA)		
Systolic	15–30	23
Diastolic	5–15	8
Mean (PAP)	10–20	15
Pulmonary artery wedge (PAWP)		
Mean	5–15	10
Left atrial (LA)	4–12	7
Left ventricular (LV)		
Systolic	90–140	120
End-diastolic (LVEDP)	4–12	7

Derived haemodynamic variables

Variable		Typical value (70 kg)
Cardiac output (CO)	$SV \times HR$	$5\,L\,min^{-1}$
Cardiac index (CI)	$CO \div BSA$	$3.2\,L\,min^{-1}\,m^{-2}$
Stroke volume (SV)	$(CO \div HR) \times 1000$	$80\,mL$
Stroke index (SI)	$SV \div BSA$	$50\,mL\,m^{-2}$
Systemic vascular resistance (SVR)	$((MAP - CVP) \div CO) \times 80$	$1000{-}1200\,dyn\,s\,cm^{-5}$ (not SI unit)
Pulmonary vascular resistance (PVR)	$((\overline{PAP} - LAP) \div CO) \times 80$	$60{-}120\,dyn\,s\,cm^{-5}$ (not SI unit)
Left ventricular stroke work index (LVSWI)	$((1.36\,(MAP - LAP)) \div 100) \times SI$	$50{-}60\,g\,m\,m^{-2}$
Rate–pressure product (RPP)	$SAP \times HR$	9600
Ejection fraction (EF)	$(ESV - EDV) \div EDV$	> 0.6

BSA, body surface area; HR, heart rate; MAP, mean arterial pressure; CVP, central venous pressure; $\overline{PAP}$, mean pulmonary arterial pressure; LAP, left atrial pressure; SAP, systolic arterial pressure; ESV, end-systolic volume; EDV, end-diastolic volume.

Vasoactive infusion regimens

Drug	Diluent	Dilution	Concentration	Infusion rate	Typical initial rate (70 kg adult)
Amiodarone	5% dextrose	300 mg in 50 mL	$6\,mg\,mL^{-1}$	Loading dose $5\,mg\,kg^{-1}$ over 1 h then 900 mg over 23 h	$25\,mL\,h^{-1}$ then $6\,mL\,h^{-1}$
Digoxin	5% dextrose 0.9% saline	250 μg in 50 mL 500 μg in 50 mL	$5\,\mu g\,mL^{-1}$ $10\,\mu g\,mL^{-1}$	250–500 μg over 30–60 min	$50\,mL\,h^{-1}$
Dobutamine	5% dextrose 0.9% saline	250 mg in 50 mL	$5\,mg\,mL^{-1}$	$0{-}25\,\mu g\,kg^{-1}\,min^{-1}$	$2\,mL\,h^{-1}$
Dopamine	5% dextrose 0.9% saline	200 mg in 50 mL	$4\,mg\,mL^{-1}$	$2{-}15\,\mu g\,kg^{-1}\,min^{-1}$	$2\,mL\,h^{-1}$
Dopexamine	5% dextrose 0.9% saline	50 mg in 50 mL	$1\,mg\,mL^{-1}$	$0.5{-}6\,\mu g\,kg^{-1}\,min^{-1}$	$2\,mL\,h^{-1}$
Epinephrine	5% dextrose 0.9% saline	5 mg in 50 mL 10 mg in 50 mL	$100\,\mu g\,mL^{-1}$ $200\,\mu g\,mL^{-1}$	$0.02{-}0.2\,\mu g\,kg^{-1}\,min^{-1}$	$5\,mL\,h^{-1}$
Enoximone	0.9% saline	100 mg in 50 mL	$2\,mg\,mL^{-1}$	$90\,\mu g\,kg^{-1}\,min^{-1}$ for 10–30 min then $5{-}20\,\mu g\,kg^{-1}\,min^{-1}$	$189\,mL\,h^{-1}$ for 10–30 min then $10\,mL\,h^{-1}$
Esmolol	5% dextrose 0.9% saline	2.5 g in 50 mL	$50\,mg\,mL^{-1}$	$50{-}200\,\mu g\,kg^{-1}\,min^{-1}$	$3\,mL\,h^{-1}$

Continued

Vasoactive infusion regimens—Cont'd

Drug	Diluent	Dilution	Concentration	Infusion rate	Typical initial rate (70 kg adult)
Glyceryl trinitrate	5% dextrose 0.9% saline	50 mg in 50 mL	1 mg mL^{-1}	0.5–12 mg h^{-1}	5 mL h^{-1}
Isoprenaline	5% dextrose D. saline	1 mg in 50 mL	20 μg mL^{-1}	0.5–10 μg min^{-1}	7 mL h^{-1}
Lidocaine	0.9% saline	500 mg in 50 mL	10 mg mL^{-1}	4 mg min^{-1} for 30 min, 2 mg min^{-1} for 2 h, then 1 mg min^{-1} for 24 h	24 mL h^{-1}
Norepinephrine	5% dextrose 0.9% saline	4 mg in 40 mL 8 mg in 40 mL	100 μg mL^{-1} 200 μg mL^{-1}	0.04–0.4 μg kg^{-1} min^{-1}	5 mL h^{-1}
Milrinone	5% dextrose 0.9% saline	10 mg in 50 mL	0.2 mg mL^{-1}	50 μg kg^{-1} min^{-1} over 10 min then 0.375–0.75 μg kg^{-1} min^{-1}	105 mL h^{-1} for 10 min then 7 mL h^{-1}
Sodium nitroprusside	5% dextrose	25 mg in 50 mL	500 μg mL^{-1}	0.3–1.5 μg kg^{-1} min^{-1}	7 mL h^{-1}

Appendix B (IVa)
Chemical pathology – biochemical values

These values are given for example only – each reporting laboratory provides reference values for its own population and method. This is especially true of enzyme assays. Values given are those obtained from Chemical Pathology in Warwick, where these are available. No inference should be made about the molecular weight of a substance by reference to US and SI values.

Name	US units	SI units
Amino acid nitrogen	4–8 mg%	3–6 mmol L^{-1}
Ammonia	80–110 µg%	<50 µmol L^{-1}
Amylase	80–180 Somogyi units%	70–300 IU L^{-1}
Base excess	± 2 mEq L^{-1}	± 2 mmol L^{-}
Bicarbonate		
Actual	22–30 mEq L^{-1}	22–30 mmol L^{-1}
Standard	21–25 mEq L^{-1}	21–25 mmol L^{-1}
Bilirubin – total	0.3–1.1 mg%	3–18 µmol L^{-1}
Buffer base (pH 7.4, P_aCO_2 5.3, Hb 15 g dL^{-1})	48 mEq L^{-1}	48 mmol L^{-1}
Calcium		
Total	8.5–10.5 mg% (4.5–5.7 mEq L^{-1})	2.25–2.6 mmol L^{-1}
Ionized	4–5 mg%	1.0–1.25 mmol L^{-1}
Chloride	95–105 mEq L^{-1}	95–105 mmol L^{-1}
Cholesterol	140–300 mg%	3.6–7.8 mmol L^{-1}
Cholinesterase, plasma (pseudocholinesterase)	Dibucaine number >80% usually normal	
	Dibucaine number <20% usually homozygote for atypical cholinesterase	
Copper	80–150 µg%	13–24 nmol L^{-1}
Urinary copper	15–50 µg per 24 h	0.2–0.8 µmol per 24 h

Continued

Name	US units	SI units
Cortisol 0900 h radioimmunoassay	9–23 µg L^{-1}	250–635 nmol L^{-1}
2400 h technique	<7.2 µg%	< 200 nmol L^{-1}
Neonatal (competitive protein-binding technique)	30 µg L^{-1}	200–650 nmol L^{-1}
		< 200 nmol L^{-1}
		330–1700 nmol L^{-1}
Creatine (phospho)kinase (CK)	100 IU L^{-1}– male	25–200 IU L^{-1}
	60 IU L^{-1} – female	25–150 IU L^{-1}
Creatinine	0.5–1.4 mg%	45–120 µmol L^{-1}
Epinephrine	100 pg mL^{-1}	0.55 nmol L^{-1}
Fibrinogen	150–400 mg%	1.5–4.0 g L^{-1}
Folate	3–20 ng mL^{-1}	3–20 µg L^{-1}
		2.1–27 nmol L^{-1}
Glucose		
Fasting	55–85 mg%	4–6 mmol L^{-1}
Postprandial	<180 mg%	<10 mmol L^{-1}
γ-Glutamyl transpeptidase	7–25 IU L^{-1}	male: <50 IU L^{-1}
		female: <30 IU L^{-1}
Hydroxybutyrate dehydrogenase (HBD)		100–240 IU L^{-1}
Iodine – total	3.5–8.0 µg L^{-1}	273–624 nmol L^{-1}
^{131}I uptake	20–50% of administered dose in 24 h	
Iron	80–160 µg%	14–30 µmol L^{-1}
Iron-binding capacity	250–400 µg%	45–69 µmol L^{-1}
Lactate	0.6–1.8 mEq L^{-1}	0.6–1.8 mmol L^{-1}
Lactate dehydrogenase	30–90 IU L^{-1}	100–300 IU L^{-1}
Lead		<1.8 µmol L^{-1}
Magnesium	1–2 mg%	
	1.5–2.0 mEq L^{-1}	0.7–1.0 mmol L^{-1}
Methaemoglobin	<3% of total haemoglobin	
Nitrogen (non-protein) (urea + urate + creatinine + creatine)	18–30 mg%	12.8–21.4 mmol L^{-1}
Norepinephrine	200 pg mL^{-1}	1.25 nmol L^{-1}
Osmolality	280–300 mosmol kg^{-1}	280–300 mmol kg^{-1}

Name	US units	SI units
Phosphate	2.0–4.5 mg%	0.8–1.4 mmol L^{-1}
	3.0–6.0 mg% (children)	1.0–1.8 mmol L^{-1} (children)
	<8.1 mg% (neonatal)	<2.6 mmol L^{-1} (neonatal)
Phosphatase		
Acid (total)	1–5 KA units%	1–9 IU L^{-1}
Acid (prostatic)		0–3 IU L^{-1}
Alkaline	3–13 KA units%	17–100 IU L^{-1}
Potassium	3.4–5.3 mEq L^{-1}	3.4–5.3 mmol L^{-1}
Protein		
Total	6.0–8.0 g%	60–80 g L^{-1}
Albumin	3.5–5.0 g%	35–50 g L^{-1}
Globulin	1.5–3.0 g%	15–30 g L^{-1}
Pyruvate	0.4–0.7 mg%	34–80 µmol L^{-1}
Sodium	133–148 mEq L^{-1}	133–148 mmol L^{-1}
Thyroxine (T$_4$)	4.7–11 µg%	52–140 nmol L^{-1}
Transaminase		
aspartate transaminase (AST)	5–40 unit mL^{-1}	5–40 IU L^{-1}
alanine transaminase (ALT)		2–53 IU L^{-1}
Transferrin	220–400 mg%	2.2–4.0 g L^{-1}
Triglycerides (fasting)	71–160 mg%	0.8–1.8 mmol L^{-1}
Tri-iodothyronine (T$_3$)	90–170 ng%	0.8–2.5 nmol L^{-1}
T$_3$ uptake	95–117%	95–117%
Urea	15–48 mg%	2.5–8.0 mmol L^{-1}
Urea nitrogen (BUN)	10–20 mg%	7.1–14.3 mmol L^{-1}
Urate		
Men	4–9.5 mg%	225–470 µmol L^{-1}
Women	3–7.5 mg%	180–390 µmol L^{-1}

Appendix B (IVb)
Conversion chart – hydrogen ion concentration to pH

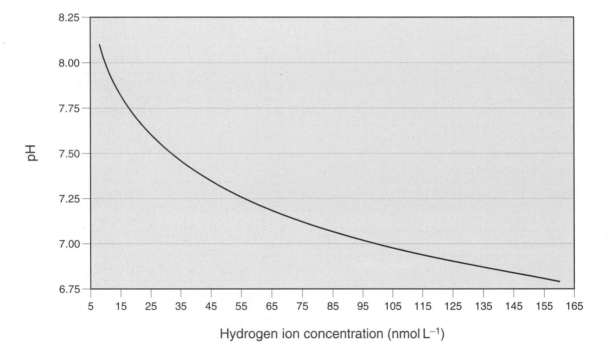

Appendix B (V)
Haematology

Normal values

Haemoglobin
Men	13.5–18.0 g dL^{-1}
Women	11.5–16.5 g dL^{-1}
10–12 years	11.5–14.8 g dL^{-1}
1 year	11.0–13.0 g dL^{-1}
3 months	9.5–12.5 g dL^{-1}
Full term	13.6–19.6 g dl^{-1}

Red blood cell count (RBC)
Men	4.5–6.0 × 10^{12} L^{-1}
Women	3.5–5.0 × 10^{12} L^{-1}

White blood cell count (WBC) 4.0–11.0 × 10^9 L^{-1}
Neutrophils	40–70%
Lymphocytes	20–45%
Monocytes	2–10%
Eosinophils	1–6%
Basophils	0–1%

Platelet count 150–400 × 10^9 L^{-1}

Reticulocyte count 0–2% of RBC

Sedimentation rate
Men	0–15 mm in 1 h
Women	0–20 mm in 1 h

Plasma viscosity 1.50–1.72 mPa s

Packed cell volume (PCV) and haematocrit (Hct)
Men	0.4–0.55
Women	0.36–0.47

Mean corpuscular volume (MCV) 76–96 fL

Mean corpuscular haemoglobin concentration (MCHC) 31–35 g dL^{-1}

Mean corpuscular haemoglobin (MCH) 27–32 pg

Coagulation tests

Activated clotting time (ACT; Haemochron type)	80–135 s
Antithrombin III	>80% normal
Bleeding time (platelet function)	2–9 min
Clotting time (largely replaced by ACT)	2–9 min
D dimers	<0.3 mg L^{-1}
Fibrinogen – plasma	1.5–4 g L^{-1}

INR (international normalized ratio warfarin therapy value)
Therapeutic range for:
Atrial fibrillation, deep venous thrombosis, pulmonary embolism, tissue heart valves	2–3
Mechanical heart valve	3–4.5

KCCT (also known as PTTK, APTT)	33–41 s
Heparin therapy value	1.5–2.5 × normal
If pregnant	1.5–2.0 × normal
Platelet count	150–400 × 10^9 L^{-1}
Prothrombin time	12–14 s
Thrombin time	circa 15 s

KCCT, kaolin cephalin clotting time; PTTK, partial thromboplastin time, kaolin; APTT, activated partial thromboplastin time.

Coagulation screen

What to check?

- Prothrombin time (PT)

- Kaolin cephalin clotting time (KCCT)

- Thrombin time (TT)

- Fibrinogen

- Platelet count

If all are normal, consider checking bleeding time and, in neonates, factor XIII concentration.

When to check?

Elective patient

- With suspicious history (bleeding after cuts, previous surgery or dental extractions, easy bruising)

- With family history of bleeding problems

- Receiving anticoagulants – warfarin, heparin or aspirin, for example

- With intercurrent illness such as obstructive jaundice, liver disease, uraemia or leukaemia

Emergency or intraoperative patient

With excessive bleeding despite apparent vascular integrity.

What to do?

Possible cause	Treatment
PT and KCCT prolonged	
Drug effect (warfarin/coumarin)	Vitamin K, FFP, coagulation concentrates
Obstructive jaundice	Vitamin K, FFP
Liver disease	Vitamin K, FFP
Haemorrhagic disease of the newborn	Vitamin K
Factor II, V, X deficiency	FFP, coagulation concentrates
If TT is also prolonged	
Fibrinogen deficiency	Cryoprecipitate, FFP
Are D-dimers increased?	
Disseminated intravascular coagulation (DIC)	Treat cause, FFP, platelets, ? antithrombin III concentrate

What to do?—Cont'd

Possible cause	Treatment
Is KCCT prolonged?	
Heparin therapy	Stop therapy, ? reverse effect with protamine
Factor VIII deficiency – haemophilia	Factor VIII concentrate: high purity
Von Willebrand's disease	Vasopressin, factor VIII concentrate: intermediate purity
Factor IX deficiency	Factor IX concentrate
Factor XI or XII deficiency	FFP
Is PT prolonged (with normal KCCT)?	
Factor VII deficiency	FFP, factor VII concentrate
Is platelet count decreased (< 100 × 10⁹ L⁻¹)?	
Peripheral destruction	
? Immune-mediated	Steroids
? DIC	Treat cause
? TTP or HUS	Platelets, FFP, ? antithrombin III concentrate, plasma exchange
Inadequate production	
Marrow failure	Platelets
Is bleeding time prolonged?	
Von Willebrand's disease	Factor VIII concentrate: intermediate purity, vasopressin
Functional platelet disorder	
Inherited	Platelets
Acquired	Platelets
Uraemia	Dialysis/haemofiltration, cryoprecipitate
Drugs	

Always consult haematology colleague when uncertain.
FFP, fresh frozen plasma; TTP, thrombotic thrombocytopenic purpura, HUS, haemolytic uraemic syndrome.

Appendix B (VI)
Fluid balance

Fluid composition of body compartments

	Typical blood volume
Infant	90 mL kg^{-1}
Child	80 mL kg^{-1}
Adult male	70 mL kg^{-1}
Adult female	60 mL kg^{-1}
Total water content (TWC)	
60% male (55% female) of body weight (18–40 years)	
55% male (46% female) of body weight (> 60 years)	
Volume of extracellular fluid 35% TWC	
Volume of intracellular fluid 65% TWC	

Intraoperative fluid requirement – adult

(1) Initial volume	1.5 mL kg^{-1} h^{-1} for duration of preoperative starvation
+ (2) Maintenance	1.5 mL kg^{-1} h^{-1}
+ (3) Operative insensible loss	e.g. 1–2 L for abdominal surgery
+ (4) Blood loss	Replace with blood when loss exceeds 20% of estimated blood volume or Hb < 8g dL^{-1}

Fluid, electrolyte and nutritional requirements

Minimum daily requirements per kilogram for adults, and children and infants. (Neonates see Appendix IXb)

	Adults (per kg)	Children and infants (per kg)
Water	30–45 mL	100–150 mL
Energy	30–50 kcal (0.15–0.21 MJ)	90–125 kcal (0.38–0.5 MJ)
Protein	0.7–1.0 g	2.2–2.5 g
Na$^+$	1–1.4 mmol	1–2.5 mmol
K$^+$	0.7–0.9 mmol	2 mmol
Ca^{2+}	0.11 mmol	0.5–1 mmol
Mg^{2+}	0.04 mmol	0.15 mmol
Fe^{2+}	1 µmol	2 µmol
Mn^{2+}	0.1 µmol	0.3 µmol
Zn^{2+}	0.7 µmol	1.0 µmol
Cu$^+$	0.07 µmol	0.3 µmol
Cl$^-$	1.3–1.9 mmol	1.8–4.3 mmol

Composition of common intravenous fluids

Name	pH	Calculated[a] osmolality	Ions (mmol L⁻¹)					CHO (g L⁻¹)	Protein (g L⁻¹)	MJ L⁻¹
			Na⁺	K⁺	Cl⁻	HCO₃⁻¹	Misc.			
Crystalloids										
Sodium chloride 0.9%	5.0	308	154	0	154	0	0	0	0	0
Glucose 5%	4.0	280	0	0	0	0	0	50	0	0.84
Glucose 4% + saline 0.18%	4.5	286	31	0	31	0	0	40	0	0.67
Glucose 5% + saline 0.45%	4.5	430	77	0	77	0	0	50	0	0.84
Lactated Ringer's (Hartmann's solution)	6.5	280	131	5	112	29 (as lact.)	Mg^{2+} 1 Ca^{2+} 1	0	0	0.038
Sodium bicarbonate 8.4%	8.0	2000	1000	0	0	1000	0	0	0	0

[a] Calculated value, assuming total dissociation of ions.

Name	pH	Oncotic pressure (mmH₂O)	Ionic content (mmol L⁻¹)				CHO (g L⁻¹)	Protein (g L⁻¹)	MJ L⁻¹	Typical half-life in plasma
			Na⁺	K⁺	Cl⁻	Misc.				
Colloids										
Gelatin (succinylated, Haemaccel)	7.4	370	145	5.1	145	Ca^{2+} 6.25 PO_4^{2-} trace SO_4^{2-} trace	0	35	0	5 h
Gelatin (polygeline, Gelofusine)	7.4	465	154	0.4	125	Ca^{2+} 0.4 Mg^{2+} 0.4	0	40	0	4 h
Dextran 70 in sodium chloride 0.9%	4–7	268	154	0	154	0	0	0	0	12 h
Dextran 70 in glucose 5%	3.5–7	268	0	0	0	0	50	0	0.84	12 h
Hetastarch (Hespan)	5.5	310	154	0	154	0	0	0	0	17 day
Pentastarch (Pentaspan)	5.0	320	154	0	154	0	0	0	0	18 h

Continued

Composition of common intravenous fluids — Cont'd

| Name | pH | Oncotic pressure (mmH$_2$O) | Ionic content (mmol L^{-1}) | | | |
			Na$^+$	K$^+$	Cl$^-$	Misc.
Blood products						
Human albumin solution (PPF 4%) (20% salt-poor solution also available – ionic content varies with manufacturer)	7.4	275	150	2	120	
Whole blood	> 6.5	Na$^+$ depends on donor values. K$^+$ increases with storage time				
Plasma-reduced blood	> 6.5	Na$^+$ depends on donor value. K$^+$ higher than in whole blood, but total quantity *per unit* is similar				
SAGM blood	> 6.5		150		150	Adenine 0.6%, glucose 2.6%, mannitol 1.6%
Accepted safe storage times at 4°C						
Heparinized blood	Only available for special applications					
Acid citrate dextrose	21 days					
Citrate phosphate dextrose	28 days					
Citrate phosphate dextrose adenine	35 days					
SAGM	35 days					

PPF, plasma protein fraction; SAGM, saline adenine glucose mannitol.

Appendix B (VII)
Renal function tests

Renal function tests

Clearance tests

Inulin clearance ≅ glomerular filtration	100–150 mL min^{-1}
Para-aminohippuric acid clearance ≅ renal plasma flow	560–830 mL min^{-1}
Creatinine clearance ≅ glomerular filtration rate (overestimates low glomerular filtration rate)	104–125 mL min^{-1}

Blood tests

Serum/plasma

Osmolality	280–300 mosmol kg^{-1}
Creatinine	45–120 µmol L^{-1}
Urea	2.7–7.0 mmol L^{-1}
Urea nitrogen	1.6–3.3 mmol L^{-1}

Urine tests

Osmolality	300–1200 mosmol kg^{-1}
Creatinine	8.85–17.7 mmol per 24 h
Sodium	50–200 mmol per 24 h

Comparative urinary values

	SG	Osmolality	U/P urea ratio	U/P osmolality
Normal	1000–1040	300–1200	>20:1	>2.0:1
Prerenal failure	>1022	>400	>20:1	>2.0:1
Renal failure				
Early	1010	<350	<14:1	<1.7:1
Late			<5:1	<1.1:1

SG, specific gravity; U, urine; P, plasma.

Appendix B (VIII)
Pulmonary function tests

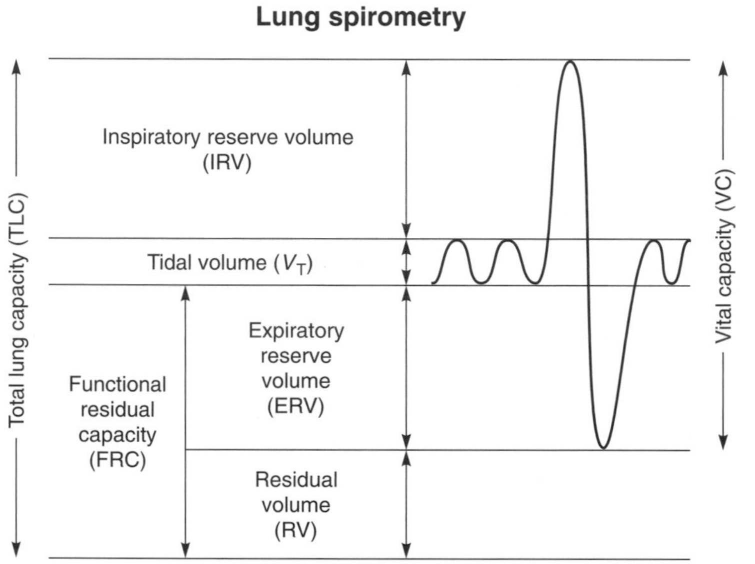

Lung spirometry

Inspiratory reserve volume (IRV)

Tidal volume (V_T)

Expiratory reserve volume (ERV)

Functional residual capacity (FRC)

Residual volume (RV)

Total lung capacity (TLC)

Vital capacity (VC)

Volumes (mL) in 60kg male

V_T	400–600
IRV	3300–3750
ERV	950–1200
FRC	2300–2600
RV	1200–1700
VC	3800–5000
TLC	5000–6500

Fig. VIII
Lung volumes in an average healthy male adult.

Commonly used abbreviations

Primary symbols

C = concentration of gas – blood phase
D = diffusing capacity
F = fractional concentration in the dry gas phase
P = partial pressure – gas
Q = volume of blood
R = respiratory exchange ratio
S = saturation of haemoglobin with oxygen or carbon dioxide
V = volume of gas
$\dot{X}$ = dot above symbol indicates 'per unit time'
$\bar{X}$ = bar above symbol indicates 'mean value'

Example: P_aO_2 = partial pressure of arterial oxygen

Secondary symbols

Usually typed as subscripts, capital letters indicate gaseous phase; lower-case letters indicate liquid phase.

A = alveolar
B = barometric
D = dead space
E = expired
I = inspired
T = tidal
a = arterial
c = capillary (pulmonary capillary)
v = venous
p = peripleural

Lung function: adult and neonatal values		
Examples	*Adult (65 kg)*	*Neonate (3 kg)*
V_D	$2.2\,mL\,kg^{-1}$	$2-3\,mL\,kg^{-1}$
V_T	$7-10\,mL\,kg^{-1}$	$5-7\,mL\,kg^{-1}$
$\dot{V}_E$	$85-100\,mL\,kg^{-1}\,min^{-1}$	$100-200\,mL\,kg^{-1}min^{-1}$
Vital capacity	$50-55\,mL\,kg^{-1}$	$33\,mL\,kg^{-1}$
Respiratory rate	$12-18\,breath\,min^{-1}$	$25-40\,breath\,min^{-1}$
P_aO_2	$12.6\,kPa\,(95\,mmHg)$	$9\,kPa\,(68\,mmHg)$
P_aCO_2	$5.3\,kPa\,(40\,mmHg)$	$4.5\,kPa\,(33\,mmHg)$

Appendix B (IX)
Paediatrics

Tracheal and tracheostomy tube size

Age (years)	TT and tracheostomy tube size ID (mm)	TT length (cm)		Age (years)	TT and tracheostomy tube size ID (mm)	TT length (cm)	
		Oral	Nasal			Oral	Nasal
Premature (by weight)							
1 kg	2.5	7		8	6.0	16	19
2 kg	3.0	8		9	6.0	16	19
3 kg	3.0/3.5	9		10	6.5	17	20
0–3 months	3.0/3.5	10		11	6.5	17	20
3–6 months	3.5	12	15	12	7.0	18	21
6–12 months	3.5	12	15	13	7.0	18	21
2	4.0	13	16	14	7.5	21	24
3	4.0	13	16	15	7.5	21	24
4	4.5	14	17	16	8.0	21	24
5	5.0	14	17	17	9.0	22	25
6	5.5	15	18	18	9.5	22	25
7	5.5	15	18	20	9.5	23	26

TT, tracheal tube; ID, internal diameter.
Below 8–10 years, non-cuffed tubes should be used.
It is always advisable to have available a tube one size smaller than calculated.

Dosage of drugs in common anaesthetic usage

Premedication

Atropine	20 µg kg^{-1}
Hyoscine	20 µg kg^{-1}
Glycopyrrolate	5 µg kg^{-1}
Diazepam	200–400 µg kg^{-1}
Alimemazine (Trimeprazine)	2 mg kg^{-1}

Intravenous induction

Propofol	3 mg kg^{-1}
Thiopental	5 mg kg^{-1}
Ketamine	2 mg kg^{-1}

Other induction routes

Ketamine intramuscular	10 mg kg^{-1}
Thiopental rectal	30 mg kg^{-1}

Neuromuscular blocking drugs

Succinylcholine	2 mg kg^{-1}
Atracurium	300–500 µg kg^{-1}
Cisatracurium	80–200 µg kg^{-1}
Mivacurium	250–400 µg kg^{-1}
Rocuronium	500–1200 µg kg^{-1}
Vecuronium	100 µg kg^{-1}
Pancuronium	80–100 µg kg^{-1}

Reversal of neuromuscular blocking drugs

Neostigmine	
Child	50 µg kg^{-1}
Neonatal	80 µg kg^{-1}
Atropine	20 µg kg^{-1}

Analgesics – intravenous/intramuscular

Morphine	200 µg kg^{-1}
Fentanyl	0.5–1.5 µg kg^{-1}
Alfentanil	2.5–5 µg kg^{-1}

Rectal

Diclofenac	2 mg kg^{-1} (for acute dosage only)

Fluid and electrolyte balance

Postoperative fluid and electrolyte requirements in infancy and childhood

Weight	Rate
Up to 10 kg	100 mL kg^{-1} day^{-1}
10–20 kg	1000 mL + (50 × [wt (kg) – 10]) mL kg^{-1} day^{-1}
20–30 kg	1500 mL + (25 × [wt (kg) – 20]) mL kg^{-1} day^{-1}

Fluid requirements in the first week of life

Day	Rate
1	0
2, 3	50 mL kg^{-1} day^{-1}
4, 5	75 mL kg^{-1} day^{-1}
6	100 mL kg^{-1} day^{-1}
7	120 mL kg^{-1} day^{-1}

Fluid and electrolyte requirements in infancy and childhood

	Age (years)										
	1 wk	1	2	3	4	5	6	7	8	9	10
Weight (kg)	3.5	10	13	15	17	19	21	23	25	28	32
Insensible water loss (mL kg^{-1} day^{-1})	30	27.5	27	26.5	26	25	24	23	22	21	20
Water requirement (mL kg^{-1} day^{-1})	120	100	100	90	90	90	70	70	70	70	70
Na$^+$ requirement (mmol kg^{-1} day^{-1})	4	3	2.5	2	2	1.9	1.9	1.9	1.8	1.75	1.7
K$^+$ requirement (mmol kg^{-1} day^{-1})	2.5	2	2	2	2	1.75	1.75	1.5	1.5	1.5	1.5

These are basal requirements. Additional fluid (10–20%) is required during major surgery, in addition to replacement of overt losses. During the postoperative period, fluid requirements are increased in the presence of pyrexia. Fluid and electrolyte balance should be adjusted after measurement of serum electrolyte concentrations and serum osmolality.

Appendix B (X)
Gas flows in anaesthetic breathing systems

System	Spontaneous ventilation	Intermittent positive-pressure ventilation
Mapleson A (Lack or Magill)	Minute ventilation (MV; theoretically V_A) 80 mL kg^{-1} min^{-1}	2.5 × MV 200 mL kg^{-1} min^{-1}
Mapleson D (Bain or coaxial Mapleson D)	2–3 × MV 150 250 mL kg^{-1} min^{-1}	70 mL kg^{-1} min^{-1} for P_aCO_2 of 5.3 kPa 100 mL kg^{-1} min^{-1} for P_aCO_2 of 4.3 kPa
Mapleson E (Ayre's T-piece)	2 × MV	As Mapleson D Minimum of 3 L min^{-1} fresh gas flow
Mapleson F (Jackson Rees modification of Ayre's T piece)	As Mapleson E	As Mapleson E

V_A, alveolar minute volume; P_aCO_2, arterial carbon dioxide tension.

Normal ventilation values for resting awake subjects

Weight (kg)	Minute volume (mL)	Tidal volume (mL)	Frequency (breath min^{-1})
Neonate 2	480	14–16	30–45
3	600	17–24	25–40
10	1680	80	21
20	3040	160	19
30	4080	240	17
40	4800	320	15
50	5200	400	13
60	5280	480	11
70	5600	560	10

Index

Page References to significant material in figure legends and tables have only been given in the absence of its concomitant mention in the text referring to that illustration. Page references in bold refer to clinical data in appendix B.

A